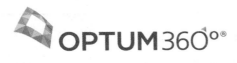

OPTUM360®

EXPERT

# 2017

# HCPCS Level II

A resourceful compilation of HCPCS codes
Supports HIPAA Compliance

**ICD-10 IS NOW.** For more resources
and training visit **Optum360Coding.com.**

D1402121

## Publisher's Notice

The Optum360 *2017 HCPCS Level II* Expert is designed to be an accurate and authoritative source of information about this government coding system. Every effort has been made to verify the accuracy of the listings, and all information is believed reliable at the time of publication. Absolute accuracy cannot be guaranteed, however. This publication is made available with the understanding that the publisher is not engaged in rendering legal or other services that require a professional license.

## Our Commitment to Accuracy

Optum360 is committed to producing accurate and reliable materials. To report corrections, please visit www.optumcoding.com/accuracy or e-mail accuracy@optum.com. You can also reach customer service by calling 1.800.464.3649, option 1.

To view Optum360 updates/correction notices, please visit http://www.optumcoding.com/ProductUpdates/

## Acknowledgments

Gregory A. Kemp, MA, *Product Manager*

Karen Schmidt, BSN, *Technical Director*

Stacy Perry, *Manager, Desktop Publishing*

Lisa Singley, *Project Manager*

Elizabeth Leibold, RHIT, *Clinical/Technical Editor*

Regina Magnani, RHIT, *Clinical/Technical Editor*

Tracy Betzler, *Senior Desktop Publishing Specialist*

Hope M. Dunn, *Senior Desktop Publishing Specialist*

Katie Russell, *Desktop Publishing Specialist*

Jean Parkinson, *Editor*

## Copyright

Property of Optum360, LLC. Optum360 and the Optum360 logo are trademarks of Optum360, LLC. All other brand or product names are trademarks or registered trademarks of their respective owner.

© 2016 Optum360, LLC. All rights reserved.

HS   ISBN 978-1-62254-201-7

## Technical Editors

### Elizabeth Leibold, RHIT

Ms. Leibold has more than 25 years of experience in the health care profession. She has served in a variety of roles, ranging from patient registration to billing and collections, and has an extensive background in both physician and hospital outpatient coding and compliance. She has worked for large health care systems and health information management services companies, and has wide-ranging experience in facility and professional component coding, along with CPT expertise in interventional procedures, infusion services, emergency department, observation, and ambulatory surgery coding. Her areas of expertise include chart-to-claim coding audits and providing staff education to both tenured and new coding staff. She is an active member of the American Health Information Management Association (AHIMA).

### Regina Magnani, RHIT

Ms. Magnani has more than 30 years of experience in the health care industry in both health information management and patient financial services. Her areas of expertise include facility revenue cycle management, patient financial services, CPT/HCPCS and ICD-10-CM coding, the outpatient prospective payment system (OPPS), and chargemaster development and maintenance. She is an active member of the Healthcare Financial Management Association (HFMA), the American Health Information Management Association (AHIMA), and the American Association of Healthcare Administrative Management (AAHAM).

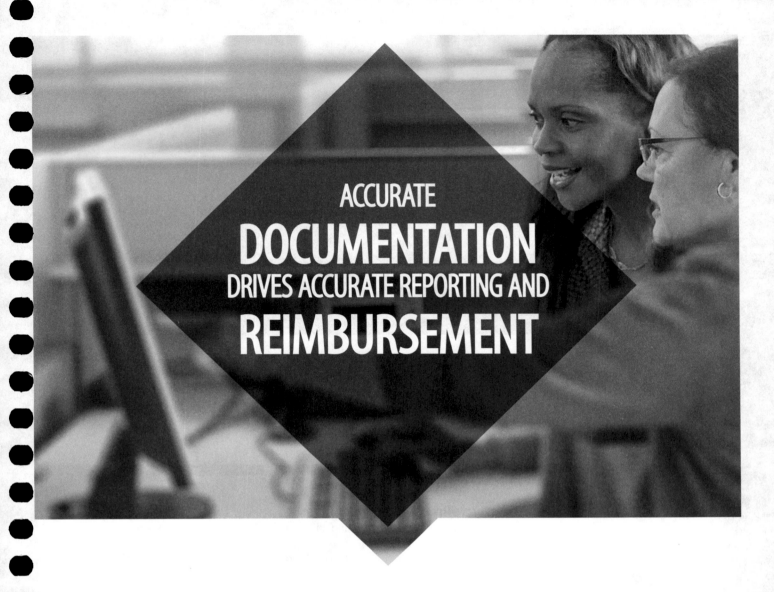

# ACCURATE
# DOCUMENTATION
## DRIVES ACCURATE REPORTING AND
# REIMBURSEMENT

Discover how breakthrough technology can strengthen your performance and provide unprecedented efficiencies to expand your CDI program. Using our clinically-based algorithms and patented LifeCode® NLP technology, Optum® CDI 3D reviews 100 percent of your records and automatically identifies those with documentation gaps and deficiencies. CDI 3D enables more timely documentation improvement, simplifies the CDI process, prepares your team for future industry demands, and positions your program for growth.

**See how Optum CDI 3D can take your program to the next level.**

**Visit:** optum360.com/CDI3D
**Call:** 1-866-223-4730
**Email:** optum360@optum.com

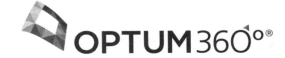

© 2016 Optum360, LLC. All rights reserved.  4/16  WF126202
U.S. Patent Nos. 6,915,254; 7,908,552; 8,682,823; 8,731,954; and other Patents Pending

# AMP IT UP

Amp it up when you turn it up with online digital coding tools.

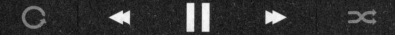

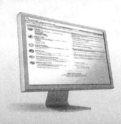

### EncoderPro.com for physicians and payers

Online digital coding look-up tool that every coder can rely on to strengthen their coding. Offering fast, detailed search capabilities in one location of over 37 Optum360 coding and referential books. Better accuracy, fewer denials, higher productivity.

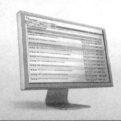

### RevenueCyclePro.com for facilities

Single source for coding, billing, coverage and reimbursement needs in facilities. Keeps you up to date with regulatory and coding changes. Online digital tool that grants access to a complete library of medical reference content and historical data. Increases efficiency across the entire revenue cycle with fast, targeted searches.

## Single code sets or all of them. Referential coding materials, guidelines and more.

### Ease of use, better accuracy, increased productivity.

Explore your options and pick the tool that best suits your needs, choosing from a wide variety available to enhance your coding and reimbursement skills and complement print products.

Learn more today about Optum360 online digital coding tools:

 **Visit:** optum360coding.com/transition

 **Call:** 1-800-464-3649, option 1

4/16   WF122348   SPRJ2861

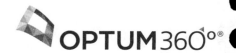

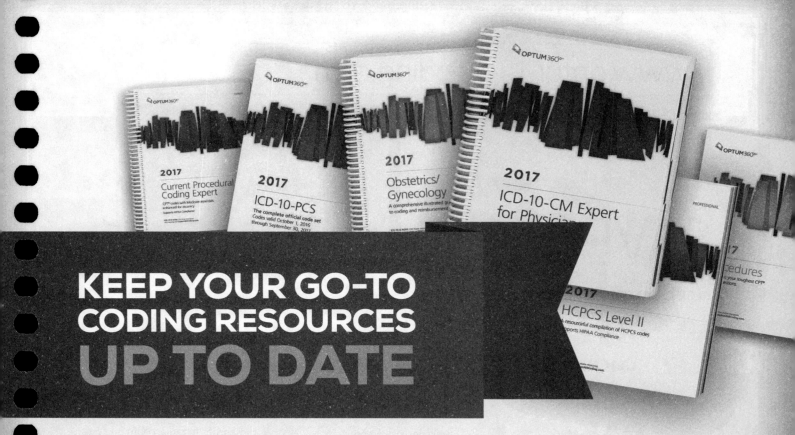

# KEEP YOUR GO-TO CODING RESOURCES
## UP TO DATE

Stay current and compliant with our 2017 edition code books. With more than 30 years in the coding industry, Optum360® is proud to be your trusted resource for coding, billing and reimbursement resources. Our 2017 editions include tools for ICD-10-CM/PCS, CPT®, HCPCS, DRG, specialty-specific coding and much more.

**SAVE UP TO 25%** ON ADDITIONAL CODING RESOURCES

 **Visit us at optum360coding.com** and enter promo code **FOBA17E4** to save 25%.

 **Call 1-800-464-3649, option 1,** and be sure to mention promo code **FOBA17E4** to save 20%.

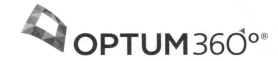

CPT is a registered trademark of the American Medical Association.
© 2016 Optum360, LLC. All rights reserved. 4/16  WF122252  SPRJ2836

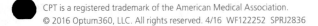

## SIMPLIFY YOUR ORDERING / MAGNIFY YOUR SAVINGS

www.optum360coding.com

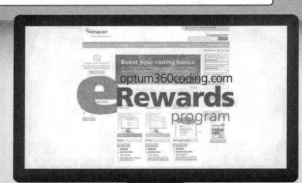

# SAVE15%
## ON YOUR NEXT ORDER WHEN YOU
### REGISTER AT OPTUM360CODING.COM

---

### 1 — CLICK

Visit optum360coding.com:

- Find the products you need quickly and easily.
- View all available formats and edition years on the same page.
- Chat live with a customer service representative.
- Visit Coding Central for expert resources, including articles, *Inside Track to ICD-10* and coding scenarios to test your knowledge.
- Shop our interactive online catalog — view product information quickly and easily and get great discounts.

### 2 — REGISTER

By registering, you'll be able to:

- Enjoy special promotions, discounts and automatic rewards.
- Get recommendations based on your order history.
- Check on shipment status and tracking.
- View order and payment history.
- Pay invoices.
- Manage your address book and ship orders to multiple locations.
- Renew your order with a single click.
- Compile a wish list of the products you want and purchase when you're ready.

### 3 — SAVE

Get 15% off your next order.

Register for an account and receive a coupon via email for 15% off your next order.

Plus, earn cash with our no-cost eRewards program.

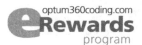

Register for an account and you're automatically enrolled in our eRewards program, where you'll get a $50 coupon for every $500 you spend.* When logged in at optum360coding.com, the eRewards meter keeps track of purchases toward your next reward.

---

## Visit us at **optum360coding.com** to register today!

*Offer valid only for customers who are NOT part of our Medallion or Partner Account programs. You must be registered at optum360coding.com to have your online purchases tracked for rewards purposes. Shipping charges and taxes still apply and cannot be used for rewards. Optum360 Coding eReward offers valid online only. © 2016 Optum360, LLC. All rights reserved. WF122408 SPRJ2826

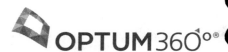

Optum360®  SIXTEENTH ANNUAL

# ESSENTIALS
CODING, BILLING & COMPLIANCE CONFERENCE

# *Level up*

## TAKE YOUR CODING KNOWLEDGE TO THE **NEXT LEVEL**.

*Visit* **OPTUM360CODING.COM/ESSENTIALS**

Only Optum360® delivers high-quality, continuing education and industry-leading content matter at this level and price.

Whether you're looking for daily tips to help make your job just a little easier, or you want to keep your skills current and relevant in this ever-changing world of coding, billing and compliance, Optum360 Essentials is truly, well, essential.

### *Register now!*

Visit | optum360coding.com/essentials

Call | 1-724-391-1004

Email | Optum360Essentials@aexp.com

### *Why attend?*

- Attend as many as 40 educational sessions, all created to be timely and relevant with what's currently happening in the industry.

- Earn as many at 16 CEUs approved by both AAPC and AHIMA.

- Stay current with updates on ICD-10-CM/PCS, HCPCS, DRG codes, HCC, PQRS, IPPS and OPPS.

- Learn about the CPT® code updates firsthand.

- Attend vetted presentations that are reviewed and approved by legal and clinical experts.

- Learn from nationally recognized experts on medical coding, billing and compliance.

- Network with a wide spectrum of medical professionals, from entry-level to expert understanding.

CPT is a registered trademark of the American Medical Association.
© 2016 Optum360, LLC. All rights reserved.  4/16  WF122314  SPRJ2858

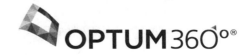

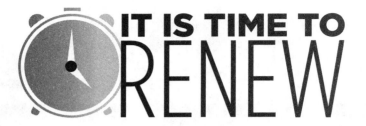

# IT IS TIME TO RENEW

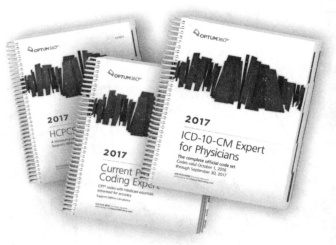

## SAVE UP TO 25%*
when you renew your coding essentials.

>> Buy 1–2 items, save 15%
Buy 3–5 items, save 20%
Buy 6+ items, save 25%

| ITEM # | TITLE<br>INDICATE THE ITEMS YOU WISH TO PURCHASE | QUANTITY | PRICE<br>PER PRODUCT | TOTAL |
|---|---|---|---|---|
| | | | | |
| | | | | |
| | | | | |
| | | | | |
| | | | | |
| | | | Subtotal | |
| | (AK, DE, HI, MT, NH & OR are exempt) | | Sales tax | |
| | 1 item $10.95 • 2–4 items $12.95 • 5+ CALL | | Shipping & handling | |
| | | | TOTAL AMOUNT ENCLOSED | |

## Save up to 25% when you renew.

 Visit **optum360coding.com** and enter the promo code below.

 Call **1-800-464-3649, option 1,** and mention the promo code below.

 Fax this order form with purchase order to **1-801-982-4033.** *Optum360 no longer accepts credit cards by fax.*

**PROMO CODE**
**FOBA17R4**

Mail this order form with payment and/or purchase order to:
**Optum360, PO Box 88050, Chicago, IL 60680-9920.**
*Optum360 no longer accepts credit cards by mail.*

Name _____

Address _____

_____

Customer number _____ Contact number _____

○ CHECK ENCLOSED (PAYABLE TO OPTUM360)

○ BILL ME   ○ P.O.# _____

( ) _____
Telephone
( ) _____
Fax
_____@_____
Email

Optum360 respects your right to privacy. We will not sell or rent your email address or fax number to anyone outside Optum360 and its business partners. If you would like to remove your name from Optum360 promotions, please call 1-800-464-3649, option 1.

*Discount does not include digital coding solutions, workers' comp, custom fee or bookstore products.

© 2016 Optum360, LLC. All rights reserved. 4/16  WF122442  SPRJ2830

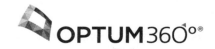

# Contents

© 2016 Optum360, LLC

# Introduction

## Organization of HCPCS

The Optum360 2017 *HCPCS Level II* Expert contains mandated changes and new codes for use as of January 1, 2017. Deleted codes have also been indicated and cross-referenced to active codes when possible. New codes have been added to the appropriate sections, eliminating the time-consuming step of looking in two places for a code. However, keep in mind that the information in this book is a reproduction of the 2017 HCPCS; additional information on coverage issues may have been provided to Medicare contractors after publication. All contractors periodically update their systems and records throughout the year. If this book does not agree with your contractor, it is either because of a mid-year update or correction, or a specific local, or regional coverage policy.

## Index

Because HCPCS is organized by code number rather than by service or supply name, the index enables the coder to locate any code without looking through individual ranges of codes. Just look up the medical or surgical supply, service, orthotic, or prosthetic in question to find the appropriate codes. This index also refers to many of the brand names by which these items are known.

## Table of Drugs and Biologicals

The brand names of drugs and biologicals listed are examples only and may not include all products available for that type. The table lists HCPCS codes from any available section including A codes, C codes, J codes, S codes, and Q codes under brand and generic names with amount, route of administration, and code numbers. While every effort is made to make the table comprehensive, it is not all-inclusive.

## Physician Quality Reporting System (PQRS)

The PQRS table is no longer published in this book. See Appendix 9 for additional information.

## Color-coded Coverage Instructions

The Optum360 *HCPCS Level II* book provides colored symbols for each coverage and reimbursement instruction. A legend to these symbols is provided on the bottom of each two-page spread.

## HOW TO USE OPTUM360 HCPCS LEVEL II BOOKS

### Blue Color Bar—Special Coverage Instructions

A blue bar for "special coverage instructions" over a code means that special coverage instructions apply to that code. These special instructions are also typically given in the form of Medicare Pub.100 reference numbers. The appendixes provide the full text of the cited Medicare Pub.100 references.

**A4336**    **Incontinence supply, urethral insert, any type, each**

### Yellow Color Bar—Carrier Discretion

Issues that are left to "carrier discretion" are covered with a yellow bar. Contact the carrier for specific coverage information on those codes.

**A9581**    **Injection, gadoxetate disodium, 1 ml**

### Pink Color Bar—Not Covered by or Invalid for Medicare

Codes that are not covered by or are invalid for Medicare are covered by a pink bar. The pertinent Medicare Internet-only Manuals (Pub. 100) reference numbers are also given explaining why a particular code is not covered. These numbers refer to the appendixes, where the Medicare references are listed.

**A4264**    **Permanent implantable contraceptive intratubal occlusion device(s) and delivery system**

Codes in the Optum360 *HCPCS Level II* follow the AMA CPT book conventions to indicate new, revised, and deleted codes.

- A black circle (●) precedes a new code.
- A black triangle (▲) precedes a code with revised terminology or rules.
- A circle (○) precedes a recycled/reinstated code.
- Codes deleted from the current active codes appear with a strike-out.

| | | |
|---|---|---|
| ● | A4337 | **Incontinence supply, rectal insert, any type, each** |
| ▲ | K0017 | **Detachable, adjustable height armrest, base, replacement only, each** |
| ○ | E1012 | **Wheelchair accessory, addition to power seating system, center mount power elevating leg rest/platform, complete system, any type, each** |
| | B9000 | ~~**Enteral nutrition infusion pump without alarm**~~ |

### ☑ Quantity Alert

Many codes in HCPCS report quantities that may not coincide with quantities available in the marketplace. For instance, a HCPCS code for an ostomy pouch with skin barrier reports each pouch, but the product is generally sold in a package of 10; "10" must be indicated in the quantity box on the CMS claim form to ensure proper reimbursement. This symbol indicates that care should be taken to verify quantities in this code. These quantity alerts do not represent Medicare Unlikely Edits (MUEs) and should not be used for MUEs.

☑ **J0120**    **Injection, tetracycline, up to 250 mg**

## ♀ Female Only

This icon identifies procedures that some payers may consider female only.

| A4280 | Adhesive skin support attachment for use with external breast prosthesis, each ♀ |

## ♂ Male Only

This icon identifies procedures that some payers may consider male only.

| A4326 | Male external catheter with integral collection chamber, anytype, each ♂ |

## Ⓐ Age Edit

This icon denotes codes intended for use with a specific age group, such as neonate, newborn, pediatric, and adult. Carefully review the code description to ensure that the code reported most appropriately reflects the patient's age.

| Q2037 | Influenza virus vaccine, split virus, when administered to individuals 3 years of age and older, for intramuscular use (FLUVIRIN) Ⓐ |

## Ⓜ Maternity

This icon identifies procedures that by definition should only be used for maternity patients generally between 12 and 55 years of age.

| H1001 | Prenatal care, at-risk enhanced service; antepartum management Ⓜ |

## A2 – Z3 ASC Payment Indicators

Codes designated as being paid by ASC groupings that were effective at the time of printing are denoted by the group number.

| G0105 | Colorectal cancer screening; colonoscopy on individual at high risk A2 |

## ♿ DMEPOS

Use this icon to identify when to consult the CMS durable medical equipment, prosthetics, orthotics, and supplies (DMEPOS) for payment of this durable medical item.

| E0988 | Manual wheelchair accessory, lever-activated, wheel drive, pair ♿ |

## ⊘ Skilled Nursing Facility (SNF)

Use this icon to identify certain items and services excluded from SNF consolidated billing. These items may be billed directly to the Medicare contractor by the provider or supplier of the service or item.

| A4653 | Peritoneal dialysis catheter anchoring device, belt, each ⊘ |

Drugs commonly reported with a code are listed underneath by brand or generic name.

| C9254 | Injection, lacosamide, 1 mg |
| | Use this code for VIMPAT. |

CMS does not use consistent terminology when a code for a specific procedure is not listed. The code description may include any of the following terms: unlisted, not otherwise classified (NOC), unspecified, unclassified, other, and miscellaneous. If unsure there is no code for the service or supply provided or used, provide adequate documentation to the payer. Check with the payer for more information.

| A0999 | Unlisted ambulance service |

For a new, revised, or deleted code, the specific effective quarter is shown to the right of the code.

| ● | Q4175[Jan] | Miroderm, per sq cm |

## OPPS Status Indicators

**A - Y** Status indicators identify how individual HCPCS Level II codes are paid or not paid under the OPPS. The same status indicator is assigned to all the codes within an ambulatory payment classification (APC). Consult the payer or resource to learn which CPT codes fall within various APCs. Status indicators for HCPCS and their definitions follow:

**A** Services furnished to a hospital outpatient that are paid under a fee schedule or payment system other than OPPS, for example:

- Ambulance Services
- Clinical Diagnostic Laboratory Services
- Non-Implantable Prosthetic and Orthotic Devices
- EPO for ESRD Patients
- Physical, Occupational, and Speech Therapy
- Routine Dialysis Services for ESRD Patients Provided in a Certified Dialysis Unit of a Hospital
- Diagnostic Mammography
- Screening Mammography

**B** Codes that are not recognized by OPPS when submitted on an outpatient hospital Part B bill type (12x and 13x)

**C** Inpatient Procedures

**E1** Items, Codes, and Services:

- That are not covered by any Medicare outpatient benefit based on statutory exclusion
- That are not covered by any Medicare outpatient benefit for reasons other than statutory exclusion
- That are not recognized by Medicare for outpatient claims but for which an alternate code for the same item or service may be available
- For which separate payment is not provided on outpatient claims

**F** Corneal Tissue Acquisition; Certain CRNA Services and Hepatitis B Vaccines

**G** Pass-Through Drugs and Biologicals

**H** Pass-Through Device Categories

**J1** Hospital Part B services paid through a comprehensive APC

**K** Nonpass-Through Drugs and Nonimplantable Biologicals, Including Therapeutic Radiopharmaceuticals

**L** Influenza Vaccine; Pneumococcal Pneumonia Vaccine

**M** Items and Services Not Billable to the Fiscal Intermediary/MAC

**N** Items and Services Packaged into APC Rates

**P** Partial Hospitalization

**Q1** STVX-Packaged Codes

**Q2** T-Packaged Codes

**Q3** Codes That May Be Paid Through a Composite APC

**R** Blood and Blood Products

**S** Significant Procedure, Not Discounted when Multiple

**T** Significant Procedure, Multiple Reduction Applies

**U** Brachytherapy Sources

**V** Clinic or Emergency Department Visit

**Y** Nonimplantable Durable Medical Equipment

| | | |
|---|---|---|
| **A** | L8440 | Prosthetic shrinker, below knee, each |
| **B** | Q4005 | Cast supplies, long arm cast, adult (11 years +), plaster |
| **C** | G0341 | Percutaneous islet cell transplant, includes portal vein catheterization and infusion |
| **E1** | A0021 | Ambulance service, outside state per mile, transport (Medicaid only) |
| **F** | V2785 | Processing, preserving and transporting corneal tissue |
| **G** | A9586 | Florbetapir F18, diagnostic, per study dose, up to 10 millicuries |
| **H** | C2623 | Catheter, transluminal angioplasty, drug-coated, non-laser |
| **K** | J1750 | Injection, iron dextran, 50 mg |
| **L** | Q2036 | Influenza virus vaccine, split virus, when administered to individuals 3 years of age and older, for intramuscular use (FLULAVAL) |
| **M** | G0333 | Pharmacy dispensing fee for inhalation drug(s); initial 30-day supply as a beneficiary |
| **N** | A4220 | Refill kit for implantable infusion pump |
| **P** | G0129 | Occupational therapy services requiring the skills of a qualified occupational therapist, furnished as a component of a partial hospitalization treatment program, per session (45 minutes or more) |
| **Q3** | C8900 | Magnetic resonance angiography with contrast, abdomen |
| **R** | P9010 | Blood (whole), for transfusion, per unit |
| **S** | G0117 | Glaucoma screening for high risk patients furnished by an optometrist or ophthalmologist |
| **T** | C9740 | Cystourethroscopy, with insertion of transprostatic implant; 4 or more implants |
| **U** | A9527 | Iodine I-125, sodium iodide solution, therapeutic, per millicurie |
| **V** | G0101 | Cervical or vaginal cancer screening; pelvic and clinical breast examination |
| **Y** | A5500 | For diabetics only, fitting (including follow-up), custom preparation and supply of off-the-shelf depth-inlay shoe manufactured to accommodate multidensity insert(s), per shoe |

## ASC Payment Indicators

**A2 – Z3** This icon identifies the ASC status payment indicators, effective January 1, 2015. They indicate how the ASC payment rate was derived and/or how the procedure, item, or service is treated under the 2015 ASC payment system. For more information about these indicators and how they affect billing, consult Optum360's *Outpatient Billing Editor*.

**A2** Surgical procedure on ASC list in CY 2007 or later; payment based on OPPS relative payment weight

**C5** Inpatient procedure

**F4** Corneal tissue acquisition, hepatitis B vaccine; paid at reasonable cost

**G2** Nonoffice-based surgical procedure added in CY 2008 or later; payment based on OPPS relative payment weight

**H2** Brachytherapy source paid separately when provided integral to a surgical procedure on ASC list; payment based on OPPS rate

**J7** Device-intensive procedure; paid at adjusted rate

**J8** Device-intensive procedure added to ASC list in CY 2008 or later; paid at adjusted rate

**K2** Drugs and biologicals paid separately when provided integral to a surgical procedure on ASC list; payment based on OPPS rate

**K7** Unclassified drugs and biologicals; payment contractor-priced

**L1** Influenza vaccine; pneumococcal vaccine; packaged item/service; no separate payment made

**L6** New Technology Intraocular Lens (NTIOL); special payment

**M5** Quality measurement code used for reporting purposes only; no payment made

**N1** Packaged service/item; no separate payment made

**P2** Office-based surgical procedure added to ASC list in CY 2008 or later with MPFS nonfacility PE RVUs; payment based on OPPS relative payment weight

**P3** Office-based surgical procedure added to ASC list in CY 2008 or later with MPFS nonfacility PE RVUs; payment based on MPFS nonfacility PE RVUs

**R2** Office-based surgical procedure added to ASC list in CY 2008 or later without MPFS nonfacility PE RVUs; payment based on OPPS relative payment weight

**Z2** Radiology service paid separately when provided integral to a surgical procedure on ASC list; payment based on OPPS relative payment weight

**Z3** Radiology service paid separately when provided integral to a surgical procedure on ASC list; payment based on MPFS nonfacility PE RVUs

---

**F4** V2785 Processing, preserving and transporting corneal tissue

**H2** A9527 Iodine I-125, sodium iodide solution, therapeutic per millicurie

**J7** C1841 Retinal prosthesis, includes all internal and external components

**K2** C9132 Prothrombin complex concentrate (human), Kcentra, per IU of Factor IX activity

**K7** C9399 Unclassified drugs or biologicals

**L1** Q2037 Influenza virus vaccine, split virus, when administered to individuals 3 years of age and older, for intramuscular use (FLUVIRIN)

**N1** C9353 Microporous collagen implantable slit tube (NeuraWrap Nerve Protector), per cm length

**Z3** G0130 Single energy x-ray absorptiometry (SEXA) bone density study, one or more sites; appendicular skeleton (peripheral) (e.g., radius, wrist, heel)

**Z2** C8911 Magnetic resonance angiography without contrast followed by with contrast, chest (excluding myocardium)

---

**CMS:** This notation precedes an instruction pertaining to this code in the CMS Internet-only Manuals (Pub 100) electronic manual or in a National Coverage Determination (NCD). These CMS sources, formerly called the Medicare Carriers Manual (MCM) and Coverage Issues Manual (CIM), present the rules for submitting these services to the federal government or its contractors and are included in the appendix of this book.

A4490 Surgical stockings above knee length, each

**CMS:** 100-02,15,110

---

**AHA:** American Hospital Association Coding Clinic for HCPCS citations help in finding expanded information about specific codes and their usage.

A4290 Sacral nerve stimulation test lead, each

**AHA:** 1Q, '02, 9

© 2016 Optum360, LLC

## About HCPCS Codes

HCPCS Level II codes are developed and maintained by the Centers for Medicare and Medicaid Services (CMS). Optum360 does not change the code descriptions other than correcting typographical errors. For 2017 there are some codes that appear to be duplicates. CMS has indicated that each of the codes is used to report a specific condition or service. At press time CMS had not provided further clarification regarding these codes. Additional information may be found on the CMS website, https://www.cms.gov/Medicare/Coding/HCPCSReleaseCodeSets/index.html or at www.optum360coding.com.

Any supplier or manufacturer can submit a request for coding modification to the HCPCS Level II national codes. A document explaining the HCPCS modification process, as well as a detailed format for submitting a recommendation for a modification to HCPCS Level II codes, is available on the HCPCS website at https://www.cms.gov/MedHCPCSGenInfo/ 01a_Application_Form_and_Instructions.asp#TopOfPage. Besides the information requested in this format, a requestor should also submit any additional descriptive material, including the manufacturer's product literature and information that is believed would be helpful in furthering CMS's understanding of the medical features of the item for which a coding modification is being recommended. The HCPCS coding review process is an ongoing, continuous process.

Requests for coding modifications should be sent to the following address:

Felicia Eggleston, CMS HCPCS Workgroup Coordinator
Centers for Medicare and Medicaid Services
C5-08-27
7500 Security Blvd
Baltimore, Maryland 21244-1850

The dental (D) codes are not included in the official 2017 HCPCS Level II code set. The American Dental Association (ADA) holds the copyright on those codes and instructed CMS to remove them. As a result, Optum360 has removed them from this product; however, Optum360 has additional resources available for customers requiring the dental codes. Please go to www.optumcoding.com or call 1.800.464.3649.

**Note:** The expanded Medically Unlikely Edit (MUE) tables containing HCPCS/CPT codes, MUE values, MUE adjudication indicators, and MUE rationale are no longer published in this book. They will be available on the Optum360 website for users of the *HCPCS Level II Expert* at www.optum360coding.com/2017HCPCSMUE.

Password: o360mue17

The table containing the Medicare national average payment (NAP) for services, supplies (DME, orthotics, prosthetics, etc.), drugs, biologicals, and nonphysician procedures using HCPCS Level II codes are available at www.optum360coding.com/2017MedAvgPay.

Password: o360map17

## How to Use HCPCS Level II

Coders should keep in mind, that the insurance companies and government do not base payment solely on what was done for the patient. They need to know why the services were performed. In addition to using the HCPCS coding system for procedures and supplies, coders must also use the ICD-10-CM coding system to denote the diagnosis. This book will not discuss ICD-10-CM codes, which can be found in a current ICD-10-CM code book for diagnosis codes. To locate a HCPCS Level II code, follow these steps:

1.  Identify the services or procedures that the patient received.

    Example:

    Patient administered PSA exam.

2.  Look up the appropriate term in the index.

    Example:

    Screening
         prostate

Coding Tip: Coders who are unable to find the procedure or service in the index can look in the table of contents for the type of procedure or device to narrow the code choices. Also, coders should remember to check the unlisted procedure guidelines for additional choices.

3.  Assign a tentative code.

    Example:

    Code G0103

    Coding Tip: To the right of the terminology, there may be a single code or multiple codes, a cross-reference, or an indication that the code has been deleted. Tentatively assign all codes listed.

4.  Locate the code or codes in the appropriate section. When multiple codes are listed in the index, be sure to read the narrative of all codes listed to find the appropriate code based on the service performed.

    Example:

    **G0103**    **Prostate cancer screening; prostate specific antigen test (PSA)**

5.  Check for color bars, symbols, notes, and references.

    Example:

    **G0103**    **Prostate cancer screening; prostate specific antigen test (PSA)**                    ♂🅰

6.  Review the appendixes for the reference definitions and other guidelines for coverage issues that apply.

7.  Determine whether any modifiers should be used.

8.  Assign the code.

    Example:

    The code assigned is G0103.

## Coding Standards
### Levels of Use

Coders may find that the same procedure is coded at two or even three levels. Which code is correct? There are certain rules to follow if this should occur.

When both a CPT and a HCPCS Level II code have virtually identical narratives for a procedure or service, the CPT code should be used. If, however, the narratives are not identical (e.g., the CPT code narrative is generic, whereas the HCPCS Level II code is specific), the Level II code should be used.

Be sure to check for a national code when a CPT code description contains an instruction to include additional information, such as describing a specific medication. For example, when billing Medicare or Medicaid for supplies, avoid using CPT code 99070 Supplies and materials (except spectacles), provided by the physician over and above those usually included with the office visit or other services rendered (list drugs, trays, supplies, or materials provided). There are many HCPCS Level II codes that specify supplies in more detail.

### Special Reports

Submit a special report with the claim when a new, unusual, or variable procedure is provided or a modifier is used. Include the following information:

*   A copy of the appropriate report (e.g., operative, x-ray), explaining the nature, extent, and need for the procedure

*   Documentation of the medical necessity of the procedure

*   Documentation of the time and effort necessary to perform the procedure

**Catheter** — continued
  transluminal — continued
    atherectomy
      directional, C1714
      rotational, C1724
    ureteral, C1758
**CBC**, G0306-G0307
**Cellular therapy**, M0075
**Cement, ostomy**, A4364
**Centrifuge, for dialysis**, E1500
**Cephalin flocculation, blood**, P2028
**Certified nurse assistant**, S9122
**Cerumen removal**, G0268
**Cervical**
  collar, L0120, L0130, L0140, L0150, L0170
  halo, L0810-L0830
  head harness/halter, E0942
  helmet, A8000-A8004
  orthotic, L0180-L0200
  traction equipment, not requiring frame, E0855
**Cervical cap contraceptive**, A4261
**Cervical-thoracic-lumbar-sacral orthotic (CTLSO)**, L0700, L0710, L1000, L1001
**Cesium-131**, C2642-C2643
**Chair**
  adjustable, dialysis, E1570
  bathtub, E0240
  commode, E0163-E0165
  lift, E0627, E0629
  rollabout, E1031
  shower or bath, E0240
  sitz bath, E0160-E0162
**Challenger manual wheelchair**, K0009
**Champion 1000 manual wheelchair**, K0004
**Champion 30000, manual wheelchair**, K0005
**CheckMate Plus blood glucose monitor**, E0607
**Chelation therapy**, M0300
  home infusion, administration, S9355
**Chemical endarterectomy**, M0300
**Chemistry and toxicology tests**, P2028-P3001
**Chemodenervation**
  vocal cord, S2340-S2341
**Chemotherapy**
  administration
    both infusion and other technique, Q0085
    home infusion, continuous, S9325-S9379, S9494-S9497
    infusion, Q0084
      continued in community, G0498
    other than infusion, Q0083
**Chemstrip bG, box of 50 blood glucose test strips**, A4253
**Chemstrip K, box of 100 ketone urine test strips**, A4250
**Chemstrip UGK, box of 100 glucose/ ketone urine test strips**, A4250
**Chest shell (cuirass)**, E0457
**Chest wrap**, E0459
**Childbirth**, S9442
  cesarean birth, S9438
  class, S9442
  early induction, G9355-G9356
  elective delivery, G9355-G9356
  Lamaze, S9436
  post-partum education, G9357-G9358
  post-partum evaluation, G9357-G9358
  post-partum screening, G9357-G9358
  preparation, S9436
  refresher, S9437
  VBAC (vaginal birth after cesarean), S9439
**Childcare**, T2026-T2027
  parents in treatment, T1009
**Chin**
  cup, cervical, L0150
  strap (for CPAP device), A7036
**Chlorhexidine**, A4248
**Chondrocyte cell harvest, arthroscopic**, S2112
**Chopart prosthetic**
  ankle, L5050, L5060
  below knee, L5100
**Chore services**, S5130-S5131
**Christian Science provider services**, S9900
**Chromic phosphate**, A9564

**Chux**, A4554
**CJR model**, G9481-G9489, G9490
**Clamp**
  external urethral, A4356
**ClarixFlo, per sq cm**, Q4155
**Classes**, S9441-S9446
  asthma, S9441
  birthing, S9442
  exercise, S9451
  infant safety, S9447
  lactation, S9443
  nutrition, S9452
  parenting, S9444
  smoking cessation, S9453
  stress management, S9454
  weight management, S9449
**Clavicle**
  splint, L3650
**Cleaning solvent, Nu-Hope**
  4 oz bottle, A4455
  16 oz bottle, A4455
**Cleanser, wound**, A6260
**Cleft palate, feeder**, S8265
**Clevis, hip orthotic**, L2570, L2600, L2610
**Clinical trials**
  lodging costs, S9994
  meals, S9996
  phase II, S9990
  phase III, S9991
  service, S9988
  transportation costs, S9992
**Clinic visit/encounter**, T1015
  hospital outpatient, G0463
  multidisciplinary, child services, T1025
**Closure device, vascular**, C1760
**Clotting time tube**, A4771
**Clubfoot wedge**, L3380
**Cochlear implant**, L8614
  battery
    alkaline, L8622
    lithium, L8623-L8624
    zinc, L8621
  headset, L8615
  microphone, L8616
  replacement, L8619
  transmitter cable, L8618
  transmitting coil, L8617
  zinc, L8621
**Coil, imaging**, C1770
**Collagen**
  implant, urinary tract, L8603
  microporous nonhuman origin, C9352-C9353
  skintest, Q3031
  wound dressing, A6021-A6024, Q4164
**Collar**
  cervical
    contour (low, standard), L0120
    multiple post, L0180-L0200
    nonadjustable foam, L0120
    Philadelphia tracheotomy, L0172
    Philly one-piece extraction, L0150
    tracheotomy, L0172
    traction, E0856
    turtle neck safety, E0942
**Colonoscopy**, G9659-G9661
  cancer screening
    patient at high risk, G0105
    patient not at high risk, G0121
  consultation, prescreening, S0285
**Coloplast**
  closed pouch, A5051
  drainable pouch, A5061
    closed, A5054
    small, A5063
  skin barrier
    4 x 4, A4362
    6 x 6, A5121
    8 x 8, A5122
    stoma cap, A5055
**Coma stimulation**, S9056
**Combo-Seat universal raised toilet seat**, E0244
**Commode**, E0160-E0171
  chair, E0163-E0165, E0170-E0171
  lift, E0172, E0625

**Commode** — continued
  pail, E0167
  seat, wheelchair, E0968
**Communication board**, E1902
**Companion care**, S5135-S5136
**Composite**
  dressing, A6203-A6205
**Comprehensive Care for Joint Replacement Model (CJR)**, G9481-G9489
  assessment, G9490
**Compressed gas system**, E0424-E0480
**Compression**
  bandage
    high, A6452
    light, A6448
    medium, A6451
  burn garment, A6501-A6512
  burn mask, A6513
  stockings, A6530-A6549
  wrap, A6545
**Compressogrip prosthetic shrinker**, L8440-L8465
**Compressor**, E0565, E0570, E0650-E0652, E0670, K0738
**Concentrator**
  oxygen, E1390-E1392
    rental, E1392
**Condom**
  female, A4268
  male, A4267
**Conductive**
  garment (for TENS), E0731
  paste or gel, A4558
**Conductivity meter (for dialysis)**, E1550
**Conference**
  interdisciplinary team, G0175
**Conforming bandage**, A6442-A6447
**Congenital torticollis orthotic**, L0112
**Congo red, blood**, P2029
**Consultation**
  telehealth, G0406-G0408, G0425-G0427, G0508-G0509
**Contact layer**, A6206-A6208
**Contact lens**, S0500, S0512-S0514, V2500-V2599
**Continent device**, A5081, A5082
**Continuous intraoperative neurophysiology monitoring**, G0453
**Continuous passive motion exercise device**, E0936
**Continuous positive airway pressure (CPAP) device**, E0601
  chin strap, A7036
  face mask, A7030-A7031
  filter, A7038-A7039
  headgear, A7035
  nasal application accessories, A7032-A7034
  oral interface, A7044
  tubing, A7037
**Contraceptive**
  cervical cap, A4261
  condom
    female, A4268
    male, A4267
  diaphragm, A4266
  foam, A4269
  gel, A4269
  hormone patch, J7304
  implant, A4264, J7306
  intratubal occlusion device, A4264
  intrauterine, copper, J7300
  Levonorgestrel, implants and supplies, J7297-J7298, J7301, J7306
  pills, S4993
  spermicide, A4269
  vaginal ring, J7303
**Contracts, maintenance, ESRD**, A4890
**Contrast material**
  high osmolar, Q9958-Q9964
  injection during MRI, A9575-A9579, Q9953
  low osmolar, Q9951, Q9965-Q9967
  nonradioactive NOC, A9698
  oral MRI, Q9954
**Controlyte, enteral nutrition**, B4155
**Coordinated care fee**
  home monitoring, G9006

**Coordinated care fee** — continued
  initial rate, G9001
  maintenance rate, G9002
  physician oversight, G9008
  risk adjusted, G9003-G9005
  scheduled team conference, G9007
**Copying fee, medical records**, S9981-S9982
**Corneal tissue processing**, V2785
**Corn, trim or remove**, S0390
**Coronary artery bypass surgery, direct**
  with coronary arterial and venous grafts
    single, each, S2208
    two arterial and single venous, S2209
  with coronary arterial grafts, only
    single, S2205
    two grafts, S2206
  with coronary venous grafts, only
    single, S2207
**Corset, spinal orthotic**, L0970-L0976
**Cough stimulation device**, E0482
**Counseling**
  alcohol, G0443
  cardiovascular disease risk, G0446
  end of life, S0257
  genetic, S0265
  lung cancer screening, G0296
  obesity, G0447
    group (2-10), G0473
  prevention
    sexually transmitted infection, G0445
**Coupling gel/paste**, A4559
**Cover, shower**
  ventricular assist device, Q0501
**Cover, wound**
  alginate dressing, A6196-A6198
  foam dressing, A6209-A6214
  hydrocolloid dressing, A6234-A6239
  hydrogel dressing, A6242-A6248
  specialty absorptive dressing, A6251-A6256
**CPAP (continuous positive airway pressure) device**, E0601
  chin strap, A7036
  exhalation port, A7045
  face mask, A7030-A7031
  headgear, A7035
  humidifier, E0561-E0562
  nasal application accessories, A7032-A7034
  oral interface, A7044
  supplies, E0470-E0472, E0561-E0562
  tubing, A7037
**Cradle, bed**, E0280
**Crisis intervention**, H2011, S9484-S9485, T2034
**Criticare HN, enteral nutrition**, B4153
**Crutch**
  substitute
    lower leg platform, E0118
**Crutches**, E0110-E0116
  accessories, A4635-A4637, E2207
  aluminum, E0114
  articulating, spring assisted, E0117
  forearm, E0111
    Ortho-Ease, E0111
  underarm, other than wood, pair, E0114
    Quikfit Custom Pack, E0114
    Red Dot, E0114
  underarm, wood, single, E0113
    Ready-for-use, E0113
  wooden, E0112
**Cryoprecipitate, each unit**, P9012
**CTLSO**, L0700, L0710, L1000-L1120
**Cuirass**, E0457
**Culture sensitivity study**, P7001
**Culture, urine, bacterial**, P7001
**Curasorb, alginate dressing**, A6196-A6199
**Cushion**
  decubitus care, E0190
  Oral/Nasal, A7029
  positioning, E0190
  wheelchair
    AK addition, L5648
    BK addition, L5646
**Custom**
  DME, K0900
  wheelchair/base, K0008, K0013
**Customized item (in addition to code for basic item)**, S1002

© 2016 Optum360, LLC

© 2016 Optum360, LLC

© 2016 Optum360, LLC

**Solution**
- calibrator, A4256
- dialysate, A4728, A4760
- enteral formulae, B4150-B4155
- parenteral nutrition, B4164-B5200

**S.O.M.I. brace**, L0190, L0200

**S.O.M.I. multiple-post collar, cervical orthotic**, L0190

**Sorbent cartridge, ESRD**, E1636

**Sorbsan, alginate dressing**, A6196-A6198

**Source**
- brachytherapy
  - gold 198, C1716
  - iodine 125, C2638-C2639
  - non-high dose rate iridium 192, C1719
  - palladium-103, C2640-C2641, C2645
  - yttrium 90, C2616

**Spacer**
- implantation spacer material, NOS
- interphalangeal joint, L8658

**Specialist Ankle Foot Orthotic**, L1930

**Specialist Closed-Back Cast Boot**, L3260

**Specialist Gaitkeeper Boot**, L3260

**Specialist Health/Post Operative Shoe**, A9270

**Specialist Heel Cups**, L3485

**Specialist Insoles**, L3510

**Specialist J-Splint Plaster Roll Immobilizer**, A4580

**Specialist Open-Back Cast Boot**, L3260

**Specialist Plaster Bandages**, A4580

**Specialist Plaster Roll Immobilizer**, A4580

**Specialist Plaster Splints**, A4580

**Specialist Pre-Formed Humeral Fracture Brace**, L3980-L3981

**Specialist Pre-Formed Ulnar Fracture Brace**, L3982

**Specialist Tibial Pre-formed Fracture Brace**, L2116

**Specialist Toe Insert for Specialist Closed-Back Cast Boot and Specialist Health/Post Operative Shoe**, A9270

**Specialized mobility technology**
- resource-intensive services, G0501

**Specialty absorptive dressing**, A6251-A6256

**Specimen**, G9291, G9295

**Spectacles**, S0504-S0510, S0516-S0518
- dispensing, S0595

**Speech and language pathologist**
- home health setting, G0153

**Speech assessment**, V5362-V5364
- speech generating device
  - software, E2511
  - supplies, E2500-E2599

**Speech generating device**, E2500

**Speech therapy**, S9128, S9152

**Spenco shoe insert, foot orthotic**, L3001

**Sperm**
- aspiration, S4028
- donor service, S4025
- sperm procurement, S4026, S4030-S4031

**Sphygmomanometer/blood pressure**, A4660

**Spinal orthotic**
- Boston type, L1200
- cervical, L0112, L0180-L0200
- cervical-thoracic-lumbar-sacral orthotic (CTLSO), L0700, L0710, L1000
- halo, L0810-L0830
- Milwaukee, L1000
- multiple post collar, L0180-L0200
- scoliosis, L1000, L1200, L1300-L1499
- torso supports, L0970-L0999

**Spirometer**
- electronic, E0487
- nonelectronic, A9284

**Splint**
- ankle, L4392-L4398, S8451
- digit, prefabricated, S8450
- dynamic, E1800, E1805, E1810, E1815
- elbow, S8452
- finger, static, Q4049
- footdrop, L4398
- halgus valgus, L3100
- long arm, Q4017-Q4020
- long leg, L4370, Q4041-Q4044
- pneumatic, L4350, L4360, L4370
- short arm, Q4021-Q4024

**Splint** — continued
- short leg, Q4045-Q4048
- Specialist Plaster Splints, A4580
- supplies, Q4051
- Thumb-O-Prene Splint, L3999
- toad finger, A4570
- wrist, S8451

**Spoke protectors, each**, K0065

**Sports supports hinged knee support**, L1832

**Standing frame system**, E0638, E0641-E0642

**Star Lumen tubing**, A4616

**Stat**
- laboratory request, S3600-S3601

**Sten, foot prosthesis**, L5972

**Stent**
- coated
  - with delivery system, C1874
  - without delivery system, C1875
  - with delivery system, C1876
  - without delivery system, C1877
- noncoronary
  - temporary, C2617, C2625

**Stent placement**
- intracoronary, C9600-C9601
  - with percutaneous transluminal coronary atherectomy, C9602-C9603

**Stereotactic radiosurgery**
- therapy, G0339, G0340

**Sterile water**, A4216-A4218

**Stimulated intrauterine insemination**, S4035

**Stimulation**
- electrical, E0740, G0281-G0283
  - acupuncture, S8930
- electromagnetic, G0295

**Stimulators**
- cough, device, E0482
- electric, supplies, A4595
- interferential current, S8130-S8131
- joint, E0762
- neuromuscular, E0744, E0745, E0764
- osteogenesis, electrical, E0747-E0749
- pelvic floor, E0740
- salivary reflex, E0755
- transcutaneous, E0770
- ultrasound, E0760

**Stocking**
- gradient compression, A6530-A6549

**Stoma**
- cap, A5055
- catheter, A5082
- cone, A4399
- plug, A5081

**Stomach tube**, B4083

**Stomahesive**
- skin barrier, A4362, A5122
- sterile wafer, A4362
- strips, A4362

**Storm Arrow power wheelchair**, K0014

**Storm Torque power wheelchair**, K0011

**Stress management class**, S9454

**Stretch device**, E1801, E1811, E1816, E1818, E1831, E1841

**Strip(s)**
- blood, A4253
- glucose test, A4253, A4772
- Nu-Hope
  - adhesive, 1 oz bottle with applicator, A4364
  - adhesive, 3 oz bottle with applicator, A4364
- urine reagent, A4250

**Stroke**, G9257-G9258

**Study**
- gastrointestinal fat absorption, S3708
- sleep, G0398-G0400

**Stump sock**, L8470-L8485

**Stylet**, A4212

**Substance abuse treatment**, T1006-T1012
- ambulatory setting, S9475
- childcare during, T1009
- couples counseling, T1006
- family counseling, T1006
- meals during, T1010
- other than tobacco, G0396, G0397
- skills development, T1012
- treatment plan, T1007

**Suction**
- wound, A9272, K0743

**Sulfamethoxazole and trimethoprim**, S0039

**Sullivan**
- CPAP, E0601

**Sumacal, enteral nutrition**, B4155

**Sunbeam moist/dry heat pad**, E0215

**Sunglass frames**, S0518

**Supplies**
- infection control NOS, S8301
- Medicare IVIG demonstration, Q2052
- miscellaneous DME, A9999
- ventricular assist device, Q0507-Q0509

**Supply/accessory/service**, A9900

**Supply fee**
- pharmacy
  - anticancer oral antiemetic or immunosuppressive drug, Q0511-Q0512
  - immunosuppressive drugs, Q0510

**Support**
- arch, L3040-L3090
- cervical, L0120
- elastic, A6530-A6549
- ongoing to maintain employment, H2025-H2026
- spinal, L0970-L0999
- vaginal, A4561-A4562

**Supported housing**, H0043-H0044

**Supportive device**
- foot pressure off loading, A9283

**Supreme bG Meter**, E0607

**Sure-Gait folding walker**, E0141, E0143

**Sure-Safe raised toilet seat**, E0244

**SureStep blood glucose monitor**, E0607

**Sur-Fit**
- closed-end pouch, A5054
- disposable convex inserts, A5093
- drainable pouch, A5063
- flange cap, A5055
- irrigation sleeve, A4397
- urostomy pouch, A5073

**Sur-Fit/Active Life tail closures**, A4421

**Surgical**
- arthroscopy
  - knee, G0289, S2112
  - shoulder, S2300
- boot, L3208-L3211
- mask, for dialysis, A4928
- procedure, return/no return to OR, G9307-G9308
- site infection, G9311-G9312
- stocking, A4490-A4510
- supplies, miscellaneous, A4649
- tray, A4550

**SurgiMend Collagen Matrix**
- fetal, C9358
- neonatal, C9360

**Survival**, G9259, G9261, G9263

**Sustacal, enteral nutrition**, B4150
- HC, B4152

**Sustagen Powder, enteral nutrition**, B4150

**Swabs, betadine or iodine**, A4247

**Swede, ACT, Cross, or Elite manual wheelchair**, K0005

**Swede Basic F# manual wheelchair**, K0004

**Swedish knee orthotic**, L1850

**Swivel adaptor**, S8186

**Syringe**, A4213
- with needle, A4206-A4209
- dialysis, A4657
- insulin, box of 100, S8490

**System2 zippered body holder**, E0700

**T**

**Table**
- bed, E0274, E0315
- sit-to-stand, E0637
- standing, E0637-E0638, E0641-E0642

**Tachdijan, Legg Perthes orthotic**, L1720

**Tamoxifen citrate**, S0187

**Tamponade**
- retinal, C1814

**Tantalum rings scleral application**, S8030

**Tape**
- nonwaterproof, A4450
- waterproof, A4452

**Taxi, nonemergency transportation**, A0100

**Tc-99 from non-highly enriched uranium**, Q9969

**Team conference**, G0175, G9007, S0220-S0221

**TechneScan**, A9512

**Technetium Tc 99**
- arcitumomab, A9568
- biscate, A9557
- depreotide, A9536
- disofenin, A9510
- exametazime, A9521, A9569
- fanolesomab, A9566
- glucepatate, A9550
- labeled red blood cells, A9560
- macroaggregated albumin, A9540
- mebrofenin, A9537
- medronate, A9503
- mertiatide, A9562
- oxidronate, A9561
- pentetate, A9539, A9567
- pertechretate, A9512
- pyrophosphate, A9538
- sestamibi, A9500
- succimer, A9551
- sulfur colloid, A9541
- teboroxime, A9501
- tetrofosmin, A9502
- tilmanocept, A9520

**Technol**
- Colles splint, L3763
- wrist and forearm splint, L3906

**Telehealth**
- consultation
  - emergency department, G0425-G0427
  - inpatient, G0406-G0408, G0425-G0427
- critical care, G0508-G0509
- facility fee, Q3014
- inpatient pharmacologic management, G0459
- transmission, T1014

**Telemonitoring**
- patient in home, includes equipment, S9110

**Television**
- amplifier, V5270
- caption decoder, V5271

**TenderCloud electric air pump**, E0182

**TenderFlo II**, E0187

**TenderGel II**, E0196

**Tenderlet lancet device**, A4258

**TenoGlide Tendon Protector Sheet**, C9356

**TENS**, A4595, E0720-E0749
- Neuro-Pulse, E0720

**Tent, oxygen**, E0455

**Terminal devices**, L6703-L6715, L6721-L6722

**Terumo disposable insulin syringes, up to 1 cc, per syringe**, A4206

**Testing**
- comparative genomic hybridization, S3870
- developmental, G0451
- drug, G0477-G0483
- genetic, S3800, S3840-S3842, S3844-S3846, S3849-S3850, S3852-S3853, S3861
- Warfarin responsiveness, genetic technique, G9143

**Test materials, home monitoring**, G0249

**Thalassemia, genetic test**
- alpha, S3845
- hemoglobin E beta, S3846

**Thallous chloride Tl 201**, A9505

**Therapeutic**
- agent, A4321
- procedures, respiratory, G0239

**Therapeutic radiopharmaceutical**
- sodium iodide I-131, A9530

**Therapy**
- activity, G0176, H2032
- beta-blocker, G9188-G9192
- infusion, Q0081
- lymphedema, S8950
- nutrition, reassessment, G0270-G0271
- respiratory, G0237-G0239

**Thermalator T-12-M**, E0239

**Thermometer**
- oral, A4931
- rectal, A4932

**Thickener, food**, B4100

© 2016 Optum360, LLC

© 2016 Optum360, LLC

## Transportation Services Including Ambulance A0021-A0999

This code range includes ground and air ambulance, nonemergency transportation (taxi, bus, automobile, wheelchair van), and ancillary transportation-related fees.

HCPCS Level II codes for ambulance services must be reported with modifiers that indicate pick-up origins and destinations. The modifier describing the arrangement (QM, QN) is listed first. The modifiers describing the origin and destination are listed second. Origin and destination modifiers are created by combining two alpha characters from the following list. Each alpha character, with the exception of X, represents either an origin or a destination. Each pair of alpha characters creates one modifier. The first position represents the origin and the second the destination. The modifiers most commonly used are:

| | |
|---|---|
| D | Diagnostic or therapeutic site other than "P" or "H" when these are used as origin codes |
| E | Residential, domiciliary, custodial facility (other than 1819 facility) |
| G | Hospital-based ESRD facility |
| H | Hospital |
| I | Site of transfer (e.g., airport or helicopter pad) between modes of ambulance transport |
| J | Free standing ESRD facility |
| N | Skilled nursing facility (SNF) |
| P | Physician's office |
| R | Residence |
| S | Scene of accident or acute event |
| X | Intermediate stop at physician's office on way to hospital (destination code only) |

Note: Modifier X can only be used as a destination code in the second position of a modifier. See S0215. For Medicaid, see T codes and T modifiers.

### Ambulance Transport and Supplies

**A0021**    **Ambulance service, outside state per mile, transport (Medicaid only)**   E

**A0080**    **Nonemergency transportation, per mile - vehicle provided by volunteer (individual or organization), with no vested interest**   E

**A0090**    **Nonemergency transportation, per mile - vehicle provided by individual (family member, self, neighbor) with vested interest**   E

**A0100**    **Nonemergency transportation; taxi**   E

**A0110**    **Nonemergency transportation and bus, intra- or interstate carrier**   E

**A0120**    **Nonemergency transportation: mini-bus, mountain area transports, or other transportation systems**   E

**A0130**    **Nonemergency transportation: wheelchair van**   E

**A0140**    **Nonemergency transportation and air travel (private or commercial) intra- or interstate**   E

**A0160**    **Nonemergency transportation: per mile - caseworker or social worker**   E

**A0170**    **Transportation ancillary: parking fees, tolls, other**   E

**A0180**    **Nonemergency transportation: ancillary: lodging-recipient**   E

**A0190**    **Nonemergency transportation: ancillary: meals, recipient**   E

**A0200**    **Nonemergency transportation: ancillary: lodging, escort**   E

**A0210**    **Nonemergency transportation: ancillary: meals, escort**   E

**A0225**    **Ambulance service, neonatal transport, base rate, emergency transport, one way**   E
      CMS: 100-04,1,10.1.4.1

**A0380**    **BLS mileage (per mile)**   E ☑
      See code(s): A0425
      CMS: 100-02,10,10.3.3; 100-04,1,10.1.4.1; 100-04,15,20.2; 100-04,15,30.2

**A0382**    **BLS routine disposable supplies**   E
      CMS: 100-02,10,30.1.1

**A0384**    **BLS specialized service disposable supplies; defibrillation (used by ALS ambulances and BLS ambulances in jurisdictions where defibrillation is permitted in BLS ambulances)**   E
      CMS: 100-02,10,30.1.1

**A0390**    **ALS mileage (per mile)**   E ☑
      See code(s): A0425
      CMS: 100-02,10,10.3.3; 100-04,1,10.1.4.1; 100-04,15,20.2; 100-04,15,30.2

**A0392**    **ALS specialized service disposable supplies; defibrillation (to be used only in jurisdictions where defibrillation cannot be performed in BLS ambulances)**   E
      CMS: 100-02,10,30.1.1

**A0394**    **ALS specialized service disposable supplies; IV drug therapy**   E
      CMS: 100-02,10,30.1.1

**A0396**    **ALS specialized service disposable supplies; esophageal intubation**   E
      CMS: 100-02,10,30.1.1

**A0398**    **ALS routine disposable supplies**   E
      CMS: 100-02,10,30.1.1

### Waiting Time

| Units | Time |
|---|---|
| 1 | 1/2 to 1 hr. |
| 2 | 1 to 1-1/2 hrs. |
| 3 | 1-1/2 to 2 hrs. |
| 4 | 2 to 2-1/2 hrs. |
| 5 | 2-1/2 to 3 hrs. |
| 6 | 3 to 3-1/2 hrs. |
| 7 | 3-1/2 to 4 hrs. |
| 8 | 4 to 4-1/2 hrs. |
| 9 | 4-1/2 to 5 hrs. |
| 10 | 5 to 5-1/2 hrs. |

**A0420**    **Ambulance waiting time (ALS or BLS), one-half (1/2) hour increments**   E
      CMS: 100-02,10,30.1.1

### Other Ambulance Services

**A0422**    **Ambulance (ALS or BLS) oxygen and oxygen supplies, life sustaining situation**   E
      CMS: 100-02,10,30.1.1

**A0424**    **Extra ambulance attendant, ground (ALS or BLS) or air (fixed or rotary winged); (requires medical review)**   E
      Pertinent documentation to evaluate medical appropriateness should be included when this code is reported.
      CMS: 100-02,10,30.1.1; 100-04,15,30.2.1

**A0425**    **Ground mileage, per statute mile**   A ☑
      CMS: 100-02,10,10.2.2; 100-02,10,10.3.3; 100-02,10,20; 100-02,10,30.1.1; 100-02,10,20; 100-04,1,10.1.4.1; 100-04,15,10.3; 100-04,15,20.2; 100-04,15,20.6; 100-04,15,30; 100-04,15,30.1.2; 100-04,15,30.2.1; 100-04,15,40
      AHA: 4Q, '12, 1

**A0426**    **Ambulance service, advanced life support, nonemergency transport, level 1 (ALS 1)**   A
      CMS: 100-02,10,10.2.2; 100-02,10,10.3.3; 100-02,10,20; 100-02,10,30.1.1; 100-02,10,20; 100-04,1,10.1.4.1; 100-04,15,10.3; 100-04,15,20.1.4; 100-04,15,30; 100-04,15,30.1.2; 100-04,15,30.2; 100-04,15,30.2.1; 100-04,15,40
      AHA: 4Q, '12, 1

| Special Coverage Instructions | Noncovered by Medicare | Carrier Discretion | ☑ Quantity Alert   ● New Code   ○ Recycled/Reinstated   ▲ Revised Code |
|---|---|---|---|

© 2016 Optum360, LLC    A2-A3 ASC Pmt    **CMS:** Pub 100    **AHA:** Coding Clinic    & DMEPOS Paid    ⊘ SNF Excluded      **A Codes — 1**

**A0427**   Ambulance service, advanced life support, emergency transport, level 1 (ALS 1 - emergency)   Ⓐ

CMS: 100-02,10,10.2.2; 100-02,10,10.3.3; 100-02,10,20; 100-02,10,30.1.1; 100-02,10.20; 100-04,1,10.1.4.1; 100-04,15,10.3; 100-04,15,20.1.4; 100-04,15,30; 100-04,15,30.1.2; 100-04,15,30.2; 100-04,15,30.2.1; 100-04,15,40

AHA: 4Q, '12, 1

**A0428**   Ambulance service, basic life support, nonemergency transport, (BLS)   Ⓐ

CMS: 100-02,10,10.2.2; 100-02,10,10.3.3; 100-02,10,20; 100-02,10,30.1.1; 100-02,10.20; 100-04,1,10.1.4.1; 100-04,15,10.3; 100-04,15,20.1.4; 100-04,15,20.6; 100-04,15,30; 100-04,15,30.1.2; 100-04,15,30.2; 100-04,15,30.2.1; 100-04,15,40

AHA: 4Q, '12, 1

**A0429**   Ambulance service, basic life support, emergency transport (BLS, emergency)   Ⓐ

CMS: 100-02,10,10.2.2; 100-02,10,10.3.3; 100-02,10,20; 100-02,10,30.1.1; 100-02,10.20; 100-04,1,10.1.4.1; 100-04,15,10.3; 100-04,15,20.1.4; 100-04,15,30; 100-04,15,30.1.2; 100-04,15,30.2; 100-04,15,30.2.1; 100-04,15,40

AHA: 4Q, '12, 1

**A0430**   Ambulance service, conventional air services, transport, one way (fixed wing)   Ⓐ

CMS: 100-02,10,10.2.2; 100-02,10,10.3.3; 100-02,10,20; 100-02,10.20; 100-04,1,10.1.4.1; 100-04,15,10.3; 100-04,15,20.1.4; 100-04,15,20.3; 100-04,15,30; 100-04,15,30.1.2; 100-04,15,30.2; 100-04,15,30.2.1; 100-04,15,40

AHA: 4Q, '12, 1

**A0431**   Ambulance service, conventional air services, transport, one way (rotary wing)   Ⓐ

CMS: 100-02,10,10.2.2; 100-02,10,10.3.3; 100-02,10,20; 100-02,10.20; 100-04,1,10.1.4.1; 100-04,15,10.3; 100-04,15,20.1.4; 100-04,15,20.3; 100-04,15,30; 100-04,15,30.1.2; 100-04,15,30.2; 100-04,15,30.2.1; 100-04,15,40

AHA: 4Q, '12, 1

**A0432**   Paramedic intercept (PI), rural area, transport furnished by a volunteer ambulance company which is prohibited by state law from billing third-party payers   Ⓐ

CMS: 100-02,10,10.2.2; 100-02,10,10.3.3; 100-02,10,20; 100-02,10,30.1.1; 100-02,10.20; 100-04,15,10.3; 100-04,15,20.1.4; 100-04,15,30; 100-04,15,30.1.2; 100-04,15,30.2; 100-04,15,30.2.1; 100-04,15,40

AHA: 4Q, '12, 1

**A0433**   Advanced life support, level 2 (ALS 2)   Ⓐ

CMS: 100-02,10,10.2.2; 100-02,10,10.3.3; 100-02,10,20; 100-02,10,30.1.1; 100-02,10.20; 100-04,15,10.3; 100-04,15,20.1.4; 100-04,15,30; 100-04,15,30.1.2; 100-04,15,30.2; 100-04,15,30.2.1; 100-04,15,40

AHA: 4Q, '12, 1

**A0434**   Specialty care transport (SCT)   Ⓐ

CMS: 100-02,10,10.2.2; 100-02,10,10.3.3; 100-02,10,20; 100-02,10,30.1.1; 100-02,10.20; 100-04,15,10.3; 100-04,15,20.1.4; 100-04,15,30; 100-04,15,30.1.2; 100-04,15,30.2; 100-04,15,30.2.1; 100-04,15,40

AHA: 4Q, '12, 1

**A0435**   Fixed wing air mileage, per statute mile   Ⓐ

CMS: 100-02,10,10.2.2; 100-02,10,10.3.3; 100-02,10,20; 100-02,10.20; 100-04,15,10.3; 100-04,15,20.1.4; 100-04,15,20.2; 100-04,15,20.3; 100-04,15,30; 100-04,15,30.1.2; 100-04,15,30.2; 100-04,15,30.2.1; 100-04,15,40

AHA: 4Q, '12, 1

**A0436**   Rotary wing air mileage, per statute mile   Ⓐ

CMS: 100-02,10,10.2.2; 100-02,10,10.3.3; 100-02,10,20; 100-02,10.20; 100-04,15,10.3; 100-04,15,20.1.4; 100-04,15,20.2; 100-04,15,20.3; 100-04,15,30; 100-04,15,30.1.2; 100-04,15,30.2; 100-04,15,30.2.1; 100-04,15,40

AHA: 4Q, '12, 1

**A0888**   Noncovered ambulance mileage, per mile (e.g., for miles traveled beyond closest appropriate facility)   Ⓔ

CMS: 100-02,10,20; 100-04,15,20.2; 100-04,15,30.1.2; 100-04,15,30.2.4

**A0998**   Ambulance response and treatment, no transport   Ⓔ

**A0999**   Unlisted ambulance service   Ⓐ

CMS: 100-02,10,10.1; 100-02,10,20

## Medical and Surgical Supplies A4206-A9999

This section covers a wide variety of medical, surgical, and some durable medical equipment (DME) related supplies and accessories. DME-related supplies, accessories, maintenance, and repair required to ensure the proper functioning of this equipment is generally covered by Medicare under the prosthetic devices provision.

### Injection Supplies

**A4206**   Syringe with needle, sterile, 1 cc or less, each   Ⓝ ☑

**A4207**   Syringe with needle, sterile 2 cc, each   Ⓝ ☑

**A4208**   Syringe with needle, sterile 3 cc, each   Ⓝ ☑

**A4209**   Syringe with needle, sterile 5 cc or greater, each   Ⓝ ☑

**A4210**   Needle-free injection device, each   Ⓔ ☑

Sometimes covered by commercial payers with preauthorization and physician letter stating need (e.g., for insulin injection in young children).

**A4211**   Supplies for self-administered injections   Ⓝ

When a drug that is usually injected by the patient (e.g., insulin or calcitonin) is injected by the physician, it is excluded from Medicare coverage unless administered in an emergency situation (e.g., diabetic coma).

**A4212**   Noncoring needle or stylet with or without catheter   Ⓝ

**A4213**   Syringe, sterile, 20 cc or greater, each   Ⓝ ☑

**A4215**   Needle, sterile, any size, each   Ⓝ

**A4216**   Sterile water, saline and/or dextrose, diluent/flush, 10 ml   Ⓝ ☑ ♿

**A4217**   Sterile water/saline, 500 ml   Ⓝ ☑ ♿ (AU)

**A4218**   Sterile saline or water, metered dose dispenser, 10 ml   Ⓝ Ⓜ ☑

**A4220**   Refill kit for implantable infusion pump   Ⓝ Ⓜ

▲ **A4221**ᴶᵃⁿ   Supplies for maintenance of non-insulin drug infusion catheter, per week (list drugs separately)   Ⓝ ♿

**A4222**   Infusion supplies for external drug infusion pump, per cassette or bag (list drugs separately)   Ⓝ ♿

**A4223**   Infusion supplies not used with external infusion pump, per cassette or bag (list drugs separately)   Ⓝ ☑

● **A4224**ᴶᵃⁿ   Supplies for maintenance of insulin infusion catheter, per week

● **A4225**ᴶᵃⁿ   Supplies for external insulin infusion pump, syringe type cartridge, sterile, each

**A4230**   Infusion set for external insulin pump, nonneedle cannula type   Ⓝ ☑

Covered by some commercial payers as ongoing supply to preauthorized pump.

**A4231**   Infusion set for external insulin pump, needle type   Ⓝ ☑

Covered by some commercial payers as ongoing supply to preauthorized pump.

**A4232**   Syringe with needle for external insulin pump, sterile, 3 cc   Ⓔ ☑

Covered by some commercial payers as ongoing supply to preauthorized pump.

---

ᴶᵃⁿ **January Update**

Special Coverage Instructions      Noncovered by Medicare      Carrier Discretion      ☑ Quantity Alert   ● New Code   ○ Recycled/Reinstated   ▲ Revised Code

**2 — A Codes**      Ⓐ Age Edit      Ⓜ Maternity Edit      ♀ Female Only      ♂ Male Only      Ⓐ-Ⓨ OPPS Status Indicators      © 2016 Optum360, LLC

## Batteries

**A4233**   Replacement battery, alkaline (other than J cell), for use with medically necessary home blood glucose monitor owned by patient, each   🄴 ☑ ♿ (NU)
CMS: 100-04,23,60.3

**A4234**   Replacement battery, alkaline, J cell, for use with medically necessary home blood glucose monitor owned by patient, each   🄴 ☑ ♿ (NU)
CMS: 100-04,23,60.3

**A4235**   Replacement battery, lithium, for use with medically necessary home blood glucose monitor owned by patient, each   🄴 ☑ ♿ (NU)
CMS: 100-04,23,60.3

**A4236**   Replacement battery, silver oxide, for use with medically necessary home blood glucose monitor owned by patient, each   🄴 ☑ ♿ (NU)
CMS: 100-04,23,60.3

## Other Supplies

**A4244**   Alcohol or peroxide, per pint   🄽 ☑

**A4245**   Alcohol wipes, per box   🄽 ☑

**A4246**   Betadine or pHisoHex solution, per pint   🄽 ☑

**A4247**   Betadine or iodine swabs/wipes, per box   🄽 ☑

**A4248**   Chlorhexidine containing antiseptic, 1 ml   🄽 🄝 ☑

**A4250**   Urine test or reagent strips or tablets (100 tablets or strips)   🄴 ☑
CMS: 100-02,15,110

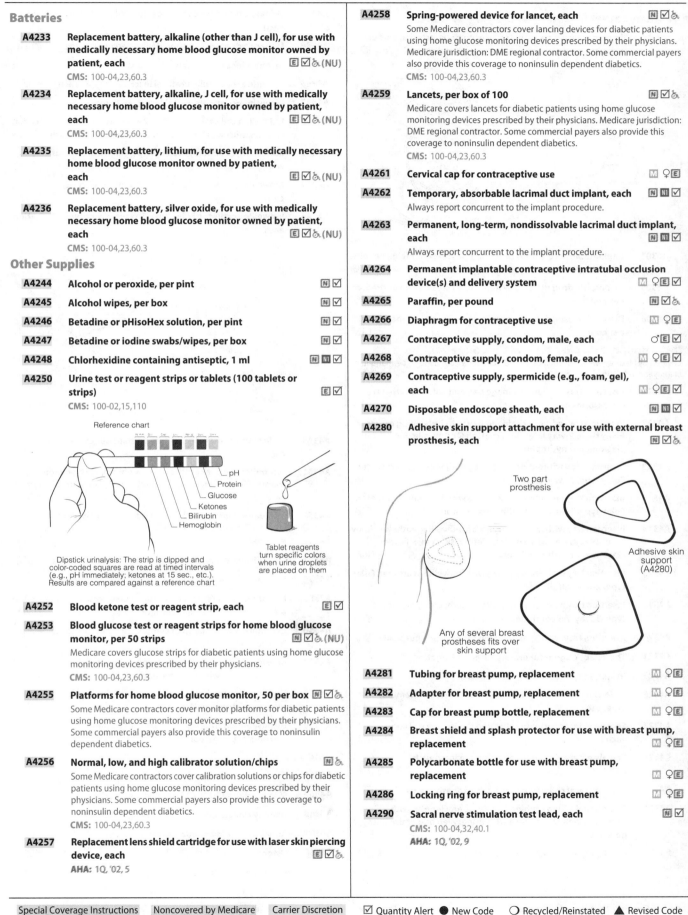

Reference chart

pH
Protein
Glucose
Ketones
Bilirubin
Hemoglobin

Dipstick urinalysis: The strip is dipped and color-coded squares are read at timed intervals (e.g., pH immediately; ketones at 15 sec., etc.). Results are compared against a reference chart

Tablet reagents turn specific colors when urine droplets are placed on them

**A4252**   Blood ketone test or reagent strip, each   🄴 ☑

**A4253**   Blood glucose test or reagent strips for home blood glucose monitor, per 50 strips   🄽 ☑ ♿ (NU)
Medicare covers glucose strips for diabetic patients using home glucose monitoring devices prescribed by their physicians.
CMS: 100-04,23,60.3

**A4255**   Platforms for home blood glucose monitor, 50 per box   🄽 ☑ ♿
Some Medicare contractors cover monitor platforms for diabetic patients using home glucose monitoring devices prescribed by their physicians. Some commercial payers also provide this coverage to noninsulin dependent diabetics.

**A4256**   Normal, low, and high calibrator solution/chips   🄽 ♿
Some Medicare contractors cover calibration solutions or chips for diabetic patients using home glucose monitoring devices prescribed by their physicians. Some commercial payers also provide this coverage to noninsulin dependent diabetics.
CMS: 100-04,23,60.3

**A4257**   Replacement lens shield cartridge for use with laser skin piercing device, each   🄴 ☑ ♿
AHA: 1Q, '02, 5

**A4258**   Spring-powered device for lancet, each   🄽 ☑ ♿
Some Medicare contractors cover lancing devices for diabetic patients using home glucose monitoring devices prescribed by their physicians. Medicare jurisdiction: DME regional contractor. Some commercial payers also provide this coverage to noninsulin dependent diabetics.
CMS: 100-04,23,60.3

**A4259**   Lancets, per box of 100   🄽 ☑ ♿
Medicare covers lancets for diabetic patients using home glucose monitoring devices prescribed by their physicians. Medicare jurisdiction: DME regional contractor. Some commercial payers also provide this coverage to noninsulin dependent diabetics.
CMS: 100-04,23,60.3

**A4261**   Cervical cap for contraceptive use   🄼 ♀🄴

**A4262**   Temporary, absorbable lacrimal duct implant, each   🄽 🄝 ☑
Always report concurrent to the implant procedure.

**A4263**   Permanent, long-term, nondissolvable lacrimal duct implant, each   🄽 🄝 ☑
Always report concurrent to the implant procedure.

**A4264**   Permanent implantable contraceptive intratubal occlusion device(s) and delivery system   🄼 ♀🄴 ☑

**A4265**   Paraffin, per pound   🄽 ☑ ♿

**A4266**   Diaphragm for contraceptive use   🄼 ♀🄴

**A4267**   Contraceptive supply, condom, male, each   ♂🄴 ☑

**A4268**   Contraceptive supply, condom, female, each   🄼 ♀🄴 ☑

**A4269**   Contraceptive supply, spermicide (e.g., foam, gel), each   🄼 ♀🄴 ☑

**A4270**   Disposable endoscope sheath, each   🄽 🄝 ☑

**A4280**   Adhesive skin support attachment for use with external breast prosthesis, each   🄽 ☑ ♿

Two part prosthesis

Adhesive skin support (A4280)

Any of several breast prostheses fits over skin support

**A4281**   Tubing for breast pump, replacement   🄼 ♀🄴

**A4282**   Adapter for breast pump, replacement   🄼 ♀

**A4283**   Cap for breast pump bottle, replacement   🄼 ♀🄴

**A4284**   Breast shield and splash protector for use with breast pump, replacement   🄼 ♀🄴

**A4285**   Polycarbonate bottle for use with breast pump, replacement   🄼 ♀🄴

**A4286**   Locking ring for breast pump, replacement   🄼 ♀🄴

**A4290**   Sacral nerve stimulation test lead, each   🄽 ☑
CMS: 100-04,32,40.1
AHA: 1Q, '02, 9

---

Special Coverage Instructions     Noncovered by Medicare     Carrier Discretion     ☑ Quantity Alert   ● New Code   ○ Recycled/Reinstated   ▲ Revised Code

© 2016 Optum360, LLC     🄐-🅩 ASC Pmt     CMS: Pub 100     AHA: Coding Clinic     ♿ DMEPOS Paid     ⊘ SNF Excluded     **A Codes — 3**

## Vascular Catheters and Drug Delivery Systems

**A4300** Implantable access catheter, (e.g., venous, arterial, epidural subarachnoid, or peritoneal, etc.) external access N N1

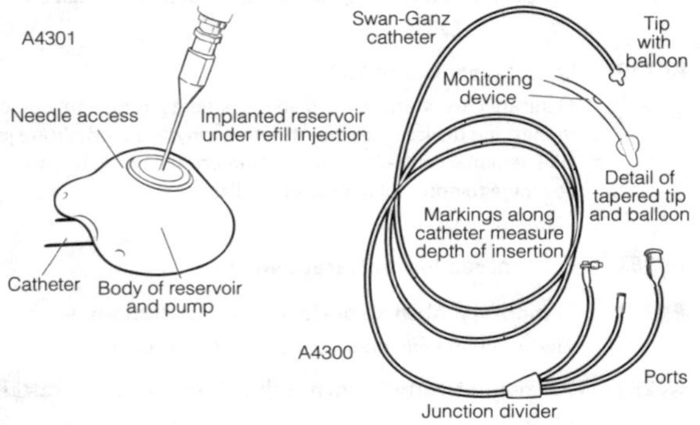
A4301
Needle access
Implanted reservoir under refill injection
Catheter
Body of reservoir and pump
Swan-Ganz catheter
Tip with balloon
Monitoring device
Detail of tapered tip and balloon
Markings along catheter measure depth of insertion
A4300
Ports
Junction divider

**A4301** Implantable access total catheter, port/reservoir (e.g., venous, arterial, epidural, subarachnoid, peritoneal, etc.) N N1

**A4305** Disposable drug delivery system, flow rate of 50 ml or greater per hour N N1 ☑

**A4306** Disposable drug delivery system, flow rate of less than 50 ml per hour N N1 ☑

## Incontinennce Appliances and Care Supplies

Covered by Medicare when the medical record indicates incontinence is permanent, or of long and indefinite duration.

**A4310** Insertion tray without drainage bag and without catheter (accessories only) N ♿

**A4311** Insertion tray without drainage bag with indwelling catheter, Foley type, 2-way latex with coating (Teflon, silicone, silicone elastomer or hydrophilic, etc.) N ♿

**A4312** Insertion tray without drainage bag with indwelling catheter, Foley type, 2-way, all silicone N ♿

**A4313** Insertion tray without drainage bag with indwelling catheter, Foley type, 3-way, for continuous irrigation N ♿

**A4314** Insertion tray with drainage bag with indwelling catheter, Foley type, 2-way latex with coating (Teflon, silicone, silicone elastomer or hydrophilic, etc.) N ♿

**A4315** Insertion tray with drainage bag with indwelling catheter, Foley type, 2-way, all silicone N ♿

**A4316** Insertion tray with drainage bag with indwelling catheter, Foley type, 3-way, for continuous irrigation N ♿

**A4320** Irrigation tray with bulb or piston syringe, any purpose N ♿

**A4321** Therapeutic agent for urinary catheter irrigation N ♿

**A4322** Irrigation syringe, bulb or piston, each N ☑ ♿

**A4326** Male external catheter with integral collection chamber, any type, each ♂ N ☑ ♿

**A4327** Female external urinary collection device; meatal cup, each ♀ N ☑ ♿

**A4328** Female external urinary collection device; pouch, each A ♀ N ☑ ♿

**A4330** Perianal fecal collection pouch with adhesive, each N ☑ ♿

**A4331** Extension drainage tubing, any type, any length, with connector/adaptor, for use with urinary leg bag or urostomy pouch, each N ☑ ♿

**A4332** Lubricant, individual sterile packet, each N ☑ ♿

**A4333** Urinary catheter anchoring device, adhesive skin attachment, each N ☑ ♿

**A4334** Urinary catheter anchoring device, leg strap, each N ☑ ♿

**A4335** Incontinence supply; miscellaneous N

**A4336** Incontinence supply, urethral insert, any type, each N ☑ ♿

**A4337** Incontinence supply, rectal insert, any type, each N

**A4338** Indwelling catheter; Foley type, 2-way latex with coating (Teflon, silicone, silicone elastomer, or hydrophilic, etc.), each N ☑ ♿

**A4340** Indwelling catheter; specialty type, (e.g., Coude, mushroom, wing, etc.), each N ☑ ♿

**A4344** Indwelling catheter, Foley type, 2-way, all silicone, each N ☑ ♿

**A4346** Indwelling catheter; Foley type, 3-way for continuous irrigation, each N ☑ ♿

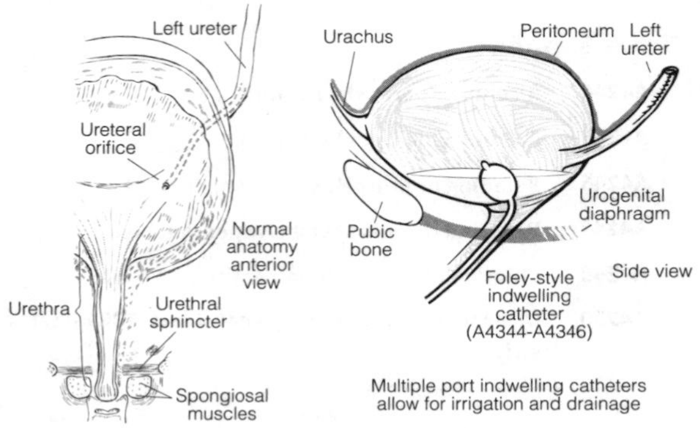
Left ureter
Ureteral orifice
Normal anatomy anterior view
Urethra
Urethral sphincter
Spongiosal muscles
Urachus
Peritoneum
Left ureter
Pubic bone
Urogenital diaphragm
Foley-style indwelling catheter (A4344-A4346)
Side view
Multiple port indwelling catheters allow for irrigation and drainage

**A4349** Male external catheter, with or without adhesive, disposable, each ♂ N ☑ ♿

**A4351** Intermittent urinary catheter; straight tip, with or without coating (Teflon, silicone, silicone elastomer, or hydrophilic, etc.), each N ☑ ♿

**A4352** Intermittent urinary catheter; Coude (curved) tip, with or without coating (Teflon, silicone, silicone elastomeric, or hydrophilic, etc.), each N ☑ ♿

**A4353** Intermittent urinary catheter, with insertion supplies N ♿

**A4354** Insertion tray with drainage bag but without catheter N ♿

**A4355** Irrigation tubing set for continuous bladder irrigation through a 3-way indwelling Foley catheter, each N ☑ ♿

**A4356** External urethral clamp or compression device (not to be used for catheter clamp), each N ☑ ♿

**A4357** Bedside drainage bag, day or night, with or without antireflux device, with or without tube, each N ☑ ♿

**A4358** Urinary drainage bag, leg or abdomen, vinyl, with or without tube, with straps, each N ☑ ♿

**A4360** Disposable external urethral clamp or compression device, with pad and/or pouch, each N ☑ ♿

## Ostomy Supplies

**A4361** Ostomy faceplate, each N ☑ ♿

**A4362** Skin barrier; solid, 4 x 4 or equivalent; each N ☑ ♿

**A4363** Ostomy clamp, any type, replacement only, each E ♿

**A4364** Adhesive, liquid or equal, any type, per oz N ☑ ♿

**A4366** Ostomy vent, any type, each N ☑ ♿

**A4367** Ostomy belt, each N ☑ ♿



© 2016 Optum360, LLC

| Code | Description | Symbols |
|------|-------------|---------|
| A4368 | Ostomy filter, any type, each | N ☑ |
| A4369 | Ostomy skin barrier, liquid (spray, brush, etc.), per oz | N ☑ &#x267F; |
| A4371 | Ostomy skin barrier, powder, per oz | N ☑ &#x267F; |
| A4372 | Ostomy skin barrier, solid 4 x 4 or equivalent, standard wear, with built-in convexity, each | N ☑ &#x267F; |
| A4373 | Ostomy skin barrier, with flange (solid, flexible or accordion), with built-in convexity, any size, each | N ☑ &#x267F; |

Barrier adheres to skin

Flange attaches to bag

Waste moves through hole in membrane

Faceplate flange and skin barrier combination (A4373)

| Code | Description | Symbols |
|------|-------------|---------|
| A4375 | Ostomy pouch, drainable, with faceplate attached, plastic, each | N ☑ &#x267F; |
| A4376 | Ostomy pouch, drainable, with faceplate attached, rubber, each | N ☑ &#x267F; |

Colostomy pouch with faceplate and drain (A4376)

| Code | Description | Symbols |
|------|-------------|---------|
| A4377 | Ostomy pouch, drainable, for use on faceplate, plastic, each | N ☑ &#x267F; |
| A4378 | Ostomy pouch, drainable, for use on faceplate, rubber, each | N ☑ &#x267F; |
| A4379 | Ostomy pouch, urinary, with faceplate attached, plastic, each | N ☑ &#x267F; |
| A4380 | Ostomy pouch, urinary, with faceplate attached, rubber, each | N ☑ &#x267F; |
| A4381 | Ostomy pouch, urinary, for use on faceplate, plastic, each | N ☑ &#x267F; |
| A4382 | Ostomy pouch, urinary, for use on faceplate, heavy plastic, each | N ☑ &#x267F; |
| A4383 | Ostomy pouch, urinary, for use on faceplate, rubber, each | N ☑ &#x267F; |
| A4384 | Ostomy faceplate equivalent, silicone ring, each | N ☑ &#x267F; |
| A4385 | Ostomy skin barrier, solid 4 x 4 or equivalent, extended wear, without built-in convexity, each | N ☑ &#x267F; |
| A4387 | Ostomy pouch, closed, with barrier attached, with built-in convexity (1 piece), each | N ☑ &#x267F; |
| A4388 | Ostomy pouch, drainable, with extended wear barrier attached, (1 piece), each | N ☑ &#x267F; |
| A4389 | Ostomy pouch, drainable, with barrier attached, with built-in convexity (1 piece), each | N ☑ &#x267F; |
| A4390 | Ostomy pouch, drainable, with extended wear barrier attached, with built-in convexity (1 piece), each | N ☑ &#x267F; |

| Code | Description | Symbols |
|------|-------------|---------|
| A4391 | Ostomy pouch, urinary, with extended wear barrier attached (1 piece), each | N ☑ &#x267F; |
| A4392 | Ostomy pouch, urinary, with standard wear barrier attached, with built-in convexity (1 piece), each | N ☑ &#x267F; |
| A4393 | Ostomy pouch, urinary, with extended wear barrier attached, with built-in convexity (1 piece), each | N ☑ &#x267F; |
| A4394 | Ostomy deodorant, with or without lubricant, for use in ostomy pouch, per fl oz | N ☑ &#x267F; |
| A4395 | Ostomy deodorant for use in ostomy pouch, solid, per tablet | N ☑ &#x267F; |
| A4396 | Ostomy belt with peristomal hernia support | N &#x267F; |
| A4397 | Irrigation supply; sleeve, each | N ☑ &#x267F; |
| A4398 | Ostomy irrigation supply; bag, each | N ☑ &#x267F; |
| A4399 | Ostomy irrigation supply; cone/catheter, with or without brush | N &#x267F; |
| A4400 | Ostomy irrigation set | N &#x267F; |
| A4402 | Lubricant, per oz | N ☑ &#x267F; |
| A4404 | Ostomy ring, each | N ☑ &#x267F; |
| A4405 | Ostomy skin barrier, nonpectin-based, paste, per oz | N ☑ &#x267F; |
| A4406 | Ostomy skin barrier, pectin-based, paste, per oz | N ☑ &#x267F; |
| A4407 | Ostomy skin barrier, with flange (solid, flexible, or accordion), extended wear, with built-in convexity, 4 x 4 in or smaller, each | N ☑ &#x267F; |
| A4408 | Ostomy skin barrier, with flange (solid, flexible or accordion), extended wear, with built-in convexity, larger than 4 x 4 in, each | N ☑ &#x267F; |
| A4409 | Ostomy skin barrier, with flange (solid, flexible or accordion), extended wear, without built-in convexity, 4 x 4 in or smaller, each | N ☑ &#x267F; |
| A4410 | Ostomy skin barrier, with flange (solid, flexible or accordion), extended wear, without built-in convexity, larger than 4 x 4 in, each | N ☑ &#x267F; |
| A4411 | Ostomy skin barrier, solid 4 x 4 or equivalent, extended wear, with built-in convexity, each | N ☑ &#x267F; |
| A4412 | Ostomy pouch, drainable, high output, for use on a barrier with flange (2 piece system), without filter, each | N ☑ &#x267F; |
| A4413 | Ostomy pouch, drainable, high output, for use on a barrier with flange (2-piece system), with filter, each | N ☑ &#x267F; |
| A4414 | Ostomy skin barrier, with flange (solid, flexible or accordion), without built-in convexity, 4 x 4 in or smaller, each | N ☑ &#x267F; |
| A4415 | Ostomy skin barrier, with flange (solid, flexible or accordion), without built-in convexity, larger than 4 x 4 in, each | N ☑ &#x267F; |
| A4416 | Ostomy pouch, closed, with barrier attached, with filter (1 piece), each | N ☑ &#x267F; |
| A4417 | Ostomy pouch, closed, with barrier attached, with built-in convexity, with filter (1 piece), each | N ☑ &#x267F; |
| A4418 | Ostomy pouch, closed; without barrier attached, with filter (1 piece), each | N ☑ &#x267F; |
| A4419 | Ostomy pouch, closed; for use on barrier with nonlocking flange, with filter (2 piece), each | N ☑ &#x267F; |
| A4420 | Ostomy pouch, closed; for use on barrier with locking flange (2 piece), each | N ☑ &#x267F; |

Special Coverage Instructions    Noncovered by Medicare    Carrier Discretion    ☑ Quantity Alert   ● New Code   ○ Recycled/Reinstated   ▲ Revised Code

© 2016 Optum360, LLC    **A2**-**Z3** ASC Pmt    **CMS:** Pub 100    **AHA:** Coding Clinic    &#x267F; DMEPOS Paid    ⊘ SNF Excluded    **A Codes — 5**

**Transportation Services Including Ambulance**

**A4421 — A4606**

| | | |
|---|---|---|
| **A4421** | Ostomy supply; miscellaneous | N |

Determine if an alternative HCPCS Level II or a CPT code better describes the service being reported. This code should be used only if a more specific code is unavailable.

**A4422** Ostomy absorbent material (sheet/pad/crystal packet) for use in ostomy pouch to thicken liquid stomal output, each  N ☑ &

**A4423** Ostomy pouch, closed; for use on barrier with locking flange, with filter (2 piece), each  N ☑ &

**A4424** Ostomy pouch, drainable, with barrier attached, with filter (1 piece), each  N ☑ &

**A4425** Ostomy pouch, drainable; for use on barrier with nonlocking flange, with filter (2-piece system), each  N ☑ &

**A4426** Ostomy pouch, drainable; for use on barrier with locking flange (2-piece system), each  N ☑ &

**A4427** Ostomy pouch, drainable; for use on barrier with locking flange, with filter (2-piece system), each  N ☑ &

**A4428** Ostomy pouch, urinary, with extended wear barrier attached, with faucet-type tap with valve (1 piece), each  N ☑ &

**A4429** Ostomy pouch, urinary, with barrier attached, with built-in convexity, with faucet-type tap with valve (1 piece), each  N ☑ &

**A4430** Ostomy pouch, urinary, with extended wear barrier attached, with built-in convexity, with faucet-type tap with valve (1 piece), each  N ☑ &

**A4431** Ostomy pouch, urinary; with barrier attached, with faucet-type tap with valve (1 piece), each  N ☑ &

**A4432** Ostomy pouch, urinary; for use on barrier with nonlocking flange, with faucet-type tap with valve (2 piece), each  N ☑ &

**A4433** Ostomy pouch, urinary; for use on barrier with locking flange (2 piece), each  N ☑ &

**A4434** Ostomy pouch, urinary; for use on barrier with locking flange, with faucet-type tap with valve (2 piece), each  N ☑ &

**A4435** Ostomy pouch, drainable, high output, with extended wear barrier (one-piece system), with or without filter, each  N &

## Miscellaneous Supplies

**A4450** Tape, nonwaterproof, per 18 sq in  N ☑ & (AU,AV,AW)
See also code A4452.

**A4452** Tape, waterproof, per 18 sq in  N ☑ & (AU,AV,AW)
See also code A4450.

**A4455** Adhesive remover or solvent (for tape, cement or other adhesive), per oz  N ☑ &

**A4456** Adhesive remover, wipes, any type, each  N ☑ &

**A4458** Enema bag with tubing, reusable  N

**A4459** Manual pump-operated enema system, includes balloon, catheter and all accessories, reusable, any type  N

**A4461** Surgical dressing holder, nonreusable, each  N ☑ &

**A4463** Surgical dressing holder, reusable, each  N ☑ &

**A4465** Nonelastic binder for extremity  N

**A4466**^Jan ~~Garment, belt, sleeve or other covering, elastic or similar stretchable material, any type, each~~
To report, see ~A4467

● **A4467**^Jan Belt, strap, sleeve, garment, or covering, any type

**A4470** Gravlee jet washer  N

**A4480** VABRA aspirator  ♀N
CMS: 100-03,230.6

**A4481** Tracheostoma filter, any type, any size, each  N ☑ &

**A4483** Moisture exchanger, disposable, for use with invasive mechanical ventilation  N &

**A4490** Surgical stockings above knee length, each  E ☑
CMS: 100-02,15,110

**A4495** Surgical stockings thigh length, each  E ☑
CMS: 100-02,15,110

**A4500** Surgical stockings below knee length, each  E ☑
CMS: 100-02,15,110

**A4510** Surgical stockings full-length, each  E ☑
CMS: 100-02,15,110

**A4520** Incontinence garment, any type, (e.g., brief, diaper), each  E ☑

**A4550** Surgical trays  B

● **A4553**^Jan Non-disposable underpads, all sizes

**A4554** Disposable underpads, all sizes  E ☑

**A4555** Electrode/transducer for use with electrical stimulation device used for cancer treatment, replacement only  E

**A4556** Electrodes (e.g., apnea monitor), per pair  N ☑ &

**A4557** Lead wires (e.g., apnea monitor), per pair  N ☑ &

**A4558** Conductive gel or paste, for use with electrical device (e.g., TENS, NMES), per oz  N ☑ &

**A4559** Coupling gel or paste, for use with ultrasound device, per oz  N ☑ &

**A4561** Pessary, rubber, any type  ♀N &

**A4562** Pessary, nonrubber, any type  ♀N &
Medicare jurisdiction: DME regional contractor.

**A4565** Slings  N &

**A4566** Shoulder sling or vest design, abduction restrainer, with or without swathe control, prefabricated, includes fitting and adjustment  E

**A4570** Splint  E
Dressings applied by a physician are included as part of the professional service.

**A4575** Topical hyperbaric oxygen chamber, disposable  E

**A4580** Cast supplies (e.g., plaster)  E
See Q4001-Q4048.

**A4590** Special casting material (e.g., fiberglass)  E
See Q4001-Q4048.

**A4595** Electrical stimulator supplies, 2 lead, per month, (e.g., TENS, NMES)  N &
CMS: 100-03,10.2

**A4600** Sleeve for intermittent limb compression device, replacement only, each  E ☑

**A4601** Lithium ion battery, rechargeable, for nonprosthetic use, replacement  E

**A4602** Replacement battery for external infusion pump owned by patient, lithium, 1.5 volt, each  N & (NU)

**A4604** Tubing with integrated heating element for use with positive airway pressure device  N & (NU)
CMS: 100-04,23,60.3; 100-04,36,50.14

**A4605** Tracheal suction catheter, closed system, each  N ☑ & (NU)

**A4606** Oxygen probe for use with oximeter device, replacement  N

---

^Jan **January Update**

Special Coverage Instructions   Noncovered by Medicare   Carrier Discretion   ☑ Quantity Alert  ● New Code   ○ Recycled/Reinstated  ▲ Revised Code

6 — A Codes   Ⓐ Age Edit   Ⓜ Maternity Edit  ♀ Female Only  ♂ Male Only  Ⓐ-Ⓨ OPPS Status Indicators   © 2016 Optum360, LLC

**A4608** Transtracheal oxygen catheter, each  N ☑ &
CMS: 100-04,23,60.3

## Supplies for Oxygen and Related Respiratory Equipment

**A4611** Battery, heavy-duty; replacement for patient-owned
ventilator  E

**A4612** Battery cables; replacement for patient-owned ventilator  E

**A4613** Battery charger; replacement for patient-owned
ventilator  E ☑

**A4614** Peak expiratory flow rate meter, hand held  N &

**A4615** Cannula, nasal  N &
CMS: 100-04,20,100.2; 100-04,23,60.3

**A4616** Tubing (oxygen), per foot  N ☑ &
CMS: 100-04,20,100.2; 100-04,23,60.3

**A4617** Mouthpiece  N &
CMS: 100-04,20,100.2; 100-04,23,60.3

**A4618** Breathing circuits  N & (NU,RR,UE)
CMS: 100-04,20,100.2

**A4619** Face tent  N & (NU)
CMS: 100-04,20,100.2

**A4620** Variable concentration mask  N &
CMS: 100-04,20,100.2; 100-04,23,60.3

**A4623** Tracheostomy, inner cannula  N &

**A4624** Tracheal suction catheter, any type other than closed system,
each  N ☑ & (NU)

**A4625** Tracheostomy care kit for new tracheostomy  N &

**A4626** Tracheostomy cleaning brush, each  N ☑ &

**A4627** Spacer, bag or reservoir, with or without mask, for use with
metered dose inhaler  E
CMS: 100-02,15,110

**A4628** Oropharyngeal suction catheter, each  N ☑ & (NU)

**A4629** Tracheostomy care kit for established tracheostomy  N &

## Replacement Supplies for DME

**A4630** Replacement batteries, medically necessary, transcutaneous
electrical stimulator, owned by patient  E ☑ & (NU)

**A4633** Replacement bulb/lamp for ultraviolet light therapy system,
each  E ☑ & (NU)

**A4634** Replacement bulb for therapeutic light box, tabletop
model  N

**A4635** Underarm pad, crutch, replacement, each  E ☑ & (NU,RR,UE)

**A4636** Replacement, handgrip, cane, crutch, or walker,
each  E ☑ & (NU,RR,UE)
CMS: 100-04,23,60.3; 100-04,36,50.15

**A4637** Replacement, tip, cane, crutch, walker, each  E ☑ & (NU,RR,UE)
CMS: 100-04,23,60.3; 100-04,36,50.15

**A4638** Replacement battery for patient-owned ear pulse generator,
each  E ☑ & (NU,RR,UE)

**A4639** Replacement pad for infrared heating pad system,
each  E ☑ & (RR)

**A4640** Replacement pad for use with medically necessary alternating
pressure pad owned by patient  E & (NU,RR,UE)

## Radiopharmaceuticals

**A4641** Radiopharmaceutical, diagnostic, not otherwise
classified  N M
CMS: 100-04,13,60.3; 100-04,13,60.3.1; 100-04,13,60.3.2
AHA: 4Q, '05, 1-6; 3Q, '04, 1-10

**A4642** Indium In-111 satumomab pendetide, diagnostic, per study
dose, up to 6 millicuries  N M ☑
Use this code for Oncoscint.
AHA: 4Q, '05, 1-6; 3Q, '04, 1-10; 2Q, '02, 8-9

## Miscellaneous Supplies

**A4648** Tissue marker, implantable, any type, each  N M ☑ ⊘
AHA: 3Q, '13

**A4649** Surgical supply; miscellaneous  N
Determine if an alternative HCPCS Level II or a CPT code better describes
the service being reported. This code should be used only if a more specific
code is unavailable.

**A4650** Implantable radiation dosimeter, each  N M ☑ ⊘

**A4651** Calibrated microcapillary tube, each  N ☑ ⊘
AHA: 1Q, '02, 5

**A4652** Microcapillary tube sealant  N ⊘
AHA: 1Q, '02, 5

## Dialysis Supplies

**A4653** Peritoneal dialysis catheter anchoring device, belt,
each  N ☑ ⊘

**A4657** Syringe, with or without needle, each  N ☑ ⊘
CMS: 100-04,13,60.7.1; 100-04,8,60.4.4; 100-04,8,60.4.6.3; 100-04,8,60.7;
100-04,8,60.7.3
AHA: 1Q, '02, 5

**A4660** Sphygmomanometer/blood pressure apparatus with cuff and
stethoscope  N ⊘

**A4663** Blood pressure cuff only  N ⊘

**A4670** Automatic blood pressure monitor  E

**A4671** Disposable cycler set used with cycler dialysis machine,
each  B ☑ ⊘

**A4672** Drainage extension line, sterile, for dialysis, each  B ☑ ⊘

**A4673** Extension line with easy lock connectors, used with
dialysis  B ⊘

**A4674** Chemicals/antiseptics solution used to clean/sterilize dialysis
equipment, per 8 oz  B ☑ ⊘

**A4680** Activated carbon filter for hemodialysis, each  N ☑ ⊘

**A4690** Dialyzer (artificial kidneys), all types, all sizes, for hemodialysis,
each  N ☑ ⊘

**A4706** Bicarbonate concentrate, solution, for hemodialysis, per
gallon  N ☑ ⊘

**A4707** Bicarbonate concentrate, powder, for hemodialysis, per
packet  N ☑ ⊘
AHA: 1Q, '02, 5

**A4708** Acetate concentrate solution, for hemodialysis, per
gallon  N ☑ ⊘
AHA: 1Q, '02, 5

**A4709** Acid concentrate, solution, for hemodialysis, per
gallon  N ☑ ⊘
AHA: 1Q, '02, 5

**A4714** Treated water (deionized, distilled, or reverse osmosis) for
peritoneal dialysis, per gallon  N ☑ ⊘

Special Coverage Instructions    Noncovered by Medicare    Carrier Discretion    ☑ Quantity Alert   ● New Code   ○ Recycled/Reinstated   ▲ Revised Code

© 2016 Optum360, LLC    A2-Z3 ASC Pmt   CMS: Pub 100   AHA: Coding Clinic   & DMEPOS Paid   ⊘ SNF Excluded                                  **A Codes — 7**

| A4719 | "Y set" tubing for peritoneal dialysis | N |
| | AHA: 1Q, '02, 5 | |
| A4720 | Dialysate solution, any concentration of dextrose, fluid volume greater than 249 cc, but less than or equal to 999 cc, for peritoneal dialysis | N ☑ ⊘ |
| | AHA: 1Q, '02, 5 | |
| A4721 | Dialysate solution, any concentration of dextrose, fluid volume greater than 999 cc but less than or equal to 1999 cc, for peritoneal dialysis | N ☑ |
| | AHA: 1Q, '02, 5 | |
| A4722 | Dialysate solution, any concentration of dextrose, fluid volume greater than 1999 cc but less than or equal to 2999 cc, for peritoneal dialysis | N ☑ |
| | AHA: 1Q, '02, 5 | |
| A4723 | Dialysate solution, any concentration of dextrose, fluid volume greater than 2999 cc but less than or equal to 3999 cc, for peritoneal dialysis | N ☑ |
| | AHA: 1Q, '02, 5 | |
| A4724 | Dialysate solution, any concentration of dextrose, fluid volume greater than 3999 cc but less than or equal to 4999 cc, for peritoneal dialysis | N ☑ ⊘ |
| | AHA: 1Q, '02, 5 | |
| A4725 | Dialysate solution, any concentration of dextrose, fluid volume greater than 4999 cc but less than or equal to 5999 cc, for peritoneal dialysis | N ☑ ⊘ |
| | AHA: 1Q, '02, 5 | |
| A4726 | Dialysate solution, any concentration of dextrose, fluid volume greater than 5999 cc, for peritoneal dialysis | N ☑ ⊘ |
| | AHA: 1Q, '02, 5 | |
| A4728 | Dialysate solution, nondextrose containing, 500 ml | B ☑ ⊘ |
| A4730 | Fistula cannulation set for hemodialysis, each | N ☑ ⊘ |
| A4736 | Topical anesthetic, for dialysis, per g | N ☑ ⊘ |
| | AHA: 1Q, '02, 5 | |
| A4737 | Injectable anesthetic, for dialysis, per 10 ml | N ☑ ⊘ |
| | AHA: 1Q, '02, 5 | |
| A4740 | Shunt accessory, for hemodialysis, any type, each | N ⊘ |
| A4750 | Blood tubing, arterial or venous, for hemodialysis, each | N ☑ ⊘ |
| A4755 | Blood tubing, arterial and venous combined, for hemodialysis, each | N ☑ ⊘ |
| A4760 | Dialysate solution test kit, for peritoneal dialysis, any type, each | N ☑ ⊘ |
| A4765 | Dialysate concentrate, powder, additive for peritoneal dialysis, per packet | N ☑ ⊘ |
| A4766 | Dialysate concentrate, solution, additive for peritoneal dialysis, per 10 ml | N ☑ ⊘ |
| | AHA: 1Q, '02, 5 | |
| A4770 | Blood collection tube, vacuum, for dialysis, per 50 | N ☑ ⊘ |
| A4771 | Serum clotting time tube, for dialysis, per 50 | N ☑ ⊘ |
| A4772 | Blood glucose test strips, for dialysis, per 50 | N ☑ ⊘ |
| A4773 | Occult blood test strips, for dialysis, per 50 | N ☑ ⊘ |
| A4774 | Ammonia test strips, for dialysis, per 50 | N ☑ ⊘ |
| A4802 | Protamine sulfate, for hemodialysis, per 50 mg | N ☑ ⊘ |
| | AHA: 1Q, '02, 5 | |
| A4860 | Disposable catheter tips for peritoneal dialysis, per 10 | N ☑ ⊘ |
| A4870 | Plumbing and/or electrical work for home hemodialysis equipment | N ⊘ |

| A4890 | Contracts, repair and maintenance, for hemodialysis equipment | N ⊘ |
| A4911 | Drain bag/bottle, for dialysis, each | N ☑ ⊘ |
| | AHA: 1Q, '02, 5 | |
| A4913 | Miscellaneous dialysis supplies, not otherwise specified | N ⊘ |
| | Pertinent documentation to evaluate medical appropriateness should be included when this code is reported. Determine if an alternative HCPCS Level II or a CPT code better describes the service being reported. This code should be used only if a more specific code is unavailable. | |
| A4918 | Venous pressure clamp, for hemodialysis, each | N ☑ ⊘ |
| A4927 | Gloves, nonsterile, per 100 | N ☑ ⊘ |
| A4928 | Surgical mask, per 20 | N ☑ ⊘ |
| | AHA: 1Q, '02, 5 | |
| A4929 | Tourniquet for dialysis, each | N ☑ ⊘ |
| | AHA: 1Q, '02, 5 | |
| A4930 | Gloves, sterile, per pair | N ☑ ⊘ |
| A4931 | Oral thermometer, reusable, any type, each | N ☑ ⊘ |
| A4932 | Rectal thermometer, reusable, any type, each | N ☑ |

## Ostomy Pouches and Supplies

| A5051 | Ostomy pouch, closed; with barrier attached (1 piece), each | N ☑ & |
| A5052 | Ostomy pouch, closed; without barrier attached (1 piece), each | N ☑ & |
| A5053 | Ostomy pouch, closed; for use on faceplate, each | N ☑ & |
| A5054 | Ostomy pouch, closed; for use on barrier with flange (2 piece), each | N ☑ & |
| A5055 | Stoma cap | N & |
| A5056 | Ostomy pouch, drainable, with extended wear barrier attached, with filter, (1 piece), each | N ☑ & |
| A5057 | Ostomy pouch, drainable, with extended wear barrier attached, with built in convexity, with filter, (1 piece), each | N ☑ & |
| A5061 | Ostomy pouch, drainable; with barrier attached, (1 piece), each | N ☑ & |
| A5062 | Ostomy pouch, drainable; without barrier attached (1 piece), each | N ☑ & |
| A5063 | Ostomy pouch, drainable; for use on barrier with flange (2-piece system), each | N ☑ & |
| A5071 | Ostomy pouch, urinary; with barrier attached (1 piece), each | N ☑ & |
| A5072 | Ostomy pouch, urinary; without barrier attached (1 piece), each | N ☑ & |
| A5073 | Ostomy pouch, urinary; for use on barrier with flange (2 piece), each | N ☑ & |
| A5081 | Stoma plug or seal, any type | N & |
| A5082 | Continent device; catheter for continent stoma | N & |
| A5083 | Continent device, stoma absorptive cover for continent stoma | N & |
| A5093 | Ostomy accessory; convex insert | N & |

## Incontinence Supplies

| A5102 | Bedside drainage bottle with or without tubing, rigid or expandable, each | N ☑ & |
| A5105 | Urinary suspensory with leg bag, with or without tube, each | N ☑ & |

| Special Coverage Instructions | Noncovered by Medicare | Carrier Discretion | ☑ Quantity Alert | ● New Code | ○ Recycled/Reinstated | ▲ Revised Code |

| | | |
|---|---|---|
| **A5112** | Urinary drainage bag, leg or abdomen, latex, with or without tube, with straps, each | N ☑ & |
| **A5113** | Leg strap; latex, replacement only, per set | E ☑ & |
| **A5114** | Leg strap; foam or fabric, replacement only, per set | E ☑ & |
| **A5120** | Skin barrier, wipes or swabs, each | N ☑ & (AU,AV) |
| **A5121** | Skin barrier; solid, 6 x 6 or equivalent, each | N ☑ & |
| **A5122** | Skin barrier; solid, 8 x 8 or equivalent, each | N ☑ & |
| **A5126** | Adhesive or nonadhesive; disk or foam pad | N & |
| **A5131** | Appliance cleaner, incontinence and ostomy appliances, per 16 oz | N ☑ & |
| **A5200** | Percutaneous catheter/tube anchoring device, adhesive skin attachment | N & |

## Diabetic Shoes, Fitting, and Modifications

According to Medicare, documentation from the prescribing physician must certify the diabetic patient has one of the following conditions: peripheral neuropathy with evidence of callus formation; history of preulcerative calluses; history of ulceration; foot deformity; previous amputation; or poor circulation. The footwear must be fitted and furnished by a podiatrist, pedorthist, orthotist, or prosthetist.

| | | |
|---|---|---|
| **A5500** | For diabetics only, fitting (including follow-up), custom preparation and supply of off-the-shelf depth-inlay shoe manufactured to accommodate multidensity insert(s), per shoe | Y ☑ & |
| | CMS: 100-02,15,140 | |
| **A5501** | For diabetics only, fitting (including follow-up), custom preparation and supply of shoe molded from cast(s) of patient's foot (custom molded shoe), per shoe | Y ☑ & |
| | CMS: 100-02,15,140 | |
| **A5503** | For diabetics only, modification (including fitting) of off-the-shelf depth-inlay shoe or custom molded shoe with roller or rigid rocker bottom, per shoe | Y ☑ & |
| | CMS: 100-02,15,140 | |
| **A5504** | For diabetics only, modification (including fitting) of off-the-shelf depth-inlay shoe or custom molded shoe with wedge(s), per shoe | Y ☑ & |
| | CMS: 100-02,15,140 | |
| **A5505** | For diabetics only, modification (including fitting) of off-the-shelf depth-inlay shoe or custom molded shoe with metatarsal bar, per shoe | Y ☑ & |
| | CMS: 100-02,15,140 | |
| **A5506** | For diabetics only, modification (including fitting) of off-the-shelf depth-inlay shoe or custom molded shoe with off-set heel(s), per shoe | Y ☑ & |
| | CMS: 100-02,15,140 | |
| **A5507** | For diabetics only, not otherwise specified modification (including fitting) of off-the-shelf depth-inlay shoe or custom molded shoe, per shoe | Y ☑ & |
| | CMS: 100-02,15,140 | |
| **A5508** | For diabetics only, deluxe feature of off-the-shelf depth-inlay shoe or custom molded shoe, per shoe | Y ☑ |
| | CMS: 100-02,15,140 | |
| **A5510** | For diabetics only, direct formed, compression molded to patient's foot without external heat source, multiple-density insert(s) prefabricated, per shoe | N ☑ |
| | CMS: 100-02,15,140 | |
| | AHA: 1Q, '02, 5 | |

| | | |
|---|---|---|
| **A5512** | For diabetics only, multiple density insert, direct formed, molded to foot after external heat source of 230 degrees Fahrenheit or higher, total contact with patient's foot, including arch, base layer minimum of 1/4 inch material of shore a 35 durometer or 3/16 inch material of shore a 40 durometer (or higher), prefabricated, each | Y ☑ & |
| **A5513** | For diabetics only, multiple density insert, custom molded from model of patient's foot, total contact with patient's foot, including arch, base layer minimum of 3/16 inch material of shore a 35 durometer or higher), includes arch filler and other shaping material, custom fabricated, each | Y ☑ & |

## Dressings

| | | |
|---|---|---|
| **A6000** | Noncontact wound-warming wound cover for use with the noncontact wound-warming device and warming card | E |
| | AHA: 1Q, '02, 5 | |
| **A6010** | Collagen based wound filler, dry form, sterile, per g of collagen | N ☑ & |
| | AHA: 1Q, '02, 5 | |
| **A6011** | Collagen based wound filler, gel/paste, per g of collagen | N ☑ & |
| **A6021** | Collagen dressing, sterile, size 16 sq in or less, each | N ☑ & |
| **A6022** | Collagen dressing, sterile, size more than 16 sq in but less than or equal to 48 sq in, each | N ☑ & |
| **A6023** | Collagen dressing, sterile, size more than 48 sq in, each | N ☑ & |
| **A6024** | Collagen dressing wound filler, sterile, per 6 in | N ☑ & |
| **A6025** | Gel sheet for dermal or epidermal application, (e.g., silicone, hydrogel, other), each | N ☑ |
| **A6154** | Wound pouch, each | N ☑ & |
| **A6196** | Alginate or other fiber gelling dressing, wound cover, sterile, pad size 16 sq in or less, each dressing | N ☑ & |
| **A6197** | Alginate or other fiber gelling dressing, wound cover, sterile, pad size more than 16 sq in but less than or equal to 48 sq in, each dressing | N ☑ & |
| **A6198** | Alginate or other fiber gelling dressing, wound cover, sterile, pad size more than 48 sq in, each dressing | N ☑ |
| **A6199** | Alginate or other fiber gelling dressing, wound filler, sterile, per 6 in | N ☑ & |
| **A6203** | Composite dressing, sterile, pad size 16 sq in or less, with any size adhesive border, each dressing | N ☑ & |
| **A6204** | Composite dressing, sterile, pad size more than 16 sq in, but less than or equal to 48 sq in, with any size adhesive border, each dressing | N ☑ & |
| **A6205** | Composite dressing, sterile, pad size more than 48 sq in, with any size adhesive border, each dressing | N ☑ |
| **A6206** | Contact layer, sterile, 16 sq in or less, each dressing | N ☑ |
| **A6207** | Contact layer, sterile, more than 16 sq in but less than or equal to 48 sq in, each dressing | N ☑ & |
| **A6208** | Contact layer, sterile, more than 48 sq in, each dressing | N ☑ |
| **A6209** | Foam dressing, wound cover, sterile, pad size 16 sq in or less, without adhesive border, each dressing | N ☑ & |
| **A6210** | Foam dressing, wound cover, sterile, pad size more than 16 sq in but less than or equal to 48 sq in, without adhesive border, each dressing | N ☑ & |
| **A6211** | Foam dressing, wound cover, sterile, pad size more than 48 sq in, without adhesive border, each dressing | N ☑ & |

Special Coverage Instructions    Noncovered by Medicare    Carrier Discretion    ☑ Quantity Alert ● New Code    ○ Recycled/Reinstated    ▲ Revised Code

© 2016 Optum360, LLC    A2-Z8 ASC Pmt    CMS: Pub 100    AHA: Coding Clinic    & DMEPOS Paid    ⊘ SNF Excluded    A Codes — 9

**A6212** Foam dressing, wound cover, sterile, pad size 16 sq in or less, with any size adhesive border, each dressing N ☑ ⟨ら⟩

**A6213** Foam dressing, wound cover, sterile, pad size more than 16 sq in but less than or equal to 48 sq in, with any size adhesive border, each dressing N ☑

**A6214** Foam dressing, wound cover, sterile, pad size more than 48 sq in, with any size adhesive border, each dressing N ☑ ⟨ら⟩

**A6215** Foam dressing, wound filler, sterile, per g N ☑

**A6216** Gauze, nonimpregnated, nonsterile, pad size 16 sq in or less, without adhesive border, each dressing N ☑

**A6217** Gauze, nonimpregnated, nonsterile, pad size more than 16 sq in but less than or equal to 48 sq in, without adhesive border, each dressing N ☑

**A6218** Gauze, nonimpregnated, nonsterile, pad size more than 48 sq in, without adhesive border, each dressing N ☑

**A6219** Gauze, nonimpregnated, sterile, pad size 16 sq in or less, with any size adhesive border, each dressing N ☑ ⟨ら⟩

**A6220** Gauze, nonimpregnated, sterile, pad size more than 16 sq in but less than or equal to 48 sq in, with any size adhesive border, each dressing N ☑ ⟨ら⟩

**A6221** Gauze, nonimpregnated, sterile, pad size more than 48 sq in, with any size adhesive border, each dressing N ☑

**A6222** Gauze, impregnated with other than water, normal saline, or hydrogel, sterile, pad size 16 sq in or less, without adhesive border, each dressing N ☑ ⟨ら⟩

**A6223** Gauze, impregnated with other than water, normal saline, or hydrogel, sterile, pad size more than 16 sq in, but less than or equal to 48 sq in, without adhesive border, each dressing N ☑

**A6224** Gauze, impregnated with other than water, normal saline, or hydrogel, sterile, pad size more than 48 sq in, without adhesive border, each dressing N ☑ ⟨ら⟩

**A6228** Gauze, impregnated, water or normal saline, sterile, pad size 16 sq in or less, without adhesive border, each dressing N ☑

**A6229** Gauze, impregnated, water or normal saline, sterile, pad size more than 16 sq in but less than or equal to 48 sq in, without adhesive border, each dressing N ☑ ⟨ら⟩

**A6230** Gauze, impregnated, water or normal saline, sterile, pad size more than 48 sq in, without adhesive border, each dressing N ☑

**A6231** Gauze, impregnated, hydrogel, for direct wound contact, sterile, pad size 16 sq in or less, each dressing N ☑ ⟨ら⟩

**A6232** Gauze, impregnated, hydrogel, for direct wound contact, sterile, pad size greater than 16 sq in, but less than or equal to 48 sq in, each dressing N ☑ ⟨ら⟩

**A6233** Gauze, impregnated, hydrogel, for direct wound contact, sterile, pad size more than 48 sq in, each dressing N ☑ ⟨ら⟩

**A6234** Hydrocolloid dressing, wound cover, sterile, pad size 16 sq in or less, without adhesive border, each dressing N ☑ ⟨ら⟩

**A6235** Hydrocolloid dressing, wound cover, sterile, pad size more than 16 sq in but less than or equal to 48 sq in, without adhesive border, each dressing N ☑ ⟨ら⟩

**A6236** Hydrocolloid dressing, wound cover, sterile, pad size more than 48 sq in, without adhesive border, each dressing N ☑ ⟨ら⟩

**A6237** Hydrocolloid dressing, wound cover, sterile, pad size 16 sq in or less, with any size adhesive border, each dressing N ☑ ⟨ら⟩

**A6238** Hydrocolloid dressing, wound cover, sterile, pad size more than 16 sq in but less than or equal to 48 sq in, with any size adhesive border, each dressing N ☑

**A6239** Hydrocolloid dressing, wound cover, sterile, pad size more than 48 sq in, with any size adhesive border, each dressing N ☑

**A6240** Hydrocolloid dressing, wound filler, paste, sterile, per oz N ☑ ⟨ら⟩

**A6241** Hydrocolloid dressing, wound filler, dry form, sterile, per g N ☑ ⟨ら⟩

**A6242** Hydrogel dressing, wound cover, sterile, pad size 16 sq in or less, without adhesive border, each dressing N ☑ ⟨ら⟩

**A6243** Hydrogel dressing, wound cover, sterile, pad size more than 16 sq in but less than or equal to 48 sq in, without adhesive border, each dressing N ☑ ⟨ら⟩

**A6244** Hydrogel dressing, wound cover, sterile, pad size more than 48 sq in, without adhesive border, each dressing N ☑ ⟨ら⟩

**A6245** Hydrogel dressing, wound cover, sterile, pad size 16 sq in or less, with any size adhesive border, each dressing N ☑ ⟨ら⟩

**A6246** Hydrogel dressing, wound cover, sterile, pad size more than 16 sq in but less than or equal to 48 sq in, with any size adhesive border, each dressing N ☑ ⟨ら⟩

**A6247** Hydrogel dressing, wound cover, sterile, pad size more than 48 sq in, with any size adhesive border, each dressing N ☑ ⟨ら⟩

**A6248** Hydrogel dressing, wound filler, gel, per fl oz N ☑ ⟨ら⟩

**A6250** Skin sealants, protectants, moisturizers, ointments, any type, any size N

Surgical dressings applied by a physician are included as part of the professional service. Surgical dressings obtained by the patient to perform homecare as prescribed by the physician are covered.

**A6251** Specialty absorptive dressing, wound cover, sterile, pad size 16 sq in or less, without adhesive border, each dressing N ☑ ⟨ら⟩

**A6252** Specialty absorptive dressing, wound cover, sterile, pad size more than 16 sq in but less than or equal to 48 sq in, without adhesive border, each dressing N ☑ ⟨ら⟩

**A6253** Specialty absorptive dressing, wound cover, sterile, pad size more than 48 sq in, without adhesive border, each dressing N ☑ ⟨ら⟩

**A6254** Specialty absorptive dressing, wound cover, sterile, pad size 16 sq in or less, with any size adhesive border, each dressing N ☑ ⟨ら⟩

**A6255** Specialty absorptive dressing, wound cover, sterile, pad size more than 16 sq in but less than or equal to 48 sq in, with any size adhesive border, each dressing N ☑ ⟨ら⟩

**A6256** Specialty absorptive dressing, wound cover, sterile, pad size more than 48 sq in, with any size adhesive border, each dressing N ☑

**A6257** Transparent film, sterile, 16 sq in or less, each dressing N ☑ ⟨ら⟩

Surgical dressings applied by a physician are included as part of the professional service. Surgical dressings obtained by the patient to perform homecare as prescribed by the physician are covered. Use this code for Polyskin, Tegaderm, and Tegaderm HP.

**A6258** Transparent film, sterile, more than 16 sq in but less than or equal to 48 sq in, each dressing N ☑ ⟨ら⟩

Surgical dressings applied by a physician are included as part of the professional service. Surgical dressings obtained by the patient to perform homecare as prescribed by the physician are covered.

---

Special Coverage Instructions     Noncovered by Medicare     Carrier Discretion     ☑ Quantity Alert   ● New Code   ○ Recycled/Reinstated   ▲ Revised Code

10 — A Codes     A Age Edit     M Maternity Edit   ♀ Female Only   ♂ Male Only   A-Y OPPS Status Indicators        © 2016 Optum360, LLC

**A6259** Transparent film, sterile, more than 48 sq in, each dressing   N ☑ &

Surgical dressings applied by a physician are included as part of the professional service. Surgical dressings obtained by the patient to perform homecare as prescribed by the physician are covered.

**A6260** Wound cleansers, any type, any size   N

Surgical dressings applied by a physician are included as part of the professional service. Surgical dressings obtained by the patient to perform homecare as prescribed by the physician are covered.

**A6261** Wound filler, gel/paste, per fl oz, not otherwise specified   N ☑

Surgical dressings applied by a physician are included as part of the professional service. Surgical dressings obtained by the patient to perform homecare as prescribed by the physician are covered.

**A6262** Wound filler, dry form, per g, not otherwise specified   N ☑

**A6266** Gauze, impregnated, other than water, normal saline, or zinc paste, sterile, any width, per linear yd   N ☑ &

Surgical dressings applied by a physician are included as part of the professional service. Surgical dressings obtained by the patient to perform homecare as prescribed by the physician are covered.

**A6402** Gauze, nonimpregnated, sterile, pad size 16 sq in or less, without adhesive border, each dressing   N ☑ &

Surgical dressings applied by a physician are included as part of the professional service. Surgical dressings obtained by the patient to perform homecare as prescribed by the physician are covered.

**A6403** Gauze, nonimpregnated, sterile, pad size more than 16 sq in, less than or equal to 48 sq in, without adhesive border, each dressing   N ☑ &

Surgical dressings applied by a physician are included as part of the professional service. Surgical dressings obtained by the patient to perform homecare as prescribed by the physician are covered.

**A6404** Gauze, nonimpregnated, sterile, pad size more than 48 sq in, without adhesive border, each dressing   N ☑

**A6407** Packing strips, nonimpregnated, sterile, up to 2 in in width, per linear yd   N ☑ &

**A6410** Eye pad, sterile, each   N ☑ &

**A6411** Eye pad, nonsterile, each   N ☑ &

**A6412** Eye patch, occlusive, each   N ☑

**A6413** Adhesive bandage, first aid type, any size, each   E ☑

**A6441** Padding bandage, nonelastic, nonwoven/nonknitted, width greater than or equal to 3 in and less than 5 in, per yd   N ☑ &

**A6442** Conforming bandage, nonelastic, knitted/woven, nonsterile, width less than 3 in, per yd   N ☑ &

**A6443** Conforming bandage, nonelastic, knitted/woven, nonsterile, width greater than or equal to 3 in and less than 5 in, per yd   N ☑ &

**A6444** Conforming bandage, nonelastic, knitted/woven, nonsterile, width greater than or equal to 5 in, per yd   N ☑ &

**A6445** Conforming bandage, nonelastic, knitted/woven, sterile, width less than 3 in, per yd   N ☑ &

**A6446** Conforming bandage, nonelastic, knitted/woven, sterile, width greater than or equal to 3 in and less than 5 in, per yd   N ☑ &

**A6447** Conforming bandage, nonelastic, knitted/woven, sterile, width greater than or equal to 5 in, per yd   N ☑ &

**A6448** Light compression bandage, elastic, knitted/woven, width less than 3 in, per yd   N ☑ &

**A6449** Light compression bandage, elastic, knitted/woven, width greater than or equal to 3 in and less than 5 in, per yd   N ☑ &

**A6450** Light compression bandage, elastic, knitted/woven, width greater than or equal to 5 in, per yd   N ☑ &

**A6451** Moderate compression bandage, elastic, knitted/woven, load resistance of 1.25 to 1.34 ft lbs at 50% maximum stretch, width greater than or equal to 3 in and less than 5 in, per yd   N ☑ &

**A6452** High compression bandage, elastic, knitted/woven, load resistance greater than or equal to 1.35 ft lbs at 50% maximum stretch, width greater than or equal to 3 in and less than 5 in, per yd   N ☑ &

**A6453** Self-adherent bandage, elastic, nonknitted/nonwoven, width less than 3 in, per yd   N ☑ &

**A6454** Self-adherent bandage, elastic, nonknitted/nonwoven, width greater than or equal to 3 in and less than 5 in, per yd   N ☑ &

**A6455** Self-adherent bandage, elastic, nonknitted/nonwoven, width greater than or equal to 5 in, per yd   N ☑ &

**A6456** Zinc paste impregnated bandage, nonelastic, knitted/woven, width greater than or equal to 3 in and less than 5 in, per yd   N ☑ &

**A6457** Tubular dressing with or without elastic, any width, per linear yd   N ☑

## Compression Garments

**A6501** Compression burn garment, bodysuit (head to foot), custom fabricated   N &

**A6502** Compression burn garment, chin strap, custom fabricated   N &

**A6503** Compression burn garment, facial hood, custom fabricated   N &

**A6504** Compression burn garment, glove to wrist, custom fabricated   N &

**A6505** Compression burn garment, glove to elbow, custom fabricated   N &

**A6506** Compression burn garment, glove to axilla, custom fabricated   N &

**A6507** Compression burn garment, foot to knee length, custom fabricated   N &

**A6508** Compression burn garment, foot to thigh length, custom fabricated   N &

**A6509** Compression burn garment, upper trunk to waist including arm openings (vest), custom fabricated   N &

**A6510** Compression burn garment, trunk, including arms down to leg openings (leotard), custom fabricated   N &

**A6511** Compression burn garment, lower trunk including leg openings (panty), custom fabricated   N &

**A6512** Compression burn garment, not otherwise classified   N

**A6513** Compression burn mask, face and/or neck, plastic or equal, custom fabricated   B &

**A6530** Gradient compression stocking, below knee, 18-30 mm Hg, each   E ☑

**A6531** Gradient compression stocking, below knee, 30-40 mm Hg, each   N ☑ & (AW)

**A6532** Gradient compression stocking, below knee, 40-50 mm Hg, each   N ☑ & (AW)

**A6533** Gradient compression stocking, thigh length, 18-30 mm Hg, each   E ☑

**A6534** Gradient compression stocking, thigh length, 30-40 mm Hg, each   E ☑

**A6535** Gradient compression stocking, thigh length, 40-50 mm Hg, each   E ☑

---

Special Coverage Instructions    Noncovered by Medicare    Carrier Discretion    ☑ Quantity Alert   ● New Code   ○ Recycled/Reinstated   ▲ Revised Code

© 2016 Optum360, LLC   A2–Z3 ASC Pmt   CMS: Pub 100   AHA: Coding Clinic   & DMEPOS Paid   ⊘ SNF Excluded   A Codes — 11

| A6536 | Gradient compression stocking, full-length/chap style, 18-30 mm Hg, each | E ☑ |
| A6537 | Gradient compression stocking, full-length/chap style, 30-40 mm Hg, each | E ☑ |
| A6538 | Gradient compression stocking, full-length/chap style, 40-50 mm Hg, each | E ☑ |
| A6539 | Gradient compression stocking, waist length, 18-30 mm Hg, each | E ☑ |
| A6540 | Gradient compression stocking, waist length, 30-40 mm Hg, each | E ☑ |
| A6541 | Gradient compression stocking, waist length, 40-50 mm Hg, each | E ☑ |
| A6544 | Gradient compression stocking, garter belt | E |
| A6545 | Gradient compression wrap, nonelastic, below knee, 30-50 mm Hg, each | N ☑ ৬ (AW) |
| A6549 | Gradient compression stocking/sleeve, not otherwise specified | E |
| A6550 | Wound care set, for negative pressure wound therapy electrical pump, includes all supplies and accessories | N ☑ ৬ |

**CMS:** 100-04,23,60.3

## Respiratory Supplies

| A7000 | Canister, disposable, used with suction pump, each | Y ☑ ৬ (NU) |
| A7001 | Canister, nondisposable, used with suction pump, each | Y ☑ ৬ (NU) |
| A7002 | Tubing, used with suction pump, each | Y ☑ ৬ (NU) |
| A7003 | Administration set, with small volume nonfiltered pneumatic nebulizer, disposable | Y ৬ (NU) |
| A7004 | Small volume nonfiltered pneumatic nebulizer, disposable | Y ৬ (NU) |
| A7005 | Administration set, with small volume nonfiltered pneumatic nebulizer, nondisposable | Y ৬ (NU) |
| A7006 | Administration set, with small volume filtered pneumatic nebulizer | Y ৬ (NU) |
| A7007 | Large volume nebulizer, disposable, unfilled, used with aerosol compressor | Y ৬ (NU) |
| A7008 | Large volume nebulizer, disposable, prefilled, used with aerosol compressor | Y ৬ (NU) |
| A7009 | Reservoir bottle, nondisposable, used with large volume ultrasonic nebulizer | Y ৬ (NU) |
| A7010 | Corrugated tubing, disposable, used with large volume nebulizer, 100 ft | Y ☑ ৬ (NU) |
| A7012 | Water collection device, used with large volume nebulizer | Y ৬ (NU) |
| A7013 | Filter, disposable, used with aerosol compressor or ultrasonic generator | Y ৬ (NU) |
| A7014 | Filter, nondisposable, used with aerosol compressor or ultrasonic generator | Y ৬ (NU) |
| A7015 | Aerosol mask, used with DME nebulizer | Y ৬ (NU) |
| A7016 | Dome and mouthpiece, used with small volume ultrasonic nebulizer | Y ৬ (NU) |
| A7017 | Nebulizer, durable, glass or autoclavable plastic, bottle type, not used with oxygen | Y ৬ (NU,RR,UE) |

| A7018 | Water, distilled, used with large volume nebulizer, 1000 ml | Y ☑ ৬ |
| A7020 | Interface for cough stimulating device, includes all components, replacement only | Y ৬ (NU) |
| A7025 | High frequency chest wall oscillation system vest, replacement for use with patient-owned equipment, each | N ☑ ৬ (RR) |
| A7026 | High frequency chest wall oscillation system hose, replacement for use with patient-owned equipment, each | Y ☑ ৬ (NU) |
| A7027 | Combination oral/nasal mask, used with continuous positive airway pressure device, each | Y ☑ ৬ (NU) |
| A7028 | Oral cushion for combination oral/nasal mask, replacement only, each | Y ☑ ৬ (NU) |
| A7029 | Nasal pillows for combination oral/nasal mask, replacement only, pair | Y ☑ ৬ (NU) |
| A7030 | Full face mask used with positive airway pressure device, each | Y ☑ ৬ (NU) |

**CMS:** 100-04,23,60.3; 100-04,36,50.14

| A7031 | Face mask interface, replacement for full face mask, each | Y ☑ ৬ (NU) |

**CMS:** 100-04,23,60.3; 100-04,36,50.14

| A7032 | Cushion for use on nasal mask interface, replacement only, each | Y ☑ ৬ (NU) |

**CMS:** 100-03,240.4; 100-04,23,60.3; 100-04,36,50.14

| A7033 | Pillow for use on nasal cannula type interface, replacement only, pair | Y ☑ ৬ (NU) |

**CMS:** 100-03,240.4; 100-04,23,60.3; 100-04,36,50.14

| A7034 | Nasal interface (mask or cannula type) used with positive airway pressure device, with or without head strap | Y ৬ (NU) |

**CMS:** 100-03,240.4; 100-04,23,60.3; 100-04,36,50.14

| A7035 | Headgear used with positive airway pressure device | Y ৬ (NU) |

**CMS:** 100-03,240.4; 100-04,23,60.3; 100-04,36,50.14

| A7036 | Chinstrap used with positive airway pressure device | Y ৬ (NU) |

**CMS:** 100-03,240.4; 100-04,23,60.3; 100-04,36,50.14

| A7037 | Tubing used with positive airway pressure device | Y ৬ (NU) |

**CMS:** 100-03,240.4; 100-04,23,60.3; 100-04,36,50.14

| A7038 | Filter, disposable, used with positive airway pressure device | Y ৬ (NU) |

**CMS:** 100-04,23,60.3; 100-04,36,50.14

| A7039 | Filter, nondisposable, used with positive airway pressure device | Y ৬ (NU) |

**CMS:** 100-04,23,60.3; 100-04,36,50.14

| A7040 | One way chest drain valve | N ৬ |
| A7041 | Water seal drainage container and tubing for use with implanted chest tube | N ৬ |
| A7044 | Oral interface used with positive airway pressure device, each | Y ☑ ৬ (NU) |

**CMS:** 100-03,240.4; 100-04,23,60.3; 100-04,36,50.14

| A7045 | Exhalation port with or without swivel used with accessories for positive airway devices, replacement only | Y ৬ (NU,RR,UE) |

**CMS:** 100-03,240.4; 100-04,23,60.3; 100-04,36,50.14

| A7046 | Water chamber for humidifier, used with positive airway pressure device, replacement, each | Y ☑ ৬ (NU) |

**CMS:** 100-04,23,60.3; 100-04,36,50.14

| A7047 | Oral interface used with respiratory suction pump, each | N ☑ ৬ (NU) |
| A7048 | Vacuum drainage collection unit and tubing kit, including all supplies needed for collection unit change, for use with implanted catheter, each | N ৬ |

---

Special Coverage Instructions        Noncovered by Medicare        Carrier Discretion        ☑ Quantity Alert  ● New Code        ○ Recycled/Reinstated   ▲ Revised Code

12 — A Codes        🅐 Age Edit   🅜 Maternity Edit   ♀ Female Only   ♂ Male Only   🅐-🆈 OPPS Status Indicators        © 2016 Optum360, LLC

## Tracheostomy Supplies

| Code | Description | |
|------|-------------|--|
| A7501 | Tracheostoma valve, including diaphragm, each | N ☑ ႕ |
| A7502 | Replacement diaphragm/faceplate for tracheostoma valve, each | N ☑ ႕ |
| A7503 | Filter holder or filter cap, reusable, for use in a tracheostoma heat and moisture exchange system, each | N ☑ ႕ |
| A7504 | Filter for use in a tracheostoma heat and moisture exchange system, each | N ☑ ႕ |
| A7505 | Housing, reusable without adhesive, for use in a heat and moisture exchange system and/or with a tracheostoma valve, each | N ☑ ႕ |
| A7506 | Adhesive disc for use in a heat and moisture exchange system and/or with tracheostoma valve, any type each | N ☑ ႕ |
| A7507 | Filter holder and integrated filter without adhesive, for use in a tracheostoma heat and moisture exchange system, each | N ☑ ႕ |
| A7508 | Housing and integrated adhesive, for use in a tracheostoma heat and moisture exchange system and/or with a tracheostoma valve, each | N ☑ ႕ |
| A7509 | Filter holder and integrated filter housing, and adhesive, for use as a tracheostoma heat and moisture exchange system, each | N ☑ ႕ |
| A7520 | Tracheostomy/laryngectomy tube, noncuffed, polyvinylchloride (PVC), silicone or equal, each | N ☑ ႕ |
| A7521 | Tracheostomy/laryngectomy tube, cuffed, polyvinylchloride (PVC), silicone or equal, each | N ☑ ႕ |
| A7522 | Tracheostomy/laryngectomy tube, stainless steel or equal (sterilizable and reusable), each | N ☑ ႕ |
| A7523 | Tracheostomy shower protector, each | N ☑ |
| A7524 | Tracheostoma stent/stud/button, each | N ☑ ႕ |
| A7525 | Tracheostomy mask, each | N ☑ ႕ |
| A7526 | Tracheostomy tube collar/holder, each | N ☑ ႕ |
| A7527 | Tracheostomy/laryngectomy tube plug/stop, each | N ☑ ႕ |

## Protective Helmet

| Code | Description | |
|------|-------------|--|
| A8000 | Helmet, protective, soft, prefabricated, includes all components and accessories | Y ႕ (NU,RR,UE) |
| A8001 | Helmet, protective, hard, prefabricated, includes all components and accessories | Y ႕ (NU,RR,UE) |
| A8002 | Helmet, protective, soft, custom fabricated, includes all components and accessories | Y ႕ (NU,RR,UE) |
| A8003 | Helmet, protective, hard, custom fabricated, includes all components and accessories | Y ႕ (NU,RR,UE) |
| A8004 | Soft interface for helmet, replacement only | Y ႕ (NU,RR,UE) |

## Other Supplies and Devices

| Code | Description | |
|------|-------------|--|
| A9150 | Nonprescription drugs | B |
| A9152 | Single vitamin/mineral/trace element, oral, per dose, not otherwise specified | E ☑ |
| A9153 | Multiple vitamins, with or without minerals and trace elements, oral, per dose, not otherwise specified | E ☑ |
| A9155 | Artificial saliva, 30 ml | B ☑ |
| A9180 | Pediculosis (lice infestation) treatment, topical, for administration by patient/caretaker | E |

**A9270** Noncovered item or service E
CMS: 100-04,11,100.1
AHA: 1Q, '14; 3Q, '04, 1-10

| Code | Description | |
|------|-------------|--|
| A9272 | Wound suction, disposable, includes dressing, all accessories and components, any type, each | E ☑ |
| A9273 | Hot water bottle, ice cap or collar, heat and/or cold wrap, any type | E |
| A9274 | External ambulatory insulin delivery system, disposable, each, includes all supplies and accessories | E ☑ |
| A9275 | Home glucose disposable monitor, includes test strips | E |
| A9276 | Sensor; invasive (e.g., subcutaneous), disposable, for use with interstitial continuous glucose monitoring system, 1 unit = 1 day supply | E ☑ |
| A9277 | Transmitter; external, for use with interstitial continuous glucose monitoring system | E |
| A9278 | Receiver (monitor); external, for use with interstitial continuous glucose monitoring system | E |
| A9279 | Monitoring feature/device, stand-alone or integrated, any type, includes all accessories, components and electronics, not otherwise classified | E |
| A9280 | Alert or alarm device, not otherwise classified | E |
| A9281 | Reaching/grabbing device, any type, any length, each | E ☑ |
| A9282 | Wig, any type, each | E ☑ |
| A9283 | Foot pressure off loading/supportive device, any type, each | E ☑ |
| A9284 | Spirometer, nonelectronic, includes all accessories | N |
| ● A9285<sup>Jan</sup> | Inversion/eversion correction device | |
| ● A9286<sup>Jan</sup> | Hygienic item or device, disposable or non-disposable, any type, each | |
| A9300 | Exercise equipment | E |

## Radiopharmaceuticals

**A9500** Technetium tc-99m sestamibi, diagnostic, per study dose N III ☑ ⊘
Use this code for Cardiolite.
AHA: 2Q, '06, 5; 4Q, '05, 1-6; 3Q, '04, 1-10

**A9501** Technetium Tc-99m teboroxime, diagnostic, per study dose N III ☑ ⊘

**A9502** Technetium Tc-99m tetrofosmin, diagnostic, per study dose N III ☑ ⊘
Use this code for Myoview.
AHA: 2Q, '06, 5; 4Q, '05, 1-6; 3Q, '04, 1-10

**A9503** Technetium Tc-99m medronate, diagnostic, per study dose, up to 30 millicuries N III ☑ ⊘
Use this code for CIS-MDP, Draximage MDP-10, Draximage MDP-25, MDP-Bracco, Technetium Tc-99m MPI-MDP.
AHA: 4Q, '05, 1-6; 3Q, '04, 1-10; 2Q, '02, 8-9

**A9504** Technetium Tc-99m apcitide, diagnostic, per study dose, up to 20 millicuries N III ☑ ⊘
Use this code for Acutect.
AHA: 4Q, '05, 1-6; 3Q, '04, 1-10; 2Q, '02, 8-9; 4Q, '01, 5

**A9505** Thallium TI-201 thallous chloride, diagnostic, per millicurie N III ☑ ⊘
Use this code for MIBG, Thallous Chloride USP.
AHA: 4Q, '05, 1-6; 3Q, '04, 1-10; 2Q, '02, 8-9

**Jan** January Update

Special Coverage Instructions    Noncovered by Medicare    Carrier Discretion    ☑ Quantity Alert    ● New Code    ○ Recycled/Reinstated    ▲ Revised Code

© 2016 Optum360, LLC    A2-Z3 ASC Pmt    CMS: Pub 100    AHA: Coding Clinic    ႕ DMEPOS Paid    ⊘ SNF Excluded

A Codes — 13

**Transportation Services Including Ambulance**

**A9507 — A9555**

**A9507** Indium In-111 capromab pendetide, diagnostic, per study dose, up to 10 millicuries  N NI ☑ ⊘
Use this code for Prostascint.
AHA: 4Q, '05, 1-6; 3Q, '04, 1-10

**A9508** Iodine I-131 iobenguane sulfate, diagnostic, per 0.5 millicurie  N NI ☑ ⊘
Use this code for MIBG.
AHA: 4Q, '05, 1-6; 3Q, '04, 1-10; 2Q, '02, 8-9

**A9509** Iodine I-123 sodium iodide, diagnostic, per millicurie  N NI ☑ ⊘

**A9510** Technetium Tc-99m disofenin, diagnostic, per study dose, up to 15 millicuries  N NI ☑ ⊘
Use this code for Hepatolite.
AHA: 4Q, '05, 1-6; 3Q, '04, 1-10

**A9512** Technetium Tc-99m pertechnetate, diagnostic, per millicurie  N NI ☑ ⊘
Use this code for Technelite, Ultra-Technelow.
AHA: 4Q, '05, 1-6; 3Q, '04, 1-10

○ **A9515**Jan Choline C-11, diagnostic, per study dose up to 20 millicuries

**A9516** Iodine I-123 sodium iodide, diagnostic, per 100 microcuries, up to 999 microcuries  N NI ☑ ⊘
AHA: 4Q, '05, 1-6; 3Q, '04, 1-10

**A9517** Iodine I-131 sodium iodide capsule(s), therapeutic, per millicurie  K ☑ ⊘
AHA: 3Q, '08, 6; 4Q, '05, 1-6; 3Q, '04, 1-10

**A9520** Technetium tc-99m, tilmanocept, diagnostic, up to 0.5 millicuries  N NI ☑

**A9521** Technetium Tc-99m exametazime, diagnostic, per study dose, up to 25 millicuries  N NI ☑ ⊘
Use this code for Ceretec.
AHA: 4Q, '05, 1-6; 3Q, '04, 1-10

**A9524** Iodine I-131 iodinated serum albumin, diagnostic, per 5 microcuries  N NI ☑ ⊘
AHA: 4Q, '05, 1-6; 3Q, '04, 1-10

**A9526** Nitrogen N-13 ammonia, diagnostic, per study dose, up to 40 millicuries  N NI ☑ ⊘
CMS: 100-04,13,60.3; 100-04,13,60.3.1; 100-04,13,60.3.2
AHA: 4Q, '05, 1-6; 3Q, '04, 1-10

**A9527** Iodine I-125, sodium iodide solution, therapeutic, per millicurie  U H2 ☑ ⊘
AHA: 3Q, '16

**A9528** Iodine I-131 sodium iodide capsule(s), diagnostic, per millicurie  N NI ☑ ⊘
AHA: 4Q, '05, 1-6; 3Q, '04, 1-10

**A9529** Iodine I-131 sodium iodide solution, diagnostic, per millicurie  N NI ☑ ⊘
AHA: 4Q, '05, 1-6; 3Q, '04, 1-10

**A9530** Iodine I-131 sodium iodide solution, therapeutic, per millicurie  K ☑ ⊘
AHA: 4Q, '05, 1-6; 3Q, '04, 1-10

**A9531** Iodine I-131 sodium iodide, diagnostic, per microcurie (up to 100 microcuries)  N NI ☑ ⊘
AHA: 4Q, '05, 1-6; 3Q, '04, 1-10

**A9532** Iodine I-125 serum albumin, diagnostic, per 5 microcuries  N NI ☑ ⊘
AHA: 4Q, '05, 1-6; 3Q, '04, 1-10

**A9536** Technetium Tc-99m depreotide, diagnostic, per study dose, up to 35 millicuries  N NI ☑ ⊘
AHA: 4Q, '05, 1-6

**A9537** Technetium Tc-99m mebrofenin, diagnostic, per study dose, up to 15 millicuries  N NI ☑ ⊘
AHA: 4Q, '05, 1-6

**A9538** Technetium Tc-99m pyrophosphate, diagnostic, per study dose, up to 25 millicuries  N NI ☑ ⊘
Use this code for CIS-PYRO, Phosphostec, Technescan Pyp Kit.
AHA: 4Q, '05, 1-6

**A9539** Technetium Tc-99m pentetate, diagnostic, per study dose, up to 25 millicuries  N NI ☑ ⊘
Use this code for AN-DTPA, DTPA, MPI-DTPA Kit-Chelate, MPI Indium DTPA IN-111, Pentate Calcium Trisodium, Pentate Zinc Trisodium.
AHA: 4Q, '05, 1-6

**A9540** Technetium Tc-99m macroaggregated albumin, diagnostic, per study dose, up to 10 millicuries  N NI ☑ ⊘
AHA: 4Q, '05, 1-6

**A9541** Technetium Tc-99m sulfur colloid, diagnostic, per study dose, up to 20 millicuries  N NI ☑ ⊘
AHA: 4Q, '05, 1-6

**A9542** Indium In-111 ibritumomab tiuxetan, diagnostic, per study dose, up to 5 millicuries  N NI ☑ ⊘
Use this code for Zevalin.
AHA: 4Q, '05, 1-6

**A9543** Yttrium Y-90 ibritumomab tiuxetan, therapeutic, per treatment dose, up to 40 millicuries  K ☑ ⊘
AHA: 4Q, '05, 1-6

~~**A9544**Jan Iodine I-131 tositumomab, diagnostic, per study dose~~

~~**A9545**Jan Iodine I-131 tositumomab, therapeutic, per treatment dose~~

**A9546** Cobalt Co-57/58, cyanocobalamin, diagnostic, per study dose, up to 1 microcurie  N NI ☑ ⊘
AHA: 4Q, '05, 1-6

**A9547** Indium In-111 oxyquinoline, diagnostic, per 0.5 millicurie  N NI ☑ ⊘
AHA: 4Q, '05, 1-6

**A9548** Indium In-111 pentetate, diagnostic, per 0.5 millicurie  N NI ☑ ⊘
AHA: 4Q, '05, 1-6

**A9550** Technetium Tc-99m sodium gluceptate, diagnostic, per study dose, up to 25 millicurie  N NI ☑ ⊘
AHA: 4Q, '05, 1-6

**A9551** Technetium Tc-99m succimer, diagnostic, per study dose, up to 10 millicuries  N NI ☑ ⊘
Use this code for MPI-DMSA Kidney Reagent.
AHA: 4Q, '05, 1-6

**A9552** Fluorodeoxyglucose F-18 FDG, diagnostic, per study dose, up to 45 millicuries  N NI ☑ ⊘
CMS: 100-03,220.6.13; 100-03,220.6.17; 100-04,13,60.15; 100-04,13,60.16; 100-04,13,60.3.2
AHA: 3Q, '08, 7, 8; 4Q, '05, 1-6

**A9553** Chromium Cr-51 sodium chromate, diagnostic, per study dose, up to 250 microcuries  N NI ☑ ⊘
Use this code for Chromitope Sodium.
AHA: 4Q, '05, 1-6

**A9554** Iodine I-125 sodium iothalamate, diagnostic, per study dose, up to 10 microcuries  N NI ☑ ⊘
Use this code for Glofil-125.
AHA: 4Q, '05, 1-6

**A9555** Rubidium Rb-82, diagnostic, per study dose, up to 60 millicuries  N NI ☑ ⊘
Use this code for Cardiogen 82.
CMS: 100-03,220.6.1; 100-04,13,60.3.2
AHA: 4Q, '05, 1-6

---

Jan **January Update**

☐ Special Coverage Instructions    ☐ Noncovered by Medicare    ☐ Carrier Discretion    ☑ Quantity Alert  ● New Code    ○ Recycled/Reinstated  ▲ Revised Code

14 — A Codes    A Age Edit  M Maternity Edit  ♀ Female Only  ♂ Male Only  A-Y OPPS Status Indicators    © 2016 Optum360, LLC

**A9556** Gallium Ga-67 citrate, diagnostic, per millicurie ☒ ☒ ☑ ⊘
AHA: 4Q, '05, 1-6

**A9557** Technetium Tc-99m bicisate, diagnostic, per study dose, up to 25 millicuries ☒ ☒ ☑ ⊘
Use this code for Neurolite.
AHA: 4Q, '05, 1-6

**A9558** Xenon Xe-133 gas, diagnostic, per 10 millicuries ☒ ☒ ☑ ⊘
AHA: 4Q, '05, 1-6

**A9559** Cobalt Co-57 cyanocobalamin, oral, diagnostic, per study dose, up to 1 microcurie ☒ ☒ ☑ ⊘
AHA: 4Q, '05, 1-6

**A9560** Technetium Tc-99m labeled red blood cells, diagnostic, per study dose, up to 30 millicuries ☒ ☒ ☑ ⊘
AHA: 3Q, '08, 7, 8; 4Q, '05, 1-6

**A9561** Technetium Tc-99m oxidronate, diagnostic, per study dose, up to 30 millicuries ☒ ☒ ☑ ⊘
Use this code for TechneScan.
AHA: 4Q, '05, 1-6

**A9562** Technetium Tc-99m mertiatide, diagnostic, per study dose, up to 15 millicuries ☒ ☒ ☑ ⊘
Use this code for TechneScan MAG-3.
AHA: 4Q, '05, 1-6

**A9563** Sodium phosphate P-32, therapeutic, per millicurie ☒ ☑ ⊘
AHA: 4Q, '05, 1-6

**A9564** Chromic phosphate P-32 suspension, therapeutic, per millicurie ☒ ☑ ⊘
Use this code for Phosphocol (P32).
AHA: 4Q, '05, 1-6

**A9566** Technetium Tc-99m fanolesomab, diagnostic, per study dose, up to 25 millicuries ☒ ☒ ☑ ⊘
AHA: 4Q, '05, 1-6

**A9567** Technetium Tc-99m pentetate, diagnostic, aerosol, per study dose, up to 75 millicuries ☒ ☒ ☑ ⊘
Use this code for AN-DTPA, DTPA, MPI-DTPA Kit-Chelate, MPI Indium DTPA IN-111, Pentate Calcium Trisodium, Pentate Zinc Trisodium.
AHA: 4Q, '05, 1-6

**A9568** Technetium Tc-99m arcitumomab, diagnostic, per study dose, up to 45 millicuries ☒ ☒ ☑ ⊘
Use this code for CEA Scan.

**A9569** Technetium Tc-99m exametazime labeled autologous white blood cells, diagnostic, per study dose ☒ ☒ ☑ ⊘
AHA: 1Q, '08, 6

**A9570** Indium In-111 labeled autologous white blood cells, diagnostic, per study dose ☒ ☒ ☑ ⊘

**A9571** Indium In-111 labeled autologous platelets, diagnostic, per study dose ☒ ☒ ☑ ⊘

**A9572** Indium In-111 pentetreotide, diagnostic, per study dose, up to 6 millicuries ☒ ☒ ☑ ⊘
Use this code for Ostreoscan.

**A9575** Injection, gadoterate meglumine, 0.1 ml ☒ ☒ ☑
Use this code for Dotarem.
AHA: 1Q, '14

**A9576** Injection, gadoteridol, (ProHance multipack), per ml ☒ ☒ ☑

**A9577** Injection, gadobenate dimeglumine (MultiHance), per ml ☒ ☒ ☑
AHA: 1Q, '08, 6

**A9578** Injection, gadobenate dimeglumine (MultiHance multipack), per ml ☒ ☒ ☑

**A9579** Injection, gadolinium-based magnetic resonance contrast agent, not otherwise specified (NOS), per ml ☒ ☒ ☑
Use this code for Omniscan, Magnevist.
AHA: 1Q, '08, 6

**A9580** Sodium fluoride F-18, diagnostic, per study dose, up to 30 millicuries ☒ ☒ ☑ ⊘
CMS: 100-03,220.6.19; 100-04,13,60.18; 100-04,13,60.3.2

**A9581** Injection, gadoxetate disodium, 1 ml ☒ ☒ ☑ ⊘
Use this code for Eovist.

**A9582** Iodine I-123 iobenguane, diagnostic, per study dose, up to 15 millicuries ☒ ☒ ☑

**A9583** Injection, gadofosveset trisodium, 1 ml ☒ ☒ ☑
Use this code for Ablavar, Vasovist.

**A9584** Iodine I-123 ioflupane, diagnostic, per study dose, up to 5 millicuries ☒ ☒ ☑
Use this code for DaTscan.

**A9585** Injection, gadobutrol, 0.1 ml ☒ ☒ ☑
Use this code for Gadavist.

**A9586** Florbetapir F18, diagnostic, per study dose, up to 10 millicuries ☒ ☒ ☑
Use this code for Amyvid.
CMS: 100-04,13,60.12; 100-04,32,60.12
AHA: 3Q, '14, 7; 1Q, '14

● **A9587**^Jan Gallium ga-68, dotatate, diagnostic, 0.1 millicurie
Use this code for Netspot.

● **A9588**^Jan Fluciclovine f-18, diagnostic, 1 millicurie
Use this code for Axumin.

● **A9597**^Jan Positron emission tomography radiopharmaceutical, diagnostic, for tumor identification, not otherwise classified

● **A9598**^Jan Positron emission tomography radiopharmaceutical, diagnostic, for non-tumor identification, not otherwise classified

▲ **A9599**^Jan Radiopharmaceutical, diagnostic, for beta-amyloid positron emission tomography (PET) imaging, per study dose, not otherwise specified ☒ ☒ ☑
CMS: 100-04,13,60.12; 100-04,32,60.12
AHA: 3Q, '14, 7; 1Q, '14

**A9600** Strontium Sr-89 chloride, therapeutic, per millicurie ☒ ☑ ⊘
Use this code for Metastron.
AHA: 4Q, '05, 1-6; 3Q, '04, 1-10; 2Q, '02, 8-9

**A9604** Samarium sm-153 lexidronam, therapeutic, per treatment dose, up to 150 millicuries ☒ ☑
Use this code for Quadramet.

**A9606** Radium RA-223 dichloride, therapeutic, per microcurie ☒
Use this code for Xofigo.

**A9698** Nonradioactive contrast imaging material, not otherwise classified, per study ☒ ☒ ⊘
AHA: 4Q, '05, 1-6

**A9699** Radiopharmaceutical, therapeutic, not otherwise classified ☒ ⊘
AHA: 4Q, '05, 1-6; 3Q, '04, 1-10

**A9700** Supply of injectable contrast material for use in echocardiography, per study ☒
AHA: 2Q, '03, 7; 4Q, '01, 5

## Miscellaneous

**A9900** Miscellaneous DME supply, accessory, and/or service component of another HCPCS code ☒

**A9901** DME delivery, set up, and/or dispensing service component of another HCPCS code ☒

---

^Jan **January Update**

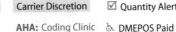 Special Coverage Instructions    Noncovered by Medicare     Carrier Discretion    ☑ Quantity Alert    ● New Code    ○ Recycled/Reinstated    ▲ Revised Code

Transportation Services Including Ambulance

A9999 — A9999

| A9999 | Miscellaneous DME supply or accessory, not otherwise specified | Y |

Special Coverage Instructions     Noncovered by Medicare     Carrier Discretion     ☑ Quantity Alert  ● New Code     ○ Recycled/Reinstated  ▲ Revised Code

16 — A Codes        Ⓐ Age Edit      Ⓜ Maternity Edit    ♀ Female Only    ♂ Male Only    Ⓐ-Ⓨ OPPS Status Indicators        © 2016 Optum360, LLC

# Enteral and Parenteral Therapy B4034-B9999

This section includes codes for supplies, formulae, nutritional solutions, and infusion pumps.

## Enteral Formulae and Enteral Medical Supplies

**B4034** Enteral feeding supply kit; syringe fed, per day, includes but not limited to feeding/flushing syringe, administration set tubing, dressings, tape ☑ ☑
CMS: 100-03,180.2; 100-04,20,160.2; 100-04,23,60.3

**B4035** Enteral feeding supply kit; pump fed, per day, includes but not limited to feeding/flushing syringe, administration set tubing, dressings, tape ☑ ☑
CMS: 100-03,180.2; 100-04,20,160.2; 100-04,23,60.3

**B4036** Enteral feeding supply kit; gravity fed, per day, includes but not limited to feeding/flushing syringe, administration set tubing, dressings, tape ☑ ☑
CMS: 100-03,180.2; 100-04,20,160.2; 100-04,23,60.3

**B4081** Nasogastric tubing with stylet ☑
CMS: 100-03,180.2; 100-04,20,160.2; 100-04,23,60.3

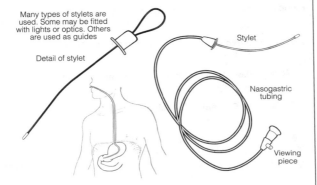

Many types of stylets are used. Some may be fitted with lights or optics. Others are used as guides

Detail of stylet

Stylet

Nasogastric tubing

Viewing piece

**B4082** Nasogastric tubing without stylet ☑
CMS: 100-03,180.2; 100-04,20,160.2; 100-04,23,60.3

**B4083** Stomach tube - Levine type ☑
CMS: 100-03,180.2; 100-04,20,160.2; 100-04,23,60.3

**B4087** Gastrostomy/jejunostomy tube, standard, any material, any type, each ☑ ☑
CMS: 100-03,180.2; 100-04,23,60.3

**B4088** Gastrostomy/jejunostomy tube, low-profile, any material, any type, each ☑ ☑
CMS: 100-03,180.2; 100-04,23,60.3

**B4100** Food thickener, administered orally, per oz ☑ ☑
CMS: 100-03,180.2

**B4102** Enteral formula, for adults, used to replace fluids and electrolytes (e.g., clear liquids), 500 ml = 1 unit ☑ ☑
CMS: 100-03,180.2

**B4103** Enteral formula, for pediatrics, used to replace fluids and electrolytes (e.g., clear liquids), 500 ml = 1 unit ☑ ☑
CMS: 100-03,180.2

**B4104** Additive for enteral formula (e.g., fiber) ☑
CMS: 100-03,180.2

**B4149** Enteral formula, manufactured blenderized natural foods with intact nutrients, includes proteins, fats, carbohydrates, vitamins and minerals, may include fiber, administered through an enteral feeding tube, 100 calories = 1 unit ☑ ☑
CMS: 100-03,180.2; 100-04,23,60.3

**B4150** Enteral formula, nutritionally complete with intact nutrients, includes proteins, fats, carbohydrates, vitamins and minerals, may include fiber, administered through an enteral feeding tube, 100 calories = 1 unit ☑ ☑
Use this code for Enrich, Ensure, Ensure HN, Ensure Powder, Isocal, Lonalac Powder, Meritene, Meritene Powder, Osmolite, Osmolite HN, Portagen Powder, Sustacal, Renu, Sustagen Powder, Travasorb.
CMS: 100-03,180.2; 100-04,20,160.2; 100-04,23,60.3

**B4152** Enteral formula, nutritionally complete, calorically dense (equal to or greater than 1.5 kcal/ml) with intact nutrients, includes proteins, fats, carbohydrates, vitamins and minerals, may include fiber, administered through an enteral feeding tube, 100 calories = 1 unit ☑ ☑
Use this code for Magnacal, Isocal HCN, Sustacal HC, Ensure Plus, Ensure Plus HN.
CMS: 100-03,180.2; 100-04,20,160.2; 100-04,23,60.3

**B4153** Enteral formula, nutritionally complete, hydrolyzed proteins (amino acids and peptide chain), includes fats, carbohydrates, vitamins and minerals, may include fiber, administered through an enteral feeding tube, 100 calories = 1 unit ☑ ☑
Use this code for Criticare HN, Vivonex t.e.n. (Total Enteral Nutrition), Vivonex HN, Vital (Vital HN), Travasorb HN, Isotein HN, Precision HN, Precision Isotonic.
CMS: 100-03,180.2; 100-04,20,160.2; 100-04,23,60.3

**B4154** Enteral formula, nutritionally complete, for special metabolic needs, excludes inherited disease of metabolism, includes altered composition of proteins, fats, carbohydrates, vitamins and/or minerals, may include fiber, administered through an enteral feeding tube, 100 calories = 1 unit ☑ ☑
Use this code for Hepatic-aid, Travasorb Hepatic, Travasorb MCT, Travasorb Renal, Traum-aid, Tramacal, Aminaid.
CMS: 100-03,180.2; 100-04,20,160.2; 100-04,23,60.3

**B4155** Enteral formula, nutritionally incomplete/modular nutrients, includes specific nutrients, carbohydrates (e.g., glucose polymers), proteins/amino acids (e.g., glutamine, arginine), fat (e.g., medium chain triglycerides) or combination, administered through an enteral feeding tube, 100 calories = 1 unit ☑ ☑
Use this code for Propac, Gerval Protein, Promix, Casec, Moducal, Controlyte, Polycose Liquid or Powder, Sumacal, Microlipids, MCT Oil, Nutri-source.
CMS: 100-03,180.2; 100-04,20,160.2; 100-04,23,60.3

**B4157** Enteral formula, nutritionally complete, for special metabolic needs for inherited disease of metabolism, includes proteins, fats, carbohydrates, vitamins and minerals, may include fiber, administered through an enteral feeding tube, 100 calories = 1 unit ☑ ☑
CMS: 100-03,180.2

**B4158** Enteral formula, for pediatrics, nutritionally complete with intact nutrients, includes proteins, fats, carbohydrates, vitamins and minerals, may include fiber and/or iron, administered through an enteral feeding tube, 100 calories = 1 unit ☑ ☑
CMS: 100-03,180.2

**B4159** Enteral formula, for pediatrics, nutritionally complete soy based with intact nutrients, includes proteins, fats, carbohydrates, vitamins and minerals, may include fiber and/or iron, administered through an enteral feeding tube, 100 calories = 1 unit ☑ ☑
CMS: 100-03,180.2

**B4160** Enteral formula, for pediatrics, nutritionally complete calorically dense (equal to or greater than 0.7 kcal/ml) with intact nutrients, includes proteins, fats, carbohydrates, vitamins and minerals, may include fiber, administered through an enteral feeding tube, 100 calories = 1 unit ☑ ☑
CMS: 100-03,180.2

Special Coverage Instructions    Noncovered by Medicare    Carrier Discretion    ☑ Quantity Alert  ● New Code    ○ Recycled/Reinstated  ▲ Revised Code

**Enteral and Parenteral Therapy**

**B4161 — B9999**

**B4161** Enteral formula, for pediatrics, hydrolyzed/amino acids and peptide chain proteins, includes fats, carbohydrates, vitamins and minerals, may include fiber, administered through an enteral feeding tube, 100 calories = 1 unit  Ⓨ ☑
CMS: 100-03,180.2

**B4162** Enteral formula, for pediatrics, special metabolic needs for inherited disease of metabolism, includes proteins, fats, carbohydrates, vitamins and minerals, may include fiber, administered through an enteral feeding tube, 100 calories = 1 unit  Ⓨ ☑
CMS: 100-03,180.2

## Parenteral Nutrition Solutions and Supplies

**B4164** Parenteral nutrition solution: carbohydrates (dextrose), 50% or less (500 ml = 1 unit), home mix  Ⓨ ☑
CMS: 100-03,180.2; 100-04,20,160.2

**B4168** Parenteral nutrition solution; amino acid, 3.5%, (500 ml = 1 unit) - home mix  Ⓨ ☑
CMS: 100-03,180.2; 100-04,20,160.2

**B4172** Parenteral nutrition solution; amino acid, 5.5% through 7%, (500 ml = 1 unit) - home mix  Ⓨ ☑
CMS: 100-03,180.2; 100-04,20,160.2

**B4176** Parenteral nutrition solution; amino acid, 7% through 8.5%, (500 ml = 1 unit) - home mix  Ⓨ ☑
CMS: 100-03,180.2; 100-04,20,160.2

**B4178** Parenteral nutrition solution: amino acid, greater than 8.5% (500 ml = 1 unit), home mix  Ⓨ ☑
CMS: 100-03,180.2; 100-04,20,160.2

**B4180** Parenteral nutrition solution: carbohydrates (dextrose), greater than 50% (500 ml = 1 unit), home mix  Ⓨ ☑
CMS: 100-03,180.2; 100-04,20,160.2

**B4185** Parenteral nutrition solution, per 10 grams lipids  Ⓑ ☑
CMS: 100-03,180.2

**B4189** Parenteral nutrition solution: compounded amino acid and carbohydrates with electrolytes, trace elements, and vitamins, including preparation, any strength, 10 to 51 g of protein, premix  Ⓨ ☑
CMS: 100-03,180.2; 100-04,20,160.2

**B4193** Parenteral nutrition solution: compounded amino acid and carbohydrates with electrolytes, trace elements, and vitamins, including preparation, any strength, 52 to 73 g of protein, premix  Ⓨ ☑
CMS: 100-03,180.2; 100-04,20,160.2

**B4197** Parenteral nutrition solution; compounded amino acid and carbohydrates with electrolytes, trace elements and vitamins, including preparation, any strength, 74 to 100 grams of protein - premix  Ⓨ ☑
CMS: 100-03,180.2; 100-04,20,160.2

**B4199** Parenteral nutrition solution; compounded amino acid and carbohydrates with electrolytes, trace elements and vitamins, including preparation, any strength, over 100 grams of protein - premix  Ⓨ ☑
CMS: 100-03,180.2; 100-04,20,160.2

**B4216** Parenteral nutrition; additives (vitamins, trace elements, Heparin, electrolytes), home mix, per day  Ⓨ
CMS: 100-03,180.2; 100-04,20,160.2

**B4220** Parenteral nutrition supply kit; premix, per day  Ⓨ
CMS: 100-03,180.2; 100-04,20,160.2

**B4222** Parenteral nutrition supply kit; home mix, per day  Ⓨ
CMS: 100-03,180.2; 100-04,20,160.2

**B4224** Parenteral nutrition administration kit, per day  Ⓨ
CMS: 100-03,180.2; 100-04,20,160.2

**B5000** Parenteral nutrition solution: compounded amino acid and carbohydrates with electrolytes, trace elements, and vitamins, including preparation, any strength, renal - Amirosyn RF, NephrAmine, RenAmine - premix  Ⓨ
Use this code for Amirosyn-RF, NephrAmine, RenAmin.
CMS: 100-03,180.2; 100-04,20,160.2

**B5100** Parenteral nutrition solution compounded amino acid and carbohydrates with electrolytes, trace elements, and vitamins, including preparation, any strength, hepatic-HepatAmine-premix  Ⓨ
Use this code for FreAmine HBC, HepatAmine.
CMS: 100-03,180.2; 100-04,20,160.2

**B5200** Parenteral nutrition solution compounded amino acid and carbohydrates with electrolytes, trace elements, and vitamins, including preparation, any strength, stress-branch chain amino acids-FreAmine-HBC-premix  Ⓨ
CMS: 100-03,180.2; 100-04,20,160.2

## Enteral and Parenteral Pumps

**B9000**ᴶᵃⁿ ~~Enteral nutrition infusion pump - without alarm~~

▲ **B9002**ᴶᵃⁿ Enteral nutrition infusion pump, any type  Ⓨ
CMS: 100-03,180.2; 100-04,20,160.2; 100-04,23,60.3

**B9004** Parenteral nutrition infusion pump, portable  Ⓨ
CMS: 100-03,180.2; 100-04,20,160.2

**B9006** Parenteral nutrition infusion pump, stationary  Ⓨ
CMS: 100-03,180.2; 100-04,20,160.2

**B9998** NOC for enteral supplies  Ⓨ
CMS: 100-03,180.2

**B9999** NOC for parenteral supplies  Ⓨ
Determine if an alternative HCPCS Level II or a CPT code better describes the service being reported. This code should be used only if a more specific code is unavailable.
CMS: 100-03,180.2

ᴶᵃⁿ **January Update**

Special Coverage Instructions    Noncovered by Medicare    Carrier Discretion    ☑ Quantity Alert  ● New Code    ○ Recycled/Reinstated  ▲ Revised Code

18 — B Codes          Ⓐ Age Edit    Ⓜ Maternity Edit    ♀ Female Only    ♂ Male Only    Ⓐ-Ⓨ OPPS Status Indicators          © 2016 Optum360, LLC

## Outpatient PPS C1713-C9899

This section reports drug, biological, and device codes that must be used by OPPS hospitals. Non-OPPS hospitals, Critical Access Hospitals (CAHs), Indian Health Service Hospitals (HIS), hospitals located in American Samoa, Guam, Saipan, or the Virgin Islands, and Maryland waiver hospitals may report these codes at their discretion. The codes can only be reported for facility (technical) services.

The C series of HCPCS may include device categories, new technology procedures, and drugs, biologicals and radiopharmaceuticals that do not have other HCPCS codes assigned. Some of these items and services are eligible for transitional pass-through payments for OPPS hospitals, have separate APC payments, or are items that are packaged. Hospitals are encouraged to report all appropriate C codes regardless of payment status.

**C1713** Anchor/screw for opposing bone-to-bone or soft tissue-to-bone (implantable) N N1
AHA: 3Q, '16; 3Q, '15, 2; 2Q, '10, 3; 3Q, '02, 4-5; 1Q, '01, 6

**C1714** Catheter, transluminal atherectomy, directional N N1
AHA: 3Q, '16; 4Q, '04, 4-5; 4Q, '03, 8; 3Q, '02, 4-5; 1Q, '01, 6

**C1715** Brachytherapy needle N N1 ⊘
AHA: 3Q, '16; 3Q, '02, 4-5; 1Q, '01, 6

**C1716** Brachytherapy source, nonstranded, gold-198, per source U H2 ☑ ⊘
AHA: 3Q, '16; 2Q, '07, 11; 4Q, '04, 8; 2Q, '04, 10; 3Q, '02, 4-5; 1Q, '01, 6

**C1717** Brachytherapy source, nonstranded, high dose rate iridium-192, per source U H2 ☑ ⊘
AHA: 3Q, '16; 2Q, '07, 11; 4Q, '04, 8; 2Q, '04, 10; 3Q, '02, 4-5; 1Q, '01, 6

**C1719** Brachytherapy source, nonstranded, nonhigh dose rate iridium-192, per source U H2 ☑ ⊘
AHA: 3Q, '16; 2Q, '07, 11; 4Q, '04, 8; 2Q, '04, 10; 3Q, '02, 4-5; 1Q, '01, 6

**C1721** Cardioverter-defibrillator, dual chamber (implantable) N N1
CMS: 100-04,14,40.8
AHA: 3Q, '16; 4Q, '04, 4-5; 3Q, '02, 4-5; 1Q, '01, 6

**C1722** Cardioverter-defibrillator, single chamber (implantable) N N1
CMS: 100-04,14,40.8
AHA: 3Q, '16; 2Q, '06, 11; 4Q, '04, 4-5; 3Q, '02, 4-5; 1Q, '01, 6

**C1724** Catheter, transluminal atherectomy, rotational N N1
AHA: 3Q, '16; 4Q, '04, 4-5; 4Q, '03, 8; 3Q, '02, 4-5; 1Q, '01, 6

**C1725** Catheter, transluminal angioplasty, non-laser (may include guidance, infusion/perfusion capability) N N1
To appropriately report drug-coated transluminal angioplasty catheters, use HCPCS code C2623.
AHA: 3Q, '16; 4Q, '04, 4-5; 4Q, '03, 8; 3Q, '02, 4-5; 1Q, '01, 6

**C1726** Catheter, balloon dilatation, nonvascular N N1
AHA: 3Q, '16; 3Q, '02, 4-5; 1Q, '01, 6

**C1727** Catheter, balloon tissue dissector, nonvascular (insertable) N N1
AHA: 3Q, '16; 3Q, '02, 4-5; 1Q, '01, 6

**C1728** Catheter, brachytherapy seed administration N N1 ⊘
AHA: 3Q, '16; 3Q, '02, 4-5; 1Q, '01, 6

**C1729** Catheter, drainage N N1
AHA: 3Q, '16; 3Q, '02, 4-5; 1Q, '01, 6

**C1730** Catheter, electrophysiology, diagnostic, other than 3D mapping (19 or fewer electrodes) N N1
AHA: 3Q, '16; 4Q, '04, 4-5; 3Q, '02, 4-5; 3Q, '01, 4-5; 1Q, '01, 6

**C1731** Catheter, electrophysiology, diagnostic, other than 3D mapping (20 or more electrodes) N N1
AHA: 3Q, '16; 4Q, '04, 4-5; 3Q, '02, 4-5; 1Q, '01, 6

**C1732** Catheter, electrophysiology, diagnostic/ablation, 3D or vector mapping N N1
AHA: 3Q, '16; 4Q, '04, 4-5; 3Q, '02, 4-5; 3Q, '01, 4-5; 1Q, '01, 6

**C1733** Catheter, electrophysiology, diagnostic/ablation, other than 3D or vector mapping, other than cool-tip N N1
AHA: 3Q, '16; 4Q, '04, 4-5; 3Q, '02, 4-5; 3Q, '01, 4-5; 1Q, '01, 6

**C1749** Endoscope, retrograde imaging/illumination colonoscope device (implantable) N N1
AHA: 3Q, '16

**C1750** Catheter, hemodialysis/peritoneal, long-term N N1
AHA: 3Q, '16; 4Q, '15, 6; 4Q, '12, 9; 4Q, '03, 8; 3Q, '02, 4-5; 1Q, '01, 6

**C1751** Catheter, infusion, inserted peripherally, centrally or midline (other than hemodialysis) N N1
AHA: 3Q, '16; 3Q, '14, 5; 4Q, '04, 4-5; 4Q, '03, 8; 3Q, '02, 4-5; 3Q, '01, 4-5; 1Q, '01, 6

**C1752** Catheter, hemodialysis/peritoneal, short-term N N1
AHA: 3Q, '16; 4Q, '03, 8; 3Q, '02, 4-5; 1Q, '01, 6

**C1753** Catheter, intravascular ultrasound N N1
AHA: 3Q, '16; 4Q, '03, 8; 3Q, '02, 4-5; 1Q, '01, 6

**C1754** Catheter, intradiscal N N1
AHA: 3Q, '16; 4Q, '03, 8; 3Q, '02, 4-5; 1Q, '01, 6

**C1755** Catheter, intraspinal N N1
AHA: 3Q, '16; 4Q, '03, 8; 3Q, '02, 4-5; 1Q, '01, 6

**C1756** Catheter, pacing, transesophageal N N1
AHA: 4Q, '03, 8; 3Q, '02, 4-5; 1Q, '01, 6

**C1757** Catheter, thrombectomy/embolectomy N N1
AHA: 3Q, '16; 4Q, '03, 8; 3Q, '02, 4-5; 1Q, '01, 6

**C1758** Catheter, ureteral N N1
AHA: 3Q, '16; 4Q, '03, 8; 3Q, '02, 4-5; 1Q, '01, 6

**C1759** Catheter, intracardiac echocardiography N N1
AHA: 3Q, '16; 4Q, '03, 8; 3Q, '02, 4-5; 3Q, '01, 4-5; 1Q, '01, 6

**C1760** Closure device, vascular (implantable/insertable) N N1
AHA: 3Q, '16; 4Q, '03, 8; 3Q, '02, 4-5; 1Q, '01, 6

**C1762** Connective tissue, human (includes fascia lata) N N1
AHA: 3Q, '16; 3Q, '15, 2; 4Q, '03, 8; 3Q, '03, 11; 3Q, '02, 4-5; 1Q, '01, 6

**C1763** Connective tissue, nonhuman (includes synthetic) N N1
AHA: 3Q, '16; 4Q, '10, 1; 2Q, '10, 3; 4Q, '03, 8; 3Q, '03, 11; 3Q, '02, 4-5; 1Q, '01, 6

**C1764** Event recorder, cardiac (implantable) N N1
CMS: 100-04,14,40.8
AHA: 3Q, '16; 2Q, '15, 8; 4Q, '03, 8; 3Q, '02, 4-5; 1Q, '01, 6

**C1765** Adhesion barrier N N1
AHA: 3Q, '16

**C1766** Introducer/sheath, guiding, intracardiac electrophysiological, steerable, other than peel-away N N1
AHA: 3Q, '16; 4Q, '04, 4-5; 3Q, '02, 4-5; 3Q, '01, 4-5

**C1767** Generator, neurostimulator (implantable), nonrechargeable N N1
CMS: 100-04,14,40.8; 100-04,32,40.1
AHA: 3Q, '16; 4Q, '06, 4; 4Q, '04, 4-5; 4Q, '03, 8; 3Q, '02, 4-5; 1Q, '02, 9; 1Q, '01, 6

**C1768** Graft, vascular N N1
AHA: 3Q, '16; 4Q, '03, 8; 3Q, '02, 4-5; 1Q, '01, 6

**C1769** Guide wire N N1
AHA: 3Q, '16; 3Q, '14, 5; 2Q, '07, 6; 4Q, '03, 8; 3Q, '02, 4-5; 3Q, '01, 4-5; 1Q, '01, 6

**C1770** Imaging coil, magnetic resonance (insertable) N N1
AHA: 3Q, '16; 4Q, '03, 8; 3Q, '02, 4-5; 1Q, '01, 6

**C1771** Repair device, urinary, incontinence, with sling graft N N1
CMS: 100-04,14,40.8
AHA: 3Q, '16; 4Q, '03, 8; 3Q, '02, 4-5; 3Q, '01, 4-5; 1Q, '01, 6

Special Coverage Instructions    Noncovered by Medicare    Carrier Discretion    ☑ Quantity Alert  ● New Code    ○ Recycled/Reinstated    ▲ Revised Code

© 2016 Optum360, LLC    A2-Z3 ASC Pmt    CMS: Pub 100    AHA: Coding Clinic    ⅋ DMEPOS Paid    ⊘ SNF Excluded

C Codes — 19

**Outpatient PPS**

**C1772 — C1886**

**C1772** Infusion pump, programmable (implantable) N N1
CMS: 100-04,14,40.8
AHA: 3Q, '16; 4Q, '04, 4-5; 3Q, '02, 4-5; 1Q, '01, 6

**C1773** Retrieval device, insertable (used to retrieve fractured medical devices) N N1
AHA: 3Q, '16; 4Q, '03, 8; 3Q, '02, 4-5; 1Q, '01, 6

**C1776** Joint device (implantable) N N1
CMS: 100-04,14,40.8
AHA: 3Q, '16; 3Q, '10, 6; 4Q, '08, 6, 8; 3Q, '02, 4-5; 3Q, '01, 4-5; 1Q, '01, 6

**C1777** Lead, cardioverter-defibrillator, endocardial single coil (implantable) N N1
AHA: 3Q, '16; 2Q, '06, 11; 4Q, '04, 4-5; 3Q, '02, 4-5; 1Q, '01, 6

**C1778** Lead, neurostimulator (implantable) N N1
CMS: 100-04,14,40.8; 100-04,32,40.1
AHA: 3Q, '16; 4Q, '11, 10; 3Q, '02, 4-5; 1Q, '02, 9; 1Q, '01, 6

**C1779** Lead, pacemaker, transvenous VDD single pass N N1
CMS: 100-04,14,40.8
AHA: 3Q, '16; 4Q, '04, 4-5; 3Q, '02, 4-5; 1Q, '01, 6

**C1780** Lens, intraocular (new technology) N N1
AHA: 3Q, '16; 3Q, '02, 4-5; 1Q, '01, 6

**C1781** Mesh (implantable) N N1
Use this code for OrthADAPT Bioimplant.
AHA: 3Q, '16; 2Q, '12, 3; 2Q, '10, 3; 2Q, '10, 2, 3; 3Q, '02, 4-5; 1Q, '01, 6

**C1782** Morcellator N N1
AHA: 3Q, '16; 3Q, '02, 4-5; 1Q, '01, 6

**C1783** Ocular implant, aqueous drainage assist device N N1
AHA: 3Q, '16

**C1784** Ocular device, intraoperative, detached retina N N1
AHA: 3Q, '16; 3Q, '02, 4-5; 1Q, '01, 6

**C1785** Pacemaker, dual chamber, rate-responsive (implantable) N N1
CMS: 100-04,14,40.8; 100-04,21,320.4.7; 100-04,32,320.4.1; 100-04,32,320.4.2; 100-04,32,320.4.4; 100-04,32,320.4.6; 100-04,32,320.4.7; 100-04,32,320.5; 100-04,32,320.6
AHA: 3Q, '16; 4Q, '03, 8; 3Q, '02, 4-5; 1Q, '01, 6

**C1786** Pacemaker, single chamber, rate-responsive (implantable) N N1
CMS: 100-04,14,40.8; 100-04,21,320.4.7; 100-04,32,320.4.1; 100-04,32,320.4.2; 100-04,32,320.4.4; 100-04,32,320.4.6; 100-04,32,320.4.7; 100-04,32,320.5; 100-04,32,320.6
AHA: 3Q, '16; 4Q, '04, 4-5; 4Q, '03, 8; 3Q, '02, 4-5; 1Q, '01, 6

**C1787** Patient programmer, neurostimulator N N1
AHA: 3Q, '16; 4Q, '03, 8; 3Q, '02, 4-5; 1Q, '01, 6

**C1788** Port, indwelling (implantable) N N1
AHA: 3Q, '16; 3Q, '14, 5; 4Q, '04, 4-5; 4Q, '03, 8; 3Q, '02, 4-5; 3Q, '01, 4-5; 1Q, '01, 6

**C1789** Prosthesis, breast (implantable) N N1
AHA: 3Q, '16; 4Q, '03, 8; 3Q, '02, 4-5; 1Q, '01, 6

**C1813** Prosthesis, penile, inflatable N N1
CMS: 100-04,14,40.8
AHA: 3Q, '16; 4Q, '03, 8; 3Q, '02, 4-5; 1Q, '01, 6

**C1814** Retinal tamponade device, silicone oil N N1
AHA: 3Q, '16; 2Q, '06, 12

**C1815** Prosthesis, urinary sphincter (implantable) N N1
CMS: 100-04,14,40.8
AHA: 3Q, '16; 4Q, '03, 8; 3Q, '02, 4-5; 1Q, '01, 6

**C1816** Receiver and/or transmitter, neurostimulator (implantable) N N1
AHA: 3Q, '16; 4Q, '03, 8; 3Q, '02, 4-5; 1Q, '01, 6

**C1817** Septal defect implant system, intracardiac N N1
AHA: 3Q, '16; 4Q, '03, 8; 3Q, '02, 4-5; 1Q, '01, 6

**C1818** Integrated keratoprosthesis N N1
AHA: 3Q, '16; 4Q, '03, 4-5

**C1819** Surgical tissue localization and excision device (implantable) N N1
AHA: 3Q, '16; 1Q, '04, 10

▲ **C1820**Apr Generator, neurostimulator (implantable), with rechargeable battery and charging system N N1
Use to report neurostimulator generators that are not high frequency.
CMS: 100-04,14,40.8; 100-04,4,10.12
AHA: 3Q, '16; 2Q, '16; 1Q, '16, 9

**C1821** Interspinous process distraction device (implantable) N N1
AHA: 3Q, '16; 2Q, '09, 1

**C1822** Generator, neurostimulator (implantable), high frequency, with rechargeable battery and charging system H J7
Use to report neurostimulator generators that are high frequency.
AHA: 3Q, '16; 2Q, '16; 1Q, '16, 9

**C1830** Powered bone marrow biopsy needle N N1
AHA: 3Q, '16; 4Q, '11, 10

**C1840** Lens, intraocular (telescopic) N N1
AHA: 3Q, '16; 3Q, '12, 10; 4Q, '11, 10

**C1841** Retinal prosthesis, includes all internal and external components N J7
AHA: 3Q, '16

**C1874** Stent, coated/covered, with delivery system N N1
AHA: 3Q, '16; 4Q, '04, 4-5; 3Q, '04, 11-13; 4Q, '03, 8; 3Q, '02, 7; 3Q, '02, 4-5; 3Q, '01, 4-5; 1Q, '01, 6

**C1875** Stent, coated/covered, without delivery system N N1
AHA: 3Q, '16; 4Q, '04, 4-5; 4Q, '03, 8; 3Q, '02, 7; 3Q, '02, 4-5; 1Q, '01, 6

**C1876** Stent, noncoated/noncovered, with delivery system N N1
AHA: 3Q, '16; 4Q, '04, 4-5; 4Q, '03, 8; 3Q, '02, 7; 3Q, '02, 4-5; 3Q, '01, 4-5; 1Q, '01, 6

**C1877** Stent, noncoated/noncovered, without delivery system N N1
AHA: 3Q, '16; 4Q, '04, 4-5; 4Q, '03, 8; 3Q, '02, 7; 3Q, '02, 4-5; 3Q, '01, 4-5; 1Q, '01, 6

**C1878** Material for vocal cord medialization, synthetic (implantable) N N1
AHA: 3Q, '16; 3Q, '02, 4-5; 1Q, '01, 6

**C1880** Vena cava filter N N1
AHA: 3Q, '16; 4Q, '03, 8; 3Q, '02, 4-5; 1Q, '01, 6

**C1881** Dialysis access system (implantable) N N1
CMS: 100-04,14,40.8
AHA: 3Q, '16; 4Q, '03, 8; 3Q, '02, 4-5; 1Q, '01, 6

**C1882** Cardioverter-defibrillator, other than single or dual chamber (implantable) N N1
CMS: 100-04,14,40.8
AHA: 3Q, '16; 2Q, '12, 9; 2Q, '06, 11; 4Q, '04, 4-5; 3Q, '02, 4-5; 1Q, '01, 6

**C1883** Adaptor/extension, pacing lead or neurostimulator lead (implantable) N N1
CMS: 100-04,32,40.1
AHA: 3Q, '16; 3Q, '02, 4-5; 1Q, '02, 9; 1Q, '01, 6

**C1884** Embolization protective system N N1
AHA: 3Q, '16; 3Q, '14, 5

**C1885** Catheter, transluminal angioplasty, laser N N1
AHA: 3Q, '16; 1Q, '16, 5; 4Q, '04, 4-5; 4Q, '03, 8; 3Q, '02, 4-5; 1Q, '01, 6

**C1886** Catheter, extravascular tissue ablation, any modality (insertable) N N1
AHA: 3Q, '16

---

Apr **April Update**

Special Coverage Instructions    Noncovered by Medicare    Carrier Discretion    ☑ Quantity Alert  ● New Code    ○ Recycled/Reinstated    ▲ Revised Code

A Age Edit    M Maternity Edit    ♀ Female Only    ♂ Male Only    A-Y OPPS Status Indicators    © 2016 Optum360, LLC

**C1887** Catheter, guiding (may include infusion/perfusion capability) N N1
AHA: 3Q, '16; 4Q, '04, 4-5; 3Q, '02, 4-5; 3Q, '01, 4-5; 1Q, '01, 6

**C1888** Catheter, ablation, noncardiac, endovascular (implantable) N N1
AHA: 3Q, '16

● **C1889**Jan Implantable/insertable device for device intensive procedure, not otherwise classified

**C1891** Infusion pump, nonprogrammable, permanent (implantable) N N1
CMS: 100-04,14,40.8
AHA: 3Q, '16; 4Q, '04, 4-5; 4Q, '03, 8; 3Q, '02, 4-5; 1Q, '01, 6

**C1892** Introducer/sheath, guiding, intracardiac electrophysiological, fixed-curve, peel-away N N1
AHA: 3Q, '16; 4Q, '04, 4-5; 3Q, '02, 4-5; 1Q, '01, 6

**C1893** Introducer/sheath, guiding, intracardiac electrophysiological, fixed-curve, other than peel-away N N1
AHA: 3Q, '16; 4Q, '04, 4-5; 3Q, '02, 4-5; 3Q, '01, 4-5; 1Q, '01, 6

**C1894** Introducer/sheath, other than guiding, other than intracardiac electrophysiological, nonlaser N N1
AHA: 3Q, '16; 3Q, '02, 4-5; 1Q, '01, 6

**C1895** Lead, cardioverter-defibrillator, endocardial dual coil (implantable) N N1
AHA: 3Q, '16; 2Q, '06, 11; 4Q, '04, 4-5; 3Q, '02, 4-5; 1Q, '01, 6

**C1896** Lead, cardioverter-defibrillator, other than endocardial single or dual coil (implantable) N N1
AHA: 3Q, '16; 2Q, '06, 11; 4Q, '04, 4-5; 3Q, '02, 4-5; 1Q, '01, 6

**C1897** Lead, neurostimulator test kit (implantable) N N1
CMS: 100-04,14,40.8; 100-04,32,40.1
AHA: 3Q, '16; 3Q, '02, 4-5; 1Q, '02, 9; 1Q, '01, 6

**C1898** Lead, pacemaker, other than transvenous VDD single pass N N1
CMS: 100-04,14,40.8
AHA: 3Q, '16; 3Q, '02, 8; 3Q, '02, 4-5; 3Q, '01, 4-5; 1Q, '01, 6

**C1899** Lead, pacemaker/cardioverter-defibrillator combination (implantable) N N1
AHA: 3Q, '16; 4Q, '04, 4-5; 3Q, '02, 4-5; 1Q, '01, 6

**C1900** Lead, left ventricular coronary venous system N N1
CMS: 100-04,14,40.8
AHA: 3Q, '16; 4Q, '04, 4-5

**C2613** Lung biopsy plug with delivery system H J7
AHA: 3Q, '16; 3Q, '15, 7

**C2614** Probe, percutaneous lumbar discectomy N N1
AHA: 3Q, '16

**C2615** Sealant, pulmonary, liquid N N1
AHA: 3Q, '16; 4Q, '03, 8; 3Q, '02, 4-5; 1Q, '01, 6

**C2616** Brachytherapy source, nonstranded, yttrium-90, per source U H2 ☑ ⊘
AHA: 3Q, '16; 2Q, '07, 11; 4Q, '04, 8; 2Q, '04, 10; 3Q, '03, 11; 3Q, '02, 4-5

**C2617** Stent, noncoronary, temporary, without delivery system N N1
AHA: 3Q, '16; 4Q, '04, 4-5; 4Q, '03, 8; 3Q, '02, 4-5; 1Q, '01, 6

**C2618** Probe/needle, cryoablation N N1
AHA: 3Q, '16; 4Q, '04, 4-5; 4Q, '03, 8; 3Q, '02, 4-5; 1Q, '01, 6

**C2619** Pacemaker, dual chamber, nonrate-responsive (implantable) N N1
CMS: 100-04,14,40.8; 100-04,21,320.4.7; 100-04,32,320.4.1; 100-04,32,320.4.2; 100-04,32,320.4.4; 100-04,32,320.4.6; 100-04,32,320.4.7; 100-04,32,320.5; 100-04,32,320.6
AHA: 3Q, '16; 3Q, '02, 4-5; 3Q, '01, 4-5; 1Q, '01, 6

**C2620** Pacemaker, single chamber, nonrate-responsive (implantable) N N1
CMS: 100-04,14,40.8; 100-04,21,320.4.7; 100-04,32,320.4.1; 100-04,32,320.4.2; 100-04,32,320.4.4; 100-04,32,320.4.6; 100-04,32,320.4.7; 100-04,32,320.5; 100-04,32,320.6
AHA: 3Q, '16; 4Q, '04, 4-5; 4Q, '03, 8; 3Q, '02, 4-5; 1Q, '01, 6

**C2621** Pacemaker, other than single or dual chamber (implantable) N N1
CMS: 100-04,14,40.8
AHA: 3Q, '16; 4Q, '03, 8; 3Q, '02, 8; 3Q, '02, 4-5; 1Q, '01, 6

**C2622** Prosthesis, penile, noninflatable N N1
CMS: 100-04,14,40.8
AHA: 3Q, '16; 4Q, '03, 8; 3Q, '02, 4-5; 1Q, '01, 6

**C2623** Catheter, transluminal angioplasty, drug-coated, non-laser H J7
AHA: 3Q, '16

**C2624** Implantable wireless pulmonary artery pressure sensor with delivery catheter, including all system components H J7
AHA: 3Q, '16; 3Q, '15, 1-2

**C2625** Stent, noncoronary, temporary, with delivery system N N1
AHA: 3Q, '16; 2Q, '15, 9; 4Q, '04, 4-5; 4Q, '03, 8; 3Q, '02, 4-5; 1Q, '01, 6

**C2626** Infusion pump, nonprogrammable, temporary (implantable) N N1
CMS: 100-04,14,40.8
AHA: 3Q, '16; 4Q, '04, 4-5; 3Q, '02, 4-5; 1Q, '01, 6

**C2627** Catheter, suprapubic/cystoscopic N N1
AHA: 3Q, '16; 4Q, '03, 8; 3Q, '02, 4-5; 1Q, '01, 6

**C2628** Catheter, occlusion N N1
AHA: 3Q, '16; 4Q, '04, 4-5; 4Q, '03, 8; 3Q, '02, 4-5; 1Q, '01, 6

**C2629** Introducer/sheath, other than guiding, other than intracardiac electrophysiological, laser N N1
AHA: 3Q, '16; 3Q, '02, 4-5; 1Q, '01, 6

**C2630** Catheter, electrophysiology, diagnostic/ablation, other than 3D or vector mapping, cool-tip N N1
AHA: 3Q, '16; 3Q, '02, 4-5; 1Q, '01, 6

**C2631** Repair device, urinary, incontinence, without sling graft N N1
CMS: 100-04,14,40.8
AHA: 3Q, '16; 4Q, '03, 8; 3Q, '02, 4-5; 1Q, '01, 6

**C2634** Brachytherapy source, nonstranded, high activity, iodine-125, greater than 1.01 mCi (NIST), per source U H2 ☑ ⊘
AHA: 3Q, '16; 2Q, '07, 11; 2Q, '05, 8; 4Q, '04, 8

**C2635** Brachytherapy source, nonstranded, high activity, palladium-103, greater than 2.2 mCi (NIST), per source U H2 ☑ ⊘
AHA: 3Q, '16; 2Q, '07, 11; 2Q, '05, 8; 4Q, '04, 8

**C2636** Brachytherapy linear source, nonstranded, palladium-103, per 1 mm U H2 ☑ ⊘
AHA: 3Q, '16; 2Q, '07, 11; 4Q, '04, 8

**C2637** Brachytherapy source, nonstranded, ytterbium-169, per source B ☑ ⊘
AHA: 3Q, '16; 2Q, '07, 11; 3Q, '05, 7

**C2638** Brachytherapy source, stranded, iodine-125, per source U H2 ☑
AHA: 3Q, '16

**C2639** Brachytherapy source, nonstranded, iodine-125, per source U H2 ☑ ⊘
AHA: 3Q, '16

**C2640** Brachytherapy source, stranded, palladium-103, per source U H2 ☑
AHA: 3Q, '16

---

Jan **January Update**

Special Coverage Instructions    Noncovered by Medicare    Carrier Discretion    ☑ Quantity Alert ● New Code    ○ Recycled/Reinstated    ▲ Revised Code

© 2016 Optum360, LLC    A2-Z3 ASC Pmt    CMS: Pub 100    AHA: Coding Clinic    ⅋ DMEPOS Paid    ⊘ SNF Excluded

**Outpatient PPS**

**C2641 — C8922**

| C2641 | Brachytherapy source, nonstranded, palladium-103, per source ☐U☐ H2 ☑ ⊘ |
|---|---|
| | AHA: 3Q, '16 |

| C2642 | Brachytherapy source, stranded, cesium-131, per source ☐U☐ H2 ☑ |
|---|---|
| | AHA: 3Q, '16 |

| C2643 | Brachytherapy source, nonstranded, cesium-131, per source ☐U☐ H2 ☑ ⊘ |
|---|---|
| | AHA: 3Q, '16 |

| C2644 | Brachytherapy source, cesium-131 chloride solution, per millicurie ☐U☐ H2 |
|---|---|
| | AHA: 3Q, '16 |

| C2645 | Brachytherapy planar source, palladium-103, per square millimeter ☐U☐ H2 |
|---|---|
| | AHA: 3Q, '16 |

| C2698 | Brachytherapy source, stranded, not otherwise specified, per source ☐U☐ H2 ☑ |
|---|---|
| | AHA: 3Q, '16 |

| C2699 | Brachytherapy source, nonstranded, not otherwise specified, per source ☐U☐ H2 ☑ |
|---|---|
| | AHA: 3Q, '16 |

| C5271 | Application of low cost skin substitute graft to trunk, arms, legs, total wound surface area up to 100 sq cm; first 25 sq cm or less wound surface area ☐T☐ G2 ☑ |
|---|---|

| C5272 | Application of low cost skin substitute graft to trunk, arms, legs, total wound surface area up to 100 sq cm; each additional 25 sq cm wound surface area, or part thereof (list separately in addition to code for primary procedure) ☐N☐ N1 ☑ |
|---|---|

| C5273 | Application of low cost skin substitute graft to trunk, arms, legs, total wound surface area greater than or equal to 100 sq cm; first 100 sq cm wound surface area, or 1% of body area of infants and children ☐T☐ G2 ☑ |
|---|---|

| C5274 | Application of low cost skin substitute graft to trunk, arms, legs, total wound surface area greater than or equal to 100 sq cm; each additional 100 sq cm wound surface area, or part thereof, or each additional 1% of body area of infants and children, or part thereof (list separately in addition to code for primary procedure) ☐N☐ N1 ☑ |
|---|---|

| C5275 | Application of low cost skin substitute graft to face, scalp, eyelids, mouth, neck, ears, orbits, genitalia, hands, feet, and/or multiple digits, total wound surface area up to 100 sq cm; first 25 sq cm or less wound surface area ☐T☐ G2 ☑ |
|---|---|

| C5276 | Application of low cost skin substitute graft to face, scalp, eyelids, mouth, neck, ears, orbits, genitalia, hands, feet, and/or multiple digits, total wound surface area up to 100 sq cm; each additional 25 sq cm wound surface area, or part thereof (list separately in addition to code for primary procedure) ☐N☐ N1 ☑ |
|---|---|

| C5277 | Application of low cost skin substitute graft to face, scalp, eyelids, mouth, neck, ears, orbits, genitalia, hands, feet, and/or multiple digits, total wound surface area greater than or equal to 100 sq cm; first 100 sq cm wound surface area, or 1% of body area of infants and children ☐T☐ G2 ☑ |
|---|---|

| C5278 | Application of low cost skin substitute graft to face, scalp, eyelids, mouth, neck, ears, orbits, genitalia, hands, feet, and/or multiple digits, total wound surface area greater than or equal to 100 sq cm; each additional 100 sq cm wound surface area, or part thereof, or each additional 1% of body area of infants and children, or part thereof (list separately in addition to code for primary procedure) ☐N☐ N1 ☑ |
|---|---|

| C8900 | Magnetic resonance angiography with contrast, abdomen ☐Q3☐ Z2 ⊘ |
|---|---|
| | CMS: 100-04,13,40.1.1; 100-04,13,40.1.2 |

| C8901 | Magnetic resonance angiography without contrast, abdomen ☐Q3☐ Z2 ⊘ |
|---|---|
| | CMS: 100-04,13,40.1.1; 100-04,13,40.1.2 |

| C8902 | Magnetic resonance angiography without contrast followed by with contrast, abdomen ☐Q3☐ Z2 ⊘ |
|---|---|
| | CMS: 100-04,13,40.1.1; 100-04,13,40.1.2 |

| C8903 | Magnetic resonance imaging with contrast, breast; unilateral ☐Q3☐ Z2 ⊘ |
|---|---|

| C8904 | Magnetic resonance imaging without contrast, breast; unilateral ☐Q3☐ Z2 ⊘ |
|---|---|

| C8905 | Magnetic resonance imaging without contrast followed by with contrast, breast; unilateral ☐Q3☐ Z2 ⊘ |
|---|---|

| C8906 | Magnetic resonance imaging with contrast, breast; bilateral ☐Q3☐ Z2 ⊘ |
|---|---|

| C8907 | Magnetic resonance imaging without contrast, breast; bilateral ☐Q3☐ Z2 ⊘ |
|---|---|

| C8908 | Magnetic resonance imaging without contrast followed by with contrast, breast; bilateral ☐Q3☐ Z2 ⊘ |
|---|---|

| C8909 | Magnetic resonance angiography with contrast, chest (excluding myocardium) ☐Q3☐ Z2 ⊘ |
|---|---|
| | CMS: 100-04,13,40.1.1; 100-04,13,40.1.2 |

| C8910 | Magnetic resonance angiography without contrast, chest (excluding myocardium) ☐Q3☐ Z2 ⊘ |
|---|---|
| | CMS: 100-04,13,40.1.1; 100-04,13,40.1.2 |

| C8911 | Magnetic resonance angiography without contrast followed by with contrast, chest (excluding myocardium) ☐Q3☐ Z2 ⊘ |
|---|---|
| | CMS: 100-04,13,40.1.1; 100-04,13,40.1.2 |

| C8912 | Magnetic resonance angiography with contrast, lower extremity ☐Q3☐ Z2 ⊘ |
|---|---|
| | CMS: 100-04,13,40.1.1; 100-04,13,40.1.2 |

| C8913 | Magnetic resonance angiography without contrast, lower extremity ☐Q3☐ Z2 ⊘ |
|---|---|
| | CMS: 100-04,13,40.1.1; 100-04,13,40.1.2 |

| C8914 | Magnetic resonance angiography without contrast followed by with contrast, lower extremity ☐Q3☐ Z2 ⊘ |
|---|---|
| | CMS: 100-04,13,40.1.1; 100-04,13,40.1.2 |

| C8918 | Magnetic resonance angiography with contrast, pelvis ☐Q3☐ Z2 ⊘ |
|---|---|
| | CMS: 100-04,13,40.1.1; 100-04,13,40.1.2 |
| | AHA: 4Q, '03, 4-5 |

| C8919 | Magnetic resonance angiography without contrast, pelvis ☐Q3☐ Z2 ⊘ |
|---|---|
| | CMS: 100-04,13,40.1.1; 100-04,13,40.1.2 |
| | AHA: 4Q, '03, 4-5 |

| C8920 | Magnetic resonance angiography without contrast followed by with contrast, pelvis ☐Q3☐ Z2 ⊘ |
|---|---|
| | CMS: 100-04,13,40.1.1; 100-04,13,40.1.2 |
| | AHA: 4Q, '03, 4-5 |

| C8921 | Transthoracic echocardiography with contrast, or without contrast followed by with contrast, for congenital cardiac anomalies; complete ☐S☐ |
|---|---|
| | CMS: 100-04,4,200.7.2 |
| | AHA: 3Q, '12, 8; 2Q, '08, 9 |

| C8922 | Transthoracic echocardiography with contrast, or without contrast followed by with contrast, for congenital cardiac anomalies; follow-up or limited study ☐S☐ |
|---|---|
| | AHA: 2Q, '08, 9 |

Special Coverage Instructions    Noncovered by Medicare    Carrier Discretion    ☑ Quantity Alert   ● New Code   ○ Recycled/Reinstated   ▲ Revised Code

22 — C Codes    ☐A☐ Age Edit   ☐M☐ Maternity Edit   ♀ Female Only   ♂ Male Only   ☐A☐-☐Y☐ OPPS Status Indicators    © 2016 Optum360, LLC

**C8923** Transthoracic echocardiography with contrast, or without contrast followed by with contrast, real-time with image documentation (2D), includes M-mode recording, when performed, complete, without spectral or color doppler echocardiography ⓢ
AHA: 2Q, '08, 9

**C8924** Transthoracic echocardiography with contrast, or without contrast followed by with contrast, real-time with image documentation (2D), includes M-mode recording when performed, follow-up or limited study ⓢ
AHA: 2Q, '08, 9

**C8925** Transesophageal echocardiography (TEE) with contrast, or without contrast followed by with contrast, real time with image documentation (2D) (with or without M-mode recording); including probe placement, image acquisition, interpretation and report ⓢ
AHA: 2Q, '08, 9

**C8926** Transesophageal echocardiography (TEE) with contrast, or without contrast followed by with contrast, for congenital cardiac anomalies; including probe placement, image acquisition, interpretation and report ⓢ
AHA: 2Q, '08, 9

**C8927** Transesophageal echocardiography (TEE) with contrast, or without contrast followed by with contrast, for monitoring purposes, including probe placement, real time 2-dimensional image acquisition and interpretation leading to ongoing (continuous) assessment of (dynamically changing) cardiac pumping function and to therapeutic measures on an immediate time basis ⓢ
AHA: 2Q, '08, 9

**C8928** Transthoracic echocardiography with contrast, or without contrast followed by with contrast, real-time with image documentation (2D), includes M-mode recording, when performed, during rest and cardiovascular stress test using treadmill, bicycle exercise and/or pharmacologically induced stress, with interpretation and report ⓢ
AHA: 2Q, '08, 9

**C8929** Transthoracic echocardiography with contrast, or without contrast followed by with contrast, real-time with image documentation (2D), includes M-mode recording, when performed, complete, with spectral doppler echocardiography, and with color flow doppler echocardiography ⓢ

**C8930** Transthoracic echocardiography, with contrast, or without contrast followed by with contrast, real-time with image documentation (2D), includes M-mode recording, when performed, during rest and cardiovascular stress test using treadmill, bicycle exercise and/or pharmacologically induced stress, with interpretation and report; including performance of continuous electrocardiographic monitoring, with physician supervision ⓢ
AHA: 3Q, '12, 8

**C8931** Magnetic resonance angiography with contrast, spinal canal and contents ⓠ₃ Z2

**C8932** Magnetic resonance angiography without contrast, spinal canal and contents ⓠ₃ Z2

**C8933** Magnetic resonance angiography without contrast followed by with contrast, spinal canal and contents ⓠ₃ Z2

**C8934** Magnetic resonance angiography with contrast, upper extremity ⓠ₃ Z2

**C8935** Magnetic resonance angiography without contrast, upper extremity ⓠ₃ Z2

**C8936** Magnetic resonance angiography without contrast followed by with contrast, upper extremity ⓠ₃ Z2

**C8957** Intravenous infusion for therapy/diagnosis; initiation of prolonged infusion (more than 8 hours), requiring use of portable or implantable pump ⓢ
CMS: 100-04,4,230.2; 100-04,4,230.2.1
AHA: 3Q, '08, 7, 8; 4Q, '05, 15

**C9113** Injection, pantoprazole sodium, per vial Ⓝ ₦1
Use this code for Protonix.
AHA: 1Q, '02, 5

**C9121** ^Jan Injection, argatroban, per 5 mg
To report, see ~J0883-J0884

**C9132** Prothrombin complex concentrate (human), Kcentra, per IU of Factor IX activity Ⓚ ₖ2 ☑

**C9137** ^Jan Injection, factor VIII (antihemophilic factor, recombinant) PEGylated, 1 IU
To report, see ~J7207

**C9138** ^Jan Injection, factor VIII (antihemophilic factor, recombinant) (Nuwiq), 1 IU
To report, see ~J7209

**C9139** ^Jan Injection, Factor IX, albumin fusion protein (recombinant), Idelvion, 1 IU
To report, see ~J7202

● **C9140** ^Jan Injection, factor VIII (antihemophilic factor, recombinant) (Afstyla), 1 IU

**C9248** Injection, clevidipine butyrate, 1 mg Ⓚ ₖ2 ☑
Use this code for Cleviprex.

**C9250** Human plasma fibrin sealant, vapor-heated, solvent-detergent (Artiss), 2 ml Ⓝ ₦1 ☑

**C9254** Injection, lacosamide, 1 mg Ⓝ ₦1 ☑
Use this code for VIMPAT.

**C9257** Injection, bevacizumab, 0.25 mg Ⓚ ₖ2 ☑
Use this code for Avastin.
CMS: 100-03,110.17
AHA: 3Q, '13

**C9275** Injection, hexaminolevulinate HCl, 100 mg, per study dose Ⓝ ₦1 ☑
Use this code for Cysview.
AHA: 2Q, '15, 9

**C9285** Lidocaine 70 mg/tetracaine 70 mg, per patch Ⓝ ₦1 ☑
Use this code for SYNERA.
AHA: 3Q, '11, 9

**C9290** Injection, bupivacaine liposome, 1 mg Ⓝ ₦1
Use this code for EXPAREL.
AHA: 2Q, '12, 7

**C9293** Injection, glucarpidase, 10 units Ⓚ ₖ2 ☑
Use this code for Voraxaze.

**C9349** ^Jan PuraPly, and PuraPly Antimicrobial, any type, per sq cm
To report, see ~Q4172

---

^Jan **January Update**

Special Coverage Instructions | Noncovered by Medicare | Carrier Discretion | ☑ Quantity Alert ● New Code ○ Recycled/Reinstated ▲ Revised Code

© 2016 Optum360, LLC | K2-Z3 ASC Pmt | CMS: Pub 100 | AHA: Coding Clinic | ☒ DMEPOS Paid | ⊘ SNF Excluded

C Codes — 23

**Outpatient PPS**

C9352 — C9604

**C9352** Microporous collagen implantable tube (NeuraGen Nerve Guide), per cm length [N] [N1] ☑
AHA: 1Q, '08, 6

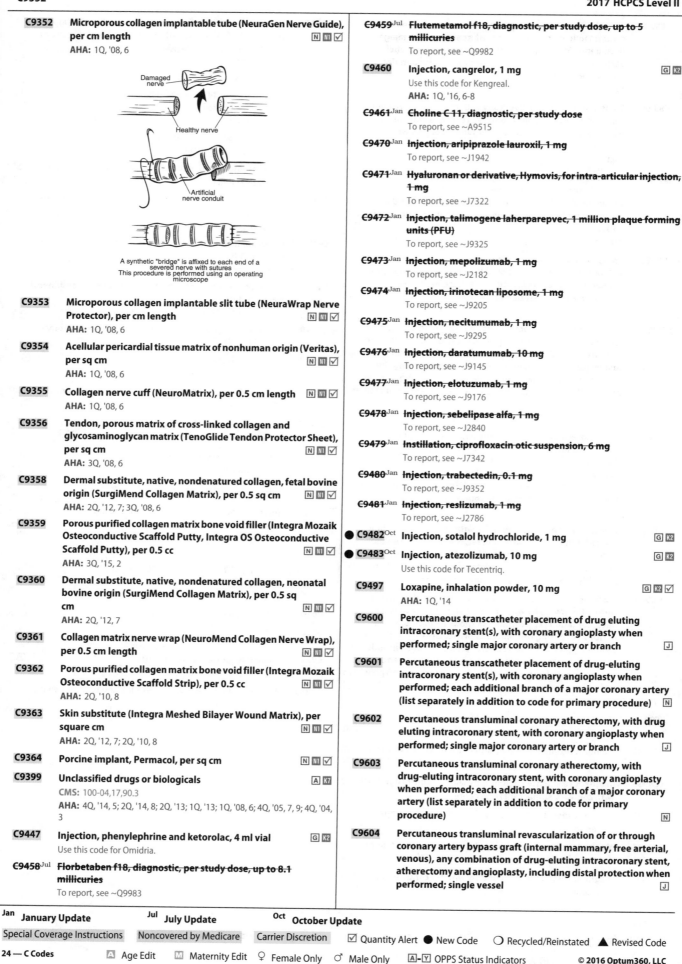

Damaged nerve

Healthy nerve

Artificial nerve conduit

A synthetic "bridge" is affixed to each end of a severed nerve with sutures
This procedure is performed using an operating microscope

**C9353** Microporous collagen implantable slit tube (NeuraWrap Nerve Protector), per cm length [N] [N1] ☑
AHA: 1Q, '08, 6

**C9354** Acellular pericardial tissue matrix of nonhuman origin (Veritas), per sq cm [N] [N1] ☑
AHA: 1Q, '08, 6

**C9355** Collagen nerve cuff (NeuroMatrix), per 0.5 cm length [N] [N1] ☑
AHA: 1Q, '08, 6

**C9356** Tendon, porous matrix of cross-linked collagen and glycosaminoglycan matrix (TenoGlide Tendon Protector Sheet), per sq cm [N] [N1] ☑
AHA: 3Q, '08, 6

**C9358** Dermal substitute, native, nondenatured collagen, fetal bovine origin (SurgiMend Collagen Matrix), per 0.5 sq cm [N] [N1] ☑
AHA: 2Q, '12, 7; 3Q, '08, 6

**C9359** Porous purified collagen matrix bone void filler (Integra Mozaik Osteoconductive Scaffold Putty, Integra OS Osteoconductive Scaffold Putty), per 0.5 cc [N] [N1] ☑
AHA: 3Q, '15, 2

**C9360** Dermal substitute, native, nondenatured collagen, neonatal bovine origin (SurgiMend Collagen Matrix), per 0.5 sq cm [N] [N1] ☑
AHA: 2Q, '12, 7

**C9361** Collagen matrix nerve wrap (NeuroMend Collagen Nerve Wrap), per 0.5 cm length [N] [N1] ☑

**C9362** Porous purified collagen matrix bone void filler (Integra Mozaik Osteoconductive Scaffold Strip), per 0.5 cc [N] [N1] ☑
AHA: 2Q, '10, 8

**C9363** Skin substitute (Integra Meshed Bilayer Wound Matrix), per square cm [N] [N1] ☑
AHA: 2Q, '12, 7; 2Q, '10, 8

**C9364** Porcine implant, Permacol, per sq cm [N] [N1] ☑

**C9399** Unclassified drugs or biologicals [A] [K7]
CMS: 100-04,17,90.3
AHA: 4Q, '14, 5; 2Q, '14, 8; 2Q, '13; 1Q, '13; 1Q, '08, 6; 4Q, '05, 7, 9; 4Q, '04, 3

**C9447** Injection, phenylephrine and ketorolac, 4 ml vial [G] [K2]
Use this code for Omidria.

~~**C9458**[Jul] Florbetaben f18, diagnostic, per study dose, up to 8.1 millicuries~~
To report, see ~Q9983

~~**C9459**[Jul] Flutemetamol f18, diagnostic, per study dose, up to 5 millicuries~~
To report, see ~Q9982

**C9460** Injection, cangrelor, 1 mg [G] [K2]
Use this code for Kengreal.
AHA: 1Q, '16, 6-8

~~**C9461**[Jan] Choline C 11, diagnostic, per study dose~~
To report, see ~A9515

~~**C9470**[Jan] Injection, aripiprazole lauroxil, 1 mg~~
To report, see ~J1942

~~**C9471**[Jan] Hyaluronan or derivative, Hymovis, for intra-articular injection, 1 mg~~
To report, see ~J7322

~~**C9472**[Jan] Injection, talimogene laherparepvec, 1 million plaque forming units (PFU)~~
To report, see ~J9325

~~**C9473**[Jan] Injection, mepolizumab, 1 mg~~
To report, see ~J2182

~~**C9474**[Jan] Injection, irinotecan liposome, 1 mg~~
To report, see ~J9205

~~**C9475**[Jan] Injection, necitumumab, 1 mg~~
To report, see ~J9295

~~**C9476**[Jan] Injection, daratumumab, 10 mg~~
To report, see ~J9145

~~**C9477**[Jan] Injection, elotuzumab, 1 mg~~
To report, see ~J9176

~~**C9478**[Jan] Injection, sebelipase alfa, 1 mg~~
To report, see ~J2840

~~**C9479**[Jan] Instillation, ciprofloxacin otic suspension, 6 mg~~
To report, see ~J7342

~~**C9480**[Jan] Injection, trabectedin, 0.1 mg~~
To report, see ~J9352

~~**C9481**[Jan] Injection, reslizumab, 1 mg~~
To report, see ~J2786

● **C9482**[Oct] Injection, sotalol hydrochloride, 1 mg [G] [K2]

● **C9483**[Oct] Injection, atezolizumab, 10 mg [G] [K2]
Use this code for Tecentriq.

**C9497** Loxapine, inhalation powder, 10 mg [G] [K2] ☑
AHA: 1Q, '14

**C9600** Percutaneous transcatheter placement of drug eluting intracoronary stent(s), with coronary angioplasty when performed; single major coronary artery or branch [J]

**C9601** Percutaneous transcatheter placement of drug-eluting intracoronary stent(s), with coronary angioplasty when performed; each additional branch of a major coronary artery (list separately in addition to code for primary procedure) [N]

**C9602** Percutaneous transluminal coronary atherectomy, with drug eluting intracoronary stent, with coronary angioplasty when performed; single major coronary artery or branch [J]

**C9603** Percutaneous transluminal coronary atherectomy, with drug-eluting intracoronary stent, with coronary angioplasty when performed; each additional branch of a major coronary artery (list separately in addition to code for primary procedure) [N]

**C9604** Percutaneous transluminal revascularization of or through coronary artery bypass graft (internal mammary, free arterial, venous), any combination of drug-eluting intracoronary stent, atherectomy and angioplasty, including distal protection when performed; single vessel [J]

---

[Jan] **January Update**   [Jul] **July Update**   [Oct] **October Update**

Special Coverage Instructions   Noncovered by Medicare   Carrier Discretion   ☑ Quantity Alert   ● New Code   ○ Recycled/Reinstated   ▲ Revised Code

24 — C Codes   [A] Age Edit   [M] Maternity Edit   ♀ Female Only   ♂ Male Only   [A]-[Y] OPPS Status Indicators   © 2016 Optum360, LLC

**C9605** Percutaneous transluminal revascularization of or through coronary artery bypass graft (internal mammary, free arterial, venous), any combination of drug-eluting intracoronary stent, atherectomy and angioplasty, including distal protection when performed; each additional branch subtended by the bypass graft (list separately in addition to code for primary procedure) N

**C9606** Percutaneous transluminal revascularization of acute total/subtotal occlusion during acute myocardial infarction, coronary artery or coronary artery bypass graft, any combination of drug-eluting intracoronary stent, atherectomy and angioplasty, including aspiration thrombectomy when performed, single vessel J

**C9607** Percutaneous transluminal revascularization of chronic total occlusion, coronary artery, coronary artery branch, or coronary artery bypass graft, any combination of drug-eluting intracoronary stent, atherectomy and angioplasty; single vessel J

**C9608** Percutaneous transluminal revascularization of chronic total occlusion, coronary artery, coronary artery branch, or coronary artery bypass graft, any combination of drug-eluting intracoronary stent, atherectomy and angioplasty; each additional coronary artery, coronary artery branch, or bypass graft (list separately in addition to code for primary procedure) N

**C9725** Placement of endorectal intracavitary applicator for high intensity brachytherapy T G2 ⊘
AHA: 3Q, '05, 7

**C9726** Placement and removal (if performed) of applicator into breast for intraoperative radiation therapy, add-on to primary breast procedure N N1
AHA: 2Q, '07, 10

**C9727** Insertion of implants into the soft palate; minimum of 3 implants T G2 ☑

**C9728** Placement of interstitial device(s) for radiation therapy/surgery guidance (e.g., fiducial markers, dosimeter), for other than the following sites (any approach): abdomen, pelvis, prostate, retroperitoneum, thorax, single or multiple S R2

**C9733** Nonophthalmic fluorescent vascular angiography Q2 N1

**C9734** Focused ultrasound ablation/therapeutic intervention, other than uterine leiomyomata, with magnetic resonance (MR) guidance T
AHA: 3Q, '13; 2Q, '13

**C9739** Cystourethroscopy, with insertion of transprostatic implant; 1 to 3 implants ♂ J G2
AHA: 2Q, '14, 8

**C9740** Cystourethroscopy, with insertion of transprostatic implant; 4 or more implants ♂ T J8
AHA: 2Q, '14, 8

**C9741** Right heart catheterization with implantation of wireless pressure sensor in the pulmonary artery, including any type of measurement, angiography, imaging supervision, interpretation, and report T
AHA: 3Q, '15, 1-2

**C9742**^Jan ~~Laryngoscopy, flexible fiberoptic, with injection into vocal cord(s), therapeutic, including diagnostic laryngoscopy, if performed~~
To report, see ~31573-31574

**C9743**^Jul ~~Injection/implantation of bulking or spacer material (any type) with or without image guidance (not to be used if a more specific code applies)~~
To report, see ~0438T

● **C9744**^Oct Ultrasound, abdominal, with contrast S Z3

**C9800**^Jan ~~Dermal injection procedure(s) for facial lipodystrophy syndrome (LDS) and provision of Radiesse or Sculptra dermal filler, including all items and supplies~~
To report, see ~G0429

**C9898** Radiolabeled product provided during a hospital inpatient stay N

**C9899** Implanted prosthetic device, payable only for inpatients who do not have inpatient coverage A

^Jan **January Update**    ^Jul **July Update**    ^Oct **October Update**

Special Coverage Instructions    Noncovered by Medicare    Carrier Discretion    ☑ Quantity Alert  ● New Code    ○ Recycled/Reinstated    ▲ Revised Code

© 2016 Optum360, LLC    A2-Z3 ASC Pmt    **CMS:** Pub 100    **AHA:** Coding Clinic    ⅋ DMEPOS Paid    ⊘ SNF Excluded    C Codes — 25

## Durable Medical Equipment E0100-E8002

E codes include durable medical equipment such as canes, crutches, walkers, commodes, decubitus care, bath and toilet aids, hospital beds, oxygen and related respiratory equipment, monitoring equipment, pacemakers, patient lifts, safety equipment, restraints, traction equipment, fracture frames, wheelchairs, and artificial kidney machines.

### Canes

**E0100** Cane, includes canes of all materials, adjustable or fixed, with tip   Y &#9855; (NU,RR,UE)

White canes for the blind are not covered under Medicare.

**E0105** Cane, quad or 3-prong, includes canes of all materials, adjustable or fixed, with tips   Y &#9855; (NU,RR,UE)

### Crutches

**E0110** Crutches, forearm, includes crutches of various materials, adjustable or fixed, pair, complete with tips and handgrips   Y ☑ &#9855; (NU,RR,UE)

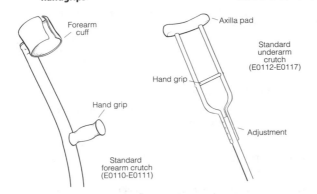

Forearm cuff

Hand grip

Standard forearm crutch (E0110-E0111)

Axilla pad

Standard underarm crutch (E0112-E0117)

Hand grip

Adjustment

**E0111** Crutch, forearm, includes crutches of various materials, adjustable or fixed, each, with tip and handgrips   Y ☑ &#9855; (NU,RR,UE)

**E0112** Crutches, underarm, wood, adjustable or fixed, pair, with pads, tips, and handgrips   Y ☑ &#9855; (NU,RR,UE)

**E0113** Crutch, underarm, wood, adjustable or fixed, each, with pad, tip, and handgrip   Y ☑ &#9855; (NU,RR,UE)

**E0114** Crutches, underarm, other than wood, adjustable or fixed, pair, with pads, tips, and handgrips   Y ☑ &#9855; (NU,RR,UE)

AHA: 2Q, '02, 1-3

**E0116** Crutch, underarm, other than wood, adjustable or fixed, with pad, tip, handgrip, with or without shock absorber, each   Y ☑ &#9855; (NU,RR,UE)

**E0117** Crutch, underarm, articulating, spring assisted, each   Y ☑ &#9855; (RR)

**E0118** Crutch substitute, lower leg platform, with or without wheels, each   E ☑

Medicare covers walkers if patient's ambulation is impaired.

### Walkers

**E0130** Walker, rigid (pickup), adjustable or fixed height   Y &#9855; (NU,RR,UE)

CMS: 100-04,23,60.3; 100-04,36,50.15

**E0135** Walker, folding (pickup), adjustable or fixed height   Y &#9855; (NU,RR,UE)

Medicare covers walkers if patient's ambulation is impaired.

CMS: 100-04,23,60.3; 100-04,36,50.15

**E0140** Walker, with trunk support, adjustable or fixed height, any type   Y &#9855; (RR)

CMS: 100-04,23,60.3; 100-04,36,50.15

**E0141** Walker, rigid, wheeled, adjustable or fixed height   Y &#9855; (NU,RR,UE)

Medicare covers walkers if patient's ambulation is impaired.

CMS: 100-04,23,60.3; 100-04,36,50.15

**E0143** Walker, folding, wheeled, adjustable or fixed height   Y &#9855; (NU,RR,UE)

Medicare covers walkers if patient's ambulation is impaired.

CMS: 100-04,23,60.3; 100-04,36,50.15

**E0144** Walker, enclosed, 4 sided framed, rigid or folding, wheeled with posterior seat   Y &#9855; (RR)

CMS: 100-04,23,60.3; 100-04,36,50.15

**E0147** Walker, heavy-duty, multiple braking system, variable wheel resistance   Y &#9855; (NU,RR,UE)

Medicare covers safety roller walkers only in patients with severe neurological disorders or restricted use of one hand. In some cases, coverage will be extended to patients with a weight exceeding the limits of a standard wheeled walker.

CMS: 100-04,23,60.3; 100-04,36,50.15

**E0148** Walker, heavy-duty, without wheels, rigid or folding, any type, each   Y ☑ &#9855; (NU,RR,UE)

CMS: 100-04,23,60.3; 100-04,36,50.15

**E0149** Walker, heavy-duty, wheeled, rigid or folding, any type   Y &#9855; (RR)

CMS: 100-04,23,60.3; 100-04,36,50.15

### Attachments

**E0153** Platform attachment, forearm crutch, each   Y ☑ &#9855; (NU,RR,UE)

**E0154** Platform attachment, walker, each   Y ☑ &#9855; (NU,RR,UE)

CMS: 100-04,23,60.3; 100-04,36,50.14; 100-04,36,50.15

**E0155** Wheel attachment, rigid pick-up walker, per pair   Y ☑ &#9855; (NU,RR,UE)

CMS: 100-04,23,60.3; 100-04,36,50.15

**E0156** Seat attachment, walker   Y &#9855; (NU,RR,UE)

CMS: 100-04,23,60.3; 100-04,36,50.14; 100-04,36,50.15

**E0157** Crutch attachment, walker, each   Y ☑ &#9855; (NU,RR,UE)

CMS: 100-04,23,60.3; 100-04,36,50.14; 100-04,36,50.15

**E0158** Leg extensions for walker, per set of 4   Y ☑ &#9855; (NU,RR,UE)

CMS: 100-04,23,60.3; 100-04,36,50.14; 100-04,36,50.15

**E0159** Brake attachment for wheeled walker, replacement, each   Y ☑ &#9855; (NU,RR,UE)

CMS: 100-04,23,60.3; 100-04,36,50.15

### Commodes

**E0160** Sitz type bath or equipment, portable, used with or without commode   Y &#9855; (NU,RR,UE)

Medicare covers sitz baths if medical record indicates that the patient has an infection or injury of the perineal area and the sitz bath is prescribed by the physician.

**E0161** Sitz type bath or equipment, portable, used with or without commode, with faucet attachment(s)   Y &#9855; (NU,RR,UE)

Medicare covers sitz baths if medical record indicates that the patient has an infection or injury of the perineal area and the sitz bath is prescribed by the physician.

**E0162** Sitz bath chair   Y &#9855; (NU,RR,UE)

Medicare covers sitz baths if medical record indicates that the patient has an infection or injury of the perineal area and the sitz bath is prescribed by the physician.

**E0163** Commode chair, mobile or stationary, with fixed arms   Y &#9855; (NU,RR,UE)

Medicare covers commodes for patients confined to their beds or rooms, for patients without indoor bathroom facilities, and to patients who cannot climb or descend the stairs necessary to reach the bathrooms in their homes.

---

Special Coverage Instructions    Noncovered by Medicare    Carrier Discretion    ☑ Quantity Alert   ● New Code   ○ Recycled/Reinstated   ▲ Revised Code

© 2016 Optum360, LLC    A2 - Z3 ASC Pmt    CMS: Pub 100    AHA: Coding Clinic    &#9855; DMEPOS Paid    ⊘ SNF Excluded

E Codes — 27

**Durable Medical Equipment**

**E0165 — E0246**

**E0165** Commode chair, mobile or stationary, with detachable arms ☒ ☒ (RR)
Medicare covers commodes for patients confined to their beds or rooms, for patients without indoor bathroom facilities, and to patients who cannot climb or descend the stairs necessary to reach the bathrooms in their homes.

**E0167** Pail or pan for use with commode chair, replacement only ☒ ☒ (NU,RR,UE)
Medicare covers commodes for patients confined to their beds or rooms, for patients without indoor bathroom facilities, and to patients who cannot climb or descend the stairs necessary to reach the bathrooms in their homes.

**E0168** Commode chair, extra wide and/or heavy-duty, stationary or mobile, with or without arms, any type, each ☒ ☑ ☒ (NU,RR,UE)

**E0170** Commode chair with integrated seat lift mechanism, electric, any type ☒ ☒ (RR)

**E0171** Commode chair with integrated seat lift mechanism, nonelectric, any type ☒ ☒ (RR)

**E0172** Seat lift mechanism placed over or on top of toilet, any type ☒

**E0175** Footrest, for use with commode chair, each ☒ ☑ ☒ (NU,RR,UE)

## Decubitus Care Equipment

**E0181** Powered pressure reducing mattress overlay/pad, alternating, with pump, includes heavy-duty ☒ ☒ (RR)
For Medicare coverage, a detailed written order must be received by the supplier before a claim is submitted.

**E0182** Pump for alternating pressure pad, for replacement only ☒ ☒ (RR)
For Medicare coverage, a detailed written order must be received by the supplier before a claim is submitted.

**E0184** Dry pressure mattress ☒ ☒ (NU,RR,UE)
For Medicare coverage, a detailed written order must be received by the supplier before a claim is submitted.

**E0185** Gel or gel-like pressure pad for mattress, standard mattress length and width ☒ ☒ (NU,RR,UE)
For Medicare coverage, a detailed written order must be received by the supplier before a claim is submitted.

**E0186** Air pressure mattress ☒ ☒ (RR)
For Medicare coverage, a detailed written order must be received by the supplier before a claim is submitted.

**E0187** Water pressure mattress ☒ ☒ (RR)
For Medicare coverage, a detailed written order must be received by the supplier before a claim is submitted.

**E0188** Synthetic sheepskin pad ☒ ☒ (NU,RR,UE)
For Medicare coverage, a detailed written order must be received by the supplier before a claim is submitted.

**E0189** Lambswool sheepskin pad, any size ☒ ☒ (NU,RR,UE)
For Medicare coverage, a detailed written order must be received by the supplier before a claim is submitted.

**E0190** Positioning cushion/pillow/wedge, any shape or size, includes all components and accessories ☒

**E0191** Heel or elbow protector, each ☒ ☑ ☒ (NU,RR,UE)

**E0193** Powered air flotation bed (low air loss therapy) ☒ ☒ (RR)
CMS: 100-04,23,60.3

**E0194** Air fluidized bed ☒ ☒ (RR)
An air fluidized bed is covered by Medicare if the patient has a stage 3 or stage 4 pressure sore and, without the bed, would require institutionalization. For Medicare coverage, a detailed written order must be received by the supplier before a claim is submitted.

**E0196** Gel pressure mattress ☒ ☒ (RR)
Medicare covers pads if physicians supervise their use in patients who have decubitus ulcers or susceptibility to them. For Medicare coverage, a detailed written order must be received by the supplier before a claim is submitted.

**E0197** Air pressure pad for mattress, standard mattress length and width ☒ ☒ (RR)
Medicare covers pads if physicians supervise their use in patients who have decubitus ulcers or susceptibility to them. For Medicare coverage, a detailed written order must be received by the supplier before a claim is submitted.

**E0198** Water pressure pad for mattress, standard mattress length and width ☒ ☒ (RR)
Medicare covers pads if physicians supervise their use in patients who have decubitus ulcers or susceptibility to them.For Medicare coverage, a detailed written order must be received by the supplier before a claim is submitted.

**E0199** Dry pressure pad for mattress, standard mattress length and width ☒ ☒ (NU,RR,UE)
Medicare covers pads if physicians supervise their use in patients who have decubitus ulcers or susceptibility to them. For Medicare coverage, a detailed written order must be received by the supplier before a claim is submitted.

## Heat/Cold Application

**E0200** Heat lamp, without stand (table model), includes bulb, or infrared element ☒ ☒ (NU,RR,UE)

**E0202** Phototherapy (bilirubin) light with photometer ☒ ☒ (RR)

**E0203** Therapeutic lightbox, minimum 10,000 lux, table top model ☒

**E0205** Heat lamp, with stand, includes bulb, or infrared element ☒ ☒ (NU,RR,UE)

**E0210** Electric heat pad, standard ☒ ☒ (NU,RR,UE)

**E0215** Electric heat pad, moist ☒ ☒ (NU,RR,UE)

**E0217** Water circulating heat pad with pump ☒ ☒ (NU,RR,UE)

**E0218** Water circulating cold pad with pump ☒

**E0221** Infrared heating pad system ☒
AHA: 1Q, '02, 5

**E0225** Hydrocollator unit, includes pads ☒ ☒ (NU,RR,UE)

**E0231** Noncontact wound-warming device (temperature control unit, AC adapter and power cord) for use with warming card and wound cover ☒
AHA: 1Q, '02, 5

**E0232** Warming card for use with the noncontact wound-warming device and noncontact wound-warming wound cover ☒
AHA: 1Q, '02, 5

**E0235** Paraffin bath unit, portable (see medical supply code A4265 for paraffin) ☒ ☒ (RR)

**E0236** Pump for water circulating pad ☒ ☒ (RR)

**E0239** Hydrocollator unit, portable ☒ ☒ (NU,RR,UE)

## Bath and Toilet Aids

**E0240** Bath/shower chair, with or without wheels, any size ☒

**E0241** Bathtub wall rail, each ☒ ☑

**E0242** Bathtub rail, floor base ☒

**E0243** Toilet rail, each ☒ ☑

**E0244** Raised toilet seat ☒

**E0245** Tub stool or bench ☒

**E0246** Transfer tub rail attachment ☒

---

Special Coverage Instructions    Noncovered by Medicare    Carrier Discretion    ☑ Quantity Alert    ● New Code    ○ Recycled/Reinstated    ▲ Revised Code

28 — E Codes    🅰 Age Edit    🅼 Maternity Edit    ♀ Female Only    ♂ Male Only    🅰-🆈 OPPS Status Indicators    © 2016 Optum360, LLC

| | | |
|---|---|---|
| **E0247** | Transfer bench for tub or toilet with or without commode opening | E |
| **E0248** | Transfer bench, heavy-duty, for tub or toilet with or without commode opening | E |
| **E0249** | Pad for water circulating heat unit, for replacement only | Y & (NU,RR,UE) |

## Hospital Beds and Accessories

**E0250** Hospital bed, fixed height, with any type side rails, with mattress     Y & (RR)
CMS: 100-04,23,60.3

**E0251** Hospital bed, fixed height, with any type side rails, without mattress     Y & (RR)
CMS: 100-04,23,60.3

**E0255** Hospital bed, variable height, hi-lo, with any type side rails, with mattress     Y & (RR)
CMS: 100-04,23,60.3

**E0256** Hospital bed, variable height, hi-lo, with any type side rails, without mattress     Y & (RR)
CMS: 100-04,23,60.3

**E0260** Hospital bed, semi-electric (head and foot adjustment), with any type side rails, with mattress     Y & (RR)
CMS: 100-04,23,60.3

**E0261** Hospital bed, semi-electric (head and foot adjustment), with any type side rails, without mattress     Y & (RR)
CMS: 100-04,23,60.3

**E0265** Hospital bed, total electric (head, foot, and height adjustments), with any type side rails, with mattress     Y & (RR)
CMS: 100-04,23,60.3

**E0266** Hospital bed, total electric (head, foot, and height adjustments), with any type side rails, without mattress     Y & (RR)
CMS: 100-04,23,60.3

**E0270** Hospital bed, institutional type includes: oscillating, circulating and Stryker frame, with mattress     E

**E0271** Mattress, innerspring     Y & (NU,RR,UE)
CMS: 100-04,23,60.3; 100-04,36,50.14

**E0272** Mattress, foam rubber     Y & (NU,RR,UE)
CMS: 100-04,23,60.3; 100-04,36,50.14

**E0273** Bed board     E

**E0274** Over-bed table     E

**E0275** Bed pan, standard, metal or plastic     Y & (NU,RR,UE)
Reusable, autoclavable bedpans are covered by Medicare for bed-confined patients.

**E0276** Bed pan, fracture, metal or plastic     Y & (NU,RR,UE)
Reusable, autoclavable bedpans are covered by Medicare for bed-confined patients.

**E0277** Powered pressure-reducing air mattress     Y & (RR)
CMS: 100-04,23,60.3

**E0280** Bed cradle, any type     Y & (NU,RR,UE)
CMS: 100-04,23,60.3; 100-04,36,50.14

**E0290** Hospital bed, fixed height, without side rails, with mattress     Y & (RR)
CMS: 100-04,23,60.3

**E0291** Hospital bed, fixed height, without side rails, without mattress     Y & (RR)
CMS: 100-04,23,60.3

**E0292** Hospital bed, variable height, hi-lo, without side rails, with mattress     Y & (RR)
CMS: 100-04,23,60.3

**E0293** Hospital bed, variable height, hi-lo, without side rails, without mattress     Y & (RR)
CMS: 100-04,23,60.3

**E0294** Hospital bed, semi-electric (head and foot adjustment), without side rails, with mattress     Y & (RR)
CMS: 100-04,23,60.3

**E0295** Hospital bed, semi-electric (head and foot adjustment), without side rails, without mattress     Y & (RR)
CMS: 100-04,23,60.3

**E0296** Hospital bed, total electric (head, foot, and height adjustments), without side rails, with mattress     Y & (RR)
CMS: 100-04,23,60.3

**E0297** Hospital bed, total electric (head, foot, and height adjustments), without side rails, without mattress     Y & (RR)
CMS: 100-04,23,60.3

**E0300** Pediatric crib, hospital grade, fully enclosed, with or without top enclosure     Y & (RR)
CMS: 100-04,23,60.3

**E0301** Hospital bed, heavy-duty, extra wide, with weight capacity greater than 350 pounds, but less than or equal to 600 pounds, with any type side rails, without mattress     Y & (RR)
CMS: 100-04,23,60.3

**E0302** Hospital bed, extra heavy-duty, extra wide, with weight capacity greater than 600 pounds, with any type side rails, without mattress     Y & (RR)
CMS: 100-04,23,60.3

**E0303** Hospital bed, heavy-duty, extra wide, with weight capacity greater than 350 pounds, but less than or equal to 600 pounds, with any type side rails, with mattress     Y & (RR)
CMS: 100-04,23,60.3

**E0304** Hospital bed, extra heavy-duty, extra wide, with weight capacity greater than 600 pounds, with any type side rails, with mattress     Y & (RR)
CMS: 100-04,23,60.3

**E0305** Bedside rails, half-length     Y & (RR)
CMS: 100-04,23,60.3

**E0310** Bedside rails, full-length     Y & (NU,RR,UE)
CMS: 100-04,23,60.3; 100-04,36,50.14

**E0315** Bed accessory: board, table, or support device, any type     E

**E0316** Safety enclosure frame/canopy for use with hospital bed, any type     Y & (RR)
CMS: 100-04,23,60.3
AHA: 1Q, '02, 5

**E0325** Urinal; male, jug-type, any material     ♂ Y & (NU,RR,UE)

**E0326** Urinal; female, jug-type, any material     A ♀ Y & (NU,RR,UE)

**E0328** Hospital bed, pediatric, manual, 360 degree side enclosures, top of headboard, footboard and side rails up to 24 in above the spring, includes mattress     Y

**E0329** Hospital bed, pediatric, electric or semi-electric, 360 degree side enclosures, top of headboard, footboard and side rails up to 24 in above the spring, includes mattress     Y

**E0350** Control unit for electronic bowel irrigation/evacuation system     E

**E0352** Disposable pack (water reservoir bag, speculum, valving mechanism, and collection bag/box) for use with the electronic bowel irrigation/evacuation system     E

**E0370** Air pressure elevator for heel     E

---

Special Coverage Instructions    Noncovered by Medicare    Carrier Discretion    ☑ Quantity Alert   ● New Code   ○ Recycled/Reinstated   ▲ Revised Code

© 2016 Optum360, LLC    A2-Z3 ASC Pmt    **CMS:** Pub 100    **AHA:** Coding Clinic   & DMEPOS Paid   ⊘ SNF Excluded     **E Codes — 29**

**Durable Medical Equipment**

**E0371 — E0550**

| | | |
|---|---|---|
| **E0371** | Nonpowered advanced pressure reducing overlay for mattress, standard mattress length and width | Y ⅋ (RR) |
| | CMS: 100-04,23,60.3 | |
| **E0372** | Powered air overlay for mattress, standard mattress length and width | Y ⅋ (RR) |
| | CMS: 100-04,23,60.3 | |
| **E0373** | Nonpowered advanced pressure reducing mattress | Y ⅋ (RR) |
| | CMS: 100-04,23,60.3 | |

## Oxygen and Related Respiratory Equipment

**E0424** Stationary compressed gaseous oxygen system, rental; includes container, contents, regulator, flowmeter, humidifier, nebulizer, cannula or mask, and tubing    Y ⅋ (RR)

For the first claim filed for home oxygen equipment or therapy, submit a certificate of medical necessity that includes the oxygen flow rate, anticipated frequency and duration of oxygen therapy, and physician signature. Medicare accepts oxygen therapy as medically necessary in cases documenting any of the following: erythocythemia with a hematocrit greater than 56 percent; a P pulmonale on EKG; or dependent edema consistent with congestive heart failure.

CMS: 100-04,20,30.6

**E0425** Stationary compressed gas system, purchase; includes regulator, flowmeter, humidifier, nebulizer, cannula or mask, and tubing    E

**E0430** Portable gaseous oxygen system, purchase; includes regulator, flowmeter, humidifier, cannula or mask, and tubing    E

**E0431** Portable gaseous oxygen system, rental; includes portable container, regulator, flowmeter, humidifier, cannula or mask, and tubing    Y ⅋ (RR)

**E0433** Portable liquid oxygen system, rental; home liquefier used to fill portable liquid oxygen containers, includes portable containers, regulator, flowmeter, humidifier, cannula or mask and tubing, with or without supply reservoir and contents gauge    Y ⅋ (RR)

**E0434** Portable liquid oxygen system, rental; includes portable container, supply reservoir, humidifier, flowmeter, refill adaptor, contents gauge, cannula or mask, and tubing    Y ⅋ (RR)

**E0435** Portable liquid oxygen system, purchase; includes portable container, supply reservoir, flowmeter, humidifier, contents gauge, cannula or mask, tubing and refill adaptor    E

**E0439** Stationary liquid oxygen system, rental; includes container, contents, regulator, flowmeter, humidifier, nebulizer, cannula or mask, & tubing    Y ⅋ (RR)

**E0440** Stationary liquid oxygen system, purchase; includes use of reservoir, contents indicator, regulator, flowmeter, humidifier, nebulizer, cannula or mask, and tubing    E

**E0441** Stationary oxygen contents, gaseous, 1 month's supply = 1 unit    Y ☑ ⅋
CMS: 100-04,20,30.6

**E0442** Stationary oxygen contents, liquid, 1 month's supply = 1 unit    Y ☑ ⅋

**E0443** Portable oxygen contents, gaseous, 1 month's supply = 1 unit    Y ☑ ⅋
CMS: 100-04,20,30.6

**E0444** Portable oxygen contents, liquid, 1 month's supply = 1 unit    Y ☑ ⅋

**E0445** Oximeter device for measuring blood oxygen levels noninvasively    N

**E0446** Topical oxygen delivery system, not otherwise specified, includes all supplies and accessories    E

**E0455** Oxygen tent, excluding croup or pediatric tents    Y

| | | |
|---|---|---|
| **E0457** | Chest shell (cuirass) | E |
| **E0459** | Chest wrap | E |
| **E0462** | Rocking bed, with or without side rails | Y ⅋ (RR) |
| **E0465** | Home ventilator, any type, used with invasive interface, (e.g., tracheostomy tube) | Y ⅋ (RR) |
| **E0466** | Home ventilator, any type, used with noninvasive interface, (e.g., mask, chest shell) | Y ⅋ (RR) |

**E0470** Respiratory assist device, bi-level pressure capability, without backup rate feature, used with noninvasive interface, e.g., nasal or facial mask (intermittent assist device with continuous positive airway pressure device)    Y ⅋ (RR)
CMS: 100-03,240.4; 100-04,23,60.3

**E0471** Respiratory assist device, bi-level pressure capability, with back-up rate feature, used with noninvasive interface, e.g., nasal or facial mask (intermittent assist device with continuous positive airway pressure device)    Y ⅋ (RR)
CMS: 100-03,240.4; 100-04,23,60.3

**E0472** Respiratory assist device, bi-level pressure capability, with backup rate feature, used with invasive interface, e.g., tracheostomy tube (intermittent assist device with continuous positive airway pressure device)    Y ⅋ (RR)
CMS: 100-03,240.4; 100-04,23,60.3

**E0480** Percussor, electric or pneumatic, home model    Y ⅋ (RR)

**E0481** Intrapulmonary percussive ventilation system and related accessories    E
AHA: 1Q, '02, 5

**E0482** Cough stimulating device, alternating positive and negative airway pressure    Y ⅋ (RR)
AHA: 1Q, '02, 5

**E0483** High frequency chest wall oscillation air-pulse generator system, (includes hoses and vest), each    Y ☑ ⅋ (RR)

**E0484** Oscillatory positive expiratory pressure device, nonelectric, any type, each    Y ☑ ⅋ (NU,RR,UE)

**E0485** Oral device/appliance used to reduce upper airway collapsibility, adjustable or nonadjustable, prefabricated, includes fitting and adjustment    Y ⅋ (NU,RR,UE)

**E0486** Oral device/appliance used to reduce upper airway collapsibility, adjustable or nonadjustable, custom fabricated, includes fitting and adjustment    Y ⅋ (NU,RR,UE)

**E0487** Spirometer, electronic, includes all accessories    N

## IPPB Machines

**E0500** IPPB machine, all types, with built-in nebulization; manual or automatic valves; internal or external power source    Y ⅋ (RR)

IPPB unit in use
Battery pack and controls
Nebulizer
Nebulizer reservoir
Oxygen supply tube

Intermittent Positive Pressure Breathing (IPPB) devices

## Humidifiers/Compressors/Nebulizers

**E0550** Humidifier, durable for extensive supplemental humidification during IPPB treatments or oxygen delivery    Y ⅋ (RR)

---

Special Coverage Instructions    Noncovered by Medicare    Carrier Discretion    ☑ Quantity Alert    ● New Code    ○ Recycled/Reinstated    ▲ Revised Code

30 — E Codes    A Age Edit    M Maternity Edit    ♀ Female Only    ♂ Male Only    A-Y OPPS Status Indicators    © 2016 Optum360, LLC

Durable Medical Equipment

E0555 — E0669

**E0555** Humidifier, durable, glass or autoclavable plastic bottle type, for use with regulator or flowmeter  Y

**E0560** Humidifier, durable for supplemental humidification during IPPB treatment or oxygen delivery  Y & (NU,RR,UE)
CMS: 100-04,23,60.3

**E0561** Humidifier, nonheated, used with positive airway pressure device  Y & (NU,RR,UE)
CMS: 100-03,240.4; 100-04,23,60.3; 100-04,36,50.14

**E0562** Humidifier, heated, used with positive airway pressure device  Y & (NU,RR,UE)
CMS: 100-03,240.4; 100-04,23,60.3; 100-04,36,50.14

**E0565** Compressor, air power source for equipment which is not self-contained or cylinder driven  Y & (RR)

**E0570** Nebulizer, with compressor  Y & (RR)

**E0572** Aerosol compressor, adjustable pressure, light duty for intermittent use  Y & (RR)

**E0574** Ultrasonic/electronic aerosol generator with small volume nebulizer  Y & (RR)

**E0575** Nebulizer, ultrasonic, large volume  Y & (RR)

**E0580** Nebulizer, durable, glass or autoclavable plastic, bottle type, for use with regulator or flowmeter  Y & (NU,RR,UE)
CMS: 100-04,23,60.3

**E0585** Nebulizer, with compressor and heater  Y & (RR)

## Pumps and Vaporizers

**E0600** Respiratory suction pump, home model, portable or stationary, electric  Y & (RR)

**E0601** Continuous positive airway pressure (CPAP) device  Y & (RR)
CMS: 100-03,240.4; 100-04,23,60.3

**E0602** Breast pump, manual, any type  M ♀ Y & (NU,RR,UE)

**E0603** Breast pump, electric (AC and/or DC), any type  M ♀ N
AHA: 1Q, '02, 5

**E0604** Breast pump, hospital grade, electric (AC and/or DC), any type  M ♀ A
AHA: 1Q, '02, 5

**E0605** Vaporizer, room type  Y & (NU,RR,UE)

**E0606** Postural drainage board  Y & (RR)

## Monitoring Devices

**E0607** Home blood glucose monitor  Y & (NU,RR,UE)
Medicare covers home blood testing devices for diabetic patients when the devices are prescribed by the patients' physicians. Many commercial payers provide this coverage to non-insulin dependent diabetics as well.

**E0610** Pacemaker monitor, self-contained, (checks battery depletion, includes audible and visible check systems)  Y & (NU,RR,UE)

**E0615** Pacemaker monitor, self-contained, checks battery depletion and other pacemaker components, includes digital/visible check systems  Y & (NU,RR,UE)

**E0616** Implantable cardiac event recorder with memory, activator, and programmer  N

**E0617** External defibrillator with integrated electrocardiogram analysis  Y & (RR)

**E0618** Apnea monitor, without recording feature  Y & (RR)

**E0619** Apnea monitor, with recording feature  Y & (RR)

**E0620** Skin piercing device for collection of capillary blood, laser, each  Y & (RR)
AHA: 1Q, '02, 5

## Patient Lifts

**E0621** Sling or seat, patient lift, canvas or nylon  Y & (NU,RR,UE)

**E0625** Patient lift, bathroom or toilet, not otherwise classified  E

▲ **E0627**Jan Seat lift mechanism, electric, any type  Y & (NU,RR,UE)
CMS: 100-04,20,100; 100-04,20,130.2; 100-04,20,130.3; 100-04,20,130.4; 100-04,20,130.5

**E0628**Jan ~~Separate seat lift mechanism for use with patient-owned furniture, electric~~
To report, see ~E0627

▲ **E0629**Jan Seat lift mechanism, non-electric, any type  Y & (NU,RR,UE)
CMS: 100-04,20,100; 100-04,20,130.2; 100-04,20,130.3; 100-04,20,130.4; 100-04,20,130.5

**E0630** Patient lift, hydraulic or mechanical, includes any seat, sling, strap(s), or pad(s)  Y & (RR)

**E0635** Patient lift, electric, with seat or sling  Y & (RR)

**E0636** Multipositional patient support system, with integrated lift, patient accessible controls  Y & (RR)

**E0637** Combination sit-to-stand frame/table system, any size including pediatric, with seat lift feature, with or without wheels  E

**E0638** Standing frame/table system, one position (e.g., upright, supine or prone stander), any size including pediatric, with or without wheels  E

**E0639** Patient lift, moveable from room to room with disassembly and reassembly, includes all components/accessories  E & (RR)

**E0640** Patient lift, fixed system, includes all components/accessories  E & (RR)

**E0641** Standing frame/table system, multi-position (e.g., 3-way stander), any size including pediatric, with or without wheels  E

**E0642** Standing frame/table system, mobile (dynamic stander), any size including pediatric  E

## Compression Devices

**E0650** Pneumatic compressor, nonsegmental home model  Y & (NU,RR,UE)

**E0651** Pneumatic compressor, segmental home model without calibrated gradient pressure  Y & (NU,RR,UE)

**E0652** Pneumatic compressor, segmental home model with calibrated gradient pressure  Y & (NU,RR,UE)

**E0655** Nonsegmental pneumatic appliance for use with pneumatic compressor, half arm  Y & (NU,RR,UE)

**E0656** Segmental pneumatic appliance for use with pneumatic compressor, trunk  Y & (RR)

**E0657** Segmental pneumatic appliance for use with pneumatic compressor, chest  Y & (RR)

**E0660** Nonsegmental pneumatic appliance for use with pneumatic compressor, full leg  Y & (NU,RR,UE)

**E0665** Nonsegmental pneumatic appliance for use with pneumatic compressor, full arm  Y & (NU,RR,UE)

**E0666** Nonsegmental pneumatic appliance for use with pneumatic compressor, half leg  Y & (NU,RR,UE)

**E0667** Segmental pneumatic appliance for use with pneumatic compressor, full leg  Y & (NU,RR,UE)

**E0668** Segmental pneumatic appliance for use with pneumatic compressor, full arm  Y & (NU,RR,UE)

**E0669** Segmental pneumatic appliance for use with pneumatic compressor, half leg  Y & (NU,RR,UE)

Jan **January Update**

Special Coverage Instructions    Noncovered by Medicare    Carrier Discretion    ☑ Quantity Alert  ● New Code  ○ Recycled/Reinstated  ▲ Revised Code

© 2016 Optum360, LLC    A2-Z3 ASC Pmt    CMS: Pub 100    AHA: Coding Clinic  & DMEPOS Paid  ⊘ SNF Excluded    E Codes — 31

**E0670** Segmental pneumatic appliance for use with pneumatic compressor, integrated, 2 full legs and trunk  Y & (NU,RR,UE)

**E0671** Segmental gradient pressure pneumatic appliance, full leg  Y & (NU,RR,UE)

**E0672** Segmental gradient pressure pneumatic appliance, full arm  Y & (NU,RR,UE)

**E0673** Segmental gradient pressure pneumatic appliance, half leg  Y & (NU,RR,UE)

**E0675** Pneumatic compression device, high pressure, rapid inflation/deflation cycle, for arterial insufficiency (unilateral or bilateral system)  Y & (RR)

**E0676** Intermittent limb compression device (includes all accessories), not otherwise specified  Y

## Ultraviolet Light

**E0691** Ultraviolet light therapy system, includes bulbs/lamps, timer and eye protection; treatment area 2 sq ft or less  Y & (NU,RR,UE)

**E0692** Ultraviolet light therapy system panel, includes bulbs/lamps, timer and eye protection, 4 ft panel  Y & (NU,RR,UE)

**E0693** Ultraviolet light therapy system panel, includes bulbs/lamps, timer and eye protection, 6 ft panel  Y & (NU,RR,UE)

**E0694** Ultraviolet multidirectional light therapy system in 6 ft cabinet, includes bulbs/lamps, timer, and eye protection  Y & (NU,RR,UE)

## Safety Equipment

**E0700** Safety equipment, device or accessory, any type  E

Fabric wrist restraint

Padded leather restraints may feature a locking device

Restraints (E0710)

Fabric gait belt for assistance in walking (E0700)

Body restraint

**E0705** Transfer device, any type, each  B ☑ & (NU,RR,UE)

**E0710** Restraints, any type (body, chest, wrist, or ankle)  E

## Nerve Stimulators and Devices

**E0720** Transcutaneous electrical nerve stimulation (TENS) device, 2 lead, localized stimulation  Y & (NU)
A Certificate of Medical Necessity is required for the purchase of a TENS. It is not required for rentals.
CMS: 100-03,10.2; 100-03,160.27; 100-03,160.7.1; 100-04,20,30.1.2

**E0730** Transcutaneous electrical nerve stimulation (TENS) device, 4 or more leads, for multiple nerve stimulation  Y & (NU)
A Certificate of Medical Necessity is required for the purchase of a TENS. It is not required for rentals.
CMS: 100-03,10.2; 100-03,160.27; 100-03,160.7.1; 100-04,20,30.1.2

**E0731** Form-fitting conductive garment for delivery of TENS or NMES (with conductive fibers separated from the patient's skin by layers of fabric)  Y & (NU)
CMS: 100-03,10.2; 100-03,160.13

▲ **E0740**<sup>Jan</sup> Non-implanted pelvic floor electrical stimulator, complete system  Y (RR)

**E0744** Neuromuscular stimulator for scoliosis  Y & (RR)

**E0745** Neuromuscular stimulator, electronic shock unit  Y & (RR)

**E0746** Electromyography (EMG), biofeedback device  N
Biofeedback therapy is covered by Medicare only for re-education of specific muscles or for treatment of incapacitating muscle spasm or weakness.

**E0747** Osteogenesis stimulator, electrical, noninvasive, other than spinal applications  Y (NU,RR,UE)
Medicare covers noninvasive osteogenic stimulation for nonunion of long bone fractures, failed fusion, or congenital pseudoarthroses.

**E0748** Osteogenesis stimulator, electrical, noninvasive, spinal applications  Y (NU,RR,UE)
Medicare covers noninvasive osteogenic stimulation as an adjunct to spinal fusion surgery for patients at high risk of pseudoarthroses due to previously failed spinal fusion, or for those undergoing fusion of three or more vertebrae.

**E0749** Osteogenesis stimulator, electrical, surgically implanted  N (RR)
Medicare covers invasive osteogenic stimulation for nonunion of long bone fractures or as an adjunct to spinal fusion surgery for patients at high risk of pseudoarthroses due to previously failed spinal fusion, or for those undergoing fusion of three or more vertebrae.
CMS: 100-04,4,190

**E0755** Electronic salivary reflex stimulator (intraoral/noninvasive)  E

**E0760** Osteogenesis stimulator, low intensity ultrasound, noninvasive  Y (NU,RR,UE)
CMS: 100-04,32,110.5

**E0761** Nonthermal pulsed high frequency radiowaves, high peak power electromagnetic energy treatment device  E

**E0762** Transcutaneous electrical joint stimulation device system, includes all accessories  B & (RR)

**E0764** Functional neuromuscular stimulation, transcutaneous stimulation of sequential muscle groups of ambulation with computer control, used for walking by spinal cord injured, entire system, after completion of training program  Y (RR)

**E0765** FDA approved nerve stimulator, with replaceable batteries, for treatment of nausea and vomiting  Y & (NU,RR,UE)

**E0766** Electrical stimulation device used for cancer treatment, includes all accessories, any type  Y

**E0769** Electrical stimulation or electromagnetic wound treatment device, not otherwise classified  B
CMS: 100-04,32,11.1

**E0770** Functional electrical stimulator, transcutaneous stimulation of nerve and/or muscle groups, any type, complete system, not otherwise specified  Y

## Infusion Supplies

**E0776** IV pole  Y & (NU,RR,UE)
CMS: 100-04,23,60.3

**E0779** Ambulatory infusion pump, mechanical, reusable, for infusion 8 hours or greater  Y & (RR)

**E0780** Ambulatory infusion pump, mechanical, reusable, for infusion less than 8 hours  Y & (NU)

**E0781** Ambulatory infusion pump, single or multiple channels, electric or battery operated, with administrative equipment, worn by patient  Y & (RR)

**E0782** Infusion pump, implantable, nonprogrammable (includes all components, e.g., pump, catheter, connectors, etc.)  N (NU,RR,UE)
CMS: 100-04,4,190

**Jan** January Update

Special Coverage Instructions    Noncovered by Medicare    Carrier Discretion    ☑ Quantity Alert  ● New Code    ○ Recycled/Reinstated  ▲ Revised Code

32 — E Codes    A Age Edit    M Maternity Edit    ♀ Female Only    ♂ Male Only    A-Y OPPS Status Indicators    © 2016 Optum360, LLC

| E0783 | Infusion pump system, implantable, programmable (includes all components, e.g., pump, catheter, connectors, etc.) | N (NU,RR,UE) |

CMS: 100-04,4,190

**E0784** External ambulatory infusion pump, insulin   Y & (RR)
Covered by some commercial payers with preauthorization.

**E0785** Implantable intraspinal (epidural/intrathecal) catheter used with implantable infusion pump, replacement   N & (KF)
CMS: 100-04,4,190

**E0786** Implantable programmable infusion pump, replacement (excludes implantable intraspinal catheter)   N (NU,RR,UE)

**E0791** Parenteral infusion pump, stationary, single, or multichannel   Y & (RR)

## Traction Equipment

**E0830** Ambulatory traction device, all types, each   N

**E0840** Traction frame, attached to headboard, cervical traction   Y & (NU,RR,UE)

**E0849** Traction equipment, cervical, free-standing stand/frame, pneumatic, applying traction force to other than mandible   Y & (RR)

**E0850** Traction stand, freestanding, cervical traction   Y & (NU,RR,UE)

**E0855** Cervical traction equipment not requiring additional stand or frame   Y & (RR)

**E0856** Cervical traction device, with inflatable air bladder(s)   Y & (RR)

**E0860** Traction equipment, overdoor, cervical   Y & (NU,RR,UE)

**E0870** Traction frame, attached to footboard, extremity traction (e.g., Buck's)   Y & (NU,RR,UE)

**E0880** Traction stand, freestanding, extremity traction (e.g., Buck's)   Y & (NU,RR,UE)

**E0890** Traction frame, attached to footboard, pelvic traction   Y & (NU,RR,UE)

**E0900** Traction stand, freestanding, pelvic traction (e.g., Buck's)   Y & (NU,RR,UE)

## Orthopedic Devices

**E0910** Trapeze bars, also known as Patient Helper, attached to bed, with grab bar   Y & (RR)
CMS: 100-04,23,60.3

**E0911** Trapeze bar, heavy-duty, for patient weight capacity greater than 250 pounds, attached to bed, with grab bar   Y & (RR)
CMS: 100-04,23,60.3

**E0912** Trapeze bar, heavy-duty, for patient weight capacity greater than 250 pounds, freestanding, complete with grab bar   Y & (RR)
CMS: 100-04,23,60.3

**E0920** Fracture frame, attached to bed, includes weights   Y & (RR)

**E0930** Fracture frame, freestanding, includes weights   Y & (RR)

**E0935** Continuous passive motion exercise device for use on knee only   Y & (RR)

**E0936** Continuous passive motion exercise device for use other than knee   E

**E0940** Trapeze bar, freestanding, complete with grab bar   Y & (RR)
CMS: 100-04,23,60.3

**E0941** Gravity assisted traction device, any type   Y & (RR)

**E0942** Cervical head harness/halter   Y & (NU,RR,UE)

**E0944** Pelvic belt/harness/boot   Y & (NU,RR,UE)

**E0945** Extremity belt/harness   Y & (NU,RR,UE)

**E0946** Fracture, frame, dual with cross bars, attached to bed, (e.g., Balken, 4 Poster)   Y & (RR)

**E0947** Fracture frame, attachments for complex pelvic traction   Y & (NU,RR,UE)

**E0948** Fracture frame, attachments for complex cervical traction   Y & (NU,RR,UE)

## Wheelchair Accessories

**E0950** Wheelchair accessory, tray, each   Y ☑ & (NU,RR,UE)
CMS: 100-04,23,60.3

**E0951** Heel loop/holder, any type, with or without ankle strap, each   Y ☑ & (NU,RR,UE)
CMS: 100-04,23,60.3

**E0952** Toe loop/holder, any type, each   Y ☑ & (NU,RR,UE)
CMS: 100-04,23,60.3

**E0955** Wheelchair accessory, headrest, cushioned, any type, including fixed mounting hardware, each   Y ☑ & (RR)
CMS: 100-04,23,60.3

**E0956** Wheelchair accessory, lateral trunk or hip support, any type, including fixed mounting hardware, each   Y ☑ & (NU,RR,UE)
CMS: 100-04,23,60.3

**E0957** Wheelchair accessory, medial thigh support, any type, including fixed mounting hardware, each   Y ☑ & (NU,RR,UE)
CMS: 100-04,23,60.3

**E0958** Manual wheelchair accessory, one-arm drive attachment, each   Y ☑ & (RR)

**E0959** Manual wheelchair accessory, adapter for amputee, each   B ☑ & (NU,RR,UE)

**E0960** Wheelchair accessory, shoulder harness/straps or chest strap, including any type mounting hardware   Y & (NU,RR,UE)
CMS: 100-04,23,60.3

**E0961** Manual wheelchair accessory, wheel lock brake extension (handle), each   B ☑ & (NU,RR,UE)

**E0966** Manual wheelchair accessory, headrest extension, each   B ☑ & (NU,RR,UE)

▲ **E0967**^Jan Manual wheelchair accessory, hand rim with projections, any type, replacement only, each   Y ☑ & (NU,RR,UE)

**E0968** Commode seat, wheelchair   Y & (RR)

**E0969** Narrowing device, wheelchair   Y & (NU,RR,UE)

**E0970** No. 2 footplates, except for elevating legrest   E
See code(s): K0037, K0042

**E0971** Manual wheelchair accessory, antitipping device, each   B ☑ & (NU,RR,UE)

**E0973** Wheelchair accessory, adjustable height, detachable armrest, complete assembly, each   B ☑ & (NU,RR,UE)
CMS: 100-04,23,60.3

**E0974** Manual wheelchair accessory, antirollback device, each   B ☑ & (NU,RR,UE)

**E0978** Wheelchair accessory, positioning belt/safety belt/pelvic strap, each   B ☑ & (NU,RR,UE)
CMS: 100-04,23,60.3

**E0980** Safety vest, wheelchair   Y & (NU,RR,UE)

**E0981** Wheelchair accessory, seat upholstery, replacement only, each   Y ☑ & (NU,RR,UE)
CMS: 100-04,23,60.3

*Durable Medical Equipment*

*E0783 — E0981*

^Jan **January Update**

Special Coverage Instructions   Noncovered by Medicare   Carrier Discretion   ☑ Quantity Alert   ● New Code   ○ Recycled/Reinstated   ▲ Revised Code

© 2016 Optum360, LLC   A2-Z3 ASC Pmt   CMS: Pub 100   AHA: Coding Clinic   & DMEPOS Paid   ⊘ SNF Excluded   E Codes — 33

**E0982** Wheelchair accessory, back upholstery, replacement only, each ☑ ☑ ♿ (NU,RR,UE)
CMS: 100-04,23,60.3

**E0983** Manual wheelchair accessory, power add-on to convert manual wheelchair to motorized wheelchair, joystick control ☑ ♿ (RR)

**E0984** Manual wheelchair accessory, power add-on to convert manual wheelchair to motorized wheelchair, tiller control ☑ ♿ (RR)

**E0985** Wheelchair accessory, seat lift mechanism ☑ ♿ (RR)

**E0986** Manual wheelchair accessory, push-rim activated power assist system ☑ ☑ ♿ (RR)

**E0988** Manual wheelchair accessory, lever-activated, wheel drive, pair ☑ ☑ ♿ (RR)

**E0990** Wheelchair accessory, elevating legrest, complete assembly, each ☑ ☑ ♿ (NU,RR,UE)
CMS: 100-04,23,60.3

**E0992** Manual wheelchair accessory, solid seat insert ☑ ♿ (NU,RR,UE)

**E0994** Armrest, each ☑ ☑ ♿ (NU,RR,UE)

▲ **E0995**^Jan Wheelchair accessory, calf rest/pad, replacement only, each ☑ ☑ ♿ (NU,RR,UE)
CMS: 100-04,23,60.3

**E1002** Wheelchair accessory, power seating system, tilt only ☑ ♿ (RR)
CMS: 100-04,23,60.3

**E1003** Wheelchair accessory, power seating system, recline only, without shear reduction ☑ ♿ (RR)
CMS: 100-04,23,60.3

**E1004** Wheelchair accessory, power seating system, recline only, with mechanical shear reduction ☑ ♿ (RR)
CMS: 100-04,23,60.3

**E1005** Wheelchair accessory, power seating system, recline only, with power shear reduction ☑ ♿ (RR)
CMS: 100-04,23,60.3

**E1006** Wheelchair accessory, power seating system, combination tilt and recline, without shear reduction ☑ ♿ (RR)
CMS: 100-04,23,60.3

**E1007** Wheelchair accessory, power seating system, combination tilt and recline, with mechanical shear reduction ☑ ♿ (RR)
CMS: 100-04,23,60.3

**E1008** Wheelchair accessory, power seating system, combination tilt and recline, with power shear reduction ☑ ♿ (RR)
CMS: 100-04,23,60.3

**E1009** Wheelchair accessory, addition to power seating system, mechanically linked leg elevation system, including pushrod and legrest, each ☑ ☑ ♿ (NU,RR,UE)
CMS: 100-04,23,60.3

**E1010** Wheelchair accessory, addition to power seating system, power leg elevation system, including legrest, pair ☑ ☑ ♿ (RR)
CMS: 100-04,23,60.3

**E1011** Modification to pediatric size wheelchair, width adjustment package (not to be dispensed with initial chair) ☑ ♿ (NU,RR,UE)

**E1012** Wheelchair accessory, addition to power seating system, center mount power elevating leg rest/platform, complete system, any type, each ☑ ♿ (RR)

**E1014** Reclining back, addition to pediatric size wheelchair ☑ ♿ (RR)

**E1015** Shock absorber for manual wheelchair, each ☑ ☑ ♿ (NU,RR,UE)

**E1016** Shock absorber for power wheelchair, each ☑ ☑ ♿ (NU,RR,UE)
CMS: 100-04,23,60.3

**E1017** Heavy-duty shock absorber for heavy-duty or extra heavy-duty manual wheelchair, each ☑ ☑ ♿ (NU,RR,UE)

**E1018** Heavy-duty shock absorber for heavy-duty or extra heavy-duty power wheelchair, each ☑ ☑ ♿ (NU,RR,UE)

**E1020** Residual limb support system for wheelchair, any type ☑ ♿ (RR)
CMS: 100-04,23,60.3

**E1028** Wheelchair accessory, manual swingaway, retractable or removable mounting hardware for joystick, other control interface or positioning accessory ☑ ♿ (RR)
CMS: 100-04,23,60.3

**E1029** Wheelchair accessory, ventilator tray, fixed ☑ ♿ (RR)
CMS: 100-04,23,60.3

**E1030** Wheelchair accessory, ventilator tray, gimbaled ☑ ♿ (RR)
CMS: 100-04,23,60.3

**E1031** Rollabout chair, any and all types with castors 5 in or greater ☑ ♿ (RR)

**E1035** Multi-positional patient transfer system, with integrated seat, operated by care giver, patient weight capacity up to and including 300 lbs ☑ ♿ (RR)
CMS: 100-02,15,110

**E1036** Multi-positional patient transfer system, extra-wide, with integrated seat, operated by caregiver, patient weight capacity greater than 300 lbs ☑ ♿ (RR)

**E1037** Transport chair, pediatric size ☑ ♿ (RR)

**E1038** Transport chair, adult size, patient weight capacity up to and including 300 pounds ☑ ♿ (RR)

**E1039** Transport chair, adult size, heavy-duty, patient weight capacity greater than 300 pounds ☑ ♿ (RR)

## Wheelchairs

**E1050** Fully-reclining wheelchair, fixed full-length arms, swing-away detachable elevating legrests ☑ ♿ (RR)

**E1060** Fully-reclining wheelchair, detachable arms, desk or full-length, swing-away detachable elevating legrests ☑ ♿ (RR)

**E1070** Fully-reclining wheelchair, detachable arms (desk or full-length) swing-away detachable footrest ☑ ♿ (RR)

**E1083** Hemi-wheelchair, fixed full-length arms, swing-away detachable elevating legrest ☑ ♿ (RR)

**E1084** Hemi-wheelchair, detachable arms desk or full-length arms, swing-away detachable elevating legrests ☑ ♿ (RR)

**E1085** Hemi-wheelchair, fixed full-length arms, swing-away detachable footrests ☑
See code(s): K0002

**E1086** Hemi-wheelchair, detachable arms, desk or full-length, swing-away detachable footrests ☑
See code(s): K0002

**E1087** High strength lightweight wheelchair, fixed full-length arms, swing-away detachable elevating legrests ☑ ♿ (RR)

**E1088** High strength lightweight wheelchair, detachable arms desk or full-length, swing-away detachable elevating legrests ☑ ♿ (RR)

**E1089** High-strength lightweight wheelchair, fixed-length arms, swing-away detachable footrest ☑
See code(s): K0004

---

^Jan **January Update**

Special Coverage Instructions   Noncovered by Medicare   Carrier Discretion   ☑ Quantity Alert   ● New Code   ○ Recycled/Reinstated   ▲ Revised Code

🅐 Age Edit   🅜 Maternity Edit   ♀ Female Only   ♂ Male Only   🅐-Ⓨ OPPS Status Indicators   © 2016 Optum360, LLC

| Code | Description | |
|---|---|---|
| **E1090** | High-strength lightweight wheelchair, detachable arms, desk or full-length, swing-away detachable footrests | E |
| | See code(s): K0004 | |
| **E1092** | Wide heavy-duty wheel chair, detachable arms (desk or full-length), swing-away detachable elevating legrests | Y ♿ (RR) |
| **E1093** | Wide heavy-duty wheelchair, detachable arms, desk or full-length arms, swing-away detachable footrest | Y ♿ (RR) |
| **E1100** | Semi-reclining wheelchair, fixed full-length arms, swing-away detachable elevating legrests | Y ♿ (RR) |
| **E1110** | Semi-reclining wheelchair, detachable arms (desk or full-length) elevating legrest | Y ♿ (RR) |
| **E1130** | Standard wheelchair, fixed full-length arms, fixed or swing-away detachable footrests | E |
| | See code(s): K0001 | |
| **E1140** | Wheelchair, detachable arms, desk or full-length, swing-away detachable footrests | E |
| | See code(s): K0001 | |
| **E1150** | Wheelchair, detachable arms, desk or full-length swing-away detachable elevating legrests | Y ♿ (RR) |
| **E1160** | Wheelchair, fixed full-length arms, swing-away detachable elevating legrests | Y ♿ (RR) |
| **E1161** | Manual adult size wheelchair, includes tilt in space | Y ♿ (RR) |
| **E1170** | Amputee wheelchair, fixed full-length arms, swing-away detachable elevating legrests | Y ♿ (RR) |
| **E1171** | Amputee wheelchair, fixed full-length arms, without footrests or legrest | Y ♿ (RR) |
| **E1172** | Amputee wheelchair, detachable arms (desk or full-length) without footrests or legrest | Y ♿ (RR) |
| **E1180** | Amputee wheelchair, detachable arms (desk or full-length) swing-away detachable footrests | Y ♿ (RR) |
| **E1190** | Amputee wheelchair, detachable arms (desk or full-length) swing-away detachable elevating legrests | Y ♿ (RR) |
| **E1195** | Heavy-duty wheelchair, fixed full-length arms, swing-away detachable elevating legrests | Y ♿ (RR) |
| **E1200** | Amputee wheelchair, fixed full-length arms, swing-away detachable footrest | Y ♿ (RR) |
| **E1220** | Wheelchair; specially sized or constructed, (indicate brand name, model number, if any) and justification | Y |
| **E1221** | Wheelchair with fixed arm, footrests | Y ♿ (RR) |
| **E1222** | Wheelchair with fixed arm, elevating legrests | Y ♿ (RR) |
| **E1223** | Wheelchair with detachable arms, footrests | Y ♿ (RR) |
| **E1224** | Wheelchair with detachable arms, elevating legrests | Y ♿ (RR) |
| **E1225** | Wheelchair accessory, manual semi-reclining back, (recline greater than 15 degrees, but less than 80 degrees), each | Y ☑ ♿ (RR) |
| **E1226** | Wheelchair accessory, manual fully reclining back, (recline greater than 80 degrees), each | B ☑ ♿ (NU,RR,UE) |
| | See also K0028 | |
| **E1227** | Special height arms for wheelchair | Y ♿ (NU,RR,UE) |
| **E1228** | Special back height for wheelchair | Y ♿ (RR) |
| **E1229** | Wheelchair, pediatric size, not otherwise specified | Y |
| **E1230** | Power operated vehicle (3- or 4-wheel nonhighway), specify brand name and model number | Y ♿ (NU,RR,UE) |
| | Prior authorization is required by Medicare for this item. | |
| **E1231** | Wheelchair, pediatric size, tilt-in-space, rigid, adjustable, with seating system | Y ♿ (NU,RR,UE) |
| **E1232** | Wheelchair, pediatric size, tilt-in-space, folding, adjustable, with seating system | Y ♿ (RR) |
| **E1233** | Wheelchair, pediatric size, tilt-in-space, rigid, adjustable, without seating system | Y ♿ (RR) |
| **E1234** | Wheelchair, pediatric size, tilt-in-space, folding, adjustable, without seating system | Y ♿ (RR) |
| **E1235** | Wheelchair, pediatric size, rigid, adjustable, with seating system | Y ♿ (RR) |
| **E1236** | Wheelchair, pediatric size, folding, adjustable, with seating system | Y ♿ (RR) |
| **E1237** | Wheelchair, pediatric size, rigid, adjustable, without seating system | Y ♿ (RR) |
| **E1238** | Wheelchair, pediatric size, folding, adjustable, without seating system | Y ♿ (RR) |
| **E1239** | Power wheelchair, pediatric size, not otherwise specified | Y |
| **E1240** | Lightweight wheelchair, detachable arms, (desk or full-length) swing-away detachable, elevating legrest | Y ♿ (RR) |
| **E1250** | Lightweight wheelchair, fixed full-length arms, swing-away detachable footrest | E |
| | See code(s): K0003 | |
| **E1260** | Lightweight wheelchair, detachable arms (desk or full-length) swing-away detachable footrest | E |
| | See code(s): K0003 | |
| **E1270** | Lightweight wheelchair, fixed full-length arms, swing-away detachable elevating legrests | Y ♿ (RR) |
| **E1280** | Heavy-duty wheelchair, detachable arms (desk or full-length) elevating legrests | Y ♿ (RR) |
| **E1285** | Heavy-duty wheelchair, fixed full-length arms, swing-away detachable footrest | E |
| | See code(s): K0006 | |
| **E1290** | Heavy-duty wheelchair, detachable arms (desk or full-length) swing-away detachable footrest | E |
| | See code(s): K0006 | |
| **E1295** | Heavy-duty wheelchair, fixed full-length arms, elevating legrest | Y ♿ (RR) |
| **E1296** | Special wheelchair seat height from floor | Y ♿ (NU,RR,UE) |
| **E1297** | Special wheelchair seat depth, by upholstery | Y ♿ (NU,RR,UE) |
| **E1298** | Special wheelchair seat depth and/or width, by construction | Y ♿ (NU,RR,UE) |

## Whirlpool - Equipment

| Code | Description | |
|---|---|---|
| **E1300** | Whirlpool, portable (overtub type) | E |
| **E1310** | Whirlpool, nonportable (built-in type) | Y ♿ (NU,RR,UE) |

## Additional Oxygen Related Equipment

| Code | Description | |
|---|---|---|
| **E1352** | Oxygen accessory, flow regulator capable of positive inspiratory pressure | Y |
| **E1353** | Regulator | Y ♿ |
| | CMS: 100-04,23,60.3 | |
| **E1354** | Oxygen accessory, wheeled cart for portable cylinder or portable concentrator, any type, replacement only, each | Y ☑ |
| **E1355** | Stand/rack | Y ♿ |
| | CMS: 100-04,23,60.3 | |
| **E1356** | Oxygen accessory, battery pack/cartridge for portable concentrator, any type, replacement only, each | Y ☑ |

---

Special Coverage Instructions    Noncovered by Medicare    Carrier Discretion    ☑ Quantity Alert   ● New Code   ○ Recycled/Reinstated   ▲ Revised Code

© 2016 Optum360, LLC    A2-Z3 ASC Pmt    CMS: Pub 100    AHA: Coding Clinic    ♿ DMEPOS Paid    ⊘ SNF Excluded     E Codes — 35

| | | |
|---|---|---|
| E1357 | Oxygen accessory, battery charger for portable concentrator, any type, replacement only, each | Y ☑ |
| E1358 | Oxygen accessory, DC power adapter for portable concentrator, any type, replacement only, each | Y ☑ |
| E1372 | Immersion external heater for nebulizer | Y ⚬ (NU,RR,UE) |
| E1390 | Oxygen concentrator, single delivery port, capable of delivering 85 percent or greater oxygen concentration at the prescribed flow rate | Y ⚬ (RR) |
| E1391 | Oxygen concentrator, dual delivery port, capable of delivering 85 percent or greater oxygen concentration at the prescribed flow rate, each | Y ☑ ⚬ (RR) |
| E1392 | Portable oxygen concentrator, rental | Y ⚬ (RR) |
| E1399 | Durable medical equipment, miscellaneous<br>CMS: 100-04,32,110.5 | Y |
| E1405 | Oxygen and water vapor enriching system with heated delivery<br>CMS: 100-04,20,20; 100-04,20,20.4 | Y ⚬ (RR) |
| E1406 | Oxygen and water vapor enriching system without heated delivery<br>CMS: 100-04,20,20; 100-04,20,20.4 | Y ⚬ (RR) |

## Artificial Kidney Machines and Accessories

| | | |
|---|---|---|
| E1500 | Centrifuge, for dialysis<br>AHA: 1Q, '02, 5 | A ⃠ |
| E1510 | Kidney, dialysate delivery system kidney machine, pump recirculating, air removal system, flowrate meter, power off, heater and temperature control with alarm, IV poles, pressure gauge, concentrate container | A ⃠ |
| E1520 | Heparin infusion pump for hemodialysis | A ⃠ |
| E1530 | Air bubble detector for hemodialysis, each, replacement | A ☑ ⃠ |
| E1540 | Pressure alarm for hemodialysis, each, replacement | A ☑ ⃠ |
| E1550 | Bath conductivity meter for hemodialysis, each | A ☑ ⃠ |
| E1560 | Blood leak detector for hemodialysis, each, replacement | A ☑ ⃠ |
| E1570 | Adjustable chair, for ESRD patients | A ⃠ |
| E1575 | Transducer protectors/fluid barriers, for hemodialysis, any size, per 10 | A ☑ ⃠ |
| E1580 | Unipuncture control system for hemodialysis | A ⃠ |
| E1590 | Hemodialysis machine | A ⃠ |
| E1592 | Automatic intermittent peritoneal dialysis system | A ⃠ |
| E1594 | Cycler dialysis machine for peritoneal dialysis | A ⃠ |
| E1600 | Delivery and/or installation charges for hemodialysis equipment | A ⃠ |
| E1610 | Reverse osmosis water purification system, for hemodialysis | A ⃠ |
| E1615 | Deionizer water purification system, for hemodialysis | A ⃠ |
| E1620 | Blood pump for hemodialysis, replacement | A ⃠ |
| E1625 | Water softening system, for hemodialysis | A ⃠ |
| E1630 | Reciprocating peritoneal dialysis system | A ⃠ |
| E1632 | Wearable artificial kidney, each | A ☑ ⃠ |
| E1634 | Peritoneal dialysis clamps, each | B ☑ |
| E1635 | Compact (portable) travel hemodialyzer system | A ⃠ |
| E1636 | Sorbent cartridges, for hemodialysis, per 10 | A ☑ ⃠ |

| | | |
|---|---|---|
| E1637 | Hemostats, each<br>AHA: 1Q, '02, 5 | A ☑ ⃠ |
| E1639 | Scale, each<br>AHA: 1Q, '02, 5 | A ☑ ⃠ |
| E1699 | Dialysis equipment, not otherwise specified | A ⃠ |

## Jaw Motion Rehabilitation System and Accessories

| | | |
|---|---|---|
| E1700 | Jaw motion rehabilitation system<br>Medicare jurisdiction: local contractor. | Y ⚬ (RR) |
| E1701 | Replacement cushions for jaw motion rehabilitation system, package of 6<br>Medicare jurisdiction: local contractor. | Y ☑ ⚬ |
| E1702 | Replacement measuring scales for jaw motion rehabilitation system, package of 200<br>Medicare jurisdiction: local contractor. | Y ☑ ⚬ |

## Flexion/Extension Device

| | | |
|---|---|---|
| E1800 | Dynamic adjustable elbow extension/flexion device, includes soft interface material | Y ⚬ (RR) |
| E1801 | Static progressive stretch elbow device, extension and/or flexion, with or without range of motion adjustment, includes all components and accessories<br>AHA: 1Q, '02, 5 | Y ⚬ (RR) |
| E1802 | Dynamic adjustable forearm pronation/supination device, includes soft interface material | Y ⚬ (RR) |
| E1805 | Dynamic adjustable wrist extension/flexion device, includes soft interface material | Y ⚬ (RR) |
| E1806 | Static progressive stretch wrist device, flexion and/or extension, with or without range of motion adjustment, includes all components and accessories<br>AHA: 1Q, '02, 5 | Y ⚬ (RR) |
| E1810 | Dynamic adjustable knee extension/flexion device, includes soft interface material | Y ⚬ (RR) |
| E1811 | Static progressive stretch knee device, extension and/or flexion, with or without range of motion adjustment, includes all components and accessories<br>AHA: 1Q, '02, 5 | Y ⚬ (RR) |
| E1812 | Dynamic knee, extension/flexion device with active resistance control | Y ⚬ (RR) |
| E1815 | Dynamic adjustable ankle extension/flexion device, includes soft interface material | Y ⚬ (RR) |
| E1816 | Static progressive stretch ankle device, flexion and/or extension, with or without range of motion adjustment, includes all components and accessories<br>AHA: 1Q, '02, 5 | Y ⚬ (RR) |
| E1818 | Static progressive stretch forearm pronation/supination device, with or without range of motion adjustment, includes all components and accessories<br>AHA: 1Q, '02, 5 | Y ⚬ (RR) |
| E1820 | Replacement soft interface material, dynamic adjustable extension/flexion device | Y ⚬ (NU,RR,UE) |
| E1821 | Replacement soft interface material/cuffs for bi-directional static progressive stretch device<br>AHA: 1Q, '02, 5 | Y ⚬ (NU,RR,UE) |
| E1825 | Dynamic adjustable finger extension/flexion device, includes soft interface material | Y ⚬ (RR) |
| E1830 | Dynamic adjustable toe extension/flexion device, includes soft interface material | Y ⚬ (RR) |

Special Coverage Instructions    Noncovered by Medicare    Carrier Discretion    ☑ Quantity Alert ● New Code ⚬ Recycled/Reinstated ▲ Revised Code

36 — E Codes    A Age Edit    M Maternity Edit    ♀ Female Only    ♂ Male Only    A-Y OPPS Status Indicators    © 2016 Optum360, LLC

**E1831** Static progressive stretch toe device, extension and/or flexion, with or without range of motion adjustment, includes all components and accessories ☐ & (RR)

**E1840** Dynamic adjustable shoulder flexion/abduction/rotation device, includes soft interface material ☐ & (RR)
AHA: 1Q, '02, 5

**E1841** Static progressive stretch shoulder device, with or without range of motion adjustment, includes all components and accessories ☐ & (RR)

## Other Devices

**E1902** Communication board, nonelectronic augmentative or alternative communication device ☐
AHA: 1Q, '02, 5

**E2000** Gastric suction pump, home model, portable or stationary, electric ☐ & (RR)
AHA: 1Q, '02, 5

**E2100** Blood glucose monitor with integrated voice synthesizer ☐ & (NU,RR,UE)
AHA: 1Q, '02, 5

**E2101** Blood glucose monitor with integrated lancing/blood sample ☐ & (NU,RR,UE)
AHA: 1Q, '02, 5

**E2120** Pulse generator system for tympanic treatment of inner ear endolymphatic fluid ☐ & (RR)

## DME Wheelchair Accessory

**E2201** Manual wheelchair accessory, nonstandard seat frame, width greater than or equal to 20 in and less than 24 in ☐ ☑ & (NU,RR,UE)

**E2202** Manual wheelchair accessory, nonstandard seat frame width, 24-27 in ☐ ☑ & (NU,RR,UE)

**E2203** Manual wheelchair accessory, nonstandard seat frame depth, 20 to less than 22 in ☐ ☑ & (NU,RR,UE)

**E2204** Manual wheelchair accessory, nonstandard seat frame depth, 22 to 25 in ☐ ☑ & (NU,RR,UE)

**E2205** Manual wheelchair accessory, handrim without projections (includes ergonomic or contoured), any type, replacement only, each ☐ ☑ & (NU,RR,UE)

▲ **E2206**ᴶᵃⁿ Manual wheelchair accessory, wheel lock assembly, complete, replacement only, each ☐ ☑ & (NU,RR,UE)

**E2207** Wheelchair accessory, crutch and cane holder, each ☐ ☑ & (NU,RR,UE)

**E2208** Wheelchair accessory, cylinder tank carrier, each ☐ ☑ & (NU,RR,UE)
CMS: 100-04,23,60.3

**E2209** Accessory, arm trough, with or without hand support, each ☐ ☑ & (NU,RR,UE)
CMS: 100-04,23,60.3

**E2210** Wheelchair accessory, bearings, any type, replacement only, each ☐ ☑ & (NU,RR,UE)
CMS: 100-04,23,60.3

**E2211** Manual wheelchair accessory, pneumatic propulsion tire, any size, each ☐ ☑ & (NU,RR,UE)

**E2212** Manual wheelchair accessory, tube for pneumatic propulsion tire, any size, each ☐ ☑ & (NU,RR,UE)

**E2213** Manual wheelchair accessory, insert for pneumatic propulsion tire (removable), any type, any size, each ☐ ☑ & (NU,RR,UE)

**E2214** Manual wheelchair accessory, pneumatic caster tire, any size, each ☐ ☑ & (NU,RR,UE)

**E2215** Manual wheelchair accessory, tube for pneumatic caster tire, any size, each ☐ ☑ & (NU,RR,UE)

**E2216** Manual wheelchair accessory, foam filled propulsion tire, any size, each ☐ ☑ & (NU,RR,UE)

**E2217** Manual wheelchair accessory, foam filled caster tire, any size, each ☐ ☑ & (NU,RR,UE)

**E2218** Manual wheelchair accessory, foam propulsion tire, any size, each ☐ ☑ & (NU,RR,UE)

**E2219** Manual wheelchair accessory, foam caster tire, any size, each ☐ ☑ & (NU,RR,UE)

▲ **E2220**ᴶᵃⁿ Manual wheelchair accessory, solid (rubber/plastic) propulsion tire, any size, replacement only, each ☐ ☑ & (NU,RR,UE)

▲ **E2221**ᴶᵃⁿ Manual wheelchair accessory, solid (rubber/plastic) caster tire (removable), any size, replacement only, each ☐ ☑ & (NU,RR,UE)

▲ **E2222**ᴶᵃⁿ Manual wheelchair accessory, solid (rubber/plastic) caster tire with integrated wheel, any size, replacement only, each ☐ ☑ & (NU,RR,UE)

▲ **E2224**ᴶᵃⁿ Manual wheelchair accessory, propulsion wheel excludes tire, any size, replacement only, each ☐ ☑ & (NU,RR,UE)

**E2225** Manual wheelchair accessory, caster wheel excludes tire, any size, replacement only, each ☐ ☑ & (NU,RR,UE)

**E2226** Manual wheelchair accessory, caster fork, any size, replacement only, each ☐ ☑ & (NU,RR,UE)

**E2227** Manual wheelchair accessory, gear reduction drive wheel, each ☐ ☑ & (RR)

**E2228** Manual wheelchair accessory, wheel braking system and lock, complete, each ☐ ☑ & (RR)

**E2230** Manual wheelchair accessory, manual standing system ☐

**E2231** Manual wheelchair accessory, solid seat support base (replaces sling seat), includes any type mounting hardware ☐ & (NU,RR,UE)

**E2291** Back, planar, for pediatric size wheelchair including fixed attaching hardware ☐

**E2292** Seat, planar, for pediatric size wheelchair including fixed attaching hardware ☐

**E2293** Back, contoured, for pediatric size wheelchair including fixed attaching hardware ☐

**E2294** Seat, contoured, for pediatric size wheelchair including fixed attaching hardware ☐

**E2295** Manual wheelchair accessory, for pediatric size wheelchair, dynamic seating frame, allows coordinated movement of multiple positioning features ☐

**E2300** Wheelchair accessory, power seat elevation system, any type ☐

**E2301** Wheelchair accessory, power standing system, any type ☐

**E2310** Power wheelchair accessory, electronic connection between wheelchair controller and one power seating system motor, including all related electronics, indicator feature, mechanical function selection switch, and fixed mounting hardware ☐ & (RR)
CMS: 100-04,23,60.3

**E2311** Power wheelchair accessory, electronic connection between wheelchair controller and 2 or more power seating system motors, including all related electronics, indicator feature, mechanical function selection switch, and fixed mounting hardware ☐ & (RR)
CMS: 100-04,23,60.3

ᴶᵃⁿ January Update

Special Coverage Instructions   Noncovered by Medicare   Carrier Discretion   ☑ Quantity Alert ● New Code   ○ Recycled/Reinstated   ▲ Revised Code

© 2016 Optum360, LLC   A2-Z3 ASC Pmt   CMS: Pub 100   AHA: Coding Clinic   & DMEPOS Paid   ⊘ SNF Excluded   E Codes — 37

Durable Medical Equipment

E1831 — E2311

**Durable Medical Equipment**

**E2312** Power wheelchair accessory, hand or chin control interface, mini-proportional remote joystick, proportional, including fixed mounting hardware ☑ & (RR)

**E2313** Power wheelchair accessory, harness for upgrade to expandable controller, including all fasteners, connectors and mounting hardware, each ☑ ☑ & (RR)

**E2321** Power wheelchair accessory, hand control interface, remote joystick, nonproportional, including all related electronics, mechanical stop switch, and fixed mounting hardware ☑ & (RR)
CMS: 100-04,23,60.3

**E2322** Power wheelchair accessory, hand control interface, multiple mechanical switches, nonproportional, including all related electronics, mechanical stop switch, and fixed mounting hardware ☑ & (RR)
CMS: 100-04,23,60.3

**E2323** Power wheelchair accessory, specialty joystick handle for hand control interface, prefabricated ☑ & (NU,RR,UE)
CMS: 100-04,23,60.3

**E2324** Power wheelchair accessory, chin cup for chin control interface ☑ & (NU,RR,UE)
CMS: 100-04,23,60.3

**E2325** Power wheelchair accessory, sip and puff interface, nonproportional, including all related electronics, mechanical stop switch, and manual swingaway mounting hardware ☑ & (RR)
CMS: 100-04,23,60.3

**E2326** Power wheelchair accessory, breath tube kit for sip and puff interface ☑ & (RR)
CMS: 100-04,23,60.3

**E2327** Power wheelchair accessory, head control interface, mechanical, proportional, including all related electronics, mechanical direction change switch, and fixed mounting hardware ☑ & (RR)
CMS: 100-04,23,60.3

**E2328** Power wheelchair accessory, head control or extremity control interface, electronic, proportional, including all related electronics and fixed mounting hardware ☑ & (RR)
CMS: 100-04,23,60.3

**E2329** Power wheelchair accessory, head control interface, contact switch mechanism, nonproportional, including all related electronics, mechanical stop switch, mechanical direction change switch, head array, and fixed mounting hardware ☑ & (RR)
CMS: 100-04,23,60.3

**E2330** Power wheelchair accessory, head control interface, proximity switch mechanism, nonproportional, including all related electronics, mechanical stop switch, mechanical direction change switch, head array, and fixed mounting hardware ☑ & (RR)
CMS: 100-04,23,60.3

**E2331** Power wheelchair accessory, attendant control, proportional, including all related electronics and fixed mounting hardware ☑

**E2340** Power wheelchair accessory, nonstandard seat frame width, 20-23 in ☑ ☑ & (NU,RR,UE)

**E2341** Power wheelchair accessory, nonstandard seat frame width, 24-27 in ☑ ☑ & (NU,RR,UE)

**E2342** Power wheelchair accessory, nonstandard seat frame depth, 20 or 21 in ☑ ☑ & (NU,RR,UE)

**E2343** Power wheelchair accessory, nonstandard seat frame depth, 22-25 in ☑ ☑ & (NU,RR,UE)

**E2351** Power wheelchair accessory, electronic interface to operate speech generating device using power wheelchair control interface ☑ & (NU,RR,UE)
CMS: 100-04,23,60.3

**E2358** Power wheelchair accessory, group 34 nonsealed lead acid battery, each ☑ ☑

**E2359** Power wheelchair accessory, group 34 sealed lead acid battery, each (e.g., gel cell, absorbed glass mat) ☑ & (NU,RR,UE)

**E2360** Power wheelchair accessory, 22 NF nonsealed lead acid battery, each ☑ ☑ & (NU,RR,UE)

**E2361** Power wheelchair accessory, 22 NF sealed lead acid battery, each (e.g., gel cell, absorbed glassmat) ☑ ☑ & (NU,RR,UE)
CMS: 100-04,23,60.3

**E2362** Power wheelchair accessory, group 24 nonsealed lead acid battery, each ☑ ☑ & (NU,RR,UE)

**E2363** Power wheelchair accessory, group 24 sealed lead acid battery, each (e.g., gel cell, absorbed glassmat) ☑ ☑ & (NU,RR,UE)
CMS: 100-04,23,60.3

**E2364** Power wheelchair accessory, U-1 nonsealed lead acid battery, each ☑ ☑ & (NU,RR,UE)

**E2365** Power wheelchair accessory, U-1 sealed lead acid battery, each (e.g., gel cell, absorbed glassmat) ☑ ☑ & (NU,RR,UE)
CMS: 100-04,23,60.3

**E2366** Power wheelchair accessory, battery charger, single mode, for use with only one battery type, sealed or nonsealed, each ☑ ☑ & (NU,RR,UE)
CMS: 100-04,23,60.3

**E2367** Power wheelchair accessory, battery charger, dual mode, for use with either battery type, sealed or nonsealed, each ☑ ☑ & (NU,RR,UE)
CMS: 100-04,23,60.3

**E2368** Power wheelchair component, drive wheel motor, replacement only ☑ & (RR)
CMS: 100-04,23,60.3

**E2369** Power wheelchair component, drive wheel gear box, replacement only ☑ & (RR)
CMS: 100-04,23,60.3

**E2370** Power wheelchair component, integrated drive wheel motor and gear box combination, replacement only ☑ & (RR)
CMS: 100-04,23,60.3

**E2371** Power wheelchair accessory, group 27 sealed lead acid battery, (e.g., gel cell, absorbed glassmat), each ☑ ☑ & (NU,RR,UE)
CMS: 100-04,23,60.3

**E2372** Power wheelchair accessory, group 27 nonsealed lead acid battery, each ☑ ☑ & (NU,RR,UE)

**E2373** Power wheelchair accessory, hand or chin control interface, compact remote joystick, proportional, including fixed mounting hardware ☑ & (RR)
CMS: 100-04,23,60.3

**E2374** Power wheelchair accessory, hand or chin control interface, standard remote joystick (not including controller), proportional, including all related electronics and fixed mounting hardware, replacement only ☑ & (RR)
CMS: 100-04,23,60.3

**E2375** Power wheelchair accessory, nonexpandable controller, including all related electronics and mounting hardware, replacement only ☑ & (RR)
CMS: 100-04,23,60.3

**E2376** Power wheelchair accessory, expandable controller, including all related electronics and mounting hardware, replacement only  Y & (RR)
CMS: 100-04,23,60.3

**E2377** Power wheelchair accessory, expandable controller, including all related electronics and mounting hardware, upgrade provided at initial issue  Y & (RR)
CMS: 100-04,23,60.3

**E2378** Power wheelchair component, actuator, replacement only  Y & (RR)
CMS: 100-04,23,60.3

**E2381** Power wheelchair accessory, pneumatic drive wheel tire, any size, replacement only, each  Y ☑ & (NU,RR,UE)
CMS: 100-04,23,60.3

**E2382** Power wheelchair accessory, tube for pneumatic drive wheel tire, any size, replacement only, each  Y ☑ & (NU,RR,UE)
CMS: 100-04,23,60.3

**E2383** Power wheelchair accessory, insert for pneumatic drive wheel tire (removable), any type, any size, replacement only, each  Y ☑ & (NU,RR,UE)
CMS: 100-04,23,60.3

**E2384** Power wheelchair accessory, pneumatic caster tire, any size, replacement only, each  Y ☑ & (NU,RR,UE)
CMS: 100-04,23,60.3

**E2385** Power wheelchair accessory, tube for pneumatic caster tire, any size, replacement only, each  Y ☑ & (NU,RR,UE)
CMS: 100-04,23,60.3

**E2386** Power wheelchair accessory, foam filled drive wheel tire, any size, replacement only, each  Y ☑ & (NU,RR,UE)
CMS: 100-04,23,60.3

**E2387** Power wheelchair accessory, foam filled caster tire, any size, replacement only, each  Y ☑ & (NU,RR,UE)
CMS: 100-04,23,60.3

**E2388** Power wheelchair accessory, foam drive wheel tire, any size, replacement only, each  Y ☑ & (NU,RR,UE)
CMS: 100-04,23,60.3

**E2389** Power wheelchair accessory, foam caster tire, any size, replacement only, each  Y ☑ & (NU,RR,UE)
CMS: 100-04,23,60.3

**E2390** Power wheelchair accessory, solid (rubber/plastic) drive wheel tire, any size, replacement only, each  Y ☑ & (NU,RR,UE)
CMS: 100-04,23,60.3

**E2391** Power wheelchair accessory, solid (rubber/plastic) caster tire (removable), any size, replacement only, each  Y ☑ & (NU,RR,UE)
CMS: 100-04,23,60.3

**E2392** Power wheelchair accessory, solid (rubber/plastic) caster tire with integrated wheel, any size, replacement only, each  Y ☑ & (NU,RR,UE)
CMS: 100-04,23,60.3

**E2394** Power wheelchair accessory, drive wheel excludes tire, any size, replacement only, each  Y ☑ & (NU,RR,UE)
CMS: 100-04,23,60.3

**E2395** Power wheelchair accessory, caster wheel excludes tire, any size, replacement only, each  Y ☑ & (NU,RR,UE)
CMS: 100-04,23,60.3

**E2396** Power wheelchair accessory, caster fork, any size, replacement only, each  Y ☑ & (NU,RR,UE)
CMS: 100-04,23,60.3

**E2397** Power wheelchair accessory, lithium-based battery, each  Y ☑ & (NU,RR,UE)

## Wound Therapy

**E2402** Negative pressure wound therapy electrical pump, stationary or portable  Y & (RR)
CMS: 100-04,23,60.3

## Speech Generating Device

**E2500** Speech generating device, digitized speech, using prerecorded messages, less than or equal to 8 minutes recording time  Y ☑ & (NU,RR,UE)

**E2502** Speech generating device, digitized speech, using prerecorded messages, greater than 8 minutes but less than or equal to 20 minutes recording time  Y ☑ & (NU,RR,UE)

**E2504** Speech generating device, digitized speech, using prerecorded messages, greater than 20 minutes but less than or equal to 40 minutes recording time  Y ☑ & (NU,RR,UE)

**E2506** Speech generating device, digitized speech, using prerecorded messages, greater than 40 minutes recording time  Y ☑ & (NU,RR,UE)

**E2508** Speech generating device, synthesized speech, requiring message formulation by spelling and access by physical contact with the device  Y & (NU,RR,UE)

**E2510** Speech generating device, synthesized speech, permitting multiple methods of message formulation and multiple methods of device access  Y & (NU,RR,UE)

**E2511** Speech generating software program, for personal computer or personal digital assistant  Y & (NU,RR,UE)

**E2512** Accessory for speech generating device, mounting system  Y & (NU,RR,UE)

**E2599** Accessory for speech generating device, not otherwise classified  Y

## Wheelchair Cushion

**E2601** General use wheelchair seat cushion, width less than 22 in, any depth  Y & (NU,RR,UE)
CMS: 100-04,23,60.3

**E2602** General use wheelchair seat cushion, width 22 in or greater, any depth  Y & (NU,RR,UE)
CMS: 100-04,23,60.3

**E2603** Skin protection wheelchair seat cushion, width less than 22 in, any depth  Y & (NU,RR,UE)
CMS: 100-04,23,60.3

**E2604** Skin protection wheelchair seat cushion, width 22 in or greater, any depth  Y & (NU,RR,UE)
CMS: 100-04,23,60.3

**E2605** Positioning wheelchair seat cushion, width less than 22 in, any depth  Y & (NU,RR,UE)
CMS: 100-04,23,60.3

**E2606** Positioning wheelchair seat cushion, width 22 in or greater, any depth  Y & (NU,RR,UE)
CMS: 100-04,23,60.3

**E2607** Skin protection and positioning wheelchair seat cushion, width less than 22 in, any depth  Y & (NU,RR,UE)
CMS: 100-04,23,60.3

**E2608** Skin protection and positioning wheelchair seat cushion, width 22 in or greater, any depth  Y & (NU,RR,UE)
CMS: 100-04,23,60.3

**E2609** Custom fabricated wheelchair seat cushion, any size  Y

**E2610** Wheelchair seat cushion, powered  B

**Durable Medical Equipment**

**E2611 — E8002**

**E2611** General use wheelchair back cushion, width less than 22 in, any height, including any type mounting hardware  Y & (NU,RR,UE)
CMS: 100-04,23,60.3

**E2612** General use wheelchair back cushion, width 22 in or greater, any height, including any type mounting hardware  Y & (NU,RR,UE)
CMS: 100-04,23,60.3

**E2613** Positioning wheelchair back cushion, posterior, width less than 22 in, any height, including any type mounting hardware  Y & (NU,RR,UE)
CMS: 100-04,23,60.3

**E2614** Positioning wheelchair back cushion, posterior, width 22 in or greater, any height, including any type mounting hardware  Y & (NU,RR,UE)
CMS: 100-04,23,60.3

**E2615** Positioning wheelchair back cushion, posterior-lateral, width less than 22 in, any height, including any type mounting hardware  Y & (NU,RR,UE)
CMS: 100-04,23,60.3

**E2616** Positioning wheelchair back cushion, posterior-lateral, width 22 in or greater, any height, including any type mounting hardware  Y & (NU,RR,UE)
CMS: 100-04,23,60.3

**E2617** Custom fabricated wheelchair back cushion, any size, including any type mounting hardware  Y

**E2619** Replacement cover for wheelchair seat cushion or back cushion, each  Y ☑ & (NU,RR,UE)
CMS: 100-04,23,60.3

**E2620** Positioning wheelchair back cushion, planar back with lateral supports, width less than 22 in, any height, including any type mounting hardware  Y & (NU,RR,UE)
CMS: 100-04,23,60.3

**E2621** Positioning wheelchair back cushion, planar back with lateral supports, width 22 in or greater, any height, including any type mounting hardware  Y & (NU,RR,UE)
CMS: 100-04,23,60.3

**E2622** Skin protection wheelchair seat cushion, adjustable, width less than 22 in, any depth  Y & (NU,RR,UE)

**E2623** Skin protection wheelchair seat cushion, adjustable, width 22 in or greater, any depth  Y & (NU,RR,UE)

**E2624** Skin protection and positioning wheelchair seat cushion, adjustable, width less than 22 in, any depth  Y & (NU,RR,UE)

**E2625** Skin protection and positioning wheelchair seat cushion, adjustable, width 22 in or greater, any depth  Y & (NU,RR,UE)

## Wheelchair Arm Support

**E2626** Wheelchair accessory, shoulder elbow, mobile arm support attached to wheelchair, balanced, adjustable  Y & (NU,RR,UE)

**E2627** Wheelchair accessory, shoulder elbow, mobile arm support attached to wheelchair, balanced, adjustable Rancho type  Y & (NU,RR,UE)

**E2628** Wheelchair accessory, shoulder elbow, mobile arm support attached to wheelchair, balanced, reclining  Y & (NU,RR,UE)

**E2629** Wheelchair accessory, shoulder elbow, mobile arm support attached to wheelchair, balanced, friction arm support (friction dampening to proximal and distal joints)  Y & (NU,RR,UE)

**E2630** Wheelchair accessory, shoulder elbow, mobile arm support, monosuspension arm and hand support, overhead elbow forearm hand sling support, yoke type suspension support  Y & (NU,RR,UE)

**E2631** Wheelchair accessory, addition to mobile arm support, elevating proximal arm  Y & (NU,RR,UE)

**E2632** Wheelchair accessory, addition to mobile arm support, offset or lateral rocker arm with elastic balance control  Y & (NU,RR,UE)

**E2633** Wheelchair accessory, addition to mobile arm support, supinator  Y & (NU,RR,UE)

## Gait Trainer

**E8000** Gait trainer, pediatric size, posterior support, includes all accessories and components  E

**E8001** Gait trainer, pediatric size, upright support, includes all accessories and components  E

**E8002** Gait trainer, pediatric size, anterior support, includes all accessories and components  E

---

Special Coverage Instructions   Noncovered by Medicare   Carrier Discretion   ☑ Quantity Alert  ● New Code   ○ Recycled/Reinstated  ▲ Revised Code

40 — E Codes          A Age Edit   M Maternity Edit   ♀ Female Only   ♂ Male Only   A-Y OPPS Status Indicators          © 2016 Optum360, LLC

## Procedures/Professional Services (Temporary) G0008-G9686

The G codes are used to identify professional health care procedures and services that would otherwise be coded in CPT but for which there are no CPT codes. Please refer to your CPT book for possible alternate code(s).

### Immunization Administration

**G0008** **Administration of influenza virus vaccine** Ⓢ
CMS: 100-02,12,40.11; 100-02,15,50.4.4.2; 100-04,18,10.2.1;
100-04,18,10.2.2.1; 100-04,18,10.2.5.2; 100-04,18,10.3.1.1; 100-04,18,10.4;
100-04,18,10.4.1; 100-04,18,10.4.2; 100-04,18,10.4.3
AHA: 2Q, '09, 1; 2Q, '06, 5; 2Q, '03, 7

**G0009** **Administration of pneumococcal vaccine** Ⓢ
CMS: 100-02,12,40.11; 100-02,15,50.4.4.2; 100-04,18,10.2.1;
100-04,18,10.2.2.1; 100-04,18,10.3.1.1; 100-04,18,10.4; 100-04,18,10.4.1;
100-04,18,10.4.2; 100-04,18,10.4.3
AHA: 2Q, '09, 1; 2Q, '03, 7

**G0010** **Administration of hepatitis B vaccine** Ⓢ
CMS: 100-02,12,40.11; 100-02,15,50.4.4.2; 100-04,18,10.2.1;
100-04,18,10.2.2.1; 100-04,18,10.3.1.1

### Semen Analysis

**G0027** **Semen analysis; presence and/or motility of sperm excluding Huhner** ♂ Ⓠ

### Screening Services

**G0101** **Cervical or vaginal cancer screening; pelvic and clinical breast examination** Ⓐ ♀ Ⓥ ⊘
G0101 can be reported with an E/M code when a separately identifiable E/M service was provided.
CMS: 100-03,210.2
AHA: 4Q, '02, 8; 3Q, '01, 6; 3Q, '01, 3

**G0102** **Prostate cancer screening; digital rectal examination** ♂ Ⓝ ⊘

**G0103** **Prostate cancer screening; prostate specific antigen test (PSA)** ♂ Ⓐ

**G0104** **Colorectal cancer screening; flexible sigmoidoscopy** Ⓣ ⒫3 ⊘
Medicare covers colorectal screening for cancer via flexible sigmoidoscopy once every four years for patients 50 years or older.
CMS: 100-02,15,280.2.2; 100-04,18,60; 100-04,18,60.1; 100-04,18,60.1.1;
100-04,18,60.2; 100-04,18,60.2.1; 100-04,18,60.6; 100-04,18,60.7
AHA: 2Q, '09, 1

**G0105** **Colorectal cancer screening; colonoscopy on individual at high risk** Ⓣ ⒜2 ⊘
An individual with ulcerative enteritis or a history of a malignant neoplasm of the lower gastrointestinal tract is considered at high-risk for colorectal cancer, as defined by CMS.
CMS: 100-02,15,280.2.2; 100-04,18,60; 100-04,18,60.1; 100-04,18,60.1.1;
100-04,18,60.2; 100-04,18,60.2.1; 100-04,18,60.6; 100-04,18,60.7;
100-04,18,60.8
AHA: 2Q, '09, 1

**G0106** **Colorectal cancer screening; alternative to G0104, screening sigmoidoscopy, barium enema** Ⓢ
CMS: 100-02,15,280.2.2; 100-04,18,60; 100-04,18,60.1; 100-04,18,60.1.1;
100-04,18,60.2; 100-04,18,60.2.1; 100-04,18,60.6; 100-04,18,60.7
AHA: 2Q, '09, 1

**G0108** **Diabetes outpatient self-management training services, individual, per 30 minutes** Ⓐ ☑ ⊘
CMS: 100-02,15,300; 100-02,15,300.2; 100-02,15,300.3; 100-02,15,300.4;
100-04,12*; 100-04,12,190.3; 100-04,12,190.3.6; 100-04,12,190.7;
100-04,18,120.1; 100-04,4,300.6; 100-04,9,181

**G0109** **Diabetes outpatient self-management training services, group session (2 or more), per 30 minutes** Ⓐ ☑ ⊘
CMS: 100-02,15,300.2; 100-04,12*; 100-04,12,190.3; 100-04,12,190.3.6;
100-04,12,190.7; 100-04,4,300.6; 100-04,9,181

**G0117** **Glaucoma screening for high risk patients furnished by an optometrist or ophthalmologist** Ⓢ ⊘
CMS: 100-02,15,280.1; 100-04,18,70.1.1
AHA: 1Q, '02, 5; 1Q, '02, 4; 3Q, '01, 12

**G0118** **Glaucoma screening for high risk patient furnished under the direct supervision of an optometrist or ophthalmologist** Ⓢ ⊘
CMS: 100-02,15,280.1; 100-04,18,70.1.1
AHA: 1Q, '02, 5; 1Q, '02, 4; 3Q, '01, 12

**G0120** **Colorectal cancer screening; alternative to G0105, screening colonoscopy, barium enema** Ⓢ
CMS: 100-02,15,280.2.2; 100-04,18,60; 100-04,18,60.1; 100-04,18,60.1.1;
100-04,18,60.2; 100-04,18,60.2.1; 100-04,18,60.6; 100-04,18,60.7;
100-04,18,60.8

**G0121** **Colorectal cancer screening; colonoscopy on individual not meeting criteria for high risk** Ⓣ ⒜2 ⊘
CMS: 100-02,15,280.2.2; 100-04,18,60; 100-04,18,60.1; 100-04,18,60.1.1;
100-04,18,60.2; 100-04,18,60.2.1; 100-04,18,60.6
AHA: 3Q, '01, 12

**G0122** **Colorectal cancer screening; barium enema** Ⓔ
CMS: 100-04,18,60; 100-04,18,60.2; 100-04,18,60.2.1; 100-04,18,60.6;
100-04,18,60.7; 100-04,18,60.8

**G0123** **Screening cytopathology, cervical or vaginal (any reporting system), collected in preservative fluid, automated thin layer preparation, screening by cytotechnologist under physician supervision** Ⓐ ♀ Ⓐ
See also P3000-P3001.
CMS: 100-03,210.2.1; 100-04,18,30.2.1; 100-04,18,30.5; 100-04,18,30.6

**G0124** **Screening cytopathology, cervical or vaginal (any reporting system), collected in preservative fluid, automated thin layer preparation, requiring interpretation by physician** Ⓐ ♀ Ⓑ ⊘
See also P3000-P3001.
CMS: 100-03,210.2.1; 100-04,18,30.2.1; 100-04,18,30.5; 100-04,18,30.6

### Miscellaneous Services

**G0127** **Trimming of dystrophic nails, any number** ⓪1 ⊘
CMS: 100-02,15,290

**G0128** **Direct (face-to-face with patient) skilled nursing services of a registered nurse provided in a comprehensive outpatient rehabilitation facility, each 10 minutes beyond the first 5 minutes** Ⓑ ☑ ⊘
CMS: 100-02,12,30.1; 100-02,12,40.8; 100-04,5,100.3; 100-04,5,20.4

**G0129** **Occupational therapy services requiring the skills of a qualified occupational therapist, furnished as a component of a partial hospitalization treatment program, per session (45 minutes or more)** Ⓟ ☑
AHA: 4Q, '12, 11-14

**G0130** **Single energy x-ray absorptiometry (SEXA) bone density study, one or more sites; appendicular skeleton (peripheral) (e.g., radius, wrist, heel)** Ⓢ ⓩ3
CMS: 100-04,13,30.1.3.1

**G0141** **Screening cytopathology smears, cervical or vaginal, performed by automated system, with manual rescreening, requiring interpretation by physician** Ⓐ ♀ Ⓑ ⊘
CMS: 100-03,210.2.1; 100-04,18,30.2.1; 100-04,18,30.5; 100-04,18,30.6

**G0143** **Screening cytopathology, cervical or vaginal (any reporting system), collected in preservative fluid, automated thin layer preparation, with manual screening and rescreening by cytotechnologist under physician supervision** Ⓐ ♀ Ⓐ
CMS: 100-03,210.2.1; 100-04,18,30.2.1; 100-04,18,30.5; 100-04,18,30.6

Special Coverage Instructions    Noncovered by Medicare    Carrier Discretion    ☑ Quantity Alert    ● New Code    ○ Recycled/Reinstated    ▲ Revised Code

© 2016 Optum360, LLC    ⒜2-ⓩ3 ASC Pmt    CMS: Pub 100    AHA: Coding Clinic    ⓺ DMEPOS Paid    ⊘ SNF Excluded    G Codes — 41

**G0144**  Screening cytopathology, cervical or vaginal (any reporting system), collected in preservative fluid, automated thin layer preparation, with screening by automated system, under physician supervision  Ⓐ ♀Ⓐ
CMS: 100-03,210.2.1; 100-04,18,30.2.1; 100-04,18,30.5; 100-04,18,30.6

**G0145**  Screening cytopathology, cervical or vaginal (any reporting system), collected in preservative fluid, automated thin layer preparation, with screening by automated system and manual rescreening under physician supervision  Ⓐ ♀Ⓐ
CMS: 100-03,210.2.1; 100-04,18,30.2.1; 100-04,18,30.5; 100-04,18,30.6

**G0147**  Screening cytopathology smears, cervical or vaginal, performed by automated system under physician supervision  Ⓐ ♀Ⓐ
CMS: 100-03,210.2.1; 100-04,18,30.2.1; 100-04,18,30.5; 100-04,18,30.6

**G0148**  Screening cytopathology smears, cervical or vaginal, performed by automated system with manual rescreening  Ⓐ ♀Ⓐ
CMS: 100-03,210.2.1; 100-04,18,30.2.1; 100-04,18,30.5; 100-04,18,30.6

**G0151**  Services performed by a qualified physical therapist in the home health or hospice setting, each 15 minutes  Ⓑ ☑
CMS: 100-04,10,40.2; 100-04,11,10; 100-04,11,30.3

**G0152**  Services performed by a qualified occupational therapist in the home health or hospice setting, each 15 minutes  Ⓑ ☑
CMS: 100-04,10,40.2; 100-04,11,10; 100-04,11,30.3

**G0153**  Services performed by a qualified speech-language pathologist in the home health or hospice setting, each 15 minutes  Ⓑ ☑
CMS: 100-04,10,40.2; 100-04,11,10; 100-04,11,30.3

**G0155**  Services of clinical social worker in home health or hospice settings, each 15 minutes  Ⓑ ☑
CMS: 100-04,10,40.2; 100-04,11,10; 100-04,11,30.3

**G0156**  Services of home health/hospice aide in home health or hospice settings, each 15 minutes  Ⓑ ☑
CMS: 100-04,10,40.2; 100-04,11,10; 100-04,11,30.3

**G0157**  Services performed by a qualified physical therapist assistant in the home health or hospice setting, each 15 minutes  Ⓑ ☑
CMS: 100-04,10,40.2; 100-04,11,10

**G0158**  Services performed by a qualified occupational therapist assistant in the home health or hospice setting, each 15 minutes  Ⓑ ☑
CMS: 100-04,10,40.2; 100-04,11,10

**G0159**  Services performed by a qualified physical therapist, in the home health setting, in the establishment or delivery of a safe and effective physical therapy maintenance program, each 15 minutes  Ⓑ ☑
CMS: 100-04,10,40.2

**G0160**  Services performed by a qualified occupational therapist, in the home health setting, in the establishment or delivery of a safe and effective occupational therapy maintenance program, each 15 minutes  Ⓑ ☑
CMS: 100-04,10,40.2

**G0161**  Services performed by a qualified speech-language pathologist, in the home health setting, in the establishment or delivery of a safe and effective speech-language pathology maintenance program, each 15 minutes  Ⓑ ☑
CMS: 100-04,10,40.2

**G0162**  Skilled services by a registered nurse (RN) for management and evaluation of the plan of care; each 15 minutes (the patient's underlying condition or complication requires an RN to ensure that essential nonskilled care achieves its purpose in the home health or hospice setting)  Ⓑ ☑
CMS: 100-04,10,40.2; 100-04,11,10

**G0163**^Jan  ~~Skilled services of a licensed nurse (LPN or RN) for the observation and assessment of the patient's condition, each 15 minutes (the change in the patient's condition requires skilled nursing personnel to identify and evaluate the patient's need for possible modification of treatment in the home health or hospice setting)~~

**G0164**^Jan  ~~Skilled services of a licensed nurse (LPN or RN), in the training and/or education of a patient or family member, in the home health or hospice setting, each 15 minutes~~

**G0166**  External counterpulsation, per treatment session  Ⓠ ☑ ⃠
CMS: 100-04,32,130; 100-04,32,130.1

**G0168**  Wound closure utilizing tissue adhesive(s) only  Ⓑ ⃠
AHA: 1Q, '05, 5; 4Q, '01, 10; 3Q, '01, 13

**G0175**  Scheduled interdisciplinary team conference (minimum of 3 exclusive of patient care nursing staff) with patient present  Ⓥ
CMS: 100-04,4,160
AHA: 3Q, '01, 6; 3Q, '01, 3

**G0176**  Activity therapy, such as music, dance, art or play therapies not for recreation, related to the care and treatment of patient's disabling mental health problems, per session (45 minutes or more)  Ⓟ
CMS: 100-04,4,260.5
AHA: 4Q, '12, 11-14

**G0177**  Training and educational services related to the care and treatment of patient's disabling mental health problems per session (45 minutes or more)  Ⓝ
CMS: 100-01,3,30; 100-01,3,30.3
AHA: 4Q, '12, 11-14

**G0179**  Physician re-certification for Medicare-covered home health services under a home health plan of care (patient not present), including contacts with home health agency and review of reports of patient status required by physicians to affirm the initial implementation of the plan of care that meets patient's needs, per re-certification period  Ⓜ ⃠
CMS: 100-04,12,180; 100-04,12,180.1

**G0180**  Physician certification for Medicare-covered home health services under a home health plan of care (patient not present), including contacts with home health agency and review of reports of patient status required by physicians to affirm the initial implementation of the plan of care that meets patient's needs, per certification period  Ⓜ ⃠
CMS: 100-04,12,180; 100-04,12,180.1

**G0181**  Physician supervision of a patient receiving Medicare-covered services provided by a participating home health agency (patient not present) requiring complex and multidisciplinary care modalities involving regular physician development and/or revision of care plans, review of subsequent reports of patient status, review of laboratory and other studies, communication (including telephone calls) with other health care professionals involved in the patient's care, integration of new information into the medical treatment plan and/or adjustment of medical therapy, within a calendar month, 30 minutes or more  Ⓜ ⃠
CMS: 100-04,12,180; 100-04,12,180.1
AHA: 2Q, '15, 10

^Jan **January Update**

Special Coverage Instructions   Noncovered by Medicare   Carrier Discretion   ☑ Quantity Alert  ● New Code  ○ Recycled/Reinstated  ▲ Revised Code

42 — G Codes   Ⓐ Age Edit   Ⓜ Maternity Edit   ♀ Female Only   ♂ Male Only   Ⓐ-Ⓨ OPPS Status Indicators   © 2016 Optum360, LLC

**G0182** Physician supervision of a patient under a Medicare-approved hospice (patient not present) requiring complex and multidisciplinary care modalities involving regular physician development and/or revision of care plans, review of subsequent reports of patient status, review of laboratory and other studies, communication (including telephone calls) with other health care professionals involved in the patient's care, integration of new information into the medical treatment plan and/or adjustment of medical therapy, within a calendar month, 30 minutes or more  Ⓜ ⊘

CMS: 100-04,11,40.1.3.1; 100-04,12,180; 100-04,12,180.1
AHA: 2Q, '15, 10

**G0186** Destruction of localized lesion of choroid (for example, choroidal neovascularization); photocoagulation, feeder vessel technique (one or more sessions)  Ⓣ 🄬 ⊘

▲ **G0202**·Jan Screening mammography, bilateral (2-view study of each breast), including computer-aided detection (CAD) when performed  Ⓐ ♀Ⓐ ⊘

CMS: 100-04,18,20; 100-04,18,20.2; 100-04,18,20.2.2; 100-04,18,20.5; 100-04,7,80.2
AHA: 2Q, '03, 5; 1Q, '03, 7; 1Q, '02, 3

▲ **G0204**·Jan Diagnostic mammography, including computer-aided detection (CAD) when performed; bilateral  Ⓐ

CMS: 100-04,18,20; 100-04,18,20.2; 100-04,18,20.2.2; 100-04,18,20.4; 100-04,18,20.5
AHA: 3Q, '13; 2Q, '03, 5; 1Q, '03, 7

▲ **G0206**·Jan Diagnostic mammography, including computer-aided detection (CAD) when performed; unilateral  Ⓐ

CMS: 100-04,18,20; 100-04,18,20.2.2; 100-04,18,20.4; 100-04,18,20.5
AHA: 3Q, '13; 4Q, '10, 4; 2Q, '03, 5; 1Q, '03, 7

**G0219** PET imaging whole body; melanoma for noncovered indications  Ⓔ

CMS: 100-03,220.6.10; 100-03,220.6.12; 100-03,220.6.17; 100-03,220.6.3; 100-03,220.6.4; 100-03,220.6.6; 100-03,220.6.7; 100-04,13,60; 100-04,13,60.16
AHA: 1Q, '02, 5; 1Q, '02, 10; 2Q, '01, 5

**G0235** PET imaging, any site, not otherwise specified  Ⓔ

CMS: 100-03,220.6.10; 100-03,220.6.12; 100-03,220.6.13; 100-03,220.6.17; 100-03,220.6.2; 100-03,220.6.3; 100-03,220.6.4; 100-03,220.6.5; 100-03,220.6.6; 100-03,220.6.7; 100-03,220.6.9; 100-04,13,60; 100-04,13,60.13; 100-04,13,60.14; 100-04,13,60.16; 100-04,13,60.17
AHA: 1Q, '07, 6

**G0237** Therapeutic procedures to increase strength or endurance of respiratory muscles, face-to-face, one-on-one, each 15 minutes (includes monitoring)  🄌 ☑ ⊘

CMS: 100-02,12,30.1; 100-02,12,40.5
AHA: 1Q, '02, 5

**G0238** Therapeutic procedures to improve respiratory function, other than described by G0237, one-on-one, face-to-face, per 15 minutes (includes monitoring)  🄌 ☑

CMS: 100-02,12,30.1; 100-02,12,40.5
AHA: 1Q, '02, 5

**G0239** Therapeutic procedures to improve respiratory function or increase strength or endurance of respiratory muscles, 2 or more individuals (includes monitoring)  🄌

CMS: 100-02,12,30.1; 100-02,12,40.5
AHA: 1Q, '02, 5

**G0245** Initial physician evaluation and management of a diabetic patient with diabetic sensory neuropathy resulting in a loss of protective sensation (LOPS) which must include: (1) the diagnosis of LOPS, (2) a patient history, (3) a physical examination that consists of at least the following elements: (a) visual inspection of the forefoot, hindfoot, and toe web spaces, (b) evaluation of a protective sensation, (c) evaluation of foot structure and biomechanics, (d) evaluation of vascular status and skin integrity, and (e) evaluation and recommendation of footwear, and (4) patient education  Ⓥ ⊘

CMS: 100-04,32,80.2; 100-04,32,80.3; 100-04,32,80.6; 100-04,32,80.8
AHA: 4Q, '02, 9-10; 3Q, '02, 11

**G0246** Follow-up physician evaluation and management of a diabetic patient with diabetic sensory neuropathy resulting in a loss of protective sensation (LOPS) to include at least the following: (1) a patient history, (2) a physical examination that includes: (a) visual inspection of the forefoot, hindfoot, and toe web spaces, (b) evaluation of protective sensation, (c) evaluation of foot structure and biomechanics, (d) evaluation of vascular status and skin integrity, and (e) evaluation and recommendation of footwear, and (3) patient education  Ⓥ ⊘

CMS: 100-03,70.2.1; 100-04,32,80; 100-04,32,80.2; 100-04,32,80.3; 100-04,32,80.6; 100-04,32,80.8
AHA: 4Q, '02, 9-10; 3Q, '02, 11

**G0247** Routine foot care by a physician of a diabetic patient with diabetic sensory neuropathy resulting in a loss of protective sensation (LOPS) to include the local care of superficial wounds (i.e., superficial to muscle and fascia) and at least the following, if present: (1) local care of superficial wounds, (2) debridement of corns and calluses, and (3) trimming and debridement of nails  🄌 ⊘

CMS: 100-03,70.2.1; 100-04,32,80; 100-04,32,80.2; 100-04,32,80.3; 100-04,32,80.6; 100-04,32,80.8
AHA: 4Q, '02, 9-10; 3Q, '02, 11

**G0248** Demonstration, prior to initiation of home INR monitoring, for patient with either mechanical heart valve(s), chronic atrial fibrillation, or venous thromboembolism who meets Medicare coverage criteria, under the direction of a physician; includes: face-to-face demonstration of use and care of the INR monitor, obtaining at least one blood sample, provision of instructions for reporting home INR test results, and documentation of patient's ability to perform testing and report results  Ⓥ

CMS: 100-03,190.11; 100-04,32,60.4.1; 100-04,32,80
AHA: 4Q, '02, 9-10; 3Q, '02, 11

**G0249** Provision of test materials and equipment for home INR monitoring of patient with either mechanical heart valve(s), chronic atrial fibrillation, or venous thromboembolism who meets Medicare coverage criteria; includes: provision of materials for use in the home and reporting of test results to physician; testing not occurring more frequently than once a week; testing materials, billing units of service include 4 tests  Ⓥ ☑

CMS: 100-03,190.11; 100-04,32,60.4.1
AHA: 4Q, '02, 9-10; 3Q, '02, 11

**G0250** Physician review, interpretation, and patient management of home INR testing for patient with either mechanical heart valve(s), chronic atrial fibrillation, or venous thromboembolism who meets Medicare coverage criteria; testing not occurring more frequently than once a week; billing units of service include 4 tests  Ⓜ ☑ ⊘

CMS: 100-03,190.11; 100-04,32,60.4.1
AHA: 4Q, '02, 9-10; 3Q, '02, 11

**G0252** PET imaging, full and partial-ring PET scanners only, for initial diagnosis of breast cancer and/or surgical planning for breast cancer (e.g., initial staging of axillary lymph nodes)  Ⓔ

CMS: 100-03,220.6.10; 100-03,220.6.3; 100-04,13,60; 100-04,13,60.16
AHA: 1Q, '07, 6; 4Q, '02, 9-10

---

Jan **January Update**

Special Coverage Instructions    Noncovered by Medicare    Carrier Discretion    ☑ Quantity Alert  ● New Code    ○ Recycled/Reinstated    ▲ Revised Code

© 2016 Optum360, LLC    🄐-🅉 ASC Pmt    CMS: Pub 100    AHA: Coding Clinic    ⅄ DMEPOS Paid    ⊘ SNF Excluded    **G Codes — 43**

**G0255** Current perception threshold/sensory nerve conduction test, (SNCT) per limb, any nerve ☐E
AHA: 4Q, '02, 9-10

**G0257** Unscheduled or emergency dialysis treatment for an ESRD patient in a hospital outpatient department that is not certified as an ESRD facility ☐S
CMS: 100-04,4,200.2; 100-04,8,60.4.7
AHA: 3Q, '14, 4; 1Q, '03, 7; 4Q, '02, 9-10

**G0259** Injection procedure for sacroiliac joint; arthrography ☐N
AHA: 4Q, '02, 9-10

**G0260** Injection procedure for sacroiliac joint; provision of anesthetic, steroid and/or other therapeutic agent, with or without arthrography ☐T ☐A2
AHA: 4Q, '02, 9-10

**G0268** Removal of impacted cerumen (one or both ears) by physician on same date of service as audiologic function testing ☐N ⊘
AHA: 2Q, '16; 1Q, '03, 11

**G0269** Placement of occlusive device into either a venous or arterial access site, postsurgical or interventional procedure (e.g., angioseal plug, vascular plug) ☐N ⊘
AHA: 4Q, '12, 10; 3Q, '11, 3; 4Q, '10, 6

**G0270** Medical nutrition therapy; reassessment and subsequent intervention(s) following second referral in same year for change in diagnosis, medical condition or treatment regimen (including additional hours needed for renal disease), individual, face-to-face with the patient, each 15 minutes ☐A ☑ ⊘
CMS: 100-02,15,270.2; 100-04,12*; 100-04,12,190.3; 100-04,12,190.7; 100-04,9,182

**G0271** Medical nutrition therapy, reassessment and subsequent intervention(s) following second referral in same year for change in diagnosis, medical condition, or treatment regimen (including additional hours needed for renal disease), group (2 or more individuals), each 30 minutes ☐A ☑ ⊘
CMS: 100-04,9,182

**G0276** Blinded procedure for lumbar stenosis, percutaneous image-guided lumbar decompression (PILD) or placebo-control, performed in an approved coverage with evidence development (CED) clinical trial ☐J ☐G2
CMS: 100-04,32,330.1; 100-04,32,330.2

**G0277** Hyperbaric oxygen under pressure, full body chamber, per 30 minute interval ☐S
AHA: 3Q, '15, 7

**G0278** Iliac and/or femoral artery angiography, nonselective, bilateral or ipsilateral to catheter insertion, performed at the same time as cardiac catheterization and/or coronary angiography, includes positioning or placement of the catheter in the distal aorta or ipsilateral femoral or iliac artery, injection of dye, production of permanent images, and radiologic supervision and interpretation (List separately in addition to primary procedure) ☐N ⊘
AHA: 3Q, '11, 3; 4Q, '06, 8

**G0279** Diagnostic digital breast tomosynthesis, unilateral or bilateral (List separately in addition to G0204 or G0206) ☐A
CMS: 100-04,18,20.2; 100-04,18,20.2.2

**G0281** Electrical stimulation, (unattended), to one or more areas, for chronic Stage III and Stage IV pressure ulcers, arterial ulcers, diabetic ulcers, and venous stasis ulcers not demonstrating measurable signs of healing after 30 days of conventional care, as part of a therapy plan of care ☐A
CMS: 100-04,32,11.1
AHA: 2Q, '03, 7; 1Q, '03, 7

**G0282** Electrical stimulation, (unattended), to one or more areas, for wound care other than described in G0281 ☐E
CMS: 100-04,32,11.1
AHA: 2Q, '03, 7; 1Q, '03, 7

**G0283** Electrical stimulation (unattended), to one or more areas for indication(s) other than wound care, as part of a therapy plan of care ☐A
AHA: 2Q, '09, 1; 2Q, '03, 7; 1Q, '03, 7

**G0288** Reconstruction, computed tomographic angiography of aorta for surgical planning for vascular surgery ☐N

**G0289** Arthroscopy, knee, surgical, for removal of loose body, foreign body, debridement/shaving of articular cartilage (chondroplasty) at the time of other surgical knee arthroscopy in a different compartment of the same knee ☐N ⊘
AHA: 2Q, '03, 9

**G0293** Noncovered surgical procedure(s) using conscious sedation, regional, general, or spinal anesthesia in a Medicare qualifying clinical trial, per day ☐01 ☑
AHA: 4Q, '02, 9-10

**G0294** Noncovered procedure(s) using either no anesthesia or local anesthesia only, in a Medicare qualifying clinical trial, per day ☐01 ☑
AHA: 4Q, '02, 9-10

**G0295** Electromagnetic therapy, to one or more areas, for wound care other than described in G0329 or for other uses ☐E
AHA: 1Q, '03, 7

**G0296** Counseling visit to discuss need for lung cancer screening using low dose CT scan (LDCT) (service is for eligibility determination and shared decision making) ☐S
CMS: 100-04,18,220; 100-04,18,220.1; 100-04,18,220.2; 100-04,18,220.3; 100-04,18,220.5

**G0297** Low dose CT scan (LDCT) for lung cancer screening ☐S
CMS: 100-04,18,220; 100-04,18,220.1; 100-04,18,220.2; 100-04,18,220.3; 100-04,18,220.5

**G0299** Direct skilled nursing services of a registered nurse (RN) in the home health or hospice setting, each 15 minutes ☐B
CMS: 100-04,10,40.2; 100-04,11,30.3

**G0300** Direct skilled nursing services of a licensed practical nurse (lpn) in the home health or hospice setting, each 15 minutes ☐B
CMS: 100-04,10,40.2; 100-04,11,30.3

**G0302** Preoperative pulmonary surgery services for preparation for LVRS, complete course of services, to include a minimum of 16 days of services ☐S ☑

**G0303** Preoperative pulmonary surgery services for preparation for LVRS, 10 to 15 days of services ☐S ☑

**G0304** Preoperative pulmonary surgery services for preparation for LVRS, 1 to 9 days of services ☐S ☑

**G0305** Postdischarge pulmonary surgery services after LVRS, minimum of 6 days of services ☐S ☑

**G0306** Complete CBC, automated (HgB, HCT, RBC, WBC, without platelet count) and automated WBC differential count ☐Q
CMS: 100-02,11,20.2

**G0307** Complete (CBC), automated (HgB, Hct, RBC, WBC; without platelet count) ☐Q
CMS: 100-02,11,20.2

**G0328** Colorectal cancer screening; fecal occult blood test, immunoassay, 1-3 simultaneous determinations ☐A
CMS: 100-02,15,280.2.2; 100-04,16,70.8; 100-04,18,60; 100-04,18,60.1; 100-04,18,60.1.1; 100-04,18,60.2; 100-04,18,60.2.1; 100-04,18,60.6; 100-04,18,60.7
AHA: 2Q, '12, 9

Special Coverage Instructions    Noncovered by Medicare    Carrier Discretion    ☑ Quantity Alert  ● New Code    ○ Recycled/Reinstated  ▲ Revised Code

44 — G Codes        ☐A Age Edit   ☐M Maternity Edit   ♀ Female Only   ♂ Male Only   ☐A-Y OPPS Status Indicators        © 2016 Optum360, LLC

**G0329** Electromagnetic therapy, to one or more areas for chronic Stage III and Stage IV pressure ulcers, arterial ulcers, diabetic ulcers and venous stasis ulcers not demonstrating measurable signs of healing after 30 days of conventional care as part of a therapy plan of care Ⓐ
CMS: 100-04,32,11.2

**G0333** Pharmacy dispensing fee for inhalation drug(s); initial 30-day supply as a beneficiary Ⓜ

**G0337** Hospice evaluation and counseling services, preelection Ⓑ
CMS: 100-04,11,10; 100-04,11,10.1

**G0339** Image guided robotic linear accelerator-based stereotactic radiosurgery, complete course of therapy in one session or first session of fractionated treatment Ⓑ⊘
AHA: 4Q, '13; 1Q, '04, 6

**G0340** Image guided robotic linear accelerator-based stereotactic radiosurgery, delivery including collimator changes and custom plugging, fractionated treatment, all lesions, per session, second through fifth sessions, maximum 5 sessions per course of treatment Ⓑ⊘
AHA: 4Q, '13; 1Q, '04, 6

**G0341** Percutaneous islet cell transplant, includes portal vein catheterization and infusion Ⓒ⊘
CMS: 100-04,32,70

**G0342** Laparoscopy for islet cell transplant, includes portal vein catheterization and infusion Ⓒ⊘
CMS: 100-04,32,70

**G0343** Laparotomy for islet cell transplant, includes portal vein catheterization and infusion Ⓒ⊘
CMS: 100-04,32,70

**G0364** Bone marrow aspiration performed with bone marrow biopsy through the same incision on the same date of service Ⓝ⊘
AHA: 3Q, '12, 6

**G0365** Vessel mapping of vessels for hemodialysis access (services for preoperative vessel mapping prior to creation of hemodialysis access using an autogenous hemodialysis conduit, including arterial inflow and venous outflow) Ⓢ P2

**G0372** Physician service required to establish and document the need for a power mobility device Ⓜ⊘
CMS: 100-04,12,30.6.15.4

## Observation/Emergency Department Services

**G0378** Hospital observation service, per hour Ⓝ
CMS: 100-02,6,20.6; 100-04,01,50.3.2; 100-04,4,290.1; 100-04,4,290.2.2; 100-04,4,290.4.1; 100-04,4,290.4.2; 100-04,4,290.4.3; 100-04,4,290.5.1; 100-04,4,290.5.2; 100-04,4,290.5.3
AHA: 4Q, '05, 7, 9

**G0379** Direct admission of patient for hospital observation care Ⓙ
CMS: 100-02,6,20.6; 100-04,4,290.4.1; 100-04,4,290.4.2; 100-04,4,290.4.3; 100-04,4,290.5.1; 100-04,4,290.5.2; 100-04,4,290.5.3
AHA: 4Q, '05, 7, 9

**G0380** Level 1 hospital emergency department visit provided in a type B emergency department; (the ED must meet at least one of the following requirements: (1) it is licensed by the state in which it is located under applicable state law as an emergency room or emergency department; (2) it is held out to the public (by name, posted signs, advertising, or other means) as a place that provides care for emergency medical conditions on an urgent basis without requiring a previously scheduled appointment; or (3) during the calendar year immediately preceding the calendar year in which a determination under 42 CFR 489.24 is being made, based on a representative sample of patient visits that occurred during that calendar year, it provides at least one-third of all of its outpatient visits for the treatment of emergency medical conditions on an urgent basis without requiring a previously scheduled appointment) Ⓙ
CMS: 100-04,4,160
AHA: 4Q, '13; 1Q, '09, 1; 4Q, '07, 1

**G0381** Level 2 hospital emergency department visit provided in a type B emergency department; (the ED must meet at least one of the following requirements: (1) it is licensed by the state in which it is located under applicable state law as an emergency room or emergency department; (2) it is held out to the public (by name, posted signs, advertising, or other means) as a place that provides care for emergency medical conditions on an urgent basis without requiring a previously scheduled appointment; or (3) during the calendar year immediately preceding the calendar year in which a determination under 42 CFR 489.24 is being made, based on a representative sample of patient visits that occurred during that calendar year, it provides at least one-third of all of its outpatient visits for the treatment of emergency medical conditions on an urgent basis without requiring a previously scheduled appointment) Ⓙ
CMS: 100-04,4,160
AHA: 4Q, '13; 1Q, '09, 1; 4Q, '07, 1

**G0382** Level 3 hospital emergency department visit provided in a type B emergency department; (the ED must meet at least one of the following requirements: (1) it is licensed by the state in which it is located under applicable state law as an emergency room or emergency department; (2) it is held out to the public (by name, posted signs, advertising, or other means) as a place that provides care for emergency medical conditions on an urgent basis without requiring a previously scheduled appointment; or (3) during the calendar year immediately preceding the calendar year in which a determination under 42 CFR 489.24 is being made, based on a representative sample of patient visits that occurred during that calendar year, it provides at least one-third of all of its outpatient visits for the treatment of emergency medical conditions on an urgent basis without requiring a previously scheduled appointment) Ⓙ
CMS: 100-04,4,160
AHA: 4Q, '13; 1Q, '09, 1; 4Q, '07, 1

**G0383** Level 4 hospital emergency department visit provided in a type B emergency department; (the ED must meet at least one of the following requirements: (1) it is licensed by the state in which it is located under applicable state law as an emergency room or emergency department; (2) it is held out to the public (by name, posted signs, advertising, or other means) as a place that provides care for emergency medical conditions on an urgent basis without requiring a previously scheduled appointment; or (3) during the calendar year immediately preceding the calendar year in which a determination under 42 CFR 489.24 is being made, based on a representative sample of patient visits that occurred during that calendar year, it provides at least one-third of all of its outpatient visits for the treatment of emergency medical conditions on an urgent basis without requiring a previously scheduled appointment) Ⓙ
CMS: 100-04,4,160
AHA: 4Q, '13; 1Q, '09, 1; 4Q, '07, 1

**G0384** Level 5 hospital emergency department visit provided in a type B emergency department; (the ED must meet at least one of the following requirements: (1) it is licensed by the state in which it is located under applicable state law as an emergency room or emergency department; (2) it is held out to the public (by name, posted signs, advertising, or other means) as a place that provides care for emergency medical conditions on an urgent basis without requiring a previously scheduled appointment; or (3) during the calendar year immediately preceding the calendar year in which a determination under 42 CFR 489.24 is being made, based on a representative sample of patient visits that occurred during that calendar year, it provides at least one-third of all of its outpatient visits for the treatment of emergency medical conditions on an urgent basis without requiring a previously scheduled appointment) J
**CMS:** 100-04,4,160; 100-04,4,290.5.1
**AHA:** 4Q, '13; 1Q, '09, 1; 4Q, '07, 1

## Other Services

**G0389**[Jan] ~~Ultrasound B-scan and/or real time with image documentation; for abdominal aortic aneurysm (AAA) screening~~

**G0390** Trauma response team associated with hospital critical care service S
**CMS:** 100-04,4,160.1

## Alcohol or Substance Abuse

**G0396** Alcohol and/or substance (other than tobacco) abuse structured assessment (e.g., AUDIT, DAST), and brief intervention 15 to 30 minutes S ☑ ⊘
**CMS:** 100-02,15,270.2; 100-04,12*; 100-04,12,190.3; 100-04,12,190.7; 100-04,4,200.6

**G0397** Alcohol and/or substance (other than tobacco) abuse structured assessment (e.g., AUDIT, DAST), and intervention, greater than 30 minutes S ☑ ⊘
**CMS:** 100-02,15,270.2; 100-04,12*; 100-04,12,190.3; 100-04,12,190.7; 100-04,4,200.6

## Home Sleep Study

**G0398** Home sleep study test (HST) with type II portable monitor, unattended; minimum of 7 channels: EEG, EOG, EMG, ECG/heart rate, airflow, respiratory effort and oxygen saturation S
**CMS:** 100-03,240.4
**AHA:** 3Q, '08, 5

**G0399** Home sleep test (HST) with type III portable monitor, unattended; minimum of 4 channels: 2 respiratory movement/airflow, 1 ECG/heart rate and 1 oxygen saturation S
**CMS:** 100-03,240.4
**AHA:** 3Q, '08, 5

**G0400** Home sleep test (HST) with type IV portable monitor, unattended; minimum of 3 channels S
**CMS:** 100-03,240.4
**AHA:** 3Q, '08, 5

## Initial Physical Exam

**G0402** Initial preventive physical examination; face-to-face visit, services limited to new beneficiary during the first 12 months of Medicare enrollment V ⊘
**CMS:** 100-04,12,100.1.1; 100-04,12,80.1; 100-04,18,140.6; 100-04,18,80; 100-04,18,80.1; 100-04,18,80.2; 100-04,18,80.3.3; 100-04,18,80.4; 100-04,9,150
**AHA:** 4Q, '09, 7

**G0403** Electrocardiogram, routine ECG with 12 leads; performed as a screening for the initial preventive physical examination with interpretation and report M
**CMS:** 100-04,12,80.1; 100-04,18,80; 100-04,18,80.1; 100-04,18,80.2

**G0404** Electrocardiogram, routine ECG with 12 leads; tracing only, without interpretation and report, performed as a screening for the initial preventive physical examination S
**CMS:** 100-04,12,80.1; 100-04,18,80; 100-04,18,80.1; 100-04,18,80.2; 100-04,18,80.3.3

**G0405** Electrocardiogram, routine ECG with 12 leads; interpretation and report only, performed as a screening for the initial preventive physical examination B ⊘
**CMS:** 100-04,12,80.1; 100-04,18,80; 100-04,18,80.1; 100-04,18,80.2

## Follow-up Telehealth

**G0406** Follow-up inpatient consultation, limited, physicians typically spend 15 minutes communicating with the patient via telehealth B ⊘
**CMS:** 100-02,15,270.2; 100-04,12*; 100-04,12,190.3; 100-04,12,190.3.1; 100-04,12,190.3.3; 100-04,12,190.3.5; 100-04,12,190.7

**G0407** Follow-up inpatient consultation, intermediate, physicians typically spend 25 minutes communicating with the patient via telehealth B ⊘
**CMS:** 100-02,15,270.2; 100-04,12*; 100-04,12,190.3; 100-04,12,190.3.1; 100-04,12,190.3.3; 100-04,12,190.3.5; 100-04,12,190.7

**G0408** Follow-up inpatient consultation, complex, physicians typically spend 35 minutes communicating with the patient via telehealth B ⊘
**CMS:** 100-02,15,270.2; 100-04,12*; 100-04,12,190.3; 100-04,12,190.3.1; 100-04,12,190.3.3; 100-04,12,190.3.5; 100-04,12,190.7

## Psychological Services

**G0409** Social work and psychological services, directly relating to and/or furthering the patient's rehabilitation goals, each 15 minutes, face-to-face; individual (services provided by a CORF qualified social worker or psychologist in a CORF) B ☑
**CMS:** 100-02,12,30.1; 100-04,5,100.11; 100-04,5,100.4

**G0410** Group psychotherapy other than of a multiple-family group, in a partial hospitalization setting, approximately 45 to 50 minutes P
**AHA:** 4Q, '12, 11-14; 4Q, '09, 9

**G0411** Interactive group psychotherapy, in a partial hospitalization setting, approximately 45 to 50 minutes P
**AHA:** 4Q, '12, 11-14; 4Q, '09, 9

## Fracture Care

**G0412** Open treatment of iliac spine(s), tuberosity avulsion, or iliac wing fracture(s), unilateral or bilateral for pelvic bone fracture patterns which do not disrupt the pelvic ring, includes internal fixation, when performed C ⊘

**G0413** Percutaneous skeletal fixation of posterior pelvic bone fracture and/or dislocation, for fracture patterns which disrupt the pelvic ring, unilateral or bilateral, (includes ilium, sacroiliac joint and/or sacrum) T ⊘

**G0414** Open treatment of anterior pelvic bone fracture and/or dislocation for fracture patterns which disrupt the pelvic ring, unilateral or bilateral, includes internal fixation when performed (includes pubic symphysis and/or superior/inferior rami) C ⊘

**G0415** Open treatment of posterior pelvic bone fracture and/or dislocation, for fracture patterns which disrupt the pelvic ring, unilateral or bilateral, includes internal fixation, when performed (includes ilium, sacroiliac joint and/or sacrum) C ⊘

## Surgical Pathology

**G0416** Surgical pathology, gross and microscopic examinations, for prostate needle biopsy, any method ♂ Z
**AHA:** 2Q, '13

---

[Jan] **January Update**

Special Coverage Instructions    Noncovered by Medicare    Carrier Discretion    ☑ Quantity Alert ● New Code    ○ Recycled/Reinstated ▲ Revised Code

**46 — G Codes**    A Age Edit    M Maternity Edit    ♀ Female Only    ♂ Male Only    A-Y OPPS Status Indicators    © 2016 Optum360, LLC

## Educational Services

**G0420**  Face-to-face educational services related to the care of chronic kidney disease; individual, per session, per one hour  Ⓐ ☑ ⊘
CMS: 100-02,15,200; 100-02,15,270.2; 100-02,15,310; 100-02,15,310.1; 100-02,15,310.2; 100-02,15,310.4; 100-02,15,310.5; 100-02,32,20.2; 100-04,12*; 100-04,12,190.3; 100-04,12,190.7

**G0421**  Face-to-face educational services related to the care of chronic kidney disease; group, per session, per one hour  Ⓐ ☑ ⊘
CMS: 100-02,15,200; 100-02,15,270.2; 100-02,15,310; 100-02,15,310.1; 100-02,15,310.2; 100-02,15,310.4; 100-02,15,310.5; 100-02,32,20.2; 100-04,12*; 100-04,12,190.3; 100-04,12,190.7

## Cardiac and Pulmonary Rehabilitation

**G0422**  Intensive cardiac rehabilitation; with or without continuous ECG monitoring with exercise, per session  Ⓢ ☑ ⊘
CMS: 100-02,15,232; 100-04,32,140.2.2.1; 100-04,32,140.2.2.2; 100-04,32,140.3; 100-04,32,140.3.1; 100-08,10,2.2.8; 100-08,15,4.2.8

**G0423**  Intensive cardiac rehabilitation; with or without continuous ECG monitoring; without exercise, per session  Ⓢ ☑ ⊘
CMS: 100-02,15,232; 100-04,32,140.2.2.1; 100-04,32,140.2.2.2; 100-04,32,140.3; 100-04,32,140.3.1; 100-08,10,2.2.8; 100-08,15,4.2.8

**G0424**  Pulmonary rehabilitation, including exercise (includes monitoring), one hour, per session, up to 2 sessions per day  Ⓠ₁ ☑ ⊘
CMS: 100-02,15,231; 100-04,32,140.4; 100-04,32,140.4.1

## Inpatient Telehealth

**G0425**  Telehealth consultation, emergency department or initial inpatient, typically 30 minutes communicating with the patient via telehealth  Ⓑ ☑ ⊘
CMS: 100-02,15,270.2; 100-04,12*; 100-04,12,190.3; 100-04,12,190.3.1; 100-04,12,190.3.2; 100-04,12,190.7

**G0426**  Telehealth consultation, emergency department or initial inpatient, typically 50 minutes communicating with the patient via telehealth  Ⓑ ☑ ⊘
CMS: 100-02,15,270.2; 100-04,12*; 100-04,12,190.3; 100-04,12,190.3.1; 100-04,12,190.3.2; 100-04,12,190.7

**G0427**  Telehealth consultation, emergency department or initial inpatient, typically 70 minutes or more communicating with the patient via telehealth  Ⓑ ☑ ⊘
CMS: 100-02,15,270.2; 100-04,12*; 100-04,12,190.3; 100-04,12,190.3.1; 100-04,12,190.3.2; 100-04,12,190.7

## Defect Fillers

**G0428**  Collagen meniscus implant procedure for filling meniscal defects (e.g., CMI, collagen scaffold, Menaflex)  Ⓔ
CMS: 100-03,150.12

**G0429**  Dermal filler injection(s) for the treatment of facial lipodystrophy syndrome (LDS) (e.g., as a result of highly active antiretroviral therapy)  Ⓑ
CMS: 100-03,250.5; 100-04,32,260.1; 100-04,32,260.2.1; 100-04,32,260.2.2

## Laboratory Services

**G0432**  Infectious agent antibody detection by enzyme immunoassay (EIA) technique, HIV-1 and/or HIV-2, screening  Ⓐ
CMS: 100-03,190.14; 100-03,190.9; 100-03,210.7; 100-04,18,130; 100-04,18,130.1; 100-04,18,130.2; 100-04,18,130.3; 100-04,18,130.4; 100-04,18,130.5

**G0433**  Infectious agent antibody detection by enzyme-linked immunosorbent assay (ELISA) technique, HIV-1 and/or HIV-2, screening  Ⓐ
CMS: 100-03,190.14; 100-03,190.9; 100-03,210.7; 100-04,16,70.8; 100-04,18,130; 100-04,18,130.1; 100-04,18,130.2; 100-04,18,130.3; 100-04,18,130.4; 100-04,18,130.5

**G0435**  Infectious agent antigen detection by rapid antibody test of oral mucosa transudate, HIV-1 or HIV-2, screening  Ⓐ
CMS: 100-03,190.14; 100-03,190.9; 100-03,210.7; 100-04,18,130; 100-04,18,130.1; 100-04,18,130.2; 100-04,18,130.3; 100-04,18,130.4; 100-04,18,130.5

## Counseling and Wellness Visit

**G0436**ᴼᶜᵗ  ~~Smoking and tobacco cessation counseling visit for the asymptomatic patient; intermediate, greater than 3 minutes, up to 10 minutes~~
To report, see ~99406

**G0437**ᴼᶜᵗ  ~~Smoking and tobacco cessation counseling visit for the asymptomatic patient; intensive, greater than 10 minutes~~
To report, see ~99407

**G0438**  Annual wellness visit; includes a personalized prevention plan of service (PPS), initial visit  Ⓐ
CMS: 100-02,15,280.5; 100-02,15,280.5.1; 100-04,12,100.1.1; 100-04,18,140; 100-04,18,140.1; 100-04,18,140.5; 100-04,18,140.6; 100-04,18,140.8

**G0439**  Annual wellness visit, includes a personalized prevention plan of service (PPS), subsequent visit  Ⓐ
CMS: 100-02,15,280.5; 100-02,15,280.5.1; 100-04,12,100.1.1; 100-04,18,140; 100-04,18,140.1; 100-04,18,140.5; 100-04,18,140.6; 100-04,18,140.8

## Other Services

**G0442**  Annual alcohol misuse screening, 15 minutes  Ⓢ ☑
CMS: 100-02,15,270.2; 100-03,210.8; 100-04,12*; 100-04,12,190.3; 100-04,12,190.7; 100-04,18,180; 100-04,18,180.1; 100-04,18,180.2; 100-04,18,180.3; 100-04,18,180.4; 100-04,18,180.5; 100-04,32,180.4; 100-04,32,180.5

**G0443**  Brief face-to-face behavioral counseling for alcohol misuse, 15 minutes  Ⓢ ☑
CMS: 100-02,15,270.2; 100-03,210.8; 100-04,12*; 100-04,12,190.3; 100-04,12,190.7; 100-04,18,180; 100-04,18,180.1; 100-04,18,180.2; 100-04,18,180.3; 100-04,18,180.4; 100-04,18,180.5; 100-04,32,180.4; 100-04,32,180.5

**G0444**  Annual depression screening, 15 minutes  Ⓢ ☑
CMS: 100-02,15,270.2; 100-04,12*; 100-04,12,190.3; 100-04,12,190.7; 100-04,18,190.0; 100-04,18,190.1; 100-04,18,190.2; 100-04,18,190.3

**G0445**  Semiannual high intensity behavioral counseling to prevent STIs, individual, face-to-face, includes education skills training & guidance on how to change sexual behavior  Ⓢ ☑
CMS: 100-02,15,270.2; 100-03,210.10; 100-04,12*; 100-04,12,190.3; 100-04,12,190.7; 100-04,18,170.1; 100-04,18,170.2; 100-04,18,170.3; 100-04,18,170.4; 100-04,18,170.4.1; 100-04,18,170.5

**G0446**  Annual, face-to-face intensive behavioral therapy for cardiovascular disease, individual, 15 minutes  Ⓢ ☑
CMS: 100-02,15,270.2; 100-03,210.11; 100-04,12*; 100-04,12,190.3; 100-04,12,190.7; 100-04,18,160; 100-04,18,160.1; 100-04,18,160.2.1; 100-04,18,160.2.2; 100-04,18,160.3; 100-04,18,160.4; 100-04,18,160.5
AHA: 2Q, '12, 8

**G0447**  Face-to-face behavioral counseling for obesity, 15 minutes  Ⓢ ☑
CMS: 100-02,15,270.2; 100-03,210.12; 100-04,12*; 100-04,12,190.3; 100-04,12,190.7; 100-04,18,200; 100-04,18,200.1; 100-04,18,200.2; 100-04,18,200.3; 100-04,18,200.4; 100-04,18,200.5

**G0448**  Insertion or replacement of a permanent pacing cardioverter-defibrillator system with transvenous lead(s), single or dual chamber with insertion of pacing electrode, cardiac venous system, for left ventricular pacing  Ⓑ

**G0451**  Development testing, with interpretation and report, per standardized instrument form  Ⓣ₃
CMS: 100-01,3,30; 100-01,3,30.3

---

ᴼᶜᵗ **October Update**

Special Coverage Instructions   Noncovered by Medicare   Carrier Discretion   ☑ Quantity Alert   ● New Code   ○ Recycled/Reinstated   ▲ Revised Code

© 2016 Optum360, LLC   Ⓐ₂-Ⓩ₃ ASC Pmt   CMS: Pub 100   AHA: Coding Clinic   ⅋ DMEPOS Paid   ⊘ SNF Excluded   G Codes — 47

## Molecular Pathology

**G0452** Molecular pathology procedure; physician interpretation and report ☐B

## Neurophysiology Monitoring

**G0453** Continuous intraoperative neurophysiology monitoring, from outside the operating room (remote or nearby), per patient, (attention directed exclusively to one patient) each 15 minutes (list in addition to primary procedure) ☐N

## Documentaton and Preparation

**G0454** Physician documentation of face-to-face visit for durable medical equipment determination performed by nurse practitioner, physician assistant or clinical nurse specialist ☐B

**G0455** Preparation with instillation of fecal microbiota by any method, including assessment of donor specimen ☐
AHA: 3Q, '13

## Prostate Brachytherapy

**G0458** Low dose rate (LDR) prostate brachytherapy services, composite rate ♂☐B☐

## Inpatient Telehealth Pharmacologic Management

**G0459** Inpatient telehealth pharmacologic management, including prescription, use, and review of medication with no more than minimal medical psychotherapy ☐B
CMS: 100-02,15,270.2; 100-04,12*; 100-04,12,190.3; 100-04,12,190.7
AHA: 2Q, '13

## Other Wound/Ulcer Care

**G0460** Autologous platelet rich plasma for chronic wounds/ulcers, including phlebotomy, centrifugation, and all other preparatory procedures, administration and dressings, per treatment ☐T
CMS: 100-03,270.3; 100-04,32,11.3.1; 100-04,32,11.3.2; 100-04,32,11.3.3; 100-04,32,11.3.4; 100-04,32,11.3.5; 100-04,32,11.3.6

## Hospital Outpatient Visit

**G0463** Hospital outpatient clinic visit for assessment and management of a patient ☐J
CMS: 100-04,4,290.5.1; 100-04,4,290.5.3; 100-04,6,20.1.1.2
AHA: 4Q, '14, 2

## Federally Qualified Health Center Visits

**G0466** Federally qualified health center (FQHC) visit, new patient ☐A

**G0467** Federally qualified health center (FQHC) visit, established patient ☐A

**G0468** Federally qualified health center (FQHC) visit, initial preventive physical exam (IPPE) or annual wellness visit (AWV) ☐A

**G0469** Federally qualified health center (FQHC) visit, mental health, new patient ☐A

**G0470** Federally qualified health center (FQHC) visit, mental health, established patient ☐A

## HHA and SNF Specimen Collection

**G0471** Collection of venous blood by venipuncture or urine sample by catheterization from an individual in a skilled nursing facility (SNF) or by a laboratory on behalf of a home health agency (HHA) ☐A
CMS: 100-04,16,60.1.4

## Hepatitis C Screening

**G0472** Hepatitis C antibody screening for individual at high risk and other covered indication(s) ☐A
CMS: 100-03,210.13; 100-04,18,210; 100-04,18,210.2; 100-04,18,210.3; 100-04,18,210.4

## Behavioral Counseling

**G0473** Face-to-face behavioral counseling for obesity, group (2-10), 30 minutes ☐S
CMS: 100-04,18,200.1; 100-04,18,200.2; 100-04,18,200.3; 100-04,18,200.4; 100-04,18,200.5

## Screening Measures

**G0475** HIV antigen/antibody, combination assay, screening ☐A
CMS: 100-03,210.7; 100-04,18,130.1; 100-04,18,130.2; 100-04,18,130.3; 100-04,18,130.5

**G0476** Infectious agent detection by nucleic acid (DNA or RNA); human papillomavirus HPV), high-risk types (e.g., 16, 18, 31, 33, 35, 39, 45, 51, 52, 56, 58, 59, 68) for cervical cancer screening, must be performed in addition to pap test ☐A
CMS: 100-03,210.2.1; 100-04,18,30.2.1; 100-04,18,30.5; 100-04,18,30.6

## Drug Testing

**G0477** Drug test(s), presumptive, any number of drug classes; any number of devices or procedures, (e.g., immunoassay) capable of being read by direct optical observation only (e.g., dipsticks, cups, cards, cartridges), includes sample validation when performed, per date of service ☐Q

**G0478** Drug test(s), presumptive, any number of drug classes; any number of devices or procedures, (e.g., immunoassay) read by instrument-assisted direct optical observation (e.g., dipsticks, cups, cards, cartridges), includes sample validation when performed, per date of service ☐Q

**G0479** Drug test(s), presumptive, any number of drug classes; any number of devices or procedures by instrumented chemistry analyzers utilizing immunoassay, enzyme assay, TOF, MALDI, LDTD, DESI, DART, GHPC, GC mass spectrometry), includes sample validation when performed, per date of service ☐Q

**G0480** Drug test(s), definitive, utilizing drug identification methods able to identify individual drugs and distinguish between structural isomers (but not necessarily stereoisomers), including, but not limited to, GC/MS (any type, single or tandem) and LC/MS (any type, single or tandem and excluding immunoassays (e.g., IA, EIA, ELISA, EMIT, FPIA) and enzymatic methods (e.g., alcohol dehydrogenase)); qualitative or quantitative, all sources(s), includes specimen validity testing, per day, 1-7 drug class(es), including metabolite(s) if performed ☐Q

**G0481** Drug test(s), definitive, utilizing drug identification methods able to identify individual drugs and distinguish between structural isomers (but not necessarily stereoisomers), including, but not limited to, GC/MS (any type, single or tandem) and LC/MS (any type, single or tandem and excluding immunoassays (e.g., IA, EIA, ELISA, EMIT, FPIA) and enzymatic methods (e.g., alcohol dehydrogenase)); qualitative or quantitative, all sources(s), includes specimen validity testing, per day, 8-14 drug class(es), including metabolite(s) if performed ☐Q

**G0482** Drug test(s), definitive, utilizing drug identification methods able to identify individual drugs and distinguish between structural isomers (but not necessarily stereoisomers), including, but not limited to, GC/MS (any type, single or tandem) and LC/MS (any type, single or tandem and excluding immunoassays (e.g., IA, EIA, ELISA, EMIT, FPIA) and enzymatic methods (e.g., alcohol dehydrogenase)); qualitative or quantitative, all sources(s), includes specimen validity testing, per day, 15-21 drug class(es), including metabolite(s) if performed ☐Q

Special Coverage Instructions   Noncovered by Medicare   Carrier Discretion   ☑ Quantity Alert ● New Code ○ Recycled/Reinstated ▲ Revised Code

48 — G Codes   ☐ Age Edit   ☐ Maternity Edit   ♀ Female Only   ♂ Male Only   ☐-Ⓨ OPPS Status Indicators   © 2016 Optum360, LLC

**G0483** Drug test(s), definitive, utilizing drug identification methods able to identify individual drugs and distinguish between structural isomers (but not necessarily stereoisomers), including, but not limited to, GC/MS (any type, single or tandem) and LC/MS (any type, single or tandem and excluding immunoassays (e.g., IA, EIA, ELISA, EMIT, FPIA) and enzymatic methods (e.g., alcohol dehydrogenase)); qualitative or quantitative, all sources(s), includes specimen validity testing, per day, 22 or more drug class(es), including metabolite(s) if performed ☒

## Home Health Nursing Visit

● **G0490**<sup>Oct</sup> Face-to-face home health nursing visit by a Rural Health Clinic (RHC) or Federally Qualified Health Center (FQHC) in an area with a shortage of home health agencies (services limited to RN or LPN only) Ⓐ

## Dialysis Procedures

● **G0491**<sup>Jan</sup> Dialysis procedure at a Medicare certified ESRD facility for acute kidney injury without ESRD

● **G0492**<sup>Jan</sup> Dialysis procedure with single evaluation by a physician or other qualified health care professional for acute kidney injury without ESRD

## Skilled Nursing Services

● **G0493**<sup>Jan</sup> Skilled services of a registered nurse (RN) for the observation and assessment of the patient's condition, each 15 minutes (the change in the patient's condition requires skilled nursing personnel to identify and evaluate the patient's need for possible modification of treatment in the home health or hospice setting)

● **G0494**<sup>Jan</sup> Skilled services of a licensed practical nurse (LPN) for the observation and assessment of the patient's condition, each 15 minutes (the change in the patient's condition requires skilled nursing personnel to identify and evaluate the patient's need for possible modification of treatment in the home health or hospice setting)

● **G0495**<sup>Jan</sup> Skilled services of a registered nurse (RN), in the training and/or education of a patient or family member, in the home health or hospice setting, each 15 minutes

● **G0496**<sup>Jan</sup> Skilled services of a licensed practical nurse (LPN), in the training and/or education of a patient or family member, in the home health or hospice setting, each 15 minutes

## Chemotherapy Infusion

● **G0498**<sup>Oct</sup> Chemotherapy administration, intravenous infusion technique; initiation of infusion in the office/clinic setting using office/clinic pump/supplies, with continuation of the infusion in the community setting (e.g., home, domiciliary, rest home or assisted living) using a portable pump provided by the office/clinic, includes follow up office/clinic visit at the conclusion of the infusion

## Hepatitis B Screening

● **G0499**<sup>Jan</sup> Hepatitis B screening in non-pregnant, high risk individual includes hepatitis B surface antigen (HBSAG) followed by a neutralizing confirmatory test for initially reactive results, and antibodies to HBSAG (anti-HBS) and hepatitis B core antigen (anti-HBC)

## Moderate Sedation

● **G0500**<sup>Jan</sup> Moderate sedation services provided by the same physician or other qualified health care professional performing a gastrointestinal endoscopic service that sedation supports, requiring the presence of an independent trained observer to assist in the monitoring of the patient's level of consciousness and physiological status; initial 15 minutes of intra-service time; patient age 5 years or older (additional time may be reported with 99153, as appropriate)

## Mobility-Assistive Technology

● **G0501**<sup>Jan</sup> Resource-intensive services for patients for whom the use of specialized mobility-assistive technology (such as adjustable height chairs or tables, patient lift, and adjustable padded leg supports) is medically necessary and used during the provision of an office/outpatient, evaluation and management visit (list separately in addition to primary service)

## Psychiatric Care Management

● **G0502**<sup>Jan</sup> Initial psychiatric collaborative care management, first 70 minutes in the first calendar month of behavioral health care manager activities, in consultation with a psychiatric consultant, and directed by the treating physician or other qualified health care professional, with the following required elements: outreach to and engagement in treatment of a patient directed by the treating physician or other qualified health care professional; initial assessment of the patient, including administration of validated rating scales, with the development of an individualized treatment plan; review by the psychiatric consultant with modifications of the plan if recommended; entering patient in a registry and tracking patient follow-up and progress using the registry, with appropriate documentation, and participation in weekly caseload consultation with the psychiatric consultant; and provision of brief interventions using evidence-based techniques such as behavioral activation, motivational interviewing, and other focused treatment strategies

● **G0503**<sup>Jan</sup> Subsequent psychiatric collaborative care management, first 60 minutes in a subsequent month of behavioral health care manager activities, in consultation with a psychiatric consultant, and directed by the treating physician or other qualified health care professional, with the following required elements: tracking patient follow-up and progress using the registry, with appropriate documentation; participation in weekly caseload consultation with the psychiatric consultant; ongoing collaboration with and coordination of the patient's mental health care with the treating physician or other qualified health care professional and any other treating mental health providers; additional review of progress and recommendations for changes in treatment, as indicated, including medications, based on recommendations provided by the psychiatric consultant; provision of brief interventions using evidence-based techniques such as behavioral activation, motivational interviewing, and other focused treatment strategies; monitoring of patient outcomes using validated rating scales; and relapse prevention planning with patients as they achieve remission of symptoms and/or other treatment goals and are prepared for discharge from active treatment

● **G0504**<sup>Jan</sup> Initial or subsequent psychiatric collaborative care management, each additional 30 minutes in a calendar month of behavioral health care manager activities, in consultation with a psychiatric consultant, and directed by the treating physician or other qualified health care professional (list separately in addition to code for primary procedure); (use G0504 in conjunction with G0502, G0503)

## Cognitive Impairment

● **G0505**<sup>Jan</sup> Cognition and functional assessment using standardized instruments with development of recorded care plan for the patient with cognitive impairment, history obtained from patient and/or caregiver, in office or other outpatient setting or home or domiciliary or rest home

## Care Management Services

● **G0506**<sup>Jan</sup> Comprehensive assessment of and care planning for patients requiring chronic care management services (list separately in addition to primary monthly care management service)

---

<sup>Jan</sup> **January Update**   <sup>Oct</sup> **October Update**

Special Coverage Instructions   Noncovered by Medicare   Carrier Discretion   ☑ Quantity Alert   ● New Code   ○ Recycled/Reinstated   ▲ Revised Code

© 2016 Optum360, LLC   Ⓑ-Ⓩ ASC Pmt   **CMS:** Pub 100   **AHA:** Coding Clinic   ♿ DMEPOS Paid   ⊘ SNF Excluded

G Codes — 49

● **G0507**[Jan] Care management services for behavioral health conditions, at least 20 minutes of clinical staff time, directed by a physician or other qualified health care professional, per calendar month, with the following required elements: initial assessment or follow-up monitoring, including the use of applicable validated rating scales; behavioral health care planning in relation to behavioral/psychiatric health problems, including revision for patients who are not progressing or whose status changes; facilitating and coordinating treatment such as psychotherapy, pharmacotherapy, counseling and/or psychiatric consultation; and continuity of care with a designated member of the care team

## Telehealth Consultation

● **G0508**[Jan] Telehealth consultation, critical care, initial, physicians typically spend 60 minutes communicating with the patient and providers via telehealth

● **G0509**[Jan] Telehealth consultation, critical care, subsequent, physicians typically spend 50 minutes communicating with the patient and providers via telehealth

## Quality Measures

G0913 Improvement in visual function achieved within 90 days following cataract surgery Ⓜ

G0914 Patient care survey was not completed by patient Ⓜ

G0915 Improvement in visual function not achieved within 90 days following cataract surgery Ⓜ

G0916 Satisfaction with care achieved within 90 days following cataract surgery Ⓜ

G0917 Patient satisfaction survey was not completed by patient Ⓜ

G0918 Satisfaction with care not achieved within 90 days following cataract surgery Ⓜ

## Medication

G3001[Jan] ~~Administration and supply of tositumomab, 450 mg~~

## Radiation Therapy

G6001 Ultrasonic guidance for placement of radiation therapy fields Ⓑ

G6002 Stereoscopic x-ray guidance for localization of target volume for the delivery of radiation therapy Ⓑ

G6003 Radiation treatment delivery, single treatment area, single port or parallel opposed ports, simple blocks or no blocks: up to 5 mev Ⓑ

G6004 Radiation treatment delivery, single treatment area, single port or parallel opposed ports, simple blocks or no blocks: 6-10 mev Ⓑ

G6005 Radiation treatment delivery, single treatment area, single port or parallel opposed ports, simple blocks or no blocks: 11-19 mev Ⓑ

G6006 Radiation treatment delivery, single treatment area, single port or parallel opposed ports, simple blocks or no blocks: 20 mev or greater Ⓑ

G6007 Radiation treatment delivery, 2 separate treatment areas, 3 or more ports on a single treatment area, use of multiple blocks: up to 5 mev Ⓑ

G6008 Radiation treatment delivery, 2 separate treatment areas, 3 or more ports on a single treatment area, use of multiple blocks: 6-10 mev Ⓑ

G6009 Radiation treatment delivery, 2 separate treatment areas, 3 or more ports on a single treatment area, use of multiple blocks: 11-19 mev Ⓑ

G6010 Radiation treatment delivery, 2 separate treatment areas, 3 or more ports on a single treatment area, use of multiple blocks: 20 mev or greater Ⓑ

G6011 Radiation treatment delivery, 3 or more separate treatment areas, custom blocking, tangential ports, wedges, rotational beam, compensators, electron beam; up to 5 mev Ⓑ

G6012 Radiation treatment delivery, 3 or more separate treatment areas, custom blocking, tangential ports, wedges, rotational beam, compensators, electron beam; 6-10 mev Ⓑ

G6013 Radiation treatment delivery, 3 or more separate treatment areas, custom blocking, tangential ports, wedges, rotational beam, compensators, electron beam; 11-19 mev Ⓑ

G6014 Radiation treatment delivery, 3 or more separate treatment areas, custom blocking, tangential ports, wedges, rotational beam, compensators, electron beam; 20 mev or greater Ⓑ

G6015 Intensity modulated treatment delivery, single or multiple fields/arcs, via narrow spatially and temporally modulated beams, binary, dynamic MLC, per treatment session Ⓑ

G6016 Compensator-based beam modulation treatment delivery of inverse planned treatment using 3 or more high resolution (milled or cast) compensator, convergent beam modulated fields, per treatment session Ⓑ

G6017 Intra-fraction localization and tracking of target or patient motion during delivery of radiation therapy (e.g., 3D positional tracking, gating, 3D surface tracking), each fraction of treatment Ⓑ

## Quality Measures

G8395 Left ventricular ejection fraction (LVEF) ≥ 40% or documentation as normal or mildly depressed left ventricular systolic function Ⓜ

G8396 Left ventricular ejection fraction (LVEF) not performed or documented Ⓜ

G8397 Dilated macular or fundus exam performed, including documentation of the presence or absence of macular edema and level of severity of retinopathy Ⓜ

G8398 Dilated macular or fundus exam not performed Ⓜ

G8399 Patient with documented results of a central dual-energy x-ray absorptiometry (DXA) ever being performed Ⓜ

G8400 Patient with central dual-energy x-ray absorptiometry (DXA) results not documented, reason not given Ⓜ

G8401[Jan] ~~Clinician documented that patient was not an eligible candidate for screening~~

G8404 Lower extremity neurological exam performed and documented Ⓜ

G8405 Lower extremity neurological exam not performed Ⓜ

G8410 Footwear evaluation performed and documented Ⓜ

G8415 Footwear evaluation was not performed Ⓜ

G8416 Clinician documented that patient was not an eligible candidate for footwear evaluation measure Ⓜ

G8417 BMI is documented above normal parameters and a follow-up plan is documented Ⓜ

G8418 BMI is documented below normal parameters and a follow-up plan is documented Ⓜ

G8419 BMI documented outside normal parameters, no follow-up plan documented, no reason given Ⓜ

G8420 BMI is documented within normal parameters and no follow-up plan is required Ⓜ

---

**Jan** January Update

Special Coverage Instructions   Noncovered by Medicare   Carrier Discretion   ☑ Quantity Alert   ● New Code   ○ Recycled/Reinstated   ▲ Revised Code

50 — G Codes   Ⓐ Age Edit   Ⓜ Maternity Edit   ♀ Female Only   ♂ Male Only   Ⓐ-Ⓨ OPPS Status Indicators   © 2016 Optum360, LLC

**G8421**   BMI not documented and no reason is given   [M]

**G8422**   BMI not documented, documentation the patient is not eligible for BMI calculation

▲ **G8427**^Jan   Eligible clinician attests to documenting in the medical record they obtained, updated, or reviewed the patient's current medications   [M]

▲ **G8428**^Jan   Current list of medications not documented as obtained, updated, or reviewed by the eligible clinician, reason not given   [M]

▲ **G8430**^Jan   Eligible clinician attests to documenting in the medical record the patient is not eligible for a current list of medications being obtained, updated, or reviewed by the eligible clinician   [M]

▲ **G8431**^Jan   Screening for depression is documented as being positive and a follow-up plan is documented   [M]

▲ **G8432**^Jan   Depression screening not documented, reason not given   [M]

▲ **G8433**^Jan   Screening for depression not completed, documented reason   [M]

**G8442**   Pain assessment not documented as being performed, documentation the patient is not eligible for a pain assessment using a standardized tool   [M]

**G8450**   Beta-blocker therapy prescribed   [M]

**G8451**   Beta-blocker therapy for LVEF < 40% not prescribed for reasons documented by the clinician (e.g., low blood pressure, fluid overload, asthma, patients recently treated with an intravenous positive inotropic agent, allergy, intolerance, other medical reasons, patient declined, other patient reasons, or other reasons attributable to the healthcare system)   [M]

**G8452**   Beta-blocker therapy not prescribed   [M]

~~**G8458**^Jan Clinician documented that patient is not an eligible candidate for genotype testing; patient not receiving antiviral treatment for hepatitis C during the measurement period (e.g., genotype test done prior to the reporting period, patient declines, patient not a candidate for antiviral treatment)~~

~~**G8460**^Jan Clinician documented that patient is not an eligible candidate for quantitative RNA testing at week 12; patient not receiving antiviral treatment for hepatitis C~~

~~**G8461**^Jan Patient receiving antiviral treatment for hepatitis C during the measurement period~~

**G8465**   High or very high risk of recurrence of prostate cancer   [M]

**G8473**   Angiotensin converting enzyme (ACE) inhibitor or angiotensin receptor blocker (ARB) therapy prescribed   [M]

**G8474**   Angiotensin converting enzyme (ACE) inhibitor or angiotensin receptor blocker (ARB) therapy not prescribed for reasons documented by the clinician (e.g., allergy, intolerance, pregnancy, renal failure due to ACE inhibitor, diseases of the aortic or mitral valve, other medical reasons) or (e.g., patient declined, other patient reasons) or (e.g., lack of drug availability, other reasons attributable to the health care system)   [M]

**G8475**   Angiotensin converting enzyme (ACE) inhibitor or angiotensin receptor blocker (ARB) therapy not prescribed, reason not given   [M]

**G8476**   Most recent blood pressure has a systolic measurement of < 140 mm Hg and a diastolic measurement of < 90 mm Hg   [M]

**G8477**   Most recent blood pressure has a systolic measurement of >=140 mm Hg and/or a diastolic measurement of >=90 mm Hg   [M]

**G8478**   Blood pressure measurement not performed or documented, reason not given   [M]

**G8482**   Influenza immunization administered or previously received   [M]

**G8483**   Influenza immunization was not administered for reasons documented by clinician (e.g., patient allergy or other medical reasons, patient declined or other patient reasons, vaccine not available or other system reasons)   [M]

**G8484**   Influenza immunization was not administered, reason not given   [M]

~~**G8485**^Jan I intend to report the diabetes mellitus (DM) measures group~~

~~**G8486**^Jan I intend to report the preventive care measures group~~

~~**G8487**^Jan I intend to report the chronic kidney disease (CKD) measures group~~

~~**G8489**^Jan I intend to report the coronary artery disease (CAD) measures group~~

~~**G8490**^Jan I intend to report the rheumatoid arthritis (RA) measures group~~

~~**G8491**^Jan I intend to report the HIV/AIDS measures group~~

~~**G8494**^Jan All quality actions for the applicable measures in the diabetes mellitus (DM) measures group have been performed for this patient~~

~~**G8495**^Jan All quality actions for the applicable measures in the chronic kidney disease (CKD) measures group have been performed for this patient~~

~~**G8496**^Jan All quality actions for the applicable measures in the preventive care measures group have been performed for this patient~~

~~**G8497**^Jan All quality actions for the applicable measures in the coronary artery bypass graft (CABG) measures group have been performed for this patient~~

~~**G8498**^Jan All quality actions for the applicable measures in the coronary artery disease (CAD) measures group have been performed for this patient~~

~~**G8499**^Jan All quality actions for the applicable measures in the rheumatoid arthritis (RA) measures group have been performed for this patient~~

~~**G8500**^Jan All quality actions for the applicable measures in the HIV/AIDS measures group have been performed for this patient~~

**G8506**   Patient receiving angiotensin converting enzyme (ACE) inhibitor or angiotensin receptor blocker (ARB) therapy   [M]

**G8509**   Pain assessment documented as positive using a standardized tool, follow-up plan not documented, reason not given   [M]

▲ **G8510**^Jan   Screening for depression is documented as negative, a follow-up plan is not required   [M]

▲ **G8511**^Jan   Screening for depression documented as positive, follow-up plan not documented, reason not given   [M]

**G8535**   Elder maltreatment screen not documented; documentation that patient not eligible for the elder maltreatment screen   [M]

**G8536**   No documentation of an elder maltreatment screen, reason not given   [M]

**G8539**   Functional outcome assessment documented as positive using a standardized tool and a care plan based on identified deficiencies on the date of functional outcome assessment, is documented   [M]

**G8540**   Functional outcome assessment not documented as being performed, documentation the patient is not eligible for a functional outcome assessment using a standardized tool   [M]

**G8541**   Functional outcome assessment using a standardized tool, not documented, reason not given   [M]

**G8542**   Functional outcome assessment using a standardized tool is documented; no functional deficiencies identified, care plan not required   [M]

^Jan **January Update**

Special Coverage Instructions    Noncovered by Medicare    Carrier Discretion    ☑ Quantity Alert   ● New Code   ○ Recycled/Reinstated   ▲ Revised Code

© 2016 Optum360, LLC    A2-Z3 ASC Pmt    CMS: Pub 100    AHA: Coding Clinic    ☒ DMEPOS Paid    ⊘ SNF Excluded

**G8543** Documentation of a positive functional outcome assessment using a standardized tool; care plan not documented, reason not given ☒M

**G8544**<sup>Jan</sup> ~~I intend to report the coronary artery bypass graft (CABG) measures group~~

**G8545**<sup>Jan</sup> ~~I intend to report the hepatitis C measures group~~

**G8548**<sup>Jan</sup> ~~I intend to report the heart failure (HF) measures group~~

**G8549**<sup>Jan</sup> ~~All quality actions for the applicable measures in the hepatitis C measures group have been performed for this patient~~

**G8551**<sup>Jan</sup> ~~All quality actions for the applicable measures in the heart failure (HF) measures group have been performed for this patient~~

**G8559** Patient referred to a physician (preferably a physician with training in disorders of the ear) for an otologic evaluation ☒M

**G8560** Patient has a history of active drainage from the ear within the previous 90 days ☒M

**G8561** Patient is not eligible for the referral for otologic evaluation for patients with a history of active drainage measure ☒M

**G8562** Patient does not have a history of active drainage from the ear within the previous 90 days ☒M

**G8563** Patient not referred to a physician (preferably a physician with training in disorders of the ear) for an otologic evaluation, reason not given ☒M

**G8564** Patient was referred to a physician (preferably a physician with training in disorders of the ear) for an otologic evaluation, reason not specified) ☒M

**G8565** Verification and documentation of sudden or rapidly progressive hearing loss ☒M

**G8566** Patient is not eligible for the "referral for otologic evaluation for sudden or rapidly progressive hearing loss" measure ☒M

**G8567** Patient does not have verification and documentation of sudden or rapidly progressive hearing loss ☒M

**G8568** Patient was not referred to a physician (preferably a physician with training in disorders of the ear) for an otologic evaluation, reason not given ☒M

**G8569** Prolonged postoperative intubation (> 24 hrs) required ☒M

**G8570** Prolonged postoperative intubation (> 24 hrs) not required ☒M

**G8571** Development of deep sternal wound infection/mediastinitis within 30 days postoperatively ☒M

**G8572** No deep sternal wound infection/mediastinitis ☒M

**G8573** Stroke following isolated CABG surgery ☒M

**G8574** No stroke following isolated CABG surgery ☒M

**G8575** Developed postoperative renal failure or required dialysis ☒M

**G8576** No postoperative renal failure/dialysis not required ☒M

**G8577** Re-exploration required due to mediastinal bleeding with or without tamponade, graft occlusion, valve dysfunction or other cardiac reason ☒M

**G8578** Re-exploration not required due to mediastinal bleeding with or without tamponade, graft occlusion, valve dysfunction or other cardiac reason ☒M

▲ **G8598**<sup>Jan</sup> Aspirin or another antiplatelet therapy used ☒M

▲ **G8599**<sup>Jan</sup> Aspirin or another antiplatelet therapy not used, reason not given ☒M

**G8600** IV tPA initiated within 3 hours (≤ 180 minutes) of time last known well ☒M

**G8601** IV tPA not initiated within 3 hours (≤ 180 minutes) of time last known well for reasons documented by clinician ☒M

**G8602** IV tPA not initiated within 3 hours (≤ 180 minutes) of time last known well, reason not given ☒M

**G8627** Surgical procedure performed within 30 days following cataract surgery for major complications (e.g., retained nuclear fragments, endophthalmitis, dislocated or wrong power iol, retinal detachment, or wound dehiscence) ☒M

**G8628** Surgical procedure not performed within 30 days following cataract surgery for major complications (e.g., retained nuclear fragments, endophthalmitis, dislocated or wrong power iol, retinal detachment, or wound dehiscence) ☒M

**G8633** Pharmacologic therapy (other than minerals/vitamins) for osteoporosis prescribed ☒M

**G8634**<sup>Jan</sup> ~~Clinician documented patient not an eligible candidate to receive pharmacologic therapy for osteoporosis~~

**G8635** Pharmacologic therapy for osteoporosis was not prescribed, reason not given ☒M

**G8645**<sup>Jan</sup> ~~I intend to report the asthma measures group~~

**G8646**<sup>Jan</sup> ~~All quality actions for the applicable measures in the asthma measures group have been performed for this patient~~

**G8647** Risk-adjusted functional status change residual score for the knee successfully calculated and the score was equal to zero (0) or greater than zero (> 0) ☒M ☑

**G8648** Risk-adjusted functional status change residual score for the knee successfully calculated and the score was less than zero (< 0) ☒M ☑

▲ **G8649**<sup>Jan</sup> Risk-adjusted functional status change residual scores for the knee not measured because the patient did not complete FOTO's status survey near discharge, not appropriate ☒M

**G8650** Risk-adjusted functional status change residual scores for the knee not measured because the patient did not complete FOTO's functional intake on admission and/or follow up status survey near discharge, reason not given ☒M

**G8651** Risk-adjusted functional status change residual score for the hip successfully calculated and the score was equal to zero (0) or greater than zero (> 0) ☒M ☑

**G8652** Risk-adjusted functional status change residual score for the hip successfully calculated and the score was less than zero (< 0) ☒M ☑

▲ **G8653**<sup>Jan</sup> Risk-adjusted functional status change residual scores for the hip not measured because the patient did not complete follow up status survey near discharge, patient not appropriate ☒M

**G8654** Risk-adjusted functional status change residual scores for the hip not measured because the patient did not complete FOTO's functional intake on admission and/or follow up status survey near discharge, reason not given ☒M

▲ **G8655**<sup>Jan</sup> Risk-adjusted functional status change residual score for the foot or ankle successfully calculated and the score was equal to zero (0) or greater than zero ( > 0) ☒M ☑

▲ **G8656**<sup>Jan</sup> Risk-adjusted functional status change residual score for the foot or ankle successfully calculated and the score was less than zero (< 0) ☒M ☑

▲ **G8657**<sup>Jan</sup> Risk-adjusted functional status change residual scores for the foot or ankle not measured because the patient did not complete FOTO's status survey near discharge, patient not appropriate ☒M

<sup>Jan</sup> **January Update**

Special Coverage Instructions    Noncovered by Medicare    Carrier Discretion    ☑ Quantity Alert    ● New Code    ○ Recycled/Reinstated    ▲ Revised Code

**52 — G Codes**    🅰 Age Edit    Ⓜ Maternity Edit    ♀ Female Only    ♂ Male Only    🅰-🆈 OPPS Status Indicators    © 2016 Optum360, LLC

▲ **G8658**^Jan Risk-adjusted functional status change residual scores for the foot or ankle not measured because the patient did not complete FOTO's functional intake on admission and/or follow-up status survey near discharge, reason not given  Ⓜ

▲ **G8659**^Jan Risk-adjusted functional status change residual score for the lumbar impairment successfully calculated and the score was equal to zero (0) or greater than zero (> 0)  Ⓜ ☑

▲ **G8660**^Jan Risk-adjusted functional status change residual score for the lumbar impairment successfully calculated and the score was less than zero (< 0)  Ⓜ ☑

▲ **G8661**^Jan Risk-adjusted functional status change residual scores for the lumbar impairment not measured because the patient did not complete FOTO's status survey near discharge, patient not appropriate  Ⓜ

▲ **G8662**^Jan Risk-adjusted functional status change residual scores for the lumbar impairment not measured because the patient did not complete FOTO's functional intake on admission and/or follow-up status survey near discharge, reason not given  Ⓜ

**G8663** Risk-adjusted functional status change residual score for the shoulder successfully calculated and the score was equal to zero (0) or greater than zero (> 0)  Ⓜ ☑

**G8664** Risk-adjusted functional status change residual score for the shoulder successfully calculated and the score was less than zero (< 0)  Ⓜ ☑

▲ **G8665**^Jan Risk-adjusted functional status change residual scores for the shoulder not measured because the patient did not complete FOTO's functional status survey near discharge, patient not appropriate  Ⓜ

**G8666** Risk-adjusted functional status change residual scores for the shoulder not measured because the patient did not complete FOTO's functional intake on admission and/or follow up status survey near discharge, reason not given  Ⓜ

**G8667** Risk-adjusted functional status change residual score for the elbow, wrist or hand successfully calculated and the score was equal to zero (0) or greater than zero (> 0)  Ⓜ ☑

**G8668** Risk-adjusted functional status change residual score for the elbow, wrist or hand successfully calculated and the score was less than zero (< 0)  Ⓜ ☑

▲ **G8669**^Jan Risk-adjusted functional status change residual scores for the elbow, wrist or hand not measured because the patient did not complete FOTO's functional follow-up status survey near discharge, patient not appropriate  Ⓜ

**G8670** Risk-adjusted functional status change residual scores for the elbow, wrist or hand not measured because the patient did not complete FOTO's functional intake on admission and/or follow up status survey near discharge, reason not given  Ⓜ

▲ **G8671**^Jan Risk-adjusted functional status change residual score for the neck, cranium, mandible, thoracic spine, ribs, or other general orthopaedic impairment successfully calculated and the score was equal to zero (0) or greater than zero (> 0)  Ⓜ ☑

▲ **G8672**^Jan Risk-adjusted functional status change residual score for the neck, cranium, mandible, thoracic spine, ribs, or other general orthopaedic impairment successfully calculated and the score was less than zero (< 0)  Ⓜ ☑

▲ **G8673**^Jan Risk-adjusted functional status change residual scores for the neck, cranium, mandible, thoracic spine, ribs, or other general orthopaedic impairment not measured because the patient did not complete FOTO's functional follow-up status survey near discharge, patient not appropriate  Ⓜ

▲ **G8674**^Jan Risk-adjusted functional status change residual scores for the neck, cranium, mandible, thoracic spine, ribs, or other general orthopaedic impairment not measured because the patient did not complete FOTO's functional intake on admission and/or follow-up status survey near discharge, reason not given  Ⓜ

**G8694** Left ventricular ejection fraction (LVEF) < 40%  Ⓜ ☑

**G8696** Antithrombotic therapy prescribed at discharge  Ⓜ

▲ **G8697**^Jan Antithrombotic therapy not prescribed for documented reasons (e.g., patient had stroke during hospital stay, patient expired during inpatient stay, other medical reason(s)); (e.g., patient left against medical advice, other patient reason(s))  Ⓜ

**G8698** Antithrombotic therapy was not prescribed at discharge, reason not given  Ⓜ

**G8708** Patient not prescribed or dispensed antibiotic  Ⓜ

**G8709** Patient prescribed or dispensed antibiotic for documented medical reason(s) (e.g., intestinal infection, pertussis, bacterial infection, lyme disease, otitis media, acute sinusitis, acute pharyngitis, acute tonsillitis, chronic sinusitis, infection of the pharynx/larynx/tonsils/adenoids, prostatitis, cellulitis, mastoiditis, or bone infections, acute lymphadenitis, impetigo, skin staph infections, pneumonia/gonococcal infections, venereal disease (syphilis, chlamydia, inflammatory diseases (female reproductive organs)), infections of the kidney, cystitis or UTI, and acne)  Ⓜ

**G8710** Patient prescribed or dispensed antibiotic  Ⓜ

**G8711** Prescribed or dispensed antibiotic  Ⓜ

**G8712** Antibiotic not prescribed or dispensed  Ⓜ

**G8721** PT category (primary tumor), PN category (regional lymph nodes), and histologic grade were documented in pathology report  Ⓜ

**G8722** Documentation of medical reason(s) for not including the PT category, the PN category or the histologic grade in the pathology report (e.g., re-excision without residual tumor; non-carcinomasanal canal)  Ⓜ

**G8723** Specimen site is other than anatomic location of primary tumor  Ⓜ

**G8724** PT category, PN category and histologic grade were not documented in the pathology report, reason not given  Ⓜ

**G8725**^Jan ~~Fasting lipid profile performed (triglycerides, LDL-C, HDL-C and total cholesterol)~~

**G8726**^Jan ~~Clinician has documented reason for not performing fasting lipid profile (e.g., patient declined, other patient reasons)~~

**G8728**^Jan ~~Fasting lipid profile not performed, reason not given~~

**G8730** Pain assessment documented as positive using a standardized tool and a follow-up plan is documented  Ⓜ

**G8731** Pain assessment using a standardized tool is documented as negative, no follow-up plan required  Ⓜ

**G8732** No documentation of pain assessment, reason not given  Ⓜ

**G8733** Elder maltreatment screen documented as positive and a follow-up plan is documented  Ⓜ

**G8734** Elder maltreatment screen documented as negative, no follow-up required  Ⓜ

**G8735** Elder maltreatment screen documented as positive, follow-up plan not documented, reason not given  Ⓜ

---

^Jan **January Update**

Special Coverage Instructions    Noncovered by Medicare    Carrier Discretion    ☑ Quantity Alert   ● New Code   ○ Recycled/Reinstated   ▲ Revised Code

© 2016 Optum360, LLC    **A2-Z3** ASC Pmt    **CMS:** Pub 100    **AHA:** Coding Clinic    ⅋ DMEPOS Paid    ⊘ SNF Excluded    **G Codes — 53**

**Procedures/Professional Services (Temporary)**

**G8749 — G8858**

**G8749** Absence of signs of melanoma (cough, dyspnea, tenderness, localized neurologic signs such as weakness, jaundice or any other sign suggesting systemic spread) or absence of symptoms of melanoma (pain, paresthesia, or any other symptom suggesting the possibility of systemic spread of melanoma) M

**G8752** Most recent systolic blood pressure < 140 mm Hg M ☑

**G8753** Most recent systolic blood pressure ≥ 140 mm Hg M ☑

**G8754** Most recent diastolic blood pressure < 90 mm Hg M ☑

**G8755** Most recent diastolic blood pressure ≥ 90 mm Hg M ☑

**G8756** No documentation of blood pressure measurement, reason not given M

~~G8757~~ Jan ~~All quality actions for the applicable measures in the chronic obstructive pulmonary disease (COPD) measures group have been performed for this patient~~

~~G8758~~ Jan ~~All quality actions for the applicable measures in the inflammatory bowel disease (IBD) measures group have been performed for this patient~~

~~G8759~~ Jan ~~All quality actions for the applicable measures in the sleep apnea measures group have been performed for this patient~~

~~G8761~~ Jan ~~All quality actions for the applicable measures in the dementia measures group have been performed for this patient~~

~~G8762~~ Jan ~~All quality actions for the applicable measures in the Parkinson's disease measures group have been performed for this patient~~

~~G8765~~ Jan ~~All quality actions for the applicable measures in the cataract measures group have been performed for this patient~~

**G8783** Normal blood pressure reading documented, follow-up not required M

~~G8784~~ Jan ~~Patient not eligible (e.g., documentation the patient is not eligible due to active diagnosis of hypertension, patient refuses, urgent or emergent situation)~~

**G8785** Blood pressure reading not documented, reason not given M

**G8797** Specimen site other than anatomic location of esophagus M

**G8798** Specimen site other than anatomic location of prostate M

**G8806** Performance of transabdominal or transvaginal ultrasound A ♀ M

**G8807** Transabdominal or transvaginal ultrasound not performed for reasons documented by clinician (e.g., patient has visited the ED multiple times within 72 hours, patient has a documented intrauterine pregnancy (IUP) A ♀ M

**G8808** Performance of trans-abdominal or trans-vaginal ultrasound not ordered, reason not given (e.g., patient has visited the ED multiple times with no documentation of a trans-abdominal or trans-vaginal ultrasound within ED or from referring eligible professional) A ♀ M

**G8809** Rh immune globulin (RhoGam) ordered M ♀ M

**G8810** Rh-immunoglobulin (RhoGAM) not ordered for reasons documented by clinician (e.g., patient had prior documented receipt of RhoGAM within 12 weeks, patient refusal) M ♀ M

**G8811** Documentation Rh immunoglobulin (Rhogam) was not ordered, reason not specified M ♀ M

▲ **G8815** Jan Documented reason in the medical records for why the statin therapy was not prescribed (i.e., lower extremity bypass was for a patient with non-artherosclerotic disease) M

**G8816** Statin medication prescribed at discharge M

**G8817** Statin therapy not prescribed at discharge, reason not given M

**G8818** Patient discharge to home no later than postoperative day #7 M

**G8825** Patient not discharged to home by postoperative day #7 M

**G8826** Patient discharged to home no later than postoperative day #2 following EVAR M

**G8833** Patient not discharged to home by postoperative day #2 following EVAR M

**G8834** Patient discharged to home no later than postoperative day #2 following CEA M

**G8838** Patient not discharged to home by postoperative day #2 following CEA M

**G8839** Sleep apnea symptoms assessed, including presence or absence of snoring and daytime sleepiness M

**G8840** Documentation of reason(s) for not documenting an assessment of sleep symptoms (e.g., patient didn't have initial daytime sleepiness, patient visited between initial testing and initiation of therapy) M

**G8841** Sleep apnea symptoms not assessed, reason not given M

**G8842** Apnea hypopnea index (AHI) or respiratory disturbance index (RDI) measured at the time of initial diagnosis M

**G8843** Documentation of reason(s) for not measuring an apnea hypopnea index (AHI) or a respiratory disturbance index (RDI) at the time of initial diagnosis (e.g., psychiatric disease, dementia, patient declined, financial, insurance coverage, test ordered but not yet completed) M

**G8844** Apnea hypopna index (AHI) or respiratory disturbance index (RDI) not measured at the time of initial diagnosis, reason not given M

**G8845** Positive airway pressure therapy prescribed M

**G8846** Moderate or severe obstructive sleep apnea (apnea hypopnea index (AHI) or respiratory disturbance index (RDI) of 15 or greater) M ☑

~~G8848~~ Jan ~~Mild obstructive sleep apnea (apnea hypopnea index (AHI) or respiratory disturbance index (RDI) of less than 15)~~

**G8849** Documentation of reason(s) for not prescribing positive airway pressure therapy (e.g., patient unable to tolerate, alternative therapies use, patient declined, financial, insurance coverage) M

**G8850** Positive airway pressure therapy not prescribed, reason not given M

**G8851** Objective measurement of adherence to positive airway pressure therapy, documented M

**G8852** Positive airway pressure therapy prescribed M

~~G8853~~ Jan ~~Positive airway pressure therapy not prescribed~~

**G8854** Documentation of reason(s) for not objectively measuring adherence to positive airway pressure therapy (e.g., patient did not bring data from continuous positive airway pressure (CPAP), therapy not yet initiated, not available on machine) M

**G8855** Objective measurement of adherence to positive airway pressure therapy not performed, reason not given M

**G8856** Referral to a physician for an otologic evaluation performed M

**G8857** Patient is not eligible for the referral for otologic evaluation measure (e.g., patients who are already under the care of a physician for acute or chronic dizziness) M

**G8858** Referral to a physician for an otologic evaluation not performed, reason not given M

---

Jan **January Update**

Special Coverage Instructions      Noncovered by Medicare      Carrier Discretion      ☑ Quantity Alert   ● New Code   ○ Recycled/Reinstated   ▲ Revised Code

**G8861** Within the past 2 years, central dual-energy x-ray absorptiometry (DXA) ordered and documented, review of systems and medication history or pharmacologic therapy (other than minerals/vitamins) for osteoporosis prescribed Ⓜ

**G8863** Patients not assessed for risk of bone loss, reason not given Ⓜ

**G8864** Pneumococcal vaccine administered or previously received Ⓜ

**G8865** Documentation of medical reason(s) for not administering or previously receiving pneumococcal vaccine (e.g., patient allergic reaction, potential adverse drug reaction) Ⓜ

**G8866** Documentation of patient reason(s) for not administering or previously receiving pneumococcal vaccine (e.g., patient refusal) Ⓜ

**G8867** Pneumococcal vaccine not administered or previously received, reason not given Ⓜ

**G8868**^Jan ~~Patients receiving a first course of anti-TNF therapy~~

**G8869** Patient has documented immunity to hepatitis B and is receiving a first course of anti-TNF therapy Ⓜ

**G8872** Excised tissue evaluated by imaging intraoperatively to confirm successful inclusion of targeted lesion Ⓜ

**G8873** Patients with needle localization specimens which are not amenable to intraoperative imaging such as MRI needle wire localization, or targets which are tentatively identified on mammogram or ultrasound which do not contain a biopsy marker but which can be verified on intraoperative inspection or pathology (e.g., needle biopsy site where the biopsy marker is remote from the actual biopsy site) Ⓜ

**G8874** Excised tissue not evaluated by imaging intraoperatively to confirm successful inclusion of targeted lesion Ⓜ

**G8875** Clinician diagnosed breast cancer preoperatively by a minimally invasive biopsy method Ⓜ

**G8876** Documentation of reason(s) for not performing minimally invasive biopsy to diagnose breast cancer preoperatively (e.g., lesion too close to skin, implant, chest wall, etc., lesion could not be adequately visualized for needle biopsy, patient condition prevents needle biopsy [weight, breast thickness, etc.], duct excision without imaging abnormality, prophylactic mastectomy, reduction mammoplasty, excisional biopsy performed by another physician) Ⓜ

**G8877** Clinician did not attempt to achieve the diagnosis of breast cancer preoperatively by a minimally invasive biopsy method, reason not given Ⓜ

**G8878** Sentinel lymph node biopsy procedure performed Ⓜ

**G8879** Clinically node negative (T1N0M0 or T2N0M0) invasive breast cancer Ⓜ

**G8880** Documentation of reason(s) sentinel lymph node biopsy not performed (e.g., reasons could include but not limited to; non-invasive cancer, incidental discovery of breast cancer on prophylactic mastectomy, incidental discovery of breast cancer on reduction mammoplasty, pre-operative biopsy proven lymph node (LN) metastases, inflammatory carcinoma, stage 3 locally advanced cancer, recurrent invasive breast cancer, patient refusal after informed consent) Ⓜ

**G8881** Stage of breast cancer is greater than T1N0M0 or T2N0M0 Ⓜ

**G8882** Sentinel lymph node biopsy procedure not performed, reason not given Ⓜ

**G8883** Biopsy results reviewed, communicated, tracked and documented Ⓜ

**G8884** Clinician documented reason that patient's biopsy results were not reviewed Ⓜ

**G8885** Biopsy results not reviewed, communicated, tracked or documented Ⓜ

**G8898**^Jan ~~I intend to report the chronic obstructive pulmonary disease (COPD) measures group~~

**G8899**^Jan ~~I intend to report the inflammatory bowel disease (IBD) measures group~~

**G8900**^Jan ~~I intend to report the sleep apnea measures group~~

**G8902**^Jan ~~I intend to report the dementia measures group~~

**G8903**^Jan ~~I intend to report the Parkinson's disease measures group~~

**G8906**^Jan ~~I intend to report the cataract measures group~~

**G8907** Patient documented not to have experienced any of the following events: a burn prior to discharge; a fall within the facility; wrong site/side/patient/procedure/implant event; or a hospital transfer or hospital admission upon discharge from the facility Ⓜ

**G8908** Patient documented to have received a burn prior to discharge Ⓜ

**G8909** Patient documented not to have received a burn prior to discharge Ⓜ

**G8910** Patient documented to have experienced a fall within ASC Ⓜ

**G8911** Patient documented not to have experienced a fall within ambulatory surgery center Ⓜ

**G8912** Patient documented to have experienced a wrong site, wrong side, wrong patient, wrong procedure or wrong implant event Ⓜ

**G8913** Patient documented not to have experienced a wrong site, wrong side, wrong patient, wrong procedure or wrong implant event Ⓜ

**G8914** Patient documented to have experienced a hospital transfer or hospital admission upon discharge from ASC Ⓜ

**G8915** Patient documented not to have experienced a hospital transfer or hospital admission upon discharge from ASC Ⓜ

**G8916** Patient with preoperative order for IV antibiotic surgical site infection (SSI) prophylaxis, antibiotic initiated on time Ⓜ

**G8917** Patient with preoperative order for IV antibiotic surgical site infection (SSI) prophylaxis, antibiotic not initiated on time Ⓜ

**G8918** Patient without preoperative order for IV antibiotic surgical site infection (SSI) prophylaxis Ⓜ

**G8923** Left ventricular ejection fraction (LVEF) < 40% or documentation of moderately or severely depressed left ventricular systolic function Ⓜ

▲ **G8924**^Jan Spirometry test results demonstrate FEV1/FVC < 70%, FEV < 60% predicted and patient has COPD symptoms (e.g., dyspnea, cough/sputum, wheezing)

▲ **G8925**^Jan Spirometry test results demonstrate FEV1 >= 60%, FEV1/FVC >= 70%, predicted or patient does not have COPD symptoms Ⓜ

**G8926** Spirometry test not performed or documented, reason not given Ⓜ

**G8927**^Jan ~~Adjuvant chemotherapy referred, prescribed or previously received for AJCC stage III, colon cancer~~

^Jan **January Update**

Special Coverage Instructions    Noncovered by Medicare    Carrier Discretion    ☑ Quantity Alert  ● New Code    ○ Recycled/Reinstated  ▲ Revised Code

© 2016 Optum360, LLC    A2-Z3 ASC Pmt    CMS: Pub 100    AHA: Coding Clinic    �DMEPOS Paid    ⊘ SNF Excluded    G Codes — 55

~~**G8928**^Jan **Adjuvant chemotherapy not prescribed or previously received, for documented reasons (e.g., medical co-morbidities, diagnosis date more than 5 years prior to the current visit date, patient's diagnosis date is within 120 days of the end of the 12 month reporting period, patient's cancer has metastasized, medical contraindication/allergy, poor performance status, other medical reasons, patient refusal, other patient reasons, patient is currently enrolled in a clinical trial that precludes prescription of chemotherapy, other system reasons)**~~

~~**G8929**^Jan **Adjuvant chemotherapy not prescribed or previously received, reason not given**~~

**G8934** Left ventricular ejection fraction (LVEF) < 40% or documentation of moderately or severely depressed left ventricular systolic function  M

**G8935** Clinician prescribed angiotensin converting enzyme (ACE) inhibitor or angiotensin receptor blocker (ARB) therapy  M

**G8936** Clinician documented that patient was not an eligible candidate for angiotensin converting enzyme (ACE) inhibitor or angiotensin receptor blocker (ARB) therapy (e.g., allergy, intolerance, pregnancy, renal failure due to ACE inhibitor, diseases of the aortic or mitral valve, other medical reasons) or (e.g., patient declined, other patient reasons) or (e.g., lack of drug availability, other reasons attributable to the health care system)  M

**G8937** Clinician did not prescribe angiotensin converting enzyme (ACE) inhibitor or angiotensin receptor blocker (ARB) therapy, reason not given  M

**G8938** BMI is documented as being outside of normal limits, follow-up plan is not documented, documentation the patient is not eligible  M

**G8939** Pain assessment documented as positive, follow-up plan not documented, documentation the patient is not eligible  M

~~**G8940**^Jan **Screening for clinical depression documented as positive, a follow-up plan not documented, documentation stating the patient is not eligible**~~

**G8941** Elder maltreatment screen documented as positive, follow-up plan not documented, documentation the patient is not eligible  M

**G8942** Functional outcomes assessment using a standardized tool is documented within the previous 30 days and care plan, based on identified deficiencies on the date of the functional outcome assessment, is documented  M

**G8944** AJCC melanoma cancer stage 0 through IIC melanoma  M

**G8946** Minimally invasive biopsy method attempted but not diagnostic of breast cancer (e.g., high risk lesion of breast such as atypical ductal hyperplasia, lobular neoplasia, atypical lobular hyperplasia, lobular carcinoma in situ, atypical columnar hyperplasia, flat epithelial atypia, radial scar, complex sclerosing lesion, papillary lesion, or any lesion with spindle cells)  M

**G8947** One or more neuropsychiatric symptoms  M

**G8950** Prehypertensive or hypertensive blood pressure reading documented, and the indicated follow-up is documented  M

**G8952** Prehypertensive or hypertensive blood pressure reading documented, indicated follow-up not documented, reason not given  M

~~**G8953**^Jan **All quality actions for the applicable measures in the oncology measures group have been performed for this patient**~~

**G8955** Most recent assessment of adequacy of volume management documented  M

**G8956** Patient receiving maintenance hemodialysis in an outpatient dialysis facility  M

**G8958** Assessment of adequacy of volume management not documented, reason not given  M

**G8959** Clinician treating major depressive disorder communicates to clinician treating comorbid condition  M

**G8960** Clinician treating major depressive disorder did not communicate to clinician treating comorbid condition, reason not given  M

**G8961** Cardiac stress imaging test primarily performed on low-risk surgery patient for preoperative evaluation within 30 days preceding this surgery  M

**G8962** Cardiac stress imaging test performed on patient for any reason including those who did not have low risk surgery or test that was performed more than 30 days preceding low risk surgery  M

**G8963** Cardiac stress imaging performed primarily for monitoring of asymptomatic patient who had PCI wihin 2 years  M

**G8964** Cardiac stress imaging test performed primarily for any other reason than monitoring of asymptomatic patient who had PCI wthin 2 years (e.g., symptomatic patient, patient greater than 2 years since PCI, initial evaluation, etc.)  M

**G8965** Cardiac stress imaging test primarily performed on low CHD risk patient for initial detection and risk assessment  M

**G8966** Cardiac stress imaging test performed on symptomatic or higher than low CHD risk patient or for any reason other than initial detection and risk assessment  M

**G8967** Warfarin or another oral anticoagulant that is FDA approved prescribed  M

▲ **G8968**^Jan Documentation of medical reason(s) for not prescribing warfarin or another oral anticoagulant that is FDA approved for the prevention of thromboembolism (e.g., allergy, risk of bleeding, other medical reasons)  M

**G8969** Documentation of patient reason(s) for not prescribing warfarin or another oral anticoagulant that is FDA approved (e.g., economic, social, and/or religious impediments, noncompliance patient refusal, other patient reasons)  M

**G8970** No risk factors or one moderate risk factor for thromboembolism  M

**G8971** Warfarin or another oral anticoagulant that is FDA approved not prescribed, reason not given  M

**G8972** One or more high risk factors for thromboembolism or more than one moderate risk factor for thromboembolism  M

**G8973** Most recent hemoglobin (HgB) level < 10 g/dl  M

**G8974** Hemoglobin level measurement not documented, reason not given  M

**G8975** Documentation of medical reason(s) for patient having a hemoglobin level < 10 g/dl (e.g., patients who have nonrenal etiologies of anemia [e.g., sickle cell anemia or other hemoglobinopathies, hypersplenism, primary bone marrow disease, anemia related to chemotherapy for diagnosis of malignancy, postoperative bleeding, active bloodstream or peritoneal infection], other medical reasons)  M

**G8976** Most recent hemoglobin (HgB) level >= 10 g/dl  M

~~**G8977**^Jan **I intend to report the oncology measures group**~~

## Functional Limitation

**G8978** Mobility: walking and moving around functional limitation, current status, at therapy episode outset and at reporting intervals  E
CMS: 100-04,5,10.6

^Jan **January Update**

Special Coverage Instructions   Noncovered by Medicare   Carrier Discretion   ☑ Quantity Alert ● New Code ○ Recycled/Reinstated ▲ Revised Code

56 — G Codes   A Age Edit   M Maternity Edit   ♀ Female Only   ♂ Male Only   A-Y OPPS Status Indicators   © 2016 Optum360, LLC

**G8979** Mobility: walking and moving around functional limitation, projected goal status, at therapy episode outset, at reporting intervals, and at discharge or to end reporting E
CMS: 100-04,5,10.6

**G8980** Mobility: walking and moving around functional limitation, discharge status, at discharge from therapy or to end reporting E
CMS: 100-04,5,10.6

**G8981** Changing and maintaining body position functional limitation, current status, at therapy episode outset and at reporting intervals E
CMS: 100-04,5,10.6

**G8982** Changing and maintaining body position functional limitation, projected goal status, at therapy episode outset, at reporting intervals, and at discharge or to end reporting E
CMS: 100-04,5,10.6

**G8983** Changing and maintaining body position functional limitation, discharge status, at discharge from therapy or to end reporting E
CMS: 100-04,5,10.6

**G8984** Carrying, moving and handling objects functional limitation, current status, at therapy episode outset and at reporting intervals E
CMS: 100-04,5,10.6

**G8985** Carrying, moving and handling objects, projected goal status, at therapy episode outset, at reporting intervals, and at discharge or to end reporting E
CMS: 100-04,5,10.6

**G8986** Carrying, moving and handling objects functional limitation, discharge status, at discharge from therapy or to end reporting E
CMS: 100-04,5,10.6

**G8987** Self care functional limitation, current status, at therapy episode outset and at reporting intervals E
CMS: 100-04,5,10.6

**G8988** Self care functional limitation, projected goal status, at therapy episode outset, at reporting intervals, and at discharge or to end reporting E
CMS: 100-04,5,10.6

**G8989** Self care functional limitation, discharge status, at discharge from therapy or to end reporting E
CMS: 100-04,5,10.6

**G8990** Other physical or occupational therapy primary functional limitation, current status, at therapy episode outset and at reporting intervals E
CMS: 100-04,5,10.6

**G8991** Other physical or occupational therapy primary functional limitation, projected goal status, at therapy episode outset, at reporting intervals, and at discharge or to end reporting E
CMS: 100-04,5,10.6

**G8992** Other physical or occupational therapy primary functional limitation, discharge status, at discharge from therapy or to end reporting E
CMS: 100-04,5,10.6

**G8993** Other physical or occupational therapy subsequent functional limitation, current status, at therapy episode outset and at reporting intervals E
CMS: 100-04,5,10.6

**G8994** Other physical or occupational therapy subsequent functional limitation, projected goal status, at therapy episode outset, at reporting intervals, and at discharge or to end reporting E
CMS: 100-04,5,10.6

**G8995** Other physical or occupational therapy subsequent functional limitation, discharge status, at discharge from therapy or to end reporting E

**G8996** Swallowing functional limitation, current status at therapy episode outset and at reporting intervals E
CMS: 100-04,5,10.6

**G8997** Swallowing functional limitation, projected goal status, at therapy episode outset, at reporting intervals, and at discharge or to end reporting E
CMS: 100-04,5,10.6

**G8998** Swallowing functional limitation, discharge status, at discharge from therapy or to end reporting E
CMS: 100-04,5,10.6

**G8999** Motor speech functional limitation, current status at therapy episode outset and at reporting intervals E
CMS: 100-04,5,10.6

## Coordinated Care

**G9001** Coordinated care fee, initial rate B

**G9002** Coordinated care fee (Level 1) B

**G9003** Coordinated care fee, risk adjusted high, initial B

**G9004** Coordinated care fee, risk adjusted low, initial B

**G9005** Coordinated care fee risk adjusted maintenance B

**G9006** Coordinated care fee, home monitoring B

**G9007** Coordinated care fee, scheduled team conference B

**G9008** Coordinated care fee, physician coordinated care oversight services B

**G9009** Coordinated care fee, risk adjusted maintenance, level 3 B

**G9010** Coordinated care fee, risk adjusted maintenance, level 4 B

**G9011** Coordinated care fee, risk adjusted maintenance, Level 5 B

**G9012** Other specified case management service not elsewhere classified B

## Demonstration Project

**G9013** ESRD demo basic bundle Level I E

**G9014** ESRD demo expanded bundle including venous access and related services E

**G9016** Smoking cessation counseling, individual, in the absence of or in addition to any other evaluation and management service, per session (6-10 minutes) [demo project code only] E ☑
CMS: 100-03,210.4

**G9017** Amantadine HCl, oral, per 100 mg (for use in a Medicare-approved demonstration project) A ☑

**G9018** Zanamivir, inhalation powder, administered through inhaler, per 10 mg (for use in a Medicare-approved demonstration project) A ☑

**G9019** Oseltamivir phosphate, oral, per 75 mg (for use in a Medicare-approved demonstration project) A ☑

**G9020** Rimantadine HCl, oral, per 100 mg (for use in a Medicare-approved demonstration project) A ☑

**G9033** Amantadine HCl, oral brand, per 100 mg (for use in a Medicare-approved demonstration project) A ☑

**G9034** Zanamivir, inhalation powder, administered through inhaler, brand, per 10 mg (for use in a Medicare-approved demonstration project) A ☑

**G9035** Oseltamivir phosphate, oral, brand, per 75 mg (for use in a Medicare-approved demonstration project) A ☑

---

Special Coverage Instructions    Noncovered by Medicare    Carrier Discretion    ☑ Quantity Alert    ● New Code    ○ Recycled/Reinstated    ▲ Revised Code

**G9036** Rimantadine HCl, oral, brand, per 100 mg (for use in a Medicare-approved demonstration project) Ⓐ ☑

**G9050** Oncology; primary focus of visit; work-up, evaluation, or staging at the time of cancer diagnosis or recurrence (for use in a Medicare-approved demonstration project) Ⓔ

**G9051** Oncology; primary focus of visit; treatment decision-making after disease is staged or restaged, discussion of treatment options, supervising/coordinating active cancer-directed therapy or managing consequences of cancer-directed therapy (for use in a Medicare-approved demonstration project) Ⓔ

**G9052** Oncology; primary focus of visit; surveillance for disease recurrence for patient who has completed definitive cancer-directed therapy and currently lacks evidence of recurrent disease; cancer-directed therapy might be considered in the future (for use in a Medicare-approved demonstration project) Ⓔ

**G9053** Oncology; primary focus of visit; expectant management of patient with evidence of cancer for whom no cancer-directed therapy is being administered or arranged at present; cancer-directed therapy might be considered in the future (for use in a Medicare-approved demonstration project) Ⓔ

**G9054** Oncology; primary focus of visit; supervising, coordinating or managing care of patient with terminal cancer or for whom other medical illness prevents further cancer treatment; includes symptom management, end-of-life care planning, management of palliative therapies (for use in a Medicare-approved demonstration project) Ⓔ

**G9055** Oncology; primary focus of visit; other, unspecified service not otherwise listed (for use in a Medicare-approved demonstration project) Ⓔ

**G9056** Oncology; practice guidelines; management adheres to guidelines (for use in a Medicare-approved demonstration project) Ⓔ

**G9057** Oncology; practice guidelines; management differs from guidelines as a result of patient enrollment in an institutional review board-approved clinical trial (for use in a Medicare-approved demonstration project) Ⓔ

**G9058** Oncology; practice guidelines; management differs from guidelines because the treating physician disagrees with guideline recommendations (for use in a Medicare-approved demonstration project) Ⓔ

**G9059** Oncology; practice guidelines; management differs from guidelines because the patient, after being offered treatment consistent with guidelines, has opted for alternative treatment or management, including no treatment (for use in a Medicare-approved demonstration project) Ⓔ

**G9060** Oncology; practice guidelines; management differs from guidelines for reason(s) associated with patient comorbid illness or performance status not factored into guidelines (for use in a Medicare-approved demonstration project) Ⓔ

**G9061** Oncology; practice guidelines; patient's condition not addressed by available guidelines (for use in a Medicare-approved demonstration project) Ⓔ

**G9062** Oncology; practice guidelines; management differs from guidelines for other reason(s) not listed (for use in a Medicare-approved demonstration project) Ⓔ

**G9063** Oncology; disease status; limited to nonsmall cell lung cancer; extent of disease initially established as Stage I (prior to neoadjuvant therapy, if any) with no evidence of disease progression, recurrence, or metastases (for use in a Medicare-approved demonstration project) Ⓜ

**G9064** Oncology; disease status; limited to nonsmall cell lung cancer; extent of disease initially established as Stage II (prior to neoadjuvant therapy, if any) with no evidence of disease progression, recurrence, or metastases (for use in a Medicare-approved demonstration project) Ⓜ

**G9065** Oncology; disease status; limited to nonsmall cell lung cancer; extent of disease initially established as Stage III a (prior to neoadjuvant therapy, if any) with no evidence of disease progression, recurrence, or metastases (for use in a Medicare-approved demonstration project) Ⓜ

**G9066** Oncology; disease status; limited to nonsmall cell lung cancer; Stage III B-IV at diagnosis, metastatic, locally recurrent, or progressive (for use in a Medicare-approved demonstration project) Ⓜ

**G9067** Oncology; disease status; limited to nonsmall cell lung cancer; extent of disease unknown, staging in progress, or not listed (for use in a Medicare-approved demonstration project) Ⓜ

**G9068** Oncology; disease status; limited to small cell and combined small cell/nonsmall cell; extent of disease initially established as limited with no evidence of disease progression, recurrence, or metastases (for use in a Medicare-approved demonstration project) Ⓜ

**G9069** Oncology; disease status; small cell lung cancer, limited to small cell and combined small cell/nonsmall cell; extensive Stage at diagnosis, metastatic, locally recurrent, or progressive (for use in a Medicare-approved demonstration project) Ⓜ

**G9070** Oncology; disease status; small cell lung cancer, limited to small cell and combined small cell/nonsmall; extent of disease unknown, staging in progress, or not listed (for use in a Medicare-approved demonstration project) Ⓜ

**G9071** Oncology; disease status; invasive female breast cancer (does not include ductal carcinoma in situ); adenocarcinoma as predominant cell type; stage I or stage IIA-IIB; or T3, N1, M0; and ER and/or PR positive; with no evidence of disease progression, recurrence, or metastases (for use in a Medicare-approved demonstration project) ♀Ⓜ

**G9072** Oncology; disease status; invasive female breast cancer (does not include ductal carcinoma in situ); adenocarcinoma as predominant cell type; stage I, or stage IIA-IIB; or T3, N1, M0; and ER and PR negative; with no evidence of disease progression, recurrence, or metastases (for use in a Medicare-approved demonstration project) ♀Ⓜ

**G9073** Oncology; disease status; invasive female breast cancer (does not include ductal carcinoma in situ); adenocarcinoma as predominant cell type; stage IIIA-IIIB; and not T3, N1, M0; and ER and/or PR positive; with no evidence of disease progression, recurrence, or metastases (for use in a Medicare-approved demonstration project) ♀Ⓜ

**G9074** Oncology; disease status; invasive female breast cancer (does not include ductal carcinoma in situ); adenocarcinoma as predominant cell type; stage IIIA-IIIB; and not T3, N1, M0; and ER and PR negative; with no evidence of disease progression, recurrence, or metastases (for use in a Medicare-approved demonstration project) ♀Ⓜ

**G9075** Oncology; disease status; invasive female breast cancer (does not include ductal carcinoma in situ); adenocarcinoma as predominant cell type; M1 at diagnosis, metastatic, locally recurrent, or progressive (for use in a Medicare-approved demonstration project) ♀Ⓜ

**G9077** Oncology; disease status; prostate cancer, limited to adenocarcinoma as predominant cell type; T1-T2C and Gleason 2-7 and PSA < or equal to 20 at diagnosis with no evidence of disease progression, recurrence, or metastases (for use in a Medicare-approved demonstration project) ♂Ⓜ

Special Coverage Instructions    Noncovered by Medicare    Carrier Discretion    ☑ Quantity Alert  ● New Code    ○ Recycled/Reinstated  ▲ Revised Code

58 — G Codes    Ⓐ Age Edit    Ⓜ Maternity Edit    ♀ Female Only    ♂ Male Only    Ⓐ-Ⓨ OPPS Status Indicators    © 2016 Optum360, LLC

**G9078** Oncology; disease status; prostate cancer, limited to adenocarcinoma as predominant cell type; T2 or T3a Gleason 8-10 or PSA > 20 at diagnosis with no evidence of disease progression, recurrence, or metastases (for use in a Medicare-approved demonstration project) ♂ Ⓜ

**G9079** Oncology; disease status; prostate cancer, limited to adenocarcinoma as predominant cell type; T3B-T4, any N; any T, N1 at diagnosis with no evidence of disease progression, recurrence, or metastases (for use in a Medicare-approved demonstration project) ♂ Ⓜ

**G9080** Oncology; disease status; prostate cancer, limited to adenocarcinoma; after initial treatment with rising PSA or failure of PSA decline (for use in a Medicare-approved demonstration project) ♂ Ⓜ

**G9083** Oncology; disease status; prostate cancer, limited to adenocarcinoma; extent of disease unknown, staging in progress, or not listed (for use in a Medicare-approved demonstration project) ♂ Ⓜ

**G9084** Oncology; disease status; colon cancer, limited to invasive cancer, adenocarcinoma as predominant cell type; extent of disease initially established as T1-3, N0, M0 with no evidence of disease progression, recurrence or metastases (for use in a Medicare-approved demonstration project) Ⓜ

**G9085** Oncology; disease status; colon cancer, limited to invasive cancer, adenocarcinoma as predominant cell type; extent of disease initially established as T4, N0, M0 with no evidence of disease progression, recurrence, or metastases (for use in a Medicare-approved demonstration project) Ⓜ

**G9086** Oncology; disease status; colon cancer, limited to invasive cancer, adenocarcinoma as predominant cell type; extent of disease initially established as T1-4, N1-2, M0 with no evidence of disease progression, recurrence, or metastases (for use in a Medicare-approved demonstration project) Ⓜ

**G9087** Oncology; disease status; colon cancer, limited to invasive cancer, adenocarcinoma as predominant cell type; M1 at diagnosis, metastatic, locally recurrent, or progressive with current clinical, radiologic, or biochemical evidence of disease (for use in a Medicare-approved demonstration project) Ⓜ

**G9088** Oncology; disease status; colon cancer, limited to invasive cancer, adenocarcinoma as predominant cell type; M1 at diagnosis, metastatic, locally recurrent, or progressive without current clinical, radiologic, or biochemical evidence of disease (for use in a Medicare-approved demonstration project) Ⓜ

**G9089** Oncology; disease status; colon cancer, limited to invasive cancer, adenocarcinoma as predominant cell type; extent of disease unknown, staging in progress or not listed (for use in a Medicare-approved demonstration project) Ⓜ

**G9090** Oncology; disease status; rectal cancer, limited to invasive cancer, adenocarcinoma as predominant cell type; extent of disease initially established as T1-2, N0, M0 (prior to neoadjuvant therapy, if any) with no evidence of disease progression, recurrence, or metastases (for use in a Medicare-approved demonstration project) Ⓜ

**G9091** Oncology; disease status; rectal cancer, limited to invasive cancer, adenocarcinoma as predominant cell type; extent of disease initially established as T3, N0, M0 (prior to neoadjuvant therapy, if any) with no evidence of disease progression, recurrence, or metastases (for use in a Medicare-approved demonstration project) Ⓜ

**G9092** Oncology; disease status; rectal cancer, limited to invasive cancer, adenocarcinoma as predominant cell type; extent of disease initially established as T1-3, N1-2, M0 (prior to neoadjuvant therapy, if any) with no evidence of disease progression, recurrence or metastases (for use in a Medicare-approved demonstration project) Ⓜ

**G9093** Oncology; disease status; rectal cancer, limited to invasive cancer, adenocarcinoma as predominant cell type; extent of disease initially established as T4, any N, M0 (prior to neoadjuvant therapy, if any) with no evidence of disease progression, recurrence, or metastases (for use in a Medicare-approved demonstration project) Ⓜ

**G9094** Oncology; disease status; rectal cancer, limited to invasive cancer, adenocarcinoma as predominant cell type; M1 at diagnosis, metastatic, locally recurrent, or progressive (for use in a Medicare-approved demonstration project) Ⓜ

**G9095** Oncology; disease status; rectal cancer, limited to invasive cancer, adenocarcinoma as predominant cell type; extent of disease unknown, staging in progress or not listed (for use in a Medicare-approved demonstration project) Ⓜ

**G9096** Oncology; disease status; esophageal cancer, limited to adenocarcinoma or squamous cell carcinoma as predominant cell type; extent of disease initially established as T1-T3, N0-N1 or NX (prior to neoadjuvant therapy, if any) with no evidence of disease progression, recurrence, or metastases (for use in a Medicare-approved demonstration project) Ⓜ

**G9097** Oncology; disease status; esophageal cancer, limited to adenocarcinoma or squamous cell carcinoma as predominant cell type; extent of disease initially established as T4, any N, M0 (prior to neoadjuvant therapy, if any) with no evidence of disease progression, recurrence, or metastases (for use in a Medicare-approved demonstration project) Ⓜ

**G9098** Oncology; disease status; esophageal cancer, limited to adenocarcinoma or squamous cell carcinoma as predominant cell type; M1 at diagnosis, metastatic, locally recurrent, or progressive (for use in a Medicare-approved demonstration project) Ⓜ

**G9099** Oncology; disease status; esophageal cancer, limited to adenocarcinoma or squamous cell carcinoma as predominant cell type; extent of disease unknown, staging in progress, or not listed (for use in a Medicare-approved demonstration project) Ⓜ

**G9100** Oncology; disease status; gastric cancer, limited to adenocarcinoma as predominant cell type; post R0 resection (with or without neoadjuvant therapy) with no evidence of disease recurrence, progression, or metastases (for use in a Medicare-approved demonstration project) Ⓜ

**G9101** Oncology; disease status; gastric cancer, limited to adenocarcinoma as predominant cell type; post R1 or R2 resection (with or without neoadjuvant therapy) with no evidence of disease progression, or metastases (for use in a Medicare-approved demonstration project) Ⓜ

**G9102** Oncology; disease status; gastric cancer, limited to adenocarcinoma as predominant cell type; clinical or pathologic M0, unresectable with no evidence of disease progression, or metastases (for use in a Medicare-approved demonstration project) Ⓜ

**G9103** Oncology; disease status; gastric cancer, limited to adenocarcinoma as predominant cell type; clinical or pathologic M1 at diagnosis, metastatic, locally recurrent, or progressive (for use in a Medicare-approved demonstration project) Ⓜ

Special Coverage Instructions    Noncovered by Medicare    Carrier Discretion    ☑ Quantity Alert    ● New Code    ○ Recycled/Reinstated    ▲ Revised Code

© 2016 Optum360, LLC    A2-Z3 ASC Pmt    CMS: Pub 100    AHA: Coding Clinic    ⅋ DMEPOS Paid    ⊘ SNF Excluded    G Codes — 59

**Procedures/Professional Services (Temporary)**

**G9104 — G9137**

**G9104** Oncology; disease status; gastric cancer, limited to adenocarcinoma as predominant cell type; extent of disease unknown, staging in progress, or not listed (for use in a Medicare-approved demonstration project) Ⓜ

**G9105** Oncology; disease status; pancreatic cancer, limited to adenocarcinoma as predominant cell type; post R0 resection without evidence of disease progression, recurrence, or metastases (for use in a Medicare-approved demonstration project) Ⓜ

**G9106** Oncology; disease status; pancreatic cancer, limited to adenocarcinoma; post R1 or R2 resection with no evidence of disease progression, or metastases (for use in a Medicare-approved demonstration project) Ⓜ

**G9107** Oncology; disease status; pancreatic cancer, limited to adenocarcinoma; unresectable at diagnosis, M1 at diagnosis, metastatic, locally recurrent, or progressive (for use in a Medicare-approved demonstration project) Ⓜ

**G9108** Oncology; disease status; pancreatic cancer, limited to adenocarcinoma; extent of disease unknown, staging in progress, or not listed (for use in a Medicare-approved demonstration project) Ⓜ

**G9109** Oncology; disease status; head and neck cancer, limited to cancers of oral cavity, pharynx and larynx with squamous cell as predominant cell type; extent of disease initially established as T1-T2 and N0, M0 (prior to neoadjuvant therapy, if any) with no evidence of disease progression, recurrence, or metastases (for use in a Medicare-approved demonstration project) Ⓜ

**G9110** Oncology; disease status; head and neck cancer, limited to cancers of oral cavity, pharynx and larynx with squamous cell as predominant cell type; extent of disease initially established as T3-4 and/or N1-3, M0 (prior to neoadjuvant therapy, if any) with no evidence of disease progression, recurrence, or metastases (for use in a Medicare-approved demonstration project) Ⓜ

**G9111** Oncology; disease status; head and neck cancer, limited to cancers of oral cavity, pharynx and larynx with squamous cell as predominant cell type; M1 at diagnosis, metastatic, locally recurrent, or progressive (for use in a Medicare-approved demonstration project) Ⓜ

**G9112** Oncology; disease status; head and neck cancer, limited to cancers of oral cavity, pharynx and larynx with squamous cell as predominant cell type; extent of disease unknown, staging in progress, or not listed (for use in a Medicare-approved demonstration project) Ⓜ

**G9113** Oncology; disease status; ovarian cancer, limited to epithelial cancer; pathologic stage 1A-B (Grade 1) without evidence of disease progression, recurrence, or metastases (for use in a Medicare-approved demonstration project) ♀ Ⓜ

**G9114** Oncology; disease status; ovarian cancer, limited to epithelial cancer; pathologic stage IA-B (grade 2-3); or stage IC (all grades); or stage II; without evidence of disease progression, recurrence, or metastases (for use in a Medicare-approved demonstration project) ♀ Ⓜ

**G9115** Oncology; disease status; ovarian cancer, limited to epithelial cancer; pathologic stage III-IV; without evidence of progression, recurrence, or metastases (for use in a Medicare-approved demonstration project) ♀ Ⓜ

**G9116** Oncology; disease status; ovarian cancer, limited to epithelial cancer; evidence of disease progression, or recurrence, and/or platinum resistance (for use in a Medicare-approved demonstration project) ♀ Ⓜ

**G9117** Oncology; disease status; ovarian cancer, limited to epithelial cancer; extent of disease unknown, staging in progress, or not listed (for use in a Medicare-approved demonstration project) ♀ Ⓜ

**G9123** Oncology; disease status; chronic myelogenous leukemia, limited to Philadelphia chromosome positive and/or BCR-ABL positive; chronic phase not in hematologic, cytogenetic, or molecular remission (for use in a Medicare-approved demonstration project) Ⓜ

**G9124** Oncology; disease status; chronic myelogenous leukemia, limited to Philadelphia chromosome positive and /or BCR-ABL positive; accelerated phase not in hematologic cytogenetic, or molecular remission (for use in a Medicare-approved demonstration project) Ⓜ

**G9125** Oncology; disease status; chronic myelogenous leukemia, limited to Philadelphia chromosome positive and/or BCR-ABL positive; blast phase not in hematologic, cytogenetic, or molecular remission (for use in a Medicare-approved demonstration project) Ⓜ

**G9126** Oncology; disease status; chronic myelogenous leukemia, limited to Philadelphia chromosome positive and/or BCR-ABL positive; in hematologic, cytogenetic, or molecular remission (for use in a Medicare-approved demonstration project) Ⓜ

**G9128** Oncology; disease status; limited to multiple myeloma, systemic disease; smoldering, stage I (for use in a Medicare-approved demonstration project) Ⓜ

**G9129** Oncology; disease status; limited to multiple myeloma, systemic disease; stage II or higher (for use in a Medicare-approved demonstration project) Ⓜ

**G9130** Oncology; disease status; limited to multiple myeloma, systemic disease; extent of disease unknown, staging in progress, or not listed (for use in a Medicare-approved demonstration project) Ⓜ

**G9131** Oncology; disease status; invasive female breast cancer (does not include ductal carcinoma in situ); adenocarcinoma as predominant cell type; extent of disease unknown, staging in progress, or not listed (for use in a Medicare-approved demonstration project) ♀ Ⓜ

**G9132** Oncology; disease status; prostate cancer, limited to adenocarcinoma; hormone-refractory/androgen-independent (e.g., rising PSA on antiandrogen therapy or postorchiectomy); clinical metastases (for use in a Medicare-approved demonstration project) ♂ Ⓜ

**G9133** Oncology; disease status; prostate cancer, limited to adenocarcinoma; hormone-responsive; clinical metastases or M1 at diagnosis (for use in a Medicare-approved demonstration project) ♂ Ⓜ

**G9134** Oncology; disease status; non-Hodgkin's lymphoma, any cellular classification; Stage I, II at diagnosis, not relapsed, not refractory (for use in a Medicare-approved demonstration project) Ⓜ

**G9135** Oncology; disease status; non-Hodgkin's lymphoma, any cellular classification; Stage III, IV, not relapsed, not refractory (for use in a Medicare-approved demonstration project) Ⓜ

**G9136** Oncology; disease status; non-Hodgkin's lymphoma, transformed from original cellular diagnosis to a second cellular classification (for use in a medicare-approved demonstration project) Ⓜ

**G9137** Oncology; disease status; non-Hodgkin's lymphoma, any cellular classification; relapsed/refractory (for use in a medicare-approved demonstration project) Ⓜ

Special Coverage Instructions    Noncovered by Medicare    Carrier Discretion    ☑ Quantity Alert  ● New Code    ○ Recycled/Reinstated  ▲ Revised Code

**60 — G Codes**    Ⓐ Age Edit   Ⓜ Maternity Edit   ♀ Female Only   ♂ Male Only   Ⓐ-Ⓨ OPPS Status Indicators      © 2016 Optum360, LLC

**G9138**   Oncology; disease status; non-Hodgkin's lymphoma, any cellular classification; diagnostic evaluation, stage not determined, evaluation of possible relapse or nonresponse to therapy, or not listed (for use in a Medicare-approved demonstration project)   M

**G9139**   Oncology; disease status; chronic myelogenous leukemia, limited to Philadelphia chromosome positive and/or BCR-ABL positive; extent of disease unknown, staging in progress, not listed (for use in a Medicare-approved demonstration project)   M

**G9140**   Frontier extended stay clinic demonstration; for a patient stay in a clinic approved for the CMS demonstration project; the following measures should be present: the stay must be equal to or greater than 4 hours; weather or other conditions must prevent transfer or the case falls into a category of monitoring and observation cases that are permitted by the rules of the demonstration; there is a maximum frontier extended stay clinic (FESC) visit of 48 hours, except in the case when weather or other conditions prevent transfer; payment is made on each period up to 4 hours, after the first 4 hours   A ☑

## Warfarin Testing

**G9143**   Warfarin responsiveness testing by genetic technique using any method, any number of specimen(s)   N
CMS: 100-03,90.1; 100-04,32,250.1; 100-04,32,250.2

## Outpatient IV Insulin TX

**G9147**   Outpatient Intravenous Insulin Treatment (OIVIT) either pulsatile or continuous, by any means, guided by the results of measurements for: respiratory quotient; and/or, urine urea nitrogen (UUN); and/or, arterial, venous or capillary glucose; and/or potassium concentration   E
CMS: 100-03,40.7; 100-04,4,320.1; 100-04,4,320.2

## Quality Assurance

**G9148**   National Committee for Quality Assurance-Level 1 medical home   M

**G9149**   National Committee for Quality Assurance-Level 2 medical home   M

**G9150**   National Committee for Quality Assurance-Level 3 medical home   M

**G9151**   MAPCP Demonstration-state provided services   M

**G9152**   MAPCP Demonstration-Community Health Teams   M

**G9153**   MAPCP Demonstration-Physician Incentive Pool   M

## Wheelchair Evaluation

**G9156**   Evaluation for wheelchair requiring face-to-face visit with physician   M

## Monitor

**G9157**   Transesophageal Doppler used for cardiac monitoring   B
CMS: 100-04,32,310; 100-04,32,310.10.3; 100-04,32,310.2

## Functional Limitation

**G9158**   Motor speech functional limitation, discharge status, at discharge from therapy or to end reporting   E
CMS: 100-04,5,10.6

**G9159**   Spoken language comprehension functional limitation, current status at therapy episode outset and at reporting intervals   E
CMS: 100-04,5,10.6

**G9160**   Spoken language comprehension functional limitation, projected goal status at therapy episode outset, at reporting intervals, and at discharge or to end reporting   E
CMS: 100-04,5,10.6

**G9161**   Spoken language comprehension functional limitation, discharge status, at discharge from therapy or to end reporting   E
CMS: 100-04,5,10.6

**G9162**   Spoken language expression functional limitation, current status at therapy episode outset and at reporting intervals   E
CMS: 100-04,5,10.6

**G9163**   Spoken language expression functional limitation, projected goal status at therapy episode outset, at reporting intervals, and at discharge or to end reporting   E
CMS: 100-04,5,10.6

**G9164**   Spoken language expression functional limitation, discharge status at discharge from therapy or to end reporting   E
CMS: 100-04,5,10.6

**G9165**   Attention functional limitation, current status at therapy episode outset and at reporting intervals   E
CMS: 100-04,5,10.6

**G9166**   Attention functional limitation, projected goal status at therapy episode outset, at reporting intervals, and at discharge or to end reporting   E
CMS: 100-04,5,10.6

**G9167**   Attention functional limitation, discharge status at discharge from therapy or to end reporting   E
CMS: 100-04,5,10.6

**G9168**   Memory functional limitation, current status at therapy episode outset and at reporting intervals   E
CMS: 100-04,5,10.6

**G9169**   Memory functional limitation, projected goal status at therapy episode outset, at reporting intervals, and at discharge or to end reporting   E
CMS: 100-04,5,10.6

**G9170**   Memory functional limitation, discharge status at discharge from therapy or to end reporting   E
CMS: 100-04,5,10.6

**G9171**   Voice functional limitation, current status at therapy episode outset and at reporting intervals   E
CMS: 100-04,5,10.6

**G9172**   Voice functional limitation, projected goal status at therapy episode outset, at reporting intervals, and at discharge or to end reporting   E
CMS: 100-04,5,10.6

**G9173**   Voice functional limitation, discharge status at discharge from therapy or to end reporting   E
CMS: 100-04,5,10.6

**G9174**   Other speech language pathology functional limitation, current status at therapy episode outset and at reporting intervals   E
CMS: 100-04,5,10.6

**G9175**   Other speech language pathology functional limitation, projected goal status at therapy episode outset, at reporting intervals, and at discharge or to end reporting   E
CMS: 100-04,5,10.6

**G9176**   Other speech language pathology functional limitation, discharge status at discharge from therapy or to end reporting   E
CMS: 100-04,5,10.6

**G9186**   Motor speech functional limitation, projected goal status at therapy episode outset, at reporting intervals, and at discharge or to end reporting   E
CMS: 100-04,5,10.6

Special Coverage Instructions   Noncovered by Medicare   Carrier Discretion   ☑ Quantity Alert   ● New Code   ○ Recycled/Reinstated   ▲ Revised Code

© 2016 Optum360, LLC   A2-Z3 ASC Pmt   CMS: Pub 100   AHA: Coding Clinic   ⅘ DMEPOS Paid   ⊘ SNF Excluded   G Codes — 61

**Procedures/Professional Services (Temporary)**

**G9187 — G9232**

## BPCI Services

**G9187** Bundled payments for care improvement initiative home visit for patient assessment performed by a qualified health care professional for individuals not considered homebound including, but not limited to, assessment of safety, falls, clinical status, fluid status, medication reconciliation/management, patient compliance with orders/plan of care, performance of activities of daily living, appropriateness of care setting; (for use only in the Medicare-approved bundled payments for care improvement initiative); may not be billed for a 30-day period covered by a transitional care management code  E

## Miscellaneous Quality Measures

**G9188** Beta-blocker therapy not prescribed, reason not given  M

**G9189** Beta-blocker therapy prescribed or currently being taken  M

**G9190** Documentation of medical reason(s) for not prescribing beta-blocker therapy (e.g., allergy, intolerance, other medical reasons)  M

**G9191** Documentation of patient reason(s) for not prescribing beta-blocker therapy (e.g., patient declined, other patient reasons)  M

**G9192** Documentation of system reason(s) for not prescribing beta-blocker therapy (e.g., other reasons attributable to the health care system)  M

**G9196** Documentation of medical reason(s) for not ordering a first or second generation cephalosporin for antimicrobial prophylaxis (e.g., patients enrolled in clinical trials, patients with documented infection prior to surgical procedure of interest, patients who were receiving antibiotics more than 24 hours prior to surgery [except colon surgery patients taking oral prophylactic antibiotics], patients who were receiving antibiotics within 24 hours prior to arrival [except colon surgery patients taking oral prophylactic antibiotics], other medical reason(s))  M

**G9197** Documentation of order for first or second generation cephalosporin for antimicrobial prophylaxis  M

**G9198** Order for first or second generation cephalosporin for antimicrobial prophylaxis was not documented, reason not given  M

**G9203**Jan RNA testing for hepatitis C documented as performed within 12 months prior to initiation of antiviral treatment for hepatitis C

**G9204**Jan RNA testing for hepatitis C was not documented as performed within 12 months prior to initiation of antiviral treatment for hepatitis C, reason not given

**G9205**Jan Patient starting antiviral treatment for hepatitis C during the measurement period

**G9206**Jan Patient starting antiviral treatment for hepatitis C during the measurement period

**G9207**Jan Hepatitis C genotype testing documented as performed within 12 months prior to initiation of antiviral treatment for hepatitis C

**G9208**Jan Hepatitis C genotype testing was not documented as performed within 12 months prior to initiation of antiviral treatment for hepatitis C, reason not given

**G9209**Jan Hepatitis C quantitative RNA testing documented as performed between 4-12 weeks after the initiation of antiviral treatment

**G9210**Jan Hepatitis C quantitative RNA testing not performed between 4-12 weeks after the initiation of antiviral treatment for documented reason(s) (e.g., patients whose treatment was discontinued during the testing period prior to testing, other medical reasons, patient declined, other patient reasons)

**G9211**Jan Hepatitis C quantitative RNA testing was not documented as performed between 4-12 weeks after the initiation of antiviral treatment, reason not given

**G9212** DSM-IVTM criteria for major depressive disorder documented at the initial evaluation  M

**G9213** DSM-IV-TR criteria for major depressive disorder not documented at the initial evaluation, reason not otherwise specified  M

**G9217**Jan PCP prophylaxis was not prescribed within 3 months of low CD4+ cell count below 200 cells/mm3, reason not given

**G9219**Jan Pneumocystis jiroveci pneumonia prophylaxis not prescribed within 3 months of low CD4+ cell count below 200 cells/mm3 for medical reason (i.e., patient's CD4+ cell count above threshold within 3 months after CD4+ cell count below threshold, indicating that the patient's CD4+ levels are within an acceptable range and the patient does not require PCP prophylaxis)

**G9222**Jan Pneumocystis jiroveci pneumonia prophylaxis prescribed wthin 3 months of low CD4+ cell count below 200 cells/mm3

**G9223** Pneumocystis jiroveci pneumonia prophylaxis prescribed within 3 months of low CD4+ cell count below 500 cells/mm3 or a CD4 percentage below 15%  M

**G9225** Foot exam was not performed, reason not given  M

▲ **G9226**Jan Foot examination performed (includes examination through visual inspection, sensory exam with 10-g monofilament plus testing any one of the following: vibration using 128-Hz tuning fork, pinprick sensation, ankle reflexes, or vibration perception threshold, and pulse exam; report when all of the 3 components are completed)  M

**G9227** Functional outcome assessment documented, care plan not documented, documented the patient is not eligible for a care plan  M

**G9228** Chlamydia, gonorrhea and syphilis screening results documented (report when results are present for all of the 3 screenings)  M

▲ **G9229**Jan Chlamydia, gonorrhea, and syphilis screening results not documented (patient refusal is the only allowed exception)  M

**G9230** Chlamydia, gonorrhea, and syphilis not screened, reason not given  M

▲ **G9231**Jan Documentation of end stage renal disease (ESRD), dialysis, renal transplant before or during the measurement period or pregnancy during the measurement period  M

▲ **G9232**Jan Clinician treating major depressive disorder did not communicate to clinician treating comorbid condition for specified patient reason (e.g., patient is unable to communicate the diagnosis of a comorbid condition; the patient is unwilling to communicate the diagnosis of a comorbid condition; or the patient is unaware of the comorbid condition, or any other specified patient reason)  M

**G9233**Jan All quality actions for the applicable measures in the total knee replacement measures group have been performed for this patient

**G9234**Jan I intend to report the total knee replacement measures group

**G9235**Jan All quality actions for the applicable measures in the general surgery measures group have been performed for this patient

**G9236**Jan All quality actions for the applicable measures in the optimizing patient exposure to ionizing radiation measures group have been performed for this patient

**G9237**Jan I intend to report the general surgery measures group

**G9238**Jan I intend to report the optimizing patient exposure to ionizing radiation measures group

---

Jan  **January Update**

Special Coverage Instructions       Noncovered by Medicare       Carrier Discretion       ☑ Quantity Alert  ● New Code       ○ Recycled/Reinstated   ▲ Revised Code

62 — G Codes        A Age Edit       M Maternity Edit      ♀ Female Only      ♂ Male Only      A-Y OPPS Status Indicators          © 2016 Optum360, LLC

▲ **G9239**ᴶᵃⁿ Documentation of reasons for patient initiaiting maintenance hemodialysis with a catheter as the mode of vascular access (e.g., patient has a maturing AVF/AVG, time-limited trial of hemodialysis, other medical reasons, patient declined AVF/AVG, other patient reasons, patient followed by reporting nephrologist for fewer than 90 days, other system reasons) Ⓜ

**G9240** Patient whose mode of vascular access is a catheter at the time maintenance hemodialysis is initiated Ⓜ

**G9241** Patient whose mode of vascular access is not a catheter at the time maintenance hemodialysis is initiated Ⓜ

**G9242** Documentation of viral load equal to or greater than 200 copies/ml or viral load not performed Ⓜ

**G9243** Documentation of viral load less than 200 copies/ml Ⓜ

**G9244**ᴶᵃⁿ ~~Antiretroviral thereapy not prescribed~~

**G9245**ᴶᵃⁿ ~~Antiretroviral therapy prescribed~~

**G9246** Patient did not have at least one medical visit in each 6 month period of the 24 month measurement period, with a minimum of 60 days between medical visits Ⓜ

**G9247** Patient had at least one medical visit in each 6 month period of the 24 month measurement period, with a minimum of 60 days between medical visits Ⓜ

**G9250** Documentation of patient pain brought to a comfortable level within 48 hours from initial assessment Ⓜ

**G9251** Documentation of patient with pain not brought to a comfortable level within 48 hours from initial assessment Ⓜ

**G9254** Documentation of patient discharged to home later than post-operative day 2 following CAS Ⓜ

**G9255** Documentation of patient discharged to home no later than post operative day 2 following CAS Ⓜ

**G9256** Documentation of patient death following CAS Ⓜ

**G9257** Documentation of patient stroke following CAS Ⓜ

**G9258** Documentation of patient stroke following CEA Ⓜ

**G9259** Documentation of patient survival and absence of stroke following CAS Ⓜ

**G9260** Documentation of patient death following CEA Ⓜ

**G9261** Documentation of patient survival and absence of stroke following CEA Ⓜ

**G9262** Documentation of patient death in the hospital following endovascular AAA repair Ⓜ

**G9263** Documentation of patient survival in the hospital following endovascular AAA repair Ⓜ

▲ **G9264**ᴶᵃⁿ Documentation of patient receiving maintenance hemodialysis for greater than or equal to 90 days with a catheter for documented reasons (e.g., other medical reasons, patient declined AVF/AVG, other patient reasons) Ⓜ

**G9265** Patient receiving maintenance hemodialysis for greater than or equal to 90 days with a catheter as the mode of vascular access Ⓜ

**G9266** Patient receiving maintenance hemodialysis for greater than or equal to 90 days without a catheter as the mode of vascular access Ⓜ

**G9267** Documentation of patient with one or more complications or mortality within 30 days Ⓜ

**G9268** Documentation of patient with one or more complications within 90 days Ⓜ

**G9269** Documentation of patient without one or more complications and without mortality within 30 days Ⓜ

**G9270** Documentation of patient without one or more complications within 90 days Ⓜ

**G9273** Blood pressure has a systolic value of < 140 and a diastolic value of < 90 Ⓜ

**G9274** Blood pressure has a systolic value of = 140 and a diastolic value of = 90 or systolic value < 140 and diastolic value = 90 or systolic value = 140 and diastolic value < 90 Ⓜ

**G9275** Documentation that patient is a current non-tobacco user Ⓜ

**G9276** Documentation that patient is a current tobacco user Ⓜ

**G9277** Documentation that the patient is on daily aspirin or antiplatelet or has documentation of a valid contraindication or exception to aspirin/antiplatelet; contraindications/exceptions include anticoagulant use, allergy to aspirin or antiplatelets, history of gastrointestinal bleed and bleeding disorder. Additionally, the following exceptions documented by the physician as a reason for not taking daily aspirin or antiplatelet are acceptable (use of nonsteroidal antiinflammatory agents, documented risk for drug interaction, uncontrolled hypertension defined as >180 systolic or >110 diastolic or gastroesophageal reflux) Ⓜ

**G9278** Documentation that the patient is not on daily aspirin or anti-platelet regimen Ⓜ

**G9279** Pneumococcal screening performed and documentation of vaccination received prior to discharge Ⓜ

**G9280** Pneumococcal vaccination not administered prior to discharge, reason not specified Ⓜ

**G9281** Screening performed and documentation that vaccination not indicated/patient refusal Ⓜ

**G9282** Documentation of medical reason(s) for not reporting the histological type or NSCLC-NOS classification with an explanation (e.g., biopsy taken for other purposes in a patient with a history of non-small cell lung cancer or other documented medical reasons) Ⓜ

**G9283** Non-small cell lung cancer biopsy and cytology specimen report documents classification into specific histologic type or classified as NSCLC-NOS with an explanation Ⓜ

**G9284** Non-small cell lung cancer biopsy and cytology specimen report does not document classification into specific histologic type or classified as NSCLC-NOS with an explanation Ⓜ

**G9285** Specimen site other than anatomic location of lung or is not classified as non-small cell lung cancer Ⓜ

**G9286** Antibiotic regimen prescribed within 10 days after onset of symptoms Ⓜ

**G9287** Antibiotic regimen not prescribed within 10 days after onset of symptoms Ⓜ

**G9288** Documentation of medical reason(s) for not reporting the histological type or nsclc-nos classification with an explanation (e.g., a solitary fibrous tumor in a person with a history of non-small cell carcinoma or other documented medical reasons) Ⓜ

**G9289** Non-small cell lung cancer biopsy and cytology specimen report documents classification into specific histologic type or classified as NSCLC-NOS with an explanation Ⓜ

**G9290** Non-small cell lung cancer biopsy and cytology specimen report does not document classification into specific histologic type or classified as NSCLC-NOS with an explanation Ⓜ

**G9291** Specimen site other than anatomic location of lung, is not classified as non-small cell lung cancer or classified as NSCLC-NOS Ⓜ

ᴶᵃⁿ **January Update**

Special Coverage Instructions    Noncovered by Medicare    Carrier Discretion    ☑ Quantity Alert  ● New Code    ○ Recycled/Reinstated    ▲ Revised Code

© 2016 Optum360, LLC    **A²-Z³** ASC Pmt    **CMS:** Pub 100    **AHA:** Coding Clinic    ☍ DMEPOS Paid    ⊘ SNF Excluded    **G Codes — 63**

**G9292** Documentation of medical reason(s) for not reporting PT category and a statement on thickness and ulceration and for PT1, mitotic rate (e.g., negative skin biopsies in a patient with a history of melanoma or other documented medical reasons) Ⓜ

**G9293** Pathology report does not include the PT category and a statement on thickness and ulceration and for PT1, mitotic rate Ⓜ

**G9294** Pathology report includes the PT category and a statement on thickness and ulceration and for PT1, mitotic rate Ⓜ

**G9295** Specimen site other than anatomic cutaneous location Ⓜ

**G9296** Patients with documented shared decision-making including discussion of conservative (non-surgical) therapy (e.g., NSAIDs, analgesics, weight loss, exercise, injections) prior to the procedure Ⓜ

**G9297** Shared decision-making including discussion of conservative (non-surgical) therapy (e.g., NSAIDs, analgesics, weight loss, exercise, injections) prior to the procedure, not documented, reason not given Ⓜ

**G9298** Patients who are evaluated for venous thromboembolic and cardiovascular risk factors within 30 days prior to the procedure (e.g., history of DVT, PE, MI, arrhythmia and stroke) Ⓜ

**G9299** Patients who are not evaluated for venous thromboembolic and cardiovascular risk factors within 30 days prior to the procedure including (e.g., history of DVT, PE, MI, arrhythmia and stroke, reason not given) Ⓜ

**G9300** Documentation of medical reason(s) for not completely infusing the prophylactic antibiotic prior to the inflation of the proximal tourniquet (e.g., a tourniquet was not used) Ⓜ

**G9301** Patients who had the prophylactic antibiotic completely infused prior to the inflation of the proximal tourniquet Ⓜ

**G9302** Prophylactic antibiotic not completely infused prior to the inflation of the proximal tourniquet, reason not given Ⓜ

**G9303** Operative report does not identify the prosthetic implant specifications including the prosthetic implant manufacturer, the brand name of the prosthetic implant and the size of each prosthetic implant, reason not given Ⓜ

**G9304** Operative report identifies the prosthetic implant specifications including the prosthetic implant manufacturer, the brand name of the prosthetic implant and the size of each prosthetic implant Ⓜ

**G9305** Intervention for presence of leak of endoluminal contents through an anastomosis not required Ⓜ

**G9306** Intervention for presence of leak of endoluminal contents through an anastomosis required Ⓜ

▲ **G9307**^Jan No return to the operating room for a surgical procedure, for complications of the principal operative procedure, within 30 days of the principal operative procedure Ⓜ

▲ **G9308**^Jan Unplanned return to the operating room for a surgical procedure, for complications of the principal operative procedure, within 30 days of the principal operative procedure Ⓜ

**G9309** No unplanned hospital readmission within 30 days of principal procedure Ⓜ

**G9310** Unplanned hospital readmission within 30 days of principal procedure Ⓜ

**G9311** No surgical site infection Ⓜ

**G9312** Surgical site infection Ⓜ

**G9313** Amoxicillin, with or without clavulanate, not prescribed as first line antibiotic at the time of diagnosis for documented reason (e.g., cystic fibrosis, immotile cilia disorders, ciliary dyskinesia, immune deficiency, prior history of sinus surgery within the past 12 months, and anatomic abnormalities, such as deviated nasal septum, resistant organisms, allergy to medication, recurrent sinusitis, chronic sinusitis, or other reasons) Ⓜ

**G9314** Amoxicillin, with or without clavulanate, not prescribed as first line antibiotic at the time of diagnosis, reason not given Ⓜ

**G9315** Documentation amoxicillin, with or without clavulanate, prescribed as a first line antibiotic at the time of diagnosis Ⓜ

**G9316** Documentation of patient-specific risk assessment with a risk calculator based on multi-institutional clinical data, the specific risk calculator used, and communication of risk assessment from risk calculator with the patient or family Ⓜ

**G9317** Documentation of patient-specific risk assessment with a risk calculator based on multi-institutional clinical data, the specific risk calculator used, and communication of risk assessment from risk calculator with the patient or family not completed Ⓜ

**G9318** Imaging study named according to standardized nomenclature Ⓜ

**G9319** Imaging study not named according to standardized nomenclature, reason not given Ⓜ

**G9321** Count of previous CT (any type of CT) and cardiac nuclear medicine (myocardial perfusion) studies documented in the 12-month period prior to the current study Ⓜ

**G9322** Count of previous CT and cardiac nuclear medicine (myocardial perfusion) studies not documented in the 12-month period prior to the current study, reason not given Ⓜ

**G9324**^Jan ~~All necessary data elements not included, reason not given~~

▲ **G9326**^Jan CT studies performed not reported to a radiation dose index registry that is capable of collecting at a minimum all necessary data elements, reason not given Ⓜ

▲ **G9327**^Jan CT studies performed reported to a radiation dose index registry that is capable of collecting at a minimum all necessary data elements Ⓜ

**G9329** DICOM format image data available to non-affiliated external health care facilities or entities on a secure, media free, reciprocally searchable basis with patient authorization for at least a 12-month period after the study not documented in final report, reason not given Ⓜ

**G9340** Final report documented that DICOM format image data available to non-affiliated external healthcare facilities or entities on a secure, media free, reciprocally searchable basis with patient authorization for at least a 12-month period after the study Ⓜ

**G9341** Search conducted for prior patient CT studies completed at non-affiliated external health care facilities or entities within the past 12-months and are available through a secure, authorized, media-free, shared archive prior to an imaging study being performed Ⓜ

**G9342** Search not conducted prior to an imaging study being performed for prior patient CT studies completed at non-affiliated external health care facilities or entities within the past 12 months and are available through a secure, authorized, media-free, shared archive, reason not given Ⓜ

---

^Jan **January Update**

Special Coverage Instructions    Noncovered by Medicare    Carrier Discretion    ☑ Quantity Alert  ● New Code    ○ Recycled/Reinstated    ▲ Revised Code

**64 — G Codes**    🅐 Age Edit    Ⓜ Maternity Edit    ♀ Female Only    ♂ Male Only    🅐-Ⓨ OPPS Status Indicators    © 2016 Optum360, LLC

**G9344** Due to system reasons search not conducted for DICOM format images for prior patient CT imaging studies completed at non-affiliated external health care facilities or entities within the past 12 months that are available through a secure, authorized, media-free, shared archive (e.g., non-affiliated external health care facilities or entities does not have archival abilities through a shared archival system) Ⓜ

**G9345** Follow-up recommendations documented according to recommended guidelines for incidentally detected pulmonary nodules (e.g., follow-up CT imaging studies needed or that no follow-up is needed) based at a minimum on nodule size and patient risk factors Ⓜ

**G9347** Follow-up recommendations not documented according to recommended guidelines for incidentally detected pulmonary nodules, reason not given Ⓜ

**G9348** CT scan of the paranasal sinuses ordered at the time of diagnosis for documented reasons (e.g., persons with sinusitis symptoms lasting at least 7 to 10 days, antibiotic resistance, immunocompromised, recurrent sinusitis, acute frontal sinusitis, acute sphenoid sinusitis, periorbital cellulitis, or other medical) Ⓜ

**G9349** Documentation of a CT scan of the paranasal sinuses ordered at the time of diagnosis or received within 28 days after date of diagnosis Ⓜ

**G9350** CT scan of the paranasal sinuses not ordered at the time of diagnosis or received within 28 days after date of diagnosis Ⓜ

**G9351** More than one CT scan of the paranasal sinuses ordered or received within 90 days after diagnosis Ⓜ

**G9352** More than one CT scan of the paranasal sinuses ordered or received within 90 days after the date of diagnosis, reason not given Ⓜ

**G9353** More than one CT scan of the paranasal sinuses ordered or received within 90 days after the date of diagnosis for documented reasons (e.g., patients with complications, second CT obtained prior to surgery, other medical reasons) Ⓜ

**G9354** One CT scan or no CT scan of the paranasal sinuses ordered within 90 days after the date of diagnosis Ⓜ

**G9355** Elective delivery or early induction not performed Ⓜ

**G9356** Elective delivery or early induction performed Ⓜ

**G9357** Post-partum screenings, evaluations and education performed Ⓜ

**G9358** Post-partum screenings, evaluations and education not performed Ⓜ

▲ **G9359**[Jan] Documentation of negative or managed positive TB screen with further evidence that TB is not active within one year of patient visit Ⓜ

**G9360** No documentation of negative or managed positive TB screen Ⓜ

▲ **G9361**[Jan] Medical indication for induction [documentation of reason(s) for elective delivery (c-section) or early induction (e.g., hemorrhage and placental complications, hypertension, preeclampsia and eclampsia, rupture of membranes-premature or prolonged, maternal conditions complicating pregnancy/delivery, fetal conditions complicating pregnancy/delivery, late pregnancy, prior uterine surgery, or participation in clinical trial)] Ⓜ

**G9364** Sinusitis caused by, or presumed to be caused by, bacterial infection Ⓜ

**G9365** One high-risk medication ordered Ⓜ

**G9366** One high-risk medication not ordered Ⓜ

**G9367** At least two different high-risk medications ordered Ⓜ

**G9368** At least two different high-risk medications not ordered Ⓜ

**G9380** Patient offered assistance with end of life issues during the measurement period Ⓜ

▲ **G9381**[Jan] Documentation of medical reason(s) for not offering assistance with end of life issues (e.g., patient in hospice care, patient in terminal phase) during the measurement period Ⓜ

**G9382** Patient not offered assistance with end of life issues during the measurement period Ⓜ

**G9383** Patient received screening for HCV infection within the 12 month reporting period Ⓜ

**G9384** Documentation of medical reason(s) for not receiving annual screening for HCV infection (e.g., decompensated cirrhosis indicating advanced disease [i.e., ascites, esophageal variceal bleeding, hepatic encephalopathy], hepatocellular carcinoma, waitlist for organ transplant, limited life expectancy, other medical reasons) Ⓜ

**G9385** Documentation of patient reason(s) for not receiving annual screening for HCV infection (e.g., patient declined, other patient reasons) Ⓜ

**G9386** Screening for HCV infection not received within the 12 month reporting period, reason not given Ⓜ

**G9389** Unplanned rupture of the posterior capsule requiring vitrectomy during cataract surgery Ⓜ

**G9390** No unplanned rupture of the posterior capsule requiring vitrectomy during cataract surgery Ⓜ

**G9393** Patient with an initial PHQ-9 score greater than nine who achieves remission at twelve months as demonstrated by a twelve month (+/- 30 days) PHQ-9 score of less than five Ⓜ

**G9394** Patient who had a diagnosis of bipolar disorder or personality disorder, death, permanent nursing home resident or receiving hospice or palliative care any time during the measurement or assessment period Ⓜ

**G9395** Patient with an initial PHQ-9 score greater than nine who did not achieve remission at twelve months as demonstrated by a twelve month (+/- 30 days) PHQ-9 score greater than or equal to five Ⓜ

**G9396** Patient with an initial PHQ-9 score greater than nine who was not assessed for remission at twelve months (+/- 30 days) Ⓜ

**G9399** Documentation in the patient record of a discussion between the physician/clinician and the patient that includes all of the following: treatment choices appropriate to genotype, risks and benefits, evidence of effectiveness, and patient preferences toward the outcome of the treatment Ⓜ

**G9400** Documentation of medical or patient reason(s) for not discussing treatment options; medical reasons: patient is not a candidate for treatment due to advanced physical or mental health comorbidity (including active substance use); currently receiving antiviral treatment; successful antiviral treatment (with sustained virologic response) prior to reporting period; other documented medical reasons; patient reasons: patient unable or unwilling to participate in the discussion or other patient reasons Ⓜ

**G9401** No documentation in the patient record of a discussion between the physician or other qualified health care professional and the patient that includes all of the following: treatment choices appropriate to genotype, risks and benefits, evidence of effectiveness, and patient preferences toward treatment Ⓜ

**G9402** Patient received follow-up on the date of discharge or within 30 days after discharge Ⓜ

[Jan] **January Update**

Special Coverage Instructions   Noncovered by Medicare   Carrier Discretion   ☑ Quantity Alert   ● New Code   ○ Recycled/Reinstated   ▲ Revised Code

© 2016 Optum360, LLC   A2-Z8 ASC Pmt   **CMS:** Pub 100   **AHA:** Coding Clinic   ☒ DMEPOS Paid   ⊘ SNF Excluded   **G Codes — 65**

**Procedures/Professional Services (Temporary)**

**G9403 — G9455**

**G9403** Clinician documented reason patient was not able to complete 30-day follow-up from acute inpatient setting discharge (e.g., patient death prior to follow-up visit, patient non-compliant for visit follow-up) Ⓜ

**G9404** Patient did not receive follow-up on the date of discharge or within 30 days after discharge Ⓜ

**G9405** Patient received follow-up within 7 days from discharge Ⓜ

**G9406** Clinician documented reason patient was not able to complete 7 day follow-up from acute inpatient setting discharge (i.e., patient death prior to follow-up visit, patient non-compliance for visit follow-up) Ⓜ

**G9407** Patient did not receive follow-up on or within 7 days after discharge Ⓜ

**G9408** Patients with cardiac tamponade and/or pericardiocentesis occurring within 30 days Ⓜ

**G9409** Patients without cardiac tamponade and/or pericardiocentesis occurring within 30 days Ⓜ

**G9410** Patient admitted within 180 days, status post CIED implantation, replacement, or revision with an infection requiring device removal or surgical revision Ⓜ

**G9411** Patient not admitted within 180 days, status post CIED implantation, replacement, or revision with an infection requiring device removal or surgical revision Ⓜ

**G9412** Patient admitted within 180 days, status post CIED implantation, replacement, or revision with an infection requiring device removal or surgical revision Ⓜ

**G9413** Patient not admitted within 180 days, status post CIED implantation, replacement, or revision with an infection requiring device removal or surgical revision Ⓜ

**G9414** Patient had one dose of meningococcal vaccine on or between the patient's 11th and 13th birthdays Ⓜ

**G9415** Patient did not have one dose of meningococcal vaccine on or between the patient's 11th and 13th birthdays Ⓜ

▲ **G9416**[Jan] Patient had one tetanus, diphtheria toxoids and acellular pertussis vaccine (TDaP) on or between the patient's 10th and 13th birthdays Ⓜ

▲ **G9417**[Jan] Patient did not have one tetanus, diphtheria toxoids and acellular pertussis vaccine (TDaP) on or between the patient's 10th and 13th birthdays Ⓜ

**G9418** Primary non-small cell lung cancer biopsy and cytology specimen report documents classification into specific histologic type or classified as NSCLC-NOS with an explanation Ⓜ

**G9419** Documentation of medical reason(s) for not including the histological type or NSCLC-NOS classification with an explanation (e.g., biopsy taken for other purposes in a patient with a history of primary nonsmall cell lung cancer or other documented medical reasons) Ⓜ

**G9420** Specimen site other than anatomic location of lung or is not classified as primary non-small cell lung cancer Ⓜ

**G9421** Primary non-small cell lung cancer biopsy and cytology specimen report does not document classification into specific histologic type or classified as NSCLC-NOS with an explanation Ⓜ

**G9422** Non-small cell lung cancer biopsy and cytology specimen report documents classification into specific histologic type or classified as NSCLC-NOS with an explanation Ⓜ

▲ **G9423**[Jan] Documentation of medical reason for not including PT category, PN category and histologic type [for patient with appropriate exclusion criteria (e.g., metastatic disease, benign tumors, malignant tumors other than carcinomas, inadequate surgical specimens) Ⓜ

▲ **G9424**[Jan] Specimen site other than anatomic location of lung, or classified as NSCLC-NOS Ⓜ

**G9425** Non-small cell lung cancer biopsy and cytology specimen report does not document classification into specific histologic type or classified as NSCLC-NOS with an explanation Ⓜ

**G9426** Improvement in median time from ED arrival to initial ED oral or parenteral pain medication administration performed for ED admitted patients Ⓜ

**G9427** Improvement in median time from ED arrival to initial ED oral or parenteral pain medication administration not performed for ED admitted patients Ⓜ

**G9428** Pathology report includes the PT category and a statement on thickness and ulceration and for PT1, mitotic rate Ⓜ

**G9429** Documentation of medical reason(s) for not including pT category and a statement on thickness and ulceration and for pT1, mitotic rate (e.g., negative skin biopsies in a patient with a history of melanoma or other documented medical reasons) Ⓜ

**G9430** Specimen site other than anatomic cutaneous location Ⓜ

**G9431** Pathology report does not include the PT category and a statement on thickness and ulceration and for PT1, mitotic rate Ⓜ

**G9432** Asthma well-controlled based on the ACT, C-ACT, ACQ, or ATAQ score and results documented Ⓜ

**G9434** Asthma not well-controlled based on the ACT, C-ACT, ACQ, or ATAQ score, or specified asthma control tool not used, reason not given Ⓜ

**G9435**[Jan] ~~Aspirin prescribed at discharge~~

**G9436**[Jan] ~~Aspirin not prescribed for documented reasons (e.g., allergy, medical intolerance, history of bleed)~~

**G9437**[Jan] ~~Aspirin not prescribed at discharge~~

**G9438**[Jan] ~~P2Y inhibitor prescribed at discharge~~

**G9439**[Jan] ~~P2Y inhibitor not prescribed for documented reasons (e.g., allergy, medical intolerance, history of bleed)~~

**G9440**[Jan] ~~P2Y inhibitor not prescribed at discharge~~

**G9441**[Jan] ~~Statin prescribed at discharge~~

**G9442**[Jan] ~~Statin not prescribed for documented reasons (e.g., allergy, medical intolerance)~~

**G9443**[Jan] ~~Statin not prescribed at discharge~~

**G9448** Patients who were born in the years 1945-1965 Ⓜ

**G9449** History of receiving blood transfusions prior to 1992 Ⓐ Ⓜ

**G9450** History of injection drug use Ⓜ

**G9451** Patient received one-time screening for HCV infection Ⓜ

**G9452** Documentation of medical reason(s) for not receiving one-time screening for HCV infection (e.g., decompensated cirrhosis indicating advanced disease [i.e., ascites, esophageal variceal bleeding, hepatic encephalopathy], hepatocellular carcinoma, waitlist for organ transplant, limited life expectancy, other medical reasons) Ⓜ

**G9453** Documentation of patient reason(s) for not receiving one-time screening for HCV infection (e.g., patient declined, other patient reasons) Ⓜ

**G9454** One-time screening for HCV infection not received within 12-month reporting period and no documentation of prior screening for HCV infection, reason not given Ⓜ

**G9455** Patient underwent abdominal imaging with ultrasound, contrast enhanced CT or contrast MRI for HCC Ⓜ

---

[Jan] **January Update**

Special Coverage Instructions     Noncovered by Medicare     Carrier Discretion     ☑ Quantity Alert  ● New Code     ○ Recycled/Reinstated  ▲ Revised Code

66 — G Codes          Ⓐ Age Edit     Ⓜ Maternity Edit    ♀ Female Only    ♂ Male Only    Ⓐ-Ⓨ OPPS Status Indicators          © 2016 Optum360, LLC

**G9456** Documentation of medical or patient reason(s) for not ordering or performing screening for HCC. Medical reason: comorbid medical conditions with expected survival < 5 years, hepatic decompensation and not a candidate for liver transplantation, or other medical reasons; patient reasons: patient declined or other patient reasons (e.g., cost of tests, time related to accessing testing equipment) M

**G9457** Patient did not undergo abdominal imaging and did not have a documented reason for not undergoing abdominal imaging in the reporting period M

**G9458** Patient documented as tobacco user and received tobacco cessation intervention (must include at least one of the following: advice given to quit smoking or tobacco use, counseling on the benefits of quitting smoking or tobacco use, assistance with or referral to external smoking or tobacco cessation support programs, or current enrollment in smoking or tobacco use cessation program) if identified as a tobacco user M

**G9459** Currently a tobacco non-user M

**G9460** Tobacco assessment or tobacco cessation intervention not performed, reason not given M

**G9463**Jan ~~I intend to report the sinusitis measures group~~

**G9464**Jan ~~All quality actions for the applicable measures in the sinusitis measures group have been performed for this patient~~

**G9465**Jan ~~I intend to report the acute otitis externa (AOE) measures group~~

**G9466**Jan ~~All quality actions for the applicable measures in the AOE measures group have been performed for this patient~~

**G9467**Jan ~~Patients who have received or are receiving corticosteroids greater than or equal to 10 mg/day of prednisone equivalents for 60 or greater consecutive days or a single prescription equating to 600 mg prednisone or greater for all fills within the last twelve months~~

**G9468** Patient not receiving corticosteroids greater than or equal to 10 mg/day of prednisone equivalents for 60 or greater consecutive days or a single prescription equating to 600 mg prednisone or greater for all fills M

**G9469** Patients who have received or are receiving corticosteroids greater than or equal to 10 mg/day of prednisone equivalents for 60 or greater consecutive days or a single prescription equating to 600 mg prednisone or greater for all fills M

**G9470** Patients not receiving corticosteroids greater than or equal to 10 mg/day of prednisone equivalents for 60 or greater consecutive days or a single prescription equating to 600 mg prednisone or greater for all fills M

**G9471** Within the past 2 years, central dual-energy x-ray absorptiometry (DXA) not ordered or documented M

**G9472** Within the past 2 years, central dual-energy x-ray absorptiometry (DXA) not ordered and documented, no review of systems and no medication history or pharmacologic therapy (other than minerals/vitamins) for osteoporosis prescribed M

## Hospice Services

**G9473** Services performed by chaplain in the hospice setting, each 15 minutes B

**G9474** Services performed by dietary counselor in the hospice setting, each 15 minutes B

**G9475** Services performed by other counselor in the hospice setting, each 15 minutes B

**G9476** Services performed by volunteer in the hospice setting, each 15 minutes B

**G9477** Services performed by care coordinator in the hospice setting, each 15 minutes B

**G9478** Services performed by other qualified therapist in the hospice setting, each 15 minutes B

**G9479** Services performed by qualified pharmacist in the hospice setting, each 15 minutes B

## Medicare Care Choice Model Program

**G9480** Admission to Medicare care choice model program (MCCM) B

## Comprehensive Care for Joint Replacement Model

● **G9481**Apr Remote in-home visit for the evaluation and management of a new patient for use only in the Medicare-approved Comprehensive Care for Joint Replacement Model, which requires these 3 key components: A problem focused history; A problem focused examination; Straightforward medical decision making, furnished in real time using interactive audio and video technology. Counseling and coordination of care with other physicians, other qualified health care professionals or agencies are provided consistent with the nature of the problem(s) and the needs of the patient or the family or both. Usually, the presenting problem(s) are self-limited or minor. Typically, 10 minutes are spent with the patient or family or both via real time, audio and video intercommunications technology. B

● **G9482**Apr Remote in-home visit for the evaluation and management of a new patient for use only in the Medicare-approved Comprehensive Care for Joint Replacement Model, which requires these 3 key components: An expanded problem focused history; An expanded problem focused examination; Straightforward medical decision making, furnished in real time using interactive audio and video technology. Counseling and coordination of care with other physicians, other qualified health care professionals or agencies are provided consistent with the nature of the problem(s) and the needs of the patient or the family or both. Usually, the presenting problem(s) are of low to moderate severity. Typically, 20 minutes are spent with the patient or family or both via real time, audio and video intercommunications technology. B

● **G9483**Apr Remote in-home visit for the evaluation and management of a new patient for use only in the Medicare-approved Comprehensive Care for Joint Replacement Model, which requires these 3 key components: A detailed history; A detailed examination; Medical decision making of low complexity, furnished in real time using interactive audio and video technology. Counseling and coordination of care with other physicians, other qualified health care professionals or agencies are provided consistent with the nature of the problem(s) and the needs of the patient or the family or both. Usually, the presenting problem(s) are of moderate severity. Typically, 30 minutes are spent with the patient or family or both via real time, audio and video intercommunications technology. B

● **G9484**Apr Remote in-home visit for the evaluation and management of a new patient for use only in the Medicare-approved Comprehensive Care for Joint Replacement Model, which requires these 3 key components: A comprehensive history; A comprehensive examination; Medical decision making of moderate complexity, furnished in real time using interactive audio and video technology. Counseling and coordination of care with other physicians, other qualified health care professionals or agencies are provided consistent with the nature of the problem(s) and the needs of the patient or the family or both. Usually, the presenting problem(s) are of moderate to high severity. Typically, 45 minutes are spent with the patient or family or both via real time, audio and video intercommunications technology. B

---

Jan **January Update**    Apr **April Update**

Special Coverage Instructions    Noncovered by Medicare    Carrier Discretion    ☑ Quantity Alert    ● New Code    ○ Recycled/Reinstated    ▲ Revised Code

© 2016 Optum360, LLC    12-23 ASC Pmt    CMS: Pub 100    AHA: Coding Clinic    ⅋ DMEPOS Paid    ⊘ SNF Excluded    G Codes — 67

● **G9485**Apr Remote in-home visit for the evaluation and management of a new patient for use only in the Medicare-approved Comprehensive Care for Joint Replacement Model, which requires these 3 key components: A comprehensive history; A comprehensive examination; Medical decision making of high complexity, furnished in real time using interactive audio and video technology. Counseling and coordination of care with other physicians, other qualified health care professionals or agencies are provided consistent with the nature of the problem(s) and the needs of the patient or the family or both. Usually, the presenting problem(s) are of moderate to high severity. Typically, 60 minutes are spent with the patient or family or both via real time, audio and video intercommunications technology. Ⓑ

● **G9486**Apr Remote in-home visit for the evaluation and management of an established patient for use only in the Medicare-approved Comprehensive Care for Joint Replacement Model, which requires at least 2 of the following 3 key components: A problem focused history; A problem focused examination; Straightforward medical decision making, furnished in real time using interactive audio and video technology. Counseling and coordination of care with other physicians, other qualified health care professionals or agencies are provided consistent with the nature of the problem(s) and the needs of the patient or the family or both. Usually, the presenting problem(s) are self limited or minor. Typically, 10 minutes are spent with the patient or family or both via real time, audio and video intercommunications technology. Ⓑ

● **G9487**Apr Remote in-home visit for the evaluation and management of an established patient for use only in the Medicare-approved Comprehensive Care for Joint Replacement Model, which requires at least 2 of the following 3 key components: An expanded problem focused history; An expanded problem focused examination; Medical decision making of low complexity, furnished in real time using interactive audio and video technology. Counseling and coordination of care with other physicians, other qualified health care professionals or agencies are provided consistent with the nature of the problem(s) and the needs of the patient or the family or both. Usually, the presenting problem(s) are of low to moderate severity. Typically, 15 minutes are spent with the patient or family or both via real time, audio and video intercommunications technology. Ⓑ

● **G9488**Apr Remote in-home visit for the evaluation and management of an established patient for use only in the Medicare-approved Comprehensive Care for Joint Replacement Model, which requires at least 2 of the following 3 key components: A detailed history; A detailed examination; Medical decision making of moderate complexity, furnished in real time using interactive audio and video technology. Counseling and coordination of care with other physicians, other qualified health care professionals or agencies are provided consistent with the nature of the problem(s) and the needs of the patient or the family or both. Usually, the presenting problem(s) are of moderate to high severity. Typically, 25 minutes are spent with the patient or family or both via real time, audio and video intercommunications technology. Ⓑ

● **G9489**Apr Remote in-home visit for the evaluation and management of an established patient for use only in the Medicare-approved Comprehensive Care for Joint Replacement Model, which requires at least 2 of the following 3 key components: A comprehensive history; A comprehensive examination; Medical decision making of high complexity, furnished in real time using interactive audio and video technology. Counseling and coordination of care with other physicians, other qualified health care professionals or agencies are provided consistent with the nature of the problem(s) and the needs of the patient or the family or both. Usually, the presenting problem(s) are of moderate to high severity. Typically, 40 minutes are spent with the patient or family or both via real time, audio and video intercommunications technology. Ⓑ

● **G9490**Apr Comprehensive Care for Joint Replacement Model, home visit for patient assessment performed by clinical staff for an individual not considered homebound, including, but not necessarily limited to patient assessment of clinical status, safety/fall prevention, functional status/ambulation, medication reconciliation/management, compliance with orders/plan of care, performance of activities of daily living, and ensuring beneficiary connections to community and other services (for use only in the Medicare-approved Comprehensive Care for Joint Replacement Model); may not be billed for a 30 day period covered by a transitional care management code. Ⓑ

**Quality Measures**

**G9496** Documentation of reason for not detecting adenoma(s) or other neoplasm. (e.g., neoplasm detected is only diagnosed as traditional serrated adenoma, sessile serrated polyp, or sessile serrated adenoma) Ⓜ

▲ **G9497**Jan Received instruction from the anesthesiologist or proxy prior to the day of surgery to abstain from smoking on the day of surgery Ⓜ

**G9498** Antibiotic regimen prescribed Ⓜ

**G9499**Jan ~~Patient did not start or is not receiving antiviral treatment for hepatitis C during the measurement period~~

▲ **G9500**Jan Radiation exposure indices, or exposure time and number of fluorographic images in final report for procedures using fluoroscopy, documented Ⓜ

▲ **G9501**Jan Radiation exposure indices, or exposure time and number of fluorographic images not documented in final report for procedure using fluoroscopy, reason not given Ⓜ

**G9502** Documentation of medical reason for not performing foot exam (i.e., patients who have had either a bilateral amputation above or below the knee, or both a left and right amputation above or below the knee before or during the measurement period) Ⓜ

**G9503** Patient taking tamsulosin hydrochloride ♂ Ⓜ

**G9504** Documented reason for not assessing hepatitis B virus (HBV) status (e.g., patient not receiving a first course of anti-TNF therapy, patient declined) within one year prior to first course of anti-TNF therapy Ⓜ

**G9505** Antibiotic regimen prescribed within 10 days after onset of symptoms for documented medical reason Ⓜ

**G9506** Biologic immune response modifier prescribed Ⓜ

Jan **January Update**        Apr **April Update**

Special Coverage Instructions    Noncovered by Medicare    Carrier Discretion    ☑ Quantity Alert  ● New Code    ○ Recycled/Reinstated  ▲ Revised Code

**68 — G Codes**        Ⓐ Age Edit    Ⓜ Maternity Edit    ♀ Female Only    ♂ Male Only    Ⓐ-Ⓨ OPPS Status Indicators    © 2016 Optum360, LLC

**G9507** Documentation that the patient is on a statin medication or has documentation of a valid contraindication or exception to statin medications; contraindications/exceptions that can be defined by diagnosis codes include pregnancy during the measurement period, active liver disease, rhabdomyolysis, end stage renal disease on dialysis and heart failure; provider documented contraindications/exceptions include breastfeeding during the measurement period, woman of child-bearing age not actively taking birth control, allergy to statin, drug interaction (HIV protease inhibitors, nefazodone, cyclosporine, gemfibrozil, and danazol) and intolerance (with supporting documentation of trying a statin at least once within the last 5 years or diagnosis codes for myositis or toxic myopathy related to drugs) M

**G9508** Documentation that the patient is not on a statin medication M

**G9509** Remission at twelve months as demonstrated by a twelve month (+/-30 days) PHQ-9 score of less than 5 M

**G9510** Remission at twelve months not demonstrated by a twelve month (+/-30 days) PHQ-9 score of less than five; either PHQ-9 score was not assessed or is greater than or equal to 5 M

**G9511** Index date PHQ-9 score greater than 9 documented during the twelve month denominator identification period M

**G9512** Individual had a PDC of 0.8 or greater M

**G9513** Individual did not have a PDC of 0.8 or greater M

**G9514** Patient required a return to the operating room within 90 days of surgery M

**G9515** Patient did not require a return to the operating room within 90 days of surgery M

**G9516** Patient achieved an improvement in visual acuity, from their preoperative level, within 90 days of surgery M

**G9517** Patient did not achieve an improvement in visual acuity, from their preoperative level, within 90 days of surgery, reason not given M

**G9518** Documentation of active injection drug use M

▲ **G9519**Jan Patient achieves final refraction (spherical equivalent) +/- 0.5 diopters of their planned refraction within 90 days of surgery M

▲ **G9520**Jan Patient does not achieve final refraction (spherical equivalent) +/- 0.5 diopters of their planned refraction within 90 days of surgery M

**G9521** Total number of emergency department visits and inpatient hospitalizations less than two in the past 12 months M

**G9522** Total number of emergency department visits and inpatient hospitalizations equal to or greater than two in the past 12 months or patient not screened, reason not given M

**G9523** Patient discontinued from hemodialysis or peritoneal dialysis M

## Hospice Care

**G9524** Patient was referred to hospice care M

**G9525** Documentation of patient reason(s) for not referring to hospice care (e.g., patient declined, other patient reasons) M

**G9526** Patient was not referred to hospice care, reason not given M

## Blunt Head Trauma

**G9529** Patient with minor blunt head trauma had an appropriate indication(s) for a head CT M

**G9530** Patient presented within 24 hours of a minor blunt head trauma with a GCS score of 15 and had a head CT ordered for trauma by an emergency care provider M

▲ **G9531**Jan Patient has documentation of ventricular shunt, brain tumor, multisystem trauma, pregnancy, or is currently taking an antiplatelet medication including: ASA/dipyridamole, clopidogrel, prasugrel, ticlopidine, ticagrelor or cilstazol) M

▲ **G9532**Jan Patient's head injury occurred greater than 24 hours before presentation to the emergency department, or has a GCS score less than 15 or does not have a GCS score documented, or had a head CT for trauma ordered by someone other than an emergency care provider, or was ordered for a reason other than trauma M

**G9533** Patient with minor blunt head trauma did not have an appropriate indication(s) for a head CT M

**G9534** Advanced brain imaging (CTA, CT, MRA or MRI) was not ordered M

**G9535** Patients with a normal neurological examination M

**G9536** Documentation of medical reason(s) for ordering an advanced brain imaging study (i.e., patient has an abnormal neurological examination; patient has the coexistence of seizures, or both; recent onset of severe headache; change in the type of headache; signs of increased intracranial pressure (e.g., papilledema, absent venous pulsations on funduscopic examination, altered mental status, focal neurologic deficits, signs of meningeal irritation); HIV-positive patients with a new type of headache; immunocompromised patient with unexplained headache symptoms; patient on coagulopathy/anticoagulation or antiplatelet therapy; very young patients with unexplained headache symptoms) M

**G9537** Documentation of system reason(s) for ordering an advanced brain imaging study (i.e., needed as part of a clinical trial; other clinician ordered the study) M

**G9538** Advanced brain imaging (CTA, CT, MRA or MRI) was ordered M

## Miscellaneous Quality Measures

**G9539** Intent for potential removal at time of placement M

**G9540** Patient alive 3 months post procedure M

**G9541** Filter removed within 3 months of placement M

**G9542** Documented reassessment for the appropriateness of filter removal within 3 months of placement M

**G9543** Documentation of at least two attempts to reach the patient to arrange a clinical reassessment for the appropriateness of filter removal within 3 months of placement M

**G9544** Patients that do not have the filter removed, documented reassessment for the appropriateness of filter removal, or documentation of at least two attempts to reach the patient to arrange a clinical reassessment for the appropriateness of filter removal within 3 months of placement M

▲ **G9547**Jan Incidental finding: liver lesion <= 0.5 cm, cystic kidney lesion < 1.0 cm or adrenal lesion <= 1.0 cm M

**G9548** Final reports for abdominal imaging studies with follow-up imaging recommended M

▲ **G9549**Jan Documentation of medical reason(s) that follow-up imaging is indicated (e.g., patient has a known malignancy that can metastasize, other medical reason(s) such as fever in an immunocompromised patient) M

**G9550** Final reports for abdominal imaging studies with follow-up imaging not recommended M

▲ **G9551**Jan Final reports for abdominal imaging studies without an incidentally found lesion noted: liver lesion <= 0.5 cm, cystic kidney lesion < 1.0 cm or adrenal lesion <= 1.0 cm noted or no lesion found M

Jan   January Update

Special Coverage Instructions   Noncovered by Medicare   Carrier Discretion   ☑ Quantity Alert   ● New Code   ○ Recycled/Reinstated   ▲ Revised Code

© 2016 Optum360, LLC   A2-Z8 ASC Pmt   CMS: Pub 100   AHA: Coding Clinic   ⅙ DMEPOS Paid   ⊘ SNF Excluded

G Codes — 69

| | | |
|---|---|---|
| G9552 | Incidental thyroid nodule < 1.0 cm noted in report | M |
| G9553 | Prior thyroid disease diagnosis | M |
| ▲ G9554 ^Jan | Final reports for CT, CTA, MRI or MRA of the chest or neck or ultrasound of the neck with follow-up imaging recommended | M |
| ▲ G9555 ^Jan | Documentation of medical reason(s) for recommending follow up imaging (e.g., patient has multiple endocrine neoplasia, patient has cervical lymphadenopathy, other medical reason(s)) | M |
| ▲ G9556 ^Jan | Final reports for CT, CTA, MRI or MRA of the chest or neck or ultrasound of the neck with follow-up imaging not recommended | M |
| ▲ G9557 ^Jan | Final reports for CT, CTA, MRI or MRA studies of the chest or neck or ultrasound of the neck without an incidentally found thyroid nodule < 1.0 cm noted or no nodule found | M |
| G9558 | Patient treated with a beta-lactam antibiotic as definitive therapy | M |
| G9559 | Documentation of medical reason(s) for not prescribing a beta-lactam antibiotic (e.g., allergy, intolerance to beta-lactam antibiotics) | M |
| G9560 | Patient not treated with a beta-lactam antibiotic as definitive therapy, reason not given | M |

## Opiate Therapy

| | | |
|---|---|---|
| G9561 | Patients prescribed opiates for longer than six weeks | M |
| G9562 | Patients who had a follow-up evaluation conducted at least every three months during opioid therapy | M |
| G9563 | Patients who did not have a follow-up evaluation conducted at least every three months during opioid therapy | M |
| G9572 ^Jan | ~~Index date PHQ-score greater than 9 documented during the twelve month denominator identification period~~ | |
| G9573 | Remission at six months as demonstrated by a six month (+/-30 days) PHQ-9 score of less than five | |
| G9574 | Remission at six months not demonstrated by a six month (+/-30 days) PHQ-9 score of less than five; either PHQ-9 score was not assessed or is greater than or equal to five | M |
| G9577 | Patients prescribed opiates for longer than six weeks | M |
| G9578 | Documentation of signed opioid treatment agreement at least once during opioid therapy | M |
| G9579 | No documentation of a signed opioid treatment agreement at least once during opioid therapy | M |

## Stroke Therapy

| | | |
|---|---|---|
| G9580 | Door to puncture time of less than 2 hours | M |
| G9581 ^Jan | ~~Door to puncture time of greater than 2 hours for reasons documented by clinician (e.g., patients who are transferred from one institution to another with a known diagnosis of CVA for endovascular stroke treatment; hospitalized patients with newly diagnosed CVA considered for endovascular stroke treatment)~~ | |
| G9582 | Door to puncture time of greater than 2 hours, no reason given | M |

## Opiate Therapy

| | | |
|---|---|---|
| G9583 | Patients prescribed opiates for longer than six weeks | M |
| G9584 | Patient evaluated for risk of misuse of opiates by using a brief validated instrument (e.g., opioid risk tool, SOAAP-R) or patient interviewed at least once during opioid therapy | M |
| G9585 | Patient not evaluated for risk of misuse of opiates by using a brief validated instrument (e.g., opioid risk tool, SOAAP-R) or patient not interviewed at least once during opioid therapy | M |

## Blunt Head Trauma

| | | |
|---|---|---|
| G9593 | Pediatric patient with minor blunt head trauma classified as low risk according to the PECARN prediction rules | M |
| G9594 | Patient presented within 24 hours of a minor blunt head trauma with a GCS score of 15 and had a head CT ordered for trauma by an emergency care provider | M |
| ▲ G9595 ^Jan | Patient has documentation of ventricular shunt, brain tumor, coagulopathy, including thrombocytopenia | M |
| ▲ G9596 ^Jan | Pediatric patient's head injury occurred greater than 24 hours before presentation to the emergency department, or has a GCS score less than 15 or does not have a GCS score documented, or had a head CT for trauma ordered by someone other than an emergency care provider, or was ordered for a reason other than trauma | M |
| G9597 | Pediatric patient with minor blunt head trauma not classified as low risk according to the PECARN prediction rules | M |

## Aortic Aneurysm

| | | |
|---|---|---|
| G9598 | Aortic aneurysm 5.5-5.9 cm maximum diameter on centerline formatted CT or minor diameter on axial formatted CT | M |
| G9599 | Aortic aneurysm 6.0 cm or greater maximum diameter on centerline formatted CT or minor diameter on axial formatted CT | M |
| G9600 | Symptomatic AAAS that required urgent/emergent (nonelective) repair | M |

## Discharge to Home

| | | |
|---|---|---|
| G9601 | Patient discharge to home no later than postoperative day #7 | M |
| G9602 | Patient not discharged to home by postoperative day #7 | M |

## Patient Survey

| | | |
|---|---|---|
| G9603 | Patient survey score improved from baseline following treatment | M |
| G9604 | Patient survey results not available | M |
| G9605 | Patient survey score did not improve from baseline following treatment | M |

## Intraoperative Cystoscopy

| | | |
|---|---|---|
| G9606 | Intraoperative cystoscopy performed to evaluate for lower tract injury | M |
| ▲ G9607 ^Jan | Documented medical reasons for not performing intraoperative cystoscopy (e.g., urethral pathology precluding cystoscopy, any patient who has a congenital or acquired absence of the urethra) | M |
| G9608 | Intraoperative cystoscopy not performed to evaluate for lower tract injury | M |

## Aspirin/Antiplatelet Therapy

| | | |
|---|---|---|
| ▲ G9609 ^Jan | Documentation of an order for antiplatelet agents | M |
| ▲ G9610 ^Jan | Documentation of medical reason(s) in the patient's record for not ordering antiplatelet agents | M |
| ▲ G9611 ^Jan | Order for antiplatelet agents was not documented in the patient's record, reason not given | M |

## Colonoscopy Documentation

| | | |
|---|---|---|
| G9612 | Photodocumentation of one or more cecal landmarks to establish a complete examination | M |

---

^Jan **January Update**

Special Coverage Instructions    Noncovered by Medicare    Carrier Discretion    ☑ Quantity Alert    ● New Code    ○ Recycled/Reinstated    ▲ Revised Code

70 — G Codes    A Age Edit    M Maternity Edit    ♀ Female Only    ♂ Male Only    A-Y OPPS Status Indicators    © 2016 Optum360, LLC

G9613  Documentation of postsurgical anatomy (e.g., right hemicolectomy, ileocecal resection, etc.) Ⓜ

G9614  No photodocumentation of cecal landmarks to establish a complete examination Ⓜ

## Preoperative Assessment

G9615  Preoperative assessment documented Ⓜ

G9616  Documentation of reason(s) for not documenting a preoperative assessment (e.g., patient with a gynecologic or other pelvic malignancy noted at the time of surgery) Ⓜ

G9617  Preoperative assessment not documented, reason not given Ⓜ

## Uterine Malignancy Screening

G9618  Documentation of screening for uterine malignancy or those that had an ultrasound and/or endometrial sampling of any kind ♀ Ⓜ

G9619Jan  ~~Documentation of reason(s) for not screening for uterine malignancy (e.g., prior hysterectomy)~~

G9620  Patient not screened for uterine malignancy, or those that have not had an ultrasound and/or endometrial sampling of any kind, reason not given ♀ Ⓜ

## Alcohol Use

G9621  Patient identified as an unhealthy alcohol user when screened for unhealthy alcohol use using a systematic screening method and received brief counseling

G9622  Patient not identified as an unhealthy alcohol user when screened for unhealthy alcohol use using a systematic screening method Ⓜ

G9623  Documentation of medical reason(s) for not screening for unhealthy alcohol use (e.g., limited life expectancy, other medical reasons) Ⓜ

G9624  Patient not screened for unhealthy alcohol screening using a systematic screening method or patient did not receive brief counseling, reason not given Ⓜ

## Bladder/Ureter Injury

▲ G9625Jan  Patient sustained bladder injury at the time of surgery or discovered subsequently up to 1 month postsurgery Ⓜ

▲ G9626Jan  Documented medical reason for not reporting bladder injury (e.g., gynecologic or other pelvic malignancy documented, concurrent surgery involving bladder pathology, injury that occurs during urinary incontinence procedure, patient death from nonmedical causes not related to surgery, patient died during procedure without evidence of bladder injury) Ⓜ

▲ G9627Jan  Patient did not sustain bladder injury at the time of surgery nor discovered subsequently up to 1 month postsurgery Ⓜ

▲ G9628Jan  Patient sustained bowel injury at the time of surgery or discovered subsequently up to 1 month postsurgery Ⓜ

▲ G9629Jan  Documented medical reasons for not reporting bowel injury (e.g., gynecologic or other pelvic malignancy documented, planned (e.g., not due to an unexpected bowel injury) resection and/or re-anastomosis of bowel, or patient death from nonmedical causes not related to surgery, patient died during procedure without evidence of bowel injury) Ⓜ

▲ G9630Jan  Patient did not sustain a bowel injury at the time of surgery nor discovered subsequently up to 1 month postsurgery Ⓜ

G9631  Patient sustained ureter injury at the time of surgery or discovered subsequently up to 1 month postsurgery Ⓜ

▲ G9632Jan  Documented medical reasons for not reporting ureter injury (e.g., gynecologic or other pelvic malignancy documented, concurrent surgery involving bladder pathology, injury that occurs during a urinary incontinence procedure, patient death from nonmedical causes not related to surgery, patient died during procedure without evidence of ureter injury) Ⓜ

▲ G9633Jan  Patient did not sustain ureter injury at the time of surgery nor discovered subsequently up to 1 month postsurgery Ⓜ

## Health-Related Quality of Life

G9634  Health-related quality of life assessed with tool during at least two visits and quality of life score remained the same or improved Ⓜ

G9635  Health-related quality of life not assessed with tool for documented reason(s) (e.g., patient has a cognitive or neuropsychiatric impairment that impairs his/her ability to complete the HRQOL survey, patient has the inability to read and/or write in order to complete the HRQOL questionnaire) Ⓜ

G9636  Health-related quality of life not assessed with tool during at least two visits or quality of life score declined Ⓜ

## Quality Measures

G9637  Final reports with documentation of one or more dose reduction techniques (e.g., automated exposure control, adjustment of the mA and/or kVp according to patient size, use of iterative reconstruction technique) Ⓜ

G9638  Final reports without documentation of one or more dose reduction techniques (e.g., automated exposure control, adjustment of the mA and/or kVp according to patient size, use of iterative reconstruction technique) Ⓜ

G9639  Major amputation or open surgical bypass not required within 48 hours of the index endovascular lower extremity revascularization procedure Ⓜ

G9640  Documentation of planned hybrid or staged procedure Ⓜ

G9641  Major amputation or open surgical bypass required within 48 hours of the index endovascular lower extremity revascularization procedure Ⓜ

▲ G9642Jan  Current smokers (e.g., cigarette, cigar, pipe, e-cigarette or marijuana) Ⓜ

G9643  Elective surgery Ⓜ

G9644  Patients who abstained from smoking prior to anesthesia on the day of surgery or procedure Ⓜ

G9645  Patients who did not abstain from smoking prior to anesthesia on the day of surgery or procedure Ⓜ

G9646  Patients with 90 day MRS score of 0 to 2 Ⓜ

G9647  Patients in whom MRS score could not be obtained at 90 day follow-up Ⓜ

G9648  Patients with 90 day MRS score greater than 2 Ⓜ

## Psoriasis Therapy

G9649  Psoriasis assessment tool documented meeting any one of the specified benchmarks (e.g., (PGA; 6-point scale), body surface area (BSA), psoriasis area and severity index (PASI) and/or dermatology life quality index) (DLQI)) Ⓜ

G9650Jan  ~~Documentation that the patient declined therapy change or has documented contraindications (e.g., experienced adverse effects or lack of efficacy with all other therapy options) in order to achieve better disease control as measured by PGA, BSA, PASI, or DLQI~~

Jan  January Update

Special Coverage Instructions    Noncovered by Medicare    Carrier Discretion    ☑ Quantity Alert    ● New Code    ○ Recycled/Reinstated    ▲ Revised Code

© 2016 Optum360, LLC    A2-Z3 ASC Pmt    CMS: Pub 100    AHA: Coding Clinic    & DMEPOS Paid    ⊘ SNF Excluded    G Codes — 71

**G9651** Psoriasis assessment tool documented not meeting any one of the specified benchmarks (e.g., (PGA; 6-point scale), body surface area (BSA), psoriasis area and severity index (PASI) and/or dermatology life quality index) (DLQI)) or psoriasis assessment tool not documented ☒ M

**G9652**Jan ~~Patient has been treated with a systemic or biologic medication for psoriasis for at least six months~~

**G9653**Jan ~~Patient has not been treated with a systemic or biologic medication for psoriasis for at least six months~~

## Anesthesia Services

**G9654** Monitored anesthesia care (MAC) M

**G9655** A transfer of care protocol or handoff tool/checklist that includes the required key handoff elements is used M

**G9656** Patient transferred directly from anesthetizing location to PACU M

**G9657**Jan ~~Transfer of care during an anesthetic or to the intensive care unit~~

**G9658** A transfer of care protocol or handoff tool/checklist that includes the required key handoff elements is not used M

## Reason for Colonoscopy

**G9659** Patients greater than 85 years of age who did not have a history of colorectal cancer or valid medical reason for the colonoscopy, including: iron deficiency anemia, lower gastrointestinal bleeding, Crohn's disease (i.e., regional enteritis), familial adenomatous polyposis, lynch syndrome (i.e., hereditary nonpolyposis colorectal cancer), inflammatory bowel disease, ulcerative colitis, abnormal finding of gastrointestinal tract, or changes in bowel habits M

**G9660** Documentation of medical reason(s) for a colonoscopy performed on a patient greater than 85 years of age (e.g., last colonoscopy incomplete, last colonoscopy had inadequate prep, iron deficiency anemia, lower gastrointestinal bleeding, Crohn's disease (i.e., regional enteritis), familial history of adenomatous polyposis, lynch syndrome (i.e., hereditary nonpolyposis colorectal cancer), inflammatory bowel disease, ulcerative colitis, abnormal finding of gastrointestinal tract, or changes in bowel habits) M

**G9661** Patients greater than 85 years of age who received a routine colonoscopy for a reason other than the following: an assessment of signs/symptoms of GI tract illness, and/or the patient is considered high risk, and/or to follow-up on previously diagnosed advance lesions M

## Statin Therapy

**G9662** Previously diagnosed or have an active diagnosis of clinical ASCVD M

**G9663** Any fasting or direct LDL-C laboratory test result = 190 mg/dl M

**G9664** Patients who are currently statin therapy users or received an order (prescription) for statin therapy M

**G9665** Patients who are not currently statin therapy users or did not receive an order (prescription) for statin therapy M

**G9666** The highest fasting or direct LDL-C laboratory test result of 70/189 mg/dl in the measurement period or two years prior to the beginning of the measurement period M

**G9667**Jan ~~Documentation of medical reason(s) for not currently being a statin therapy user or receive an order (prescription) for statin therapy (e.g., patient with adverse effect, allergy or intolerance to statin medication therapy, patients who have an active diagnosis of pregnancy or who are breastfeeding, patients who are receiving palliative care, patients with active liver disease or hepatic disease or insufficiency, patients with end stage renal disease (ESRD), and patients with diabetes who have a fasting or direct LDL-C laboratory test result < 70 mg/dl and are not taking statin therapy)~~

## Multiple Chronic Conditions

**G9669**Jan ~~I intend to report the multiple chronic conditions measures group~~

**G9670**Jan ~~All quality actions for the applicable measures in the multiple chronic conditions measures group have been performed for this patient~~

## Diabetic Retinopathy

**G9671**Jan ~~I intend to report the diabetic retinopathy measures group~~

**G9672**Jan ~~All quality actions for the applicable measures in the diabetic retinopathy measures group have been performed for this patient~~

## Cardiovascular Measures

**G9673**Jan ~~I intend to report the cardiovascular prevention measures group~~

**G9674** Patients with clinical ASCVD diagnosis M

**G9675** Patients who have ever had a fasting or direct laboratory result of LDL-C = 190 mg/dl M

**G9676** Patients aged 40 to 75 years at the beginning of the measurement period with type 1 or type 2 diabetes and with an LDL-C result of 70/189 mg/dl recorded as the highest fasting or direct laboratory test result in the measurement year or during the two years prior to the beginning of the measurement period M

**G9677**Jan ~~All quality actions for the applicable measures in the cardiovascular prevention measures group have been performed for this patient~~

## Oncology Demonstration Project

● **G9678**Apr Oncology Care Model (OCM) Monthly Enhanced Oncology Services (MEOS) payment for enhanced care management services for OCM beneficiaries. MEOS covers care management services for Medicare beneficiaries in a 6-month OCM Episode of Care triggered by the administration of chemotherapy. Enhanced care management services include services driven by the OCM practice requirements, including: 24/7 clinician access, use of an ONC-certified Electronic Health Record, utilization of data for quality improvement, patient navigation, documentation of care plans, and use of clinical guidelines. B
G9678 may only be billed for OCM beneficiaries by OCM practitioners.

## Nursing Facility Care

● **G9679**Oct Onsite acute care treatment of a nursing facility resident with pneumonia. May only be billed once per day per beneficiary M

● **G9680**Oct Onsite acute care treatment of a nursing facility resident with CHF. May only be billed once per day per beneficiary M

● **G9681**Oct Onsite acute care treatment of a nursing facility resident with COPD or asthma. May only be billed once per day per beneficiary M

● **G9682**Oct Onsite acute care treatment of a nursing facility resident with a skin infection. May only be billed once per day per beneficiary M

**Jan** January Update   **Apr** April Update   **Oct** October Update

Special Coverage Instructions   Noncovered by Medicare   Carrier Discretion   ☑ Quantity Alert   ● New Code   ○ Recycled/Reinstated   ▲ Revised Code

72 — G Codes   A Age Edit   M Maternity Edit   ♀ Female Only   ♂ Male Only   A-Y OPPS Status Indicators   © 2016 Optum360, LLC

● G9683<sup>Oct</sup> Onsite acute care treatment of a nursing facility resident with fluid or electrolyte disorder or dehydration (similar pattern). May only be billed once per day per beneficiary ▢M

● G9684<sup>Oct</sup> Onsite acute care treatment of a nursing facility resident for a UTI. May only be billed once per day per beneficiary ▢M

● G9685<sup>Oct</sup> Evaluation and management of a beneficiary's acute change in condition in a nursing facility ▢B

● G9686<sup>Oct</sup> Onsite nursing facility conference, that is separate and distinct from an Evaluation and Management visit, including qualified practitioner and at least one member of the nursing facility interdisciplinary care team ▢B

## Other Quality Measures

● G9687<sup>Jan</sup> Hospice services provided to patient any time during the measurement period

● G9688<sup>Jan</sup> Patients using hospice services any time during the measurement period

● G9689<sup>Jan</sup> Patient admitted for performance of elective carotid intervention

● G9690<sup>Jan</sup> Patient receiving hospice services any time during the measurement period

● G9691<sup>Jan</sup> Patient had hospice services any time during the measurement period

● G9692<sup>Jan</sup> Hospice services received by patient any time during the measurement period

● G9693<sup>Jan</sup> Patient use of hospice services any time during the measurement period

● G9694<sup>Jan</sup> Hospice services utilized by patient any time during the measurement period

● G9695<sup>Jan</sup> Long-acting inhaled bronchodilator prescribed

● G9696<sup>Jan</sup> Documentation of medical reason(s) for not prescribing a long-acting inhaled bronchodilator

● G9697<sup>Jan</sup> Documentation of patient reason(s) for not prescribing a long-acting inhaled bronchodilator

● G9698<sup>Jan</sup> Documentation of system reason(s) for not prescribing a long-acting inhaled bronchodilator

● G9699<sup>Jan</sup> Long-acting inhaled bronchodilator not prescribed, reason not otherwise specified

● G9700<sup>Jan</sup> Patients who use hospice services any time during the measurement period

● G9701<sup>Jan</sup> Children who are taking antibiotics in the 30 days prior to the date of the encounter during which the diagnosis was established

● G9702<sup>Jan</sup> Patients who use hospice services any time during the measurement period

● G9703<sup>Jan</sup> Children who are taking antibiotics in the 30 days prior to the diagnosis of pharyngitis

● G9704<sup>Jan</sup> AJCC breast cancer stage I: T1 mic or T1a documented

● G9705<sup>Jan</sup> AJCC breast cancer stage I: T1b (tumor > 0.5 cm but <= 1 cm in greatest dimension) documented

● G9706<sup>Jan</sup> Low (or very low) risk of recurrence, prostate cancer

● G9707<sup>Jan</sup> Patient received hospice services any time during the measurement period

● G9708<sup>Jan</sup> Women who had a bilateral mastectomy or who have a history of a bilateral mastectomy or for whom there is evidence of a right and a left unilateral mastectomy

● G9709<sup>Jan</sup> Hospice services used by patient any time during the measurement period

● G9710<sup>Jan</sup> Patient was provided hospice services any time during the measurement period

● G9711<sup>Jan</sup> Patients with a diagnosis or past history of total colectomy or colorectal cancer

● G9712<sup>Jan</sup> Documentation of medical reason(s) for prescribing or dispensing antibiotic (e.g., intestinal infection, pertussis, bacterial infection, lyme disease, otitis media, acute sinusitis, acute pharyngitis, acute tonsillitis, chronic sinusitis, infection of the pharynx/larynx/tonsils/adenoids, prostatitis, cellulitis/mastoiditis/bone infections, acute lymphadenitis, impetigo, skin staph infections, pneumonia, gonococcal infections/venereal disease (syphilis, chlamydia, inflammatory diseases [female reproductive organs]), infections of the kidney, cystitis/UTI, acne, HIV disease/asymptomatic HIV, cystic fibrosis, disorders of the immune system, malignancy neoplasms, chronic bronchitis, emphysema, bronchiectasis, extrinsic allergic alveolitis, chronic airway obstruction, chronic obstructive asthma, pneumoconiosis and other lung disease due to external agents, other diseases of the respiratory system, and tuberculosis

● G9713<sup>Jan</sup> Patients who use hospice services any time during the measurement period

● G9714<sup>Jan</sup> Patient is using hospice services any time during the measurement period

● G9715<sup>Jan</sup> Patients who use hospice services any time during the measurement period

● G9716<sup>Jan</sup> BMI is documented as being outside of normal limits, follow-up plan is not completed for documented reason

● G9717<sup>Jan</sup> Documentation stating the patient has an active diagnosis of depression or has diagnosed bipolar disorder, therefore screening or follow-up not required

● G9718<sup>Jan</sup> Hospice services for patient provided any time during the measurement period

● G9719<sup>Jan</sup> Patient is not ambulatory, bed ridden, immobile, confined to chair, wheelchair bound, dependent on helper pushing wheelchair, independent in wheelchair or minimal help in wheelchair

● G9720<sup>Jan</sup> Hospice services for patient occurred any time during the measurement period

● G9721<sup>Jan</sup> Patient not ambulatory, bed ridden, immobile, confined to chair, wheelchair bound, dependent on helper pushing wheelchair, independent in wheelchair or minimal help in wheelchair

● G9722<sup>Jan</sup> Documented history of renal failure or baseline serum creatinine = 4.0 mg/dl; renal transplant recipients are not considered to have preoperative renal failure, unless, since transplantation the CR has been or is 4.0 or higher

● G9723<sup>Jan</sup> Hospice services for patient received any time during the measurement period

● G9724<sup>Jan</sup> Patients who had documentation of use of anticoagulant medications overlapping the measurement year

● G9725<sup>Jan</sup> Patients who use hospice services any time during the measurement period

● G9726<sup>Jan</sup> Patient refused to participate

● G9727<sup>Jan</sup> Patient unable to complete the FOTO knee intake PROM at admission and discharge due to blindness, illiteracy, severe mental incapacity or language incompatibility and an adequate proxy is not available

● G9728<sup>Jan</sup> Patient refused to participate

● G9729<sup>Jan</sup> Patient unable to complete the FOTO hip intake PROM at admission and discharge due to blindness, illiteracy, severe mental incapacity or language incompatibility and an adequate proxy is not available

<sup>Jan</sup> January Update    <sup>Oct</sup> October Update

Special Coverage Instructions    Noncovered by Medicare    Carrier Discretion    ☑ Quantity Alert   ● New Code   ○ Recycled/Reinstated   ▲ Revised Code

© 2016 Optum360, LLC    A2-Z3 ASC Pmt    CMS: Pub 100    AHA: Coding Clinic    ⅄ DMEPOS Paid    ⊘ SNF Excluded

G Codes — 73

**Procedures/Professional Services (Temporary)**

**G9730 — G9780**

● **G9730**Jan Patient refused to participate

● **G9731**Jan Patient unable to complete the FOTO foot or ankle intake PROM at admission and discharge due to blindness, illiteracy, severe mental incapacity or language incompatibility and an adequate proxy is not available

● **G9732**Jan Patient refused to participate

● **G9733**Jan Patient unable to complete the FOTO lumbar intake PROM at admission and discharge due to blindness, illiteracy, severe mental incapacity or language incompatibility and an adequate proxy is not available

● **G9734**Jan Patient refused to participate

● **G9735**Jan Patient unable to complete the FOTO shoulder intake PROM at admission and discharge due to blindness, illiteracy, severe mental incapacity or language incompatibility and an adequate proxy is not available

● **G9736**Jan Patient refused to participate

● **G9737**Jan Patient unable to complete the FOTO elbow, wrist or hand intake PROM at admission and discharge due to blindness, illiteracy, severe mental incapacity or language incompatibility and an adequate proxy is not available

● **G9738**Jan Patient refused to participate

● **G9739**Jan Patient unable to complete the FOTO general orthopedic intake PROM at admission and discharge due to blindness, illiteracy, severe mental incapacity or language incompatibility and an adequate proxy is not available

● **G9740**Jan Hospice services given to patient any time during the measurement period

● **G9741**Jan Patients who use hospice services any time during the measurement period

● **G9742**Jan Psychiatric symptoms assessed

● **G9743**Jan Psychiatric symptoms not assessed, reason not otherwise specified

● **G9744**Jan Patient not eligible due to active diagnosis of hypertension

● **G9745**Jan Documented reason for not screening or recommending a follow-up for high blood pressure

● **G9746**Jan Patient has mitral stenosis or prosthetic heart valves or patient has transient or reversible cause of AF (e.g., pneumonia, hyperthyroidism, pregnancy, cardiac surgery)

● **G9747**Jan Patient is undergoing palliative dialysis with a catheter

● **G9748**Jan Patient approved by a qualified transplant program and scheduled to receive a living donor kidney transplant

● **G9749**Jan Patient is undergoing palliative dialysis with a catheter

● **G9750**Jan Patient approved by a qualified transplant program and scheduled to receive a living donor kidney transplant

● **G9751**Jan Patient died at any time during the 24-month measurement period

● **G9752**Jan Emergency surgery

● **G9753**Jan Documentation of medical reason for not conducting a search for DICOM format images for prior patient CT imaging studies completed at non-affiliated external healthcare facilities or entities within the past 12 months that are available through a secure, authorized, media-free, shared archive (e.g., trauma, acute myocardial infarction, stroke, aortic aneurysm where time is of the essence)

● **G9754**Jan A finding of an incidental pulmonary nodule

● **G9755**Jan Documentation of medical reason(s) that follow-up imaging is indicated (e.g., patient has a known malignancy that can metastasize, other medical reason(s)

● **G9756**Jan Surgical procedures that included the use of silicone oil

● **G9757**Jan Surgical procedures that included the use of silicone oil

● **G9758**Jan Patient in hospice and in terminal phase

● **G9759**Jan History of preoperative posterior capsule rupture

● **G9760**Jan Patients who use hospice services any time during the measurement period

● **G9761**Jan Patients who use hospice services any time during the measurement period

● **G9762**Jan Patient had at least three HPV vaccines on or between the patient's 9th and 13th birthdays

● **G9763**Jan Patient did not have at least three HPV vaccines on or between the patient's 9th and 13th birthdays

● **G9764**Jan Patient has been treated with an oral systemic or biologic medication for psoriasis

● **G9765**Jan Documentation that the patient declined therapy change, has documented contraindications, or has not been treated with an oral systemic or biologic for at least six consecutive months (e.g., experienced adverse effects or lack of efficacy with all other therapy options) in order to achieve better disease control as measured by PGA, BSA, PASI, or DLQI

● **G9766**Jan Patients who are transferred from one institution to another with a known diagnosis of CVA for endovascular stroke treatment

● **G9767**Jan Hospitalized patients with newly diagnosed CVA considered for endovascular stroke treatment

● **G9768**Jan Patients who utilize hospice services any time during the measurement period

● **G9769**Jan Patient had a bone mineral density test in the past two years or received osteoporosis medication or therapy in the past 12 months

● **G9770**Jan Peripheral nerve block (PNB)

● **G9771**Jan At least 1 body temperature measurement equal to or greater than 35.5 degrees celsius (or 95.9 degrees fahrenheit) achieved within the 30 minutes immediately before or the 15 minutes immediately after anesthesia end time

● **G9772**Jan Documentation of one of the following medical reason(s) for not achieving at least 1 body temperature measurement equal to or greater than 35.5 degrees celsius (or 95.9 degrees fahrenheit) achieved within the 30 minutes immediately before or the 15 minutes immediately after anesthesia end time (e.g., emergency cases, intentional hypothermia, etc.)

● **G9773**Jan At least 1 body temperature measurement equal to or greater than 35.5 degrees celsius (or 95.9 degrees fahrenheit) not achieved within the 30 minutes immediately before or the 15 minutes immediately after anesthesia end time

● **G9774**Jan Patients who have had a hysterectomy

● **G9775**Jan Patient received at least 2 prophylactic pharmacologic anti-emetic agents of different classes preoperatively and/or intraoperatively

● **G9776**Jan Documentation of medical reason for not receiving at least 2 prophylactic pharmacologic anti-emetic agents of different classes preoperatively and/or intraoperatively (e.g., intolerance or other medical reason)

● **G9777**Jan Patient did not receive at least 2 prophylactic pharmacologic anti-emetic agents of different classes preoperatively and/or intraoperatively

● **G9778**Jan Patients who have a diagnosis of pregnancy

● **G9779**Jan Patients who are breastfeeding

● **G9780**Jan Patients who have a diagnosis of rhabdomyolysis

---

**Jan** **January Update**

Special Coverage Instructions  Noncovered by Medicare  Carrier Discretion  ☑ Quantity Alert  ● New Code  ○ Recycled/Reinstated  ▲ Revised Code

74 — G Codes  Ⓐ Age Edit  Ⓜ Maternity Edit  ♀ Female Only  ♂ Male Only  Ⓐ-Ⓨ OPPS Status Indicators  © 2016 Optum360, LLC

● **G9781**<sup>Jan</sup> Documentation of medical reason(s) for not currently being a statin therapy user or receive an order (prescription) for statin therapy (e.g., patient with adverse effect, allergy or intolerance to statin medication therapy, patients who are receiving palliative care, patients with active liver disease or hepatic disease or insufficiency, and patients with end stage renal disease (ESRD))

● **G9782**<sup>Jan</sup> History of or active diagnosis of familial or pure hypercholesterolemia

● **G9783**<sup>Jan</sup> Documentation of patients with diabetes who have a most recent fasting or direct LDL- C laboratory test result < 70 mg/dl and are not taking statin therapy

● **G9784**<sup>Jan</sup> Pathologists/dermatopathologists providing a second opinion on a biopsy

● **G9785**<sup>Jan</sup> Pathology report diagnosing cutaneous basal cell carcinoma or squamous cell carcinoma (to include in situ disease) sent from the pathologist/dermatopathologist to the biopsying clinician for review within 7 business days from the time when the tissue specimen was received by the pathologist

● **G9786**<sup>Jan</sup> Pathology report diagnosing cutaneous basal cell carcinoma or squamous cell carcinoma (to include in situ disease) was not sent from the pathologist/dermatopathologist to the biopsying clinician for review within 7 business days from the time when the tissue specimen was received by the pathologist

● **G9787**<sup>Jan</sup> Patient alive as of the last day of the measurement year

● **G9788**<sup>Jan</sup> Most recent BP is less than or equal to 140/90 mm Hg

● **G9789**<sup>Jan</sup> Blood pressure recorded during inpatient stays, emergency room visits, urgent care visits, and patient self-reported BP's (home and health fair BP results)

● **G9790**<sup>Jan</sup> Most recent BP is greater than 140/90 mm Hg, or blood pressure not documented

● **G9791**<sup>Jan</sup> Most recent tobacco status is tobacco free

● **G9792**<sup>Jan</sup> Most recent tobacco status is not tobacco free

● **G9793**<sup>Jan</sup> Patient is currently on a daily aspirin or other antiplatelet

● **G9794**<sup>Jan</sup> Documentation of medical reason(s) for not on a daily aspirin or other antiplatelet (e.g., history of gastrointestinal bleed or intra-cranial bleed or documentation of active anticoagulant use during the measurement period

● **G9795**<sup>Jan</sup> Patient is not currently on a daily aspirin or other antiplatelet

● **G9796**<sup>Jan</sup> Patient is currently on a statin therapy

● **G9797**<sup>Jan</sup> Patient is not on a statin therapy

● **G9798**<sup>Jan</sup> Discharge(s) for AMI between July 1 of the year prior measurement year to June 30 of the measurement period

● **G9799**<sup>Jan</sup> Patients with a medication dispensing event indicator of a history of asthma any time during the patient's history through the end of the measure period

● **G9800**<sup>Jan</sup> Patients who are identified as having an intolerance or allergy to beta-blocker therapy

● **G9801**<sup>Jan</sup> Hospitalizations in which the patient was transferred directly to a non-acute care facility for any diagnosis

● **G9802**<sup>Jan</sup> Patients who use hospice services any time during the measurement period

● **G9803**<sup>Jan</sup> Patient prescribed a 180-day course of treatment with beta-blockers post discharge for AMI

● **G9804**<sup>Jan</sup> Patient was not prescribed a 180-day course of treatment with beta-blockers post discharge for AMI

● **G9805**<sup>Jan</sup> Patients who use hospice services any time during the measurement period

● **G9806**<sup>Jan</sup> Patients who received cervical cytology or an HPV test

● **G9807**<sup>Jan</sup> Patients who did not receive cervical cytology or an HPV test

● **G9808**<sup>Jan</sup> Any patients who had no asthma controller medications dispensed during the measurement year

● **G9809**<sup>Jan</sup> Patients who use hospice services any time during the measurement period

● **G9810**<sup>Jan</sup> Patient achieved a PDC of at least 75% for their asthma controller medication

● **G9811**<sup>Jan</sup> Patient did not achieve a PDC of at least 75% for their asthma controller medication

● **G9812**<sup>Jan</sup> Patient died including all deaths occurring during the hospitalization in which the operation was performed, even if after 30 days, and those deaths occurring after discharge from the hospital, but within 30 days of the procedure

● **G9813**<sup>Jan</sup> Patient did not die within 30 days of the procedure or during the index hospitalization

● **G9814**<sup>Jan</sup> Death occurring during hospitalization

● **G9815**<sup>Jan</sup> Death did not occur during hospitalization

● **G9816**<sup>Jan</sup> Death occurring 30 days post procedure

● **G9817**<sup>Jan</sup> Death did not occur 30 days post procedure

● **G9818**<sup>Jan</sup> Documentation of sexual activity

● **G9819**<sup>Jan</sup> Patients who use hospice services any time during the measurement period

● **G9820**<sup>Jan</sup> Documentation of a chlamydia screening test with proper follow-up

● **G9821**<sup>Jan</sup> No documentation of a chlamydia screening test with proper follow-up

● **G9822**<sup>Jan</sup> Women who had an endometrial ablation procedure during the year prior to the index date (exclusive of the index date)

● **G9823**<sup>Jan</sup> Endometrial sampling or hysteroscopy with biopsy and results documented

● **G9824**<sup>Jan</sup> Endometrial sampling or hysteroscopy with biopsy and results not documented

● **G9825**<sup>Jan</sup> HER2/neu negative or undocumented/unknown

● **G9826**<sup>Jan</sup> Patient transferred to practice after initiation of chemotherapy

● **G9827**<sup>Jan</sup> HER2-targeted therapies not administered during the initial course of treatment

● **G9828**<sup>Jan</sup> HER2-targeted therapies administered during the initial course of treatment

● **G9829**<sup>Jan</sup> Breast adjuvant chemotherapy administered

● **G9830**<sup>Jan</sup> HER2/neu positive

● **G9831**<sup>Jan</sup> AJCC stage at breast cancer diagnosis = II or III

● **G9832**<sup>Jan</sup> AJCC stage at breast cancer diagnosis = I (Ia or Ib) and T-stage at breast cancer diagnosis does not equal = T1, T1a, T1b

● **G9833**<sup>Jan</sup> Patient transfer to practice after initiation of chemotherapy

● **G9834**<sup>Jan</sup> Patient has metastatic disease at diagnosis

● **G9835**<sup>Jan</sup> Trastuzumab administered within 12 months of diagnosis

● **G9836**<sup>Jan</sup> Reason for not administering trastuzumab documented (e.g., patient declined, patient died, patient transferred, contraindication or other clinical exclusion, neoadjuvant chemotherapy or radiation not complete)

● **G9837**<sup>Jan</sup> Trastuzumab not administered within 12 months of diagnosis

● **G9838**<sup>Jan</sup> Patient has metastatic disease at diagnosis

● **G9839**<sup>Jan</sup> Anti-EGFR monoclonal antibody therapy

---

<sup>Jan</sup> **January Update**

Special Coverage Instructions    Noncovered by Medicare    Carrier Discretion    ☑ Quantity Alert  ● New Code  ○ Recycled/Reinstated  ▲ Revised Code

© 2016 Optum360, LLC   A2-Z3 ASC Pmt   CMS: Pub 100   AHA: Coding Clinic   ♿ DMEPOS Paid   ⊘ SNF Excluded

- ● G9840<sup>Jan</sup> KRAS gene mutation testing performed before initiation of anti-EGFR MoAb
- ● G9841<sup>Jan</sup> KRAS gene mutation testing not performed before initiation of anti-EGFR MoAb
- ● G9842<sup>Jan</sup> Patient has metastatic disease at diagnosis
- ● G9843<sup>Jan</sup> KRAS gene mutation
- ● G9844<sup>Jan</sup> Patient did not receive anti-EGFR monoclonal antibody therapy
- ● G9845<sup>Jan</sup> Patient received anti-EGFR monoclonal antibody therapy
- ● G9846<sup>Jan</sup> Patients who died from cancer
- ● G9847<sup>Jan</sup> Patient received chemotherapy in the last 14 days of life
- ● G9848<sup>Jan</sup> Patient did not receive chemotherapy in the last 14 days of life
- ● G9849<sup>Jan</sup> Patients who died from cancer
- ● G9850<sup>Jan</sup> Patient had more than one emergency department visit in the last 30 days of life
- ● G9851<sup>Jan</sup> Patient had one or less emergency department visits in the last 30 days of life
- ● G9852<sup>Jan</sup> Patients who died from cancer
- ● G9853<sup>Jan</sup> Patient admitted to the ICU in the last 30 days of life
- ● G9854<sup>Jan</sup> Patient was not admitted to the ICU in the last 30 days of life
- ● G9855<sup>Jan</sup> Patients who died from cancer
- ● G9856<sup>Jan</sup> Patient was not admitted to hospice
- ● G9857<sup>Jan</sup> Patient admitted to hospice
- ● G9858<sup>Jan</sup> Patient enrolled in hospice
- ● G9859<sup>Jan</sup> Patients who died from cancer
- ● G9860<sup>Jan</sup> Patient spent less than three days in hospice care
- ● G9861<sup>Jan</sup> Patient spent greater than or equal to three days in hospice care
- ● G9862<sup>Jan</sup> Documentation of medical reason(s) for not recommending at least a 10 year follow-up interval (e.g., inadequate prep, familial or personal history of colonic polyps, patient had no adenoma and age is = 66 years old, or life expectancy < 10 years old, other medical reasons)

Jan  January Update

Special Coverage Instructions    Noncovered by Medicare    Carrier Discretion    ☑ Quantity Alert    ● New Code    ○ Recycled/Reinstated    ▲ Revised Code

76 — G Codes    Ⓐ Age Edit    Ⓜ Maternity Edit    ♀ Female Only    ♂ Male Only    Ⓐ-Ⓨ OPPS Status Indicators    © 2016 Optum360, LLC

## Alcohol and Drug Abuse Treatment Services H0001-H2037

The H codes are used by those state Medicaid agencies that are mandated by state law to establish separate codes for identifying mental health services that include alcohol and drug treatment services.

**H0001** Alcohol and/or drug assessment

**H0002** Behavioral health screening to determine eligibility for admission to treatment program

**H0003** Alcohol and/or drug screening; laboratory analysis of specimens for presence of alcohol and/or drugs

**H0004** Behavioral health counseling and therapy, per 15 minutes ☑

**H0005** Alcohol and/or drug services; group counseling by a clinician

**H0006** Alcohol and/or drug services; case management

**H0007** Alcohol and/or drug services; crisis intervention (outpatient)

**H0008** Alcohol and/or drug services; subacute detoxification (hospital inpatient)

**H0009** Alcohol and/or drug services; acute detoxification (hospital inpatient)

**H0010** Alcohol and/or drug services; subacute detoxification (residential addiction program inpatient)

**H0011** Alcohol and/or drug services; acute detoxification (residential addiction program inpatient)

**H0012** Alcohol and/or drug services; subacute detoxification (residential addiction program outpatient)

**H0013** Alcohol and/or drug services; acute detoxification (residential addiction program outpatient)

**H0014** Alcohol and/or drug services; ambulatory detoxification

**H0015** Alcohol and/or drug services; intensive outpatient (treatment program that operates at least 3 hours/day and at least 3 days/week and is based on an individualized treatment plan), including assessment, counseling; crisis intervention, and activity therapies or education

**H0016** Alcohol and/or drug services; medical/somatic (medical intervention in ambulatory setting)

**H0017** Behavioral health; residential (hospital residential treatment program), without room and board, per diem ☑

**H0018** Behavioral health; short-term residential (nonhospital residential treatment program), without room and board, per diem ☑

**H0019** Behavioral health; long-term residential (nonmedical, nonacute care in a residential treatment program where stay is typically longer than 30 days), without room and board, per diem ☑

**H0020** Alcohol and/or drug services; methadone administration and/or service (provision of the drug by a licensed program)

**H0021** Alcohol and/or drug training service (for staff and personnel not employed by providers)

**H0022** Alcohol and/or drug intervention service (planned facilitation)

**H0023** Behavioral health outreach service (planned approach to reach a targeted population)

**H0024** Behavioral health prevention information dissemination service (one-way direct or nondirect contact with service audiences to affect knowledge and attitude)

**H0025** Behavioral health prevention education service (delivery of services with target population to affect knowledge, attitude and/or behavior)

**H0026** Alcohol and/or drug prevention process service, community-based (delivery of services to develop skills of impactors)

**H0027** Alcohol and/or drug prevention environmental service (broad range of external activities geared toward modifying systems in order to mainstream prevention through policy and law)

**H0028** Alcohol and/or drug prevention problem identification and referral service (e.g., student assistance and employee assistance programs), does not include assessment

**H0029** Alcohol and/or drug prevention alternatives service (services for populations that exclude alcohol and other drug use e.g., alcohol free social events)

**H0030** Behavioral health hotline service

**H0031** Mental health assessment, by nonphysician

**H0032** Mental health service plan development by nonphysician

**H0033** Oral medication administration, direct observation

**H0034** Medication training and support, per 15 minutes ☑

**H0035** Mental health partial hospitalization, treatment, less than 24 hours ☑

**H0036** Community psychiatric supportive treatment, face-to-face, per 15 minutes ☑

**H0037** Community psychiatric supportive treatment program, per diem ☑

**H0038** Self-help/peer services, per 15 minutes ☑

**H0039** Assertive community treatment, face-to-face, per 15 minutes ☑

**H0040** Assertive community treatment program, per diem ☑

**H0041** Foster care, child, nontherapeutic, per diem Ⓐ ☑

**H0042** Foster care, child, nontherapeutic, per month Ⓐ ☑

**H0043** Supported housing, per diem ☑

**H0044** Supported housing, per month ☑

**H0045** Respite care services, not in the home, per diem ☑

**H0046** Mental health services, not otherwise specified

**H0047** Alcohol and/or other drug abuse services, not otherwise specified

**H0048** Alcohol and/or other drug testing: collection and handling only, specimens other than blood

**H0049** Alcohol and/or drug screening

**H0050** Alcohol and/or drug services, brief intervention, per 15 minutes ☑

**H1000** Prenatal care, at-risk assessment Ⓜ ♀
AHA: 1Q, '02, 5

**H1001** Prenatal care, at-risk enhanced service; antepartum management Ⓜ ♀
AHA: 1Q, '02, 5

**H1002** Prenatal care, at risk enhanced service; care coordination Ⓜ ♀
AHA: 1Q, '02, 5

**H1003** Prenatal care, at-risk enhanced service; education Ⓜ ♀
AHA: 1Q, '02, 5

**H1004** Prenatal care, at-risk enhanced service; follow-up home visit Ⓜ ♀
AHA: 1Q, '02, 5

**H1005** Prenatal care, at-risk enhanced service package (includes H1001-H1004) Ⓜ ♀
AHA: 1Q, '02, 5

**H1010** Nonmedical family planning education, per session ☑

Special Coverage Instructions    Noncovered by Medicare    Carrier Discretion    ☑ Quantity Alert ● New Code    ○ Recycled/Reinstated    ▲ Revised Code

© 2016 Optum360, LLC    A2-Z3 ASC Pmt    CMS: Pub 100    AHA: Coding Clinic    DMEPOS Paid    ⊘ SNF Excluded    H Codes — 77

**Alcohol and Drug Abuse Treatments**

**H1011 — H2037**

| Code | Description | |
|------|-------------|---|
| H1011 | Family assessment by licensed behavioral health professional for state defined purposes | |
| H2000 | Comprehensive multidisciplinary evaluation | |
| H2001 | Rehabilitation program, per 1/2 day | ☑ |
| H2010 | Comprehensive medication services, per 15 minutes | ☑ |
| H2011 | Crisis intervention service, per 15 minutes | ☑ |
| H2012 | Behavioral health day treatment, per hour | ☑ |
| H2013 | Psychiatric health facility service, per diem | ☑ |
| H2014 | Skills training and development, per 15 minutes | ☑ |
| H2015 | Comprehensive community support services, per 15 minutes | ☑ |
| H2016 | Comprehensive community support services, per diem | ☑ |
| H2017 | Psychosocial rehabilitation services, per 15 minutes | ☑ |
| H2018 | Psychosocial rehabilitation services, per diem | ☑ |
| H2019 | Therapeutic behavioral services, per 15 minutes | ☑ |
| H2020 | Therapeutic behavioral services, per diem | ☑ |
| H2021 | Community-based wrap-around services, per 15 minutes | ☑ |
| H2022 | Community-based wrap-around services, per diem | ☑ |
| H2023 | Supported employment, per 15 minutes | ☑ |
| H2024 | Supported employment, per diem | ☑ |
| H2025 | Ongoing support to maintain employment, per 15 minutes | ☑ |
| H2026 | Ongoing support to maintain employment, per diem | ☑ |
| H2027 | Psychoeducational service, per 15 minutes | ☑ |
| H2028 | Sexual offender treatment service, per 15 minutes | ☑ |
| H2029 | Sexual offender treatment service, per diem | ☑ |
| H2030 | Mental health clubhouse services, per 15 minutes | ☑ |
| H2031 | Mental health clubhouse services, per diem | ☑ |
| H2032 | Activity therapy, per 15 minutes | ☑ |
| H2033 | Multisystemic therapy for juveniles, per 15 minutes | ☑ |
| H2034 | Alcohol and/or drug abuse halfway house services, per diem | ☑ |
| H2035 | Alcohol and/or other drug treatment program, per hour | ☑ |
| H2036 | Alcohol and/or other drug treatment program, per diem | ☑ |
| H2037 | Developmental delay prevention activities, dependent child of client, per 15 minutes | Ⓐ ☑ |

Special Coverage Instructions    Noncovered by Medicare    Carrier Discretion    ☑ Quantity Alert   ● New Code   ○ Recycled/Reinstated   ▲ Revised Code

78 — H Codes    Ⓐ Age Edit    Ⓜ Maternity Edit    ♀ Female Only    ♂ Male Only    Ⓐ-Ⓨ OPPS Status Indicators    © 2016 Optum360, LLC

## J Codes Drugs J0120-J8499

J codes include drugs that ordinarily cannot be self-administered, chemotherapy drugs, immunosuppressive drugs, inhalation solutions, and other miscellaneous drugs and solutions

### Miscellaneous Drugs

**J0120** Injection, tetracycline, up to 250 mg ☒ ☒ ☑

**J0129** Injection, abatacept, 10 mg (code may be used for Medicare when drug administered under the direct supervision of a physician, not for use when drug is self-administered) ☒ ☒ ☑
Use this code for Orencia.

**J0130** Injection abciximab, 10 mg ☒ ☒ ☑
Use this code for ReoPro.

**J0131** Injection, acetaminophen, 10 mg ☒ ☒ ☑
Use this code for OFIRMEV.

**J0132** Injection, acetylcysteine, 100 mg ☒ ☒ ☑
Use this code for Acetadote.

**J0133** Injection, acyclovir, 5 mg ☒ ☒ ☑
Use this code for Zovirax.

**J0135** Injection, adalimumab, 20 mg ☒ ☒ ☑
Use this code for Humira.
AHA: 3Q, '05, 7, 9; 2Q, '05, 11

**J0153** Injection, adenosine, 1 mg (not to be used to report any adenosine phosphate compounds) ☒ ☒ ☑
Use this code for Adenocard, Adenoscan.
AHA: 1Q, '15, 6

**J0171** Injection, Adrenalin, epinephrine, 0.1 mg ☒ ☒ ☑

**J0178** Injection, aflibercept, 1 mg ☒ ☒ ☑
Use this code for Eylea.

**J0180** Injection, agalsidase beta, 1 mg ☒ ☒ ☑
Use this code for Fabrazyme.
AHA: 2Q, '05, 11

**J0190** Injection, biperiden lactate, per 5 mg ☒ ☑

**J0200** Injection, alatrofloxacin mesylate, 100 mg ☒ ☒ ☑
CMS: 100-02,15,50.5

**J0202** Injection, alemtuzumab, 1 mg ☒ ☒
Use this code for Lemtrada.
AHA: 1Q, '16, 6-8

**J0205** Injection, alglucerase, per 10 units ☒ ☑
Use this code for Ceredase.
AHA: 2Q, '05, 11

**J0207** Injection, amifostine, 500 mg ☒ ☒ ☑
Use this code for Ethyol.

**J0210** Injection, methyldopate HCl, up to 250 mg ☒ ☒ ☑
Use this code for Aldomet.

**J0215** Injection, alefacept, 0.5 mg ☒ ☒ ☑
Use this for Amevive.

**J0220** Injection, alglucosidase alfa, 10 mg, not otherwise specified ☒ ☒ ☑
Use this code for Myozyme.
AHA: 2Q, '13; 1Q, '08, 6

**J0221** Injection, alglucosidase alfa, (Lumizyme), 10 mg ☒ ☒ ☑
AHA: 2Q, '13

**J0256** Injection, alpha 1-proteinase inhibitor (human), not otherwise specified, 10 mg ☒ ☒ ☑
Use this code for Aralast, Aralast NP, Prolastin C, Zemira.
AHA: 2Q, '13; 2Q, '05, 11

**J0257** Injection, alpha 1 proteinase inhibitor (human), (GLASSIA), 10 mg ☒ ☒ ☑

**J0270** Injection, alprostadil, 1.25 mcg (code may be used for Medicare when drug administered under the direct supervision of a physician, not for use when drug is self-administered) ☒
Use this code for Alprostadil, Caverject, Edex, Prostin VR Pediatric.

**J0275** Alprostadil urethral suppository (code may be used for Medicare when drug administered under the direct supervision of a physician, not for use when drug is self-administered) ☒
Use this code for Muse.

**J0278** Injection, amikacin sulfate, 100 mg ☒ ☒ ☑
Use this code for Amikin.

**J0280** Injection, aminophyllin, up to 250 mg ☒ ☒ ☑
AHA: 4Q, '05, 1-6

**J0282** Injection, amiodarone HCl, 30 mg ☒ ☒ ☑
Use this code for Cordarone IV.

**J0285** Injection, amphotericin B, 50 mg ☒ ☒ ☑
Use this for Amphocin, Fungizone.

**J0287** Injection, amphotericin B lipid complex, 10 mg ☒ ☒ ☑
Use this code for Abelcet.

**J0288** Injection, amphotericin B cholesteryl sulfate complex, 10 mg ☒ ☒ ☑
Use this code for Amphotec.

**J0289** Injection, amphotericin B liposome, 10 mg ☒ ☒ ☑
Use this code for Ambisome.

**J0290** Injection, ampicillin sodium, 500 mg ☒ ☒ ☑

**J0295** Injection, ampicillin sodium/sulbactam sodium, per 1.5 g ☒ ☒ ☑
Use this code for Unasyn.

**J0300** Injection, amobarbital, up to 125 mg ☒ ☒ ☑
Use this code for Amytal.

**J0330** Injection, succinylcholine chloride, up to 20 mg ☒ ☒ ☑
Use this code for Anectine, Quelicin.

**J0348** Injection, anidulafungin, 1 mg ☒ ☒ ☑
Use this code for Eraxis.

**J0350** Injection, anistreplase, per 30 units ☒ ☑
Use this code for Eminase.

**J0360** Injection, hydralazine HCl, up to 20 mg ☒ ☒ ☑

**J0364** Injection, apomorphine HCl, 1 mg ☒ ☑
Use this code for Apokyn.

**J0365** Injection, aprotinin, 10,000 kiu ☒ ☑
Use this code for Trasylol.

**J0380** Injection, metaraminol bitartrate, per 10 mg ☒ ☒ ☑
Use this code for Aramine.

**J0390** Injection, chloroquine HCl, up to 250 mg ☒ ☒ ☑
Use this code for Aralen.

**J0395** Injection, arbutamine HCl, 1 mg ☒ ☑

**J0400** Injection, aripiprazole, intramuscular, 0.25 mg ☒ ☒ ☑
Use this code for Abilify.
AHA: 1Q, '08, 6

**J0401** Injection, aripiprazole, extended release, 1 mg ☒ ☒ ☑
Use this code for the Abilify Maintena kit.
AHA: 1Q, '14

**J0456** Injection, azithromycin, 500 mg ☒ ☒ ☑
Use this code for Zithromax.
CMS: 100-02,15,50.5

---

Special Coverage Instructions    Noncovered by Medicare    Carrier Discretion    ☑ Quantity Alert   ● New Code   ○ Recycled/Reinstated   ▲ Revised Code

© 2016 Optum360, LLC    ☒-☒ ASC Pmt    CMS: Pub 100    AHA: Coding Clinic    ⅃ DMEPOS Paid    ⊘ SNF Excluded    J Codes — 79

| Code | Description | Indicators |
|------|-------------|------------|
| J0461 | **Injection, atropine sulfate, 0.01 mg**<br>Use this code for AtroPen. | N N1 ☑ |
| J0470 | **Injection, dimercaprol, per 100 mg**<br>Use this code for BAL. | N N1 ☑ |
| J0475 | **Injection, baclofen, 10 mg**<br>Use this code for Lioresal, Gablofen. | K K2 ☑ |
| J0476 | **Injection, baclofen, 50 mcg for intrathecal trial**<br>Use this code for Lioresal, Gablofen. | K K2 ☑ |
| J0480 | **Injection, basiliximab, 20 mg**<br>Use this code for Simulect. | K K2 |
| J0485 | **Injection, belatacept, 1 mg**<br>Use this code for Nulojix. | K K2 ☑ |
| J0490 | **Injection, belimumab, 10 mg**<br>Use this code for BENLYSTA. | K K2 ☑ |
| J0500 | **Injection, dicyclomine HCl, up to 20 mg**<br>Use this code for Bentyl. | N N1 ☑ |
| J0515 | **Injection, benztropine mesylate, per 1 mg**<br>Use this code for Cogentin. | N N1 ☑ |
| J0520 | **Injection, bethanechol chloride, Myotonachol or Urecholine, up to 5 mg** | N N1 ☑ |
| J0558 | **Injection, penicillin G benzathine and penicillin G procaine, 100,000 units**<br>Use this code for Bicillin CR, Bicillin CR 900/300, Bicillin CR Tubex. | N N1 ☑ |
| J0561 | **Injection, penicillin G benzathine, 100,000 units**<br>AHA: 2Q, '13 | K K2 ☑ |
| ○ J0570^Jan | **Buprenorphine implant, 74.2 mg**<br>Use this code for Probuphine. | |
| J0571 | **Buprenorphine, oral, 1 mg**<br>Use this code for Subutex.<br>AHA: 1Q, '15, 6 | E |
| J0572 | **Buprenorphine/naloxone, oral, less than or equal to 3 mg buprenorphine**<br>Use this code for Bunavail, Suboxone, Zubsolv.<br>AHA: 1Q, '15, 6 | E ☑ |
| ▲ J0573^Jan | **Buprenorphine/naloxone, oral, greater than 3 mg, but less than or equal to 6 mg buprenorphine**<br>Use this code for Bunavail, Suboxone, Zubsolv.<br>AHA: 1Q, '16, 6-8; 1Q, '15, 6 | E ☑ |
| J0574 | **Buprenorphine/naloxone, oral, greater than 6 mg, but less than or equal to 10 mg buprenorphine**<br>Use this code for Bunavail, Suboxone.<br>AHA: 1Q, '16, 6-8; 1Q, '15, 6 | E ☑ |
| J0575 | **Buprenorphine/naloxone, oral, greater than 10 mg buprenorphine**<br>Use this code for Suboxone.<br>AHA: 1Q, '16, 6-8; 1Q, '15, 6 | E ☑ |
| J0583 | **Injection, bivalirudin, 1 mg**<br>Use this code for Angiomax. | N N1 ☑ |
| J0585 | **Injection, onabotulinumtoxinA, 1 unit**<br>Use this code for Botox, Botox Cosmetic. | K K2 ☑ |
| J0586 | **Injection, abobotulinumtoxinA, 5 units**<br>Use this code for Dysport. | K K2 ☑ |
| J0587 | **Injection, rimabotulinumtoxinB, 100 units**<br>Use this code for Myobloc.<br>AHA: 2Q, '02, 8-9; 1Q, '02, 5 | K K2 ☑ |
| J0588 | **Injection, incobotulinumtoxinA, 1 unit**<br>Use this code for XEOMIN. | K K2 ☑ |
| J0592 | **Injection, buprenorphine HCl, 0.1 mg**<br>Use this code for Buprenex. | N N1 ☑ |
| J0594 | **Injection, busulfan, 1 mg**<br>Use this code for Busulfex. | K K2 ☑ |
| J0595 | **Injection, butorphanol tartrate, 1 mg**<br>Use this code for Stadol.<br>AHA: 2Q, '05, 11 | N N1 ☑ |
| J0596 | **Injection, C1 esterase inhibitor (recombinant), Ruconest, 10 units** | G K2 |
| J0597 | **Injection, C-1 esterase inhibitor (human), Berinert, 10 units** | K K2 ☑ |
| J0598 | **Injection, C-1 esterase inhibitor (human), Cinryze, 10 units** | K K2 ☑ |
| J0600 | **Injection, edetate calcium disodium, up to 1,000 mg**<br>Use this code for Calcium Disodium Versenate, Calcium EDTA. | K K2 ☑ |
| J0610 | **Injection, calcium gluconate, per 10 ml** | N N1 ☑ |
| J0620 | **Injection, calcium glycerophosphate and calcium lactate, per 10 ml** | N N1 ☑ |
| J0630 | **Injection, calcitonin salmon, up to 400 units**<br>Use this code for Calcimar, Miacalcin.<br>CMS: 100-04,10,90.1 | K K2 ☑ |
| J0636 | **Injection, calcitriol, 0.1 mcg**<br>Use this code for Calcijex. | N N1 ☑ |
| J0637 | **Injection, caspofungin acetate, 5 mg**<br>Use this code for Cancidas. | K K2 |
| J0638 | **Injection, canakinumab, 1 mg**<br>Use this code for ILARIS. | K K2 |
| J0640 | **Injection, leucovorin calcium, per 50 mg**<br>AHA: 1Q, '09, 10 | N N1 ☑ |
| J0641 | **Injection, levoleucovorin calcium, 0.5 mg**<br>Use this code for Fusilev. | K K2 ☑ |
| J0670 | **Injection, mepivacaine HCl, per 10 ml**<br>Use this code for Carbocaine, Polocaine, Isocaine HCl, Scandonest | N N1 ☑ |
| J0690 | **Injection, cefazolin sodium, 500 mg** | N N1 ☑ |
| J0692 | **Injection, cefepime HCl, 500 mg**<br>AHA: 1Q, '02, 5 | N N1 ☑ |
| J0694 | **Injection, cefoxitin sodium, 1 g** | N N1 ☑ |
| J0695 | **Injection, ceftolozane 50 mg and tazobactam 25 mg**<br>Use this code for Zerbaxa. | G K2 |
| J0696 | **Injection, ceftriaxone sodium, per 250 mg** | N N1 ☑ |
| J0697 | **Injection, sterile cefuroxime sodium, per 750 mg** | N N1 ☑ |
| J0698 | **Injection, cefotaxime sodium, per g** | N N1 ☑ |
| J0702 | **Injection, betamethasone acetate 3 mg and betamethasone sodium phosphate 3 mg** | N N1 ☑ |
| J0706 | **Injection, caffeine citrate, 5 mg**<br>AHA: 2Q, '02, 8-9; 1Q, '02, 5 | N N1 ☑ |
| J0710 | **Injection, cephapirin sodium, up to 1 g** | E ☑ |
| J0712 | **Injection, ceftaroline fosamil, 10 mg** | K K2 ☑ |
| J0713 | **Injection, ceftazidime, per 500 mg** | N N1 ☑ |
| J0714 | **Injection, ceftazidime and avibactam, 0.5 g/0.125 g**<br>Use this code for Avycaz.<br>AHA: 1Q, '16, 6-8 | K K2 |
| J0715 | **Injection, ceftizoxime sodium, per 500 mg** | N N1 ☑ |
| J0716 | **Injection, Centruroides immune f(ab)2, up to 120 mg** | K K2 ☑ |

**Jan** **January Update**

Special Coverage Instructions   Noncovered by Medicare   Carrier Discretion   ☑ Quantity Alert ● New Code ○ Recycled/Reinstated ▲ Revised Code

80 — J Codes   A Age Edit  M Maternity Edit  ♀ Female Only  ♂ Male Only  A-Y OPPS Status Indicators  © 2016 Optum360, LLC

**J0717** Injection, certolizumab pegol, 1 mg (code may be used for Medicare when drug administered under the direct supervision of a physician, not for use when drug is self administered) K K2 ☑
AHA: 1Q, '14

**J0720** Injection, chloramphenicol sodium succinate, up to 1 g K K2 ☑

**J0725** Injection, chorionic gonadotropin, per 1,000 USP units K K2 ☑

**J0735** Injection, clonidine HCl, 1 mg N N1 ☑

**J0740** Injection, cidofovir, 375 mg K K2 ☑

**J0743** Injection, cilastatin sodium; imipenem, per 250 mg N N1 ☑

**J0744** Injection, ciprofloxacin for intravenous infusion, 200 mg N N1 ☑
AHA: 1Q, '02, 5

**J0745** Injection, codeine phosphate, per 30 mg N N1 ☑

**J0760**^Jan ~~Injection, colchicine, per 1 mg~~

**J0770** Injection, colistimethate sodium, up to 150 mg N N1 ☑

**J0775** Injection, collagenase, clostridium histolyticum, 0.01 mg K K2 ☑

**J0780** Injection, prochlorperazine, up to 10 mg N N1 ☑

**J0795** Injection, corticorelin ovine triflutate, 1 mcg K K2 ☑

**J0800** Injection, corticotropin, up to 40 units K K2 ☑

**J0833** Injection, cosyntropin, not otherwise specified, 0.25 mg K K2 ☑
AHA: 2Q, '13

**J0834** Injection, cosyntropin (Cortrosyn), 0.25 mg N N1 ☑

**J0840** Injection, crotalidae polyvalent immune fab (ovine), up to 1 g K K2 ☑

**J0850** Injection, cytomegalovirus immune globulin intravenous (human), per vial K K2 ☑

**J0875** Injection, dalbavancin, 5 mg G K2
Use this code for Dalvance.

**J0878** Injection, daptomycin, 1 mg K K2 ☑
Use this code for Cubicin.
AHA: 2Q, '05, 11

**J0881** Injection, darbepoetin alfa, 1 mcg (non-ESRD use) K K2 ☑
Use this code for Aranesp.
CMS: 100-03,110.21; 100-04,17,80.12

**J0882** Injection, darbepoetin alfa, 1 mcg (for ESRD on dialysis) K ☑ ⊘
Use this code for Aranesp.
CMS: 100-04,13,60.7.1; 100-04,8,60.4; 100-04,8,60.4.1; 100-04,8,60.4.2; 100-04,8,60.4.5.1; 100-04,8,60.4.6.3; 100-04,8,60.4.6.4; 100-04,8,60.4.6.5; 100-04,8,60.7

● **J0883**^Jan Injection, argatroban, 1 mg (for non-ESRD use)

● **J0884**^Jan Injection, argatroban, 1 mg (for ESRD on dialysis)

**J0885** Injection, epoetin alfa, (for non-ESRD use), 1000 units K K2 ☑
Use this code for Epogen/Procrit.
CMS: 100-03,110.21; 100-04,17,80.12
AHA: 2Q, '06, 4, 5

**J0887** Injection, epoetin beta, 1 microgram, (for ESRD on dialysis) K
Use this code for Mircera.
AHA: 1Q, '15, 6

**J0888** Injection, epoetin beta, 1 microgram, (for non-ESRD use) E N1
Use this code for Mircera.
AHA: 1Q, '15, 6

**J0890** Injection, peginesatide, 0.1 mg (for ESRD on dialysis) E ☑
Use this code for Omontys.
CMS: 100-04,8,60.4; 100-04,8,60.4.1; 100-04,8,60.4.2; 100-04,8,60.4.5.1; 100-04,8,60.4.7

**J0894** Injection, decitabine, 1 mg K K2 ☑ ⊘
Use this code for Dacogen.

**J0895** Injection, deferoxamine mesylate, 500 mg N N1 ☑
Use this code for Desferal.

**J0897** Injection, denosumab, 1 mg K K2 ☑
Use this code for XGEVA, Prolia.
AHA: 1Q, '16, 5

**J0945** Injection, brompheniramine maleate, per 10 mg N N1 ☑

**J1000** Injection, depo-estradiol cypionate, up to 5 mg N N1 ☑
Use this code for depGynogen, Depogen, Estradiol Cypionate.

**J1020** Injection, methylprednisolone acetate, 20 mg N N1 ☑
Use this code for Depo-Medrol.
AHA: 2Q, '09, 9; 3Q, '05, 10

**J1030** Injection, methylprednisolone acetate, 40 mg N N1 ☑
Use this code for DepoMedalone40, Depo-Medrol, Sano-Drol.
AHA: 2Q, '09, 9; 3Q, '05, 10

**J1040** Injection, methylprednisolone acetate, 80 mg N N1 ☑
Use this code for Cortimed, DepMedalone, DepoMedalone 80, Depo-Medrol, Duro Cort, Methylcotolone, Pri-Methylate, Sano-Drol.
AHA: 2Q, '09, 9

**J1050** Injection, medroxyprogesterone acetate, 1 mg N N1 ☑

**J1071** Injection, testosterone cypionate, 1 mg N N1
Use this code for Depo-testosterone.
AHA: 2Q, '15, 7; 1Q, '15, 6

**J1094** Injection, dexamethasone acetate, 1 mg N N1
Use this code for Cortastat LA, Dalalone L.A., Dexamethasone Acetate Anhydrous, Dexone LA.

**J1100** Injection, dexamethasone sodium phosphate, 1 mg N N1 ☑
Use this code for Cortastat, Dalalone, Decaject, Dexone, Solurex, Adrenocort, Primethasone, Dexasone, Dexim, Medidex, Spectro-Dex.

**J1110** Injection, dihydroergotamine mesylate, per 1 mg N N1 ☑
Use this code for D.H.E. 45.

**J1120** Injection, acetazolamide sodium, up to 500 mg N N1 ☑
Use this code for Diamox.
AHA: 4Q, '05, 1-6; 3Q, '04, 1-10

○ **J1130**^Jan Injection, diclofenac sodium, 0.5 mg
Use this code for Dyloject.

**J1160** Injection, digoxin, up to 0.5 mg K K2 ☑
Use this code for Lanoxin.
AHA: 4Q, '05, 1-6

**J1162** Injection, digoxin immune fab (ovine), per vial K K2 ☑
Use this code for Digibind, Digifab.

**J1165** Injection, phenytoin sodium, per 50 mg N N1 ☑
Use this code for Dilantin.

**J1170** Injection, hydromorphone, up to 4 mg N N1 ☑
Use this code for Dilaudid, Dilaudid-HP.

**J1180** Injection, dyphylline, up to 500 mg E ☑

**J1190** Injection, dexrazoxane HCl, per 250 mg K K2 ☑
Use this code for Zinecard.

---

**Jan** January Update

Special Coverage Instructions    Noncovered by Medicare    Carrier Discretion    ☑ Quantity Alert  ● New Code    ○ Recycled/Reinstated  ▲ Revised Code

© 2016 Optum360, LLC    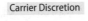 ASC Pmt    **CMS:** Pub 100    **AHA:** Coding Clinic  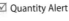 DMEPOS Paid    ⊘ SNF Excluded    **J Codes — 81**

**Drugs Administered Other Than Oral Method**

**J1200 — J1556**

**J1200** **Injection, diphenhydramine HCl, up to 50 mg** N N1 ☑
Use this code for Benadryl, Benahist 10, Benahist 50, Benoject-10, Benoject-50, Bena-D 10, Bena-D 50, Nordryl, Dihydrex, Dimine, Diphenacen-50, Hyrexin-50, Truxadryl, Wehdryl.
**AHA:** 1Q, '02, 1-2

**J1205** **Injection, chlorothiazide sodium, per 500 mg** K K2 ☑
Use this code for Diuril Sodium.

**J1212** **Injection, DMSO, dimethyl sulfoxide, 50%, 50 ml** K K2 ☑
Use this code for Rimso 50. DMSO is covered only as a treatment of interstitial cystitis.

**J1230** **Injection, methadone HCl, up to 10 mg** N N1 ☑
Use this code for Dolophine HCl.

**J1240** **Injection, dimenhydrinate, up to 50 mg** N N1 ☑
Use this code for Dramamine, Dinate, Dommanate, Dramanate, Dramilin, Dramocen, Dramoject, Dymenate, Hydrate, Marmine, Wehamine.

**J1245** **Injection, dipyridamole, per 10 mg** N N1 ☑
Use this code for Persantine IV.
**AHA:** 4Q, '05, 1-6; 3Q, '04, 1-10

**J1250** **Injection, Dobutamine HCl, per 250 mg** N N1 ☑
**AHA:** 4Q, '05, 1-6; 3Q, '04, 1-10

**J1260** **Injection, dolasetron mesylate, 10 mg** N N1 ☑
Use this code for Anzemet.

**J1265** **Injection, dopamine HCl, 40 mg** N N1 ☑
**AHA:** 4Q, '05, 1-6

**J1267** **Injection, doripenem, 10 mg** N N1
Use this code for Doribax.

**J1270** **Injection, doxercalciferol, 1 mcg** N N1 ☑
Use this code for Hectorol.
**AHA:** 1Q, '02, 5

**J1290** **Injection, ecallantide, 1 mg** K K2 ☑
Use this code for KALBITOR.

**J1300** **Injection, eculizumab, 10 mg** K K2 ☑
Use this code for Soliris.
**AHA:** 1Q, '08, 6

**J1320** **Injection, amitriptyline HCl, up to 20 mg** N N1 ☑
Use this code for Elavil.

**J1322** **Injection, elosulfase alfa, 1 mg** G K2
Use this code for Vimizim.
**AHA:** 1Q, '15, 6

**J1324** **Injection, enfuvirtide, 1 mg** K K2 ☑
Use this code for Fuzeon.

**J1325** **Injection, epoprostenol, 0.5 mg** N N1 ☑
Use this code for Flolan and Veletri. See K0455 for infusion pump for epoprosterol.

**J1327** **Injection, eptifibatide, 5 mg** K K2 ☑
Use this code for Integrilin.

**J1330** **Injection, ergonovine maleate, up to 0.2 mg** K K2 ☑
Medicare jurisdiction: local contractor. Use this code for Ergotrate Maleate.

**J1335** **Injection, ertapenem sodium, 500 mg** N N1 ☑
Use this code for Invanz.

**J1364** **Injection, erythromycin lactobionate, per 500 mg** K K2 ☑

**J1380** **Injection, estradiol valerate, up to 10 mg** N N1 ☑
Use this code for Delestrogen, Dioval, Dioval XX, Dioval 40, Duragen-10, Duragen-20, Duragen-40, Estradiol L.A., Estradiol L.A. 20, Estradiol L.A. 40, Gynogen L.A. 10, Gynogen L.A. 20, Gynogen L.A. 40, Valergen 10, Valergen 20, Valergen 40, Estra-L 20, Estra-L 40, L.A.E. 20.

**J1410** **Injection, estrogen conjugated, per 25 mg** K K2 ☑
Use this code for Natural Estrogenic Substance, Premarin Intravenous, Primestrin Aqueous.

**J1430** **Injection, ethanolamine oleate, 100 mg** K K2
Use this code for Ethamiolin.

**J1435** **Injection, estrone, per 1 mg** E ☑
Use this code for Estone Aqueous, Estragyn, Estro-A, Estrone, Estronol, Theelin Aqueous, Estone 5, Kestrone 5.

**J1436** **Injection, etidronate disodium, per 300 mg** N N1 ☑
Use this code for Didronel.

**J1438** **Injection, etanercept, 25 mg (code may be used for Medicare when drug administered under the direct supervision of a physician, not for use when drug is self-administered)** K K2 ☑
Use this code for Enbrel.

**J1439** **Injection, ferric carboxymaltose, 1 mg** G K2
Use this code for Injectafer.
**AHA:** 1Q, '15, 6

**J1442** **Injection, filgrastim (G-CSF), excludes biosimilars, 1 microgram** K K2 ☑
Use this code for Neupogen.
**AHA:** 1Q, '14

**J1443** **Injection, ferric pyrophosphate citrate solution, 0.1 mg of iron** N N1
Use this code for Triferic.
**AHA:** 1Q, '16, 6-8

**J1447** **Injection, tbo-filgrastim, 1 microgram** G K2
Use this code for Granix.
**AHA:** 1Q, '16, 6-8

**J1450** **Injection, fluconazole, 200 mg** N N1 ☑
Use this code for Diflucan.
**CMS:** 100-02,15,50.5; 100-02,15,50.6

**J1451** **Injection, fomepizole, 15 mg** K K2 ☑
Use this code for Antizol.
**CMS:** 100-02,15,50.6

**J1452** **Injection, fomivirsen sodium, intraocular, 1.65 mg** E ☑
Use this code for Vitravene.
**CMS:** 100-02,15,50.4.2; 100-02,15,50.6

**J1453** **Injection, fosaprepitant, 1 mg** K K2
Use this code for Emend.
**CMS:** 100-02,15,50.6

**J1455** **Injection, foscarnet sodium, per 1,000 mg** N N1 ☑
Use this code for Foscavir.
**CMS:** 100-02,15,50.6

**J1457** **Injection, gallium nitrate, 1 mg** N N1 ☑
Use this code for Ganite.
**CMS:** 100-02,15,50.6
**AHA:** 2Q, '05, 11

**J1458** **Injection, galsulfase, 1 mg** K K2 ☑
Use this code for Naglazyme.
**CMS:** 100-02,15,50.6

**J1459** **Injection, immune globulin (Privigen), intravenous, nonlyophilized (e.g., liquid), 500 mg** K K2
**CMS:** 100-02,15,50.6

**J1460** **Injection, gamma globulin, intramuscular, 1 cc** N N1 ☑
Use this code for GamaSTAN SD.
**CMS:** 100-02,15,50.6; 100-04,17,80.6

**J1556** **Injection, immune globulin (Bivigam), 500 mg** K K2 ☑
**CMS:** 100-02,15,50.6

---

Special Coverage Instructions    Noncovered by Medicare    Carrier Discretion    ☑ Quantity Alert    ● New Code    ○ Recycled/Reinstated    ▲ Revised Code

82 — J Codes    A Age Edit    M Maternity Edit    ♀ Female Only    ♂ Male Only    A-Y OPPS Status Indicators    © 2016 Optum360, LLC

| | |
|---|---|
| **J1557** | Injection, immune globulin, (Gammaplex), intravenous, nonlyophilized (e.g., liquid), 500 mg  ☒ ☒ ☑ |
| | CMS: 100-02,15,50.6 |
| **J1559** | Injection, immune globulin (Hizentra), 100 mg  ☒ ☒ ☑ |
| | CMS: 100-02,15,50.6 |
| **J1560** | Injection, gamma globulin, intramuscular, over 10 cc  ☒ ☒ ☑ |
| | Use this code for GamaSTAN SD. |
| | CMS: 100-02,15,50.6; 100-04,17,80.6 |
| **J1561** | Injection, immune globulin, (Gamunex/Gamunex-C/Gammaked), nonlyophilized (e.g., liquid), 500 mg  ☒ ☒ ☑ |
| | CMS: 100-02,15,50.6 |
| | AHA: 1Q, '08, 6 |
| **J1562** | Injection, immune globulin (Vivaglobin), 100 mg  ☒ ☑ |
| | CMS: 100-02,15,50.6 |
| **J1566** | Injection, immune globulin, intravenous, lyophilized (e.g., powder), not otherwise specified, 500 mg  ☒ ☒ ☑ |
| | Use this code for Carimune. |
| | CMS: 100-02,15,50.6 |
| | AHA: 2Q, '13 |
| **J1568** | Injection, immune globulin, (Octagam), intravenous, nonlyophilized (e.g., liquid), 500 mg  ☒ ☒ ☑ |
| | CMS: 100-02,15,50.6 |
| | AHA: 1Q, '08, 6 |
| **J1569** | Injection, immune globulin, (Gammagard liquid), nonlyophilized, (e.g., liquid), 500 mg  ☒ ☒ ☑ |
| | CMS: 100-02,15,50.6 |
| | AHA: 1Q, '08, 6 |
| **J1570** | Injection, ganciclovir sodium, 500 mg  ☒ ☒ ☑ |
| | Use this code for Cytovene. |
| **J1571** | Injection, hepatitis B immune globulin (Hepagam B), intramuscular, 0.5 ml  ☒ ☒ ☑ |
| | AHA: 3Q, '08, 7, 8; 1Q, '08, 6 |
| **J1572** | Injection, immune globulin, (Flebogamma/Flebogamma Dif), intravenous, nonlyophilized (e.g., liquid), 500 mg  ☒ ☒ ☑ |
| | AHA: 1Q, '08, 6 |
| **J1573** | Injection, hepatitis B immune globulin (Hepagam B), intravenous, 0.5 ml  ☒ ☒ ☑ |
| | AHA: 3Q, '08, 7, 8; 1Q, '08, 6 |
| **J1575** | Injection, immune globulin/hyaluronidase, 100 mg immuneglobulin  ☒ ☒ |
| | Use this code for HyQvia. |
| | AHA: 1Q, '16, 6-8 |
| **J1580** | Injection, garamycin, gentamicin, up to 80 mg  ☒ ☒ ☑ |
| | Use this code for Gentamicin Sulfate, Jenamicin. |
| **J1590**<sup>Jan</sup> | ~~Injection, gatifloxacin, 10 mg~~ |
| **J1595** | Injection, glatiramer acetate, 20 mg  ☒ ☒ ☑ |
| | Use this code for Copaxone. |
| **J1599** | Injection, immune globulin, intravenous, nonlyophilized (e.g., liquid), not otherwise specified, 500 mg  ☒ ☒ ☑ |
| | AHA: 2Q, '13 |
| **J1600** | Injection, gold sodium thiomalate, up to 50 mg  ☒ ☒ ☑ |
| | Use this code for Myochrysine. |
| | CMS: 100-04,4,20.6.4 |
| **J1602** | Injection, golimumab, 1 mg, for intravenous use  ☒ ☒ ☑ |
| | Use this code for Simponi. |
| | AHA: 1Q, '14 |
| **J1610** | Injection, glucagon HCl, per 1 mg  ☒ ☒ ☑ |
| | Use this code for Glucagen. |
| | AHA: 4Q, '05, 1-6 |
| **J1620** | Injection, gonadorelin HCl, per 100 mcg  ☒ ☑ |
| | Use this code for Factrel, Lutrepulse. |
| **J1626** | Injection, granisetron HCl, 100 mcg  ☒ ☒ ☑ |
| | Use this code for Kytril. |
| | CMS: 100-04,4,20.6.4 |
| **J1630** | Injection, haloperidol, up to 5 mg  ☒ ☒ ☑ |
| | Use this code for Haldol. |
| | CMS: 100-04,4,20.6.4 |
| **J1631** | Injection, haloperidol decanoate, per 50 mg  ☒ ☒ ☑ |
| | Use this code for Haldol Decanoate-50. |
| | CMS: 100-04,4,20.6.4 |
| **J1640** | Injection, hemin, 1 mg  ☒ ☒ ☑ |
| | Use this code for Panhematin. |
| **J1642** | Injection, heparin sodium, (heparin lock flush), per 10 units  ☒ ☒ ☑ |
| | Use this code for Hep-Lock, Hep-Lock U/P, Hep-Pak, Lok-Pak. |
| | CMS: 100-04,4,20.6.4 |
| | AHA: 4Q, '05, 1-6 |
| **J1644** | Injection, Heparin sodium, per 1000 units  ☒ ☒ ☑ |
| | Use this code for Heparin Sodium, Liquaemin Sodium. |
| | CMS: 100-04,4,20.6.4 |
| **J1645** | Injection, dalteparin sodium, per 2500 IU  ☒ ☒ ☑ |
| | Use this code for Fragmin. |
| | CMS: 100-04,4,20.6.4 |
| **J1650** | Injection, enoxaparin sodium, 10 mg  ☒ ☒ ☑ |
| | Use this code for Lovenox. |
| | CMS: 100-04,4,20.6.4 |
| **J1652** | Injection, fondaparinux sodium, 0.5 mg  ☒ ☒ ☑ |
| | Use this code for Atrixtra. |
| **J1655** | Injection, tinzaparin sodium, 1000 IU  ☒ ☑ |
| | Use this code for Innohep. |
| | CMS: 100-04,4,20.6.4 |
| | AHA: 1Q, '02, 5 |
| **J1670** | Injection, tetanus immune globulin, human, up to 250 units  ☒ ☒ ☑ |
| | Use this code for HyperTET SD. |
| **J1675** | Injection, histrelin acetate, 10 mcg  ☒ |
| | Use this code for Supprelin LA. |
| **J1700** | Injection, hydrocortisone acetate, up to 25 mg  ☒ ☒ ☑ |
| | Use this code for Hydrocortone Acetate. |
| | CMS: 100-04,4,20.6.4 |
| **J1710** | Injection, hydrocortisone sodium phosphate, up to 50 mg  ☒ ☒ ☑ |
| | Use this code for Hydrocortone Phosphate. |
| | CMS: 100-04,4,20.6.4 |
| **J1720** | Injection, hydrocortisone sodium succinate, up to 100 mg  ☒ ☒ ☑ |
| | Use this code for Solu-Cortef, A-Hydrocort. |
| | CMS: 100-04,4,20.6.4 |
| **J1725** | Injection, hydroxyprogesterone caproate, 1 mg  ☒ ♀ ☒ ☒ |
| | Use this code for Makena. |
| **J1730** | Injection, diazoxide, up to 300 mg  ☒ ☑ |
| **J1740** | Injection, ibandronate sodium, 1 mg  ☒ ☒ ☑ |
| | Use this code for Boniva. |
| **J1741** | Injection, ibuprofen, 100 mg  ☒ ☒ ☑ |
| | Use this code for Caldolor. |
| **J1742** | Injection, ibutilide fumarate, 1 mg  ☒ ☒ ☑ |
| | Use this code for Corvert. |

**Jan** **January Update**

Special Coverage Instructions    Noncovered by Medicare    Carrier Discretion    ☑ Quantity Alert    ● New Code    ○ Recycled/Reinstated    ▲ Revised Code

© 2016 Optum360, LLC    **A2**-**Z8** ASC Pmt    **CMS:** Pub 100    **AHA:** Coding Clinic    ⅃ DMEPOS Paid    ⊘ SNF Excluded    J Codes — 83

**Drugs Administered Other Than Oral Method**

**J1743 — J2175**

| | | |
|---|---|---|
| **J1743** | Injection, idursulfase, 1 mg | K K2 |
| | Use this code for Elaprase. | |
| **J1744** | Injection, icatibant, 1 mg | K K2 ☑ |
| | Use this code for Firazyr. | |
| ▲ **J1745**^Jan | Injection, infliximab, excludes biosimilar, 10 mg | K K2 ☑ |
| | Use this code for Remicade. | |
| **J1750** | Injection, iron dextran, 50 mg | K K2 |
| | Use this code for INFeD. | |
| **J1756** | Injection, iron sucrose, 1 mg | N N1 ☑ |
| | Use this code for Venofer. | |
| | CMS: 100-04,8,60.2.4.2 | |
| **J1786** | Injection, imiglucerase, 10 units | K K2 ☑ |
| | Use this code for Cerezyme. | |
| **J1790** | Injection, droperidol, up to 5 mg | N N1 ☑ |
| | Use this code for Inapsine. | |
| | CMS: 100-04,4,20.6.4 | |
| **J1800** | Injection, propranolol HCl, up to 1 mg | N N1 ☑ |
| | Use this code for Inderal. | |
| | CMS: 100-04,4,20.6.4 | |
| | AHA: 4Q, '05, 1-6 | |
| **J1810** | Injection, droperidol and fentanyl citrate, up to 2 ml ampule | E ☑ |
| | AHA: 2Q, '02, 8-9 | |
| **J1815** | Injection, insulin, per 5 units | N N1 ☑ |
| | Use this code for Humalog, Humulin, Iletin, Insulin Lispo, Lantus, Levemir, NPH, Pork insulin, Regular insulin, Ultralente, Velosulin, Humulin R, Iletin II Regular Pork, Insulin Purified Pork, Relion, Lente Iletin I, Novolin R, Humulin R U-500. | |
| | CMS: 100-04,4,20.6.4 | |
| | AHA: 4Q, '05, 1-6 | |
| **J1817** | Insulin for administration through DME (i.e., insulin pump) per 50 units | N N1 ☑ |
| | Use this code for Humalog, Humulin, Vesolin BR, Iletin II NPH Pork, Lispro-PFC, Novolin, Novolog, Novolog Flexpen, Novolog Mix, Relion Novolin. | |
| | AHA: 4Q, '05, 1-6 | |
| **J1826** | Injection, interferon beta-1a, 30 mcg | E ☑ |
| | Use this code for AVONEX, Rebif. | |
| | AHA: 4Q, '14, 6; 2Q, '11, 9 | |
| **J1830** | Injection interferon beta-1b, 0.25 mg (code may be used for Medicare when drug administered under the direct supervision of a physician, not for use when drug is self-administered) | K K2 ☑ |
| | Use this code for Betaseron. | |
| **J1833** | Injection, isavuconazonium, 1 mg | G K2 |
| | Use this code for Cresemba. | |
| **J1835** | Injection, itraconazole, 50 mg | E ☑ |
| | Use this code for Sporonox IV. | |
| | CMS: 100-04,4,20.6.4 | |
| | AHA: 1Q, '02, 5 | |
| **J1840** | Injection, kanamycin sulfate, up to 500 mg | N N1 ☑ |
| | Use this code for Kantrex. | |
| | CMS: 100-04,4,20.6.4 | |
| **J1850** | Injection, kanamycin sulfate, up to 75 mg | N N1 ☑ |
| | Use this code for Kantrex. | |
| | CMS: 100-04,4,20.6.4 | |
| | AHA: 2Q, '13 | |
| **J1885** | Injection, ketorolac tromethamine, per 15 mg | N N1 ☑ |
| | Use this code for Toradol. | |
| | CMS: 100-04,4,20.6.4 | |

| | | |
|---|---|---|
| **J1890** | Injection, cephalothin sodium, up to 1 g | N N1 ☑ |
| | CMS: 100-04,4,20.6.4 | |
| **J1930** | Injection, lanreotide, 1 mg | K K2 ☑ |
| | Use this code for Somatuline. | |
| **J1931** | Injection, laronidase, 0.1 mg | K K2 ☑ |
| | Use this code for Aldurazyme. | |
| | AHA: 2Q, '05, 11; 1Q, '05, 7, 9-10 | |
| **J1940** | Injection, furosemide, up to 20 mg | N N1 ☑ |
| | Use this code for Lasix. | |
| | CMS: 100-04,4,20.6.4 | |
| | AHA: 4Q, '05, 1-6; 3Q, '04, 1-10 | |
| ● **J1942**^Jan | Injection, aripiprazole lauroxil, 1 mg | |
| | Use this code for Aristada. | |
| **J1945** | Injection, lepirudin, 50 mg | K K2 ☑ |
| | Use this code for Refludan. | |
| | This drug is used for patients with heparin-induced thrombocytopenia. | |
| **J1950** | Injection, leuprolide acetate (for depot suspension), per 3.75 mg | K K2 ☑ |
| | Use this code for Lupron Depot-Pedi. | |
| **J1953** | Injection, levetiracetam, 10 mg | N N1 ☑ |
| | Use this code for Keppra. | |
| **J1955** | Injection, levocarnitine, per 1 g | B ☑ |
| | Use this code for Carnitor. | |
| **J1956** | Injection, levofloxacin, 250 mg | N N1 ☑ |
| | Use this code for Levaquin. | |
| | CMS: 100-04,4,20.6.4 | |
| **J1960** | Injection, levorphanol tartrate, up to 2 mg | N N1 ☑ |
| | Use this code for Levo-Dromoran. | |
| | CMS: 100-04,4,20.6.4 | |
| **J1980** | Injection, hyoscyamine sulfate, up to 0.25 mg | N N1 ☑ |
| | Use this code for Levsin. | |
| | CMS: 100-04,4,20.6.4 | |
| **J1990** | Injection, chlordiazepoxide HCl, up to 100 mg | N N1 ☑ |
| | Use this code for Librium. | |
| | CMS: 100-04,4,20.6.4 | |
| **J2001** | Injection, lidocaine HCl for intravenous infusion, 10 mg | N N1 ☑ |
| | Use this code for Xylocaine. | |
| | CMS: 100-04,4,20.6.4 | |
| **J2010** | Injection, lincomycin HCl, up to 300 mg | N N1 ☑ |
| | Use this code for Lincocin. | |
| | CMS: 100-04,4,20.6.4 | |
| **J2020** | Injection, linezolid, 200 mg | K K2 ☑ |
| | Use this code for Zyvok. | |
| | AHA: 2Q, '02, 8-9; 1Q, '02, 5 | |
| **J2060** | Injection, lorazepam, 2 mg | N N1 ☑ |
| | Use this code for Ativan. | |
| | CMS: 100-04,4,20.6.4 | |
| **J2150** | Injection, mannitol, 25% in 50 ml | N N1 ☑ |
| | Use this code for Osmitrol. | |
| | CMS: 100-04,4,20.6.4 | |
| **J2170** | Injection, mecasermin, 1 mg | N N1 ☑ |
| | Use this code for Iplex, Increlex. | |
| | CMS: 100-04,4,20.6.4 | |
| **J2175** | Injection, meperidine HCl, per 100 mg | N N1 ☑ |
| | Use this code for Demerol. | |
| | CMS: 100-04,4,20.6.4 | |

^Jan **January Update**

Special Coverage Instructions    Noncovered by Medicare    Carrier Discretion    ☑ Quantity Alert    ● New Code    ○ Recycled/Reinstated    ▲ Revised Code

84 — J Codes    A Age Edit    M Maternity Edit    ♀ Female Only    ♂ Male Only    A-Y OPPS Status Indicators    © 2016 Optum360, LLC

**J2180**  Injection, meperidine and promethazine HCl, up to 50 mg  N N1 ☑
Use this code for Mepergan Injection.
CMS: 100-04,4,20.6.4

● **J2182**^Jan  Injection, mepolizumab, 1 mg
Use this code for Nucala.

**J2185**  Injection, meropenem, 100 mg  N N1 ☑
Use this code for Merrem.
CMS: 100-04,4,20.6.4
AHA: 2Q, '05, 11

**J2210**  Injection, methylergonovine maleate, up to 0.2 mg  N N1 ☑
Use this code for Methergine.
CMS: 100-04,4,20.6.4

**J2212**  Injection, methylnaltrexone, 0.1 mg  N N1 ☑
Use this code for Relistor.

**J2248**  Injection, micafungin sodium, 1 mg  N N1 ☑
Use this code for Mycamine.

**J2250**  Injection, midazolam HCl, per 1 mg  N N1 ☑
Use this code for Versed.
CMS: 100-04,4,20.6.4

**J2260**  Injection, milrinone lactate, 5 mg  N N1 ☑
Use this code for Primacor.
CMS: 100-04,4,20.6.4

**J2265**  Injection, minocycline HCl, 1 mg  N N1 ☑
Use this code for MINOCIN.

**J2270**  Injection, morphine sulfate, up to 10 mg  N N1 ☑
Use this code for Depodur, Infumorph.
CMS: 100-04,4,20.6.4
AHA: 2Q, '13; 4Q, '05, 1-6; 3Q, '04, 1-10

**J2274**  Injection, morphine sulfate, preservative-free for epidural or intrathecal use, 10 mg  N N1 ☑
Use this code for DepoDur, Astromorph PF, Durarmorph PF.
AHA: 1Q, '15, 6

**J2278**  Injection, ziconotide, 1 mcg  K K2 ☑
Use this code for Prialt.

**J2280**  Injection, moxifloxacin, 100 mg  N N1 ☑
Use this code for Avelox.
CMS: 100-04,4,20.6.4
AHA: 2Q, '05, 11

**J2300**  Injection, nalbuphine HCl, per 10 mg  N N1 ☑
Use this code for Nubain.
CMS: 100-04,4,20.6.4

**J2310**  Injection, naloxone HCl, per 1 mg  N N1 ☑
Use this code for Narcan.

**J2315**  Injection, naltrexone, depot form, 1 mg  K K2 ☑
Use this code for Vivitrol.

**J2320**  Injection, nandrolone decanoate, up to 50 mg  K K2 ☑

**J2323**  Injection, natalizumab, 1 mg  K K2
Use this code for Tysabri.
AHA: 1Q, '08, 6

**J2325**  Injection, nesiritide, 0.1 mg  K K2 ☑
Use this code for Natrecor.
CMS: 100-03,200.1

**J2353**  Injection, octreotide, depot form for intramuscular injection, 1 mg  K K2 ☑
Use this code for Sandostatin LAR.

**J2354**  Injection, octreotide, nondepot form for subcutaneous or intravenous injection, 25 mcg  N N1 ☑
Use this code for Sandostatin.

**J2355**  Injection, oprelvekin, 5 mg  K K2 ☑
Use this code for Neumega.
AHA: 2Q, '05, 11

**J2357**  Injection, omalizumab, 5 mg  K K2 ☑
Use this code for Xolair.
AHA: 2Q, '05, 11

**J2358**  Injection, olanzapine, long-acting, 1 mg  K K2 ☑
Use this code for ZYPREXA RELPREVV.

**J2360**  Injection, orphenadrine citrate, up to 60 mg  N N1 ☑
Use this code for Norflex.

**J2370**  Injection, phenylephrine HCl, up to 1 ml  N N1 ☑

**J2400**  Injection, chloroprocaine HCl, per 30 ml  N N1 ☑
Use this code for Nesacaine, Nesacaine-MPF.

**J2405**  Injection, ondansetron HCl, per 1 mg  N N1 ☑
Use this code for Zofran.

**J2407**  Injection, oritavancin, 10 mg  G K2
Use this code for Orbactiv.

**J2410**  Injection, oxymorphone HCl, up to 1 mg  N N1 ☑
Use this code for Numorphan, Oxymorphone HCl.

**J2425**  Injection, palifermin, 50 mcg  K K2 ☑
Use this code for Kepivance.

**J2426**  Injection, paliperidone palmitate extended release, 1 mg  K K2
Use this code for INVEGA SUSTENNA.

**J2430**  Injection, pamidronate disodium, per 30 mg  N N1 ☑
Use this code for Aredia.

**J2440**  Injection, papaverine HCl, up to 60 mg  N N1 ☑

**J2460**  Injection, oxytetracycline HCl, up to 50 mg  N ☑
Use this code for Terramycin IM.

**J2469**  Injection, palonosetron HCl, 25 mcg  K K2 ☑
Use this code for Aloxi.
AHA: 2Q, '05, 11; 1Q, '05, 7, 9-10

**J2501**  Injection, paricalcitol, 1 mcg  N N1 ☑
Use this code For Zemplar.

**J2502**  Injection, pasireotide long acting, 1 mg  G K2
Use this code for Signifor LAR.

**J2503**  Injection, pegaptanib sodium, 0.3 mg  K K2
Use this code for Macugen.

**J2504**  Injection, pegademase bovine, 25 IU  K K2 ☑
Use this code for Adagen.

**J2505**  Injection, pegfilgrastim, 6 mg  K K2 ☑
Use this code for Neulasta.

**J2507**  Injection, pegloticase, 1 mg  K K2 ☑
Use this code for KRYSTEXXA.

**J2510**  Injection, penicillin G procaine, aqueous, up to 600,000 units  K K2 ☑
Use this code for Wycillin, Duracillin A.S., Pfizerpen A.S., Crysticillin 300 A.S., Crysticillin 600 A.S.

**J2513**  Injection, pentastarch, 10% solution, 100 ml  E

**J2515**  Injection, pentobarbital sodium, per 50 mg  N N1 ☑
Use this code for Nembutal Sodium Solution.

**J2540**  Injection, penicillin G potassium, up to 600,000 units  N N1 ☑
Use this code for Pfizerpen.

---

^Jan  **January Update**

Special Coverage Instructions        Noncovered by Medicare        Carrier Discretion        ☑ Quantity Alert  ● New Code        ○ Recycled/Reinstated  ▲ Revised Code

© 2016 Optum360, LLC        A2-Z3 ASC Pmt        CMS: Pub 100        AHA: Coding Clinic        ♿ DMEPOS Paid        ⊘ SNF Excluded        J Codes — 85

**Drugs Administered Other Than Oral Method**

**J2543 — J2950**

**J2543** Injection, piperacillin sodium/tazobactam sodium, 1 g/0.125 g (1.125 g) N N1 ☑
Use this code for Zosyn.

**J2545** Pentamidine isethionate, inhalation solution, FDA-approved final product, noncompounded, administered through DME, unit dose form, per 300 mg B ☑
Use this code for Nebupent, Pentam 300.

**J2547** Injection, peramivir, 1 mg G K2
Use this code for Rapivab.

**J2550** Injection, promethazine HCl, up to 50 mg N N1 ☑
Use this code for Phenergan.

**J2560** Injection, phenobarbital sodium, up to 120 mg N N1 ☑

**J2562** Injection, plerixafor, 1 mg K K2 ☑
Use this code for Mozobil.

**J2590** Injection, oxytocin, up to 10 units N N1 ☑
Use this code for Pitocin, Syntocinon.

**J2597** Injection, desmopressin acetate, per 1 mcg K K2 ☑
Use this code for DDAVP.

**J2650** Injection, prednisolone acetate, up to 1 ml N N1 ☑

**J2670** Injection, tolazoline HCl, up to 25 mg K K2 ☑

**J2675** Injection, progesterone, per 50 mg N N1
Use this code for Gesterone, Gestrin.

**J2680** Injection, fluphenazine decanoate, up to 25 mg N N1 ☑

**J2690** Injection, procainamide HCl, up to 1 g N N1 ☑
Use this code for Pronestyl.

**J2700** Injection, oxacillin sodium, up to 250 mg N N1 ☑
Use this code for Bactocill

**J2704** Injection, propofol, 10 mg N N1
Use this code for Diprivan.
**AHA:** 1Q, '15, 6

**J2710** Injection, neostigmine methylsulfate, up to 0.5 mg N N1 ☑
Use this code for Prostigmin.

**J2720** Injection, protamine sulfate, per 10 mg N N1 ☑

**J2724** Injection, protein C concentrate, intravenous, human, 10 IU K K2

**J2725** Injection, protirelin, per 250 mcg E ☑
Use this code for Thyrel TRH.

**J2730** Injection, pralidoxime chloride, up to 1 g N N1 ☑
Use this code for Protopam Chloride.

**J2760** Injection, phentolamine mesylate, up to 5 mg K K2 ☑
Use this code for Regitine.

**J2765** Injection, metoclopramide HCl, up to 10 mg N N1 ☑
Use this code for Reglan.

**J2770** Injection, quinupristin/dalfopristin, 500 mg (150/350) K K2 ☑
Use this code for Synercid.

**J2778** Injection, ranibizumab, 0.1 mg K K2 ☑
Use this code for Lucentis.
**AHA:** 1Q, '08, 6

**J2780** Injection, ranitidine HCl, 25 mg N N1 ☑
Use this code for Zantac.

**J2783** Injection, rasburicase, 0.5 mg K K2 ☑
Use this code for Elitek.
**AHA:** 2Q, '05, 11; 2Q, '04, 8

**J2785** Injection, regadenoson, 0.1 mg N N1 ☑
Use this code for Lexiscan.

● **J2786**^Jan Injection, reslizumab, 1 mg
Use this code for Cinqair.

**J2788** Injection, Rho D immune globulin, human, minidose, 50 mcg (250 i.u.) N N1 ☑
Use this code for RhoGam, MiCRhoGAM.

**J2790** Injection, Rho D immune globulin, human, full dose, 300 mcg (1500 i.u.) N N1 ☑
Use this code for RhoGam, HypRho SD.

**J2791** Injection, Rho(D) immune globulin (human), (Rhophylac), intramuscular or intravenous, 100 IU N N1
Use this for Rhophylac.
**AHA:** 1Q, '08, 6

**J2792** Injection, Rho D immune globulin, intravenous, human, solvent detergent, 100 IU K K2 ☑
Use this code for WINRho SDF.

**J2793** Injection, rilonacept, 1 mg K K2 ☑
Use this code for Arcalyst.

**J2794** Injection, risperidone, long acting, 0.5 mg K K2 ☑
Use this code for Risperdal Consta Long Acting.
**AHA:** 2Q, '05, 11; 1Q, '05, 7, 9-10

**J2795** Injection, ropivacaine HCl, 1 mg N N1 ☑
Use this code for Naropin.

**J2796** Injection, romiplostim, 10 mcg K K2 ☑
Use this code for Nplate.

**J2800** Injection, methocarbamol, up to 10 ml K K2 ☑
Use this code for Robaxin.

**J2805** Injection, sincalide, 5 mcg N N1
Use this code for Kinevac.
**AHA:** 4Q, '05, 1-6

**J2810** Injection, theophylline, per 40 mg N N1 ☑

**J2820** Injection, sargramostim (GM-CSF), 50 mcg K K2 ☑
Use this code for Leukine.

○ **J2840**^Jan Injection, sebelipase alfa, 1 mg
Use this code for Kanuma.

**J2850** Injection, secretin, synthetic, human, 1 mcg K K2 ☑

**J2860** Injection, siltuximab, 10 mg G K2
Use this code for Sylvant.

**J2910** Injection, aurothioglucose, up to 50 mg N N1 ☑
Use this code for Solganal.

**J2916** Injection, sodium ferric gluconate complex in sucrose injection, 12.5 mg N N1 ☑
**CMS:** 100-03,110.10

**J2920** Injection, methylprednisolone sodium succinate, up to 40 mg N N1 ☑
Use this code for Solu-Medrol, A-methaPred.

**J2930** Injection, methylprednisolone sodium succinate, up to 125 mg N N1 ☑
Use this code for Solu-Medrol, A-methaPred.

**J2940** Injection, somatrem, 1 mg E ☑
Use this code for Protropin.
**AHA:** 2Q, '02, 8-9; 1Q, '02, 5

**J2941** Injection, somatropin, 1 mg K K2 ☑
Use this code for Humatrope, Genotropin Nutropin, Biotropin, Genotropin, Genotropin Miniquick, Norditropin, Nutropin, Nutropin AQ, Saizen, Saizen Somatropin RDNA Origin, Serostim, Serostim RDNA Origin, Zorbtive.
**AHA:** 2Q, '02, 8-9; 1Q, '02, 5

**J2950** Injection, promazine HCl, up to 25 mg N N1 ☑
Use this code for Sparine, Prozine-50.

---

^Jan **January Update**

Special Coverage Instructions    Noncovered by Medicare    Carrier Discretion    ☑ Quantity Alert  ● New Code    ○ Recycled/Reinstated    ▲ Revised Code

86 — J Codes    A Age Edit    M Maternity Edit    ♀ Female Only    ♂ Male Only    A-Y OPPS Status Indicators    © 2016 Optum360, LLC

| Code | Description | Indicators |
|---|---|---|
| **J2993** | **Injection, reteplase, 18.1 mg** <br> Use this code for Retavase. | K K2 ☑ |
| **J2995** | **Injection, streptokinase, per 250,000 IU** <br> Use this code for Streptase. | N N1 ☑ |
| **J2997** | **Injection, alteplase recombinant, 1 mg** <br> Use this code for Activase, Cathflo. <br> AHA: 1Q, '14 | K K2 ☑ |
| **J3000** | **Injection, streptomycin, up to 1 g** <br> Use this code for Streptomycin Sulfate. | N N1 ☑ |
| **J3010** | **Injection, fentanyl citrate, 0.1 mg** <br> Use this code for Sublimaze. | N N1 ☑ |
| **J3030** | **Injection, sumatriptan succinate, 6 mg (code may be used for Medicare when drug administered under the direct supervision of a physician, not for use when drug is self-administered)** <br> Use this code for Imitrex. | N N1 ☑ |
| **J3060** | **Injection, taliglucerace alfa, 10 units** <br> Use this code for Elelyso. | K K2 ☑ |
| **J3070** | **Injection, pentazocine, 30 mg** <br> Use this code for Talwin. | K K2 ☑ |
| **J3090** | **Injection, tedizolid phosphate, 1 mg** <br> Use this code for Sivextro. | G K2 |
| **J3095** | **Injection, telavancin, 10 mg** <br> Use this code for VIBATIV. | K K2 ☑ |
| **J3101** | **Injection, tenecteplase, 1 mg** <br> Use this code for TNKase. | K K2 ☑ |
| **J3105** | **Injection, terbutaline sulfate, up to 1 mg** <br> For terbutaline in inhalation solution, see K0525 and K0526. | N N1 ☑ |
| **J3110** | **Injection, teriparatide, 10 mcg** <br> Use this code for Forteo. <br> CMS: 100-04,10,90.1 | B ☑ |
| **J3121** | **Injection, testosterone enanthate, 1 mg** <br> Use this code for Delatstryl. <br> AHA: 1Q, '15, 6 | N N1 |
| **J3145** | **Injection, testosterone undecanoate, 1 mg** <br> Use this code for Aveed. <br> AHA: 1Q, '15, 6 | G K2 |
| **J3230** | **Injection, chlorpromazine HCl, up to 50 mg** <br> Use this code for Thorazine. | N N1 ☑ |
| **J3240** | **Injection, thyrotropin alpha, 0.9 mg, provided in 1.1 mg vial** <br> Use this code for Thyrogen. <br> AHA: 4Q, '05, 1-6; 2Q, '05, 11; 3Q, '04, 1-10 | K K2 ☑ |
| **J3243** | **Injection, tigecycline, 1 mg** <br> Use this code for Tygacil. | K K2 ☑ |
| **J3246** | **Injection, tirofiban HCl, 0.25 mg** <br> Use this code for Aggrastat. <br> AHA: 1Q, '05, 7, 9-10 | K K2 ☑ |
| **J3250** | **Injection, trimethobenzamide HCl, up to 200 mg** <br> Use this code for Tigan, Tiject-20, Arrestin. | N N1 ☑ |
| **J3260** | **Injection, tobramycin sulfate, up to 80 mg** <br> Use this code for Nebcin. | N N1 ☑ |
| **J3262** | **Injection, tocilizumab, 1 mg** <br> Use this code for ACTEMRA. | K K2 ☑ |
| **J3265** | **Injection, torsemide, 10 mg/ml** <br> Use this code for Demadex, Torsemide. | N N1 ☑ |
| **J3280** | **Injection, thiethylperazine maleate, up to 10 mg** | N N1 ☑ |
| **J3285** | **Injection, treprostinil, 1 mg** <br> Use this code for Remodulin. | K K2 ☑ |
| **J3300** | **Injection, triamcinolone acetonide, preservative free, 1 mg** <br> Use this code for TRIVARIS, TRIESENCE. | K K2 |
| **J3301** | **Injection, triamcinolone acetonide, not otherwise specified, 10 mg** <br> Use this code for Kenalog-10, Kenalog-40, Tri-Kort, Kenaject-40, Cenacort A-40, Triam-A, Trilog. <br> AHA: 2Q, '13 | N N1 ☑ |
| **J3302** | **Injection, triamcinolone diacetate, per 5 mg** <br> Use this code for Aristocort, Aristocort Intralesional, Aristocort Forte, Amcort, Trilone, Cenacort Forte. | N N1 ☑ |
| **J3303** | **Injection, triamcinolone hexacetonide, per 5 mg** <br> Use this code for Aristospan Intralesional, Aristospan Intra-articular. | N N1 ☑ |
| **J3305** | **Injection, trimetrexate glucuronate, per 25 mg** <br> Use this code for Neutrexin. | N ☑ |
| **J3310** | **Injection, perphenazine, up to 5 mg** <br> Use this code for Trilafon. | N N1 ☑ |
| **J3315** | **Injection, triptorelin pamoate, 3.75 mg** <br> Use this code for Trelstar Depot, Trelstar Depot Plus Debioclip Kit, Trelstar LA. | ♂ K K2 ☑ |
| **J3320** | **Injection, spectinomycin dihydrochloride, up to 2 g** <br> Use this code for Trobicin. | E ☑ |
| **J3350** | **Injection, urea, up to 40 g** | N N1 ☑ |
| **J3355** | **Injection, urofollitropin, 75 IU** <br> Use this code for Metrodin, Bravelle, Fertinex. | K K2 |
| ▲ **J3357**Jan | **Ustekinumab, for subcutaneous injection, 1 mg** <br> Use this code for STELARA. | K K2 ☑ |
| **J3360** | **Injection, diazepam, up to 5 mg** <br> Use this code for Diastat, Dizac, Valium. <br> AHA: 2Q, '07, 6 | N N1 ☑ |
| **J3364** | **Injection, urokinase, 5,000 IU vial** <br> Use this code for Kinlytic. | N N1 ☑ |
| **J3365** | **Injection, IV, urokinase, 250,000 IU vial** <br> Use this code for Kinlytic. | K ☑ |
| **J3370** | **Injection, vancomycin HCl, 500 mg** <br> Use this code for Vancocin. | N N1 ☑ |
| **J3380** | **Injection, vedolizumab, 1 mg** <br> Use this code for Entyvio. | G K2 |
| **J3385** | **Injection, velaglucerase alfa, 100 units** <br> Use this code for VPRIV. | K K2 ☑ |
| **J3396** | **Injection, verteporfin, 0.1 mg** <br> Use this code for Visudyne. <br> CMS: 100-03,80.2; 100-03,80.2.1; 100-03,80.3; 100-03,80.3.1; 100-04,32,300; 100-04,32,300.1; 100-04,32,300.2 <br> AHA: 1Q, '05, 7, 9-10 | K K2 ☑ |
| **J3400** | **Injection, triflupromazine HCl, up to 20 mg** | E ☑ |
| **J3410** | **Injection, hydroxyzine HCl, up to 25 mg** <br> Use this code for Vistaril, Vistaject-25, Hyzine, Hyzine-50. | N N1 ☑ |
| **J3411** | **Injection, thiamine HCl, 100 mg** <br> AHA: 2Q, '05, 11 | N N1 ☑ |
| **J3415** | **Injection, pyridoxine HCl, 100 mg** <br> AHA: 2Q, '05, 11 | N N1 ☑ |

**J3420** Injection, vitamin B-12 cyanocobalamin, up to 1,000 mcg  N  N1  ☑

Use this code for Sytobex, Redisol, Rubramin PC, Betalin 12, Berubigen, Cobex, Cobal, Crystal B12, Cyano, Cyanocobalamin, Hydroxocobalamin, Hydroxycobal, Nutri-Twelve.

**J3430** Injection, phytonadione (vitamin K), per 1 mg  N  N1  ☑

Use this code for AquaMephyton, Konakion, Menadione, Phytonadione.

**J3465** Injection, voriconazole, 10 mg  K  K2  ☑

AHA: 2Q, '05, 11

**J3470** Injection, hyaluronidase, up to 150 units  N  N1  ☑

**J3471** Injection, hyaluronidase, ovine, preservative free, per 1 USP unit (up to 999 USP units)  N  N1  ☑

**J3472** Injection, hyaluronidase, ovine, preservative free, per 1,000 USP units  N  N1  ☑

**J3473** Injection, hyaluronidase, recombinant, 1 USP unit  N  N1  ☑

**J3475** Injection, magnesium sulfate, per 500 mg  N  N1  ☑

Use this code for Mag Sul, Sulfa Mag.

**J3480** Injection, potassium chloride, per 2 mEq  N  N1  ☑

**J3485** Injection, zidovudine, 10 mg  N  N1  ☑

Use this code for Retrovir, Zidovudine.

**J3486** Injection, ziprasidone mesylate, 10 mg  N  N1  ☑

Use this code for Geodon.

AHA: 2Q, '05, 11

**J3489** Injection, zoledronic acid, 1 mg  K  K2  ☑

Use this code for Reclast and Zometa.

**J3490** Unclassified drugs  N  N1

CMS: 100-03,1,110.22; 100-03,110.22; 100-04,10,90.1; 100-04,32,280.1; 100-04,32,280.2; 100-04,8,60.2.1.1

AHA: 3Q, '15, 7; 4Q, '14, 5; 2Q, '14, 8; 2Q, '13; 1Q, '13; 4Q, '12, 9; 2Q, '09, 1; 1Q, '08, 6; 4Q, '05, 1-6; 3Q, '04, 1-10

**J3520** Edetate disodium, per 150 mg  E  ☑

Use this code for Endrate, Disotate, Meritate, Chealamide, E.D.T.A. This drug is used in chelation therapy, a treatment for atherosclerosis that is not covered by Medicare.

**J3530** Nasal vaccine inhalation  N  N1

**J3535** Drug administered through a metered dose inhaler  E

**J3570** Laetrile, amygdalin, vitamin B-17  E

The FDA has found Laetrile to have no safe or effective therapeutic purpose.

**J3590** Unclassified biologics  N  N1

CMS: 100-03,1,110.22; 100-03,110.22; 100-04,32,280.1; 100-04,32,280.2

AHA: 3Q, '15, 7; 4Q, '12, 9

**J7030** Infusion, normal saline solution, 1,000 cc  N  N1  ☑

**J7040** Infusion, normal saline solution, sterile (500 ml=1 unit)  N  N1  ☑

**J7042** 5% dextrose/normal saline (500 ml = 1 unit)  N  N1  ☑

**J7050** Infusion, normal saline solution, 250 cc  N  N1  ☑

**J7060** 5% dextrose/water (500 ml = 1 unit)  N  N1  ☑

**J7070** Infusion, D-5-W, 1,000 cc  N  N1  ☑

**J7100** Infusion, dextran 40, 500 ml  N  N1  ☑

Use this code for Gentran, 10% LMD, Rheomacrodex.

**J7110** Infusion, dextran 75, 500 ml  N  N1  ☑

Use this code for Gentran 75.

**J7120** Ringers lactate infusion, up to 1,000 cc  N  N1  ☑

**J7121** 5% dextrose in lactated ringers infusion, up to 1000 cc  N

AHA: 1Q, '16, 6-8

**J7131** Hypertonic saline solution, 1 ml  N  N1  ☑

● **J7175**Jan Injection, factor X, (human), 1 IU

Use this code for Coagadex.

**J7178** Injection, human fibrinogen concentrate, 1 mg  K  K2  ☑

Use this code for RiaSTAP.

● **J7179**Jan Injection, von Willebrand factor (recombinant), (Vonvendi), 1 IU VWF:RCo

**J7180** Injection, factor XIII (antihemophilic factor, human), 1 IU  K  K2  ☑

Use this code for Corifact.

**J7181** Injection, factor XIII A-subunit, (recombinant), per IU  G  K2

AHA: 1Q, '15, 6

**J7182** Injection, factor VIII, (antihemophilic factor, recombinant), (NovoEight), per IU  E

AHA: 1Q, '15, 6

**J7183** Injection, von Willebrand factor complex (human), Wilate, 1 IU vWF:RCo  K  K2  ☑

**J7185** Injection, factor VIII (antihemophilic factor, recombinant) (Xyntha), per IU  K  K2  ☑

**J7186** Injection, antihemophilic factor VIII/von Willebrand factor complex (human), per factor VIII i.u.  K  K2

Use this code for Alphanate.

CMS: 100-04,17,80.4.1

**J7187** Injection, von Willebrand factor complex (Humate-P), per IU VWF:RCO  K  K2

CMS: 100-04,17,80.4.1

**J7188** Injection, factor VIII (antihemophilic factor, recombinant), per IU  K  K2

Use this code for Obizur.

AHA: 1Q, '16, 6-8

**J7189** Factor VIIa (antihemophilic factor, recombinant), per 1 mcg  K  K2  ☑

CMS: 100-04,17,80.4.1

**J7190** Factor VIII (antihemophilic factor, human) per IU  K  K2  ☑

Use this code for Koate-DVI, Monarc-M, Monoclate-P.

CMS: 100-04,17,80.4; 100-04,17,80.4.1

**J7191** Factor VIII (antihemophilic factor (porcine)), per IU  K  K2  ☑

CMS: 100-04,17,80.4; 100-04,17,80.4.1

**J7192** Factor VIII (antihemophilic factor, recombinant) per IU, not otherwise specified  K  K2  ☑

Use this code for Recombinate, Kogenate FS, Helixate FX, Advate rAHF-PFM, Antihemophilic Factor Human Method M Monoclonal Purified, Refacto.

CMS: 100-04,17,80.4; 100-04,17,80.4.1

AHA: 2Q, '13

**J7193** Factor IX (antihemophilic factor, purified, nonrecombinant) per IU  K  K2  ☑

Use this code for AlphaNine SD, Mononine.

CMS: 100-04,17,80.4; 100-04,17,80.4.1

AHA: 2Q, '02, 8-9

**J7194** Factor IX complex, per IU  K  K2  ☑

Use this code for Konyne-80, Profilnine SD, Proplex T, Proplex T, Bebulin VH, factor IX+ complex, Profilnine SD.

CMS: 100-04,17,80.4; 100-04,17,80.4.1

**J7195** Injection, factor IX (antihemophilic factor, recombinant) per IU, not otherwise specified  K  K2  ☑

Use this code for Benefix.

CMS: 100-04,17,80.4; 100-04,17,80.4.1

AHA: 2Q, '02, 8-9; 1Q, '02, 5

---

Jan **January Update**

☑ Special Coverage Instructions    Noncovered by Medicare    Carrier Discretion    ☑ Quantity Alert    ● New Code    ○ Recycled/Reinstated    ▲ Revised Code

**J7196** Injection, antithrombin recombinant, 50 IU  K K2 ☑
Use this code for ATryn.

**J7197** Antithrombin III (human), per IU  K K2 ☑
Use this code for Thrombate III, ATnativ.
**CMS:** 100-04,17,80.4.1

**J7198** Antiinhibitor, per IU  K K2 ☑
Medicare jurisdiction: local contractor. Use this code for Autoplex T, Feiba VH AICC.
**CMS:** 100-03,110.3; 100-04,17,80.4; 100-04,17,80.4.1

**J7199** Hemophilia clotting factor, not otherwise classified  B
Medicare jurisdiction: local contractor.
**CMS:** 100-04,17,80.4; 100-04,17,80.4.1
**AHA:** 2Q, '13

**J7200** Injection, factor IX, (antihemophilic factor, recombinant), Rixubis, per IU  G K2
**AHA:** 1Q, '15, 6

▲ **J7201**Jan Injection, factor IX, Fc fusion protein, (recombinant), Alprolix, 1 IU  G K2
**AHA:** 1Q, '15, 6

● **J7202**Jan Injection, factor IX, albumin fusion protein, (recombinant), Idelvion, 1 IU

**J7205** Injection, factor VIII Fc fusion protein (recombinant), per IU  G K2
Use this code for Eloctate.

● **J7207**Jan Injection, factor VIII, (antihemophilic factor, recombinant), pegylated, 1 IU
Use this code for Adynovate.

● **J7209**Jan Injection, factor VIII, (antihemophilic factor, recombinant), (Nuwiq), 1 IU

▲ **J7297**Jan Levonorgestrel-releasing intrauterine contraceptive system (Liletta), 52 mg  M ♀ E
**AHA:** 1Q, '16, 6-8

▲ **J7298**Jan Levonorgestrel-releasing intrauterine contraceptive system (Mirena), 52 mg  M ♀ E
**AHA:** 1Q, '16, 6-8

**J7300** Intrauterine copper contraceptive  E
Use this code for Paragard T380A.

▲ **J7301**Jan Levonorgestrel-releasing intrauterine contraceptive system (Skyla), 13.5 mg  M ♀ E ☑
**AHA:** 4Q, '14, 6

**J7303** Contraceptive supply, hormone containing vaginal ring, each  ♀ E ☑
Use this code for Nuvaring Vaginal Ring.

**J7304** Contraceptive supply, hormone containing patch, each  E ☑

**J7306** Levonorgestrel (contraceptive) implant system, including implants and supplies  E

**J7307** Etonogestrel (contraceptive) implant system, including implant and supplies  E
Use this code for Implanon and Nexplanon.

**J7308** Aminolevulinic acid HCl for topical administration, 20%, single unit dosage form (354 mg)  K K2 ☑
**AHA:** 2Q, '05, 11; 1Q, '02, 5

**J7309** Methyl aminolevulinate (MAL) for topical administration, 16.8%, 1 g  K K2 ☑
Use this code for Metvixia.

**J7310** Ganciclovir, 4.5 mg, long-acting implant  K K2 ☑
Use this code for Vitrasert.

**J7311** Fluocinolone acetonide, intravitreal implant  K K2
Use this code for Retisert.

**J7312** Injection, dexamethasone, intravitreal implant, 0.1 mg  K K2 ☑
Use this code for OZURDEX.

**J7313** Injection, fluocinolone acetonide, intravitreal implant, 0.01 mg  G K2
Use this code for Iluvien.

**J7315** Mitomycin, opthalmic, 0.2 mg  N N1 ☑
Use this code for Mitosol.
**AHA:** 2Q, '14, 8; 2Q, '13

**J7316** Injection, ocriplasmin, 0.125 mg  K K2 ☑
Use this code for Jetrea.

○ **J7320**Jan Hyaluronan or derivative, GenVisc 850, for intra-articular injection, 1 mg

**J7321** Hyaluronan or derivative, Hyalgan or Supartz, for intra-articular injection, per dose  K K2 ☑
**AHA:** 4Q, '12, 9; 1Q, '08, 6

○ **J7322**Jan Hyaluronan or derivative, Hymovis, for intra-articular injection, 1 mg

**J7323** Hyaluronan or derivative, Euflexxa, for intra-articular injection, per dose  K K2 ☑
**AHA:** 4Q, '12, 9; 1Q, '08, 6

**J7324** Hyaluronan or derivative, Orthovisc, for intra-articular injection, per dose  K K2 ☑
**AHA:** 4Q, '12, 9; 1Q, '08, 6

**J7325** Hyaluronan or derivative, Synvisc or Synvisc-One, for intra-articular injection, 1 mg  K K2 ☑
**AHA:** 4Q, '12, 9

**J7326** Hyaluronan or derivative, Gel-One, for intra-articular injection, per dose  K K2
**AHA:** 4Q, '12, 9

**J7327** Hyaluronan or derivative, Monovisc, for intra-articular injection, per dose  K K2
**AHA:** 1Q, '15, 6

**J7328** Hyaluronan or derivative, Gel-Syn, for intra-articular injection, 0.1 mg  E
**AHA:** 1Q, '16, 6-8

**J7330** Autologous cultured chondrocytes, implant  B ☑
Medicare jurisdiction: local contractor. Use this code for Carticel.
**AHA:** 4Q, '10, 1

**J7336** Capsaicin 8% patch, per sq cm  K K2
Use this code for Qutenza.
**AHA:** 1Q, '15, 6

▲ **J7340**Jan Carbidopa 5 mg/levodopa 20 mg enteral suspension, 100 ml  K K2
Use this code for Duopa.
**AHA:** 1Q, '16, 6-8

○ **J7342**Jan Installation, ciprofloxacin otic suspension, 6 mg
Use this code for Otipro.

**J7500** Azathioprine, oral, 50 mg  N N1 ☑
Use this code for Azasan, Imuran.
**CMS:** 100-02,15,50.5; 100-04,17,80.3

**J7501** Azathioprine, parenteral, 100 mg  K K2 ☑
**CMS:** 100-04,17,80.3

**J7502** Cyclosporine, oral, 100 mg  N N1 ☑
Use this code for Neoral, Sandimmune, Gengraf, Sangcya.
**CMS:** 100-02,15,50.5; 100-04,17,80.3

**J7503** Tacrolimus, extended release, oral, 0.25 mg  G K2
Use this code for Envarsus XR.
**AHA:** 1Q, '16, 6-8

---

Jan **January Update**

Special Coverage Instructions     Noncovered by Medicare     Carrier Discretion     ☑ Quantity Alert     ● New Code     ○ Recycled/Reinstated     ▲ Revised Code

**J7504**  **Lymphocyte immune globulin, antithymocyte globulin, equine, parenteral, 250 mg** ☒ K2 ☑
Use this code for Atgam.
CMS: 100-03,260.7; 100-04,17,80.3

**J7505**  **Muromonab-CD3, parenteral, 5 mg** ☒ ☑
Use this code for Orthoclone OKT3.
CMS: 100-04,17,80.3

**J7507**  **Tacrolimus, immediate release, oral, 1 mg** ☒ N1 ☑
Use this code for Prograf.
CMS: 100-02,15,50.5; 100-04,17,80.3

**J7508**  **Tacrolimus, extended release, (Astagraf XL), oral, 0.1 mg** ☒ K2 ☑
AHA: 1Q, '16, 6-8; 1Q, '14

**J7509**  **Methylprednisolone, oral, per 4 mg** ☒ N1 ☑
Use this code for Medrol, Methylpred.
CMS: 100-02,15,50.5; 100-04,17,80.3

**J7510**  **Prednisolone, oral, per 5 mg** ☒ N1 ☑
Use this code for Delta-Cortef, Cotolone, Pediapred, Prednoral, Prelone.
CMS: 100-02,15,50.5; 100-04,17,80.3

**J7511**  **Lymphocyte immune globulin, antithymocyte globulin, rabbit, parenteral, 25 mg** ☒ K2 ☑
Use this code for Thymoglobulin.
CMS: 100-04,17,80.3
AHA: 2Q, '02, 8-9; 1Q, '02, 5

**J7512**  **Prednisone, immediate release or delayed release, oral, 1 mg** ☒
AHA: 1Q, '16, 6-8

**J7513**  **Daclizumab, parenteral, 25 mg** ☒ K2 ☑
Use this code for Zenapax.
CMS: 100-02,15,50.5; 100-04,17,80.3
AHA: 2Q, '05, 11

**J7515**  **Cyclosporine, oral, 25 mg** ☒ N1 ☑
Use this code for Neoral, Sandimmune, Gengraf, Sangcya.
CMS: 100-04,17,80.3

**J7516**  **Cyclosporine, parenteral, 250 mg** ☒ N1 ☑
Use this code for Neoral, Sandimmune, Gengraf, Sangcya.
CMS: 100-04,17,80.3

**J7517**  **Mycophenolate mofetil, oral, 250 mg** ☒ N1 ☑
Use this code for CellCept.
CMS: 100-04,17,80.3

**J7518**  **Mycophenolic acid, oral, 180 mg** ☒ N1 ☑
Use this code for Myfortic Delayed Release.
CMS: 100-04,17,80.3.1
AHA: 2Q, '05, 11

**J7520**  **Sirolimus, oral, 1 mg** ☒ N1 ☑
Use this code for Rapamune.
CMS: 100-02,15,50.5; 100-04,17,80.3

**J7525**  **Tacrolimus, parenteral, 5 mg** ☒ K2 ☑
Use this code for Prograf.
CMS: 100-02,15,50.5; 100-04,17,80.3

**J7527**  **Everolimus, oral, 0.25 mg** ☒ N1 ☑
Use this code for Zortress, Afinitor.

**J7599**  **Immunosuppressive drug, not otherwise classified** ☒ N1
Determine if an alternative HCPCS Level II or a CPT code better describes the service being reported. This code should be used only if a more specific code is unavailable.
CMS: 100-02,15,50.5; 100-04,17,80.3
AHA: 2Q, '13

## Inhalation Drugs

**J7604**  **Acetylcysteine, inhalation solution, compounded product, administered through DME, unit dose form, per g** ☒ ☑

**J7605**  **Arformoterol, inhalation solution, FDA approved final product, noncompounded, administered through DME, unit dose form, 15 mcg** ☒ ☑

**J7606**  **Formoterol fumarate, inhalation solution, FDA approved final product, noncompounded, administered through DME, unit dose form, 20 mcg** ☒
Use this code for PERFOROMIST.

**J7607**  **Levalbuterol, inhalation solution, compounded product, administered through DME, concentrated form, 0.5 mg** ☒ ☑
CMS: 100-03,200.2

**J7608**  **Acetylcysteine, inhalation solution, FDA-approved final product, noncompounded, administered through DME, unit dose form, per g** ☒ ☑
Use this code for Acetadote, Mucomyst, Mucosil.

**J7609**  **Albuterol, inhalation solution, compounded product, administered through DME, unit dose, 1 mg** ☒ ☑

**J7610**  **Albuterol, inhalation solution, compounded product, administered through DME, concentrated form, 1 mg** ☒ ☑

**J7611**  **Albuterol, inhalation solution, FDA-approved final product, noncompounded, administered through DME, concentrated form, 1 mg** ☒ ☑
Use this code for Accuneb, Proventil, Respirol, Ventolin.
AHA: 2Q, '08, 10; 2Q, '07, 10

**J7612**  **Levalbuterol, inhalation solution, FDA-approved final product, noncompounded, administered through DME, concentrated form, 0.5 mg** ☒ ☑
Use this code for Xopenex HFA.
CMS: 100-03,200.2
AHA: 2Q, '08, 10; 2Q, '07, 10

**J7613**  **Albuterol, inhalation solution, FDA-approved final product, noncompounded, administered through DME, unit dose, 1 mg** ☒ ☑
Use this code for Accuneb, Proventil, Respirol, Ventolin.
AHA: 2Q, '08, 10; 2Q, '07, 10

**J7614**  **Levalbuterol, inhalation solution, FDA-approved final product, noncompounded, administered through DME, unit dose, 0.5 mg** ☒ ☑
Use this code for Xopenex.
CMS: 100-03,200.2
AHA: 2Q, '08, 10; 2Q, '07, 10

**J7615**  **Levalbuterol, inhalation solution, compounded product, administered through DME, unit dose, 0.5 mg** ☒ ☑
CMS: 100-03,200.2

**J7620**  **Albuterol, up to 2.5 mg and ipratropium bromide, up to 0.5 mg, FDA-approved final product, noncompounded, administered through DME** ☒ ☑

**J7622**  **Beclomethasone, inhalation solution, compounded product, administered through DME, unit dose form, per mg** ☒ ☑
Use this code for Beclovent, Beconase.
AHA: 1Q, '02, 5

**J7624**  **Betamethasone, inhalation solution, compounded product, administered through DME, unit dose form, per mg** ☒ ☑
AHA: 1Q, '02, 5

---

☑ Special Coverage Instructions    Noncovered by Medicare    Carrier Discretion    ☑ Quantity Alert  ● New Code    ○ Recycled/Reinstated    ▲ Revised Code

90 — J Codes              Ⓐ Age Edit    Ⓜ Maternity Edit    ♀ Female Only    ♂ Male Only    Ⓐ-Ⓨ OPPS Status Indicators              © 2016 Optum360, LLC

**J7626** Budesonide, inhalation solution, FDA-approved final product, noncompounded, administered through DME, unit dose form, up to 0.5 mg  M ☑
Use this code for Pulmicort, Pulmicort Flexhaler, Pulmicort Respules, Vanceril.
AHA: 1Q, '02, 5

**J7627** Budesonide, inhalation solution, compounded product, administered through DME, unit dose form, up to 0.5 mg  M ☑

**J7628** Bitolterol mesylate, inhalation solution, compounded product, administered through DME, concentrated form, per mg  M ☑

**J7629** Bitolterol mesylate, inhalation solution, compounded product, administered through DME, unit dose form, per mg  M ☑

**J7631** Cromolyn sodium, inhalation solution, FDA-approved final product, noncompounded, administered through DME, unit dose form, per 10 mg  M ☑
Use this code for Intal, Nasalcrom.

**J7632** Cromolyn sodium, inhalation solution, compounded product, administered through DME, unit dose form, per 10 mg  M ☑

**J7633** Budesonide, inhalation solution, FDA-approved final product, noncompounded, administered through DME, concentrated form, per 0.25 mg  M ☑
Use this code for Pulmicort, Pulmicort Flexhaler, Pulmicort Respules, Vanceril.

**J7634** Budesonide, inhalation solution, compounded product, administered through DME, concentrated form, per 0.25 mg  M ☑

**J7635** Atropine, inhalation solution, compounded product, administered through DME, concentrated form, per mg  M ☑

**J7636** Atropine, inhalation solution, compounded product, administered through DME, unit dose form, per mg  M ☑

**J7637** Dexamethasone, inhalation solution, compounded product, administered through DME, concentrated form, per mg  M ☑

**J7638** Dexamethasone, inhalation solution, compounded product, administered through DME, unit dose form, per mg  M ☑

**J7639** Dornase alfa, inhalation solution, FDA-approved final product, noncompounded, administered through DME, unit dose form, per mg  M ☑
Use this code for Pulmozyme.

**J7640** Formoterol, inhalation solution, compounded product, administered through DME, unit dose form, 12 mcg  E ☑

**J7641** Flunisolide, inhalation solution, compounded product, administered through DME, unit dose, per mg  M ☑
Use this code for Aerobid, Flunisolide.
AHA: 1Q, '02, 5

**J7642** Glycopyrrolate, inhalation solution, compounded product, administered through DME, concentrated form, per mg  M ☑

**J7643** Glycopyrrolate, inhalation solution, compounded product, administered through DME, unit dose form, per mg  M ☑

**J7644** Ipratropium bromide, inhalation solution, FDA-approved final product, noncompounded, administered through DME, unit dose form, per mg  M ☑
Use this code for Atrovent.

**J7645** Ipratropium bromide, inhalation solution, compounded product, administered through DME, unit dose form, per mg  M ☑

**J7647** Isoetharine HCl, inhalation solution, compounded product, administered through DME, concentrated form, per mg  M ☑

**J7648** Isoetharine HCl, inhalation solution, FDA-approved final product, noncompounded, administered through DME, concentrated form, per mg  M ☑
Use this code for Beta-2.

**J7649** Isoetharine HCl, inhalation solution, FDA-approved final product, noncompounded, administered through DME, unit dose form, per mg  M ☑

**J7650** Isoetharine HCl, inhalation solution, compounded product, administered through DME, unit dose form, per mg  M ☑

**J7657** Isoproterenol HCl, inhalation solution, compounded product, administered through DME, concentrated form, per mg  M ☑

**J7658** Isoproterenol HCl, inhalation solution, FDA-approved final product, noncompounded, administered through DME, concentrated form, per mg  M ☑
Use this code for Isuprel HCl.

**J7659** Isoproterenol HCl, inhalation solution, FDA-approved final product, noncompounded, administered through DME, unit dose form, per mg  M ☑
Use this code for Isuprel HCl.

**J7660** Isoproterenol HCl, inhalation solution, compounded product, administered through DME, unit dose form, per mg  M ☑

**J7665** Mannitol, administered through an inhaler, 5 mg  N M ☑
Use this code for ARIDOL.

**J7667** Metaproterenol sulfate, inhalation solution, compounded product, concentrated form, per 10 mg  M ☑

**J7668** Metaproterenol sulfate, inhalation solution, FDA-approved final product, noncompounded, administered through DME, concentrated form, per 10 mg  M ☑
Use this code for Alupent.

**J7669** Metaproterenol sulfate, inhalation solution, FDA-approved final product, noncompounded, administered through DME, unit dose form, per 10 mg  M ☑
Use this code for Alupent.

**J7670** Metaproterenol sulfate, inhalation solution, compounded product, administered through DME, unit dose form, per 10 mg  M ☑

**J7674** Methacholine chloride administered as inhalation solution through a nebulizer, per 1 mg  N M ☑
AHA: 2Q, '05, 11

**J7676** Pentamidine isethionate, inhalation solution, compounded product, administered through DME, unit dose form, per 300 mg  M ☑

**J7680** Terbutaline sulfate, inhalation solution, compounded product, administered through DME, concentrated form, per mg  M ☑
Use this code for Brethine.

**J7681** Terbutaline sulfate, inhalation solution, compounded product, administered through DME, unit dose form, per mg  M ☑
Use this code for Brethine.

**J7682** Tobramycin, inhalation solution, FDA-approved final product, noncompounded, unit dose form, administered through DME, per 300 mg  M ☑
Use this code for Tobi.

**J7683** Triamcinolone, inhalation solution, compounded product, administered through DME, concentrated form, per mg  M ☑
Use this code for Azmacort.

**J7684** Triamcinolone, inhalation solution, compounded product, administered through DME, unit dose form, per mg  M ☑
Use this code for Azmacort.

**J7685** Tobramycin, inhalation solution, compounded product, administered through DME, unit dose form, per 300 mg  M ☑

Special Coverage Instructions    Noncovered by Medicare    Carrier Discretion    ☑ Quantity Alert  ● New Code    ○ Recycled/Reinstated    ▲ Revised Code

© 2016 Optum360, LLC    A2-Z3 ASC Pmt    CMS: Pub 100    AHA: Coding Clinic    ♿ DMEPOS Paid    ⊘ SNF Excluded    J Codes — 91

**Chemotherapy Drugs**

**J7686 — J9043**

**J7686** Treprostinil, inhalation solution, FDA-approved final product, noncompounded, administered through DME, unit dose form, 1.74 mg ☒☑
Use this code for Tyvaso.

**J7699** NOC drugs, inhalation solution administered through DME ☒

**J7799** NOC drugs, other than inhalation drugs, administered through DME ☒ ☒
AHA: 3Q, '15, 7

**J7999** Compounded drug, not otherwise classified ☒
AHA: 1Q, '16, 6-8

**J8498** Antiemetic drug, rectal/suppository, not otherwise specified ☒
AHA: 2Q, '13

**J8499** Prescription drug, oral, nonchemotherapeutic, NOS ☒
AHA: 2Q, '13

## J Codes Chemotherapy Drugs J8501-J9999

### Oral Chemotherapy Drugs

**J8501** Aprepitant, oral, 5 mg ☒ ☒ ☑
Use this code for Emend.
CMS: 100-02,15,50.5.4; 100-03,110.18; 100-04,17,80.2.1; 100-04,17,80.2.4
AHA: 3Q, '05, 7, 9

**J8510** Busulfan, oral, 2 mg ☒ ☒ ☑
Use this code for Busulfex, Myleran.
CMS: 100-02,15,50.5; 100-04,17,80.1.1

**J8515** Cabergoline, oral, 0.25 mg ☒ ☑
Use this code for Dostinex.
CMS: 100-02,15,50.5

**J8520** Capecitabine, oral, 150 mg ☒ ☒ ☑
Use this code for Xeloda.
CMS: 100-02,15,50.5; 100-04,17,80.1.1

**J8521** Capecitabine, oral, 500 mg ☒ ☒ ☑
Use this code for Xeloda.
CMS: 100-02,15,50.5; 100-04,17,80.1.1

**J8530** Cyclophosphamide, oral, 25 mg ☒ ☒ ☑
Use this code for Cytoxan.
CMS: 100-02,15,50.5; 100-04,17,80.1.1
AHA: 1Q, '02, 1-2

**J8540** Dexamethasone, oral, 0.25 mg ☒ ☒ ☑
Use this code for Decadron.

**J8560** Etoposide, oral, 50 mg ☒ ☒ ☑
Use this code for VePesid.
CMS: 100-02,15,50.5; 100-04,17,80.1.1

**J8562** Fludarabine phosphate, oral, 10 mg ☒ ☑
Use this code for Oforta.

**J8565** Gefitinib, oral, 250 mg ☒ ☑
Use this code for Iressa.
CMS: 100-04,17,80.1.1
AHA: 4Q, '14, 6

**J8597** Antiemetic drug, oral, not otherwise specified ☒ ☒
AHA: 2Q, '13

**J8600** Melphalan, oral, 2 mg ☒ ☒ ☑
Use this code for Alkeran.
CMS: 100-02,15,50.5; 100-04,17,80.1.1

**J8610** Methotrexate, oral, 2.5 mg ☒ ☒ ☑
Use this code for Trexall, RHEUMATREX.
CMS: 100-02,15,50.5; 100-04,17,80.1.1

**J8650** Nabilone, oral, 1 mg ☒ ☒ ☑
Use this code for Cesamet.

**J8655** Netupitant 300 mg and palonosetron 0.5 mg ☒ ☒
Use this code for Akynzeo.

● **J8670**Jan Rolapitant, oral, 1 mg
Use this code for Varubi.

**J8700** Temozolomide, oral, 5 mg ☒ ☒ ☑
Use this code for Temodar.
CMS: 100-02,15,50.5

**J8705** Topotecan, oral, 0.25 mg ☒ ☒ ☑
Use this code for Hycamtin.

**J8999** Prescription drug, oral, chemotherapeutic, NOS ☒
Determine if an alternative HCPCS Level II or a CPT code better describes the service being reported. This code should be used only if a more specific code is unavailable.
CMS: 100-02,15,50.5; 100-04,17,80.1.1; 100-04,17,80.1.2
AHA: 2Q, '13

### Injectable Chemotherapy Drugs

These codes cover the cost of the chemotherapy drug only, not the administration.

**J9000** Injection, doxorubicin HCl, 10 mg ☒ ☒ ☑ ⊘
Use this code for Adriamycin PFS, Adriamycin RDF, Rubex.
AHA: 4Q, '07, 5

**J9015** Injection, aldesleukin, per single use vial ☒ ☒ ☑ ⊘
Use this code for Proleukin, IL-2, Interleukin.
AHA: 2Q, '05, 11

**J9017** Injection, arsenic trioxide, 1 mg ☒ ☒ ☑ ⊘
Use this code for Trisenox.
AHA: 2Q, '05, 11; 2Q, '02, 8-9; 1Q, '02, 5

**J9019** Injection, asparaginase (Erwinaze), 1,000 IU ☒ ☒

**J9020** Injection, asparaginase, not otherwise specified, 10,000 units ☒ ☒ ☑ ⊘
Use this code for Elspar.
AHA: 2Q, '13

**J9025** Injection, azacitidine, 1 mg ☒ ☒ ☑ ⊘
Use this code for Vidaza.

**J9027** Injection, clofarabine, 1 mg ☒ ☒ ☑ ⊘
Use this code for Clolar.

**J9031** BCG (intravesical) per instillation ☒ ☒ ☑
Use this code for Tice BCG, PACIS BCG, TheraCys.

**J9032** Injection, belinostat, 10 mg ☒ ☒
Use this code for Beleodaq.

▲ **J9033**Jan Injection, bendamustine HCl (Treanda), 1 mg ☒ ☒ ☑ ⊘

● **J9034**Jan Injection, bendamustine HCl (Bendeka), 1 mg

**J9035** Injection, bevacizumab, 10 mg ☒ ☒ ☑ ⊘
Use this code for Avastin.
CMS: 100-03,110.17
AHA: 3Q, '13; 2Q, '13; 2Q, '05, 11

**J9039** Injection, blinatumomab, 1 microgram ☒ ☒
Use this code for Blincyto.

**J9040** Injection, bleomycin sulfate, 15 units ☒ ☒ ☑ ⊘
Use this code for Blenoxane.

**J9041** Injection, bortezomib, 0.1 mg ☒ ☒ ☑ ⊘
Use this code for Velcade.
AHA: 2Q, '05, 11; 1Q, '05, 7, 9-10

**J9042** Injection, brentuximab vedotin, 1 mg ☒ ☒
Use this code for Adcentris.

**J9043** Injection, cabazitaxel, 1 mg ☒ ☒ ☑
Use this code for Jevtana.

Jan  January Update

Special Coverage Instructions    Noncovered by Medicare    Carrier Discretion    ☑ Quantity Alert  ● New Code  ○ Recycled/Reinstated  ▲ Revised Code

92 — J Codes        Ⓐ Age Edit   Ⓜ Maternity Edit   ♀ Female Only   ♂ Male Only   Ⓐ-Ⓨ OPPS Status Indicators        © 2016 Optum360, LLC

| Code | Description | Indicators |
|------|-------------|------------|
| **J9045** | **Injection, carboplatin, 50 mg** <br> Use this code for Paraplatin. | N M1 ☑ ⊘ |
| **J9047** | **Injection, carfilzomib, 1 mg** <br> Use this code for Kyprolis. | K K2 ☑ |
| **J9050** | **Injection, carmustine, 100 mg** <br> Use this code for BiCNU. | K K2 ☑ ⊘ |
| **J9055** | **Injection, cetuximab, 10 mg** <br> Use this code for Erbitux. <br> **CMS:** 100-03,110.17 <br> **AHA:** 2Q, '05, 11 | K K2 ☑ ⊘ |
| **J9060** | **Injection, cisplatin, powder or solution, 10 mg** <br> Use this code for Plantinol AQ. <br> **AHA:** 2Q, '13 | N M1 ☑ ⊘ |
| **J9065** | **Injection, cladribine, per 1 mg** <br> Use this code for Leustatin. | K K2 ☑ ⊘ |
| **J9070** | **Cyclophosphamide, 100 mg** <br> Use this code for Endoxan-Asta. | K K2 ☑ ⊘ |
| **J9098** | **Injection, cytarabine liposome, 10 mg** <br> Use this code for Depocyt. | K K2 ☑ ⊘ |
| **J9100** | **Injection, cytarabine, 100 mg** <br> Use this code for Cytosar-U, Ara-C, Tarabin CFS. | N M1 ☑ ⊘ |
| **J9120** | **Injection, dactinomycin, 0.5 mg** <br> Use this code for Cosmegen. | K K2 ☑ ⊘ |
| **J9130** | **Dacarbazine, 100 mg** <br> Use this code for DTIC-Dome. <br> **AHA:** 1Q, '08, 6 | N M1 ☑ ⊘ |
| ● **J9145**[Jan] | **Injection, daratumumab, 10 mg** <br> Use this code for Darzalex. | |
| **J9150** | **Injection, daunorubicin, 10 mg** <br> Use this code for Cerubidine. | K K2 ☑ ⊘ |
| **J9151** | **Injection, daunorubicin citrate, liposomal formulation, 10 mg** <br> Use this code for Daunoxome. | K K2 ☑ ⊘ |
| **J9155** | **Injection, degarelix, 1 mg** | K K2 ☑ |
| **J9160** | **Injection, denileukin diftitox, 300 mcg** <br> Use this code for Ontak. <br> **AHA:** 2Q, '05, 11 | E ☑ ⊘ |
| **J9165** | **Injection, diethylstilbestrol diphosphate, 250 mg** | N ☑ |
| **J9171** | **Injection, docetaxel, 1 mg** <br> Use this code for Taxotere. | K K2 ☑ ⊘ |
| **J9175** | **Injection, Elliotts' B solution, 1 ml** | N M1 ☑ |
| ● **J9176**[Jan] | **Injection, elotuzumab, 1 mg** <br> Use this code for Empliciti. | |
| **J9178** | **Injection, epirubicin HCl, 2 mg** <br> Use this code for Ellence. | N M1 ☑ ⊘ |
| **J9179** | **Injection, eribulin mesylate, 0.1 mg** <br> Use this code for Halaven. | K K2 ☑ |
| **J9181** | **Injection, etoposide, 10 mg** <br> Use this code for VePesid, Toposar. | N M1 ☑ ⊘ |
| **J9185** | **Injection, fludarabine phosphate, 50 mg** <br> Use this code for Fludara. | N M1 ☑ ⊘ |
| **J9190** | **Injection, fluorouracil, 500 mg** <br> Use this code for Adrucil. | N M1 ☑ |
| **J9200** | **Injection, floxuridine, 500 mg** <br> Use this code for FUDR. | K K2 ☑ ⊘ |
| **J9201** | **Injection, gemcitabine HCl, 200 mg** <br> Use this code for Gemzar. | N M1 ☑ ⊘ |
| **J9202** | **Goserelin acetate implant, per 3.6 mg** <br> Use this code for Zoladex. | K K2 ☑ |
| ● **J9205**[Jan] | **Injection, irinotecan liposome, 1 mg** <br> Use this code for Onivyde. | |
| **J9206** | **Injection, irinotecan, 20 mg** <br> Use this code for Camptosar. <br> **CMS:** 100-03,110.17 | N M1 ☑ ⊘ |
| **J9207** | **Injection, ixabepilone, 1 mg** <br> Use this code for IXEMPRA. | K K2 ☑ ⊘ |
| **J9208** | **Injection, ifosfamide, 1 g** <br> Use this code for IFEX, Mitoxana. | K K2 ☑ ⊘ |
| **J9209** | **Injection, mesna, 200 mg** <br> Use this code for Mesnex. | N M1 ☑ |
| **J9211** | **Injection, idarubicin HCl, 5 mg** <br> Use this code for Idamycin. | K K2 ☑ ⊘ |
| **J9212** | **Injection, interferon alfacon-1, recombinant, 1 mcg** <br> Use this code for Infergen. | N ☑ |
| **J9213** | **Injection, interferon, alfa-2a, recombinant, 3 million units** <br> Use this code for Roferon-A. | K K2 ☑ |
| **J9214** | **Injection, interferon, alfa-2b, recombinant, 1 million units** <br> Use this code for Intron A, Rebetron Kit. | K K2 ☑ |
| **J9215** | **Injection, interferon, alfa-N3, (human leukocyte derived), 250,000 IU** <br> Use this code for Alferon N. | E ☑ |
| **J9216** | **Injection, interferon, gamma 1-b, 3 million units** <br> Use this code for Actimmune. <br> **AHA:** 2Q, '05, 11 | K K2 ☑ |
| **J9217** | **Leuprolide acetate (for depot suspension), 7.5 mg** <br> Use this code for Lupron Depot, Eligard. <br> **AHA:** 3Q, '15, 3 | K K2 ☑ |
| **J9218** | **Leuprolide acetate, per 1 mg** <br> Use this code for Lupron. <br> **AHA:** 3Q, '15, 3 | N M1 ☑ |
| **J9219** | **Leuprolide acetate implant, 65 mg** <br> Use this code for Lupron Implant, Viadur. <br> **AHA:** 4Q, '01, 5 | K K2 ☑ |
| **J9225** | **Histrelin implant (Vantas), 50 mg** | K K2 ☑ ⊘ |
| **J9226** | **Histrelin implant (Supprelin LA), 50 mg** <br> **AHA:** 1Q, '08, 6 | K K2 ☑ |
| **J9228** | **Injection, ipilimumab, 1 mg** <br> Use this code for YERVOY. | K K2 ☑ |
| **J9230** | **Injection, mechlorethamine HCl, (nitrogen mustard), 10 mg** <br> Use this code for Mustargen. | K K2 ☑ ⊘ |
| **J9245** | **Injection, melphalan HCl, 50 mg** <br> Use this code for Alkeran, L-phenylalanine mustard. | K K2 ☑ ⊘ |
| **J9250** | **Methotrexate sodium, 5 mg** <br> Use this code for Folex, Folex PFS, Methotrexate LPF. | N M1 ☑ |
| **J9260** | **Methotrexate sodium, 50 mg** <br> Use this code for Folex, Folex PFS, Methotrexate LPF. | N M1 ☑ |
| **J9261** | **Injection, nelarabine, 50 mg** <br> Use this code for Arranon. | K K2 ☑ ⊘ |

[Jan] **January Update**

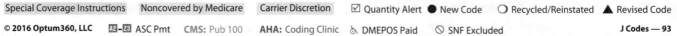

Special Coverage Instructions    Noncovered by Medicare    Carrier Discretion    ☑ Quantity Alert   ● New Code   ○ Recycled/Reinstated   ▲ Revised Code

© 2016 Optum360, LLC    A2-Z3 ASC Pmt    **CMS:** Pub 100    **AHA:** Coding Clinic    ☒ DMEPOS Paid    ⊘ SNF Excluded

**Chemotherapy Drugs**

**J9262 — J9999**

**J9262**    **Injection, omacetaxine mepesuccinate, 0.01 mg**   K K2 ☑
Use this code for Synribo.

**J9263**    **Injection, oxaliplatin, 0.5 mg**   K K2 ☑ ⊘
Use this code for Eloxatin.
**AHA:** 1Q, '09, 10

**J9264**    **Injection, paclitaxel protein-bound particles, 1 mg**   K K2 ☑ ⊘
Use this code for Abraxane.

**J9266**    **Injection, pegaspargase, per single dose vial**   K K2 ☑ ⊘
Use this code for Oncaspar.
**AHA:** 2Q, '02, 8-9

**J9267**    **Injection, paclitaxel, 1 mg**   N N1
Use this code for Taxol.
**AHA:** 1Q, '15, 6

**J9268**    **Injection, pentostatin, 10 mg**   K K2 ☑ ⊘
Use this code for Nipent.

**J9270**    **Injection, plicamycin, 2.5 mg**   N N1 ☑ ⊘
Use this code for Mithacin.

**J9271**    **Injection, pembrolizumab, 1 mg**   G K2
Use this code for Keytruda.

**J9280**    **Injection, mitomycin, 5 mg**   K K2 ☑ ⊘
Use this code for Mutamycin.
**AHA:** 2Q, '14, 8

**J9293**    **Injection, mitoxantrone HCl, per 5 mg**   K K2 ☑ ⊘
Use this code for Navantrone.

○ **J9295**^Jan    **Injection, necitumumab, 1 mg**
Use this code for Portrazza.

**J9299**    **Injection, nivolumab, 1 mg**   G K2
Use this code for Opdivo.

**J9300**    **Injection, gemtuzumab ozogamicin, 5 mg**   E ☑ ⊘
**AHA:** 2Q, '05, 11; 2Q, '02, 8-9; 1Q, '02, 5

**J9301**    **Injection, obinutuzumab, 10 mg**   G K2
Use this code for Gazyva.
**AHA:** 1Q, '15, 6

**J9302**    **Injection, ofatumumab, 10 mg**   K K2 ☑
Use this code for Arzerra.

**J9303**    **Injection, panitumumab, 10 mg**   K K2 ☑ ⊘
Use this code for Vectibix.
**AHA:** 1Q, '08, 6

**J9305**    **Injection, pemetrexed, 10 mg**   K K2 ☑ ⊘
Use this code for Alimta.
**AHA:** 2Q, '05, 11

**J9306**    **Injection, pertuzumab, 1 mg**   K K2 ☑
Use this code for Perjeta.

**J9307**    **Injection, pralatrexate, 1 mg**   K K2 ☑
Use this code for FOLOTYN.

**J9308**    **Injection, ramucirumab, 5 mg**   G K2
Use this code for Cyramza.

**J9310**    **Injection, rituximab, 100 mg**   K K2 ☑ ⊘
Use this code for RituXan.
**AHA:** 3Q, '13; 4Q, '05, 1-6; 3Q, '04, 1-10

**J9315**    **Injection, romidepsin, 1 mg**   K K2 ☑
Use this code for ISTODAX.

**J9320**    **Injection, streptozocin, 1 g**   K K2 ☑ ⊘
Use this code for Zanosar.

● **J9325**^Jan    **Injection, talimogene laherparepvec, per 1 million plaque forming units**
Use this code for Imlygic.

**J9328**    **Injection, temozolomide, 1 mg**   K K2 ☑ ⊘
Use this code for Temodar.

**J9330**    **Injection, temsirolimus, 1 mg**   K K2 ☑ ⊘
Use this code for TORISEL.

**J9340**    **Injection, thiotepa, 15 mg**   K K2 ☑ ⊘
Use this code for Thioplex.

**J9351**    **Injection, topotecan, 0.1 mg**   N N1 ☑
Use this code for Hycamtin.

● **J9352**^Jan    **Injection, trabectedin, 0.1 mg**
Use this code for Yondelis.

**J9354**    **Injection, ado-trastuzumab emtansine, 1 mg**   K K2 ☑
Use this code for Kadcyla.

**J9355**    **Injection, trastuzumab, 10 mg**   K K2 ☑ ⊘
Use this code for Herceptin.

**J9357**    **Injection, valrubicin, intravesical, 200 mg**   K K2 ☑ ⊘
Use this code for Valstar.

**J9360**    **Injection, vinblastine sulfate, 1 mg**   N N1 ☑ ⊘
Use this code for Velban.

**J9370**    **Vincristine sulfate, 1 mg**   N N1 ☑ ⊘
Use this code for Oncovin, Vincasar PFS.

**J9371**    **Injection, vincristine sulfate liposome, 1 mg**   G K2 ☑
Use this code for Marqibo kit.
**AHA:** 1Q, '14

**J9390**    **Injection, vinorelbine tartrate, 10 mg**   N N1 ☑ ⊘
Use this code for Navelbine.
**AHA:** 2Q, '05, 8

**J9395**    **Injection, fulvestrant, 25 mg**   K K2 ☑ ⊘
Use this code for Faslodex.

**J9400**    **Injection, ziv-aflibercept, 1 mg**   K K2 ☑
Use this code for Zaltrap.

**J9600**    **Injection, porfimer sodium, 75 mg**   K K2 ☑ ⊘
Use this code for Photofrin.

**J9999**    **Not otherwise classified, antineoplastic drugs**   N N1
Determine if an alternative HCPCS Level II or a CPT code better describes the service being reported. This code should be used only if a more specific code is unavailable.
**AHA:** 3Q, '15, 7; 2Q, '13; 1Q, '13; 4Q, '12, 9; 1Q, '08, 6; 1Q, '02, 1-2

---

^Jan **January Update**

Special Coverage Instructions    Noncovered by Medicare    Carrier Discretion    ☑ Quantity Alert   ● New Code   ○ Recycled/Reinstated   ▲ Revised Code

## Temporary Codes K0001-K0902

The K codes were established for use by the DME Medicare Administrative Contractors (DME MACs). The K codes are developed when the currently existing permanent national codes for supplies and certain product categories do not include the codes needed to implement a DME MAC medical review policy.

### Wheelchairs and Accessories

| K0001 | Standard wheelchair | Y & (RR) |
|---|---|---|
| K0002 | Standard hemi (low seat) wheelchair | Y & (RR) |
| K0003 | Lightweight wheelchair | Y & (RR) |
| K0004 | High strength, lightweight wheelchair | Y & (RR) |
| K0005 | Ultralightweight wheelchair | Y & (NU,RR,UE) |
| K0006 | Heavy-duty wheelchair | Y & (RR) |
| K0007 | Extra heavy-duty wheelchair | Y & (RR) |
| K0008 | Custom manual wheelchair/base | Y |
| K0009 | Other manual wheelchair/base | Y & (RR) |
| K0010 | Standard-weight frame motorized/power wheelchair | Y & (RR) |
| K0011 | Standard-weight frame motorized/power wheelchair with programmable control parameters for speed adjustment, tremor dampening, acceleration control and braking | Y & (RR) |
| K0012 | Lightweight portable motorized/power wheelchair | Y & (RR) |
| K0013 | Custom motorized/power wheelchair base | Y |
| K0014 | Other motorized/power wheelchair base | Y |
| K0015 | Detachable, nonadjustable height armrest, each | Y ☑ & (RR) |
| | CMS: 100-04,23,60.3 | |
| K0017 | Detachable, adjustable height armrest, base, replacement only, each | Y ☑ & (NU,RR,UE) |
| | CMS: 100-04,23,60.3 | |
| K0018 | Detachable, adjustable height armrest, upper portion, replacement only, each | Y ☑ & (NU,RR,UE) |
| | CMS: 100-04,23,60.3 | |
| ▲ K0019[Jan] | Arm pad, replacement only, each | Y ☑ & (NU,RR,UE) |
| | CMS: 100-04,23,60.3 | |
| K0020 | Fixed, adjustable height armrest, pair | Y ☑ & (NU,RR,UE) |
| | CMS: 100-04,23,60.3 | |
| ▲ K0037[Jan] | High mount flip-up footrest, replacement only, each | Y ☑ & (NU,RR,UE) |
| | CMS: 100-04,23,60.3 | |
| K0038 | Leg strap, each | Y ☑ & (NU,RR,UE) |
| | CMS: 100-04,23,60.3 | |
| K0039 | Leg strap, H style, each | Y ☑ & (NU,RR,UE) |
| | CMS: 100-04,23,60.3 | |
| K0040 | Adjustable angle footplate, each | Y ☑ & (NU,RR,UE) |
| | CMS: 100-04,23,60.3 | |
| K0041 | Large size footplate, each | Y ☑ & (NU,RR,UE) |
| | CMS: 100-04,23,60.3 | |
| ▲ K0042[Jan] | Standard size footplate, replacement only, each | Y ☑ & (NU,RR,UE) |
| | CMS: 100-04,23,60.3 | |
| ▲ K0043[Jan] | Footrest, lower extension tube, replacement only, each | Y ☑ & (NU,RR,UE) |
| | CMS: 100-04,23,60.3 | |
| ▲ K0044[Jan] | Footrest, upper hanger bracket, replacement only, each | Y ☑ & (NU,RR,UE) |
| | CMS: 100-04,23,60.3 | |

| ▲ K0045[Jan] | Footrest, complete assembly, replacement only, each | Y & (NU,RR,UE) |
|---|---|---|
| | CMS: 100-04,23,60.3 | |
| ▲ K0046[Jan] | Elevating legrest, lower extension tube, replacement only, each | Y ☑ & (NU,RR,UE) |
| | CMS: 100-04,23,60.3 | |
| ▲ K0047[Jan] | Elevating legrest, upper hanger bracket, replacement only, each | Y ☑ & (NU,RR,UE) |
| | CMS: 100-04,23,60.3 | |
| ▲ K0050[Jan] | Ratchet assembly, replacement only | Y & (NU,RR,UE) |
| | CMS: 100-04,23,60.3 | |
| ▲ K0051[Jan] | Cam release assembly, footrest or legrest, replacement only, each | Y ☑ & (NU,RR,UE) |
| | CMS: 100-04,23,60.3 | |
| ▲ K0052[Jan] | Swingaway, detachable footrests, replacement only, each | Y ☑ & (NU,RR,UE) |
| | CMS: 100-04,23,60.3 | |
| K0053 | Elevating footrests, articulating (telescoping), each | Y ☑ & (NU,RR,UE) |
| | CMS: 100-04,23,60.3 | |
| K0056 | Seat height less than 17 in or equal to or greater than 21 in for a high-strength, lightweight, or ultralightweight wheelchair | Y ☑ & (NU,RR,UE) |
| K0065 | Spoke protectors, each | Y ☑ & (NU,RR,UE) |
| ▲ K0069[Jan] | Rear wheel assembly, complete, with solid tire, spokes or molded, replacement only, each | Y ☑ & (NU,RR,UE) |
| ▲ K0070[Jan] | Rear wheel assembly, complete, with pneumatic tire, spokes or molded, replacement only, each | Y ☑ & (RR) |
| ▲ K0071[Jan] | Front caster assembly, complete, with pneumatic tire, replacement only, each | Y ☑ & (NU,RR,UE) |
| ▲ K0072[Jan] | Front caster assembly, complete, with semi-pneumatic tire, replacement only, each | Y ☑ & (NU,RR,UE) |
| K0073 | Caster pin lock, each | Y ☑ & (NU,RR,UE) |
| ▲ K0077[Jan] | Front caster assembly, complete, with solid tire, replacement only, each | Y ☑ & (NU,RR,UE) |
| ▲ K0098[Jan] | Drive belt for power wheelchair, replacement only | Y ☑ & (NU,RR,UE) |
| | CMS: 100-04,23,60.3 | |
| K0105 | IV hanger, each | Y ☑ & (NU,RR,UE) |
| K0108 | Wheelchair component or accessory, not otherwise specified | Y |
| K0195 | Elevating legrests, pair (for use with capped rental wheelchair base) | Y & (RR) |
| | CMS: 100-04,23,60.3 | |

### Equipment, Replacement, Repair, Rental

| K0455 | Infusion pump used for uninterrupted parenteral administration of medication, (e.g., epoprostenol or treprostinol) | Y & (RR) |
|---|---|---|
| K0462 | Temporary replacement for patient-owned equipment being repaired, any type | Y |
| | CMS: 100-04,20,40.1 | |
| ▲ K0552[Jan] | Supplies for external non-insulin drug infusion pump, syringe type cartridge, sterile, each | Y ☑ & |
| K0601 | Replacement battery for external infusion pump owned by patient, silver oxide, 1.5 volt, each | Y ☑ & (NU) |
| | AHA: 2Q, '03, 7 | |

---

Jan  January Update

Special Coverage Instructions    Noncovered by Medicare    Carrier Discretion    ☑ Quantity Alert    ● New Code    ○ Recycled/Reinstated    ▲ Revised Code

© 2016 Optum360, LLC    A2-Z3 ASC Pmt    CMS: Pub 100    AHA: Coding Clinic    & DMEPOS Paid    ⊘ SNF Excluded

**K0602**  Replacement battery for external infusion pump owned by patient, silver oxide, 3 volt, each  Y ☑ & (NU)
AHA: 2Q, '03, 7

**K0603**  Replacement battery for external infusion pump owned by patient, alkaline, 1.5 volt, each  Y ☑ & (NU)
AHA: 2Q, '03, 7

**K0604**  Replacement battery for external infusion pump owned by patient, lithium, 3.6 volt, each  Y ☑ & (NU)
AHA: 2Q, '03, 7

**K0605**  Replacement battery for external infusion pump owned by patient, lithium, 4.5 volt, each  Y ☑ & (NU)
AHA: 2Q, '03, 7

**K0606**  Automatic external defibrillator, with integrated electrocardiogram analysis, garment type  Y (RR)
AHA: 4Q, '03, 4-5

**K0607**  Replacement battery for automated external defibrillator, garment type only, each  Y ☑ & (RR)
AHA: 4Q, '03, 4-5

**K0608**  Replacement garment for use with automated external defibrillator, each  Y ☑ & (NU,RR,UE)
AHA: 4Q, '03, 4-5

**K0609**  Replacement electrodes for use with automated external defibrillator, garment type only, each  Y ☑ & (KF)
AHA: 4Q, '03, 4-5

**K0669**  Wheelchair accessory, wheelchair seat or back cushion, does not meet specific code criteria or no written coding verification from DME PDAC  Y

**K0672**  Addition to lower extremity orthotic, removable soft interface, all components, replacement only, each  A ☑ &

**K0730**  Controlled dose inhalation drug delivery system  Y & (RR)

**K0733**  Power wheelchair accessory, 12 to 24 amp hour sealed lead acid battery, each (e.g., gel cell, absorbed glassmat)  Y & (NU,RR,UE)
CMS: 100-04,23,60.3

**K0738**  Portable gaseous oxygen system, rental; home compressor used to fill portable oxygen cylinders; includes portable containers, regulator, flowmeter, humidifier, cannula or mask, and tubing  Y & (RR)

**K0739**  Repair or nonroutine service for durable medical equipment other than oxygen equipment requiring the skill of a technician, labor component, per 15 minutes  Y ☑

**K0740**  Repair or nonroutine service for oxygen equipment requiring the skill of a technician, labor component, per 15 minutes  E ☑

**K0743**  Suction pump, home model, portable, for use on wounds  Y

**K0744**  Absorptive wound dressing for use with suction pump, home model, portable, pad size 16 sq in or less  A ☑

**K0745**  Absorptive wound dressing for use with suction pump, home model, portable, pad size more than 16 sq in but less than or equal to 48 sq in  A ☑

**K0746**  Absorptive wound dressing for use with suction pump, home model, portable, pad size greater than 48 sq in  A

## Power Operated Vehicle and Accessories

**K0800**  Power operated vehicle, group 1 standard, patient weight capacity up to and including 300 pounds  Y & (NU,RR,UE)
CMS: 100-04,12,30.6.15.4; 100-04,23,60.3

**K0801**  Power operated vehicle, group 1 heavy-duty, patient weight capacity 301 to 450 pounds  Y & (NU,RR,UE)
CMS: 100-04,12,30.6.15.4; 100-04,23,60.3

**K0802**  Power operated vehicle, group 1 very heavy-duty, patient weight capacity 451 to 600 pounds  Y & (NU,RR,UE)
CMS: 100-04,12,30.6.15.4; 100-04,23,60.3

**K0806**  Power operated vehicle, group 2 standard, patient weight capacity up to and including 300 pounds  Y & (NU,RR,UE)
CMS: 100-04,12,30.6.15.4; 100-04,23,60.3

**K0807**  Power operated vehicle, group 2 heavy-duty, patient weight capacity 301 to 450 pounds  Y & (NU,RR,UE)
CMS: 100-04,12,30.6.15.4; 100-04,23,60.3

**K0808**  Power operated vehicle, group 2 very heavy-duty, patient weight capacity 451 to 600 pounds  Y & (NU,RR,UE)
CMS: 100-04,12,30.6.15.4; 100-04,23,60.3

**K0812**  Power operated vehicle, not otherwise classified  Y
CMS: 100-04,12,30.6.15.4

## Power Wheelchairs

**K0813**  Power wheelchair, group 1 standard, portable, sling/solid seat and back, patient weight capacity up to and including 300 pounds  Y & (RR)
CMS: 100-04,23,60.3

**K0814**  Power wheelchair, group 1 standard, portable, captain's chair, patient weight capacity up to and including 300 pounds  Y & (RR)
CMS: 100-04,23,60.3

**K0815**  Power wheelchair, group 1 standard, sling/solid seat and back, patient weight capacity up to and including 300 pounds  Y & (RR)
CMS: 100-04,23,60.3

**K0816**  Power wheelchair, group 1 standard, captain's chair, patient weight capacity up to and including 300 pounds  Y & (RR)
CMS: 100-04,23,60.3

**K0820**  Power wheelchair, group 2 standard, portable, sling/solid seat/back, patient weight capacity up to and including 300 pounds  Y & (RR)
CMS: 100-04,23,60.3

**K0821**  Power wheelchair, group 2 standard, portable, captain's chair, patient weight capacity up to and including 300 pounds  Y & (RR)
CMS: 100-04,23,60.3

**K0822**  Power wheelchair, group 2 standard, sling/solid seat/back, patient weight capacity up to and including 300 pounds  Y & (RR)
CMS: 100-04,23,60.3

**K0823**  Power wheelchair, group 2 standard, captain's chair, patient weight capacity up to and including 300 pounds  Y & (RR)
CMS: 100-04,23,60.3

**K0824**  Power wheelchair, group 2 heavy-duty, sling/solid seat/back, patient weight capacity 301 to 450 pounds  Y & (RR)
CMS: 100-04,23,60.3

**K0825**  Power wheelchair, group 2 heavy-duty, captain's chair, patient weight capacity 301 to 450 pounds  Y & (RR)
CMS: 100-04,23,60.3

**K0826**  Power wheelchair, group 2 very heavy-duty, sling/solid seat/back, patient weight capacity 451 to 600 pounds  Y & (RR)
CMS: 100-04,23,60.3

**K0827**  Power wheelchair, group 2 very heavy-duty, captain's chair, patient weight capacity 451 to 600 pounds  Y & (RR)
CMS: 100-04,23,60.3

---

Special Coverage Instructions   Noncovered by Medicare   Carrier Discretion   ☑ Quantity Alert  ● New Code   ○ Recycled/Reinstated  ▲ Revised Code

96 — K Codes   A Age Edit   M Maternity Edit   ♀ Female Only   ♂ Male Only   A-Y OPPS Status Indicators   © 2016 Optum360, LLC

| | | |
|---|---|---|
| **K0828** | Power wheelchair, group 2 extra heavy-duty, sling/solid seat/back, patient weight capacity 601 pounds or more | Ⓨ 🏍 (RR) |
| | CMS: 100-04,23,60.3 | |
| **K0829** | Power wheelchair, group 2 extra heavy-duty, captain's chair, patient weight 601 pounds or more | Ⓨ 🏍 (RR) |
| | CMS: 100-04,23,60.3 | |
| **K0830** | Power wheelchair, group 2 standard, seat elevator, sling/solid seat/back, patient weight capacity up to and including 300 pounds | Ⓨ |
| **K0831** | Power wheelchair, group 2 standard, seat elevator, captain's chair, patient weight capacity up to and including 300 pounds | Ⓨ |
| **K0835** | Power wheelchair, group 2 standard, single power option, sling/solid seat/back, patient weight capacity up to and including 300 pounds | Ⓨ 🏍 (RR) |
| | CMS: 100-04,23,60.3 | |
| **K0836** | Power wheelchair, group 2 standard, single power option, captain's chair, patient weight capacity up to and including 300 pounds | Ⓨ 🏍 (RR) |
| | CMS: 100-04,23,60.3 | |
| **K0837** | Power wheelchair, group 2 heavy-duty, single power option, sling/solid seat/back, patient weight capacity 301 to 450 pounds | Ⓨ 🏍 (RR) |
| | CMS: 100-04,23,60.3 | |
| **K0838** | Power wheelchair, group 2 heavy-duty, single power option, captain's chair, patient weight capacity 301 to 450 pounds | Ⓨ 🏍 (RR) |
| | CMS: 100-04,23,60.3 | |
| **K0839** | Power wheelchair, group 2 very heavy-duty, single power option sling/solid seat/back, patient weight capacity 451 to 600 pounds | Ⓨ 🏍 (RR) |
| | CMS: 100-04,23,60.3 | |
| **K0840** | Power wheelchair, group 2 extra heavy-duty, single power option, sling/solid seat/back, patient weight capacity 601 pounds or more | Ⓨ 🏍 (RR) |
| | CMS: 100-04,23,60.3 | |
| **K0841** | Power wheelchair, group 2 standard, multiple power option, sling/solid seat/back, patient weight capacity up to and including 300 pounds | Ⓨ 🏍 (RR) |
| | CMS: 100-04,23,60.3 | |
| **K0842** | Power wheelchair, group 2 standard, multiple power option, captain's chair, patient weight capacity up to and including 300 pounds | Ⓨ 🏍 (RR) |
| | CMS: 100-04,23,60.3 | |
| **K0843** | Power wheelchair, group 2 heavy-duty, multiple power option, sling/solid seat/back, patient weight capacity 301 to 450 pounds | Ⓨ 🏍 (RR) |
| | CMS: 100-04,23,60.3 | |
| **K0848** | Power wheelchair, group 3 standard, sling/solid seat/back, patient weight capacity up to and including 300 pounds | Ⓨ 🏍 (RR) |
| | CMS: 100-04,23,60.3 | |
| **K0849** | Power wheelchair, group 3 standard, captain's chair, patient weight capacity up to and including 300 pounds | Ⓨ 🏍 (RR) |
| | CMS: 100-04,23,60.3 | |
| **K0850** | Power wheelchair, group 3 heavy-duty, sling/solid seat/back, patient weight capacity 301 to 450 pounds | Ⓨ 🏍 (RR) |
| | CMS: 100-04,23,60.3 | |
| **K0851** | Power wheelchair, group 3 heavy-duty, captain's chair, patient weight capacity 301 to 450 pounds | Ⓨ 🏍 (RR) |
| | CMS: 100-04,23,60.3 | |
| **K0852** | Power wheelchair, group 3 very heavy-duty, sling/solid seat/back, patient weight capacity 451 to 600 pounds | Ⓨ 🏍 (RR) |
| | CMS: 100-04,23,60.3 | |
| **K0853** | Power wheelchair, group 3 very heavy-duty, captain's chair, patient weight capacity 451 to 600 pounds | Ⓨ 🏍 (RR) |
| | CMS: 100-04,23,60.3 | |
| **K0854** | Power wheelchair, group 3 extra heavy-duty, sling/solid seat/back, patient weight capacity 601 pounds or more | Ⓨ 🏍 (RR) |
| | CMS: 100-04,23,60.3 | |
| **K0855** | Power wheelchair, group 3 extra heavy-duty, captain's chair, patient weight capacity 601 pounds or more | Ⓨ 🏍 (RR) |
| | CMS: 100-04,23,60.3 | |
| **K0856** | Power wheelchair, group 3 standard, single power option, sling/solid seat/back, patient weight capacity up to and including 300 pounds | Ⓨ 🏍 (RR) |
| | CMS: 100-04,23,60.3 | |
| **K0857** | Power wheelchair, group 3 standard, single power option, captain's chair, patient weight capacity up to and including 300 pounds | Ⓨ 🏍 (RR) |
| | CMS: 100-04,23,60.3 | |
| **K0858** | Power wheelchair, group 3 heavy-duty, single power option, sling/solid seat/back, patient weight capacity 301 to 450 pounds | Ⓨ 🏍 (RR) |
| | CMS: 100-04,23,60.3 | |
| **K0859** | Power wheelchair, group 3 heavy-duty, single power option, captain's chair, patient weight capacity 301 to 450 pounds | Ⓨ 🏍 (RR) |
| | CMS: 100-04,23,60.3 | |
| **K0860** | Power wheelchair, group 3 very heavy-duty, single power option, sling/solid seat/back, patient weight capacity 451 to 600 pounds | Ⓨ 🏍 (RR) |
| | CMS: 100-04,23,60.3 | |
| **K0861** | Power wheelchair, group 3 standard, multiple power option, sling/solid seat/back, patient weight capacity up to and including 300 pounds | Ⓨ 🏍 (RR) |
| | CMS: 100-04,23,60.3 | |
| **K0862** | Power wheelchair, group 3 heavy-duty, multiple power option, sling/solid seat/back, patient weight capacity 301 to 450 pounds | Ⓨ 🏍 (RR) |
| | CMS: 100-04,23,60.3 | |
| **K0863** | Power wheelchair, group 3 very heavy-duty, multiple power option, sling/solid seat/back, patient weight capacity 451 to 600 pounds | Ⓨ 🏍 (RR) |
| | CMS: 100-04,23,60.3 | |
| **K0864** | Power wheelchair, group 3 extra heavy-duty, multiple power option, sling/solid seat/back, patient weight capacity 601 pounds or more | Ⓨ 🏍 (RR) |
| | CMS: 100-04,23,60.3 | |
| **K0868** | Power wheelchair, group 4 standard, sling/solid seat/back, patient weight capacity up to and including 300 pounds | Ⓨ |
| **K0869** | Power wheelchair, group 4 standard, captain's chair, patient weight capacity up to and including 300 pounds | Ⓨ |
| **K0870** | Power wheelchair, group 4 heavy-duty, sling/solid seat/back, patient weight capacity 301 to 450 pounds | Ⓨ |
| **K0871** | Power wheelchair, group 4 very heavy-duty, sling/solid seat/back, patient weight capacity 451 to 600 pounds | Ⓨ |

Special Coverage Instructions    Noncovered by Medicare    Carrier Discretion    ☑ Quantity Alert ● New Code    ○ Recycled/Reinstated ▲ Revised Code

© 2016 Optum360, LLC    A2-Z3 ASC Pmt    CMS: Pub 100    AHA: Coding Clinic    🏍 DMEPOS Paid    ⊘ SNF Excluded    K Codes — 97

**K0877** Power wheelchair, group 4 standard, single power option, sling/solid seat/back, patient weight capacity up to and including 300 pounds ☒Y

**K0878** Power wheelchair, group 4 standard, single power option, captain's chair, patient weight capacity up to and including 300 pounds ☒Y

**K0879** Power wheelchair, group 4 heavy-duty, single power option, sling/solid seat/back, patient weight capacity 301 to 450 pounds ☒Y

**K0880** Power wheelchair, group 4 very heavy-duty, single power option, sling/solid seat/back, patient weight 451 to 600 pounds ☒Y

**K0884** Power wheelchair, group 4 standard, multiple power option, sling/solid seat/back, patient weight capacity up to and including 300 pounds ☒Y

**K0885** Power wheelchair, group 4 standard, multiple power option, captain's chair, patient weight capacity up to and including 300 pounds ☒Y

**K0886** Power wheelchair, group 4 heavy-duty, multiple power option, sling/solid seat/back, patient weight capacity 301 to 450 pounds ☒Y

**K0890** Power wheelchair, group 5 pediatric, single power option, sling/solid seat/back, patient weight capacity up to and including 125 pounds ☒Y

**K0891** Power wheelchair, group 5 pediatric, multiple power option, sling/solid seat/back, patient weight capacity up to and including 125 pounds ☒Y

**K0898** Power wheelchair, not otherwise classified ☒Y

**K0899** Power mobility device, not coded by DME PDAC or does not meet criteria ☒Y
CMS: 100-04,12,30.6.15.4

## Other DME

**K0900** Customized durable medical equipment, other than wheelchair ☒Y

**K0901**[Jan] ~~Knee orthosis (KO), single upright, thigh and calf, with adjustable flexion and extension joint (unicentric or polycentric), medial-lateral and rotation control, with or without varus/valgus adjustment, prefabricated, off-the-shelf~~
To report, see ~L1851

**K0902**[Jan] ~~Knee orthosis (KO), double upright, thigh and calf, with adjustable flexion and extension joint (unicentric or polycentric), medial-lateral and rotation control, with or without varus/valgus adjustment, prefabricated, off-the-shelf~~
To report, see ~L1852

[Jan] **January Update**

Special Coverage Instructions    Noncovered by Medicare    Carrier Discretion    ☑ Quantity Alert  ● New Code    ○ Recycled/Reinstated    ▲ Revised Code

98 — K Codes    Ⓐ Age Edit    Ⓜ Maternity Edit    ♀ Female Only    ♂ Male Only    Ⓐ-Ⓨ OPPS Status Indicators    © 2016 Optum360, LLC

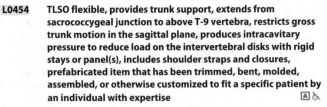

## Orthotic Procedures and Devices L0112-L4631

L codes include orthotic and prosthetic procedures and devices, as well as scoliosis equipment, orthopedic shoes, and prosthetic implants.

### Cervical

**L0112** Cranial cervical orthotic, congenital torticollis type, with or without soft interface material, adjustable range of motion joint, custom fabricated Ⓐ ♿

**L0113** Cranial cervical orthotic, torticollis type, with or without joint, with or without soft interface material, prefabricated, includes fitting and adjustment Ⓐ ♿

**L0120** Cervical, flexible, nonadjustable, prefabricated, off-the-shelf (foam collar) Ⓐ ♿

**L0130** Cervical, flexible, thermoplastic collar, molded to patient Ⓐ ♿

**L0140** Cervical, semi-rigid, adjustable (plastic collar) Ⓐ ♿

**L0150** Cervical, semi-rigid, adjustable molded chin cup (plastic collar with mandibular/occipital piece) Ⓐ ♿

**L0160** Cervical, semi-rigid, wire frame occipital/mandibular support, prefabricated, off-the-shelf Ⓐ ♿

**L0170** Cervical, collar, molded to patient model Ⓐ ♿

**L0172** Cervical, collar, semi-rigid thermoplastic foam, two-piece, prefabricated, off-the-shelf Ⓐ ♿

**L0174** Cervical, collar, semi-rigid, thermoplastic foam, two piece with thoracic extension, prefabricated, off-the-shelf Ⓐ ♿

### Multiple Post Collar

**L0180** Cervical, multiple post collar, occipital/mandibular supports, adjustable Ⓐ ♿

**L0190** Cervical, multiple post collar, occipital/mandibular supports, adjustable cervical bars (SOMI, Guilford, Taylor types) Ⓐ ♿

**L0200** Cervical, multiple post collar, occipital/mandibular supports, adjustable cervical bars, and thoracic extension Ⓐ ♿

### Thoracic

**L0220** Thoracic, rib belt, custom fabricated Ⓐ ♿

**L0450** TLSO, flexible, provides trunk support, upper thoracic region, produces intracavitary pressure to reduce load on the intervertebral disks with rigid stays or panel(s), includes shoulder straps and closures, prefabricated, off-the-shelf Ⓐ ♿

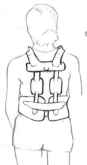

TLSO brace with adjustable straps and pads (L0450). The model at right and similar devices such as the Boston brace are molded polymer over foam and may be bivalve (front and back components)

Thoracic lumbar sacral orthosis (TLSO)

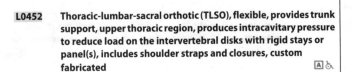

**L0452** Thoracic-lumbar-sacral orthotic (TLSO), flexible, provides trunk support, upper thoracic region, produces intracavitary pressure to reduce load on the intervertebral disks with rigid stays or panel(s), includes shoulder straps and closures, custom fabricated Ⓐ ♿

**L0454** TLSO flexible, provides trunk support, extends from sacrococcygeal junction to above T-9 vertebra, restricts gross trunk motion in the sagittal plane, produces intracavitary pressure to reduce load on the intervertebral disks with rigid stays or panel(s), includes shoulder straps and closures, prefabricated item that has been trimmed, bent, molded, assembled, or otherwise customized to fit a specific patient by an individual with expertise Ⓐ ♿

**L0455** TLSO, flexible, provides trunk support, extends from sacrococcygeal junction to above T-9 vertebra, restricts gross trunk motion in the sagittal plane, produces intracavitary pressure to reduce load on the intervertebral disks with rigid stays or panel(s), includes shoulder straps and closures, prefabricated, off-the-shelf Ⓐ ♿

**L0456** TLSO, flexible, provides trunk support, thoracic region, rigid posterior panel and soft anterior apron, extends from the sacrococcygeal junction and terminates just inferior to the scapular spine, restricts gross trunk motion in the sagittal plane, produces intracavitary pressure to reduce load on the intervertebral disks, includes straps and closures, prefabricated item that has been trimmed, bent, molded, assembled, or otherwise customized to fit a specific patient by an individual with expertise Ⓐ ♿

**L0457** TLSO, flexible, provides trunk support, thoracic region, rigid posterior panel and soft anterior apron, extends from the sacrococcygeal junction and terminates just inferior to the scapular spine, restricts gross trunk motion in the sagittal plane, produces intracavitary pressure to reduce load on the intervertebral disks, includes straps and closures, prefabricated, off-the-shelf Ⓐ ♿

**L0458** Thoracic-lumbar-sacral orthotic (TLSO), triplanar control, modular segmented spinal system, 2 rigid plastic shells, posterior extends from the sacrococcygeal junction and terminates just inferior to the scapular spine, anterior extends from the symphysis pubis to the xiphoid, soft liner, restricts gross trunk motion in the sagittal, coronal, and transverse planes, lateral strength is provided by overlapping plastic and stabilizing closures, includes straps and closures, prefabricated, includes fitting and adjustment Ⓐ ♿

**L0460** TLSO, triplanar control, modular segmented spinal system, two rigid plastic shells, posterior extends from the sacrococcygeal junction and terminates just inferior to the scapular spine, anterior extends from the symphysis pubis to the sternal notch, soft liner, restricts gross trunk motion in the sagittal, coronal, and transverse planes, lateral strength is provided by overlapping plastic and stabilizing closures, includes straps and closures, prefabricated item that has been trimmed, bent, molded, assembled, or otherwise customized to fit a specific patient by an individual with expertise Ⓐ ♿

**L0462** Thoracic-lumbar-sacral orthotic (TLSO), triplanar control, modular segmented spinal system, 3 rigid plastic shells, posterior extends from the sacrococcygeal junction and terminates just inferior to the scapular spine, anterior extends from the symphysis pubis to the sternal notch, soft liner, restricts gross trunk motion in the sagittal, coronal, and transverse planes, lateral strength is provided by overlapping plastic and stabilizing closures, includes straps and closures, prefabricated, includes fitting and adjustment Ⓐ ♿

L0112 — L0462

Special Coverage Instructions — Noncovered by Medicare — Carrier Discretion — ☑ Quantity Alert — ● New Code — ○ Recycled/Reinstated — ▲ Revised Code

© 2016 Optum360, LLC — Ⓐ²-Ⓩ³ ASC Pmt — CMS: Pub 100 — AHA: Coding Clinic — ♿ DMEPOS Paid — ⊘ SNF Excluded

L Codes — 99

**L0464** Thoracic-lumbar-sacral orthotic (TLSO), triplanar control, modular segmented spinal system, 4 rigid plastic shells, posterior extends from sacrococcygeal junction and terminates just inferior to scapular spine, anterior extends from symphysis pubis to the sternal notch, soft liner, restricts gross trunk motion in sagittal, coronal, and transverse planes, lateral strength is provided by overlapping plastic and stabilizing closures, includes straps and closures, prefabricated, includes fitting and adjustment [A] &

**L0466** TLSO, sagittal control, rigid posterior frame and flexible soft anterior apron with straps, closures and padding, restricts gross trunk motion in sagittal plane, produces intracavitary pressure to reduce load on intervertebral disks, prefabricated item that has been trimmed, bent, molded, assembled, or otherwise customized to fit a specific patient by an individual with expertise [A] &

**L0467** TLSO, sagittal control, rigid posterior frame and flexible soft anterior apron with straps, closures and padding, restricts gross trunk motion in sagittal plane, produces intracavitary pressure to reduce load on intervertebral disks, prefabricated, off-the-shelf [A] &

**L0468** TLSO, sagittal-coronal control, rigid posterior frame and flexible soft anterior apron with straps, closures and padding, extends from sacrococcygeal junction over scapulae, lateral strength provided by pelvic, thoracic, and lateral frame pieces, restricts gross trunk motion in sagittal, and coronal planes, produces intracavitary pressure to reduce load on intervertebral disks, prefabricated item that has been trimmed, bent, molded, assembled, or otherwise customized to fit a specific patient by an individual with expertise [A] &

**L0469** TLSO, sagittal-coronal control, rigid posterior frame and flexible soft anterior apron with straps, closures and padding, extends from sacrococcygeal junction over scapulae, lateral strength provided by pelvic, thoracic, and lateral frame pieces, restricts gross trunk motion in sagittal and coronal planes, produces intracavitary pressure to reduce load on intervertebral disks, prefabricated, off-the-shelf [A] &

**L0470** Thoracic-lumbar-sacral orthotic (TLSO), triplanar control, rigid posterior frame and flexible soft anterior apron with straps, closures and padding extends from sacrococcygeal junction to scapula, lateral strength provided by pelvic, thoracic, and lateral frame pieces, rotational strength provided by subclavicular extensions, restricts gross trunk motion in sagittal, coronal, and transverse planes, provides intracavitary pressure to reduce load on the intervertebral disks, includes fitting and shaping the frame, prefabricated, includes fitting and adjustment [A] &

**L0472** Thoracic-lumbar-sacral orthotic (TLSO), triplanar control, hyperextension, rigid anterior and lateral frame extends from symphysis pubis to sternal notch with 2 anterior components (one pubic and one sternal), posterior and lateral pads with straps and closures, limits spinal flexion, restricts gross trunk motion in sagittal, coronal, and transverse planes, includes fitting and shaping the frame, prefabricated, includes fitting and adjustment [A] &

**L0480** Thoracic-lumbar-sacral orthotic (TLSO), triplanar control, 1 piece rigid plastic shell without interface liner, with multiple straps and closures, posterior extends from sacrococcygeal junction and terminates just inferior to scapular spine, anterior extends from symphysis pubis to sternal notch, anterior or posterior opening, restricts gross trunk motion in sagittal, coronal, and transverse planes, includes a carved plaster or CAD-CAM model, custom fabricated [A] &

**L0482** Thoracic-lumbar-sacral orthotic (TLSO), triplanar control, 1 piece rigid plastic shell with interface liner, multiple straps and closures, posterior extends from sacrococcygeal junction and terminates just inferior to scapular spine, anterior extends from symphysis pubis to sternal notch, anterior or posterior opening, restricts gross trunk motion in sagittal, coronal, and transverse planes, includes a carved plaster or CAD-CAM model, custom fabricated [A] &

**L0484** Thoracic-lumbar-sacral orthotic (TLSO), triplanar control, 2 piece rigid plastic shell without interface liner, with multiple straps and closures, posterior extends from sacrococcygeal junction and terminates just inferior to scapular spine, anterior extends from symphysis pubis to sternal notch, lateral strength is enhanced by overlapping plastic, restricts gross trunk motion in the sagittal, coronal, and transverse planes, includes a carved plaster or CAD-CAM model, custom fabricated [A] &

**L0486** Thoracic-lumbar-sacral orthotic (TLSO), triplanar control, 2 piece rigid plastic shell with interface liner, multiple straps and closures, posterior extends from sacrococcygeal junction and terminates just inferior to scapular spine, anterior extends from symphysis pubis to sternal notch, lateral strength is enhanced by overlapping plastic, restricts gross trunk motion in the sagittal, coronal, and transverse planes, includes a carved plaster or CAD-CAM model, custom fabricated [A] &

**L0488** Thoracic-lumbar-sacral orthotic (TLSO), triplanar control, 1 piece rigid plastic shell with interface liner, multiple straps and closures, posterior extends from sacrococcygeal junction and terminates just inferior to scapular spine, anterior extends from symphysis pubis to sternal notch, anterior or posterior opening, restricts gross trunk motion in sagittal, coronal, and transverse planes, prefabricated, includes fitting and adjustment [A] &

**L0490** Thoracic-lumbar-sacral orthotic (TLSO), sagittal-coronal control, 1 piece rigid plastic shell, with overlapping reinforced anterior, with multiple straps and closures, posterior extends from sacrococcygeal junction and terminates at or before the T-9 vertebra, anterior extends from symphysis pubis to xiphoid, anterior opening, restricts gross trunk motion in sagittal and coronal planes, prefabricated, includes fitting and adjustment [A] &

**L0491** Thoracic-lumbar-sacral orthotic (TLSO), sagittal-coronal control, modular segmented spinal system, 2 rigid plastic shells, posterior extends from the sacrococcygeal junction and terminates just inferior to the scapular spine, anterior extends from the symphysis pubis to the xiphoid, soft liner, restricts gross trunk motion in the sagittal and coronal planes, lateral strength is provided by overlapping plastic and stabilizing closures, includes straps and closures, prefabricated, includes fitting and adjustment [A] &

**L0492** Thoracic-lumbar-sacral orthotic (TLSO), sagittal-coronal control, modular segmented spinal system, 3 rigid plastic shells, posterior extends from the sacrococcygeal junction and terminates just inferior to the scapular spine, anterior extends from the symphysis pubis to the xiphoid, soft liner, restricts gross trunk motion in the sagittal and coronal planes, lateral strength is provided by overlapping plastic and stabilizing closures, includes straps and closures, prefabricated, includes fitting and adjustment [A] &

## Cervical-Thoracic-Lumbar-Sacral Orthotic

**L0621** Sacroiliac orthosis, flexible, provides pelvic-sacral support, reduces motion about the sacroiliac joint, includes straps, closures, may include pendulous abdomen design, prefabricated, off-the-shelf [A] &

---

Special Coverage Instructions    Noncovered by Medicare    Carrier Discretion    ☑ Quantity Alert   ● New Code    ○ Recycled/Reinstated   ▲ Revised Code

   [A] Age Edit   [M] Maternity Edit   ♀ Female Only   ♂ Male Only   [A]-[Y] OPPS Status Indicators    © 2016 Optum360, LLC

**L0622** Sacroiliac orthotic, flexible, provides pelvic-sacral support, reduces motion about the sacroiliac joint, includes straps, closures, may include pendulous abdomen design, custom fabricated   A &

**L0623** Sacroiliac orthosis, provides pelvic-sacral support, with rigid or semi-rigid panels over the sacrum and abdomen, reduces motion about the sacroiliac joint, includes straps, closures, may include pendulous abdomen design, prefabricated, off-the-shelf   A &

**L0624** Sacroiliac orthotic, provides pelvic-sacral support, with rigid or semi-rigid panels placed over the sacrum and abdomen, reduces motion about the sacroiliac joint, includes straps, closures, may include pendulous abdomen design, custom fabricated   A &

**L0625** Lumbar orthosis, flexible, provides lumbar support, posterior extends from L-1 to below L-5 vertebra, produces intracavitary pressure to reduce load on the intervertebral discs, includes straps, closures, may include pendulous abdomen design, shoulder straps, stays, prefabricated, off-the-shelf   A &

**L0626** Lumbar orthosis, sagittal control, with rigid posterior panel(s), posterior extends from L-1 to below L-5 vertebra, produces intracavitary pressure to reduce load on the intervertebral discs, includes straps, closures, may include padding, stays, shoulder straps, pendulous abdomen design, prefabricated item that has been trimmed, bent, molded, assembled, or otherwise customized to fit a specific patient by an individual with expertise   A &

**L0627** Lumbar orthosis, sagittal control, with rigid anterior and posterior panels, posterior extends from L-1 to below L-5 vertebra, produces intracavitary pressure to reduce load on the intervertebral discs, includes straps, closures, may include padding, shoulder straps, pendulous abdomen design, prefabricated item that has been trimmed, bent, molded, assembled, or otherwise customized to fit a specific patient by an individual with expertise   A &

**L0628** Lumbar-sacral orthosis, flexible, provides lumbo-sacral support, posterior extends from sacrococcygeal junction to T-9 vertebra, produces intracavitary pressure to reduce load on the intervertebral discs, includes straps, closures, may include stays, shoulder straps, pendulous abdomen design, prefabricated, off-the-shelf   A &

**L0629** Lumbar-sacral orthotic, flexible, provides lumbo-sacral support, posterior extends from sacrococcygeal junction to T-9 vertebra, produces intracavitary pressure to reduce load on the intervertebral discs, includes straps, closures, may include stays, shoulder straps, pendulous abdomen design, custom fabricated   A &

**L0630** Lumbar-sacral orthosis, sagittal control, with rigid posterior panel(s), posterior extends from sacrococcygeal junction to T-9 vertebra, produces intracavitary pressure to reduce load on the intervertebral discs, includes straps, closures, may include padding, stays, shoulder straps, pendulous abdomen design, prefabricated item that has been trimmed, bent, molded, assembled, or otherwise customized to fit a specific patient by an individual with expertise   A &

**L0631** Lumbar-sacral orthosis, sagittal control, with rigid anterior and posterior panels, posterior extends from sacrococcygeal junction to T-9 vertebra, produces intracavitary pressure to reduce load on the intervertebral discs, includes straps, closures, may include padding, shoulder straps, pendulous abdomen design, prefabricated item that has been trimmed, bent, molded, assembled, or otherwise customized to fit a specific patient by an individual with expertise   A &

**L0632** Lumbar-sacral orthotic (LSO), sagittal control, with rigid anterior and posterior panels, posterior extends from sacrococcygeal junction to T-9 vertebra, produces intracavitary pressure to reduce load on the intervertebral discs, includes straps, closures, may include padding, shoulder straps, pendulous abdomen design, custom fabricated   A &

**L0633** Lumbar-sacral orthosis, sagittal-coronal control, with rigid posterior frame/panel(s), posterior extends from sacrococcygeal junction to T-9 vertebra, lateral strength provided by rigid lateral frame/panels, produces intracavitary pressure to reduce load on intervertebral discs, includes straps, closures, may include padding, stays, shoulder straps, pendulous abdomen design, prefabricated item that has been trimmed, bent, molded, assembled, or otherwise customized to fit a specific patient by an individual with expertise   A &

**L0634** Lumbar-sacral orthotic (LSO), sagittal-coronal control, with rigid posterior frame/panel(s), posterior extends from sacrococcygeal junction to T-9 vertebra, lateral strength provided by rigid lateral frame/panel(s), produces intracavitary pressure to reduce load on intervertebral discs, includes straps, closures, may include padding, stays, shoulder straps, pendulous abdomen design, custom fabricated   A &

**L0635** Lumbar-sacral orthotic (LSO), sagittal-coronal control, lumbar flexion, rigid posterior frame/panel(s), lateral articulating design to flex the lumbar spine, posterior extends from sacrococcygeal junction to T-9 vertebra, lateral strength provided by rigid lateral frame/panel(s), produces intracavitary pressure to reduce load on intervertebral discs, includes straps, closures, may include padding, anterior panel, pendulous abdomen design, prefabricated, includes fitting and adjustment   A &

**L0636** Lumbar-sacral orthotic (LSO), sagittal-coronal control, lumbar flexion, rigid posterior frame/panels, lateral articulating design to flex the lumbar spine, posterior extends from sacrococcygeal junction to T-9 vertebra, lateral strength provided by rigid lateral frame/panels, produces intracavitary pressure to reduce load on intervertebral discs, includes straps, closures, may include padding, anterior panel, pendulous abdomen design, custom fabricated   A &

**L0637** Lumbar-sacral orthosis, sagittal-coronal control, with rigid anterior and posterior frame/panels, posterior extends from sacrococcygeal junction to T-9 vertebra, lateral strength provided by rigid lateral frame/panels, produces intracavitary pressure to reduce load on intervertebral discs, includes straps, closures, may include padding, shoulder straps, pendulous abdomen design, prefabricated item that has been trimmed, bent, molded, assembled, or otherwise customized to fit a specific patient by an individual with expertise   A &

**L0638** Lumbar-sacral orthotic (LSO), sagittal-coronal control, with rigid anterior and posterior frame/panels, posterior extends from sacrococcygeal junction to T-9 vertebra, lateral strength provided by rigid lateral frame/panels, produces intracavitary pressure to reduce load on intervertebral discs, includes straps, closures, may include padding, shoulder straps, pendulous abdomen design, custom fabricated   A &

**L0639** Lumbar-sacral orthosis, sagittal-coronal control, rigid shell(s)/panel(s), posterior extends from sacrococcygeal junction to T-9 vertebra, anterior extends from symphysis pubis to xyphoid, produces intracavitary pressure to reduce load on the intervertebral discs, overall strength is provided by overlapping rigid material and stabilizing closures, includes straps, closures, may include soft interface, pendulous abdomen design, prefabricated item that has been trimmed, bent, molded, assembled, or otherwise customized to fit a specific patient by an individual with expertise   A &

---

Special Coverage Instructions    Noncovered by Medicare    Carrier Discretion    ☑ Quantity Alert  ● New Code    ○ Recycled/Reinstated    ▲ Revised Code

© 2016 Optum360, LLC    A2–Z3 ASC Pmt    CMS: Pub 100    AHA: Coding Clinic    & DMEPOS Paid    ⊘ SNF Excluded    L Codes — 101

**L0640** Lumbar-sacral orthotic (LSO), sagittal-coronal control, rigid shell(s)/panel(s), posterior extends from sacrococcygeal junction to T-9 vertebra, anterior extends from symphysis pubis to xyphoid, produces intracavitary pressure to reduce load on the intervertebral discs, overall strength is provided by overlapping rigid material and stabilizing closures, includes straps, closures, may include soft interface, pendulous abdomen design, custom fabricated [A] [&]

**L0641** Lumbar orthosis, sagittal control, with rigid posterior panel(s), posterior extends from L-1 to below L-5 vertebra, produces intracavitary pressure to reduce load on the intervertebral discs, includes straps, closures, may include padding, stays, shoulder straps, pendulous abdomen design, prefabricated, off-the-shelf [A] [&]

**L0642** Lumbar orthosis, sagittal control, with rigid anterior and posterior panels, posterior extends from L-1 to below L-5 vertebra, produces intracavitary pressure to reduce load on the intervertebral discs, includes straps, closures, may include padding, shoulder straps, pendulous abdomen design, prefabricated, off-the-shelf [A] [&]

**L0643** Lumbar-sacral orthosis, sagittal control, with rigid posterior panel(s), posterior extends from sacrococcygeal junction to T-9 vertebra, produces intracavitary pressure to reduce load on the intervertebral discs, includes straps, closures, may include padding, stays, shoulder straps, pendulous abdomen design, prefabricated, off-the-shelf [A] [&]

**L0648** Lumbar-sacral orthosis, sagittal control, with rigid anterior and posterior panels, posterior extends from sacrococcygeal junction to T-9 vertebra, produces intracavitary pressure to reduce load on the intervertebral discs, includes straps, closures, may include padding, shoulder straps, pendulous abdomen design, prefabricated, off-the-shelf [A] [&]

**L0649** Lumbar-sacral orthosis, sagittal-coronal control, with rigid posterior frame/panel(s), posterior extends from sacrococcygeal junction to T-9 vertebra, lateral strength provided by rigid lateral frame/panels, produces intracavitary pressure to reduce load on intervertebral discs, includes straps, closures, may include padding, stays, shoulder straps, pendulous abdomen design, prefabricated, off-the-shelf [A] [&]

**L0650** Lumbar-sacral orthosis, sagittal-coronal control, with rigid anterior and posterior frame/panel(s), posterior extends from sacrococcygeal junction to T-9 vertebra, lateral strength provided by rigid lateral frame/panel(s), produces intracavitary pressure to reduce load on intervertebral discs, includes straps, closures, may include padding, shoulder straps, pendulous abdomen design, prefabricated, off-the-shelf [A] [&]

**L0651** Lumbar-sacral orthosis, sagittal-coronal control, rigid shell(s)/panel(s), posterior extends from sacrococcygeal junction to T-9 vertebra, anterior extends from symphysis pubis to xyphoid, produces intracavitary pressure to reduce load on the intervertebral discs, overall strength is provided by overlapping rigid material and stabilizing closures, includes straps, closures, may include soft interface, pendulous abdomen design, prefabricated, off-the-shelf [A] [&]

**L0700** Cervical-thoracic-lumbar-sacral orthotic (CTLSO), anterior-posterior-lateral control, molded to patient model, (Minerva type) [A] [&]

**L0710** Cervical-thoracic-lumbar-sacral orthotic (CTLSO), anterior-posterior-lateral-control, molded to patient model, with interface material, (Minerva type) [A] [&]

## Halo Procedure

**L0810** Halo procedure, cervical halo incorporated into jacket vest [A] [&]

**L0820** Halo procedure, cervical halo incorporated into plaster body jacket [A] [&]

**L0830** Halo procedure, cervical halo incorporated into Milwaukee type orthotic [A] [&]

**L0859** Addition to halo procedure, magnetic resonance image compatible systems, rings and pins, any material [A] [&]

**L0861** Addition to halo procedure, replacement liner/interface material [A] [&]

## Additions to Spinal Orthotic

**L0970** Thoracic-lumbar-sacral orthotic (TLSO), corset front [A] [&]

**L0972** Lumbar-sacral orthotic (LSO), corset front [A] [&]

**L0974** Thoracic-lumbar-sacral orthotic (TLSO), full corset [A] [&]

**L0976** Lumbar-sacral orthotic (LSO), full corset [A] [&]

**L0978** Axillary crutch extension [A] [&]

**L0980** Peroneal straps, prefabricated, off-the-shelf, pair [A] [☑] [&]

**L0982** Stocking supporter grips, prefabricated, off-the-shelf, set of four (4) [A] [☑] [&]

**L0984** Protective body sock, prefabricated, off-the-shelf, each [A] [☑] [&]

**L0999** Addition to spinal orthotic, not otherwise specified [A]

Determine if an alternative HCPCS Level II or a CPT code better describes the service being reported. This code should be used only if a more specific code is unavailable.

## Orthotic Devices - Scoliosis Procedures

The orthotic care of scoliosis differs from other orthotic care in that the treatment is more dynamic in nature and uses continual modification of the orthosis to the patient's changing condition. This coding structure uses the proper names - or eponyms - of the procedures because they have historic and universal acceptance in the profession. It should be recognized that variations to the basic procedures described by the founders/developers are accepted in various medical and orthotic practices throughout the country. All procedures include model of patient when indicated.

**L1000** Cervical-thoracic-lumbar-sacral orthotic (CTLSO) (Milwaukee), inclusive of furnishing initial orthotic, including model [A] [&]

Cervical component

A variety of configurations are available for the Milwaukee brace (L1000)

Thoracic component

Axilla sling (L1010)

Lumbar-sacral component

Milwaukee-style braces; cervical thoracic lumbar sacral orthosis (CTSLO)

**L1001** Cervical-thoracic-lumbar-sacral orthotic (CTLSO), immobilizer, infant size, prefabricated, includes fitting and adjustment [A] [A] [&]

**L1005** Tension based scoliosis orthotic and accessory pads, includes fitting and adjustment [A] [&]
AHA: 1Q, '02, 5

**L1010** Addition to cervical-thoracic-lumbar-sacral orthotic (CTLSO) or scoliosis orthotic, axilla sling [A] [&]

**L1020** Addition to cervical-thoracic-lumbar-sacral orthotic (CTLSO) or scoliosis orthotic, kyphosis pad [A] [&]

**L1025** Addition to cervical-thoracic-lumbar-sacral orthotic (CTLSO) or scoliosis orthotic, kyphosis pad, floating [A] [&]

---

Special Coverage Instructions   Noncovered by Medicare   Carrier Discretion   ☑ Quantity Alert   ● New Code   ○ Recycled/Reinstated   ▲ Revised Code

[A] Age Edit   [M] Maternity Edit   ♀ Female Only   ♂ Male Only   [A]-[Y] OPPS Status Indicators   © 2016 Optum360, LLC

**L1030** Addition to cervical-thoracic-lumbar-sacral orthotic (CTLSO) or scoliosis orthotic, lumbar bolster pad   Ⓐ ♿

**L1040** Addition to cervical-thoracic-lumbar-sacral orthotic (CTLSO) or scoliosis orthotic, lumbar or lumbar rib pad   Ⓐ ♿

**L1050** Addition to cervical-thoracic-lumbar-sacral orthotic (CTLSO) or scoliosis orthotic, sternal pad   Ⓐ ♿

**L1060** Addition to cervical-thoracic-lumbar-sacral orthotic (CTLSO) or scoliosis orthotic, thoracic pad   Ⓐ ♿

**L1070** Addition to cervical-thoracic-lumbar-sacral orthotic (CTLSO) or scoliosis orthotic, trapezius sling   Ⓐ ♿

**L1080** Addition to cervical-thoracic-lumbar-sacral orthotic (CTLSO) or scoliosis orthotic, outrigger   Ⓐ ♿

**L1085** Addition to cervical-thoracic-lumbar-sacral orthotic (CTLSO) or scoliosis orthotic, outrigger, bilateral with vertical extensions   Ⓐ ♿

**L1090** Addition to cervical-thoracic-lumbar-sacral orthotic (CTLSO) or scoliosis orthotic, lumbar sling   Ⓐ ♿

**L1100** Addition to cervical-thoracic-lumbar-sacral orthotic (CTLSO) or scoliosis orthotic, ring flange, plastic or leather   Ⓐ ♿

**L1110** Addition to cervical-thoracic-lumbar-sacral orthotic (CTLSO) or scoliosis orthotic, ring flange, plastic or leather, molded to patient model   Ⓐ ♿

**L1120** Addition to cervical-thoracic-lumbar-sacral orthotic (CTLSO), scoliosis orthotic, cover for upright, each   Ⓐ ☑ ♿

## Thoracic-Lumbar-Sacral Orthotic (TLSO) (Low Profile)

**L1200** Thoracic-lumbar-sacral orthotic (TLSO), inclusive of furnishing initial orthotic only   Ⓐ ♿

**L1210** Addition to thoracic-lumbar-sacral orthotic (TLSO), (low profile), lateral thoracic extension   Ⓐ ♿

**L1220** Addition to thoracic-lumbar-sacral orthotic (TLSO), (low profile), anterior thoracic extension   Ⓐ ♿

**L1230** Addition to thoracic-lumbar-sacral orthotic (TLSO), (low profile), Milwaukee type superstructure   Ⓐ ♿

**L1240** Addition to thoracic-lumbar-sacral orthotic (TLSO), (low profile), lumbar derotation pad   Ⓐ ♿

**L1250** Addition to thoracic-lumbar-sacral orthotic (TLSO), (low profile), anterior ASIS pad   Ⓐ ♿

**L1260** Addition to thoracic-lumbar-sacral orthotic (TLSO), (low profile), anterior thoracic derotation pad   Ⓐ ♿

**L1270** Addition to thoracic-lumbar-sacral orthotic (TLSO), (low profile), abdominal pad   Ⓐ ♿

**L1280** Addition to thoracic-lumbar-sacral orthotic (TLSO), (low profile), rib gusset (elastic), each   Ⓐ ☑ ♿

**L1290** Addition to thoracic-lumbar-sacral orthotic (TLSO), (low profile), lateral trochanteric pad   Ⓐ ♿

## Other Scoliosis Procedures

**L1300** Other scoliosis procedure, body jacket molded to patient model   Ⓐ ♿

**L1310** Other scoliosis procedure, postoperative body jacket   Ⓐ ♿

**L1499** Spinal orthotic, not otherwise specified   Ⓐ

Determine if an alternative HCPCS Level II or a CPT code better describes the service being reported. This code should be used only if a more specific code is unavailable.

## Hip Orthotic (HO) - Flexible

**L1600** Hip orthosis, abduction control of hip joints, flexible, Frejka type with cover, prefabricated item that has been trimmed, bent, molded, assembled, or otherwise customized to fit a specific patient by an inidividual with expertise   Ⓐ ♿

**L1610** Hip orthosis, abduction control of hip joints, flexible, (Frejka cover only), prefabricated item that has been trimmed, bent, molded, assembled, or otherwise customized to fit a specific patient by an individual with expertise   Ⓐ ♿

**L1620** Hip orthosis, abduction control of hip joints, flexible, (Pavlik harness), prefabricated item that has been trimmed, bent, molded, assembled, or otherwise customized to fit a specific patient by an individual with expertise   Ⓐ ♿

**L1630** Hip orthotic (HO), abduction control of hip joints, semi-flexible (Von Rosen type), custom fabricated   Ⓐ ♿

**L1640** Hip orthotic (HO), abduction control of hip joints, static, pelvic band or spreader bar, thigh cuffs, custom fabricated   Ⓐ ♿

**L1650** Hip orthotic (HO), abduction control of hip joints, static, adjustable, (Ilfled type), prefabricated, includes fitting and adjustment   Ⓐ ♿

**L1652** Hip orthotic, bilateral thigh cuffs with adjustable abductor spreader bar, adult size, prefabricated, includes fitting and adjustment, any type   Ⓐ ♿

**L1660** Hip orthotic (HO), abduction control of hip joints, static, plastic, prefabricated, includes fitting and adjustment   Ⓐ ♿

**L1680** Hip orthotic (HO), abduction control of hip joints, dynamic, pelvic control, adjustable hip motion control, thigh cuffs (Rancho hip action type), custom fabricated   Ⓐ ♿

**L1685** Hip orthosis (HO), abduction control of hip joint, postoperative hip abduction type, custom fabricated   Ⓐ ♿

**L1686** Hip orthotic (HO), abduction control of hip joint, postoperative hip abduction type, prefabricated, includes fitting and adjustment   Ⓐ ♿

**L1690** Combination, bilateral, lumbo-sacral, hip, femur orthotic providing adduction and internal rotation control, prefabricated, includes fitting and adjustment   Ⓐ ♿

## Legg Perthes

**L1700** Legg Perthes orthotic, (Toronto type), custom fabricated   Ⓐ ♿

**L1710** Legg Perthes orthotic, (Newington type), custom fabricated   Ⓐ ♿

**L1720** Legg Perthes orthotic, trilateral, (Tachdijan type), custom fabricated   Ⓐ ♿

**L1730** Legg Perthes orthotic, (Scottish Rite type), custom fabricated   Ⓐ ♿

**L1755** Legg Perthes orthotic, (Patten bottom type), custom fabricated   Ⓐ ♿

## Knee Orthotic

**L1810** Knee orthosis, elastic with joints, prefabricated item that has been trimmed, bent, molded, assembled, or otherwise customized to fit a specific patient by an individual with expertise   Ⓐ ♿

**L1812** Knee orthosis, elastic with joints, prefabricated, off-the-shelf   Ⓐ ♿

**L1820** Knee orthotic, elastic with condylar pads and joints, with or without patellar control, prefabricated, includes fitting and adjustment   Ⓐ ♿

**L1830** Knee orthosis, immobilizer, canvas longitudinal, prefabricated, off-the-shelf   Ⓐ ♿

---

Special Coverage Instructions    Noncovered by Medicare    Carrier Discretion    ☑ Quantity Alert   ● New Code   ○ Recycled/Reinstated   ▲ Revised Code

© 2016 Optum360, LLC   A2–Z3 ASC Pmt   **CMS:** Pub 100   **AHA:** Coding Clinic   ♿ DMEPOS Paid   ⊘ SNF Excluded     **L Codes — 103**

**Orthotic Devices and Procedures**

**L1831 — L1971**

**L1831** Knee orthotic, locking knee joint(s), positional orthotic, prefabricated, includes fitting and adjustment    [A] &

**L1832** Knee orthosis, adjustable knee joints (unicentric or polycentric), positional orthosis, rigid support, prefabricated item that has been trimmed, bent, molded, assembled, or otherwise customized to fit a specific patient by an individual with expertise    [A] &

**L1833** Knee orthosis, adjustable knee joints (unicentric or polycentric), positional orthosis, rigid support, prefabricated, off-the shelf    [A] &

**L1834** Knee orthotic (KO), without knee joint, rigid, custom fabricated    [A] &

**L1836** Knee orthosis, rigid, without joint(s), includes soft interface material, prefabricated, off-the-shelf    [A] &

**L1840** Knee orthotic (KO), derotation, medial-lateral, anterior cruciate ligament, custom fabricated    [A] &

**L1843** Knee orthosis, single upright, thigh and calf, with adjustable flexion and extension joint (unicentric or polycentric), medial-lateral and rotation control, with or without varus/valgus adjustment, prefabricated item that has been trimmed, bent, molded, assembled, or otherwise customized to fit a specific patient by an individual with expertise    [A] &

**L1844** Knee orthotic (KO), single upright, thigh and calf, with adjustable flexion and extension joint (unicentric or polycentric), medial-lateral and rotation control, with or without varus/valgus adjustment, custom fabricated    [A] &

**L1845** Knee orthosis, double upright, thigh and calf, with adjustable flexion and extension joint (unicentric or polycentric), medial-lateral and rotation control, with or without varus/valgus adjustment, prefabricated item that has been trimmed, bent, molded, assembled, or otherwise customized to fit a specific patient by an individual with expertise    [A] &

**L1846** Knee orthotic, double upright, thigh and calf, with adjustable flexion and extension joint (unicentric or polycentric), medial-lateral and rotation control, with or without varus/valgus adjustment, custom fabricated    [A] &

**L1847** Knee orthosis, double upright with adjustable joint, with inflatable air support chamber(s), prefabricated item that has been trimmed, bent, molded, assembled, or otherwise customized to fit a specific patient by an individual with expertise    [A] &

**L1848** Knee orthosis, double upright with adjustable joint, with inflatable air support chamber(s), prefabricated, off-the-shelf    [A] &

**L1850** Knee orthosis, swedish type, prefabricated, off-the-shelf    [A] &

● **L1851**[Jan] Knee orthosis (KO), single upright, thigh and calf, with adjustable flexion and extension joint (unicentric or polycentric), medial-lateral and rotation control, with or without varus/valgus adjustment, prefabricated, off-the-shelf

● **L1852**[Jan] Knee orthosis (KO), double upright, thigh and calf, with adjustable flexion and extension joint (unicentric or polycentric), medial-lateral and rotation control, with or without varus/valgus adjustment, prefabricated, off-the-shelf

**L1860** Knee orthotic (KO), modification of supracondylar prosthetic socket, custom fabricated (SK)    [A] &

## Ankle-Foot Orthotic (AFO)

**L1900** Ankle-foot orthotic (AFO), spring wire, dorsiflexion assist calf band, custom fabricated    [A] &

**L1902** Ankle orthosis, ankle gauntlet or similar, with or without joints, prefabricated, off-the-shelf    [A] &

**L1904** Ankle orthosis, ankle gauntlet or similar, with or without joints, custom fabricated    [A] &

▲ **L1906**[Jan] Ankle foot orthosis, multiligamentous ankle support, prefabricated, off-the-shelf    [A] &

**L1907** Ankle orthosis, supramalleolar with straps, with or without interface/pads, custom fabricated    [A] &

**L1910** Ankle-foot orthotic (AFO), posterior, single bar, clasp attachment to shoe counter, prefabricated, includes fitting and adjustment    [A] &

**L1920** Ankle-foot orthotic (AFO), single upright with static or adjustable stop (Phelps or Perlstein type), custom fabricated    [A] &

**L1930** Ankle-foot orthotic (AFO), plastic or other material, prefabricated, includes fitting and adjustment    [A] &

Ankle foot orthotic (AFO), plastic or other material (L1930)

Flexible carbon component

Foot component may fit inside shoe

**L1932** Ankle-foot orthotic (AFO), rigid anterior tibial section, total carbon fiber or equal material, prefabricated, includes fitting and adjustment    [A] &

**L1940** Ankle-foot orthotic (AFO), plastic or other material, custom fabricated    [A] &

**L1945** Ankle-foot orthotic (AFO), plastic, rigid anterior tibial section (floor reaction), custom fabricated    [A] &

Rigid tibial anterior floor reaction; ankle-foot orthosis (AFO) (L1945)

Spiral; ankle-foot orthosis (AFO) (L1950)

**L1950** Ankle-foot orthotic (AFO), spiral, (Institute of Rehabilitative Medicine type), plastic, custom fabricated    [A] &

**L1951** Ankle-foot orthotic (AFO), spiral, (Institute of rehabilitative Medicine type), plastic or other material, prefabricated, includes fitting and adjustment    [A] &

**L1960** Ankle-foot orthotic (AFO), posterior solid ankle, plastic, custom fabricated    [A] &

**L1970** Ankle-foot orthotic (AFO), plastic with ankle joint, custom fabricated    [A] &

**L1971** Ankle-foot orthotic (AFO), plastic or other material with ankle joint, prefabricated, includes fitting and adjustment    [A] &

---

[Jan] **January Update**

Special Coverage Instructions      Noncovered by Medicare      Carrier Discretion      ☑ Quantity Alert   ● New Code   ○ Recycled/Reinstated   ▲ Revised Code

104 — L Codes      [A] Age Edit   [M] Maternity Edit   ♀ Female Only   ♂ Male Only   [A]-[Y] OPPS Status Indicators      © 2016 Optum360, LLC

**L1980** Ankle-foot orthotic (AFO), single upright free plantar dorsiflexion, solid stirrup, calf band/cuff (single bar 'BK' orthotic), custom fabricated  A &

**L1990** Ankle-foot orthotic (AFO), double upright free plantar dorsiflexion, solid stirrup, calf band/cuff (double bar 'BK' orthotic), custom fabricated  A &

## Knee-Ankle-Foot Orthotic (KAFO) - Or Any Combination

**L2000** Knee-ankle-foot orthotic (KAFO), single upright, free knee, free ankle, solid stirrup, thigh and calf bands/cuffs (single bar 'AK' orthotic), custom fabricated  A &

**L2005** Knee-ankle-foot orthotic (KAFO), any material, single or double upright, stance control, automatic lock and swing phase release, any type activation, includes ankle joint, any type, custom fabricated  A &

**L2010** Knee-ankle-foot orthotic (KAFO), single upright, free ankle, solid stirrup, thigh and calf bands/cuffs (single bar 'AK' orthotic), without knee joint, custom fabricated  A &

**L2020** Knee-ankle-foot orthotic (KAFO), double upright, free ankle, solid stirrup, thigh and calf bands/cuffs (double bar 'AK' orthotic), custom fabricated  A &

**L2030** Knee-ankle-foot orthotic (KAFO), double upright, free ankle, solid stirrup, thigh and calf bands/cuffs, (double bar 'AK' orthotic), without knee joint, custom fabricated  A &

**L2034** Knee-ankle-foot orthotic (KAFO), full plastic, single upright, with or without free motion knee, medial-lateral rotation control, with or without free motion ankle, custom fabricated  A &

**L2035** Knee-ankle-foot orthotic (KAFO), full plastic, static (pediatric size), without free motion ankle, prefabricated, includes fitting and adjustment  A &

**L2036** Knee-ankle-foot orthotic (KAFO), full plastic, double upright, with or without free motion knee, with or without free motion ankle, custom fabricated  A &

**L2037** Knee-ankle-foot orthotic (KAFO), full plastic, single upright, with or without free motion knee, with or without free motion ankle, custom fabricated  A &

**L2038** Knee-ankle-foot orthotic (KAFO), full plastic, with or without free motion knee, multi-axis ankle, custom fabricated  A &

## Torsion Control: Hip-Knee-Ankle-Foot Orthotic (HKAFO)

**L2040** Hip-knee-ankle-foot orthotic (HKAFO), torsion control, bilateral rotation straps, pelvic band/belt, custom fabricated  A &

**L2050** Hip-knee-ankle-foot orthotic (HKAFO), torsion control, bilateral torsion cables, hip joint, pelvic band/belt, custom fabricated  A &

**L2060** Hip-knee-ankle-foot orthotic (HKAFO), torsion control, bilateral torsion cables, ball bearing hip joint, pelvic band/ belt, custom fabricated  A &

**L2070** Hip-knee-ankle-foot orthotic (HKAFO), torsion control, unilateral rotation straps, pelvic band/belt, custom fabricated  A &

**L2080** Hip-knee-ankle-foot orthotic (HKAFO), torsion control, unilateral torsion cable, hip joint, pelvic band/belt, custom fabricated  A &

**L2090** Hip-knee-ankle-foot orthotic (HKAFO), torsion control, unilateral torsion cable, ball bearing hip joint, pelvic band/ belt, custom fabricated  A &

**L2106** Ankle-foot orthotic (AFO), fracture orthotic, tibial fracture cast orthotic, thermoplastic type casting material, custom fabricated  A &

**L2108** Ankle-foot orthotic (AFO), fracture orthotic, tibial fracture cast orthotic, custom fabricated  A &

**L2112** Ankle-foot orthotic (AFO), fracture orthotic, tibial fracture orthotic, soft, prefabricated, includes fitting and adjustment  A &

**L2114** Ankle-foot orthotic (AFO), fracture orthotic, tibial fracture orthotic, semi-rigid, prefabricated, includes fitting and adjustment  A &

**L2116** Ankle-foot orthotic (AFO), fracture orthotic, tibial fracture orthotic, rigid, prefabricated, includes fitting and adjustment  A &

**L2126** Knee-ankle-foot orthotic (KAFO), fracture orthotic, femoral fracture cast orthotic, thermoplastic type casting material, custom fabricated  A &

**L2128** Knee-ankle-foot orthotic (KAFO), fracture orthotic, femoral fracture cast orthotic, custom fabricated  A &

**L2132** Knee-ankle-foot orthotic (KAFO), fracture orthotic, femoral fracture cast orthotic, soft, prefabricated, includes fitting and adjustment  A &

**L2134** Knee-ankle-foot orthotic (KAFO), fracture orthotic, femoral fracture cast orthotic, semi-rigid, prefabricated, includes fitting and adjustment  A &

**L2136** Knee-ankle-foot orthotic (KAFO), fracture orthotic, femoral fracture cast orthotic, rigid, prefabricated, includes fitting and adjustment  A &

## Additions to Fracture Orthotic

**L2180** Addition to lower extremity fracture orthotic, plastic shoe insert with ankle joints  A &

**L2182** Addition to lower extremity fracture orthotic, drop lock knee joint  A &

**L2184** Addition to lower extremity fracture orthotic, limited motion knee joint  A &

**L2186** Addition to lower extremity fracture orthotic, adjustable motion knee joint, Lerman type  A &

**L2188** Addition to lower extremity fracture orthotic, quadrilateral brim  A &

**L2190** Addition to lower extremity fracture orthotic, waist belt  A &

**L2192** Addition to lower extremity fracture orthotic, hip joint, pelvic band, thigh flange, and pelvic belt  A &

## Additions to Lower Extremity Orthotic: Shoe-Ankle-Shin-Knee

**L2200** Addition to lower extremity, limited ankle motion, each joint  A ☑ &

**L2210** Addition to lower extremity, dorsiflexion assist (plantar flexion resist), each joint  A ☑ &

**L2220** Addition to lower extremity, dorsiflexion and plantar flexion assist/resist, each joint  A ☑ &

**L2230** Addition to lower extremity, split flat caliper stirrups and plate attachment  A &

**L2232** Addition to lower extremity orthotic, rocker bottom for total contact ankle-foot orthotic (AFO), for custom fabricated orthotic only  A &

**L2240** Addition to lower extremity, round caliper and plate attachment  A &

**L2250** Addition to lower extremity, foot plate, molded to patient model, stirrup attachment  A &

**L2260** Addition to lower extremity, reinforced solid stirrup (Scott-Craig type)  A &

**L2265** Addition to lower extremity, long tongue stirrup  A &

---

Special Coverage Instructions    Noncovered by Medicare    Carrier Discretion    ☑ Quantity Alert   ● New Code   ○ Recycled/Reinstated   ▲ Revised Code

© 2016 Optum360, LLC    A2–Z3 ASC Pmt    CMS: Pub 100    AHA: Coding Clinic    & DMEPOS Paid    ⊘ SNF Excluded    L Codes — 105

**Orthotic Devices and Procedures**

**L2270 — L2800**

| Code | Description | |
|------|-------------|---|
| L2270 | Addition to lower extremity, varus/valgus correction (T) strap, padded/lined or malleolus pad | Ⓐ &#9855; |
| L2275 | Addition to lower extremity, varus/valgus correction, plastic modification, padded/lined | Ⓐ &#9855; |
| L2280 | Addition to lower extremity, molded inner boot | Ⓐ &#9855; |
| L2300 | Addition to lower extremity, abduction bar (bilateral hip involvement), jointed, adjustable | Ⓐ &#9855; |
| L2310 | Addition to lower extremity, abduction bar, straight | Ⓐ &#9855; |
| L2320 | Addition to lower extremity, nonmolded lacer, for custom fabricated orthotic only | Ⓐ &#9855; |
| L2330 | Addition to lower extremity, lacer molded to patient model, for custom fabricated orthotic only | Ⓐ &#9855; |
| L2335 | Addition to lower extremity, anterior swing band | Ⓐ &#9855; |
| L2340 | Addition to lower extremity, pretibial shell, molded to patient model | Ⓐ &#9855; |
| L2350 | Addition to lower extremity, prosthetic type, (BK) socket, molded to patient model, (used for PTB, AFO orthoses) | Ⓐ &#9855; |
| L2360 | Addition to lower extremity, extended steel shank | Ⓐ &#9855; |
| L2370 | Addition to lower extremity, Patten bottom | Ⓐ &#9855; |
| L2375 | Addition to lower extremity, torsion control, ankle joint and half solid stirrup | Ⓐ &#9855; |
| L2380 | Addition to lower extremity, torsion control, straight knee joint, each joint | Ⓐ ☑ &#9855; |
| L2385 | Addition to lower extremity, straight knee joint, heavy-duty, each joint | Ⓐ ☑ &#9855; |
| L2387 | Addition to lower extremity, polycentric knee joint, for custom fabricated knee-ankle-foot orthotic (KAFO), each joint | Ⓐ ☑ &#9855; |
| L2390 | Addition to lower extremity, offset knee joint, each joint | Ⓐ ☑ &#9855; |
| L2395 | Addition to lower extremity, offset knee joint, heavy-duty, each joint | Ⓐ ☑ &#9855; |
| L2397 | Addition to lower extremity orthotic, suspension sleeve | Ⓐ &#9855; |

## Additions to Straight Knee or Offset Knee Joints

| Code | Description | |
|------|-------------|---|
| L2405 | Addition to knee joint, drop lock, each | Ⓐ ☑ &#9855; |
| L2415 | Addition to knee lock with integrated release mechanism (bail, cable, or equal), any material, each joint | Ⓐ ☑ &#9855; |
| L2425 | Addition to knee joint, disc or dial lock for adjustable knee flexion, each joint | Ⓐ ☑ &#9855; |
| L2430 | Addition to knee joint, ratchet lock for active and progressive knee extension, each joint | Ⓐ ☑ &#9855; |
| L2492 | Addition to knee joint, lift loop for drop lock ring | Ⓐ &#9855; |

## Additions: Thigh/Weight Bearing - Gluteal/Ischial Weight Bearing

| Code | Description | |
|------|-------------|---|
| L2500 | Addition to lower extremity, thigh/weight bearing, gluteal/ischial weight bearing, ring | Ⓐ &#9855; |
| L2510 | Addition to lower extremity, thigh/weight bearing, quadri-lateral brim, molded to patient model | Ⓐ &#9855; |
| L2520 | Addition to lower extremity, thigh/weight bearing, quadri-lateral brim, custom fitted | Ⓐ &#9855; |
| L2525 | Addition to lower extremity, thigh/weight bearing, ischial containment/narrow M-L brim molded to patient model | Ⓐ &#9855; |
| L2526 | Addition to lower extremity, thigh/weight bearing, ischial containment/narrow M-L brim, custom fitted | Ⓐ &#9855; |

| Code | Description | |
|------|-------------|---|
| L2530 | Addition to lower extremity, thigh/weight bearing, lacer, nonmolded | Ⓐ &#9855; |
| L2540 | Addition to lower extremity, thigh/weight bearing, lacer, molded to patient model | Ⓐ &#9855; |
| L2550 | Addition to lower extremity, thigh/weight bearing, high roll cuff | Ⓐ &#9855; |

## Additions: Pelvic and Thoracic Control

| Code | Description | |
|------|-------------|---|
| L2570 | Addition to lower extremity, pelvic control, hip joint, Clevis type 2 position joint, each | Ⓐ ☑ &#9855; |
| L2580 | Addition to lower extremity, pelvic control, pelvic sling | Ⓐ &#9855; |
| L2600 | Addition to lower extremity, pelvic control, hip joint, Clevis type, or thrust bearing, free, each | Ⓐ ☑ &#9855; |
| L2610 | Addition to lower extremity, pelvic control, hip joint, Clevis or thrust bearing, lock, each | Ⓐ ☑ &#9855; |
| L2620 | Addition to lower extremity, pelvic control, hip joint, heavy-duty, each | Ⓐ ☑ &#9855; |
| L2622 | Addition to lower extremity, pelvic control, hip joint, adjustable flexion, each | Ⓐ ☑ &#9855; |
| L2624 | Addition to lower extremity, pelvic control, hip joint, adjustable flexion, extension, abduction control, each | Ⓐ ☑ &#9855; |
| L2627 | Addition to lower extremity, pelvic control, plastic, molded to patient model, reciprocating hip joint and cables | Ⓐ &#9855; |
| L2628 | Addition to lower extremity, pelvic control, metal frame, reciprocating hip joint and cables | Ⓐ &#9855; |
| L2630 | Addition to lower extremity, pelvic control, band and belt, unilateral | Ⓐ &#9855; |
| L2640 | Addition to lower extremity, pelvic control, band and belt, bilateral | Ⓐ &#9855; |
| L2650 | Addition to lower extremity, pelvic and thoracic control, gluteal pad, each | Ⓐ &#9855; |
| L2660 | Addition to lower extremity, thoracic control, thoracic band | Ⓐ &#9855; |
| L2670 | Addition to lower extremity, thoracic control, paraspinal uprights | Ⓐ &#9855; |
| L2680 | Addition to lower extremity, thoracic control, lateral support uprights | Ⓐ &#9855; |

## Additions: General

| Code | Description | |
|------|-------------|---|
| L2750 | Addition to lower extremity orthotic, plating chrome or nickel, per bar | Ⓐ ☑ &#9855; |
| L2755 | Addition to lower extremity orthotic, high strength, lightweight material, all hybrid lamination/prepreg composite, per segment, for custom fabricated orthotic only | Ⓐ &#9855; |
| L2760 | Addition to lower extremity orthotic, extension, per extension, per bar (for lineal adjustment for growth) | Ⓐ ☑ &#9855; |
| L2768 | Orthotic side bar disconnect device, per bar<br>AHA: 1Q, '02, 5 | Ⓐ ☑ &#9855; |
| L2780 | Addition to lower extremity orthotic, noncorrosive finish, per bar | Ⓐ ☑ &#9855; |
| L2785 | Addition to lower extremity orthotic, drop lock retainer, each | Ⓐ ☑ &#9855; |
| L2795 | Addition to lower extremity orthotic, knee control, full kneecap | Ⓐ &#9855; |
| L2800 | Addition to lower extremity orthotic, knee control, knee cap, medial or lateral pull, for use with custom fabricated orthotic only | Ⓐ &#9855; |

---

Special Coverage Instructions     Noncovered by Medicare     Carrier Discretion     ☑ Quantity Alert  ● New Code   ○ Recycled/Reinstated   ▲ Revised Code

**L2810** Addition to lower extremity orthotic, knee control, condylar pad  A &

**L2820** Addition to lower extremity orthotic, soft interface for molded plastic, below knee section  A &

**L2830** Addition to lower extremity orthotic, soft interface for molded plastic, above knee section  A &

**L2840** Addition to lower extremity orthotic, tibial length sock, fracture or equal, each  A ☑ &

**L2850** Addition to lower extremity orthotic, femoral length sock, fracture or equal, each  A ☑ &

**L2861** Addition to lower extremity joint, knee or ankle, concentric adjustable torsion style mechanism for custom fabricated orthotics only, each  E ☑

**L2999** Lower extremity orthotic, not otherwise specified  A
Determine if an alternative HCPCS Level II or a CPT code better describes the service being reported. This code should be used only if a more specific code is unavailable.

## Orthopedic Footwear

### Inserts

**L3000** Foot insert, removable, molded to patient model, UCB type, Berkeley shell, each  A ☑ &

**L3001** Foot, insert, removable, molded to patient model, Spenco, each  A ☑ &

**L3002** Foot insert, removable, molded to patient model, Plastazote or equal, each  A ☑ &

**L3003** Foot insert, removable, molded to patient model, silicone gel, each  A ☑ &

**L3010** Foot insert, removable, molded to patient model, longitudinal arch support, each  A ☑ &

**L3020** Foot insert, removable, molded to patient model, longitudinal/metatarsal support, each  A ☑ &

**L3030** Foot insert, removable, formed to patient foot, each  A ☑ &

**L3031** Foot, insert/plate, removable, addition to lower extremity orthotic, high strength, lightweight material, all hybrid lamination/prepreg composite, each  A ☑ &

### Arch Support, Removable, Premolded

**L3040** Foot, arch support, removable, premolded, longitudinal, each  A ☑ &

**L3050** Foot, arch support, removable, premolded, metatarsal, each  A ☑ &

**L3060** Foot, arch support, removable, premolded, longitudinal/metatarsal, each  A ☑ &

### Arch Support, Nonremovable, Attached to Shoe

**L3070** Foot, arch support, nonremovable, attached to shoe, longitudinal, each  A ☑ &

**L3080** Foot, arch support, nonremovable, attached to shoe, metatarsal, each  A ☑ &

**L3090** Foot, arch support, nonremovable, attached to shoe, longitudinal/metatarsal, each  A ☑ &

**L3100** Hallus-valgus night dynamic splint, prefabricated, off-the-shelf  A &

## Abduction and Rotation Bars

**L3140** Foot, abduction rotation bar, including shoes  A &

A Denis-Browne style splint is a bar that can be applied by strapping or mounted on a shoe. This type of splint generally corrects congenital conditions such as genu varus

Denis-Browne splint

The angle may be adjusted on a plate on the sole of the shoe

**L3150** Foot, abduction rotation bar, without shoes  A &

**L3160** Foot, adjustable shoe-styled positioning device  A

**L3170** Foot, plastic, silicone or equal, heel stabilizer, prefabricated, off-the-shelf, each  A ☑ &

## Orthopedic Shoes and Boots

**L3201** Orthopedic shoe, Oxford with supinator or pronator, infant  A A

**L3202** Orthopedic shoe, Oxford with supinator or pronator, child  A A

**L3203** Orthopedic shoe, Oxford with supinator or pronator, junior  A A

**L3204** Orthopedic shoe, hightop with supinator or pronator, infant  A A

**L3206** Orthopedic shoe, hightop with supinator or pronator, child  A A

**L3207** Orthopedic shoe, hightop with supinator or pronator, junior  A A

**L3208** Surgical boot, each, infant  A A ☑

**L3209** Surgical boot, each, child  A A ☑

**L3211** Surgical boot, each, junior  A A ☑

**L3212** Benesch boot, pair, infant  A A ☑

**L3213** Benesch boot, pair, child  A A ☑

**L3214** Benesch boot, pair, junior  A A ☑

**L3215** Orthopedic footwear, ladies shoe, oxford, each  A ♀ E ☑

**L3216** Orthopedic footwear, ladies shoe, depth inlay, each  A ♀ E ☑

**L3217** Orthopedic footwear, ladies shoe, hightop, depth inlay, each  A ♀ E ☑

**L3219** Orthopedic footwear, mens shoe, oxford, each  A ♂ E ☑

**L3221** Orthopedic footwear, mens shoe, depth inlay, each  A ♂ E ☑

**L3222** Orthopedic footwear, mens shoe, hightop, depth inlay, each  A ♂ E ☑

**L3224** Orthopedic footwear, woman's shoe, oxford, used as an integral part of a brace (orthotic)  ♀ A &

**L3225** Orthopedic footwear, man's shoe, oxford, used as an integral part of a brace (orthotic)  ♂ A &

**L3230** Orthopedic footwear, custom shoe, depth inlay, each  A ☑

**L3250** Orthopedic footwear, custom molded shoe, removable inner mold, prosthetic shoe, each  A ☑

---

Special Coverage Instructions   Noncovered by Medicare   Carrier Discretion   ☑ Quantity Alert   ● New Code   ○ Recycled/Reinstated   ▲ Revised Code

**Orthotic Devices and Procedures**

**L3251 — L3740**

| | | |
|---|---|---|
| L3251 | Foot, shoe molded to patient model, silicone shoe, each | Ⓐ ☑ |
| L3252 | Foot, shoe molded to patient model, Plastazote (or similar), custom fabricated, each | Ⓐ ☑ |
| L3253 | Foot, molded shoe, Plastazote (or similar), custom fitted, each | Ⓐ ☑ |
| L3254 | Nonstandard size or width | Ⓐ |
| L3255 | Nonstandard size or length | Ⓐ |
| L3257 | Orthopedic footwear, additional charge for split size | Ⓐ |
| L3260 | Surgical boot/shoe, each | Ⓔ ☑ |
| L3265 | Plastazote sandal, each | Ⓐ ☑ |

## Shoe Modification - Lifts

| | | |
|---|---|---|
| L3300 | Lift, elevation, heel, tapered to metatarsals, per in | Ⓐ ☑ &#9855; |
| L3310 | Lift, elevation, heel and sole, neoprene, per in | Ⓐ ☑ &#9855; |
| L3320 | Lift, elevation, heel and sole, cork, per in | Ⓐ ☑ |
| L3330 | Lift, elevation, metal extension (skate) | Ⓐ &#9855; |
| L3332 | Lift, elevation, inside shoe, tapered, up to one-half in | Ⓐ ☑ &#9855; |
| L3334 | Lift, elevation, heel, per in | Ⓐ ☑ &#9855; |

## Shoe Modification - Wedges

| | | |
|---|---|---|
| L3340 | Heel wedge, SACH | Ⓐ &#9855; |
| L3350 | Heel wedge | Ⓐ &#9855; |
| L3360 | Sole wedge, outside sole | Ⓐ &#9855; |
| L3370 | Sole wedge, between sole | Ⓐ &#9855; |
| L3380 | Clubfoot wedge | Ⓐ &#9855; |
| L3390 | Outflare wedge | Ⓐ &#9855; |
| L3400 | Metatarsal bar wedge, rocker | Ⓐ &#9855; |
| L3410 | Metatarsal bar wedge, between sole | Ⓐ &#9855; |
| L3420 | Full sole and heel wedge, between sole | Ⓐ &#9855; |

## Shoe Modifications - Heels

| | | |
|---|---|---|
| L3430 | Heel, counter, plastic reinforced | Ⓐ &#9855; |
| L3440 | Heel, counter, leather reinforced | Ⓐ &#9855; |
| L3450 | Heel, SACH cushion type | Ⓐ &#9855; |
| L3455 | Heel, new leather, standard | Ⓐ &#9855; |
| L3460 | Heel, new rubber, standard | Ⓐ &#9855; |
| L3465 | Heel, Thomas with wedge | Ⓐ &#9855; |
| L3470 | Heel, Thomas extended to ball | Ⓐ &#9855; |
| L3480 | Heel, pad and depression for spur | Ⓐ &#9855; |
| L3485 | Heel, pad, removable for spur | Ⓐ |

## Miscellaneous Shoe Additions

| | | |
|---|---|---|
| L3500 | Orthopedic shoe addition, insole, leather | Ⓐ &#9855; |
| L3510 | Orthopedic shoe addition, insole, rubber | Ⓐ &#9855; |
| L3520 | Orthopedic shoe addition, insole, felt covered with leather | Ⓐ &#9855; |
| L3530 | Orthopedic shoe addition, sole, half | Ⓐ &#9855; |
| L3540 | Orthopedic shoe addition, sole, full | Ⓐ &#9855; |
| L3550 | Orthopedic shoe addition, toe tap, standard | Ⓐ &#9855; |
| L3560 | Orthopedic shoe addition, toe tap, horseshoe | Ⓐ &#9855; |
| L3570 | Orthopedic shoe addition, special extension to instep (leather with eyelets) | Ⓐ &#9855; |
| L3580 | Orthopedic shoe addition, convert instep to Velcro closure | Ⓐ &#9855; |
| L3590 | Orthopedic shoe addition, convert firm shoe counter to soft counter | Ⓐ &#9855; |
| L3595 | Orthopedic shoe addition, March bar | Ⓐ &#9855; |

## Transfer or Replacement

| | | |
|---|---|---|
| L3600 | Transfer of an orthosis from one shoe to another, caliper plate, existing | Ⓐ &#9855; |
| L3610 | Transfer of an orthosis from one shoe to another, caliper plate, new | Ⓐ &#9855; |
| L3620 | Transfer of an orthosis from one shoe to another, solid stirrup, existing | Ⓐ &#9855; |
| L3630 | Transfer of an orthosis from one shoe to another, solid stirrup, new | Ⓐ &#9855; |
| L3640 | Transfer of an orthosis from one shoe to another, Dennis Browne splint (Riveton), both shoes | Ⓐ &#9855; |
| L3649 | Orthopedic shoe, modification, addition or transfer, not otherwise specified | Ⓐ |

L3649 — Determine if an alternative HCPCS Level II or a CPT code better describes the service being reported. This code should be used only if a more specific code is unavailable.

## Shoulder Orthotic (SO)

| | | |
|---|---|---|
| L3650 | Shoulder orthosis, figure of eight design abduction restrainer, prefabricated, off-the-shelf | Ⓐ &#9855; |
| L3660 | Shoulder orthosis, figure of eight design abduction restrainer, canvas and webbing, prefabricated, off-the-shelf | Ⓐ &#9855; |
| L3670 | Shoulder orthosis, acromio/clavicular (canvas and webbing type), prefabricated, off-the-shelf | Ⓐ &#9855; |
| L3671 | Shoulder orthotic (SO), shoulder joint design, without joints, may include soft interface, straps, custom fabricated, includes fitting and adjustment | Ⓐ &#9855; |
| L3674 | Shoulder orthotic, abduction positioning (airplane design), thoracic component and support bar, with or without nontorsion joint/turnbuckle, may include soft interface, straps, custom fabricated, includes fitting and adjustment | Ⓐ &#9855; |
| L3675 | Shoulder orthosis, vest type abduction restrainer, canvas webbing type or equal, prefabricated, off-the-shelf | Ⓐ &#9855; |
| L3677 | Shoulder orthosis, shoulder joint design, without joints, may include soft interface, straps, prefabricated item that has been trimmed, bent, molded, assembled, or otherwise customized to fit a specific patient by an individual with expertise | Ⓐ |

L3677 — **AHA:** 1Q, '02, 5

| | | |
|---|---|---|
| L3678 | Shoulder orthosis, shoulder joint design, without joints, may include soft interface, straps, prefabricated, off-the-shelf | Ⓐ |

## Elbow Orthotic (EO)

| | | |
|---|---|---|
| L3702 | Elbow orthotic (EO), without joints, may include soft interface, straps, custom fabricated, includes fitting and adjustment | Ⓐ &#9855; |
| L3710 | Elbow orthosis, elastic with metal joints, prefabricated, off-the-shelf | Ⓐ &#9855; |
| L3720 | Elbow orthotic (EO), double upright with forearm/arm cuffs, free motion, custom fabricated | Ⓐ &#9855; |
| L3730 | Elbow orthotic (EO), double upright with forearm/arm cuffs, extension/ flexion assist, custom fabricated | Ⓐ &#9855; |
| L3740 | Elbow orthotic (EO), double upright with forearm/arm cuffs, adjustable position lock with active control, custom fabricated | Ⓐ &#9855; |

---

Special Coverage Instructions    Noncovered by Medicare    Carrier Discretion        ☑ Quantity Alert  ● New Code    ○ Recycled/Reinstated    ▲ Revised Code

**L3760** Elbow orthotic (EO), with adjustable position locking joint(s), prefabricated, includes fitting and adjustments, any type  A &

**L3762** Elbow orthosis, rigid, without joints, includes soft interface material, prefabricated, off-the-shelf  A &

**L3763** Elbow-wrist-hand orthotic (EWHO), rigid, without joints, may include soft interface, straps, custom fabricated, includes fitting and adjustment  A &

**L3764** Elbow-wrist-hand orthotic (EWHO), includes one or more nontorsion joints, elastic bands, turnbuckles, may include soft interface, straps, custom fabricated, includes fitting and adjustment  A &

**L3765** Elbow-wrist-hand-finger orthotic (EWHFO), rigid, without joints, may include soft interface, straps, custom fabricated, includes fitting and adjustment  A &

**L3766** Elbow-wrist-hand-finger orthotic (EWHFO), includes one or more nontorsion joints, elastic bands, turnbuckles, may include soft interface, straps, custom fabricated, includes fitting and adjustment  A &

## Wrist-Hand-Finger Orthotic (WHFO)

**L3806** Wrist-hand-finger orthotic (WHFO), includes one or more nontorsion joint(s), turnbuckles, elastic bands/springs, may include soft interface material, straps, custom fabricated, includes fitting and adjustment  A &

**L3807** Wrist hand finger orthosis, without joint(s), prefabricated item that has been trimmed, bent, molded, assembled, or otherwise customized to fit a specific patient by an individual with expertise  A &

**L3808** Wrist-hand-finger orthotic (WHFO), rigid without joints, may include soft interface material; straps, custom fabricated, includes fitting and adjustment  A &

**L3809** Wrist hand finger orthosis, without joint(s), prefabricated, off-the-shelf, any type  A &

## Additions to Upper Extremity Orthotic

**L3891** Addition to upper extremity joint, wrist or elbow, concentric adjustable torsion style mechanism for custom fabricated orthotics only, each  E ☑

## Dynamic Flexor Hinge, Reciprocal Wrist Extension/Flexion, Finger Flexion/Extension

**L3900** Wrist-hand-finger orthotic (WHFO), dynamic flexor hinge, reciprocal wrist extension/ flexion, finger flexion/extension, wrist or finger driven, custom fabricated  A &

**L3901** Wrist-hand-finger orthotic (WHFO), dynamic flexor hinge, reciprocal wrist extension/ flexion, finger flexion/extension, cable driven, custom fabricated  A &

## External Power

**L3904** Wrist-hand-finger orthotic (WHFO), external powered, electric, custom fabricated  A &

## Other Upper Extremity Orthotics

**L3905** Wrist-hand orthotic (WHO), includes one or more nontorsion joints, elastic bands, turnbuckles, may include soft interface, straps, custom fabricated, includes fitting and adjustment  A &

**L3906** Wrist-hand orthosis (WHO), without joints, may include soft interface, straps, custom fabricated, includes fitting and adjustment  A &

**L3908** Wrist hand orthosis, wrist extension control cock-up, non molded, prefabricated, off-the-shelf  A &

**L3912** Hand finger orthosis (HFO), flexion glove with elastic finger control, prefabricated, off-the-shelf  A &

**L3913** Hand finger orthotic (HFO), without joints, may include soft interface, straps, custom fabricated, includes fitting and adjustment  A &

**L3915** Wrist hand orthosis, includes one or more nontorsion joint(s), elastic bands, turnbuckles, may include soft interface, straps, prefabricated item that has been trimmed, bent, molded, assembled, or otherwise customized to fit a specific patient by an individual with expertise  A &

**L3916** Wrist hand orthosis, includes one or more nontorsion joint(s), elastic bands, turnbuckles, may include soft interface, straps, prefabricated, off-the-shelf  A &

**L3917** Hand orthosis, metacarpal fracture orthosis, prefabricated item that has been trimmed, bent, molded, assembled, or otherwise customized to fit a specific patient by an individual with expertise  A &

**L3918** Hand orthosis, metacarpal fracture orthosis, prefabricated, off-the-shelf  A &

**L3919** Hand orthotic (HO), without joints, may include soft interface, straps, custom fabricated, includes fitting and adjustment  A &

**L3921** Hand finger orthotic (HFO), includes one or more nontorsion joints, elastic bands, turnbuckles, may include soft interface, straps, custom fabricated, includes fitting and adjustment  A &

**L3923** Hand finger orthosis, without joints, may include soft interface, straps, prefabricated item that has been trimmed, bent, molded, assembled, or otherwise customized to fit a specific patient by an individual with expertise  A &

**L3924** Hand finger orthosis, without joints, may include soft interface, straps, prefabricated, off-the-shelf  A &

**L3925** Finger orthosis, proximal interphalangeal (PIP)/distal interphalangeal (DIP), non-torsion joint/spring, extension/flexion, may include soft interface material, prefabricated, off-the-shelf  A &

**L3927** Finger orthosis, proximal interphalangeal (PIP)/distal interphalangeal (DIP), without joint/spring, extension/flexion (e.g., static or ring type), may include soft interface material, prefabricated, off-the-shelf  A &

**L3929** Hand finger orthosis, includes one or more nontorsion joint(s), turnbuckles, elastic bands/springs, may include soft interface material, straps, prefabricated item that has been trimmed, bent, molded, assembled, or otherwise customized to fit a specific patient by an individual with expertise  A &

**L3930** Hand finger orthosis, includes one or more nontorsion joint(s), turnbuckles, elastic bands/springs, may include soft interface material, straps, prefabricated, off-the-shelf  A &

**L3931** Wrist-hand-finger orthotic (WHFO), includes one or more nontorsion joint(s), turnbuckles, elastic bands/springs, may include soft interface material, straps, prefabricated, includes fitting and adjustment  A &

**L3933** Finger orthotic (FO), without joints, may include soft interface, custom fabricated, includes fitting and adjustment  A &

**L3935** Finger orthotic, nontorsion joint, may include soft interface, custom fabricated, includes fitting and adjustment  A &

**L3956** Addition of joint to upper extremity orthotic, any material; per joint  A ☑ &

Special Coverage Instructions    Noncovered by Medicare    Carrier Discretion    ☑ Quantity Alert    ● New Code    ○ Recycled/Reinstated    ▲ Revised Code

© 2016 Optum360, LLC    M-Z ASC Pmt    CMS: Pub 100    AHA: Coding Clinic    & DMEPOS Paid    ⊘ SNF Excluded    L Codes — 109

**Orthotic Devices and Procedures**

**L3960 — L4398**

## Shoulder, Elbow, Wrist, Hand Orthotic

**L3960** Shoulder-elbow-wrist-hand orthotic (SEWHO), abduction positioning, airplane design, prefabricated, includes fitting and adjustment Ⓐ &

**L3961** Shoulder elbow wrist hand orthotic (SEWHO), shoulder cap design, without joints, may include soft interface, straps, custom fabricated, includes fitting and adjustment Ⓐ &

**L3962** Shoulder-elbow-wrist-hand orthotic (SEWHO), abduction positioning, Erb's palsy design, prefabricated, includes fitting and adjustment Ⓐ &

**L3967** Shoulder-elbow-wrist-hand orthotic (SEWHO), abduction positioning (airplane design), thoracic component and support bar, without joints, may include soft interface, straps, custom fabricated, includes fitting and adjustment Ⓐ &

## Additions to Mobile Arm Supports

**L3971** Shoulder-elbow-wrist-hand orthotic (SEWHO), shoulder cap design, includes one or more nontorsion joints, elastic bands, turnbuckles, may include soft interface, straps, custom fabricated, includes fitting and adjustment Ⓐ &

**L3973** Shoulder-elbow-wrist-hand orthotic (SEWHO), abduction positioning (airplane design), thoracic component and support bar, includes one or more nontorsion joints, elastic bands, turnbuckles, may include soft interface, straps, custom fabricated, includes fitting and adjustment Ⓐ &

**L3975** Shoulder-elbow-wrist-hand-finger orthotic (SEWHO), shoulder cap design, without joints, may include soft interface, straps, custom fabricated, includes fitting and adjustment Ⓐ &

**L3976** Shoulder-elbow-wrist-hand-finger orthotic (SEWHO), abduction positioning (airplane design), thoracic component and support bar, without joints, may include soft interface, straps, custom fabricated, includes fitting and adjustment Ⓐ &

**L3977** Shoulder-elbow-wrist-hand-finger orthotic (SEWHO), shoulder cap design, includes one or more nontorsion joints, elastic bands, turnbuckles, may include soft interface, straps, custom fabricated, includes fitting and adjustment Ⓐ &

**L3978** Shoulder-elbow-wrist-hand-finger orthotic (SEWHO), abduction positioning (airplane design), thoracic component and support bar, includes one or more nontorsion joints, elastic bands, turnbuckles, may include soft interface, straps, custom fabricated, includes fitting and adjustment Ⓐ &

## Fracture Orthotic

**L3980** Upper extremity fracture orthotic, humeral, prefabricated, includes fitting and adjustment Ⓐ &

**L3981** Upper extremity fracture orthosis, humeral, prefabricated, includes shoulder cap design, with or without joints, forearm section, may include soft interface, straps, includes fitting and adjustments Ⓐ &

**L3982** Upper extremity fracture orthotic, radius/ulnar, prefabricated, includes fitting and adjustment Ⓐ &

**L3984** Upper extremity fracture orthotic, wrist, prefabricated, includes fitting and adjustment Ⓐ &

**L3995** Addition to upper extremity orthotic, sock, fracture or equal, each Ⓐ ☑ &

**L3999** Upper limb orthotic, not otherwise specified Ⓐ

## Repairs

**L4000** Replace girdle for spinal orthotic (cervical-thoracic-lumbar-sacral orthotic (CTLSO) or spinal orthotic SO) Ⓐ &

**L4002** Replacement strap, any orthotic, includes all components, any length, any type Ⓐ &

**L4010** Replace trilateral socket brim Ⓐ &

**L4020** Replace quadrilateral socket brim, molded to patient model Ⓐ &

**L4030** Replace quadrilateral socket brim, custom fitted Ⓐ &

**L4040** Replace molded thigh lacer, for custom fabricated orthotic only Ⓐ &

**L4045** Replace nonmolded thigh lacer, for custom fabricated orthotic only Ⓐ &

**L4050** Replace molded calf lacer, for custom fabricated orthotic only Ⓐ &

**L4055** Replace nonmolded calf lacer, for custom fabricated orthotic only Ⓐ &

**L4060** Replace high roll cuff Ⓐ &

**L4070** Replace proximal and distal upright for KAFO Ⓐ &

**L4080** Replace metal bands KAFO, proximal thigh Ⓐ &

**L4090** Replace metal bands KAFO-AFO, calf or distal thigh Ⓐ &

**L4100** Replace leather cuff KAFO, proximal thigh Ⓐ &

**L4110** Replace leather cuff KAFO-AFO, calf or distal thigh Ⓐ &

**L4130** Replace pretibial shell Ⓐ &

**L4205** Repair of orthotic device, labor component, per 15 minutes Ⓐ ☑

**L4210** Repair of orthotic device, repair or replace minor parts Ⓐ

## Miscellaneous Lower Limb Supports

**L4350** Ankle control orthosis, stirrup style, rigid, includes any type interface (e.g., pneumatic, gel), prefabricated, off-the-shelf Ⓐ &

**L4360** Walking boot, pneumatic and/or vacuum, with or without joints, with or without interface material, prefabricated item that has been trimmed, bent, molded, assembled, or otherwise customized to fit a specific patient by an individual with expertise Ⓐ &

**L4361** Walking boot, pneumatic and/or vacuum, with or without joints, with or without interface material, prefabricated, off-the-shelf Ⓐ &

**L4370** Pneumatic full leg splint, prefabricated, off-the-shelf Ⓐ &

**L4386** Walking boot, non-pneumatic, with or without joints, with or without interface material, prefabricated item that has been trimmed, bent, molded, assembled, or otherwise customized to fit a specific patient by an individual with expertise Ⓐ &

**L4387** Walking boot, non-pneumatic, with or without joints, with or without interface material, prefabricated, off-the-shelf Ⓐ &

**L4392** Replacement, soft interface material, static AFO Ⓐ &

**L4394** Replace soft interface material, foot drop splint Ⓐ &

**L4396** Static or dynamic ankle foot orthosis, including soft interface material, adjustable for fit, for positioning, may be used for minimal ambulation, prefabricated item that has been trimmed, bent, molded, assembled, or otherwise customized to fit a specific patient by an individual with expertise Ⓐ &

**L4397** Static or dynamic ankle foot orthosis, including soft interface material, adjustable for fit, for positioning, may be used for minimal ambulation, prefabricated, off-the-shelf Ⓐ &

**L4398** Foot drop splint, recumbent positioning device, prefabricated, off-the-shelf Ⓐ &

---

Special Coverage Instructions   Noncovered by Medicare   Carrier Discretion   ☑ Quantity Alert   ● New Code   ○ Recycled/Reinstated   ▲ Revised Code

110 — L Codes   Ⓐ Age Edit   Ⓜ Maternity Edit   ♀ Female Only   ♂ Male Only   Ⓐ-Ⓨ OPPS Status Indicators   © 2016 Optum360, LLC

**L4631** Ankle-foot orthotic, walking boot type, varus/valgus correction, rocker bottom, anterior tibial shell, soft interface, custom arch support, plastic or other material, includes straps and closures, custom fabricated [A] ♿

## Prosthetic Procedures L5000-L9900

The codes in this section are considered as "base" or "basic procedures or prosthetics" and may be modified by listing items/procedures or special materials from the "additions" sections and adding them to the base procedure.

### Partial Foot

**L5000** Partial foot, shoe insert with longitudinal arch, toe filler [A] ♿

**L5010** Partial foot, molded socket, ankle height, with toe filler [A] ♿

**L5020** Partial foot, molded socket, tibial tubercle height, with toe filler [A] ♿

### Ankle

**L5050** Ankle, Symes, molded socket, SACH foot [A] ⊘ ♿

**L5060** Ankle, Symes, metal frame, molded leather socket, articulated ankle/foot [A] ⊘ ♿

### Below Knee

**L5100** Below knee, molded socket, shin, SACH foot [A] ⊘ ♿

**L5105** Below knee, plastic socket, joints and thigh lacer, SACH foot [A] ⊘ ♿

### Knee Disarticulation

**L5150** Knee disarticulation (or through knee), molded socket, external knee joints, shin, SACH foot [A] ⊘ ♿

**L5160** Knee disarticulation (or through knee), molded socket, bent knee configuration, external knee joints, shin, SACH foot [A] ⊘ ♿

### Above Knee

**L5200** Above knee, molded socket, single axis constant friction knee, shin, SACH foot [A] ⊘ ♿

**L5210** Above knee, short prosthesis, no knee joint (stubbies), with foot blocks, no ankle joints, each [A] ☑ ⊘ ♿

**L5220** Above knee, short prosthesis, no knee joint (stubbies), with articulated ankle/foot, dynamically aligned, each [A] ☑ ⊘ ♿

**L5230** Above knee, for proximal femoral focal deficiency, constant friction knee, shin, SACH foot [A] ⊘ ♿

### Hip Disarticulation

**L5250** Hip disarticulation, Canadian type; molded socket, hip joint, single axis constant friction knee, shin, SACH foot [A] ⊘ ♿

**L5270** Hip disarticulation, tilt table type; molded socket, locking hip joint, single axis constant friction knee, shin, SACH foot [A] ⊘ ♿

### Hemipelvectomy

**L5280** Hemipelvectomy, Canadian type; molded socket, hip joint, single axis constant friction knee, shin, SACH foot [A] ⊘ ♿

**L5301** Below knee, molded socket, shin, SACH foot, endoskeletal system [A] ⊘ ♿
AHA: 1Q, '02, 5

**L5312** Knee disarticulation (or through knee), molded socket, single axis knee, pylon, SACH foot, endoskeletal system [A] ♿

**L5321** Above knee, molded socket, open end, SACH foot, endoskeletal system, single axis knee [A] ⊘ ♿
AHA: 1Q, '02, 5

**L5331** Hip disarticulation, Canadian type, molded socket, endoskeletal system, hip joint, single axis knee, SACH foot [A] ⊘ ♿
AHA: 1Q, '02, 5

**L5341** Hemipelvectomy, Canadian type, molded socket, endoskeletal system, hip joint, single axis knee, SACH foot [A] ⊘ ♿
AHA: 1Q, '02, 5

### Immediate Postsurgical or Early Fitting Procedures

**L5400** Immediate postsurgical or early fitting, application of initial rigid dressing, including fitting, alignment, suspension, and one cast change, below knee [A] ☑ ♿

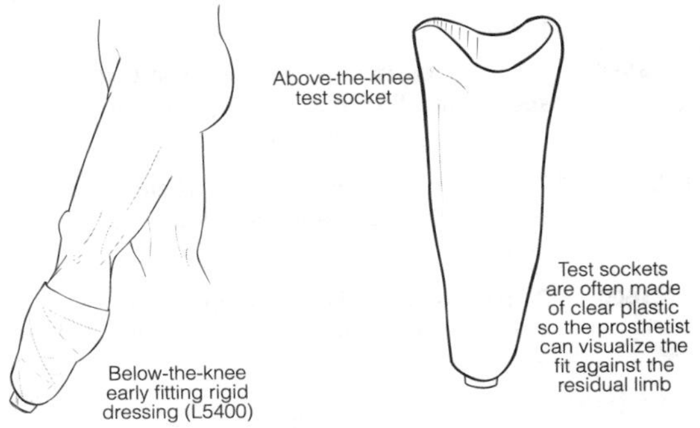
Above-the-knee test socket
Test sockets are often made of clear plastic so the prosthetist can visualize the fit against the residual limb
Below-the-knee early fitting rigid dressing (L5400)

**L5410** Immediate postsurgical or early fitting, application of initial rigid dressing, including fitting, alignment and suspension, below knee, each additional cast change and realignment [A] ☑ ♿

**L5420** Immediate postsurgical or early fitting, application of initial rigid dressing, including fitting, alignment and suspension and one cast change AK or knee disarticulation [A] ☑ ♿

**L5430** Immediate postsurgical or early fitting, application of initial rigid dressing, including fitting, alignment and suspension, AK or knee disarticulation, each additional cast change and realignment [A] ☑ ♿

**L5450** Immediate postsurgical or early fitting, application of nonweight bearing rigid dressing, below knee [A] ♿

**L5460** Immediate postsurgical or early fitting, application of nonweight bearing rigid dressing, above knee [A] ♿

### Initial Prosthesis

**L5500** Initial, below knee PTB type socket, nonalignable system, pylon, no cover, SACH foot, plaster socket, direct formed [A] ⊘ ♿

**L5505** Initial, above knee, knee disarticulation, ischial level socket, nonalignable system, pylon, no cover, SACH foot, plaster socket, direct formed [A] ⊘ ♿

### Preparatory Prosthesis

**L5510** Preparatory, below knee PTB type socket, nonalignable system, pylon, no cover, SACH foot, plaster socket, molded to model [A] ⊘ ♿

**L5520** Preparatory, below knee PTB type socket, nonalignable system, pylon, no cover, SACH foot, thermoplastic or equal, direct formed [A] ⊘ ♿

**L5530** Preparatory, below knee PTB type socket, nonalignable system, pylon, no cover, SACH foot, thermoplastic or equal, molded to model [A] ⊘ ♿

**L5535** Preparatory, below knee PTB type socket, nonalignable system, no cover, SACH foot, prefabricated, adjustable open end socket [A] ⊘ ♿

**L5540** Preparatory, below knee PTB type socket, nonalignable system, pylon, no cover, SACH foot, laminated socket, molded to model [A] ⊘ ♿

**L5560** Preparatory, above knee, knee disarticulation, ischial level socket, nonalignable system, pylon, no cover, SACH foot, plaster socket, molded to model [A] ⊘ ♿


© 2016 Optum360, LLC

**L5570** Preparatory, above knee - knee disarticulation, ischial level socket, nonalignable system, pylon, no cover, SACH foot, thermoplastic or equal, direct formed Ⓐ⊘♿

**L5580** Preparatory, above knee, knee disarticulation, ischial level socket, nonalignable system, pylon, no cover, SACH foot, thermoplastic or equal, molded to model Ⓐ⊘♿

**L5585** Preparatory, above knee - knee disarticulation, ischial level socket, nonalignable system, pylon, no cover, SACH foot, prefabricated adjustable open end socket Ⓐ⊘♿

**L5590** Preparatory, above knee, knee disarticulation, ischial level socket, nonalignable system, pylon, no cover, SACH foot, laminated socket, molded to model Ⓐ⊘♿

**L5595** Preparatory, hip disarticulation/hemipelvectomy, pylon, no cover, SACH foot, thermoplastic or equal, molded to patient model Ⓐ⊘♿

**L5600** Preparatory, hip disarticulation/hemipelvectomy, pylon, no cover, SACH foot, laminated socket, molded to patient model Ⓐ⊘♿

## Additions

### Additions: Lower Extremity

**L5610** Addition to lower extremity, endoskeletal system, above knee, hydracadence system Ⓐ⊘♿

**L5611** Addition to lower extremity, endoskeletal system, above knee, knee disarticulation, 4-bar linkage, with friction swing phase control Ⓐ⊘♿

**L5613** Addition to lower extremity, endoskeletal system, above knee, knee disarticulation, 4-bar linkage, with hydraulic swing phase control Ⓐ⊘♿

**L5614** Addition to lower extremity, exoskeletal system, above knee-knee disarticulation, 4 bar linkage, with pneumatic swing phase control Ⓐ⊘♿

**L5616** Addition to lower extremity, endoskeletal system, above knee, universal multiplex system, friction swing phase control Ⓐ⊘♿

**L5617** Addition to lower extremity, quick change self-aligning unit, above knee or below knee, each Ⓐ☑♿

### Additions: Test Sockets

**L5618** Addition to lower extremity, test socket, Symes Ⓐ⊘♿

**L5620** Addition to lower extremity, test socket, below knee Ⓐ⊘♿

**L5622** Addition to lower extremity, test socket, knee disarticulation Ⓐ⊘♿

**L5624** Addition to lower extremity, test socket, above knee Ⓐ⊘♿

**L5626** Addition to lower extremity, test socket, hip disarticulation Ⓐ⊘♿

**L5628** Addition to lower extremity, test socket, hemipelvectomy Ⓐ⊘♿

**L5629** Addition to lower extremity, below knee, acrylic socket Ⓐ⊘♿

### Additions: Socket Variations

**L5630** Addition to lower extremity, Symes type, expandable wall socket Ⓐ⊘♿

**L5631** Addition to lower extremity, above knee or knee disarticulation, acrylic socket Ⓐ⊘♿

**L5632** Addition to lower extremity, Symes type, PTB brim design socket Ⓐ⊘♿

**L5634** Addition to lower extremity, Symes type, posterior opening (Canadian) socket Ⓐ⊘♿

**L5636** Addition to lower extremity, Symes type, medial opening socket Ⓐ⊘♿

**L5637** Addition to lower extremity, below knee, total contact Ⓐ⊘♿

**L5638** Addition to lower extremity, below knee, leather socket Ⓐ⊘♿

**L5639** Addition to lower extremity, below knee, wood socket Ⓐ⊘♿

**L5640** Addition to lower extremity, knee disarticulation, leather socket Ⓐ⊘♿

**L5642** Addition to lower extremity, above knee, leather socket Ⓐ⊘♿

**L5643** Addition to lower extremity, hip disarticulation, flexible inner socket, external frame Ⓐ⊘♿

**L5644** Addition to lower extremity, above knee, wood socket Ⓐ⊘♿

**L5645** Addition to lower extremity, below knee, flexible inner socket, external frame Ⓐ⊘♿

**L5646** Addition to lower extremity, below knee, air, fluid, gel or equal, cushion socket Ⓐ⊘♿

**L5647** Addition to lower extremity, below knee, suction socket Ⓐ⊘♿

**L5648** Addition to lower extremity, above knee, air, fluid, gel or equal, cushion socket Ⓐ⊘♿

**L5649** Addition to lower extremity, ischial containment/narrow M-L socket Ⓐ⊘♿

**L5650** Additions to lower extremity, total contact, above knee or knee disarticulation socket Ⓐ⊘♿

**L5651** Addition to lower extremity, above knee, flexible inner socket, external frame Ⓐ⊘♿

**L5652** Addition to lower extremity, suction suspension, above knee or knee disarticulation socket Ⓐ⊘♿

**L5653** Addition to lower extremity, knee disarticulation, expandable wall socket Ⓐ⊘♿

### Additions: Socket Insert and Suspension

**L5654** Addition to lower extremity, socket insert, Symes, (Kemblo, Pelite, Aliplast, Plastazote or equal) Ⓐ⊘♿

**L5655** Addition to lower extremity, socket insert, below knee (Kemblo, Pelite, Aliplast, Plastazote or equal) Ⓐ⊘♿

**L5656** Addition to lower extremity, socket insert, knee disarticulation (Kemblo, Pelite, Aliplast, Plastazote or equal) Ⓐ⊘♿

**L5658** Addition to lower extremity, socket insert, above knee (Kemblo, Pelite, Aliplast, Plastazote or equal) Ⓐ⊘♿

**L5661** Addition to lower extremity, socket insert, multidurometer Symes Ⓐ⊘♿

**L5665** Addition to lower extremity, socket insert, multidurometer, below knee Ⓐ⊘♿

**L5666** Addition to lower extremity, below knee, cuff suspension Ⓐ⊘♿

**L5668** Addition to lower extremity, below knee, molded distal cushion Ⓐ⊘♿

Special Coverage Instructions    Noncovered by Medicare    Carrier Discretion    ☑ Quantity Alert   ● New Code   ○ Recycled/Reinstated   ▲ Revised Code

112 — L Codes    Ⓐ Age Edit    Ⓜ Maternity Edit    ♀ Female Only    ♂ Male Only    Ⓐ-Ⓨ OPPS Status Indicators    © 2016 Optum360, LLC

**L5670** Addition to lower extremity, below knee, molded supracondylar suspension (PTS or similar) A ⊘ ㅎ

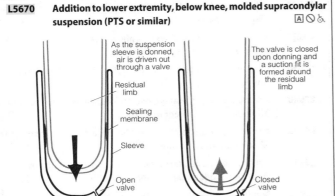

**L5671** Addition to lower extremity, below knee/above knee suspension locking mechanism (shuttle, lanyard, or equal), excludes socket insert A ⊘ ㅎ

AHA: 1Q, '02, 5

**L5672** Addition to lower extremity, below knee, removable medial brim suspension A ⊘ ㅎ

**L5673** Addition to lower extremity, below knee/above knee, custom fabricated from existing mold or prefabricated, socket insert, silicone gel, elastomeric or equal, for use with locking mechanism A ⊘ ㅎ

**L5676** Additions to lower extremity, below knee, knee joints, single axis, pair A ☑ ⊘ ㅎ

**L5677** Additions to lower extremity, below knee, knee joints, polycentric, pair A ☑ ⊘ ㅎ

**L5678** Additions to lower extremity, below knee, joint covers, pair A ☑ ⊘ ㅎ

**L5679** Addition to lower extremity, below knee/above knee, custom fabricated from existing mold or prefabricated, socket insert, silicone gel, elastomeric or equal, not for use with locking mechanism A ⊘ ㅎ

**L5680** Addition to lower extremity, below knee, thigh lacer, nonmolded A ⊘ ㅎ

**L5681** Addition to lower extremity, below knee/above knee, custom fabricated socket insert for congenital or atypical traumatic amputee, silicone gel, elastomeric or equal, for use with or without locking mechanism, initial only (for other than initial, use code L5673 or L5679) A ⊘ ㅎ

**L5682** Addition to lower extremity, below knee, thigh lacer, gluteal/ischial, molded A ⊘ ㅎ

**L5683** Addition to lower extremity, below knee/above knee, custom fabricated socket insert for other than congenital or atypical traumatic amputee, silicone gel, elastomeric or equal, for use with or without locking mechanism, initial only (for other than initial, use code L5673 or L5679) A ⊘ ㅎ

**L5684** Addition to lower extremity, below knee, fork strap A ⊘ ㅎ

**L5685** Addition to lower extremity prosthesis, below knee, suspension/sealing sleeve, with or without valve, any material, each A ⊘ ㅎ

**L5686** Addition to lower extremity, below knee, back check (extension control) A ⊘ ㅎ

**L5688** Addition to lower extremity, below knee, waist belt, webbing A ⊘ ㅎ

**L5690** Addition to lower extremity, below knee, waist belt, padded and lined A ⊘ ㅎ

**L5692** Addition to lower extremity, above knee, pelvic control belt, light A ⊘ ㅎ

**L5694** Addition to lower extremity, above knee, pelvic control belt, padded and lined A ⊘ ㅎ

**L5695** Addition to lower extremity, above knee, pelvic control, sleeve suspension, neoprene or equal, each A ☑ ⊘ ㅎ

**L5696** Addition to lower extremity, above knee or knee disarticulation, pelvic joint A ⊘ ㅎ

**L5697** Addition to lower extremity, above knee or knee disarticulation, pelvic band A ⊘ ㅎ

**L5698** Addition to lower extremity, above knee or knee disarticulation, Silesian bandage A ⊘ ㅎ

**L5699** All lower extremity prostheses, shoulder harness A ⊘ ㅎ

## Replacements

**L5700** Replacement, socket, below knee, molded to patient model A ⊘ ㅎ

**L5701** Replacement, socket, above knee/knee disarticulation, including attachment plate, molded to patient model A ⊘ ㅎ

**L5702** Replacement, socket, hip disarticulation, including hip joint, molded to patient model A ⊘ ㅎ

**L5703** Ankle, Symes, molded to patient model, socket without solid ankle cushion heel (SACH) foot, replacement only A ⊘ ㅎ

**L5704** Custom shaped protective cover, below knee A ⊘ ㅎ

**L5705** Custom shaped protective cover, above knee A ⊘ ㅎ

**L5706** Custom shaped protective cover, knee disarticulation A ⊘ ㅎ

**L5707** Custom shaped protective cover, hip disarticulation A ⊘ ㅎ

## Additions: Exoskeletal Knee-Shin System

**L5710** Addition, exoskeletal knee-shin system, single axis, manual lock A ⊘ ㅎ

**L5711** Additions exoskeletal knee-shin system, single axis, manual lock, ultra-light material A ⊘ ㅎ

**L5712** Addition, exoskeletal knee-shin system, single axis, friction swing and stance phase control (safety knee) A ⊘ ㅎ

**L5714** Addition, exoskeletal knee-shin system, single axis, variable friction swing phase control A ⊘ ㅎ

**L5716** Addition, exoskeletal knee-shin system, polycentric, mechanical stance phase lock A ⊘ ㅎ

**L5718** Addition, exoskeletal knee-shin system, polycentric, friction swing and stance phase control A ⊘ ㅎ

**L5722** Addition, exoskeletal knee-shin system, single axis, pneumatic swing, friction stance phase control A ⊘ ㅎ

**L5724** Addition, exoskeletal knee-shin system, single axis, fluid swing phase control A ⊘ ㅎ

**L5726** Addition, exoskeletal knee-shin system, single axis, external joints, fluid swing phase control A ⊘ ㅎ

**L5728** Addition, exoskeletal knee-shin system, single axis, fluid swing and stance phase control A ⊘ ㅎ

**L5780** Addition, exoskeletal knee-shin system, single axis, pneumatic/hydra pneumatic swing phase control A ⊘ ㅎ

**L5781** Addition to lower limb prosthesis, vacuum pump, residual limb volume management and moisture evacuation system A ⊘ ㅎ

**L5782** Addition to lower limb prosthesis, vacuum pump, residual limb volume management and moisture evacuation system, heavy-duty A ⊘ ㅎ

Special Coverage Instructions | Noncovered by Medicare | Carrier Discretion | ☑ Quantity Alert | ● New Code | ○ Recycled/Reinstated | ▲ Revised Code

© 2016 Optum360, LLC | A2-Z3 ASC Pmt | CMS: Pub 100 | AHA: Coding Clinic | ㅎ DMEPOS Paid | ⊘ SNF Excluded | L Codes — 113

**Prosthetic Procedures**

**L5785 — L5976**

## Component Modification

**L5785**   Addition, exoskeletal system, below knee, ultra-light material (titanium, carbon fiber or equal)   Ⓐ ⊘ ♿

**L5790**   Addition, exoskeletal system, above knee, ultra-light material (titanium, carbon fiber or equal)   Ⓐ ⊘ ♿

**L5795**   Addition, exoskeletal system, hip disarticulation, ultra-light material (titanium, carbon fiber or equal)   Ⓐ ⊘ ♿

## Additions: Endoskeletal Knee-Shin System

**L5810**   Addition, endoskeletal knee-shin system, single axis, manual lock   Ⓐ ⊘ ♿

**L5811**   Addition, endoskeletal knee-shin system, single axis, manual lock, ultra-light material   Ⓐ ⊘ ♿

**L5812**   Addition, endoskeletal knee-shin system, single axis, friction swing and stance phase control (safety knee)   Ⓐ ⊘ ♿

**L5814**   Addition, endoskeletal knee-shin system, polycentric, hydraulic swing phase control, mechanical stance phase lock   Ⓐ ⊘ ♿

**L5816**   Addition, endoskeletal knee-shin system, polycentric, mechanical stance phase lock   Ⓐ ⊘ ♿

**L5818**   Addition, endoskeletal knee-shin system, polycentric, friction swing and stance phase control   Ⓐ ⊘ ♿

**L5822**   Addition, endoskeletal knee-shin system, single axis, pneumatic swing, friction stance phase control   Ⓐ ⊘ ♿

**L5824**   Addition, endoskeletal knee-shin system, single axis, fluid swing phase control   Ⓐ ⊘ ♿

**L5826**   Addition, endoskeletal knee-shin system, single axis, hydraulic swing phase control, with miniature high activity frame   Ⓐ ⊘ ♿

**L5828**   Addition, endoskeletal knee-shin system, single axis, fluid swing and stance phase control   Ⓐ ⊘ ♿

**L5830**   Addition, endoskeletal knee-shin system, single axis, pneumatic/swing phase control   Ⓐ ⊘ ♿

**L5840**   Addition, endoskeletal knee-shin system, 4-bar linkage or multiaxial, pneumatic swing phase control   Ⓐ ⊘ ♿

**L5845**   Addition, endoskeletal knee-shin system, stance flexion feature, adjustable   Ⓐ ⊘ ♿

**L5848**   Addition to endoskeletal knee-shin system, fluid stance extension, dampening feature, with or without adjustability   Ⓐ ⊘ ♿

**L5850**   Addition, endoskeletal system, above knee or hip disarticulation, knee extension assist   Ⓐ ⊘ ♿

**L5855**   Addition, endoskeletal system, hip disarticulation, mechanical hip extension assist   Ⓐ ⊘ ♿

**L5856**   Addition to lower extremity prosthesis, endoskeletal knee-shin system, microprocessor control feature, swing and stance phase, includes electronic sensor(s), any type   Ⓐ ⊘ ♿

**L5857**   Addition to lower extremity prosthesis, endoskeletal knee-shin system, microprocessor control feature, swing phase only, includes electronic sensor(s), any type   Ⓐ ⊘ ♿

**L5858**   Addition to lower extremity prosthesis, endoskeletal knee shin system, microprocessor control feature, stance phase only, includes electronic sensor(s), any type   Ⓐ ⊘ ♿

**L5859**   Addition to lower extremity prosthesis, endoskeletal knee-shin system, powered and programmable flexion/extension assist control, includes any type motor(s)   Ⓐ ♿

**L5910**   Addition, endoskeletal system, below knee, alignable system   Ⓐ ⊘ ♿

**L5920**   Addition, endoskeletal system, above knee or hip disarticulation, alignable system   Ⓐ ⊘ ♿

**L5925**   Addition, endoskeletal system, above knee, knee disarticulation or hip disarticulation, manual lock   Ⓐ ⊘ ♿

**L5930**   Addition, endoskeletal system, high activity knee control frame   Ⓐ ⊘ ♿

**L5940**   Addition, endoskeletal system, below knee, ultra-light material (titanium, carbon fiber or equal)   Ⓐ ⊘ ♿

**L5950**   Addition, endoskeletal system, above knee, ultra-light material (titanium, carbon fiber or equal)   Ⓐ ⊘ ♿

**L5960**   Addition, endoskeletal system, hip disarticulation, ultra-light material (titanium, carbon fiber or equal)   Ⓐ ⊘ ♿

**L5961**   Addition, endoskeletal system, polycentric hip joint, pneumatic or hydraulic control, rotation control, with or without flexion and/or extension control   Ⓐ ♿

**L5962**   Addition, endoskeletal system, below knee, flexible protective outer surface covering system   Ⓐ ⊘ ♿

**L5964**   Addition, endoskeletal system, above knee, flexible protective outer surface covering system   Ⓐ ⊘ ♿

**L5966**   Addition, endoskeletal system, hip disarticulation, flexible protective outer surface covering system   Ⓐ ⊘ ♿

**L5968**   Addition to lower limb prosthesis, multiaxial ankle with swing phase active dorsiflexion feature   Ⓐ ⊘ ♿

**L5969**   Addition, endoskeletal ankle-foot or ankle system, power assist, includes any type motor(s)   Ⓐ

**L5970**   All lower extremity prostheses, foot, external keel, SACH foot   Ⓐ ⊘ ♿

**L5971**   All lower extremity prostheses, solid ankle cushion heel (SACH) foot, replacement only   Ⓐ ⊘ ♿

**L5972**   All lower extremity prostheses, foot, flexible keel   Ⓐ ⊘ ♿

**L5973**   Endoskeletal ankle foot system, microprocessor controlled feature, dorsiflexion and/or plantar flexion control, includes power source   Ⓐ ⊘ ♿

**L5974**   All lower extremity prostheses, foot, single axis ankle/foot   Ⓐ ⊘ ♿

Foot prosthesis (L5974)

Energy storing foot (L5976)

Carbon

**L5975**   All lower extremity prostheses, combination single axis ankle and flexible keel foot   Ⓐ ⊘ ♿

**L5976**   All lower extremity prostheses, energy storing foot (Seattle Carbon Copy II or equal)   Ⓐ ⊘ ♿

Special Coverage Instructions   Noncovered by Medicare   Carrier Discretion   ☑ Quantity Alert   ● New Code   ○ Recycled/Reinstated   ▲ Revised Code
Ⓐ Age Edit   Ⓜ Maternity Edit   ♀ Female Only   ♂ Male Only   Ⓐ-Ⓨ OPPS Status Indicators   © 2016 Optum360, LLC

**L5978** All lower extremity prostheses, foot, multiaxial ankle/foot ⒶⓈ⅋

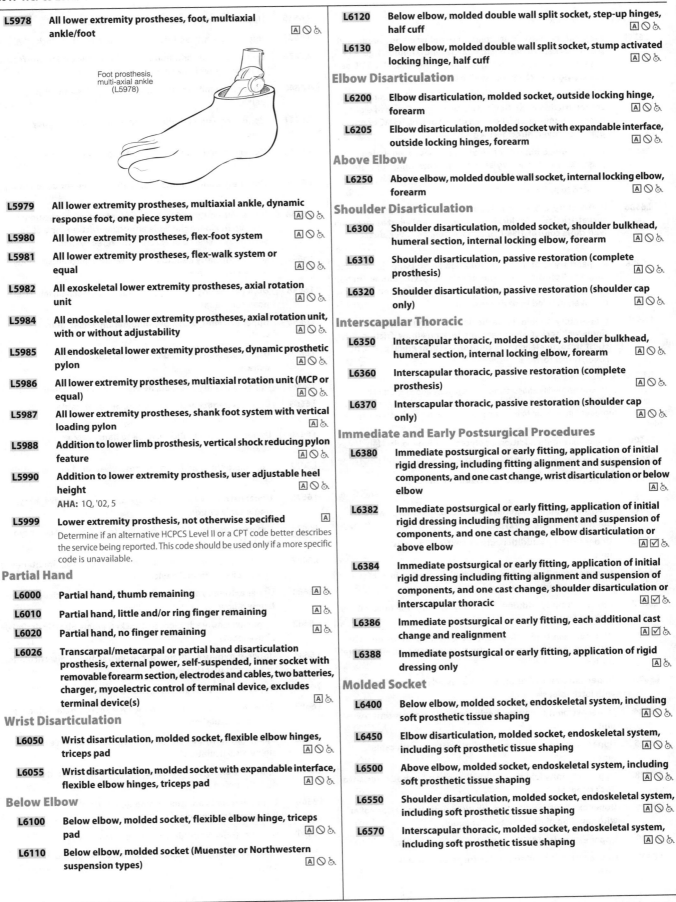

Foot prosthesis, multi-axial ankle (L5978)

**L5979** All lower extremity prostheses, multiaxial ankle, dynamic response foot, one piece system ⒶⓈ⅋

**L5980** All lower extremity prostheses, flex-foot system ⒶⓈ⅋

**L5981** All lower extremity prostheses, flex-walk system or equal ⒶⓈ⅋

**L5982** All exoskeletal lower extremity prostheses, axial rotation unit ⒶⓈ⅋

**L5984** All endoskeletal lower extremity prostheses, axial rotation unit, with or without adjustability ⒶⓈ⅋

**L5985** All endoskeletal lower extremity prostheses, dynamic prosthetic pylon ⒶⓈ⅋

**L5986** All lower extremity prostheses, multiaxial rotation unit (MCP or equal) ⒶⓈ⅋

**L5987** All lower extremity prostheses, shank foot system with vertical loading pylon ⒶⓈ⅋

**L5988** Addition to lower limb prosthesis, vertical shock reducing pylon feature ⒶⓈ⅋

**L5990** Addition to lower extremity prosthesis, user adjustable heel height ⒶⓈ⅋

AHA: 1Q, '02, 5

**L5999** Lower extremity prosthesis, not otherwise specified Ⓐ

Determine if an alternative HCPCS Level II or a CPT code better describes the service being reported. This code should be used only if a more specific code is unavailable.

## Partial Hand

**L6000** Partial hand, thumb remaining Ⓐ⅋

**L6010** Partial hand, little and/or ring finger remaining Ⓐ⅋

**L6020** Partial hand, no finger remaining Ⓐ⅋

**L6026** Transcarpal/metacarpal or partial hand disarticulation prosthesis, external power, self-suspended, inner socket with removable forearm section, electrodes and cables, two batteries, charger, myoelectric control of terminal device, excludes terminal device(s) Ⓐ⅋

## Wrist Disarticulation

**L6050** Wrist disarticulation, molded socket, flexible elbow hinges, triceps pad ⒶⓈ⅋

**L6055** Wrist disarticulation, molded socket with expandable interface, flexible elbow hinges, triceps pad ⒶⓈ⅋

## Below Elbow

**L6100** Below elbow, molded socket, flexible elbow hinge, triceps pad ⒶⓈ⅋

**L6110** Below elbow, molded socket (Muenster or Northwestern suspension types) ⒶⓈ⅋

**L6120** Below elbow, molded double wall split socket, step-up hinges, half cuff ⒶⓈ⅋

**L6130** Below elbow, molded double wall split socket, stump activated locking hinge, half cuff ⒶⓈ⅋

## Elbow Disarticulation

**L6200** Elbow disarticulation, molded socket, outside locking hinge, forearm ⒶⓈ⅋

**L6205** Elbow disarticulation, molded socket with expandable interface, outside locking hinges, forearm ⒶⓈ⅋

## Above Elbow

**L6250** Above elbow, molded double wall socket, internal locking elbow, forearm ⒶⓈ⅋

## Shoulder Disarticulation

**L6300** Shoulder disarticulation, molded socket, shoulder bulkhead, humeral section, internal locking elbow, forearm ⒶⓈ⅋

**L6310** Shoulder disarticulation, passive restoration (complete prosthesis) ⒶⓈ⅋

**L6320** Shoulder disarticulation, passive restoration (shoulder cap only) ⒶⓈ⅋

## Interscapular Thoracic

**L6350** Interscapular thoracic, molded socket, shoulder bulkhead, humeral section, internal locking elbow, forearm ⒶⓈ⅋

**L6360** Interscapular thoracic, passive restoration (complete prosthesis) ⒶⓈ⅋

**L6370** Interscapular thoracic, passive restoration (shoulder cap only) ⒶⓈ⅋

## Immediate and Early Postsurgical Procedures

**L6380** Immediate postsurgical or early fitting, application of initial rigid dressing, including fitting alignment and suspension of components, and one cast change, wrist disarticulation or below elbow Ⓐ⅋

**L6382** Immediate postsurgical or early fitting, application of initial rigid dressing including fitting alignment and suspension of components, and one cast change, elbow disarticulation or above elbow Ⓐ☑⅋

**L6384** Immediate postsurgical or early fitting, application of initial rigid dressing including fitting alignment and suspension of components, and one cast change, shoulder disarticulation or interscapular thoracic Ⓐ☑⅋

**L6386** Immediate postsurgical or early fitting, each additional cast change and realignment Ⓐ☑⅋

**L6388** Immediate postsurgical or early fitting, application of rigid dressing only Ⓐ⅋

## Molded Socket

**L6400** Below elbow, molded socket, endoskeletal system, including soft prosthetic tissue shaping ⒶⓈ⅋

**L6450** Elbow disarticulation, molded socket, endoskeletal system, including soft prosthetic tissue shaping ⒶⓈ⅋

**L6500** Above elbow, molded socket, endoskeletal system, including soft prosthetic tissue shaping ⒶⓈ⅋

**L6550** Shoulder disarticulation, molded socket, endoskeletal system, including soft prosthetic tissue shaping ⒶⓈ⅋

**L6570** Interscapular thoracic, molded socket, endoskeletal system, including soft prosthetic tissue shaping ⒶⓈ⅋

Special Coverage Instructions    Noncovered by Medicare    Carrier Discretion    ☑ Quantity Alert   ● New Code   ○ Recycled/Reinstated   ▲ Revised Code

© 2016 Optum360, LLC    Ⓜ-Ⓩ ASC Pmt    CMS: Pub 100    AHA: Coding Clinic    ⅋ DMEPOS Paid    Ⓢ SNF Excluded    L Codes — 115

## Preparatory Socket

**L6580** Preparatory, wrist disarticulation or below elbow, single wall plastic socket, friction wrist, flexible elbow hinges, figure of eight harness, humeral cuff, Bowden cable control, USMC or equal pylon, no cover, molded to patient model   Ⓐ ⊘ ♿

**L6582** Preparatory, wrist disarticulation or below elbow, single wall socket, friction wrist, flexible elbow hinges, figure of eight harness, humeral cuff, Bowden cable control, USMC or equal pylon, no cover, direct formed   Ⓐ ⊘ ♿

**L6584** Preparatory, elbow disarticulation or above elbow, single wall plastic socket, friction wrist, locking elbow, figure of eight harness, fair lead cable control, USMC or equal pylon, no cover, molded to patient model   Ⓐ ⊘ ♿

**L6586** Preparatory, elbow disarticulation or above elbow, single wall socket, friction wrist, locking elbow, figure of eight harness, fair lead cable control, USMC or equal pylon, no cover, direct formed   Ⓐ ⊘ ♿

**L6588** Preparatory, shoulder disarticulation or interscapular thoracic, single wall plastic socket, shoulder joint, locking elbow, friction wrist, chest strap, fair lead cable control, USMC or equal pylon, no cover, molded to patient model   Ⓐ ⊘ ♿

**L6590** Preparatory, shoulder disarticulation or interscapular thoracic, single wall socket, shoulder joint, locking elbow, friction wrist, chest strap, fair lead cable control, USMC or equal pylon, no cover, direct formed   Ⓐ ⊘ ♿

## Additions: Upper Limb

The following procedures/modifications/components may be added to other base procedures. The items in this section should reflect the additional complexity of each modification procedure, in addition to the base procedure, at the time of the original order.

**L6600** Upper extremity additions, polycentric hinge, pair   Ⓐ ☑ ⊘ ♿

**L6605** Upper extremity additions, single pivot hinge, pair   Ⓐ ☑ ⊘ ♿

**L6610** Upper extremity additions, flexible metal hinge, pair   Ⓐ ☑ ⊘ ♿

**L6611** Addition to upper extremity prosthesis, external powered, additional switch, any type   Ⓐ ⊘ ♿

**L6615** Upper extremity addition, disconnect locking wrist unit   Ⓐ ⊘ ♿

**L6616** Upper extremity addition, additional disconnect insert for locking wrist unit, each   Ⓐ ☑ ⊘ ♿

**L6620** Upper extremity addition, flexion/extension wrist unit, with or without friction   Ⓐ ⊘ ♿

**L6621** Upper extremity prosthesis addition, flexion/extension wrist with or without friction, for use with external powered terminal device   Ⓐ ⊘ ♿

**L6623** Upper extremity addition, spring assisted rotational wrist unit with latch release   Ⓐ ⊘ ♿

**L6624** Upper extremity addition, flexion/extension and rotation wrist unit   Ⓐ ⊘ ♿

**L6625** Upper extremity addition, rotation wrist unit with cable lock   Ⓐ ⊘ ♿

**L6628** Upper extremity addition, quick disconnect hook adapter, Otto Bock or equal   Ⓐ ⊘ ♿

**L6629** Upper extremity addition, quick disconnect lamination collar with coupling piece, Otto Bock or equal   Ⓐ ⊘ ♿

**L6630** Upper extremity addition, stainless steel, any wrist   Ⓐ ⊘ ♿

**L6632** Upper extremity addition, latex suspension sleeve, each   Ⓐ ☑ ⊘ ♿

**L6635** Upper extremity addition, lift assist for elbow   Ⓐ ⊘ ♿

**L6637** Upper extremity addition, nudge control elbow lock   Ⓐ ⊘ ♿

**L6638** Upper extremity addition to prosthesis, electric locking feature, only for use with manually powered elbow   Ⓐ ⊘ ♿

**L6640** Upper extremity additions, shoulder abduction joint, pair   Ⓐ ☑ ⊘ ♿

**L6641** Upper extremity addition, excursion amplifier, pulley type   Ⓐ ⊘ ♿

**L6642** Upper extremity addition, excursion amplifier, lever type   Ⓐ ⊘ ♿

**L6645** Upper extremity addition, shoulder flexion-abduction joint, each   Ⓐ ☑ ⊘ ♿

**L6646** Upper extremity addition, shoulder joint, multipositional locking, flexion, adjustable abduction friction control, for use with body powered or external powered system   Ⓐ ⊘ ♿

**L6647** Upper extremity addition, shoulder lock mechanism, body powered actuator   Ⓐ ⊘ ♿

**L6648** Upper extremity addition, shoulder lock mechanism, external powered actuator   Ⓐ ⊘ ♿

**L6650** Upper extremity addition, shoulder universal joint, each   Ⓐ ☑ ⊘ ♿

**L6655** Upper extremity addition, standard control cable, extra   Ⓐ ⊘ ♿

**L6660** Upper extremity addition, heavy-duty control cable   Ⓐ ⊘ ♿

**L6665** Upper extremity addition, Teflon, or equal, cable lining   Ⓐ ⊘ ♿

**L6670** Upper extremity addition, hook to hand, cable adapter   Ⓐ ⊘ ♿

**L6672** Upper extremity addition, harness, chest or shoulder, saddle type   Ⓐ ⊘ ♿

**L6675** Upper extremity addition, harness, (e.g., figure of eight type), single cable design   Ⓐ ⊘ ♿

**L6676** Upper extremity addition, harness, (e.g., figure of eight type), dual cable design   Ⓐ ⊘ ♿

**L6677** Upper extremity addition, harness, triple control, simultaneous operation of terminal device and elbow   Ⓐ ⊘ ♿

**L6680** Upper extremity addition, test socket, wrist disarticulation or below elbow   Ⓐ ⊘ ♿

**L6682** Upper extremity addition, test socket, elbow disarticulation or above elbow   Ⓐ ⊘ ♿

**L6684** Upper extremity addition, test socket, shoulder disarticulation or interscapular thoracic   Ⓐ ⊘ ♿

**L6686** Upper extremity addition, suction socket   Ⓐ ⊘ ♿

**L6687** Upper extremity addition, frame type socket, below elbow or wrist disarticulation   Ⓐ ⊘ ♿

**L6688** Upper extremity addition, frame type socket, above elbow or elbow disarticulation   Ⓐ ⊘ ♿

**L6689** Upper extremity addition, frame type socket, shoulder disarticulation   Ⓐ ⊘ ♿

**L6690** Upper extremity addition, frame type socket, interscapular-thoracic   Ⓐ ⊘ ♿

**L6691** Upper extremity addition, removable insert, each   Ⓐ ☑ ⊘ ♿

**L6692** Upper extremity addition, silicone gel insert or equal, each   Ⓐ ☑ ⊘ ♿

Special Coverage Instructions    Noncovered by Medicare    Carrier Discretion    ☑ Quantity Alert   ● New Code   ○ Recycled/Reinstated   ▲ Revised Code

116 — L Codes    Ⓐ Age Edit   Ⓜ Maternity Edit   ♀ Female Only   ♂ Male Only   Ⓐ-Ⓨ OPPS Status Indicators    © 2016 Optum360, LLC

**L6693**   Upper extremity addition, locking elbow, forearm counterbalance    A ⊘ ♿

**L6694**   Addition to upper extremity prosthesis, below elbow/above elbow, custom fabricated from existing mold or prefabricated, socket insert, silicone gel, elastomeric or equal, for use with locking mechanism    A ⊘ ♿

**L6695**   Addition to upper extremity prosthesis, below elbow/above elbow, custom fabricated from existing mold or prefabricated, socket insert, silicone gel, elastomeric or equal, not for use with locking mechanism    A ⊘ ♿

**L6696**   Addition to upper extremity prosthesis, below elbow/above elbow, custom fabricated socket insert for congenital or atypical traumatic amputee, silicone gel, elastomeric or equal, for use with or without locking mechanism, initial only (for other than initial, use code L6694 or L6695)    A ⊘ ♿

**L6697**   Addition to upper extremity prosthesis, below elbow/above elbow, custom fabricated socket insert for other than congenital or atypical traumatic amputee, silicone gel, elastomeric or equal, for use with or without locking mechanism, initial only (for other than initial, use code L6694 or L6695)    A ⊘ ♿

**L6698**   Addition to upper extremity prosthesis, below elbow/above elbow, lock mechanism, excludes socket insert    A ⊘ ♿

## Terminal Device

**L6703**   Terminal device, passive hand/mitt, any material, any size    A ⊘ ♿

**L6704**   Terminal device, sport/recreational/work attachment, any material, any size    A ⊘ ♿

**L6706**   Terminal device, hook, mechanical, voluntary opening, any material, any size, lined or unlined    A ⊘ ♿

**L6707**   Terminal device, hook, mechanical, voluntary closing, any material, any size, lined or unlined    A ⊘ ♿

**L6708**   Terminal device, hand, mechanical, voluntary opening, any material, any size    A ⊘ ♿

**L6709**   Terminal device, hand, mechanical, voluntary closing, any material, any size    A ⊘ ♿

**L6711**   Terminal device, hook, mechanical, voluntary opening, any material, any size, lined or unlined, pediatric    A ♿

**L6712**   Terminal device, hook, mechanical, voluntary closing, any material, any size, lined or unlined, pediatric    A ♿

**L6713**   Terminal device, hand, mechanical, voluntary opening, any material, any size, pediatric    A ♿

**L6714**   Terminal device, hand, mechanical, voluntary closing, any material, any size, pediatric    A ♿

**L6715**   Terminal device, multiple articulating digit, includes motor(s), initial issue or replacement    A ♿

**L6721**   Terminal device, hook or hand, heavy-duty, mechanical, voluntary opening, any material, any size, lined or unlined    A ♿

**L6722**   Terminal device, hook or hand, heavy-duty, mechanical, voluntary closing, any material, any size, lined or unlined    A ♿

## Addition to Terminal Device

**L6805**   Addition to terminal device, modifier wrist unit    A ⊘ ♿

**L6810**   Addition to terminal device, precision pinch device    A ⊘ ♿

**L6880**   Electric hand, switch or myoelectric controlled, independently articulating digits, any grasp pattern or combination of grasp patterns, includes motor(s)    A ♿

**L6881**   Automatic grasp feature, addition to upper limb electric prosthetic terminal device    A ⊘ ♿

    AHA: 1Q, '02, 5

**L6882**   Microprocessor control feature, addition to upper limb prosthetic terminal device    A ⊘ ♿

    AHA: 1Q, '02, 5

## Replacement Socket

**L6883**   Replacement socket, below elbow/wrist disarticulation, molded to patient model, for use with or without external power    A ⊘ ♿

**L6884**   Replacement socket, above elbow/elbow disarticulation, molded to patient model, for use with or without external power    A ⊘ ♿

**L6885**   Replacement socket, shoulder disarticulation/interscapular thoracic, molded to patient model, for use with or without external power    A ⊘ ♿

## Hand Restoration

**L6890**   Addition to upper extremity prosthesis, glove for terminal device, any material, prefabricated, includes fitting and adjustment    A ♿

**L6895**   Addition to upper extremity prosthesis, glove for terminal device, any material, custom fabricated    A ♿

**L6900**   Hand restoration (casts, shading and measurements included), partial hand, with glove, thumb or one finger remaining    A ♿

**L6905**   Hand restoration (casts, shading and measurements included), partial hand, with glove, multiple fingers remaining    A ♿

**L6910**   Hand restoration (casts, shading and measurements included), partial hand, with glove, no fingers remaining    A ♿

**L6915**   Hand restoration (shading and measurements included), replacement glove for above    A ♿

## External Power

**L6920**   Wrist disarticulation, external power, self-suspended inner socket, removable forearm shell, Otto Bock or equal switch, cables, 2 batteries and 1 charger, switch control of terminal device    A ⊘ ♿

**L6925**   Wrist disarticulation, external power, self-suspended inner socket, removable forearm shell, Otto Bock or equal electrodes, cables, 2 batteries and one charger, myoelectronic control of terminal device    A ⊘ ♿

**L6930**   Below elbow, external power, self-suspended inner socket, removable forearm shell, Otto Bock or equal switch, cables, 2 batteries and one charger, switch control of terminal device    A ⊘ ♿

**L6935**   Below elbow, external power, self-suspended inner socket, removable forearm shell, Otto Bock or equal electrodes, cables, 2 batteries and one charger, myoelectronic control of terminal device    A ⊘ ♿

**L6940**   Elbow disarticulation, external power, molded inner socket, removable humeral shell, outside locking hinges, forearm, Otto Bock or equal switch, cables, 2 batteries and one charger, switch control of terminal device    A ⊘ ♿

**L6945**   Elbow disarticulation, external power, molded inner socket, removable humeral shell, outside locking hinges, forearm, Otto Bock or equal electrodes, cables, 2 batteries and one charger, myoelectronic control of terminal device    A ⊘ ♿

**L6950**   Above elbow, external power, molded inner socket, removable humeral shell, internal locking elbow, forearm, Otto Bock or equal switch, cables, 2 batteries and one charger, switch control of terminal device    A ⊘ ♿

Special Coverage Instructions    Noncovered by Medicare    Carrier Discretion    ☑ Quantity Alert   ● New Code   ○ Recycled/Reinstated   ▲ Revised Code

© 2016 Optum360, LLC    N-Z ASC Pmt    CMS: Pub 100    AHA: Coding Clinic    ♿ DMEPOS Paid    ⊘ SNF Excluded     L Codes — 117

**Prosthetic Procedures**

**L6955 — L8039**

**L6955** Above elbow, external power, molded inner socket, removable humeral shell, internal locking elbow, forearm, Otto Bock or equal electrodes, cables, 2 batteries and one charger, myoelectronic control of terminal device  Ⓐ⊘♿

**L6960** Shoulder disarticulation, external power, molded inner socket, removable shoulder shell, shoulder bulkhead, humeral section, mechanical elbow, forearm, Otto Bock or equal switch, cables, 2 batteries and one charger, switch control of terminal device  Ⓐ⊘♿

**L6965** Shoulder disarticulation, external power, molded inner socket, removable shoulder shell, shoulder bulkhead, humeral section, mechanical elbow, forearm, Otto Bock or equal electrodes, cables, 2 batteries and one charger, myoelectronic control of terminal device  Ⓐ⊘♿

**L6970** Interscapular-thoracic, external power, molded inner socket, removable shoulder shell, shoulder bulkhead, humeral section, mechanical elbow, forearm, Otto Bock or equal switch, cables, 2 batteries and one charger, switch control of terminal device  Ⓐ⊘♿

**L6975** Interscapular-thoracic, external power, molded inner socket, removable shoulder shell, shoulder bulkhead, humeral section, mechanical elbow, forearm, Otto Bock or equal electrodes, cables, 2 batteries and one charger, myoelectronic control of terminal device  Ⓐ⊘♿

### Electric Hand and Accessories

**L7007** Electric hand, switch or myoelectric controlled, adult  ⒶⒶ⊘♿

**L7008** Electric hand, switch or myoelectric, controlled, pediatric  ⒶⒶ⊘♿

**L7009** Electric hook, switch or myoelectric controlled, adult  ⒶⒶ⊘♿

**L7040** Prehensile actuator, switch controlled  Ⓐ⊘♿

**L7045** Electric hook, switch or myoelectric controlled, pediatric  Ⓐ⊘♿

### Electronic Elbow and Accessories

**L7170** Electronic elbow, Hosmer or equal, switch controlled  Ⓐ⊘♿

**L7180** Electronic elbow, microprocessor sequential control of elbow and terminal device  Ⓐ⊘♿

**L7181** Electronic elbow, microprocessor simultaneous control of elbow and terminal device  Ⓐ⊘♿

**L7185** Electronic elbow, adolescent, Variety Village or equal, switch controlled  Ⓐ⊘♿

**L7186** Electronic elbow, child, Variety Village or equal, switch controlled  Ⓐ⊘♿

**L7190** Electronic elbow, adolescent, Variety Village or equal, myoelectronically controlled  Ⓐ⊘♿

**L7191** Electronic elbow, child, Variety Village or equal, myoelectronically controlled  Ⓐ⊘♿

### Electronic Wrist and Accessories

**L7259** Electronic wrist rotator, any type  Ⓐ♿

### Battery Components

**L7360** Six volt battery, each  Ⓐ☑♿

**L7362** Battery charger, 6 volt, each  Ⓐ☑⊘♿

**L7364** Twelve volt battery, each  Ⓐ☑⊘♿

**L7366** Battery charger, twelve volt, each  Ⓐ☑⊘♿

**L7367** Lithium ion battery, rechargeable, replacement  Ⓐ⊘♿

**L7368** Lithium ion battery charger, replacement only  Ⓐ⊘♿

### Additions to Upper Extremity Prosthesis

**L7400** Addition to upper extremity prosthesis, below elbow/wrist disarticulation, ultralight material (titanium, carbon fiber or equal)  Ⓐ⊘♿

**L7401** Addition to upper extremity prosthesis, above elbow disarticulation, ultralight material (titanium, carbon fiber or equal)  Ⓐ⊘♿

**L7402** Addition to upper extremity prosthesis, shoulder disarticulation/interscapular thoracic, ultralight material (titanium, carbon fiber or equal)  Ⓐ⊘♿

**L7403** Addition to upper extremity prosthesis, below elbow/wrist disarticulation, acrylic material  Ⓐ⊘♿

**L7404** Addition to upper extremity prosthesis, above elbow disarticulation, acrylic material  Ⓐ⊘♿

**L7405** Addition to upper extremity prosthesis, shoulder disarticulation/interscapular thoracic, acrylic material  Ⓐ⊘♿

**L7499** Upper extremity prosthesis, not otherwise specified  Ⓐ

### Repairs

**L7510** Repair of prosthetic device, repair or replace minor parts  Ⓐ
Medicare jurisdiction: local contractor if repair of implanted prosthetic device.

**L7520** Repair prosthetic device, labor component, per 15 minutes  Ⓐ☑
Medicare jurisdiction: local contractor if repair of implanted prosthetic device.

### Donning Sleeve

**L7600** Prosthetic donning sleeve, any material, each  Ⓔ☑

### Male Prosthetic

**L7900** Male vacuum erection system  ♂Ⓔ

**L7902** Tension ring, for vacuum erection device, any type, replacement only, each  ♂Ⓔ

### Breast Prosthesis

**L8000** Breast prosthesis, mastectomy bra, without integrated breast prosthesis form, any size, any type  ♀Ⓐ♿

**L8001** Breast prosthesis, mastectomy bra, with integrated breast prosthesis form, unilateral, any size, any type  ♀Ⓐ♿
AHA: 1Q, '02, 5

**L8002** Breast prosthesis, mastectomy bra, with integrated breast prosthesis form, bilateral, any size, any type  ♀Ⓐ♿
AHA: 1Q, '02, 5

**L8010** Breast prosthesis, mastectomy sleeve  ♀Ⓐ

**L8015** External breast prosthesis garment, with mastectomy form, post mastectomy  ♀Ⓐ♿

**L8020** Breast prosthesis, mastectomy form  ♀Ⓐ♿

**L8030** Breast prosthesis, silicone or equal, without integral adhesive  ♀Ⓐ

**L8031** Breast prosthesis, silicone or equal, with integral adhesive  Ⓐ♿

**L8032** Nipple prosthesis, reusable, any type, each  Ⓐ☑♿

**L8035** Custom breast prosthesis, post mastectomy, molded to patient model  ♀Ⓐ♿

**L8039** Breast prosthesis, not otherwise specified  ♀Ⓐ

Special Coverage Instructions   Noncovered by Medicare   Carrier Discretion   ☑ Quantity Alert ● New Code ○ Recycled/Reinstated ▲ Revised Code
Ⓐ Age Edit   Ⓜ Maternity Edit   ♀ Female Only   ♂ Male Only   Ⓐ-Ⓨ OPPS Status Indicators   © 2016 Optum360, LLC

## Face and Ear Prosthesis

**L8040**    Nasal prosthesis, provided by a nonphysician   A &#9855; (KM,KN)

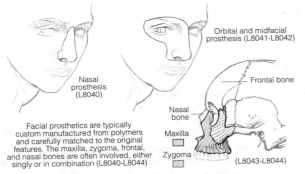

Orbital and midfacial prosthesis (L8041-L8042)

Nasal prosthesis (L8040)

Frontal bone

Nasal bone

Maxilla

Zygoma

(L8043-L8044)

Facial prosthetics are typically custom manufactured from polymers and carefully matched to the original features. The maxilla, zygoma, frontal, and nasal bones are often involved, either singly or in combination (L8040-L8044).

**L8041**    Midfacial prosthesis, provided by a nonphysician   A &#9855; (KM,KN)

**L8042**    Orbital prosthesis, provided by a nonphysician   A &#9855; (KM,KN)

**L8043**    Upper facial prosthesis, provided by a nonphysician   A &#9855; (KM,KN)

**L8044**    Hemi-facial prosthesis, provided by a nonphysician   A &#9855; (KM,KN)

**L8045**    Auricular prosthesis, provided by a nonphysician   A &#9855; (KM,KN)

**L8046**    Partial facial prosthesis, provided by a nonphysician   A &#9855; (KM,KN)

**L8047**    Nasal septal prosthesis, provided by a nonphysician   A &#9855; (KM,KN)

**L8048**    Unspecified maxillofacial prosthesis, by report, provided by a nonphysician   A

**L8049**    Repair or modification of maxillofacial prosthesis, labor component, 15 minute increments, provided by a nonphysician   A

## Trusses

**L8300**    Truss, single with standard pad   A &#9855;

**L8310**    Truss, double with standard pads   A &#9855;

**L8320**    Truss, addition to standard pad, water pad   A &#9855;

**L8330**    Truss, addition to standard pad, scrotal pad   ♂ A &#9855;

## Prosthetic Socks

**L8400**    Prosthetic sheath, below knee, each   A ☑ &#9855;

**L8410**    Prosthetic sheath, above knee, each   A ☑ &#9855;

**L8415**    Prosthetic sheath, upper limb, each   A ☑ &#9855;

**L8417**    Prosthetic sheath/sock, including a gel cushion layer, below knee or above knee, each   A ☑ &#9855;

**L8420**    Prosthetic sock, multiple ply, below knee, each   A ☑ &#9855;

**L8430**    Prosthetic sock, multiple ply, above knee, each   A ☑ &#9855;

**L8435**    Prosthetic sock, multiple ply, upper limb, each   A ☑ &#9855;

**L8440**    Prosthetic shrinker, below knee, each   A ☑ &#9855;

**L8460**    Prosthetic shrinker, above knee, each   A ☑ &#9855;

**L8465**    Prosthetic shrinker, upper limb, each   A ☑ &#9855;

**L8470**    Prosthetic sock, single ply, fitting, below knee, each   A ☑ &#9855;

**L8480**    Prosthetic sock, single ply, fitting, above knee, each   A ☑ &#9855;

**L8485**    Prosthetic sock, single ply, fitting, upper limb, each   A ☑ &#9855;

**L8499**    Unlisted procedure for miscellaneous prosthetic services   A

Determine if an alternative HCPCS Level II or a CPT code better describes the service being reported. This code should be used only if a more specific code is unavailable.

## Larynx and Trachea Prothetics and Accessories

**L8500**    Artificial larynx, any type   A &#9855;

**L8501**    Tracheostomy speaking valve   A &#9855;

**L8505**    Artificial larynx replacement battery/accessory, any type   A
**AHA:** 1Q, '02, 5

**L8507**    Tracheo-esophageal voice prosthesis, patient inserted, any type, each   A ☑ &#9855;
**AHA:** 1Q, '02, 5

**L8509**    Tracheo-esophageal voice prosthesis, inserted by a licensed health care provider, any type   A &#9855;
**AHA:** 1Q, '02, 5

**L8510**    Voice amplifier   A &#9855;
**AHA:** 1Q, '02, 5

**L8511**    Insert for indwelling tracheoesophageal prosthesis, with or without valve, replacement only, each   A ☑ &#9855;

**L8512**    Gelatin capsules or equivalent, for use with tracheoesophageal voice prosthesis, replacement only, per 10   A ☑ &#9855;

**L8513**    Cleaning device used with tracheoesophageal voice prosthesis, pipet, brush, or equal, replacement only, each   A ☑ &#9855;

**L8514**    Tracheoesophageal puncture dilator, replacement only, each   A ☑ &#9855;

**L8515**    Gelatin capsule, application device for use with tracheoesophageal voice prosthesis, each   A ☑ &#9855;

## Breast Implant

**L8600**    Implantable breast prosthesis, silicone or equal   ♀ N &#9855;

Medicare covers implants inserted in post-mastectomy reconstruction in a breast cancer patient. Always report concurrent to the implant procedure.
**CMS:** 100-04,4,190

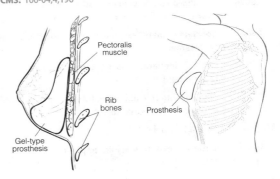

Pectoralis muscle

Rib bones

Prosthesis

Gel-type prosthesis

## Bulking Agents

**L8603**    Injectable bulking agent, collagen implant, urinary tract, 2.5 ml syringe, includes shipping and necessary supplies   N ☑ &#9855;
**CMS:** 100-04,4,190

**L8604**    Injectable bulking agent, dextranomer/hyaluronic acid copolymer implant, urinary tract, 1 ml, includes shipping and necessary supplies   N ☑

**L8605**    Injectable bulking agent, dextranomer/hyaluronic acid copolymer implant, anal canal, 1 ml, includes shipping and necessary supplies   N &#9855;

**L8606**    Injectable bulking agent, synthetic implant, urinary tract, 1 ml syringe, includes shipping and necessary supplies   N ☑ &#9855;

**L8607**    Injectable bulking agent for vocal cord medialization, 0.1 ml, includes shipping and necessary supplies   N &#9855;

---

Special Coverage Instructions    Noncovered by Medicare    Carrier Discretion    ☑ Quantity Alert   ● New Code   ○ Recycled/Reinstated   ▲ Revised Code

© 2016 Optum360, LLC    A2-Z3 ASC Pmt    CMS: Pub 100    AHA: Coding Clinic    &#9855; DMEPOS Paid    ⊘ SNF Excluded    L Codes — 119

**Prosthetic Procedures**

L8609 — L8695

## Eye and Ear Implants and Accessories

**L8609** Artificial cornea ⬛&

**L8610** Ocular implant ⬛&
CMS: 100-04,4,190

**L8612** Aqueous shunt ⬛&
CMS: 100-04,4,190

**L8613** Ossicula implant ⬛&
CMS: 100-04,4,190

**L8614** Cochlear device, includes all internal and external components ⬛&
A cochlear implant is covered by Medicare when the patient has bilateral sensorineural deafness.
CMS: 100-04,14,40.8; 100-04,4,190
AHA: 3Q, '16; 4Q, '03, 8; 3Q, '02, 4-5; 1Q, '01, 6

**L8615** Headset/headpiece for use with cochlear implant device, replacement Ⓐ&

**L8616** Microphone for use with cochlear implant device, replacement Ⓐ&

**L8617** Transmitting coil for use with cochlear implant device, replacement Ⓐ&

**L8618** Transmitter cable for use with cochlear implant device, replacement Ⓐ&

**L8619** Cochlear implant, external speech processor and controller, integrated system, replacement Ⓐ&
Medicare jurisdiction: local contractor.

**L8621** Zinc air battery for use with cochlear implant device and auditory osseointegrated sound processors, replacement, each Ⓐ☑&

**L8622** Alkaline battery for use with cochlear implant device, any size, replacement, each Ⓐ☑&

**L8623** Lithium ion battery for use with cochlear implant device speech processor, other than ear level, replacement, each Ⓐ☑&

**L8624** Lithium ion battery for use with cochlear implant device speech processor, ear level, replacement, each Ⓐ☑&

**L8627** Cochlear implant, external speech processor, component, replacement Ⓐ&

**L8628** Cochlear implant, external controller component, replacement Ⓐ&

**L8629** Transmitting coil and cable, integrated, for use with cochlear implant device, replacement Ⓐ&

## Upper Extremity Implants

**L8630** Metacarpophalangeal joint implant ⬛&
CMS: 100-04,4,190

Bone is cut at the MP joint (arthroplasty)

Bone may be hollowed out in both metacarpal and phalangeal sides in preparation for a prosthesis

Prosthetic joint implant

Prosthesis in place

Metacarpophalangeal prosthetic implant

**L8631** Metacarpal phalangeal joint replacement, 2 or more pieces, metal (e.g., stainless steel or cobalt chrome), ceramic-like material (e.g., pyrocarbon), for surgical implantation (all sizes, includes entire system) ⬛&

## Lower Extremity Implants

**L8641** Metatarsal joint implant ⬛&
CMS: 100-04,4,190

**L8642** Hallux implant ⬛&
CMS: 100-04,4,190

## Interphalangeal Implants

**L8658** Interphalangeal joint spacer, silicone or equal, each ⬛☑&
CMS: 100-04,4,190

**L8659** Interphalangeal finger joint replacement, 2 or more pieces, metal (e.g., stainless steel or cobalt chrome), ceramic-like material (e.g., pyrocarbon) for surgical implantation, any size ⬛&

## Cardiovascular Implant

**L8670** Vascular graft material, synthetic, implant ⬛&
CMS: 100-04,4,190

## Neurostimulator and Accessories

**L8679** Implantable neurostimulator, pulse generator, any type ⬛&

**L8680** Implantable neurostimulator electrode, each Ⓔ☑

**L8681** Patient programmer (external) for use with implantable programmable neurostimulator pulse generator, replacement only Ⓐ&

**L8682** Implantable neurostimulator radiofrequency receiver ⬛&

**L8683** Radiofrequency transmitter (external) for use with implantable neurostimulator radiofrequency receiver Ⓐ&

**L8684** Radiofrequency transmitter (external) for use with implantable sacral root neurostimulator receiver for bowel and bladder management, replacement Ⓐ&

**L8685** Implantable neurostimulator pulse generator, single array, rechargeable, includes extension Ⓔ

**L8686** Implantable neurostimulator pulse generator, single array, nonrechargeable, includes extension Ⓔ

**L8687** Implantable neurostimulator pulse generator, dual array, rechargeable, includes extension Ⓔ

**L8688** Implantable neurostimulator pulse generator, dual array, nonrechargeable, includes extension Ⓔ

**L8689** External recharging system for battery (internal) for use with implantable neurostimulator, replacement only Ⓐ&

## Miscellaneous Prosthetics and Accessories

**L8690** Auditory osseointegrated device, includes all internal and external components ⬛&
CMS: 100-04,14,40.8
AHA: 3Q, '16

**L8691** Auditory osseointegrated device, external sound processor, replacement Ⓐ&

**L8692** Auditory osseointegrated device, external sound processor, used without osseointegration, body worn, includes headband or other means of external attachment Ⓔ

**L8693** Auditory osseointegrated device abutment, any length, replacement only Ⓐ&

**L8695** External recharging system for battery (external) for use with implantable neurostimulator, replacement only Ⓐ&

Prosthetic Procedures

| | |
|---|---|
| **L8696** | **Antenna (external) for use with implantable diaphragmatic/phrenic nerve stimulation device, replacement, each** A &#9855; |
| **L8699** | **Prosthetic implant, not otherwise specified** N |
| | Determine if an alternative HCPCS Level II or a CPT code better describes the service being reported. This code should be used only if a more specific code is unavailable. |
| | **CMS:** 100-04,4,190 |
| | **AHA:** 3Q, '15, 2 |
| **L9900** | **Orthotic and prosthetic supply, accessory, and/or service component of another HCPCS L code** N |

L8696 — L9900

Special Coverage Instructions    Noncovered by Medicare    Carrier Discretion    &#9745; Quantity Alert   &#9679; New Code   &#9711; Recycled/Reinstated   &#9650; Revised Code

© 2016 Optum360, LLC    A2-Z3 ASC Pmt    **CMS:** Pub 100    **AHA:** Coding Clinic   &#9855; DMEPOS Paid   &#8709; SNF Excluded     **L Codes — 121**

## Medical Services M0075-M0301

### Other Medical Services

M codes include office services, cellular therapy, prolotherapy, intragastric hypothermia, IV chelation therapy, and fabric wrapping of an abdominal aneurysm.

**M0075** **Cellular therapy**      E

The therapeutic efficacy of injecting foreign proteins has not been established.

**M0076** **Prolotherapy**      E

The therapeutic efficacy of prolotherapy and joint sclerotherapy has not been established.

**M0100** **Intragastric hypothermia using gastric freezing**      E

Code with caution: This procedure is considered obsolete.

### Cardiovascular Services

**M0300** **IV chelation therapy (chemical endarterectomy)**      E

Chelation therapy is considered experimental in the United States.

**CMS:** 100-03,20.21; 100-03,20.22

**M0301** **Fabric wrapping of abdominal aneurysm**      E

Code with caution: This procedure has largely been replaced with more effective treatment modalities. Submit documentation.

Special Coverage Instructions    Noncovered by Medicare    Carrier Discretion    ☑ Quantity Alert ● New Code   ○ Recycled/Reinstated ▲ Revised Code

© 2016 Optum360, LLC    A2-Z3 ASC Pmt    **CMS:** Pub 100    **AHA:** Coding Clinic   ⅄ DMEPOS Paid    ⊘ SNF Excluded

M Codes — 123

**Pathology And Laboratory Services**

**P2028 — P9046**

# Pathology and Laboratory Services P2028-P9615

P codes include chemistry, toxicology, and microbiology tests, screening Papanicolaou procedures, and various blood products.

## Chemistry and Toxicology Tests

**P2028** **Cephalin floculation, blood** Ⓐ
Code with caution: This test is considered obsolete. Submit documentation.

**P2029** **Congo red, blood** Ⓐ
Code with caution: This test is considered obsolete. Submit documentation.

**P2031** **Hair analysis (excluding arsenic)** Ⓔ

**P2033** **Thymol turbidity, blood** Ⓐ
Code with caution: This test is considered obsolete. Submit documentation.

**P2038** **Mucoprotein, blood (seromucoid) (medical necessity procedure)** Ⓐ
Code with caution: This test is considered obsolete. Submit documentation.

## Pathology Screening Tests

**P3000** **Screening Papanicolaou smear, cervical or vaginal, up to 3 smears, by technician under physician supervision** Ⓐ ♀Ⓐ
One Pap test is covered by Medicare every two years, unless the physician suspects cervical abnormalities and shortens the interval. See also G0123-G0124.
**CMS:** 100-02,15,280.4; 100-03,210.2.1; 100-04,18,30.2.1; 100-04,18,30.5; 100-04,18,30.6

**P3001** **Screening Papanicolaou smear, cervical or vaginal, up to 3 smears, requiring interpretation by physician** Ⓐ ♀Ⓑ⊘
One Pap test is covered by Medicare every two years, unless the physician suspects cervical abnormalities and shortens the interval. See also G0123-G0124.
**CMS:** 100-02,15,280.4; 100-03,210.2.1; 100-04,18,30.2.1; 100-04,18,30.5; 100-04,18,30.6

## Microbiology Tests

**P7001** **Culture, bacterial, urine; quantitative, sensitivity study** Ⓔ

## Miscellaneous

**P9010** **Blood (whole), for transfusion, per unit** Ⓡ ☑
**CMS:** 100-01,3,20.5; 100-01,3,20.5.2; 100-01,3,20.5.3; 100-02,1,10; 100-04,3,40.2.2
**AHA:** 3Q, '04, 11-13

**P9011** **Blood, split unit** Ⓡ ☑
**CMS:** 100-01,3,20.5; 100-01,3,20.5.2; 100-01,3,20.5.3; 100-02,1,10; 100-04,3,40.2.2; 100-04,4,231.4
**AHA:** 2Q, '05, 1-3; 3Q, '04, 11-13

**P9012** **Cryoprecipitate, each unit** Ⓡ ☑
**CMS:** 100-02,1,10; 100-04,3,40.2.2
**AHA:** 3Q, '04, 11-13

**P9016** **Red blood cells, leukocytes reduced, each unit** Ⓡ ☑
**CMS:** 100-02,1,10; 100-04,3,40.2.2
**AHA:** 4Q, '04, 2; 3Q, '04, 11-13

**P9017** **Fresh frozen plasma (single donor), frozen within 8 hours of collection, each unit** Ⓡ ☑
**CMS:** 100-02,1,10; 100-04,3,40.2.2
**AHA:** 3Q, '04, 11-13

**P9019** **Platelets, each unit** Ⓡ ☑
**CMS:** 100-02,1,10; 100-04,3,40.2.2
**AHA:** 3Q, '04, 11-13

**P9020** **Platelet rich plasma, each unit** Ⓡ ☑
**CMS:** 100-04,3,40.2.2
**AHA:** 3Q, '04, 11-13

**P9021** **Red blood cells, each unit** Ⓡ ☑
**CMS:** 100-01,3,20.5; 100-01,3,20.5.2; 100-01,3,20.5.3; 100-02,1,10; 100-04,3,40.2.2
**AHA:** 4Q, '04, 2; 3Q, '04, 11-13

**P9022** **Red blood cells, washed, each unit** Ⓡ ☑
**CMS:** 100-01,3,20.5; 100-01,3,20.5.2; 100-01,3,20.5.3; 100-02,1,10; 100-04,3,40.2.2
**AHA:** 3Q, '04, 11-13

**P9023** **Plasma, pooled multiple donor, solvent/detergent treated, frozen, each unit** Ⓡ ☑
**CMS:** 100-02,1,10; 100-04,3,40.2.2
**AHA:** 3Q, '04, 11-13

**P9031** **Platelets, leukocytes reduced, each unit** Ⓡ ☑
**CMS:** 100-02,1,10; 100-04,3,40.2.2
**AHA:** 3Q, '04, 11-13

**P9032** **Platelets, irradiated, each unit** Ⓡ ☑
**CMS:** 100-02,1,10; 100-04,3,40.2.2
**AHA:** 2Q, '05, 1-3; 3Q, '04, 11-13

**P9033** **Platelets, leukocytes reduced, irradiated, each unit** Ⓡ ☑
**CMS:** 100-02,1,10; 100-04,3,40.2.2
**AHA:** 2Q, '05, 1-3; 3Q, '04, 11-13

**P9034** **Platelets, pheresis, each unit** Ⓡ ☑
**CMS:** 100-02,1,10; 100-04,3,40.2.2
**AHA:** 3Q, '04, 11-13

**P9035** **Platelets, pheresis, leukocytes reduced, each unit** Ⓡ ☑
**CMS:** 100-02,1,10; 100-04,3,40.2.2
**AHA:** 3Q, '04, 11-13

**P9036** **Platelets, pheresis, irradiated, each unit** Ⓡ ☑
**CMS:** 100-02,1,10; 100-04,3,40.2.2
**AHA:** 2Q, '05, 1-3; 3Q, '04, 11-13

**P9037** **Platelets, pheresis, leukocytes reduced, irradiated, each unit** Ⓡ ☑
**CMS:** 100-02,1,10; 100-04,3,40.2.2
**AHA:** 2Q, '05, 1-3; 3Q, '04, 11-13

**P9038** **Red blood cells, irradiated, each unit** Ⓡ ☑
**CMS:** 100-01,3,20.5; 100-01,3,20.5.2; 100-01,3,20.5.3; 100-02,1,10; 100-04,3,40.2.2
**AHA:** 2Q, '05, 1-3; 3Q, '04, 11-13

**P9039** **Red blood cells, deglycerolized, each unit** Ⓡ ☑
**CMS:** 100-02,1,10; 100-04,3,40.2.2
**AHA:** 3Q, '04, 11-13

**P9040** **Red blood cells, leukocytes reduced, irradiated, each unit** Ⓡ ☑
**CMS:** 100-02,1,10; 100-04,3,40.2.2
**AHA:** 2Q, '05, 1-3; 3Q, '04, 11-13

**P9041** **Infusion, albumin (human), 5%, 50 ml** Ⓚ ⓚ² ☑
**CMS:** 100-02,1,10; 100-04,3,40.2.2
**AHA:** 3Q, '04, 11-13

**P9043** **Infusion, plasma protein fraction (human), 5%, 50 ml** Ⓡ ☑
**CMS:** 100-02,1,10; 100-04,3,40.2.2
**AHA:** 3Q, '04, 11-13

**P9044** **Plasma, cryoprecipitate reduced, each unit** Ⓡ ☑
**CMS:** 100-02,1,10; 100-04,3,40.2.2
**AHA:** 3Q, '04, 11-13

**P9045** **Infusion, albumin (human), 5%, 250 ml** Ⓚ ⓚ² ☑
**CMS:** 100-02,1,10; 100-04,3,40.2.2
**AHA:** 3Q, '04, 11-13; 1Q, '02, 5

**P9046** **Infusion, albumin (human), 25%, 20 ml** Ⓚ ⓚ² ☑
**CMS:** 100-02,1,10; 100-04,3,40.2.2
**AHA:** 3Q, '04, 11-13; 1Q, '02, 5

Special Coverage Instructions ▪ Noncovered by Medicare ▪ Carrier Discretion ▪ ☑ Quantity Alert ● New Code ○ Recycled/Reinstated ▲ Revised Code

124 — P Codes ▪ Ⓐ Age Edit ▪ Ⓜ Maternity Edit ▪ ♀ Female Only ▪ ♂ Male Only ▪ Ⓐ-Ⓨ OPPS Status Indicators ▪ © 2016 Optum360, LLC

**P9047**   Infusion, albumin (human), 25%, 50 ml   K K2 ☑
CMS: 100-02,1,10; 100-04,3,40.2.2
AHA: 3Q, '04, 11-13; 1Q, '02, 5

**P9048**   Infusion, plasma protein fraction (human), 5%, 250 ml   R ☑
CMS: 100-02,1,10; 100-04,3,40.2.2
AHA: 3Q, '04, 11-13; 1Q, '02, 5

**P9050**   Granulocytes, pheresis, each unit   R ☑
CMS: 100-02,1,10; 100-03,110.5; 100-04,3,40.2.2
AHA: 3Q, '04, 11-13; 1Q, '02, 5

**P9051**   Whole blood or red blood cells, leukocytes reduced, CMV-negative, each unit   R ☑
CMS: 100-02,1,10; 100-04,3,40.2.2
AHA: 3Q, '04, 11-13

**P9052**   Platelets, HLA-matched leukocytes reduced, apheresis/pheresis, each unit   R ☑
CMS: 100-02,1,10; 100-04,3,40.2.2
AHA: 3Q, '04, 11-13

**P9053**   Platelets, pheresis, leukocytes reduced, CMV-negative, irradiated, each unit   R ☑
CMS: 100-02,1,10; 100-04,3,40.2.2
AHA: 2Q, '05, 1-3; 3Q, '04, 11-13

**P9054**   Whole blood or red blood cells, leukocytes reduced, frozen, deglycerol, washed, each unit   R ☑
CMS: 100-02,1,10; 100-04,3,40.2.2
AHA: 3Q, '04, 11-13

**P9055**   Platelets, leukocytes reduced, CMV-negative, apheresis/pheresis, each unit   R ☑
CMS: 100-02,1,10; 100-04,3,40.2.2
AHA: 3Q, '04, 11-13

**P9056**   Whole blood, leukocytes reduced, irradiated, each unit   R ☑
CMS: 100-02,1,10; 100-04,3,40.2.2
AHA: 2Q, '05, 1-3; 3Q, '04, 11-13

**P9057**   Red blood cells, frozen/deglycerolized/washed, leukocytes reduced, irradiated, each unit   R ☑
CMS: 100-02,1,10; 100-04,3,40.2.2
AHA: 2Q, '05, 1-3; 3Q, '04, 11-13

**P9058**   Red blood cells, leukocytes reduced, CMV-negative, irradiated, each unit   R ☑
CMS: 100-02,1,10; 100-04,3,40.2.2
AHA: 2Q, '05, 1-3; 3Q, '04, 11-13

**P9059**   Fresh frozen plasma between 8-24 hours of collection, each unit   R ☑
CMS: 100-02,1,10; 100-04,3,40.2.2
AHA: 3Q, '04, 11-13

**P9060**   Fresh frozen plasma, donor retested, each unit   R ☑
CMS: 100-02,1,10; 100-04,3,40.2.2
AHA: 3Q, '04, 11-13

**P9070**   Plasma, pooled multiple donor, pathogen reduced, frozen, each unit   R
AHA: 1Q, '16, 7

**P9071**   Plasma (single donor), pathogen reduced, frozen, each unit   R
AHA: 1Q, '16, 7

▲ **P9072**^Jan   Platelets, pheresis, pathogen reduced or rapid bacterial tested, each unit   R
AHA: 1Q, '16, 7

**P9603**   Travel allowance, one way in connection with medically necessary laboratory specimen collection drawn from homebound or nursing homebound patient; prorated miles actually travelled   A ☑
CMS: 100-04,16,60; 100-04,16,60.2

**P9604**   Travel allowance, one way in connection with medically necessary laboratory specimen collection drawn from homebound or nursing homebound patient; prorated trip charge   A ☑
CMS: 100-04,16,60; 100-04,16,60.2

**P9612**   Catheterization for collection of specimen, single patient, all places of service   A
CMS: 100-04,16,60
AHA: 2Q, '09, 1; 3Q, '07, 5

**P9615**   Catheterization for collection of specimen(s) (multiple patients)   N
CMS: 100-04,16,60; 100-04,16,60.1.4

---

^Jan **January Update**

Special Coverage Instructions    Noncovered by Medicare    Carrier Discretion    ☑ Quantity Alert    ● New Code    ○ Recycled/Reinstated    ▲ Revised Code

© 2016 Optum360, LLC    A2-Z3 ASC Pmt    CMS: Pub 100    AHA: Coding Clinic    ♿ DMEPOS Paid    ⊘ SNF Excluded    P Codes — 125

**Temporary Codes**

Q0035 — Q0174

## Q Codes (Temporary) Q0035-Q9983

Temporary Q codes are used to pay health care providers for supplies, drugs, and biologicals to which no permanent code has been assigned.

**Q0035 Cardiokymography** ⬚

Covered only in conjunction with electrocardiographic stress testing in male patients with atypical angina or nonischemic chest pain, or female patients with angina.

**Q0081 Infusion therapy, using other than chemotherapeutic drugs, per visit** 🅱 ☑

**AHA:** 1Q, '05, 7, 9-10; 4Q, '04, 6; 2Q, '04, 11; 1Q, '04, 4-5; 4Q, '02, 6-7; 2Q, '02, 8-9; 2Q, '02; 1Q, '02, 7

**Q0083 Chemotherapy administration by other than infusion technique only (e.g., subcutaneous, intramuscular, push), per visit** 🅱 ☑

**AHA:** 1Q, '05, 7, 9-10; 4Q, '04, 6; 1Q, '04, 4-5; 1Q, '02, 7; 1Q, '02, 1-2

**Q0084 Chemotherapy administration by infusion technique only, per visit** 🅱 ☑

**AHA:** 1Q, '05, 7, 9-10; 4Q, '04, 6; 2Q, '04, 11; 1Q, '04, 4-5; 1Q, '02, 7; 1Q, '02, 1-2

**Q0085 Chemotherapy administration by both infusion technique and other technique(s) (e.g. subcutaneous, intramuscular, push), per visit** 🅱 ☑

**AHA:** 4Q, '04, 6; 1Q, '04, 4-5; 1Q, '02, 7; 1Q, '02, 1-2

**Q0091 Screening Papanicolaou smear; obtaining, preparing and conveyance of cervical or vaginal smear to laboratory** 🅰 ♀🆂 ⊘

One pap test is covered by Medicare every two years for low risk patients and every one year for high risk patients. Q0091 can be reported with an E/M code when a separately identifiable E/M service is provided.

**CMS:** 100-02,15,280.4; 100-03,210.2.1; 100-04,18,30.2.1; 100-04,18,30.5; 100-04,18,30.6

**AHA:** 4Q, '08, 3; 4Q, '02, 8

**Q0092 Set-up portable x-ray equipment** 🅽

**CMS:** 100-04,13,90.4

**Q0111 Wet mounts, including preparations of vaginal, cervical or skin specimens** 🅰

**Q0112 All potassium hydroxide (KOH) preparations** 🅰

**Q0113 Pinworm examinations** 🅰

**Q0114 Fern test** ♀🅰

**Q0115 Postcoital direct, qualitative examinations of vaginal or cervical mucous** 🅰 ♀🅰

**Q0138 Injection, ferumoxytol, for treatment of iron deficiency anemia, 1 mg (non-ESRD use)** 🅺 🅺2 ☑

Use this code for Feraheme.

**Q0139 Injection, ferumoxytol, for treatment of iron deficiency anemia, 1 mg (for ESRD on dialysis)** 🅺 ☑

Use this code for Feraheme.

**Q0144 Azithromycin dihydrate, oral, capsules/powder, 1 g** 🅴 ☑

Use this code for Zithromax, Zithromax Z-PAK.

**Q0161 Chlorpromazine hydrochloride, 5 mg, oral, FDA approved prescription anti-emetic, for use as a complete therapeutic substitute for an IV anti-emetic at the time of chemotherapy treatment, not to exceed a 48 hour dosage regimen** 🅽 🎚 ☑

**CMS:** 100-02,15,50.5.4; 100-03,110.18; 100-04,17,80.2.1

**AHA:** 1Q, '14

**Q0162 Ondansetron 1 mg, oral, FDA approved prescription antiemetic, for use as a complete therapeutic substitute for an IV antiemetic at the time of chemotherapy treatment, not to exceed a 48 hour dosage regimen** 🅽 🎚 ☑

Use this code for Zofran, Zuplenz.

**CMS:** 100-02,15,50.5.4; 100-03,110.18; 100-04,17,80.2.1

**Q0163 Diphenhydramine HCl, 50 mg, oral, FDA approved prescription antiemetic, for use as a complete therapeutic substitute for an IV antiemetic at time of chemotherapy treatment not to exceed a 48-hour dosage regimen** 🅽 🎚 ☑

See also J1200. Medicare covers at the time of chemotherapy if regimen doesn't exceed 48 hours. Submit on the same claim as the chemotherapy. Use this code for Truxadryl.

**CMS:** 100-02,15,50.5.4; 100-03,110.18; 100-04,17,80.2.1

**AHA:** 2Q, '12, 9; 1Q, '08, 1; 1Q, '02, 1-2

**Q0164 Prochlorperazine maleate, 5 mg, oral, FDA approved prescription antiemetic, for use as a complete therapeutic substitute for an IV antiemetic at the time of chemotherapy treatment, not to exceed a 48-hour dosage regimen** 🅽 🎚 ☑

Medicare covers at the time of chemotherapy if regimen doesn't exceed 48 hours. Submit on the same claim as the chemotherapy. Use this code for Compazine.

**CMS:** 100-02,15,50.5.4; 100-03,110.18; 100-04,17,80.2.1

**AHA:** 1Q, '08, 1

**Q0166 Granisetron HCl, 1 mg, oral, FDA approved prescription antiemetic, for use as a complete therapeutic substitute for an IV antiemetic at the time of chemotherapy treatment, not to exceed a 24-hour dosage regimen** 🅽 🎚 ☑

Medicare covers at the time of chemotherapy if regimen doesn't exceed 48 hours. Submit on the same claim as the chemotherapy. Use this code for Kytril.

**CMS:** 100-02,15,50.5.4; 100-03,110.18; 100-04,17,80.2.1

**AHA:** 1Q, '08, 1

**Q0167 Dronabinol, 2.5 mg, oral, FDA approved prescription antiemetic, for use as a complete therapeutic substitute for an IV antiemetic at the time of chemotherapy treatment, not to exceed a 48-hour dosage regimen** 🅽 🎚 ☑

Medicare covers at the time of chemotherapy if regimen doesn't exceed 48 hours. Submit on the same claim as the chemotherapy. Use this code for Marinol.

**CMS:** 100-02,15,50.5.4; 100-03,110.18; 100-04,17,80.2.1

**AHA:** 1Q, '08, 1

**Q0169 Promethazine HCl, 12.5 mg, oral, FDA approved prescription antiemetic, for use as a complete therapeutic substitute for an IV antiemetic at the time of chemotherapy treatment, not to exceed a 48-hour dosage regimen** 🅽 🎚 ☑

Medicare covers at the time of chemotherapy if regimen doesn't exceed 48 hours. Submit on the same claim as the chemotherapy. Use this code for Phenergan, Amergan.

**CMS:** 100-02,15,50.5.4; 100-03,110.18; 100-04,17,80.2.1

**AHA:** 1Q, '08, 1

**Q0173 Trimethobenzamide HCl, 250 mg, oral, FDA approved prescription antiemetic, for use as a complete therapeutic substitute for an IV antiemetic at the time of chemotherapy treatment, not to exceed a 48-hour dosage regimen** 🅽 🎚 ☑

Medicare covers at the time of chemotherapy if regimen doesn't exceed 48 hours. Submit on the same claim as the chemotherapy. Use this code for Tebamide, T-Gen, Ticon, Tigan, Triban, Thimazide.

**CMS:** 100-02,15,50.5.4; 100-03,110.18; 100-04,17,80.2.1

**AHA:** 1Q, '08, 1

**Q0174 Thiethylperazine maleate, 10 mg, oral, FDA approved prescription antiemetic, for use as a complete therapeutic substitute for an IV antiemetic at the time of chemotherapy treatment, not to exceed a 48-hour dosage regimen** 🅽 ☑

Medicare covers at the time of chemotherapy if regimen doesn't exceed 48 hours. Submit on the same claim as the chemotherapy.

**CMS:** 100-02,15,50.5.4; 100-03,110.18; 100-04,17,80.2.1

**AHA:** 1Q, '08, 1

---

Special Coverage Instructions    Noncovered by Medicare    Carrier Discretion    ☑ Quantity Alert    ● New Code    ○ Recycled/Reinstated    ▲ Revised Code

126 — Q Codes (Temporary)    🅰 Age Edit    🅼 Maternity Edit    ♀ Female Only    ♂ Male Only    🅰-Y OPPS Status Indicators    © 2016 Optum360, LLC

**Q0175** Perphenazine, 4 mg, oral, FDA approved prescription antiemetic, for use as a complete therapeutic substitute for an IV antiemetic at the time of chemotherapy treatment, not to exceed a 48 hour dosage regimen  N III ☑

Medicare covers at the time of chemotherapy if regimen doesn't exceed 48 hours. Submit on the same claim as the chemotherapy. Use this code for Trilifon.

**CMS:** 100-02,15,50.5.4; 100-03,110.18; 100-04,17,80.2.1
**AHA:** 1Q, '08, 1

**Q0177** Hydroxyzine pamoate, 25 mg, oral, FDA approved prescription antiemetic, for use as a complete therapeutic substitute for an IV antiemetic at the time of chemotherapy treatment, not to exceed a 48-hour dosage regimen  N III ☑

Medicare covers at the time of chemotherapy if regimen doesn't exceed 48 hours. Submit on the same claim as the chemotherapy. Use this code for Vistaril.

**CMS:** 100-02,15,50.5.4; 100-03,110.18; 100-04,17,80.2.1
**AHA:** 1Q, '08, 1

**Q0180** Dolasetron mesylate, 100 mg, oral, FDA approved prescription antiemetic, for use as a complete therapeutic substitute for an IV antiemetic at the time of chemotherapy treatment, not to exceed a 24-hour dosage regimen  N III ☑

Medicare covers at the time of chemotherapy if regimen doesn't exceed 24 hours. Submit on the same claim as the chemotherapy. Use this code for Anzemet.

**CMS:** 100-02,15,50.5.4; 100-03,110.18; 100-04,17,80.2.1
**AHA:** 1Q, '08, 1

**Q0181** Unspecified oral dosage form, FDA approved prescription antiemetic, for use as a complete therapeutic substitute for an IV antiemetic at the time of chemotherapy treatment, not to exceed a 48-hour dosage regimen  N III

Medicare covers at the time of chemotherapy if regimen doesn't exceed 48-hours. Submit on the same claim as the chemotherapy.

**CMS:** 100-02,15,50.5.4; 100-03,110.18; 100-04,17,80.2.1
**AHA:** 2Q, '12, 9; 1Q, '08, 1

**Q0478** Power adapter for use with electric or electric/pneumatic ventricular assist device, vehicle type  A ☿

**Q0479** Power module for use with electric or electric/pneumatic ventricular assist device, replacement only  A ☿

**Q0480** Driver for use with pneumatic ventricular assist device, replacement only  A ☿
**AHA:** 3Q, '05, 1-2

**Q0481** Microprocessor control unit for use with electric ventricular assist device, replacement only  A ☿
**AHA:** 3Q, '05, 1-2

**Q0482** Microprocessor control unit for use with electric/pneumatic combination ventricular assist device, replacement only  A ☿
**AHA:** 3Q, '05, 1-2

**Q0483** Monitor/display module for use with electric ventricular assist device, replacement only  A ☿
**AHA:** 3Q, '05, 1-2

**Q0484** Monitor/display module for use with electric or electric/pneumatic ventricular assist device, replacement only  A ☿
**AHA:** 3Q, '05, 1-2

**Q0485** Monitor control cable for use with electric ventricular assist device, replacement only  A ☿
**AHA:** 3Q, '05, 1-2

**Q0486** Monitor control cable for use with electric/pneumatic ventricular assist device, replacement only  A ☿
**AHA:** 3Q, '05, 1-2

**Q0487** Leads (pneumatic/electrical) for use with any type electric/pneumatic ventricular assist device, replacement only  A ☿
**AHA:** 3Q, '05, 1-2

**Q0488** Power pack base for use with electric ventricular assist device, replacement only  A
**AHA:** 3Q, '05, 1-2

**Q0489** Power pack base for use with electric/pneumatic ventricular assist device, replacement only  A ☿
**AHA:** 3Q, '05, 1-2

**Q0490** Emergency power source for use with electric ventricular assist device, replacement only  A ☿
**AHA:** 3Q, '05, 1-2

**Q0491** Emergency power source for use with electric/pneumatic ventricular assist device, replacement only  A ☿
**AHA:** 3Q, '05, 1-2

**Q0492** Emergency power supply cable for use with electric ventricular assist device, replacement only  A ☿
**AHA:** 3Q, '05, 1-2

**Q0493** Emergency power supply cable for use with electric/pneumatic ventricular assist device, replacement only  A ☿
**AHA:** 3Q, '05, 1-2

**Q0494** Emergency hand pump for use with electric or electric/pneumatic ventricular assist device, replacement only  A ☿
**AHA:** 3Q, '05, 1-2

**Q0495** Battery/power pack charger for use with electric or electric/pneumatic ventricular assist device, replacement only  A ☿
**AHA:** 3Q, '05, 1-2

**Q0496** Battery, other than lithium-ion, for use with electric or electric/pneumatic ventricular assist device, replacement only  A ☿
**AHA:** 3Q, '05, 1-2

**Q0497** Battery clips for use with electric or electric/pneumatic ventricular assist device, replacement only  A ☿
**AHA:** 3Q, '05, 1-2

**Q0498** Holster for use with electric or electric/pneumatic ventricular assist device, replacement only  A ☿
**AHA:** 3Q, '05, 1-2

**Q0499** Belt/vest/bag for use to carry external peripheral components of any type ventricular assist device, replacement only  A ☿
**AHA:** 3Q, '05, 1-2

**Q0500** Filters for use with electric or electric/pneumatic ventricular assist device, replacement only  A ☑ ☿

The base unit for this code is for each filter.
**AHA:** 3Q, '05, 1-2

**Q0501** Shower cover for use with electric or electric/pneumatic ventricular assist device, replacement only  A ☿
**AHA:** 3Q, '05, 1-2

**Q0502** Mobility cart for pneumatic ventricular assist device, replacement only  A ☿
**AHA:** 3Q, '05, 1-2

**Q0503** Battery for pneumatic ventricular assist device, replacement only, each  A ☑ ☿
**AHA:** 3Q, '05, 1-2

**Q0504** Power adapter for pneumatic ventricular assist device, replacement only, vehicle type  A ☿
**AHA:** 3Q, '05, 1-2

**Q0506** Battery, lithium-ion, for use with electric or electric/pneumatic ventricular assist device, replacement only  A ☿

Special Coverage Instructions    Noncovered by Medicare    Carrier Discretion    ☑ Quantity Alert    ● New Code    ○ Recycled/Reinstated    ▲ Revised Code

© 2016 Optum360, LLC    N2–N3 ASC Pmt    **CMS:** Pub 100    **AHA:** Coding Clinic    ☿ DMEPOS Paid    ⊘ SNF Excluded    Q Codes (Temporary) — 127

**Temporary Codes**

Q0507 — Q4007

**Q0507** Miscellaneous supply or accessory for use with an external ventricular assist device [A]
CMS: 100-04,32,320.3.5

**Q0508** Miscellaneous supply or accessory for use with an implanted ventricular assist device [A]
CMS: 100-04,32,320.3.5

**Q0509** Miscellaneous supply or accessory for use with any implanted ventricular assist device for which payment was not made under Medicare Part A [A]
CMS: 100-04,32,320.3.5

**Q0510** Pharmacy supply fee for initial immunosuppressive drug(s), first month following transplant [B]

**Q0511** Pharmacy supply fee for oral anticancer, oral antiemetic, or immunosuppressive drug(s); for the first prescription in a 30-day period [B]

**Q0512** Pharmacy supply fee for oral anticancer, oral antiemetic, or immunosuppressive drug(s); for a subsequent prescription in a 30-day period [B]

**Q0513** Pharmacy dispensing fee for inhalation drug(s); per 30 days [B]

**Q0514** Pharmacy dispensing fee for inhalation drug(s); per 90 days [B]

**Q0515** Injection, sermorelin acetate, 1 mcg [E] ☑

**Q1004** New technology, intraocular lens, category 4 as defined in Federal Register notice [E]

**Q1005** New technology, intraocular lens, category 5 as defined in Federal Register notice [E]

**Q2004** Irrigation solution for treatment of bladder calculi, for example renacidin, per 500 ml [N] [N1] ☑

**Q2009** Injection, fosphenytoin, 50 mg phenytoin equivalent [N] [N1] ☑
Use this code for Cerebyx.

**Q2017** Injection, teniposide, 50 mg [K] [K2] ☑
Use this code for Vumon.

**Q2026** Injection, Radiesse, 0.1 ml [B] ☑
CMS: 100-03,250.5; 100-04,32,260.1; 100-04,32,260.2.1; 100-04,32,260.2.2

**Q2028** Injection, sculptra, 0.5 mg [B] ☑
CMS: 100-04,32,260.2.2
AHA: 1Q, '14

**Q2034** Influenza virus vaccine, split virus, for intramuscular use (Agriflu) [L] [L1]
CMS: 100-04,18,10.1.2
AHA: 3Q, '12, 10

**Q2035** Influenza virus vaccine, split virus, when administered to individuals 3 years of age and older, for intramuscular use (AFLURIA) [A] [L] [L1]
CMS: 100-02,15,50.4.4.2; 100-04,18,10.1.2

**Q2036** Influenza virus vaccine, split virus, when administered to individuals 3 years of age and older, for intramuscular use (FLULAVAL) [A] [L] [L1]
CMS: 100-02,15,50.4.4.2; 100-04,18,10.1.2

**Q2037** Influenza virus vaccine, split virus, when administered to individuals 3 years of age and older, for intramuscular use (FLUVIRIN) [A] [L] [L1]
CMS: 100-02,15,50.4.4.2; 100-04,18,10.1.2

**Q2038** Influenza virus vaccine, split virus, when administered to individuals 3 years of age and older, for intramuscular use (Fluzone) [A] [L] [L1]
CMS: 100-02,15,50.4.4.2; 100-04,18,10.1.2

▲ **Q2039**^Jan Influenza virus vaccine, not otherwise specified [A] [L] [L1]
CMS: 100-02,15,50.4.4.2; 100-04,18,10.1.2

**Q2043** Sipuleucel-T, minimum of 50 million autologous cd54+ cells activated with PAP-GM-CSF, including leukapheresis and all other preparatory procedures, per infusion ♂ [K] [K2] ☑
Use this code for PROVENGE.
CMS: 100-03,1,110.22; 100-03,110.22; 100-04,32,280.1; 100-04,32,280.2; 100-04,32,280.4; 100-04,32,280.5
AHA: 2Q, '12, 7; 3Q, '11, 9

**Q2049** Injection, doxorubicin hydrochloride, liposomal, imported Lipodox, 10 mg [K] [K2] ☑
AHA: 3Q, '12, 10

**Q2050** Injection, doxorubicin hydrochloride, liposomal, not otherwise specified, 10 mg [K] [K2] ☑ ◯
AHA: 4Q, '13; 3Q, '13

**Q2052** Services, supplies and accessories used in the home under the Medicare intravenous immune globulin (IVIG) demonstration [E]
AHA: 2Q, '14, 8

**Q3001** Radioelements for brachytherapy, any type, each [B] ☑ ◯

**Q3014** Telehealth originating site facility fee [A] ◯
CMS: 100-04,12,190.5; 100-04,12,190.6

**Q3027** Injection, interferon beta-1a, 1 mcg for intramuscular use [K] [K2] ☑
Use this code for Avonex.
AHA: 1Q, '14

**Q3028** Injection, interferon beta-1a, 1 mcg for subcutaneous use [E] ☑
Use this code for Rebif.

**Q3031** Collagen skin test [N] [N1]

**Q4001** Casting supplies, body cast adult, with or without head, plaster [A] [B] &
CMS: 100-04,20,170
AHA: 2Q, '02, 1-3

**Q4002** Cast supplies, body cast adult, with or without head, fiberglass [A] [B] &
CMS: 100-04,20,170
AHA: 2Q, '02, 1-3

**Q4003** Cast supplies, shoulder cast, adult (11 years +), plaster [A] [B] &
CMS: 100-04,20,170
AHA: 2Q, '02, 1-3

**Q4004** Cast supplies, shoulder cast, adult (11 years +), fiberglass [A] [B] &
CMS: 100-04,20,170
AHA: 2Q, '02, 1-3

**Q4005** Cast supplies, long arm cast, adult (11 years +), plaster [A] [B] &
CMS: 100-04,20,170
AHA: 2Q, '02, 1-3

**Q4006** Cast supplies, long arm cast, adult (11 years +), fiberglass [A] [B] &
CMS: 100-04,20,170
AHA: 2Q, '02, 1-3

**Q4007** Cast supplies, long arm cast, pediatric (0-10 years), plaster [A] [B] &
CMS: 100-04,20,170
AHA: 2Q, '02, 1-3

^Jan **January Update**

Special Coverage Instructions    Noncovered by Medicare    Carrier Discretion    ☑ Quantity Alert   ● New Code   ◯ Recycled/Reinstated   ▲ Revised Code

**128 — Q Codes (Temporary)**    [A] Age Edit   [M] Maternity Edit   ♀ Female Only   ♂ Male Only   [A]-[Y] OPPS Status Indicators    © 2016 Optum360, LLC

| | |
|---|---|
| **Q4008** | **Cast supplies, long arm cast, pediatric (0-10 years), fiberglass** ⒶⒷ♿<br>CMS: 100-04,20,170<br>AHA: 2Q, '02, 1-3 |
| **Q4009** | **Cast supplies, short arm cast, adult (11 years +), plaster** ⒶⒷ♿<br>CMS: 100-04,20,170<br>AHA: 2Q, '02, 1-3 |
| **Q4010** | **Cast supplies, short arm cast, adult (11 years +), fiberglass** ⒶⒷ♿<br>CMS: 100-04,20,170<br>AHA: 2Q, '02, 1-3 |
| **Q4011** | **Cast supplies, short arm cast, pediatric (0-10 years), plaster** ⒶⒷ♿<br>CMS: 100-04,20,170<br>AHA: 2Q, '02, 1-3 |
| **Q4012** | **Cast supplies, short arm cast, pediatric (0-10 years), fiberglass** ⒶⒷ♿<br>CMS: 100-04,20,170<br>AHA: 2Q, '02, 1-3 |
| **Q4013** | **Cast supplies, gauntlet cast (includes lower forearm and hand), adult (11 years +), plaster** ⒶⒷ♿<br>CMS: 100-04,20,170<br>AHA: 2Q, '02, 1-3 |
| **Q4014** | **Cast supplies, gauntlet cast (includes lower forearm and hand), adult (11 years +), fiberglass** ⒶⒷ♿<br>CMS: 100-04,20,170<br>AHA: 2Q, '02, 1-3 |
| **Q4015** | **Cast supplies, gauntlet cast (includes lower forearm and hand), pediatric (0-10 years), plaster** ⒶⒷ♿<br>CMS: 100-04,20,170<br>AHA: 2Q, '02, 1-3 |
| **Q4016** | **Cast supplies, gauntlet cast (includes lower forearm and hand), pediatric (0-10 years), fiberglass** ⒶⒷ♿<br>CMS: 100-04,20,170<br>AHA: 2Q, '02, 1-3 |
| **Q4017** | **Cast supplies, long arm splint, adult (11 years +), plaster** ⒶⒷ♿<br>CMS: 100-04,20,170<br>AHA: 2Q, '02, 1-3 |
| **Q4018** | **Cast supplies, long arm splint, adult (11 years +), fiberglass** ⒶⒷ♿<br>CMS: 100-04,20,170<br>AHA: 2Q, '02, 1-3 |
| **Q4019** | **Cast supplies, long arm splint, pediatric (0-10 years), plaster** ⒶⒷ♿<br>CMS: 100-04,20,170<br>AHA: 2Q, '02, 1-3 |
| **Q4020** | **Cast supplies, long arm splint, pediatric (0-10 years), fiberglass** ⒶⒷ♿<br>CMS: 100-04,20,170<br>AHA: 2Q, '02, 1-3 |
| **Q4021** | **Cast supplies, short arm splint, adult (11 years +), plaster** ⒶⒷ♿<br>CMS: 100-04,20,170<br>AHA: 2Q, '02, 1-3 |
| **Q4022** | **Cast supplies, short arm splint, adult (11 years +), fiberglass** ⒶⒷ♿<br>CMS: 100-04,20,170<br>AHA: 2Q, '02, 1-3 |
| **Q4023** | **Cast supplies, short arm splint, pediatric (0-10 years), plaster** ⒶⒷ♿<br>CMS: 100-04,20,170<br>AHA: 2Q, '02, 1-3 |
| **Q4024** | **Cast supplies, short arm splint, pediatric (0-10 years), fiberglass** ⒶⒷ♿<br>CMS: 100-04,20,170<br>AHA: 2Q, '02, 1-3 |
| **Q4025** | **Cast supplies, hip spica (one or both legs), adult (11 years +), plaster** ⒶⒷ♿<br>CMS: 100-04,20,170<br>AHA: 2Q, '02, 1-3 |
| **Q4026** | **Cast supplies, hip spica (one or both legs), adult (11 years +), fiberglass** ⒶⒷ♿<br>CMS: 100-04,20,170<br>AHA: 2Q, '02, 1-3 |
| **Q4027** | **Cast supplies, hip spica (one or both legs), pediatric (0-10 years), plaster** ⒶⒷ♿<br>CMS: 100-04,20,170<br>AHA: 2Q, '02, 1-3 |
| **Q4028** | **Cast supplies, hip spica (one or both legs), pediatric (0-10 years), fiberglass** ⒶⒷ♿<br>CMS: 100-04,20,170<br>AHA: 2Q, '02, 1-3 |
| **Q4029** | **Cast supplies, long leg cast, adult (11 years +), plaster** ⒶⒷ♿<br>CMS: 100-04,20,170<br>AHA: 2Q, '02, 1-3 |
| **Q4030** | **Cast supplies, long leg cast, adult (11 years +), fiberglass** ⒶⒷ♿<br>CMS: 100-04,20,170<br>AHA: 2Q, '02, 1-3 |
| **Q4031** | **Cast supplies, long leg cast, pediatric (0-10 years), plaster** ⒶⒷ♿<br>CMS: 100-04,20,170<br>AHA: 2Q, '02, 1-3 |
| **Q4032** | **Cast supplies, long leg cast, pediatric (0-10 years), fiberglass** ⒶⒷ♿<br>CMS: 100-04,20,170<br>AHA: 2Q, '02, 1-3 |
| **Q4033** | **Cast supplies, long leg cylinder cast, adult (11 years +), plaster** ⒶⒷ♿<br>CMS: 100-04,20,170<br>AHA: 2Q, '02, 1-3 |
| **Q4034** | **Cast supplies, long leg cylinder cast, adult (11 years +), fiberglass** ⒶⒷ♿<br>CMS: 100-04,20,170<br>AHA: 2Q, '02, 1-3 |
| **Q4035** | **Cast supplies, long leg cylinder cast, pediatric (0-10 years), plaster** ⒶⒷ♿<br>CMS: 100-04,20,170<br>AHA: 2Q, '02, 1-3 |
| **Q4036** | **Cast supplies, long leg cylinder cast, pediatric (0-10 years), fiberglass** ⒶⒷ♿<br>CMS: 100-04,20,170<br>AHA: 2Q, '02, 1-3 |
| **Q4037** | **Cast supplies, short leg cast, adult (11 years +), plaster** ⒶⒷ♿<br>CMS: 100-04,20,170<br>AHA: 2Q, '02, 1-3 |

Temporary Codes

Q4008 — Q4037

Special Coverage Instructions    Noncovered by Medicare    Carrier Discretion    ☑ Quantity Alert    ● New Code    ○ Recycled/Reinstated    ▲ Revised Code

© 2016 Optum360, LLC    Ⓐ²–Ⓩ³ ASC Pmt    CMS: Pub 100    AHA: Coding Clinic    ♿ DMEPOS Paid    ⊘ SNF Excluded    Q Codes (Temporary) — 129

| | | |
|---|---|---|
| **Q4038** | Cast supplies, short leg cast, adult (11 years +), fiberglass | A B ♿ |
| | CMS: 100-04,20,170 | |
| | AHA: 2Q, '02, 1-3 | |
| **Q4039** | Cast supplies, short leg cast, pediatric (0-10 years), plaster | A B ♿ |
| | CMS: 100-04,20,170 | |
| | AHA: 2Q, '02, 1-3 | |
| **Q4040** | Cast supplies, short leg cast, pediatric (0-10 years), fiberglass | A B ♿ |
| | CMS: 100-04,20,170 | |
| | AHA: 2Q, '02, 1-3 | |
| **Q4041** | Cast supplies, long leg splint, adult (11 years +), plaster | A B ♿ |
| | CMS: 100-04,20,170 | |
| | AHA: 2Q, '02, 1-3 | |
| **Q4042** | Cast supplies, long leg splint, adult (11 years +), fiberglass | A B ♿ |
| | CMS: 100-04,20,170 | |
| | AHA: 2Q, '02, 1-3 | |
| **Q4043** | Cast supplies, long leg splint, pediatric (0-10 years), plaster | A B ♿ |
| | CMS: 100-04,20,170 | |
| | AHA: 2Q, '02, 1-3 | |
| **Q4044** | Cast supplies, long leg splint, pediatric (0-10 years), fiberglass | A B ♿ |
| | CMS: 100-04,20,170 | |
| | AHA: 2Q, '02, 1-3 | |
| **Q4045** | Cast supplies, short leg splint, adult (11 years +), plaster | A B ♿ |
| | CMS: 100-04,20,170 | |
| | AHA: 2Q, '02, 1-3 | |
| **Q4046** | Cast supplies, short leg splint, adult (11 years +), fiberglass | A B ♿ |
| | CMS: 100-04,20,170 | |
| | AHA: 2Q, '02, 1-3 | |
| **Q4047** | Cast supplies, short leg splint, pediatric (0-10 years), plaster | A B ♿ |
| | CMS: 100-04,20,170 | |
| | AHA: 2Q, '02, 1-3 | |
| **Q4048** | Cast supplies, short leg splint, pediatric (0-10 years), fiberglass | A B ♿ |
| | CMS: 100-04,20,170 | |
| | AHA: 2Q, '02, 1-3 | |
| **Q4049** | Finger splint, static | B ♿ |
| | CMS: 100-04,20,170 | |
| | AHA: 2Q, '07, 10; 2Q, '02, 1-3 | |
| **Q4050** | Cast supplies, for unlisted types and materials of casts | B |
| | CMS: 100-04,20,170 | |
| | AHA: 2Q, '02, 1-3 | |
| **Q4051** | Splint supplies, miscellaneous (includes thermoplastics, strapping, fasteners, padding and other supplies) | B |
| | CMS: 100-04,20,170 | |
| | AHA: 2Q, '02, 1-3 | |
| **Q4074** | Iloprost, inhalation solution, FDA-approved final product, noncompounded, administered through DME, unit dose form, up to 20 mcg | Y ☑ |
| **Q4081** | Injection, epoetin alfa, 100 units (for ESRD on dialysis) | N ☑ |
| | CMS: 100-04,8,60.4; 100-04,8,60.4.1; 100-04,8,60.4.2; 100-04,8,60.4.4; 100-04,8,60.4.4.1; 100-04,8,60.4.4.2; 100-04,8,60.4.5.1 | |

| | | |
|---|---|---|
| **Q4082** | Drug or biological, not otherwise classified, Part B drug competitive acquisition program (CAP) | B |
| **Q4100** | Skin substitute, not otherwise specified | N N1 ☑ |
| | AHA: 2Q, '12, 7; 2Q, '10, 2, 3 | |
| **Q4101** | Apligraf, per sq cm | N N1 ☑ |
| | AHA: 2Q, '12, 7; 2Q, '10, 2, 3 | |
| **Q4102** | Oasis wound matrix, per sq cm | N N1 ☑ |
| | AHA: 3Q, '12, 8; 2Q, '12, 7; 2Q, '10, 2, 3 | |
| **Q4103** | Oasis burn matrix, per sq cm | N N1 ☑ |
| | AHA: 2Q, '12, 7; 2Q, '10, 2, 3 | |
| **Q4104** | Integra bilayer matrix wound dressing (BMWD), per sq cm | N N1 ☑ |
| | AHA: 3Q, '14, 4; 2Q, '12, 7; 2Q, '10, 8; 2Q, '10, 2, 3 | |
| ▲ **Q4105**Jan | Integra dermal regeneration template (DRT) or Integra Omnigraft dermal regeneration matrix, per sq cm | N N1 ☑ |
| | AHA: 2Q, '12, 7; 2Q, '10, 8; 2Q, '10, 2, 3 | |
| **Q4106** | Dermagraft, per sq cm | N N1 ☑ |
| | AHA: 2Q, '12, 7; 2Q, '10, 2, 3 | |
| **Q4107** | GRAFTJACKET, per sq cm | N N1 ☑ |
| | AHA: 2Q, '12, 7; 2Q, '10, 2, 3 | |
| **Q4108** | Integra matrix, per sq cm | N N1 ☑ |
| | AHA: 2Q, '12, 7; 2Q, '10, 8; 2Q, '10, 2, 3 | |
| **Q4110** | PriMatrix, per sq cm | N N1 ☑ |
| | AHA: 2Q, '12, 7; 2Q, '10, 2, 3 | |
| **Q4111** | GammaGraft, per sq cm | N N1 ☑ |
| | AHA: 2Q, '12, 7; 2Q, '10, 2, 3 | |
| **Q4112** | Cymetra, injectable, 1 cc | N N1 ☑ |
| | AHA: 2Q, '12, 7; 2Q, '10, 2, 3 | |
| **Q4113** | GRAFTJACKET XPRESS, injectable, 1cc | N N1 ☑ |
| | AHA: 2Q, '12, 7; 2Q, '10, 2, 3 | |
| **Q4114** | Integra flowable wound matrix, injectable, 1 cc | N N1 ☑ |
| | AHA: 2Q, '12, 7; 2Q, '10, 8; 2Q, '10, 2, 3 | |
| **Q4115** | AlloSkin, per sq cm | N N1 ☑ |
| | AHA: 2Q, '12, 7; 2Q, '10, 2, 3 | |
| **Q4116** | AlloDerm, per sq cm | N N1 ☑ |
| | AHA: 2Q, '12, 7; 2Q, '10, 2, 3 | |
| **Q4117** | HYALOMATRIX, per sq cm | N N1 ☑ |
| **Q4118** | MatriStem micromatrix, 1 mg | N N1 ☑ |
| | AHA: 4Q, '13; 2Q, '12, 7 | |
| ~~Q4119~~Jan | ~~MatriStem wound matrix, per sq cm~~ | |
| ~~Q4120~~Jan | ~~MatriStem burn matrix, per sq cm~~ | |
| **Q4121** | TheraSkin, per sq cm | G K2 ☑ |
| | AHA: 2Q, '12, 7 | |
| **Q4122** | DermACELL, per sq cm | N N1 ☑ |
| | AHA: 2Q, '12, 7 | |
| **Q4123** | AlloSkin RT, per sq cm | N N1 ☑ |
| **Q4124** | OASIS ultra tri-layer wound matrix, per sq cm | N N1 ☑ |
| | AHA: 2Q, '12, 7 | |
| **Q4125** | ArthroFlex, per sq cm | N N1 ☑ |
| **Q4126** | MemoDerm, DermaSpan, TranZgraft or InteguPly, per sq cm | N N1 ☑ |
| **Q4127** | Talymed, per sq cm | N N1 ☑ |
| | AHA: 2Q, '13 | |
| **Q4128** | FlexHD, AllopatchHD, or Matrix HD, per sq cm | N N1 ☑ |

---

Jan   **January Update**

Special Coverage Instructions      Noncovered by Medicare      Carrier Discretion      ☑ Quantity Alert ● New Code   ○ Recycled/Reinstated   ▲ Revised Code

| Code | Description | Indicators |
|------|-------------|------------|
| Q4129<sup>Jan</sup> | Unite biomatrix, per sq cm | |
| Q4130 | Strattice TM, per sq cm <br> AHA: 2Q, '12, 7 | N N1 ☑ |
| ▲ Q4131<sup>Jan</sup> | EpiFix or Epicord, per sq cm | N N1 ☑ |
| Q4132 | Grafix Core, per sq cm | N N1 ☑ |
| Q4133 | Grafix Prime, per sq cm | N N1 ☑ |
| Q4134 | HMatrix, per sq cm | N N1 ☑ |
| Q4135 | Mediskin, per sq cm | N N1 ☑ |
| Q4136 | E-Z Derm, per sq cm | N N1 ☑ |
| Q4137 | AmnioExcel or BioDExCel, per sq cm <br> AHA: 1Q, '14 | N N1 ☑ |
| Q4138 | BioDFence DryFlex, per sq cm <br> AHA: 1Q, '14 | N N1 ☑ |
| Q4139 | AmnioMatrix or BioDMatrix, injectable, 1 cc <br> AHA: 1Q, '14 | N N1 ☑ |
| Q4140 | BioDFence, per sq cm <br> AHA: 1Q, '14 | N N1 ☑ |
| Q4141 | AlloSkin AC, per sq cm <br> AHA: 1Q, '14 | N N1 ☑ |
| Q4142 | XCM biologic tissue matrix, per sq cm <br> AHA: 1Q, '14 | N N1 ☑ |
| Q4143 | Repriza, per sq cm <br> AHA: 1Q, '14 | N N1 ☑ |
| Q4145 | EpiFix, injectable, 1 mg <br> AHA: 1Q, '14 | N N1 ☑ |
| Q4146 | Tensix, per sq cm <br> AHA: 1Q, '14 | N N1 ☑ |
| Q4147 | Architect, Architect PX, or Architect FX, extracellular matrix, per sq cm <br> AHA: 1Q, '14 | N N1 ☑ |
| Q4148 | Neox 1k, per sq cm <br> AHA: 1Q, '14 | N N1 ☑ |
| Q4149 | Excellagen, 0.1 cc <br> AHA: 1Q, '14 | N N1 ☑ |
| Q4150 | AlloWrap DS or dry, per sq cm | N N1 |
| Q4151 | AmnioBand or Guardian, per sq cm | N N1 |
| Q4152 | DermaPure, per sq cm | N N1 |
| Q4153 | Dermavest and Plurivest, per sq cm <br> AHA: 1Q, '16, 6-8 | N N1 |
| Q4154 | Biovance, per sq cm | N N1 |
| Q4155 | Neox Flo or Clarix Flo 1 mg | N N1 |
| Q4156 | Neox 100, per sq cm | N N1 |
| Q4157 | Revitalon, per sq cm | N N1 |
| Q4158 | Marigen, per sq cm | N N1 |
| Q4159 | Affinity, per sq cm | N N1 |
| Q4160 | Nushield, per sq cm | N N1 |
| Q4161 | Bio-ConneKt wound matrix, per sq cm <br> AHA: 1Q, '16, 6-8 | N |
| Q4162 | AmnioPro Flow, BioSkin Flow, BioRenew Flow, WoundEx Flow, Amniogen-A, Amniogen-C, 0.5 cc <br> AHA: 1Q, '16, 6-8 | N |

| Code | Description | Indicators |
|------|-------------|------------|
| Q4163 | AmnioPro, BioSkin, BioRenew, WoundEx, Amniogen-45, Amniogen-200, per sq cm <br> AHA: 1Q, '16, 6-8 | N |
| Q4164 | Helicoll, per sq cm <br> AHA: 1Q, '16, 6-8 | N |
| Q4165 | Keramatrix, per sq cm <br> AHA: 1Q, '16, 6-8 | N |
| ● Q4166<sup>Jan</sup> | Cytal, per sq cm | |
| ● Q4167<sup>Jan</sup> | Truskin, per sq cm | |
| ● Q4168<sup>Jan</sup> | AmnioBand, 1 mg | |
| ● Q4169<sup>Jan</sup> | Artacent wound, per sq cm | |
| ● Q4170<sup>Jan</sup> | Cygnus, per sq cm | |
| ● Q4171<sup>Jan</sup> | Interfyl, 1 mg | |
| ● Q4172<sup>Jan</sup> | PuraPly or PuraPly AM, per sq cm | |
| ● Q4173<sup>Jan</sup> | PalinGen or PalinGen XPlus, per sq cm | |
| ● Q4174<sup>Jan</sup> | PalinGen or ProMatrX, 0.36 mg per 0.25 cc | |
| ● Q4175<sup>Jan</sup> | Miroderm, per sq cm | |
| Q5001 | Hospice or home health care provided in patient's home/residence <br> CMS: 100-04,10,40.2; 100-04,11,10; 100-04,11,30.3 | B |
| Q5002 | Hospice or home health care provided in assisted living facility <br> CMS: 100-04,10,40.2; 100-04,11,10; 100-04,11,30.3 | B |
| Q5003 | Hospice care provided in nursing long-term care facility (LTC) or nonskilled nursing facility (NF) <br> CMS: 100-04,11,10; 100-04,11,30.3 | B |
| Q5004 | Hospice care provided in skilled nursing facility (SNF) <br> CMS: 100-04,11,10; 100-04,11,30.3 | B |
| Q5005 | Hospice care provided in inpatient hospital <br> CMS: 100-04,11,10; 100-04,11,30.3 | B |
| Q5006 | Hospice care provided in inpatient hospice facility <br> CMS: 100-04,11,10; 100-04,11,30.3 | B |
| Q5007 | Hospice care provided in long-term care facility <br> CMS: 100-04,11,10; 100-04,11,30.3 | B |
| Q5008 | Hospice care provided in inpatient psychiatric facility <br> CMS: 100-04,11,10; 100-04,11,30.3 | B |
| Q5009 | Hospice or home health care provided in place not otherwise specified (NOS) <br> CMS: 100-04,10,40.2; 100-04,11,10; 100-04,11,30.3 | B |
| Q5010 | Hospice home care provided in a hospice facility <br> CMS: 100-04,11,10; 100-04,11,30.3 | B |
| Q5101 | Injection, filgrastim (G-CSF), biosimilar, 1 microgram <br> Use this code for Zarxio. Also assign modifier ZA. <br> AHA: 2Q, '16; 4Q, '15, 4; 3Q, '15, 7 | G K2 |
| ● Q5102<sup>Jul</sup> | Injection, infliximab, biosimilar, 10 mg <br> Use this code for Inflectra. Also assign modifier ZB. | E |
| Q9950 | Injection, sulfur hexafluoride lipid microspheres, per ml <br> Use this code for Lumason. | G K2 |
| Q9951 | Low osmolar contrast material, 400 or greater mg/ml iodine concentration, per ml <br> AHA: 3Q, '12, 8 | N N1 ☑ |
| Q9953 | Injection, iron-based magnetic resonance contrast agent, per ml <br> AHA: 3Q, '12, 8 | N N1 ☑ |

<sup>Jan</sup> January Update  <sup>Jul</sup> July Update

Special Coverage Instructions | Noncovered by Medicare | Carrier Discretion | ☑ Quantity Alert | ● New Code | ○ Recycled/Reinstated | ▲ Revised Code

© 2016 Optum360, LLC | A2-Z3 ASC Pmt | CMS: Pub 100 | AHA: Coding Clinic | ✋ DMEPOS Paid | ⊘ SNF Excluded | Q Codes (Temporary) — 131

**Temporary Codes**

**Q9954 — Q9983**

**Q9954** Oral magnetic resonance contrast agent, per 100 ml  ⓃⓂ☑
AHA: 3Q, '12, 8

**Q9955** Injection, perflexane lipid microspheres, per ml  ⓃⓂ☑
AHA: 3Q, '12, 8

**Q9956** Injection, octafluoropropane microspheres, per ml  ⓃⓂ☑
Use this code for Optison.
AHA: 3Q, '12, 8

**Q9957** Injection, perflutren lipid microspheres, per ml  ⓃⓂ☑
Use this code for Definity.
AHA: 3Q, '12, 8

**Q9958** High osmolar contrast material, up to 149 mg/ml iodine
concentration, per ml  ⓃⓂ☑
AHA: 3Q, '12, 8; 4Q, '11, 6; 1Q, '07, 6; 3Q, '05, 7, 9

**Q9959** High osmolar contrast material, 150-199 mg/ml iodine
concentration, per ml  ⓃⓂ☑
AHA: 3Q, '12, 8; 4Q, '11, 6; 3Q, '05, 7, 9

**Q9960** High osmolar contrast material, 200-249 mg/ml iodine
concentration, per ml  ⓃⓂ☑
AHA: 3Q, '12, 8; 4Q, '11, 6; 1Q, '07, 6; 3Q, '05, 7, 9

**Q9961** High osmolar contrast material, 250-299 mg/ml iodine
concentration, per ml  ⓃⓂ☑
AHA: 3Q, '12, 8; 4Q, '11, 6; 3Q, '05, 7, 9

**Q9962** High osmolar contrast material, 300-349 mg/ml iodine
concentration, per ml  ⓃⓂ☑
AHA: 3Q, '12, 8; 4Q, '11, 6; 3Q, '05, 7, 9

**Q9963** High osmolar contrast material, 350-399 mg/ml iodine
concentration, per ml  ⓃⓂ☑
AHA: 3Q, '12, 8; 4Q, '11, 6; 3Q, '05, 7, 9

**Q9964** High osmolar contrast material, 400 or greater mg/ml iodine
concentration, per ml  ⓃⓂ☑
AHA: 3Q, '12, 8; 4Q, '11, 6; 3Q, '05, 7, 9

**Q9965** Low osmolar contrast material, 100-199 mg/ml iodine
concentration, per ml  ⓃⓂ☑
Use this code for Omnipaque 140, Omnipaque 180, Optiray 160, Optiray
140, ULTRAVIST 150.
AHA: 3Q, '12, 8; 4Q, '11, 6; 1Q, '08, 6

**Q9966** Low osmolar contrast material, 200-299 mg/ml iodine
concentration, per ml  ⓃⓂ☑
Use this code for Omnipaque 240, Optiray 240, ULTRAVIST 240.
AHA: 3Q, '12, 8; 4Q, '11, 6; 1Q, '08, 6

**Q9967** Low osmolar contrast material, 300-399 mg/ml iodine
concentration, per ml  ⓃⓂ☑
Use this code for Omnipaque 300, Omnipaque 350, Optiray, Optiray 300,
Optiray 320, Oxilan 300, Oxilan 350, ULTRAVIST 300, ULTRAVIST 370.
AHA: 3Q, '12, 8; 4Q, '11, 6; 1Q, '08, 6

**Q9968** Injection, nonradioactive, noncontrast, visualization adjunct
(e.g., methylene blue, isosulfan blue), 1 mg  ⓀⓀ²☑

**Q9969** Tc-99m from nonhighly enriched uranium source, full cost
recovery add-on, per study dose  Ⓚ☑

~~**Q9980**~~ᴶᵃⁿ ~~Hyaluronan or derivative, for intra-articular injection, 1 mg~~

~~**Q9981**~~ᴶᵃⁿ ~~Rolapitant, oral, 1 mg~~
To report, see ~J8670

● **Q9982**ᴶᵘˡ Flutemetamol F18, diagnostic, per study dose, up to 5
millicuries  ⒼⓀ²
Use this code for Vizamyl.

● **Q9983**ᴶᵘˡ Florbetaben F18, diagnostic, per study dose, up to 8.1
millicuries  ⒼⓀ²
Use this code for Neuraceq.

ᴶᵃⁿ **January Update**          ᴶᵘˡ **July Update**

Special Coverage Instructions   Noncovered by Medicare   Carrier Discretion   ☑ Quantity Alert  ● New Code   ○ Recycled/Reinstated  ▲ Revised Code

**132 — Q Codes**          🅐 Age Edit   Ⓜ Maternity Edit  ♀ Female Only  ♂ Male Only   🅐-🆈 OPPS Status Indicators        © 2016 Optum360, LLC
**(Temporary)**

## Diagnostic Radiology Services R0070-R0076

R codes are used for the transportation of portable x-ray and/or EKG equipment.

**R0070** **Transportation of portable x-ray equipment and personnel to home or nursing home, per trip to facility or location, one patient seen** Ⓑ ☑

Only a single, reasonable transportation charge is allowed for each trip the portable x-ray supplier makes to a location. When more than one patient is x-rayed at the same location, prorate the single allowable transport charge among all patients.

**CMS:** 100-04,13,90.3

**R0075** **Transportation of portable x-ray equipment and personnel to home or nursing home, per trip to facility or location, more than one patient seen** Ⓑ ☑

Only a single, reasonable transportation charge is allowed for each trip the portable x-ray supplier makes to a location. When more than one patient is x-rayed at the same location, prorate the single allowable transport charge among all patients.

**CMS:** 100-04,13,90.3

**R0076** **Transportation of portable EKG to facility or location, per patient** Ⓑ ☑

Only a single, reasonable transportation charge is allowed for each trip the portable EKG supplier makes to a location. When more than one patient is tested at the same location, prorate the single allowable transport charge among all patients.

**CMS:** 100-04,13,90.3

Special Coverage Instructions     Noncovered by Medicare     Carrier Discretion     ☑ Quantity Alert ● New Code     ○ Recycled/Reinstated     ▲ Revised Code

© 2016 Optum360, LLC     A2-Z3 ASC Pmt     CMS: Pub 100     AHA: Coding Clinic     ⅗ DMEPOS Paid     ⊘ SNF Excluded     R Codes — 133

## Temporary National Codes (Non-Medicare) S0012-S9999

The S codes are used by the Blue Cross/Blue Shield Association (BCBSA) and the Health Insurance Association of America (HIAA) to report drugs, services, and supplies for which there are no national codes but for which codes are needed by the private sector to implement policies, programs, or claims processing. They are for the purpose of meeting the particular needs of the private sector. These codes are also used by the Medicaid program, but they are not payable by Medicare.

**S0012**  **Butorphanol tartrate, nasal spray, 25 mg** ☑
Use this code for Stadol NS.

**S0014**  **Tacrine HCl, 10 mg** ☑
Use this code for Cognex.

**S0017**  **Injection, aminocaproic acid, 5 g** ☑
Use this code for Amicar.

**S0020**  **Injection, bupivicaine HCl, 30 ml** ☑
Use this code for Marcaine, Sensorcaine.

**S0021**  **Injection, cefoperazone sodium, 1 g** ☑
Use this code for Cefobid.

**S0023**  **Injection, cimetidine HCl, 300 mg** ☑
Use this code for Tagamet HCl.

**S0028**  **Injection, famotidine, 20 mg** ☑
Use this code for Pepcid.

**S0030**  **Injection, metronidazole, 500 mg** ☑
Use this code for Flagyl IV RTU.

**S0032**  **Injection, nafcillin sodium, 2 g** ☑
Use this code for Nallpen, Unipen.

**S0034**  **Injection, ofloxacin, 400 mg** ☑
Use this code for Floxin IV.

**S0039**  **Injection, sulfamethoxazole and trimethoprim, 10 ml** ☑
Use this code for Bactrim IV, Septra IV, SMZ-TMP, Sulfutrim.

**S0040**  **Injection, ticarcillin disodium and clavulanate potassium, 3.1 g** ☑
Use this code for Timentin.

**S0073**  **Injection, aztreonam, 500 mg** ☑
Use this code for Azactam.

**S0074**  **Injection, cefotetan disodium, 500 mg** ☑
Use this code for Cefotan.

**S0077**  **Injection, clindamycin phosphate, 300 mg** ☑
Use this code for Cleocin Phosphate.

**S0078**  **Injection, fosphenytoin sodium, 750 mg** ☑
Use this code for Cerebryx.

**S0080**  **Injection, pentamidine isethionate, 300 mg** ☑
Use this code for NebuPent, Pentam 300, Pentacarinat. See also code J2545.

**S0081**  **Injection, piperacillin sodium, 500 mg** ☑
Use this code for Pipracil.

**S0088**  **Imatinib, 100 mg** ☑
Use this code for Gleevec.

**S0090**  **Sildenafil citrate, 25 mg** A☑
Use this code for Viagra.

**S0091**  **Granisetron HCl, 1 mg (for circumstances falling under the Medicare statute, use Q0166)** ☑
Use this code for Kytril.

**S0092**  **Injection, hydromorphone HCl, 250 mg (loading dose for infusion pump)** ☑
Use this code for Dilaudid, Hydromophone. See also J1170.

**S0093**  **Injection, morphine sulfate, 500 mg (loading dose for infusion pump)** ☑
Use this code for Duramorph, MS Contin, Morphine Sulfate. See also J2270, J2271, J2275.

**S0104**  **Zidovudine, oral, 100 mg**
See also J3485 for Retrovir.

**S0106**  **Bupropion HCl sustained release tablet, 150 mg, per bottle of 60 tablets** ☑
Use this code for Wellbutrin SR tablets.

**S0108**  **Mercaptopurine, oral, 50 mg** ☑
Use this code for Purinethol oral.

**S0109**  **Methadone, oral, 5 mg** ☑
Use this code for Dolophine.

**S0117**  **Tretinoin, topical, 5 g** ☑

**S0119**  **Ondansetron, oral, 4 mg (for circumstances falling under the Medicare statute, use HCPCS Q code)** ☑
Use this code for Zofran, Zuplenz.

**S0122**  **Injection, menotropins, 75 IU** ☑
Use this code for Humegon, Pergonal, Repronex.

**S0126**  **Injection, follitropin alfa, 75 IU** ☑
Use this code for Gonal-F.

**S0128**  **Injection, follitropin beta, 75 IU** ♀☑
Use this code for Follistim.

**S0132**  **Injection, ganirelix acetate, 250 mcg** ♀
Use this code for Antagon.

**S0136**  **Clozapine, 25 mg** ☑
Use this code for Clozaril.

**S0137**  **Didanosine (ddI), 25 mg** ☑
Use this code for Videx.

**S0138**  **Finasteride, 5 mg** ♂☑
Use this code for Propecia (oral), Proscar (oral).

**S0139**  **Minoxidil, 10 mg** ☑

**S0140**  **Saquinavir, 200 mg** ☑
Use this code for Fortovase (oral), Invirase (oral).

**S0142**  **Colistimethate sodium, inhalation solution administered through DME, concentrated form, per mg** ☑

**S0145**  **Injection, pegylated interferon alfa-2a, 180 mcg per ml**
Use this code for Pegasys.

**S0148**  **Injection, pegylated interferon alfa-2B, 10 mcg** ☑

**S0155**  **Sterile dilutant for epoprostenol, 50 ml** ☑
Use this code for Flolan.

**S0156**  **Exemestane, 25 mg** ☑
Use this code for Aromasin.

**S0157**  **Becaplermin gel 0.01%, 0.5 gm** ☑
Use this code for Regraex Gel.

**S0160**  **Dextroamphetamine sulfate, 5 mg** ☑

**S0164**  **Injection, pantoprazole sodium, 40 mg** ☑
Use this code for Protonix IV.

**S0166**  **Injection, olanzapine, 2.5 mg** ☑
Use this code for Zyprexa.

**S0169**  **Calcitrol, 0.25 mcg** ☑
Use this code for Calcijex.

**S0170**  **Anastrozole, oral, 1 mg** ☑
Use this code for Arimidex.

---

Special Coverage Instructions    Noncovered by Medicare    Carrier Discretion    ☑ Quantity Alert  ● New Code    ○ Recycled/Reinstated   ▲ Revised Code

© 2016 Optum360, LLC    A2-Z3 ASC Pmt   **CMS:** Pub 100   **AHA:** Coding Clinic   ♿ DMEPOS Paid   ⊘ SNF Excluded    S Codes — 135

**Temporary National Codes (Non-Medicare)**

**S0171 — S0500**

| Code | Description | |
|---|---|---|
| S0171 | Injection, bumetanide, 0.5 mg | ☑ |
| | Use this code for Bumex. | |
| S0172 | Chlorambucil, oral, 2 mg | ☑ |
| | Use this code for Leukeran. | |
| S0174 | Dolasetron mesylate, oral 50 mg (for circumstances falling under the Medicare statute, use Q0180) | ☑ |
| | Use this code for Anzemet. | |
| S0175 | Flutamide, oral, 125 mg | ☑ |
| | Use this code for Eulexin. | |
| S0176 | Hydroxyurea, oral, 500 mg | ☑ |
| | Use this code for Droxia, Hydrea, Mylocel. | |
| S0177 | Levamisole HCl, oral, 50 mg | ☑ |
| | Use this code for Ergamisol. | |
| S0178 | Lomustine, oral, 10 mg | ☑ |
| | Use this code for Ceenu. | |
| S0179 | Megestrol acetate, oral, 20 mg | ☑ |
| | Use this code for Megace. | |
| S0182 | Procarbazine HCl, oral, 50 mg | ☑ |
| | Use this code for Matulane. | |
| S0183 | Prochlorperazine maleate, oral, 5 mg (for circumstances falling under the Medicare statute, use Q0164) | ☑ |
| | Use this code for Compazine. | |
| S0187 | Tamoxifen citrate, oral, 10 mg | ☑ |
| | Use this code for Nolvadex. | |
| S0189 | Testosterone pellet, 75 mg | ☑ |
| S0190 | Mifepristone, oral, 200 mg | ♀☑ |
| | Use this code for Mifoprex 200 mg oral. | |
| S0191 | Misoprostol, oral, 200 mcg | ☑ |
| S0194 | Dialysis/stress vitamin supplement, oral, 100 capsules | ☑ |
| S0197 | Prenatal vitamins, 30-day supply | ♀☑ |
| S0199 | Medically induced abortion by oral ingestion of medication including all associated services and supplies (e.g., patient counseling, office visits, confirmation of pregnancy by HCG, ultrasound to confirm duration of pregnancy, ultrasound to confirm completion of abortion) except drugs | ♀ |
| S0201 | Partial hospitalization services, less than 24 hours, per diem | |
| S0207 | Paramedic intercept, nonhospital-based ALS service (nonvoluntary), nontransport | |
| S0208 | Paramedic intercept, hospital-based ALS service (nonvoluntary), nontransport | |
| S0209 | Wheelchair van, mileage, per mile | ☑ |
| S0215 | Nonemergency transportation; mileage, per mile | ☑ |
| | See also codes A0021-A0999 for transportation. | |
| S0220 | Medical conference by a physician with interdisciplinary team of health professionals or representatives of community agencies to coordinate activities of patient care (patient is present); approximately 30 minutes | ☑ |
| S0221 | Medical conference by a physician with interdisciplinary team of health professionals or representatives of community agencies to coordinate activities of patient care (patient is present); approximately 60 minutes | ☑ |
| S0250 | Comprehensive geriatric assessment and treatment planning performed by assessment team | Ⓐ |
| S0255 | Hospice referral visit (advising patient and family of care options) performed by nurse, social worker, or other designated staff | |
| | CMS: 100-04,11,10 | |
| S0257 | Counseling and discussion regarding advance directives or end of life care planning and decisions, with patient and/or surrogate (list separately in addition to code for appropriate evaluation and management service) | |
| S0260 | History and physical (outpatient or office) related to surgical procedure (list separately in addition to code for appropriate evaluation and management service) | |
| S0265 | Genetic counseling, under physician supervision, each 15 minutes | ☑ |
| S0270 | Physician management of patient home care, standard monthly case rate (per 30 days) | ☑ |
| S0271 | Physician management of patient home care, hospice monthly case rate (per 30 days) | ☑ |
| S0272 | Physician management of patient home care, episodic care monthly case rate (per 30 days) | ☑ |
| S0273 | Physician visit at member's home, outside of a capitation arrangement | |
| S0274 | Nurse practitioner visit at member's home, outside of a capitation arrangement | |
| S0280 | Medical home program, comprehensive care coordination and planning, initial plan | |
| S0281 | Medical home program, comprehensive care coordination and planning, maintenance of plan | |
| ● S0285ᴶᵘˡ | Colonoscopy consultation performed prior to a screening colonoscopy procedure | |
| S0302 | Completed early periodic screening diagnosis and treatment (EPSDT) service (list in addition to code for appropriate evaluation and management service) | |
| S0310 | Hospitalist services (list separately in addition to code for appropriate evaluation and management service) | |
| ● S0311ᴶᵘˡ | Comprehensive management and care coordination for advanced illness, per calendar month | |
| S0315 | Disease management program; initial assessment and initiation of the program | |
| S0316 | Disease management program, follow-up/reassessment | |
| S0317 | Disease management program; per diem | ☑ |
| S0320 | Telephone calls by a registered nurse to a disease management program member for monitoring purposes; per month | |
| S0340 | Lifestyle modification program for management of coronary artery disease, including all supportive services; first quarter/stage | |
| S0341 | Lifestyle modification program for management of coronary artery disease, including all supportive services; second or third quarter/stage | |
| S0342 | Lifestyle modification program for management of coronary artery disease, including all supportive services; 4th quarter / stage | |
| S0353 | Treatment planning and care coordination management for cancer initial treatment | |
| S0354 | Treatment planning and care coordination management for cancer established patient with a change of regimen | |
| S0390 | Routine foot care; removal and/or trimming of corns, calluses and/or nails and preventive maintenance in specific medical conditions (e.g., diabetes), per visit | |
| S0395 | Impression casting of a foot performed by a practitioner other than the manufacturer of the orthotic | |
| S0400 | Global fee for extracorporeal shock wave lithotripsy treatment of kidney stone(s) | |
| S0500 | Disposable contact lens, per lens | ☑ |

Jul **July Update**

Special Coverage Instructions    Noncovered by Medicare    Carrier Discretion    ☑ Quantity Alert  ● New Code  ○ Recycled/Reinstated  ▲ Revised Code

136 — S Codes    Ⓐ Age Edit  Ⓜ Maternity Edit  ♀ Female Only  ♂ Male Only  Ⓐ-Ⓨ OPPS Status Indicators    © 2016 Optum360, LLC

| Code | Description | |
|------|-------------|---|
| S0504 | Single vision prescription lens (safety, athletic, or sunglass), per lens | ☑ |
| S0506 | Bifocal vision prescription lens (safety, athletic, or sunglass), per lens | ☑ |
| S0508 | Trifocal vision prescription lens (safety, athletic, or sunglass), per lens | ☑ |
| S0510 | Nonprescription lens (safety, athletic, or sunglass), per lens | ☑ |
| S0512 | Daily wear specialty contact lens, per lens | ☑ |
| S0514 | Color contact lens, per lens | ☑ |
| S0515 | Scleral lens, liquid bandage device, per lens | |
| S0516 | Safety eyeglass frames | |
| S0518 | Sunglasses frames | |
| S0580 | Polycarbonate lens (list this code in addition to the basic code for the lens) | |
| S0581 | Nonstandard lens (list this code in addition to the basic code for the lens) | |
| S0590 | Integral lens service, miscellaneous services reported separately | |
| S0592 | Comprehensive contact lens evaluation | |
| S0595 | Dispensing new spectacle lenses for patient supplied frame | |
| S0596 | Phakic intraocular lens for correction of refractive error | ☑ |
| S0601 | Screening proctoscopy | ♂ |
| S0610 | Annual gynecological examination, new patient | A ♀ |
| S0612 | Annual gynecological examination, established patient | A ♀ |
| S0613 | Annual gynecological examination; clinical breast examination without pelvic evaluation | ♀ |
| S0618 | Audiometry for hearing aid evaluation to determine the level and degree of hearing loss | |
| S0620 | Routine ophthalmological examination including refraction; new patient | |
| S0621 | Routine ophthalmological examination including refraction; established patient | |
| S0622 | Physical exam for college, new or established patient (list separately in addition to appropriate evaluation and management code) | |
| S0630 | Removal of sutures; by a physician other than the physician who originally closed the wound | |
| S0800 | Laser in situ keratomileusis (LASIK) | |
| S0810 | Photorefractive keratectomy (PRK) | |
| S0812 | Phototherapeutic keratectomy (PTK) | |
| S1001 | Deluxe item, patient aware (list in addition to code for basic item)<br>CMS: 100-02,1,10.1.4 | |
| S1002 | Customized item (list in addition to code for basic item) | |
| S1015 | IV tubing extension set | |
| S1016 | Non-PVC (polyvinyl chloride) intravenous administration set, for use with drugs that are not stable in PVC e.g., Paclitaxel | |
| S1030 | Continuous noninvasive glucose monitoring device, purchase (for physician interpretation of data, use CPT code) | |
| S1031 | Continuous noninvasive glucose monitoring device, rental, including sensor, sensor replacement, and download to monitor (for physician interpretation of data, use CPT code) | |
| S1034 | Artificial pancreas device system (e.g., low glucose suspend [LGS] feature) including continuous glucose monitor, blood glucose device, insulin pump and computer algorithm that communicates with all of the devices | |
| S1035 | Sensor; invasive (e.g., subcutaneous), disposable, for use with artificial pancreas device system | |
| S1036 | Transmitter; external, for use with artificial pancreas device system | |
| S1037 | Receiver (monitor); external, for use with artificial pancreas device system | |
| S1040 | Cranial remolding orthotic, pediatric, rigid, with soft interface material, custom fabricated, includes fitting and adjustment(s) | |
| S1090 | Mometasone furoate sinus implant, 370 micrograms | |
| S2053 | Transplantation of small intestine and liver allografts | |
| S2054 | Transplantation of multivisceral organs | |
| S2055 | Harvesting of donor multivisceral organs, with preparation and maintenance of allografts; from cadaver donor | |
| S2060 | Lobar lung transplantation | |
| S2061 | Donor lobectomy (lung) for transplantation, living donor | |
| S2065 | Simultaneous pancreas kidney transplantation | |
| S2066 | Breast reconstruction with gluteal artery perforator (GAP) flap, including harvesting of the flap, microvascular transfer, closure of donor site and shaping the flap into a breast, unilateral | |
| S2067 | Breast reconstruction of a single breast with "stacked" deep inferior epigastric perforator (DIEP) flap(s) and/or gluteal artery perforator (GAP) flap(s), including harvesting of the flap(s), microvascular transfer, closure of donor site(s) and shaping the flap into a breast, unilateral | |
| S2068 | Breast reconstruction with deep inferior epigastric perforator (DIEP) flap or superficial inferior epigastric artery (SIEA) flap, including harvesting of the flap, microvascular transfer, closure of donor site and shaping the flap into a breast, unilateral | |
| S2070 | Cystourethroscopy, with ureteroscopy and/or pyeloscopy; with endoscopic laser treatment of ureteral calculi (includes ureteral catheterization) | |
| S2079 | Laparoscopic esophagomyotomy (Heller type) | |
| S2080 | Laser-assisted uvulopalatoplasty (LAUP) | |
| S2083 | Adjustment of gastric band diameter via subcutaneous port by injection or aspiration of saline | |
| S2095 | Transcatheter occlusion or embolization for tumor destruction, percutaneous, any method, using yttrium-90 microspheres | |
| S2102 | Islet cell tissue transplant from pancreas; allogeneic | |
| S2103 | Adrenal tissue transplant to brain | |
| S2107 | Adoptive immunotherapy i.e. development of specific antitumor reactivity (e.g., tumor-infiltrating lymphocyte therapy) per course of treatment | |
| S2112 | Arthroscopy, knee, surgical for harvesting of cartilage (chondrocyte cells) | |
| S2115 | Osteotomy, periacetabular, with internal fixation | |
| S2117 | Arthroereisis, subtalar | |
| S2118 | Metal-on-metal total hip resurfacing, including acetabular and femoral components | |
| S2120 | Low density lipoprotein (LDL) apheresis using heparin-induced extracorporeal LDL precipitation | |
| S2140 | Cord blood harvesting for transplantation, allogeneic | |
| S2142 | Cord blood-derived stem-cell transplantation, allogeneic | |

---

Special Coverage Instructions    Noncovered by Medicare    Carrier Discretion    ☑ Quantity Alert   ● New Code   ○ Recycled/Reinstated   ▲ Revised Code

**Temporary National Codes (Non-Medicare)**

**S2150 — S3852**

**S2150** Bone marrow or blood-derived stem cells (peripheral or umbilical), allogeneic or autologous, harvesting, transplantation, and related complications; including: pheresis and cell preparation/storage; marrow ablative therapy; drugs, supplies, hospitalization with outpatient follow-up; medical/surgical, diagnostic, emergency, and rehabilitative services; and the number of days of pre and post transplant care in the global definition

**S2152** Solid organ(s), complete or segmental, single organ or combination of organs; deceased or living donor (s), procurement, transplantation, and related complications; including: drugs; supplies; hospitalization with outpatient follow-up; medical/surgical, diagnostic, emergency, and rehabilitative services, and the number of days of pre and posttransplant care in the global definition

**S2202** Echosclerotherapy

**S2205** Minimally invasive direct coronary artery bypass surgery involving mini-thoracotomy or mini-sternotomy surgery, performed under direct vision; using arterial graft(s), single coronary arterial graft

**S2206** Minimally invasive direct coronary artery bypass surgery involving mini-thoracotomy or mini-sternotomy surgery, performed under direct vision; using arterial graft(s), 2 coronary arterial grafts

**S2207** Minimally invasive direct coronary artery bypass surgery involving mini-thoracotomy or mini-sternotomy surgery, performed under direct vision; using venous graft only, single coronary venous graft

**S2208** Minimally invasive direct coronary artery bypass surgery involving mini-thoracotomy or mini-sternotomy surgery, performed under direct vision; using single arterial and venous graft(s), single venous graft

**S2209** Minimally invasive direct coronary artery bypass surgery involving mini-thoracotomy or mini-sternotomy surgery, performed under direct vision; using 2 arterial grafts and single venous graft

**S2225** Myringotomy, laser-assisted

**S2230** Implantation of magnetic component of semi-implantable hearing device on ossicles in middle ear

**S2235** Implantation of auditory brain stem implant

**S2260** Induced abortion, 17 to 24 weeks  M ♀

**S2265** Induced abortion, 25 to 28 weeks  M ♀

**S2266** Induced abortion, 29 to 31 weeks  M ♀

**S2267** Induced abortion, 32 weeks or greater  M ♀

**S2300** Arthroscopy, shoulder, surgical; with thermally-induced capsulorrhaphy

**S2325** Hip core decompression

**S2340** Chemodenervation of abductor muscle(s) of vocal cord

**S2341** Chemodenervation of adductor muscle(s) of vocal cord

**S2342** Nasal endoscopy for postoperative debridement following functional endoscopic sinus surgery, nasal and/or sinus cavity(s), unilateral or bilateral

**S2348** Decompression procedure, percutaneous, of nucleus pulposus of intervertebral disc, using radiofrequency energy, single or multiple levels, lumbar

**S2350** Diskectomy, anterior, with decompression of spinal cord and/or nerve root(s), including osteophytectomy; lumbar, single interspace

**S2351** Diskectomy, anterior, with decompression of spinal cord and/or nerve root(s), including osteophytectomy; lumbar, each additional interspace (list separately in addition to code for primary procedure)

**S2400** Repair, congenital diaphragmatic hernia in the fetus using temporary tracheal occlusion, procedure performed in utero  M ♀

**S2401** Repair, urinary tract obstruction in the fetus, procedure performed in utero  M ♀

**S2402** Repair, congenital cystic adenomatoid malformation in the fetus, procedure performed in utero  M ♀

**S2403** Repair, extralobar pulmonary sequestration in the fetus, procedure performed in utero  M ♀

**S2404** Repair, myelomeningocele in the fetus, procedure performed in utero  M ♀

**S2405** Repair of sacrococcygeal teratoma in the fetus, procedure performed in utero  M ♀

**S2409** Repair, congenital malformation of fetus, procedure performed in utero, not otherwise classified  M ♀

**S2411** Fetoscopic laser therapy for treatment of twin-to-twin transfusion syndrome  M ♀

**S2900** Surgical techniques requiring use of robotic surgical system (list separately in addition to code for primary procedure)
**AHA:** 2Q, '10, 6

**S3000** Diabetic indicator; retinal eye exam, dilated, bilateral

**S3005** Performance measurement, evaluation of patient self assessment, depression

**S3600** STAT laboratory request (situations other than S3601)

**S3601** Emergency STAT laboratory charge for patient who is homebound or residing in a nursing facility

**S3620** Newborn metabolic screening panel, includes test kit, postage and the laboratory tests specified by the state for inclusion in this panel (e.g., galactose; hemoglobin, electrophoresis; hydroxyprogesterone, 17-d; phenylanine (PKU); and thyroxine, total)  A

**S3630** Eosinophil count, blood, direct

**S3645** HIV-1 antibody testing of oral mucosal transudate

**S3650** Saliva test, hormone level; during menopause  A ♀

**S3652** Saliva test, hormone level; to assess preterm labor risk  M ♀

**S3655** Antisperm antibodies test (immunobead)  M ♀

**S3708** Gastrointestinal fat absorption study

**S3722** Dose optimization by area under the curve (AUC) analysis, for infusional 5-fluorouracil

**S3800** Genetic testing for amyotrophic lateral sclerosis (ALS)

**S3840** DNA analysis for germline mutations of the RET proto-oncogene for susceptibility to multiple endocrine neoplasia type 2

**S3841** Genetic testing for retinoblastoma

**S3842** Genetic testing for Von Hippel-Lindau disease

**S3844** DNA analysis of the connexin 26 gene (GJB2) for susceptibility to congenital, profound deafness

**S3845** Genetic testing for alpha-thalassemia

**S3846** Genetic testing for hemoglobin E beta-thalassemia

**S3849** Genetic testing for Niemann-Pick disease

**S3850** Genetic testing for sickle cell anemia

**S3852** DNA analysis for APOE epsilon 4 allele for susceptibility to Alzheimer's disease

---

 Special Coverage Instructions     Noncovered by Medicare     Carrier Discretion     ☑ Quantity Alert  ● New Code     ○ Recycled/Reinstated  ▲ Revised Code

**138 — S Codes**      A Age Edit     M Maternity Edit     ♀ Female Only     ♂ Male Only     A-Y OPPS Status Indicators          © 2016 Optum360, LLC

| | | |
|---|---|---|
| S3853 | Genetic testing for myotonic muscular dystrophy | |
| ○ S3854^Jul | Gene expression profiling panel for use in the management of breast cancer treatment AHA: 2Q, '16 | |
| S3861 | Genetic testing, sodium channel, voltage-gated, type V, alpha subunit (SCN5A) and variants for suspected Brugada Syndrome | |
| S3865 | Comprehensive gene sequence analysis for hypertrophic cardiomyopathy | |
| S3866 | Genetic analysis for a specific gene mutation for hypertrophic cardiomyopathy (HCM) in an individual with a known HCM mutation in the family | |
| S3870 | Comparative genomic hybridization (CGH) microarray testing for developmental delay, autism spectrum disorder and/or intellectual disability | |
| S3900 | Surface electromyography (EMG) | |
| S3902 | Ballistocardiogram | |
| S3904 | Masters 2 step | |
| S4005 | Interim labor facility global (labor occurring but not resulting in delivery) | M ♀ |
| S4011 | In vitro fertilization; including but not limited to identification and incubation of mature oocytes, fertilization with sperm, incubation of embryo(s), and subsequent visualization for determination of development | M ♀ |
| S4013 | Complete cycle, gamete intrafallopian transfer (GIFT), case rate | M ♀ |
| S4014 | Complete cycle, zygote intrafallopian transfer (ZIFT), case rate | M ♀ |
| S4015 | Complete in vitro fertilization cycle, not otherwise specified, case rate | M ♀ |
| S4016 | Frozen in vitro fertilization cycle, case rate | M ♀ |
| S4017 | Incomplete cycle, treatment cancelled prior to stimulation, case rate | M ♀ |
| S4018 | Frozen embryo transfer procedure cancelled before transfer, case rate | M ♀ |
| S4020 | In vitro fertilization procedure cancelled before aspiration, case rate | M ♀ |
| S4021 | In vitro fertilization procedure cancelled after aspiration, case rate | M ♀ |
| S4022 | Assisted oocyte fertilization, case rate | M ♀ |
| S4023 | Donor egg cycle, incomplete, case rate | M ♀ |
| S4025 | Donor services for in vitro fertilization (sperm or embryo), case rate | A ♀ |
| S4026 | Procurement of donor sperm from sperm bank | ♂ |
| S4027 | Storage of previously frozen embryos | M ♀ |
| S4028 | Microsurgical epididymal sperm aspiration (MESA) | A ♂ |
| S4030 | Sperm procurement and cryopreservation services; initial visit | A ♂ |
| S4031 | Sperm procurement and cryopreservation services; subsequent visit | A ♂ |
| S4035 | Stimulated intrauterine insemination (IUI), case rate | M ♀ |
| S4037 | Cryopreserved embryo transfer, case rate | M ♀ |
| S4040 | Monitoring and storage of cryopreserved embryos, per 30 days | M ♀ |
| S4042 | Management of ovulation induction (interpretation of diagnostic tests and studies, nonface-to-face medical management of the patient), per cycle | |
| S4981 | Insertion of levonorgestrel-releasing intrauterine system | ♀ |
| S4989 | Contraceptive intrauterine device (e.g., Progestacert IUD), including implants and supplies | M ♀ |
| S4990 | Nicotine patches, legend | ☑ |
| S4991 | Nicotine patches, nonlegend | ☑ |
| S4993 | Contraceptive pills for birth control | M ♀ |
| S4995 | Smoking cessation gum | |
| S5000 | Prescription drug, generic | ☑ |
| S5001 | Prescription drug, brand name | ☑ |
| S5010 | 5% dextrose and 0.45% normal saline, 1000 ml | ☑ |
| S5012 | 5% dextrose with potassium chloride, 1000 ml | ☑ |
| S5013 | 5% dextrose/0.45% normal saline with potassium chloride and magnesium sulfate, 1000 ml | ☑ |
| S5014 | 5% dextrose/0.45% normal saline with potassium chloride and magnesium sulfate, 1500 ml | ☑ |
| S5035 | Home infusion therapy, routine service of infusion device (e.g., pump maintenance) | |
| S5036 | Home infusion therapy, repair of infusion device (e.g., pump repair) | |
| S5100 | Day care services, adult; per 15 minutes | A ☑ |
| S5101 | Day care services, adult; per half day | A ☑ |
| S5102 | Day care services, adult; per diem | A ☑ |
| S5105 | Day care services, center-based; services not included in program fee, per diem | ☑ |
| S5108 | Home care training to home care client, per 15 minutes | ☑ |
| S5109 | Home care training to home care client, per session | ☑ |
| S5110 | Home care training, family; per 15 minutes | ☑ |
| S5111 | Home care training, family; per session | |
| S5115 | Home care training, nonfamily; per 15 minutes | ☑ |
| S5116 | Home care training, nonfamily; per session | ☑ |
| S5120 | Chore services; per 15 minutes | ☑ |
| S5121 | Chore services; per diem | ☑ |
| S5125 | Attendant care services; per 15 minutes | ☑ |
| S5126 | Attendant care services; per diem | ☑ |
| S5130 | Homemaker service, NOS; per 15 minutes | ☑ |
| S5131 | Homemaker service, NOS; per diem | ☑ |
| S5135 | Companion care, adult (e.g., IADL/ADL); per 15 minutes | A ☑ |
| S5136 | Companion care, adult (e.g., IADL/ADL); per diem | A ☑ |
| S5140 | Foster care, adult; per diem | A ☑ |
| S5141 | Foster care, adult; per month | A ☑ |
| S5145 | Foster care, therapeutic, child; per diem | A ☑ |
| S5146 | Foster care, therapeutic, child; per month | A ☑ |
| S5150 | Unskilled respite care, not hospice; per 15 minutes | ☑ |
| S5151 | Unskilled respite care, not hospice; per diem | ☑ |
| S5160 | Emergency response system; installation and testing | |
| S5161 | Emergency response system; service fee, per month (excludes installation and testing) | ☑ |

**Jul** **July Update**

Special Coverage Instructions    Noncovered by Medicare    Carrier Discretion    ☑ Quantity Alert ● New Code ○ Recycled/Reinstated ▲ Revised Code

© 2016 Optum360, LLC   A2-Z3 ASC Pmt   CMS: Pub 100   AHA: Coding Clinic   ⅋ DMEPOS Paid   ⊘ SNF Excluded    S Codes — 139

| Code | Description | |
|------|-------------|---|
| S5162 | Emergency response system; purchase only | |
| S5165 | Home modifications; per service | |
| S5170 | Home delivered meals, including preparation; per meal | |
| S5175 | Laundry service, external, professional; per order | |
| S5180 | Home health respiratory therapy, initial evaluation | |
| S5181 | Home health respiratory therapy, NOS, per diem | |
| S5185 | Medication reminder service, nonface-to-face; per month | ☑ |
| S5190 | Wellness assessment, performed by nonphysician | |
| S5199 | Personal care item, NOS, each | |
| S5497 | Home infusion therapy, catheter care/maintenance, not otherwise classified; includes administrative services, professional pharmacy services, care coordination, and all necessary supplies and equipment (drugs and nursing visits coded separately), per diem | ☑ |
| S5498 | Home infusion therapy, catheter care/maintenance, simple (single lumen), includes administrative services, professional pharmacy services, care coordination and all necessary supplies and equipment, (drugs and nursing visits coded separately), per diem | ☑ |
| S5501 | Home infusion therapy, catheter care/maintenance, complex (more than one lumen), includes administrative services, professional pharmacy services, care coordination, and all necessary supplies and equipment (drugs and nursing visits coded separately), per diem | ☑ |
| S5502 | Home infusion therapy, catheter care/maintenance, implanted access device, includes administrative services, professional pharmacy services, care coordination and all necessary supplies and equipment (drugs and nursing visits coded separately), per diem (use this code for interim maintenance of vascular access not currently in use) | ☑ |
| S5517 | Home infusion therapy, all supplies necessary for restoration of catheter patency or declotting | |
| S5518 | Home infusion therapy, all supplies necessary for catheter repair | |
| S5520 | Home infusion therapy, all supplies (including catheter) necessary for a peripherally inserted central venous catheter (PICC) line insertion | |
| S5521 | Home infusion therapy, all supplies (including catheter) necessary for a midline catheter insertion | |
| S5522 | Home infusion therapy, insertion of peripherally inserted central venous catheter (PICC), nursing services only (no supplies or catheter included) | |
| S5523 | Home infusion therapy, insertion of midline venous catheter, nursing services only (no supplies or catheter included) | |
| S5550 | Insulin, rapid onset, 5 units | ☑ |
| S5551 | Insulin, most rapid onset (Lispro or Aspart); 5 units | ☑ |
| S5552 | Insulin, intermediate acting (NPH or LENTE); 5 units | ☑ |
| S5553 | Insulin, long acting; 5 units | ☑ |
| S5560 | Insulin delivery device, reusable pen; 1.5 ml size | ☑ |
| S5561 | Insulin delivery device, reusable pen; 3 ml size | ☑ |
| S5565 | Insulin cartridge for use in insulin delivery device other than pump; 150 units | ☑ |
| S5566 | Insulin cartridge for use in insulin delivery device other than pump; 300 units | ☑ |
| S5570 | Insulin delivery device, disposable pen (including insulin); 1.5 ml size | ☑ |
| S5571 | Insulin delivery device, disposable pen (including insulin); 3 ml size | ☑ |
| S8030 | Scleral application of tantalum ring(s) for localization of lesions for proton beam therapy | |
| S8032 Oct | ~~Low-dose computed tomography for lung cancer screening~~ To report, see ~G0297 | |
| S8035 | Magnetic source imaging | |
| S8037 | Magnetic resonance cholangiopancreatography (MRCP) | |
| S8040 | Topographic brain mapping | |
| S8042 | Magnetic resonance imaging (MRI), low-field | |
| S8055 | Ultrasound guidance for multifetal pregnancy reduction(s), technical component (only to be used when the physician doing the reduction procedure does not perform the ultrasound, guidance is included in the CPT code for multifetal pregnancy reduction (59866) | Ⓜ ♀ |
| S8080 | Scintimammography (radioimmunoscintigraphy of the breast), unilateral, including supply of radiopharmaceutical | |
| S8085 | Fluorine-18 fluorodeoxyglucose (F-18 FDG) imaging using dual-head coincidence detection system (nondedicated PET scan) | |
| S8092 | Electron beam computed tomography (also known as ultrafast CT, cine CT) | |
| S8096 | Portable peak flow meter | |
| S8097 | Asthma kit (including but not limited to portable peak expiratory flow meter, instructional video, brochure, and/or spacer) | ☑ |
| S8100 | Holding chamber or spacer for use with an inhaler or nebulizer; without mask | |
| S8101 | Holding chamber or spacer for use with an inhaler or nebulizer; with mask | |
| S8110 | Peak expiratory flow rate (physician services) | |
| S8120 | Oxygen contents, gaseous, 1 unit equals 1 cubic foot | ☑ |
| S8121 | Oxygen contents, liquid, 1 unit equals 1 pound | ☑ |
| S8130 | Interferential current stimulator, 2 channel | |
| S8131 | Interferential current stimulator, 4 channel | |
| S8185 | Flutter device | |
| S8186 | Swivel adaptor | |
| S8189 | Tracheostomy supply, not otherwise classified | |
| S8210 | Mucus trap | |
| S8265 | Haberman feeder for cleft lip/palate | |
| S8270 | Enuresis alarm, using auditory buzzer and/or vibration device | |
| S8301 | Infection control supplies, not otherwise specified | |
| S8415 | Supplies for home delivery of infant | Ⓜ ♀ |
| S8420 | Gradient pressure aid (sleeve and glove combination), custom made | |
| S8421 | Gradient pressure aid (sleeve and glove combination), ready made | |
| S8422 | Gradient pressure aid (sleeve), custom made, medium weight | |
| S8423 | Gradient pressure aid (sleeve), custom made, heavy weight | |
| S8424 | Gradient pressure aid (sleeve), ready made | |
| S8425 | Gradient pressure aid (glove), custom made, medium weight | |
| S8426 | Gradient pressure aid (glove), custom made, heavy weight | |
| S8427 | Gradient pressure aid (glove), ready made | |
| S8428 | Gradient pressure aid (gauntlet), ready made | |
| S8429 | Gradient pressure exterior wrap | |

Oct October Update

Special Coverage Instructions    Noncovered by Medicare    Carrier Discretion    ☑ Quantity Alert  ● New Code   ○ Recycled/Reinstated  ▲ Revised Code

140 — S Codes          Ⓐ Age Edit    Ⓜ Maternity Edit    ♀ Female Only    ♂ Male Only    Ⓐ-Ⓨ OPPS Status Indicators    © 2016 Optum360, LLC

| | | |
|---|---|---|
| **S8430** | Padding for compression bandage, roll | ☑ |
| **S8431** | Compression bandage, roll | ☑ |
| **S8450** | Splint, prefabricated, digit (specify digit by use of modifier) | ☑ |

Mobile dorsal splint

Static finger splint

Slip-on splint

Various types of digit splints (S8450)

| | | |
|---|---|---|
| **S8451** | Splint, prefabricated, wrist or ankle | ☑ |
| **S8452** | Splint, prefabricated, elbow | ☑ |
| **S8460** | Camisole, postmastectomy | |
| **S8490** | Insulin syringes (100 syringes, any size) | ☑ |
| **S8930** | Electrical stimulation of auricular acupuncture points; each 15 minutes of personal one-on-one contact with patient | ☑ |
| **S8940** | Equestrian/hippotherapy, per session | |
| **S8948** | Application of a modality (requiring constant provider attendance) to one or more areas; low-level laser; each 15 minutes | ☑ |
| **S8950** | Complex lymphedema therapy, each 15 minutes | ☑ |
| **S8990** | Physical or manipulative therapy performed for maintenance rather than restoration | |
| **S8999** | Resuscitation bag (for use by patient on artificial respiration during power failure or other catastrophic event) | |
| **S9001** | Home uterine monitor with or without associated nursing services | Ⓜ ♀ |
| **S9007** | Ultrafiltration monitor | |
| **S9024** | Paranasal sinus ultrasound | |
| **S9025** | Omnicardiogram/cardiointegram | |
| **S9034** | Extracorporeal shockwave lithotripsy for gall stones (if performed with ERCP, use 43265) | |
| **S9055** | Procuren or other growth factor preparation to promote wound healing | |
| **S9056** | Coma stimulation per diem | ☑ |
| **S9061** | Home administration of aerosolized drug therapy (e.g., Pentamidine); administrative services, professional pharmacy services, care coordination, all necessary supplies and equipment (drugs and nursing visits coded separately), per diem | ☑ |
| **S9083** | Global fee urgent care centers | |
| **S9088** | Services provided in an urgent care center (list in addition to code for service) | |
| **S9090** | Vertebral axial decompression, per session | ☑ |
| **S9097** | Home visit for wound care | |
| **S9098** | Home visit, phototherapy services (e.g., Bili-lite), including equipment rental, nursing services, blood draw, supplies, and other services, per diem | ☑ |
| **S9110** | Telemonitoring of patient in their home, including all necessary equipment; computer system, connections, and software; maintenance; patient education and support; per month | |

| | | |
|---|---|---|
| **S9117** | Back school, per visit | ☑ |
| **S9122** | Home health aide or certified nurse assistant, providing care in the home; per hour | ☑ |
| **S9123** | Nursing care, in the home; by registered nurse, per hour (use for general nursing care only, not to be used when CPT codes 99500-99602 can be used) | ☑ |
| **S9124** | Nursing care, in the home; by licensed practical nurse, per hour | ☑ |
| **S9125** | Respite care, in the home, per diem | ☑ |
| **S9126** | Hospice care, in the home, per diem<br>**CMS:** 100-04,11,10 | ☑ |
| **S9127** | Social work visit, in the home, per diem | ☑ |
| **S9128** | Speech therapy, in the home, per diem | ☑ |
| **S9129** | Occupational therapy, in the home, per diem | ☑ |
| **S9131** | Physical therapy; in the home, per diem | ☑ |
| **S9140** | Diabetic management program, follow-up visit to non-MD provider | |
| **S9141** | Diabetic management program, follow-up visit to MD provider | ☑ |
| **S9145** | Insulin pump initiation, instruction in initial use of pump (pump not included) | |
| **S9150** | Evaluation by ocularist | |
| **S9152** | Speech therapy, re-evaluation | |
| **S9208** | Home management of preterm labor, including administrative services, professional pharmacy services, care coordination, and all necessary supplies or equipment (drugs and nursing visits coded separately), per diem (do not use this code with any home infusion per diem code) | Ⓜ ♀ ☑ |
| **S9209** | Home management of preterm premature rupture of membranes (PPROM), including administrative services, professional pharmacy services, care coordination, and all necessary supplies or equipment (drugs and nursing visits coded separately), per diem (do not use this code with any home infusion per diem code) | Ⓜ ♀ ☑ |
| **S9211** | Home management of gestational hypertension, includes administrative services, professional pharmacy services, care coordination and all necessary supplies and equipment (drugs and nursing visits coded separately); per diem (do not use this code with any home infusion per diem code) | Ⓜ ♀ ☑ |
| **S9212** | Home management of postpartum hypertension, includes administrative services, professional pharmacy services, care coordination, and all necessary supplies and equipment (drugs and nursing visits coded separately), per diem (do not use this code with any home infusion per diem code) | ♀ ☑ |
| **S9213** | Home management of preeclampsia, includes administrative services, professional pharmacy services, care coordination, and all necessary supplies and equipment (drugs and nursing services coded separately); per diem (do not use this code with any home infusion per diem code) | Ⓜ ♀ ☑ |
| **S9214** | Home management of gestational diabetes, includes administrative services, professional pharmacy services, care coordination, and all necessary supplies and equipment (drugs and nursing visits coded separately); per diem (do not use this code with any home infusion per diem code) | Ⓜ ♀ ☑ |
| **S9325** | Home infusion therapy, pain management infusion; administrative services, professional pharmacy services, care coordination, and all necessary supplies and equipment, (drugs and nursing visits coded separately), per diem (do not use this code with S9326, S9327 or S9328) | ☑ |

Special Coverage Instructions      Noncovered by Medicare      Carrier Discretion      ☑ Quantity Alert      ● New Code      ○ Recycled/Reinstated      ▲ Revised Code

© 2016 Optum360, LLC      A2-Z3 ASC Pmt      CMS: Pub 100      AHA: Coding Clinic      ⅊ DMEPOS Paid      ⊘ SNF Excluded

**Temporary National Codes (Non-Medicare)**

**S9326 — S9364**

**S9326** Home infusion therapy, continuous (24 hours or more) pain management infusion; administrative services, professional pharmacy services, care coordination and all necessary supplies and equipment (drugs and nursing visits coded separately), per diem ☑

**S9327** Home infusion therapy, intermittent (less than 24 hours) pain management infusion; administrative services, professional pharmacy services, care coordination, and all necessary supplies and equipment (drugs and nursing visits coded separately), per diem ☑

**S9328** Home infusion therapy, implanted pump pain management infusion; administrative services, professional pharmacy services, care coordination, and all necessary supplies and equipment (drugs and nursing visits coded separately), per diem ☑

**S9329** Home infusion therapy, chemotherapy infusion; administrative services, professional pharmacy services, care coordination, and all necessary supplies and equipment (drugs and nursing visits coded separately), per diem (do not use this code with S9330 or S9331) ☑

**S9330** Home infusion therapy, continuous (24 hours or more) chemotherapy infusion; administrative services, professional pharmacy services, care coordination, and all necessary supplies and equipment (drugs and nursing visits coded separately), per diem ☑

**S9331** Home infusion therapy, intermittent (less than 24 hours) chemotherapy infusion; administrative services, professional pharmacy services, care coordination, and all necessary supplies and equipment (drugs and nursing visits coded separately), per diem ☑

**S9335** Home therapy, hemodialysis; administrative services, professional pharmacy services, care coordination, and all necessary supplies and equipment (drugs and nursing services coded separately), per diem ☑

**S9336** Home infusion therapy, continuous anticoagulant infusion therapy (e.g., Heparin), administrative services, professional pharmacy services, care coordination and all necessary supplies and equipment (drugs and nursing visits coded separately), per diem ☑

**S9338** Home infusion therapy, immunotherapy, administrative services, professional pharmacy services, care coordination, and all necessary supplies and equipment (drugs and nursing visits coded separately), per diem ☑

**S9339** Home therapy; peritoneal dialysis, administrative services, professional pharmacy services, care coordination and all necessary supplies and equipment (drugs and nursing visits coded separately), per diem ☑

**S9340** Home therapy; enteral nutrition; administrative services, professional pharmacy services, care coordination, and all necessary supplies and equipment (enteral formula and nursing visits coded separately), per diem ☑

**S9341** Home therapy; enteral nutrition via gravity; administrative services, professional pharmacy services, care coordination, and all necessary supplies and equipment (enteral formula and nursing visits coded separately), per diem ☑

**S9342** Home therapy; enteral nutrition via pump; administrative services, professional pharmacy services, care coordination, and all necessary supplies and equipment (enteral formula and nursing visits coded separately), per diem ☑

**S9343** Home therapy; enteral nutrition via bolus; administrative services, professional pharmacy services, care coordination, and all necessary supplies and equipment (enteral formula and nursing visits coded separately), per diem ☑

**S9345** Home infusion therapy, antihemophilic agent infusion therapy (e.g., factor VIII); administrative services, professional pharmacy services, care coordination, and all necessary supplies and equipment (drugs and nursing visits coded separately), per diem ☑

**S9346** Home infusion therapy, alpha-1-proteinase inhibitor (e.g., Prolastin); administrative services, professional pharmacy services, care coordination, and all necessary supplies and equipment (drugs and nursing visits coded separately), per diem ☑

**S9347** Home infusion therapy, uninterrupted, long-term, controlled rate intravenous or subcutaneous infusion therapy (e.g., epoprostenol); administrative services, professional pharmacy services, care coordination, and all necessary supplies and equipment (drugs and nursing visits coded separately), per diem ☑

**S9348** Home infusion therapy, sympathomimetic/inotropic agent infusion therapy (e.g., Dobutamine); administrative services, professional pharmacy services, care coordination, all necessary supplies and equipment (drugs and nursing visits coded separately), per diem ☑

**S9349** Home infusion therapy, tocolytic infusion therapy; administrative services, professional pharmacy services, care coordination, and all necessary supplies and equipment (drugs and nursing visits coded separately), per diem Ⓜ ♀☑

**S9351** Home infusion therapy, continuous or intermittent antiemetic infusion therapy; administrative services, professional pharmacy services, care coordination, and all necessary supplies and equipment (drugs and visits coded separately), per diem ☑

**S9353** Home infusion therapy, continuous insulin infusion therapy; administrative services, professional pharmacy services, care coordination, and all necessary supplies and equipment (drugs and nursing visits coded separately), per diem ☑

**S9355** Home infusion therapy, chelation therapy; administrative services, professional pharmacy services, care coordination, and all necessary supplies and equipment (drugs and nursing visits coded separately), per diem ☑

**S9357** Home infusion therapy, enzyme replacement intravenous therapy; (e.g., Imiglucerase); administrative services, professional pharmacy services, care coordination, and all necessary supplies and equipment (drugs and nursing visits coded separately), per diem ☑

**S9359** Home infusion therapy, antitumor necrosis factor intravenous therapy; (e.g., Infliximab); administrative services, professional pharmacy services, care coordination, and all necessary supplies and equipment (drugs and nursing visits coded separately), per diem ☑

**S9361** Home infusion therapy, diuretic intravenous therapy; administrative services, professional pharmacy services, care coordination, and all necessary supplies and equipment (drugs and nursing visits coded separately), per diem ☑

**S9363** Home infusion therapy, antispasmotic therapy; administrative services, professional pharmacy services, care coordination, and all necessary supplies and equipment (drugs and nursing visits coded separately), per diem ☑

**S9364** Home infusion therapy, total parenteral nutrition (TPN); administrative services, professional pharmacy services, care coordination, and all necessary supplies and equipment including standard TPN formula (lipids, specialty amino acid formulas, drugs other than in standard formula and nursing visits coded separately), per diem (do not use with home infusion codes S9365-S9368 using daily volume scales) ☑

Special Coverage Instructions   Noncovered by Medicare   Carrier Discretion   ☑ Quantity Alert   ● New Code   ○ Recycled/Reinstated   ▲ Revised Code

142 — S Codes    Ⓐ Age Edit   Ⓜ Maternity Edit   ♀ Female Only   ♂ Male Only   Ⓐ-Ⓨ OPPS Status Indicators   © 2016 Optum360, LLC

**S9365** Home infusion therapy, total parenteral nutrition (TPN); 1 liter per day, administrative services, professional pharmacy services, care coordination, and all necessary supplies and equipment including standard TPN formula (lipids, specialty amino acid formulas, drugs other than in standard formula and nursing visits coded separately), per diem ☑

**S9366** Home infusion therapy, total parenteral nutrition (TPN); more than 1 liter but no more than 2 liters per day, administrative services, professional pharmacy services, care coordination, and all necessary supplies and equipment including standard TPN formula (lipids, specialty amino acid formulas, drugs other than in standard formula and nursing visits coded separately), per diem ☑

**S9367** Home infusion therapy, total parenteral nutrition (TPN); more than 2 liters but no more than 3 liters per day, administrative services, professional pharmacy services, care coordination, and all necessary supplies and equipment including standard TPN formula (lipids, specialty amino acid formulas, drugs other than in standard formula and nursing visits coded separately), per diem ☑

**S9368** Home infusion therapy, total parenteral nutrition (TPN); more than 3 liters per day, administrative services, professional pharmacy services, care coordination, and all necessary supplies and equipment including standard TPN formula (lipids, specialty amino acid formulas, drugs other than in standard formula and nursing visits coded separately), per diem ☑

**S9370** Home therapy, intermittent antiemetic injection therapy; administrative services, professional pharmacy services, care coordination, and all necessary supplies and equipment (drugs and nursing visits coded separately), per diem

**S9372** Home therapy; intermittent anticoagulant injection therapy (e.g., Heparin); administrative services, professional pharmacy services, care coordination, and all necessary supplies and equipment (drugs and nursing visits coded separately), per diem (do not use this code for flushing of infusion devices with Heparin to maintain patency)

**S9373** Home infusion therapy, hydration therapy; administrative services, professional pharmacy services, care coordination, and all necessary supplies and equipment (drugs and nursing visits coded separately), per diem (do not use with hydration therapy codes S9374-S9377 using daily volume scales)

**S9374** Home infusion therapy, hydration therapy; 1 liter per day, administrative services, professional pharmacy services, care coordination, and all necessary supplies and equipment (drugs and nursing visits coded separately), per diem

**S9375** Home infusion therapy, hydration therapy; more than 1 liter but no more than 2 liters per day, administrative services, professional pharmacy services, care coordination, and all necessary supplies and equipment (drugs and nursing visits coded separately), per diem

**S9376** Home infusion therapy, hydration therapy; more than 2 liters but no more than 3 liters per day, administrative services, professional pharmacy services, care coordination, and all necessary supplies and equipment (drugs and nursing visits coded separately), per diem

**S9377** Home infusion therapy, hydration therapy; more than 3 liters per day, administrative services, professional pharmacy services, care coordination, and all necessary supplies (drugs and nursing visits coded separately), per diem

**S9379** Home infusion therapy, infusion therapy, not otherwise classified; administrative services, professional pharmacy services, care coordination, and all necessary supplies and equipment (drugs and nursing visits coded separately), per diem

**S9381** Delivery or service to high risk areas requiring escort or extra protection, per visit

**S9401** Anticoagulation clinic, inclusive of all services except laboratory tests, per session

**S9430** Pharmacy compounding and dispensing services

**S9433** Medical food nutritionally complete, administered orally, providing 100% of nutritional intake

**S9434** Modified solid food supplements for inborn errors of metabolism

**S9435** Medical foods for inborn errors of metabolism

**S9436** Childbirth preparation/Lamaze classes, nonphysician provider, per session Ⓜ ♀ ☑

**S9437** Childbirth refresher classes, nonphysician provider, per session Ⓜ ♀

**S9438** Cesarean birth classes, nonphysician provider, per session Ⓜ ♀ ☑

**S9439** VBAC (vaginal birth after cesarean) classes, nonphysician provider, per session Ⓜ ♀ ☑

**S9441** Asthma education, nonphysician provider, per session ☑

**S9442** Birthing classes, nonphysician provider, per session Ⓜ ♀ ☑

**S9443** Lactation classes, nonphysician provider, per session Ⓜ ♀ ☑

**S9444** Parenting classes, nonphysician provider, per session ☑

**S9445** Patient education, not otherwise classified, nonphysician provider, individual, per session ☑

**S9446** Patient education, not otherwise classified, nonphysician provider, group, per session ☑

**S9447** Infant safety (including CPR) classes, nonphysician provider, per session ☑

**S9449** Weight management classes, nonphysician provider, per session ☑

**S9451** Exercise classes, nonphysician provider, per session

**S9452** Nutrition classes, nonphysician provider, per session

**S9453** Smoking cessation classes, nonphysician provider, per session

**S9454** Stress management classes, nonphysician provider, per session

**S9455** Diabetic management program, group session

**S9460** Diabetic management program, nurse visit

**S9465** Diabetic management program, dietitian visit

**S9470** Nutritional counseling, dietitian visit

**S9472** Cardiac rehabilitation program, nonphysician provider, per diem

**S9473** Pulmonary rehabilitation program, nonphysician provider, per diem

**S9474** Enterostomal therapy by a registered nurse certified in enterostomal therapy, per diem

**S9475** Ambulatory setting substance abuse treatment or detoxification services, per diem

**S9476** Vestibular rehabilitation program, nonphysician provider, per diem

**S9480** Intensive outpatient psychiatric services, per diem

**S9482** Family stabilization services, per 15 minutes ☑

**S9484** Crisis intervention mental health services, per hour ☑

**S9485** Crisis intervention mental health services, per diem

---

Special Coverage Instructions    Noncovered by Medicare    Carrier Discretion    ☑ Quantity Alert   ● New Code   ○ Recycled/Reinstated   ▲ Revised Code

© 2016 Optum360, LLC    A2-Z3 ASC Pmt    CMS: Pub 100    AHA: Coding Clinic    ♿ DMEPOS Paid    ⊘ SNF Excluded    S Codes — 143

**S9490** Home infusion therapy, corticosteroid infusion; administrative services, professional pharmacy services, care coordination, and all necessary supplies and equipment (drugs and nursing visits coded separately), per diem

**S9494** Home infusion therapy, antibiotic, antiviral, or antifungal therapy; administrative services, professional pharmacy services, care coordination, and all necessary supplies and equipment (drugs and nursing visits coded separately), per diem (do not use this code with home infusion codes for hourly dosing schedules S9497-S9504)

**S9497** Home infusion therapy, antibiotic, antiviral, or antifungal therapy; once every 3 hours; administrative services, professional pharmacy services, care coordination, and all necessary supplies and equipment (drugs and nursing visits coded separately), per diem

**S9500** Home infusion therapy, antibiotic, antiviral, or antifungal therapy; once every 24 hours; administrative services, professional pharmacy services, care coordination, and all necessary supplies and equipment (drugs and nursing visits coded separately), per diem

**S9501** Home infusion therapy, antibiotic, antiviral, or antifungal therapy; once every 12 hours; administrative services, professional pharmacy services, care coordination, and all necessary supplies and equipment (drugs and nursing visits coded separately), per diem

**S9502** Home infusion therapy, antibiotic, antiviral, or antifungal therapy; once every 8 hours, administrative services, professional pharmacy services, care coordination, and all necessary supplies and equipment (drugs and nursing visits coded separately), per diem

**S9503** Home infusion therapy, antibiotic, antiviral, or antifungal; once every 6 hours; administrative services, professional pharmacy services, care coordination, and all necessary supplies and equipment (drugs and nursing visits coded separately), per diem

**S9504** Home infusion therapy, antibiotic, antiviral, or antifungal; once every 4 hours; administrative services, professional pharmacy services, care coordination, and all necessary supplies and equipment (drugs and nursing visits coded separately), per diem

**S9529** Routine venipuncture for collection of specimen(s), single homebound, nursing home, or skilled nursing facility patient

**S9537** Home therapy; hematopoietic hormone injection therapy (e.g., erythropoietin, G-CSF, GM-CSF); administrative services, professional pharmacy services, care coordination, and all necessary supplies and equipment (drugs and nursing visits coded separately), per diem

**S9538** Home transfusion of blood product(s); administrative services, professional pharmacy services, care coordination and all necessary supplies and equipment (blood products, drugs, and nursing visits coded separately), per diem

**S9542** Home injectable therapy, not otherwise classified, including administrative services, professional pharmacy services, care coordination, and all necessary supplies and equipment (drugs and nursing visits coded separately), per diem

**S9558** Home injectable therapy; growth hormone, including administrative services, professional pharmacy services, care coordination, and all necessary supplies and equipment (drugs and nursing visits coded separately), per diem

**S9559** Home injectable therapy, interferon, including administrative services, professional pharmacy services, care coordination, and all necessary supplies and equipment (drugs and nursing visits coded separately), per diem

**S9560** Home injectable therapy; hormonal therapy (e.g., leuprolide, goserelin), including administrative services, professional pharmacy services, care coordination, and all necessary supplies and equipment (drugs and nursing visits coded separately), per diem

**S9562** Home injectable therapy, palivizumab, including administrative services, professional pharmacy services, care coordination, and all necessary supplies and equipment (drugs and nursing visits coded separately), per diem

**S9590** Home therapy, irrigation therapy (e.g., sterile irrigation of an organ or anatomical cavity); including administrative services, professional pharmacy services, care coordination, and all necessary supplies and equipment (drugs and nursing visits coded separately), per diem

**S9810** Home therapy; professional pharmacy services for provision of infusion, specialty drug administration, and/or disease state management, not otherwise classified, per hour (do not use this code with any per diem code)

**S9900** Services by a Journal-listed Christian Science practitioner for the purpose of healing, per diem

**S9901** Services by a journal-listed Christian Science nurse, per hour

**S9960** Ambulance service, conventional air services, nonemergency transport, one way (fixed wing)

**S9961** Ambulance service, conventional air service, nonemergency transport, one way (rotary wing)

**S9970** Health club membership, annual

**S9975** Transplant related lodging, meals and transportation, per diem

**S9976** Lodging, per diem, not otherwise classified

**S9977** Meals, per diem, not otherwise specified

**S9981** Medical records copying fee, administrative

**S9982** Medical records copying fee, per page                                      ☑

**S9986** Not medically necessary service (patient is aware that service not medically necessary)

**S9988** Services provided as part of a Phase I clinical trial

**S9989** Services provided outside of the United States of America (list in addition to code(s) for services(s))

**S9990** Services provided as part of a Phase II clinical trial

**S9991** Services provided as part of a Phase III clinical trial

**S9992** Transportation costs to and from trial location and local transportation costs (e.g., fares for taxicab or bus) for clinical trial participant and one caregiver/companion

**S9994** Lodging costs (e.g., hotel charges) for clinical trial participant and one caregiver/companion

**S9996** Meals for clinical trial participant and one caregiver/companion

**S9999** Sales tax

---

Special Coverage Instructions        Noncovered by Medicare        Carrier Discretion        ☑ Quantity Alert   ● New Code   ○ Recycled/Reinstated   ▲ Revised Code

144 — S Codes                    Ⓐ Age Edit      Ⓜ Maternity Edit      ♀ Female Only      ♂ Male Only      Ⓐ-Ⓨ OPPS Status Indicators        © 2016 Optum360, LLC

## National T Codes Established for State Medicaid Agencies T1000-T5999

The T codes are designed for use by Medicaid state agencies to establish codes for items for which there are no permanent national codes but for which codes are necessary to administer the Medicaid program (T codes are not accepted by Medicare but can be used by private insurers). This range of codes describes nursing and home health-related services, substance abuse treatment, and certain training-related procedures.

**T1000** Private duty/independent nursing service(s), licensed, up to 15 minutes ☑

**T1001** Nursing assessment/evaluation

**T1002** RN services, up to 15 minutes ☑

**T1003** LPN/LVN services, up to 15 minutes ☑

**T1004** Services of a qualified nursing aide, up to 15 minutes ☑

**T1005** Respite care services, up to 15 minutes ☑

**T1006** Alcohol and/or substance abuse services, family/couple counseling

**T1007** Alcohol and/or substance abuse services, treatment plan development and/or modification

**T1009** Child sitting services for children of the individual receiving alcohol and/or substance abuse services

**T1010** Meals for individuals receiving alcohol and/or substance abuse services (when meals not included in the program)

**T1012** Alcohol and/or substance abuse services, skills development

**T1013** Sign language or oral interpretive services, per 15 minutes ☑

**T1014** Telehealth transmission, per minute, professional services bill separately

**T1015** Clinic visit/encounter, all-inclusive
AHA: 1Q, '02, 5

**T1016** Case management, each 15 minutes ☑

**T1017** Targeted case management, each 15 minutes ☑

**T1018** School-based individualized education program (IEP) services, bundled

**T1019** Personal care services, per 15 minutes, not for an inpatient or resident of a hospital, nursing facility, ICF/MR or IMD, part of the individualized plan of treatment (code may not be used to identify services provided by home health aide or certified nurse assistant) ☑

**T1020** Personal care services, per diem, not for an inpatient or resident of a hospital, nursing facility, ICF/MR or IMD, part of the individualized plan of treatment (code may not be used to identify services provided by home health aide or certified nurse assistant)

**T1021** Home health aide or certified nurse assistant, per visit

**T1022** Contracted home health agency services, all services provided under contract, per day

**T1023** Screening to determine the appropriateness of consideration of an individual for participation in a specified program, project or treatment protocol, per encounter

**T1024** Evaluation and treatment by an integrated, specialty team contracted to provide coordinated care to multiple or severely handicapped children, per encounter 🅰

**T1025** Intensive, extended multidisciplinary services provided in a clinic setting to children with complex medical, physical, mental and psychosocial impairments, per diem 🅰

**T1026** Intensive, extended multidisciplinary services provided in a clinic setting to children with complex medical, physical, medical and psychosocial impairments, per hour 🅰

**T1027** Family training and counseling for child development, per 15 minutes ☑

**T1028** Assessment of home, physical and family environment, to determine suitability to meet patient's medical needs

**T1029** Comprehensive environmental lead investigation, not including laboratory analysis, per dwelling

**T1030** Nursing care, in the home, by registered nurse, per diem ☑

**T1031** Nursing care, in the home, by licensed practical nurse, per diem ☑

● **T1040**ᴶᵃⁿ Medicaid certified community behavioral health clinic services, per diem

● **T1041**ᴶᵃⁿ Medicaid certified community behavioral health clinic services, per month

**T1502** Administration of oral, intramuscular and/or subcutaneous medication by health care agency/professional, per visit ☑

**T1503** Administration of medication, other than oral and/or injectable, by a health care agency/professional, per visit ☑

**T1505** Electronic medication compliance management device, includes all components and accessories, not otherwise classified

**T1999** Miscellaneous therapeutic items and supplies, retail purchases, not otherwise classified; identify product in "remarks"

**T2001** Nonemergency transportation; patient attendant/escort

**T2002** Nonemergency transportation; per diem ☑

**T2003** Nonemergency transportation; encounter/trip

**T2004** Nonemergency transport; commercial carrier, multipass

**T2005** Nonemergency transportation; stretcher van

**T2007** Transportation waiting time, air ambulance and nonemergency vehicle, one-half (1/2) hour increments ☑

**T2010** Preadmission screening and resident review (PASRR) level I identification screening, per screen ☑

**T2011** Preadmission screening and resident review (PASRR) level II evaluation, per evaluation

**T2012** Habilitation, educational; waiver, per diem ☑

**T2013** Habilitation, educational, waiver; per hour ☑

**T2014** Habilitation, prevocational, waiver; per diem ☑

**T2015** Habilitation, prevocational, waiver; per hour ☑

**T2016** Habilitation, residential, waiver; per diem ☑

**T2017** Habilitation, residential, waiver; 15 minutes ☑

**T2018** Habilitation, supported employment, waiver; per diem ☑

**T2019** Habilitation, supported employment, waiver; per 15 minutes ☑

**T2020** Day habilitation, waiver; per diem ☑

**T2021** Day habilitation, waiver; per 15 minutes ☑

**T2022** Case management, per month ☑

**T2023** Targeted case management; per month ☑

**T2024** Service assessment/plan of care development, waiver

**T2025** Waiver services; not otherwise specified (NOS)

**T2026** Specialized childcare, waiver; per diem ☑

**T2027** Specialized childcare, waiver; per 15 minutes ☑

**T2028** Specialized supply, not otherwise specified, waiver

**T2029** Specialized medical equipment, not otherwise specified, waiver

---

ᴶᵃⁿ **January Update**

Special Coverage Instructions    Noncovered by Medicare    Carrier Discretion    ☑ Quantity Alert   ● New Code   ○ Recycled/Reinstated   ▲ Revised Code

© 2016 Optum360, LLC    🄰2-🄰3 ASC Pmt    CMS: Pub 100    AHA: Coding Clinic    ♿ DMEPOS Paid    ⊘ SNF Excluded    **T Codes — 145**

**National T Codes**

**T2030 — T5999**

| Code | Description | |
|---|---|---|
| T2030 | Assisted living, waiver; per month | ☑ |
| T2031 | Assisted living; waiver, per diem | ☑ |
| T2032 | Residential care, not otherwise specified (NOS), waiver; per month | ☑ |
| T2033 | Residential care, not otherwise specified (NOS), waiver; per diem | ☑ |
| T2034 | Crisis intervention, waiver; per diem | ☑ |
| T2035 | Utility services to support medical equipment and assistive technology/devices, waiver | |
| T2036 | Therapeutic camping, overnight, waiver; each session | ☑ |
| T2037 | Therapeutic camping, day, waiver; each session | ☑ |
| T2038 | Community transition, waiver; per service | ☑ |
| T2039 | Vehicle modifications, waiver; per service | ☑ |
| T2040 | Financial management, self-directed, waiver; per 15 minutes | ☑ |
| T2041 | Supports brokerage, self-directed, waiver; per 15 minutes | ☑ |
| T2042 | Hospice routine home care; per diem<br>CMS: 100-04,11,10 | ☑ |
| T2043 | Hospice continuous home care; per hour<br>CMS: 100-04,11,10 | ☑ |
| T2044 | Hospice inpatient respite care; per diem<br>CMS: 100-04,11,10 | ☑ |
| T2045 | Hospice general inpatient care; per diem<br>CMS: 100-04,11,10 | ☑ |
| T2046 | Hospice long-term care, room and board only; per diem<br>CMS: 100-04,11,10 | ☑ |
| T2048 | Behavioral health; long-term care residential (nonacute care in a residential treatment program where stay is typically longer than 30 days), with room and board, per diem | ☑ |
| T2049 | Nonemergency transportation; stretcher van, mileage; per mile | ☑ |
| T2101 | Human breast milk processing, storage and distribution only | ♀ |
| T4521 | Adult sized disposable incontinence product, brief/diaper, small, each | ☑ |
| T4522 | Adult sized disposable incontinence product, brief/diaper, medium, each | ☑ |
| T4523 | Adult sized disposable incontinence product, brief/diaper, large, each | ☑ |
| T4524 | Adult sized disposable incontinence product, brief/diaper, extra large, each | ☑ |
| T4525 | Adult sized disposable incontinence product, protective underwear/pull-on, small size, each | ☑ |
| T4526 | Adult sized disposable incontinence product, protective underwear/pull-on, medium size, each | ☑ |
| T4527 | Adult sized disposable incontinence product, protective underwear/pull-on, large size, each | ☑ |
| T4528 | Adult sized disposable incontinence product, protective underwear/pull-on, extra large size, each | ☑ |
| T4529 | Pediatric sized disposable incontinence product, brief/diaper, small/medium size, each | ☑ |
| T4530 | Pediatric sized disposable incontinence product, brief/diaper, large size, each | ☑ |
| T4531 | Pediatric sized disposable incontinence product, protective underwear/pull-on, small/medium size, each | ☑ |
| T4532 | Pediatric sized disposable incontinence product, protective underwear/pull-on, large size, each | ☑ |
| T4533 | Youth sized disposable incontinence product, brief/diaper, each | ☑ |
| T4534 | Youth sized disposable incontinence product, protective underwear/pull-on, each | ☑ |
| T4535 | Disposable liner/shield/guard/pad/undergarment, for incontinence, each | ☑ |
| T4536 | Incontinence product, protective underwear/pull-on, reusable, any size, each | ☑ |
| T4537 | Incontinence product, protective underpad, reusable, bed size, each | ☑ |
| T4538 | Diaper service, reusable diaper, each diaper | ☑ |
| T4539 | Incontinence product, diaper/brief, reusable, any size, each | ☑ |
| T4540 | Incontinence product, protective underpad, reusable, chair size, each | ☑ |
| T4541 | Incontinence product, disposable underpad, large, each | ☑ |
| T4542 | Incontinence product, disposable underpad, small size, each | ☑ |
| T4543 | Adult sized disposable incontinence product, protective brief/diaper, above extra large, each | ☑ |
| T4544 | Adult sized disposable incontinence product, protective underwear/pull-on, above extra large, each | |
| T5001 | Positioning seat for persons with special orthopedic needs | |
| T5999 | Supply, not otherwise specified | |

---

Special Coverage Instructions     Noncovered by Medicare     Carrier Discretion     ☑ Quantity Alert   ● New Code     ○ Recycled/Reinstated   ▲ Revised Code

146 — T Codes          🅰 Age Edit     🅼 Maternity Edit     ♀ Female Only     ♂ Male Only     🅰-🆈 OPPS Status Indicators          © 2016 Optum360, LLC

## Vision Services V2020-V2799

These V codes include vision-related supplies, including spectacles, lenses, contact lenses, prostheses, intraocular lenses, and miscellaneous lenses.

### Frames

**V2020**   Frames, purchases   Ⓐ ⚕

**V2025**   Deluxe frame   Ⓔ
CMS: 100-04,1,30.3.5

### Single Vision, Glass, or Plastic

**V2100**   Sphere, single vision, plano to plus or minus 4.00, per lens   Ⓐ ☑ ⚕

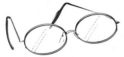

Monofocal spectacles (V2100-V2114)

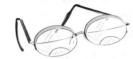

Trifocal spectacles (V2300-V2314)

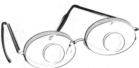

Low vision aids mounted to spectacles (V2610)

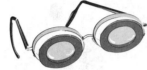

Telescopic or other compound lens fitted on spectacles as a low vision aid (V2615)

**V2101**   Sphere, single vision, plus or minus 4.12 to plus or minus 7.00d, per lens   Ⓐ ☑ ⚕

**V2102**   Sphere, single vision, plus or minus 7.12 to plus or minus 20.00d, per lens   Ⓐ ☑ ⚕

**V2103**   Spherocylinder, single vision, plano to plus or minus 4.00d sphere, 0.12 to 2.00d cylinder, per lens   Ⓐ ☑ ⚕

**V2104**   Spherocylinder, single vision, plano to plus or minus 4.00d sphere, 2.12 to 4.00d cylinder, per lens   Ⓐ ☑ ⚕

**V2105**   Spherocylinder, single vision, plano to plus or minus 4.00d sphere, 4.25 to 6.00d cylinder, per lens   Ⓐ ☑ ⚕

**V2106**   Spherocylinder, single vision, plano to plus or minus 4.00d sphere, over 6.00d cylinder, per lens   Ⓐ ☑ ⚕

**V2107**   Spherocylinder, single vision, plus or minus 4.25 to plus or minus 7.00 sphere, 0.12 to 2.00d cylinder, per lens   Ⓐ ☑ ⚕

**V2108**   Spherocylinder, single vision, plus or minus 4.25d to plus or minus 7.00d sphere, 2.12 to 4.00d cylinder, per lens   Ⓐ ☑ ⚕

**V2109**   Spherocylinder, single vision, plus or minus 4.25 to plus or minus 7.00d sphere, 4.25 to 6.00d cylinder, per lens   Ⓐ ☑ ⚕

**V2110**   Spherocylinder, single vision, plus or minus 4.25 to 7.00d sphere, over 6.00d cylinder, per lens   Ⓐ ☑ ⚕

**V2111**   Spherocylinder, single vision, plus or minus 7.25 to plus or minus 12.00d sphere, 0.25 to 2.25d cylinder, per lens   Ⓐ ☑ ⚕

**V2112**   Spherocylinder, single vision, plus or minus 7.25 to plus or minus 12.00d sphere, 2.25d to 4.00d cylinder, per lens   Ⓐ ☑ ⚕

**V2113**   Spherocylinder, single vision, plus or minus 7.25 to plus or minus 12.00d sphere, 4.25 to 6.00d cylinder, per lens   Ⓐ ☑ ⚕

**V2114**   Spherocylinder, single vision, sphere over plus or minus 12.00d, per lens   Ⓐ ☑ ⚕

**V2115**   Lenticular (myodisc), per lens, single vision   Ⓐ ☑ ⚕

**V2118**   Aniseikonic lens, single vision   Ⓐ ⚕

**V2121**   Lenticular lens, per lens, single   Ⓐ ☑ ⚕

**V2199**   Not otherwise classified, single vision lens   Ⓐ

### Bifocal, Glass, or Plastic

**V2200**   Sphere, bifocal, plano to plus or minus 4.00d, per lens   Ⓐ ☑ ⚕

**V2201**   Sphere, bifocal, plus or minus 4.12 to plus or minus 7.00d, per lens   Ⓐ ☑ ⚕

**V2202**   Sphere, bifocal, plus or minus 7.12 to plus or minus 20.00d, per lens   Ⓐ ☑ ⚕

**V2203**   Spherocylinder, bifocal, plano to plus or minus 4.00d sphere, 0.12 to 2.00d cylinder, per lens   Ⓐ ☑ ⚕

**V2204**   Spherocylinder, bifocal, plano to plus or minus 4.00d sphere, 2.12 to 4.00d cylinder, per lens   Ⓐ ☑ ⚕

**V2205**   Spherocylinder, bifocal, plano to plus or minus 4.00d sphere, 4.25 to 6.00d cylinder, per lens   Ⓐ ☑ ⚕

**V2206**   Spherocylinder, bifocal, plano to plus or minus 4.00d, over 6.00d cylinder, per lens   Ⓐ ☑ ⚕

**V2207**   Spherocylinder, bifocal, plus or minus 4.25 to plus or minus 7.00d sphere, 0.12 to 2.00d cylinder, per lens   Ⓐ ☑ ⚕

**V2208**   Spherocylinder, bifocal, plus or minus 4.25 to plus or minus 7.00d sphere, 2.12 to 4.00d cylinder, per lens   Ⓐ ☑ ⚕

**V2209**   Spherocylinder, bifocal, plus or minus 4.25 to plus or minus 7.00d sphere, 4.25 to 6.00d cylinder, per lens   Ⓐ ☑ ⚕

**V2210**   Spherocylinder, bifocal, plus or minus 4.25 to plus or minus 7.00d sphere, over 6.00d cylinder, per lens   Ⓐ ☑ ⚕

**V2211**   Spherocylinder, bifocal, plus or minus 7.25 to plus or minus 12.00d sphere, 0.25 to 2.25d cylinder, per lens   Ⓐ ☑ ⚕

**V2212**   Spherocylinder, bifocal, plus or minus 7.25 to plus or minus 12.00d sphere, 2.25 to 4.00d cylinder, per lens   Ⓐ ☑ ⚕

**V2213**   Spherocylinder, bifocal, plus or minus 7.25 to plus or minus 12.00d sphere, 4.25 to 6.00d cylinder, per lens   Ⓐ ☑ ⚕

**V2214**   Spherocylinder, bifocal, sphere over plus or minus 12.00d, per lens   Ⓐ ☑ ⚕

**V2215**   Lenticular (myodisc), per lens, bifocal   Ⓐ ☑ ⚕

**V2218**   Aniseikonic, per lens, bifocal   Ⓐ ☑ ⚕

**V2219**   Bifocal seg width over 28mm   Ⓐ ☑ ⚕

**V2220**   Bifocal add over 3.25d   Ⓐ ☑ ⚕

**V2221**   Lenticular lens, per lens, bifocal   Ⓐ ⚕

**V2299**   Specialty bifocal (by report)   Ⓐ
Pertinent documentation to evaluate medical appropriateness should be included when this code is reported.

### Trifocal, Glass, or Plastic

**V2300**   Sphere, trifocal, plano to plus or minus 4.00d, per lens   Ⓐ ☑ ⚕

**V2301**   Sphere, trifocal, plus or minus 4.12 to plus or minus 7.00d per lens   Ⓐ ☑ ⚕

**V2302**   Sphere, trifocal, plus or minus 7.12 to plus or minus 20.00, per lens   Ⓐ ☑ ⚕

**V2303**   Spherocylinder, trifocal, plano to plus or minus 4.00d sphere, 0.12 to 2.00d cylinder, per lens   Ⓐ ☑ ⚕

**V2304**   Spherocylinder, trifocal, plano to plus or minus 4.00d sphere, 2.25 to 4.00d cylinder, per lens   Ⓐ ☑ ⚕

**V2305**   Spherocylinder, trifocal, plano to plus or minus 4.00d sphere, 4.25 to 6.00 cylinder, per lens   Ⓐ ☑ ⚕

**V2306**   Spherocylinder, trifocal, plano to plus or minus 4.00d sphere, over 6.00d cylinder, per lens   Ⓐ ☑ ⚕

**V2307**   Spherocylinder, trifocal, plus or minus 4.25 to plus or minus 7.00d sphere, 0.12 to 2.00d cylinder, per lens   Ⓐ ☑ ⚕

---

Special Coverage Instructions   Noncovered by Medicare   Carrier Discretion   ☑ Quantity Alert   ● New Code   ○ Recycled/Reinstated   ▲ Revised Code

© 2016 Optum360, LLC   Ⓐ²-Ⓩ³ ASC Pmt   CMS: Pub 100   AHA: Coding Clinic   ⚕ DMEPOS Paid   ⊘ SNF Excluded

**V2308** Spherocylinder, trifocal, plus or minus 4.25 to plus or minus 7.00d sphere, 2.12 to 4.00d cylinder, per lens ☐☑♿

**V2309** Spherocylinder, trifocal, plus or minus 4.25 to plus or minus 7.00d sphere, 4.25 to 6.00d cylinder, per lens ☐☑♿

**V2310** Spherocylinder, trifocal, plus or minus 4.25 to plus or minus 7.00d sphere, over 6.00d cylinder, per lens ☐☑♿

**V2311** Spherocylinder, trifocal, plus or minus 7.25 to plus or minus 12.00d sphere, 0.25 to 2.25d cylinder, per lens ☐☑♿

**V2312** Spherocylinder, trifocal, plus or minus 7.25 to plus or minus 12.00d sphere, 2.25 to 4.00d cylinder, per lens ☐☑♿

**V2313** Spherocylinder, trifocal, plus or minus 7.25 to plus or minus 12.00d sphere, 4.25 to 6.00d cylinder, per lens ☐☑♿

**V2314** Spherocylinder, trifocal, sphere over plus or minus 12.00d, per lens ☐☑♿

**V2315** Lenticular, (myodisc), per lens, trifocal ☐☑♿

**V2318** Aniseikonic lens, trifocal ☐♿

**V2319** Trifocal seg width over 28 mm ☐☑♿

**V2320** Trifocal add over 3.25d ☐☑♿

**V2321** Lenticular lens, per lens, trifocal ☐♿

**V2399** Specialty trifocal (by report) ☐
Pertinent documentation to evaluate medical appropriateness should be included when this code is reported.

## Variable Asphericity Lens, Glass, or Plastic

**V2410** Variable asphericity lens, single vision, full field, glass or plastic, per lens ☐☑♿

**V2430** Variable asphericity lens, bifocal, full field, glass or plastic, per lens ☐☑♿

**V2499** Variable sphericity lens, other type ☐

## Contact Lens

**V2500** Contact lens, PMMA, spherical, per lens ☐☑♿

**V2501** Contact lens, PMMA, toric or prism ballast, per lens ☐☑♿

**V2502** Contact lens PMMA, bifocal, per lens ☐☑♿

**V2503** Contact lens, PMMA, color vision deficiency, per lens ☐☑♿

**V2510** Contact lens, gas permeable, spherical, per lens ☐☑♿

**V2511** Contact lens, gas permeable, toric, prism ballast, per lens ☐☑♿

**V2512** Contact lens, gas permeable, bifocal, per lens ☐☑♿

**V2513** Contact lens, gas permeable, extended wear, per lens ☐☑♿

**V2520** Contact lens, hydrophilic, spherical, per lens ☐☑♿
Hydrophilic contact lenses are covered by Medicare only for aphakic patients. Local contractor if incident to physician services.

**V2521** Contact lens, hydrophilic, toric, or prism ballast, per lens ☐☑♿
Hydrophilic contact lenses are covered by Medicare only for aphakic patients. Local contractor if incident to physician services.

**V2522** Contact lens, hydrophilic, bifocal, per lens ☐☑♿
Hydrophilic contact lenses are covered by Medicare only for aphakic patients. Local contractor if incident to physician services.

**V2523** Contact lens, hydrophilic, extended wear, per lens ☐☑♿
Hydrophilic contact lenses are covered by Medicare only for aphakic patients.

**V2530** Contact lens, scleral, gas impermeable, per lens (for contact lens modification, see 92325) ☐☑♿

**V2531** Contact lens, scleral, gas permeable, per lens (for contact lens modification, see 92325) ☐☑♿

**V2599** Contact lens, other type ☐
Local contractor if incident to physician services.

## Vision Aids

**V2600** Hand held low vision aids and other nonspectacle mounted aids ☐

**V2610** Single lens spectacle mounted low vision aids ☐

**V2615** Telescopic and other compound lens system, including distance vision telescopic, near vision telescopes and compound microscopic lens system ☐

## Prosthetic Eye

**V2623** Prosthetic eye, plastic, custom ☐♿

Implant

One type of eye implant

Reverse angle

Peg

Side view    Peg

Previously placed prosthetic receptacle

Implant

Peg hole drilled into prosthetic

**V2624** Polishing/resurfacing of ocular prosthesis ☐♿

**V2625** Enlargement of ocular prosthesis ☐♿

**V2626** Reduction of ocular prosthesis ☐♿

**V2627** Scleral cover shell ☐♿
A scleral shell covers the cornea and the anterior sclera. Medicare covers a scleral shell when it is prescribed as an artificial support to a shrunken and sightless eye or as a barrier in the treatment of severe dry eye.

**V2628** Fabrication and fitting of ocular conformer ☐♿

**V2629** Prosthetic eye, other type ☐

## Intraocular Lenses

**V2630** Anterior chamber intraocular lens Ⓝ Ⓗ ♿
The IOL must be FDA-approved for reimbursement. Medicare payment for an IOL is included in the payment for ASC facility services. Medicare jurisdiction: local contractor.

**V2631** Iris supported intraocular lens Ⓝ Ⓗ ♿
The IOL must be FDA-approved for reimbursement. Medicare payment for an IOL is included in the payment for ASC facility services. Medicare jurisdiction: local contractor.

**V2632** Posterior chamber intraocular lens Ⓝ Ⓗ ♿
The IOL must be FDA-approved for reimbursement. Medicare payment for an IOL is included in the payment for ASC facility services. Medicare jurisdiction: local contractor.
CMS: 100-04,32,120.2

## Miscellaneous

**V2700** Balance lens, per lens ☐☑♿

**V2702** Deluxe lens feature Ⓔ

**V2710** Slab off prism, glass or plastic, per lens ☐☑♿

**V2715** Prism, per lens ☐☑♿

**V2718** Press-on lens, Fresnel prism, per lens ☐☑♿

**V2730** Special base curve, glass or plastic, per lens ☐☑♿

---

Special Coverage Instructions    Noncovered by Medicare    Carrier Discretion    ☑ Quantity Alert   ● New Code    ○ Recycled/Reinstated    ▲ Revised Code

148 — V Codes    Ⓐ Age Edit    Ⓜ Maternity Edit    ♀ Female Only    ♂ Male Only    Ⓐ-Ⓨ OPPS Status Indicators    © 2016 Optum360, LLC

| V2744 | Tint, photochromatic, per lens | A ☑ & |
| V2745 | Addition to lens; tint, any color, solid, gradient or equal, excludes photochromatic, any lens material, per lens | A ☑ & |
| V2750 | Antireflective coating, per lens | A ☑ & |
| V2755 | U-V lens, per lens | A ☑ & |
| V2756 | Eye glass case | E |
| V2760 | Scratch resistant coating, per lens | E ☑ & |
| V2761 | Mirror coating, any type, solid, gradient or equal, any lens material, per lens | B ☑ |
| V2762 | Polarization, any lens material, per lens | E ☑ & |
| V2770 | Occluder lens, per lens | A ☑ & |
| V2780 | Oversize lens, per lens | A ☑ & |
| V2781 | Progressive lens, per lens | B ☑ |
| V2782 | Lens, index 1.54 to 1.65 plastic or 1.60 to 1.79 glass, excludes polycarbonate, per lens | A ☑ & |
| V2783 | Lens, index greater than or equal to 1.66 plastic or greater than or equal to 1.80 glass, excludes polycarbonate, per lens | A ☑ & |
| V2784 | Lens, polycarbonate or equal, any index, per lens | A ☑ & |

**V2785** Processing, preserving and transporting corneal tissue  F M
Medicare jurisdiction: local contractor.
**CMS:** 100-04,4,200.1

| V2786 | Specialty occupational multifocal lens, per lens | E ☑ & |

**V2787** Astigmatism correcting function of intraocular lens  E
**CMS:** 100-04,32,120.1; 100-04,32,120.2

**V2788** Presbyopia correcting function of intraocular lens  E
**CMS:** 100-04,32,120.1; 100-04,32,120.2

**V2790** Amniotic membrane for surgical reconstruction, per procedure  N N1
Medicare jurisdiction: local contractor.
**CMS:** 100-04,4,200.4

**V2797** Vision supply, accessory and/or service component of another HCPCS vision code  E

**V2799** Vision item or service, miscellaneous  A
Determine if an alternative HCPCS Level II or a CPT code better describes the service being reported. This code should be used only if a more specific code is unavailable.

## Hearing Services V5008-V5364
This range of codes describes hearing tests and related supplies and equipment, speech-language pathology screenings, and repair of augmentative communicative system.

### Hearing Services

| V5008 | Hearing screening | E |
| V5010 | Assessment for hearing aid | E |
| V5011 | Fitting/orientation/checking of hearing aid | E |
| V5014 | Repair/modification of a hearing aid | E |
| V5020 | Conformity evaluation | E |

### Monaural Hearing Aid

| V5030 | Hearing aid, monaural, body worn, air conduction | E |
| V5040 | Hearing aid, monaural, body worn, bone conduction | E |
| V5050 | Hearing aid, monaural, in the ear | E |
| V5060 | Hearing aid, monaural, behind the ear | E |

### Other Hearing Services

| V5070 | Glasses, air conduction | E |
| V5080 | Glasses, bone conduction | E |
| V5090 | Dispensing fee, unspecified hearing aid | E |
| V5095 | Semi-implantable middle ear hearing prosthesis | E |
| V5100 | Hearing aid, bilateral, body worn | E |
| V5110 | Dispensing fee, bilateral | E |

### Hearing Aids, Services, and Accessories

| V5120 | Binaural, body | E |
| V5130 | Binaural, in the ear | E |
| V5140 | Binaural, behind the ear | E |
| V5150 | Binaural, glasses | E |
| V5160 | Dispensing fee, binaural | E |
| V5170 | Hearing aid, CROS, in the ear | E |
| V5180 | Hearing aid, CROS, behind the ear | E |
| V5190 | Hearing aid, CROS, glasses | E |
| V5200 | Dispensing fee, CROS | E |
| V5210 | Hearing aid, BICROS, in the ear | E |
| V5220 | Hearing aid, BICROS, behind the ear | E |
| V5230 | Hearing aid, BICROS, glasses | E |
| V5240 | Dispensing fee, BICROS | E |

**V5241** Dispensing fee, monaural hearing aid, any type  E
**AHA:** 1Q, '02, 5

**V5242** Hearing aid, analog, monaural, CIC (completely in the ear canal)  E
**AHA:** 1Q, '02, 5

**V5243** Hearing aid, analog, monaural, ITC (in the canal)  E
**AHA:** 1Q, '02, 5

**V5244** Hearing aid, digitally programmable analog, monaural, CIC  E
**AHA:** 1Q, '02, 5

**V5245** Hearing aid, digitally programmable, analog, monaural, ITC  E
**AHA:** 1Q, '02, 5

**V5246** Hearing aid, digitally programmable analog, monaural, ITE (in the ear)  E
**AHA:** 1Q, '02, 5

**V5247** Hearing aid, digitally programmable analog, monaural, BTE (behind the ear)  E
**AHA:** 1Q, '02, 5

**V5248** Hearing aid, analog, binaural, CIC  E
**AHA:** 1Q, '02, 5

**V5249** Hearing aid, analog, binaural, ITC  E
**AHA:** 1Q, '02, 5

**V5250** Hearing aid, digitally programmable analog, binaural, CIC  E
**AHA:** 1Q, '02, 5

**V5251** Hearing aid, digitally programmable analog, binaural, ITC  E
**AHA:** 1Q, '02, 5

**V5252** Hearing aid, digitally programmable, binaural, ITE  E
**AHA:** 1Q, '02, 5

**V5253** Hearing aid, digitally programmable, binaural, BTE  E
**AHA:** 1Q, '02, 5

Special Coverage Instructions   Noncovered by Medicare   Carrier Discretion   ☑ Quantity Alert   ● New Code   ○ Recycled/Reinstated   ▲ Revised Code

© 2016 Optum360, LLC   A2-Z3 ASC Pmt   CMS: Pub 100   AHA: Coding Clinic   & DMEPOS Paid   ⊘ SNF Excluded   V Codes — 149

**V5254**  Hearing aid, digital, monaural, CIC  E
AHA: 1Q, '02, 5

**V5255**  Hearing aid, digital, monaural, ITC  E
AHA: 1Q, '02, 5

**V5256**  Hearing aid, digital, monaural, ITE  E
AHA: 1Q, '02, 5

**V5257**  Hearing aid, digital, monaural, BTE  E
AHA: 1Q, '02, 5

**V5258**  Hearing aid, digital, binaural, CIC  E
AHA: 1Q, '02, 5

**V5259**  Hearing aid, digital, binaural, ITC  E
AHA: 1Q, '02, 5

**V5260**  Hearing aid, digital, binaural, ITE  E
AHA: 1Q, '02, 5

**V5261**  Hearing aid, digital, binaural, BTE  E
AHA: 1Q, '02, 5

**V5262**  Hearing aid, disposable, any type, monaural  E
AHA: 1Q, '02, 5

**V5263**  Hearing aid, disposable, any type, binaural  E
AHA: 1Q, '02, 5

**V5264**  Ear mold/insert, not disposable, any type  E
AHA: 1Q, '02, 5

**V5265**  Ear mold/insert, disposable, any type  E
AHA: 1Q, '02, 5

**V5266**  Battery for use in hearing device  E
AHA: 1Q, '02, 5

**V5267**  Hearing aid or assistive listening device/supplies/accessories, not otherwise specified  E
AHA: 1Q, '02, 5

## Assistive Listening Device

**V5268**  Assistive listening device, telephone amplifier, any type  E
AHA: 1Q, '02, 5

**V5269**  Assistive listening device, alerting, any type  E
AHA: 1Q, '02, 5

**V5270**  Assistive listening device, television amplifier, any type  E
AHA: 1Q, '02, 5

**V5271**  Assistive listening device, television caption decoder  E
AHA: 1Q, '02, 5

**V5272**  Assistive listening device, TDD  E
AHA: 1Q, '02, 5

**V5273**  Assistive listening device, for use with cochlear implant  E
AHA: 1Q, '02, 5

**V5274**  Assistive listening device, not otherwise specified  E
AHA: 1Q, '02, 5

## Miscellaneous Hearing Services

**V5275**  Ear impression, each  E ☑
AHA: 1Q, '02, 5

**V5281**  Assistive listening device, personal FM/DM system, monaural (1 receiver, transmitter, microphone), any type  E

**V5282**  Assistive listening device, personal FM/DM system, binaural (2 receivers, transmitter, microphone), any type  E

**V5283**  Assistive listening device, personal FM/DM neck, loop induction receiver  E

**V5284**  Assistive listening device, personal FM/DM, ear level receiver  E

**V5285**  Assistive listening device, personal FM/DM, direct audio input receiver  E

**V5286**  Assistive listening device, personal blue tooth FM/DM receiver  E

**V5287**  Assistive listening device, personal FM/DM receiver, not otherwise specified  E

**V5288**  Assistive listening device, personal FM/DM transmitter assistive listening device  E

**V5289**  Assistive listening device, personal FM/DM adapter/boot coupling device for receiver, any type  E

**V5290**  Assistive listening device, transmitter microphone, any type  E

**V5298**  Hearing aid, not otherwise classified  E

**V5299**  Hearing service, miscellaneous  B ⊘
Determine if an alternative HCPCS Level II or a CPT code better describes the service being reported. This code should be used only if a more specific code is unavailable.

## Speech-Language Pathology Services

**V5336**  Repair/modification of augmentative communicative system or device (excludes adaptive hearing aid)  E
Medicare jurisdiction: DME regional contractor.

**V5362**  Speech screening  E

**V5363**  Language screening  E

**V5364**  Dysphagia screening  E

---

Special Coverage Instructions    Noncovered by Medicare    Carrier Discretion    ☑ Quantity Alert  ● New Code    ○ Recycled/Reinstated    ▲ Revised Code

150 — V Codes    A Age Edit    M Maternity Edit    ♀ Female Only    ♂ Male Only    A-Y OPPS Status Indicators    © 2016 Optum360, LLC

# Appendix 1 — Table of Drugs and Biologicals

## Introduction and Directions

The HCPCS 2017 Table of Drugs and Biologicals is designed to quickly and easily direct the user to drug names and their corresponding codes. Both generic and brand or trade names are alphabetically listed in the "Drug Name" column of the table. The associated A, C, J, K, Q, or S code is given only for the generic name of the drug. While every effort is made to make the table comprehensive, it is not all-inclusive.

The "Unit Per" column lists the stated amount for the referenced generic drug as provided by CMS. "Up to" listings are inclusive of all quantities up to and including the listed amount. All other listings are for the amount of the drug as listed. The editors recognize that the availability of some drugs in the quantities listed is dependent on many variables beyond the control of the clinical ordering clerk. The availability in your area of regularly used drugs in the most cost-effective quantities should be relayed to your third-party payers.

The "Route of Administration" column addresses the most common methods of delivering the referenced generic drug as described in current pharmaceutical literature. The official definitions for Level II drug codes generally describe administration other than by oral method. Therefore, with a handful of exceptions, oral-delivered options for most drugs are omitted from the Route of Administration column.

Intravenous administration includes all methods, such as gravity infusion, injections, and timed pushes. When several routes of administration are listed, the first listing is simply the first, or most common, method as described in current reference literature. The "VAR" posting denotes various routes of administration and is used for drugs that are commonly administered into joints, cavities, tissues, or topical applications, in addition to other parenteral administrations. Listings posted with "OTH" alert the user to other administration methods, such as suppositories or catheter injections.

Please be reminded that the Table of Drugs and Biologicals, as well as all HCPCS Level II national definitions and listings, constitutes a post-treatment medical reference for billing purposes only. Although the editors have exercised all normal precautions to ensure the accuracy of the table and related material, the use of any of this information to select medical treatment is entirely inappropriate. Do not code directly from the table. Refer to the tabular section for complete information.

See Appendix 3 for abbreviations.

| Drug Name | Unit Per | Route | Code |
|---|---|---|---|
| 10% LMD | 500 ML | IV | J7100 |
| 4-FACTOR PROTHROMBRIN COMPLEX CONCENTRATE | 1 IU | IV | C9132 |
| 5% DEXTROSE AND .45% NORMAL SALINE | 1000 ML | IV | S5010 |
| 5% DEXTROSE IN LACTATED RINGERS | 1000 CC | IV | J7121 |
| 5% DEXTROSE WITH POTASSIUM CHLORIDE | 1000 ML | IV | S5012 |
| 5% DEXTROSE/.45% NS WITH KCL AND MAG SULFATE | 1000ML | IV | S5013 |
| 5% DEXTROSE/.45% NS WITH KCL AND MAG SULFATE | 1500 ML | IV | S5014 |
| 5% DEXTROSE/NORMAL SALINE | 5% | VAR | J7042 |
| 5% DEXTROSE/WATER | 500 ML | IV | J7060 |
| A-HYDROCORT | 100 MG | IV, IM, SC | J1720 |
| A-METHAPRED | 40 MG | IM, IV | J2920 |
| A-METHAPRED | 125 MG | IM, IV | J2930 |
| ABATACEPT | 10 MG | IV | J0129 |

| Drug Name | Unit Per | Route | Code |
|---|---|---|---|
| ABCIXIMAB | 10 MG | IV | J0130 |
| ABELCET | 10 MG | IV | J0287 |
| ABILIFY | 0.25 MG | IM | J0400 |
| ABILIFY MAINTENA KIT | 1 MG | IM | J0401 |
| ABLAVAR | 1 ML | IV | A9583 |
| ABOBOTULINUMTOXINA | 5 UNITS | IM | J0586 |
| ABRAXANE | 1 MG | IV | J9264 |
| ACCELULAR PERICARDIAL TISSUE MATRIX NONHUMAN | SQ CM | OTH | C9354 |
| ACCUNEB NONCOMPOUNDED, CONCENTRATED | 1 MG | INH | J7611 |
| ACCUNEB NONCOMPOUNDED, UNIT DOSE | 1 MG | INH | J7613 |
| ACETADOTE | 100 MG | IV | J0132 |
| ACETADOTE | 1 G | INH | J7608 |
| ACETAMINOPHEN | 10 MG | IV | J0131 |
| ACETAZOLAMIDE SODIUM | 500 MG | IM, IV | J1120 |
| ACETYLCYSTEINE COMPOUNDED | PER G | INH | J7604 |
| ACETYLCYSTEINE NONCOMPOUNDED | 1 G | INH | J7608 |
| ACTEMRA | 1 MG | IV | J3262 |
| ACTHREL | 1 MCG | IV | J0795 |
| ACTIMMUNE | 3 MU | SC | J9216 |
| ACTIVASE | 1 MG | IV | J2997 |
| ACUTECT | STUDY DOSE UP TO 20 MCI | IV | A9504 |
| ACYCLOVIR | 5 MG | IV | J0133 |
| ADAGEN | 25 IU | IM | J2504 |
| ADALIMUMAB | 20 MG | SC | J0135 |
| ADCETRIS | 1 MG | IV | J9042 |
| ADENOCARD | 1 MG | IV | J0153 |
| ADENOSINE | 1 MG | IV | J0153 |
| ADENSOSCAN | 1 MG | IV | J0153 |
| ADO-TRASTUZUMAB EMTANSINE | 1 MG | IV | J9354 |
| ADRENALIN | 0.1 MG | IM, IV, SC | J0171 |
| ADRENOCORT | 1 MG | IM, IV, OTH | J1100 |
| ADRIAMYCIN | 10 MG | IV | J9000 |
| ADRUCIL | 500 MG | IV | J9190 |
| ADYNOVATE | 1 IU | IV | J7207 |
| ~~ADYNOVATE~~ | ~~IU~~ | ~~IV~~ | ~~C9137~~ |
| AEROBID | 1 MG | INH | J7641 |
| AFFINITY | SQ CM | OTH | Q4159 |
| AFINITOR | 0.25 MG | ORAL | J7527 |
| AFLIBERCEPT | 1 MG | OTH | J0178 |
| AFLURIA | EA | IM | Q2035 |

© 2016 Optum360, LLC

| Drug Name | Unit Per | Route | Code |
|---|---|---|---|
| AFSTYLA | 1 IU | IV | C9140 |
| AGALSIDASE BETA | 1 MG | IV | J0180 |
| AGGRASTAT | 12.5 MG | IM, IV | J3246 |
| AGRIFLU | UNKNOWN | IM | Q2034 |
| AKYNZEO | 300 MG/0.5 MG | ORAL | J8655 |
| AKYNZEO | 300 MG/0.5 MG | ORAL | C9448 |
| ALATROFLOXACIN MESYLATE | 100 MG | IV | J0200 |
| ALBUTEROL AND IPRATROPIUM BROMIDE NONCOMPOUNDED | 2.5MG/0.5 MG | INH | J7620 |
| ALBUTEROL COMPOUNDED, CONCENTRATED | 1 MG | INH | J7610 |
| ALBUTEROL COMPOUNDED, UNIT DOSE | 1 MG | INH | J7609 |
| ALBUTEROL NONCOMPOUNDED, UNIT DOSE | 1 MG | INH | J7613 |
| ALBUTEROL, NONCOMPOUNDED, CONCENTRATED FORM | 1 MG | INH | J7611 |
| ALDESLEUKIN | 1 VIAL | IV | J9015 |
| ALDURAZYME | 0.1 MG | IV | J1931 |
| ALEFACEPT | 0.5 MG | IV, IM | J0215 |
| ALEMTUZUMAB | 1 MG | IV | J0202 |
| ALFERON N | 250,000 IU | IM | J9215 |
| ALGLUCERASE | 10 U | IV | J0205 |
| ALGLUCOSIDASE ALFA (LUMIZYME) | 10 MG | IV | J0221 |
| ALGLUCOSIDASE ALFA NOS | 10 MG | IV | J0220 |
| ALIMTA | 10 MG | IV | J9305 |
| ALKERAN | 2 MG | ORAL | J8600 |
| ALKERAN | 50 MG | IV | J9245 |
| ALLODERM | SQ CM | OTH | Q4116 |
| ALLOGRAFT, CYMETRA | 1 CC | INJ | Q4112 |
| ALLOGRAFT, GRAFTJACKET EXPRESS | 1 CC | INJ | Q4113 |
| ALLOPATCHHD | SQ CM | OTH | Q4128 |
| ALLOSKIN | SQ CM | OTH | Q4115 |
| ALLOSKIN AC | SQ CM | OTH | Q4141 |
| ALLOSKIN RT | SQ CM | OTH | Q4123 |
| ALLOWRAP DS OR DRY | SQ CM | OTH | Q4150 |
| ALOXI | 25 MCG | IV | J2469 |
| ALPHA 1 - PROTEINASE INHIBITOR (HUMAN) NOS | 10 MG | IV | J0256 |
| ALPHA 1-PROTENIASE INHIBITOR (HUMAN) (GLASSIA) | 10 MG | IV | J0257 |
| ALPHANATE | PER FACTOR VIII IU | IV | J7186 |
| ALPHANINE SD | 1 IU | IV | J7193 |
| ALPROLIX | IU | IV | J7201 |
| ALPROSTADIL | 1.25 MCG | IV | J0270 |
| ALPROSTADIL | EA | OTH | J0275 |
| ALTEPLASE RECOMBINANT | 1 MG | IV | J2997 |
| ALUPENT, NONCOMPOUNDED, CONCENTRATED | 10 MG | INH | J7668 |

| Drug Name | Unit Per | Route | Code |
|---|---|---|---|
| ALUPENT, NONCOMPOUNDED, UNIT DOSE | 10 MG | INH | J7669 |
| AMANTADINE HCL (DEMONSTRATION PROJECT) | 100 MG | ORAL | G9017 |
| AMANTADINE HYDROCHLORIDE (BRAND NAME) (DEMONSTRTION PROJECT) | 100 MG | ORAL | G9033 |
| AMANTADINE HYDROCHLORIDE (GENERIC) | 100 MG | ORAL | G9017 |
| AMBISOME | 10 MG | IV | J0289 |
| AMCORT | 5 MG | IM | J3302 |
| AMERGAN | 12.5 MG | ORAL | Q0169 |
| AMEVIVE | 0.5 MG | IV, IM | J0215 |
| AMICAR | 5 G | IV | S0017 |
| AMIFOSTINE | 500 MG | IV | J0207 |
| AMIKACIN SULFATE | 100 MG | IM, IV | J0278 |
| AMINOCAPRIOC ACID | 5 G | IV | S0017 |
| AMINOPHYLLINE | 250 MG | IV | J0280 |
| AMIODARONE HCL | 30 MG | IV | J0282 |
| AMITRIPTYLINE HCL | 20 MG | IM | J1320 |
| AMMONIA N-13 | STUDY DOSE UP TO 40 MCI | IV | A9526 |
| AMNIOBAND | 1 MG | OTH | Q4168 |
| AMNIOBAND | SQ CM | OTH | Q4151 |
| AMNIOEXCEL | SQ CM | OTH | Q4137 |
| AMNIOGEN-A | 0.5 CC | OTH | Q4162 |
| AMNIOGEN-C | 0.5 CC | OTH | Q4162 |
| AMNIOMATRIX | 1 CC | OTH | Q4139 |
| AMNIOPRO | SQ CM | OTH | Q4163 |
| AMNIOPRO FLOW | 0.5 CC | OTH | Q4162 |
| AMOBARBITAL | 125 MG | IM, IV | J0300 |
| AMPHOCIN | 50 MG | IV | J0285 |
| AMPHOTEC | 10 MG | IV | J0287 |
| AMPHOTERICIN B | 50 MG | IV | J0285 |
| AMPHOTERICIN B CHOLESTERYL SULFATE COMPLEX | 10 MG | IV | J0288 |
| AMPHOTERICIN B LIPID COMPLEX | 10 MG | IV | J0287 |
| AMPHOTERICIN B LIPOSOME | 10 MG | IV | J0289 |
| AMPICILLIN SODIUM | 500 MG | IM, IV | J0290 |
| AMPICILLIN SODIUM/SULBACTAM SODIUM | 1.5 G | IM, IV | J0295 |
| AMYGDALIN | VAR | INJ | J3570 |
| AMYTAL | 125 MG | IM, IV | J0300 |
| AMYVID | UP TO 10 MILLICUIRES | IV | A9586 |
| AN-DTPA DIAGNOSTIC | STUDY DOSE UP TO 25 MCI | IV | A9539 |
| AN-DTPA THERAPEUTIC | STUDY DOSE UP TO 25 MCI | INH | A9567 |
| ANASCORP | UP TO 120 MG | IV | J0716 |
| ANASTROZOLE | 1 MG | ORAL | S0170 |

| Drug Name | Unit Per | Route | Code |
|---|---|---|---|
| ANCEF | 500 MG | IM, IV | J0690 |
| ANECTINE | 20 MG | IM, IV | J0330 |
| ANGIOMAX | 1 MG | IV | J0583 |
| ANIDULAFUNGIN | 1 MG | IV | J0348 |
| ANISTREPLASE | 30 U | IV | J0350 |
| ANTAGON | 250 MCG | SC | S0132 |
| ANTI-INHIBITOR | 1 IU | IV | J7198 |
| ANTI-THYMOCYTE GLOBULIN,EQUINE | 250 MG | OTH | J7504 |
| ANTIEMETIC NOC | VAR | ORAL | Q0181 |
| ANTIEMETIC DRUG NOC | VAR | OTH | J8498 |
| ANTIEMETIC DRUG NOS | VAR | ORAL | J8597 |
| ANTIHEMOPHILIC FACTOR HUMAN METHOD M MONOCLONAL PURIFIED | 1 IU | IV | J7192 |
| ANTIHEMOPHILIC FACTOR PORCINE | 1 IU | IV | J7191 |
| ANTIHEMOPHILIC FACTOR VIII, XYNTHA, RECOMBINANT | 1 IU | IV | J7185 |
| ANTIHEMOPHILIC FACTOR VIII/VON WILLEBRAND FACTOR COMPLEX, HUMAN | PER FACTOR VIII IU | IV | J7186 |
| ANTITHROMBIN III | 1 IU | IV | J7195 |
| ANTITHROMBIN RECOMBINANT | 50 IU | IV | J7196 |
| ANTIZOL | 15 MG | IV | J1451 |
| ANZEMET | 10 MG | IV | J1260 |
| ANZEMET | 100 MG | ORAL | Q0180 |
| ANZEMET | 50 MG | ORAL | S0174 |
| APLIGRAF | SQ CM | OTH | Q4101 |
| APOKYN | 1 MG | SC | J0364 |
| APOMORPHINE HYDROCHLORIDE | 1 MG | SC | J0364 |
| APREPITANT | 5 MG | ORAL | J8501 |
| APROTININ | 10,000 KIU | IV | J0365 |
| AQUAMEPHYTON | 1 MG | IM, SC, IV | J3430 |
| ARA-C | 100 MG | SC, IV | J9100 |
| ARALEN | UP TO 250 MG | IM, IV | J0390 |
| ARAMINE | 10 MG | IV, IM, SC | J0380 |
| ARANESP, ESRD USE | 1 MCG | SC, IV | J0882 |
| ARANESP, NON-ESRD USE | 1 MCG | SC, IV | J0881 |
| ARBUTAMINE HCL | 1 MG | IV | J0395 |
| ARCALYST | 1 MG | SC | J2793 |
| ARCHITECT EXTRACELLULAR MATRIX | SQ CM | OTH | Q4147 |
| AREDIA | 30 MG | IV | J2430 |
| ARFORMOTEROL | 15 MCG | INH | J7605 |
| ARGATROBAN | 1 MG | IV | J0883 |
| ARGATROBAN | 1 MG | IV | J0884 |
| ARIDOL | 5 MG | INH | J7665 |
| ARIMIDEX | 1 MG | ORAL | S0170 |
| ARIPIPRAZOLE | 0.25 MG | IM | J0400 |
| ~~ARIPIPRAZOLE LAUROXIL~~ | ~~MG~~ | ~~IM~~ | ~~C9470~~ |
| ARIPIPRAZOLE LAUROXIL | 1 MG | IM | J1942 |

| Drug Name | Unit Per | Route | Code |
|---|---|---|---|
| ARIPIPRAZOLE, EXTENDED RELEASE | 1 MG | IM | J0401 |
| ARISTADA | 1 MG | IM | J1942 |
| ~~ARISTADA~~ | ~~MG~~ | ~~IM~~ | ~~C9470~~ |
| ARISTOCORT | 5 MG | IM | J3302 |
| ARISTOCORTE FORTE | 5 MG | IM | J3302 |
| ARISTOCORTE INTRALESIONAL | 5 MG | OTH | J3302 |
| ARISTOSPAN | 5 MG | VAR | J3303 |
| ARIXTRA | 0.5 MG | SC | J1652 |
| AROMASIN | 25 MG | ORAL | S0156 |
| ARRANON | 50 MG | IV | J9261 |
| ARRESTIN | 200 MG | IM | J3250 |
| ARSENIC TRIOXIDE | 1 MG | IV | J9017 |
| ARTACENT WOUND | SQ CM | OTH | Q4169 |
| ARTHROFLEX | SQ CM | OTH | Q4125 |
| ARTISS FIBRIN SEALANT | 2 ML | OTH | C9250 |
| ARZERRA | 10 MG | IV | J9302 |
| ASPARAGINASE | 10,000 U | IM, IV, SC | J9020 |
| ASPARAGINASE | 1,000 IU | IM,IV,SC | J9019 |
| ASTAGRAF XL | 0.1 MG | ORAL | J7508 |
| ASTRAMORPH PF | 10 MG | OTH | J2274 |
| ATEZOLIZUMAB | 10 MG | IV | C9483 |
| ATGAM | 250 MG | OTH | J7504 |
| ATIVAN | 2 MG | IM, IV | J2060 |
| ATOPICLAIR | ANY SIZE | OTH | A6250 |
| ATROPEN | 0.01 MG | IM | J0461 |
| ATROPINE SULFATE | 0.01 MG | IM, IV, SC | J0461 |
| ATROPINE, COMPOUNDED, CONCENTRATED | I MG | INH | J7635 |
| ATROPINE, COMPOUNDED, UNIT DOSE | 1 MG | INH | J7636 |
| ATROVENT, NONCOMPOUNDED, UNIT DOSE | 1 MG | INH | J7644 |
| ATRYN | 50 IU | IV | J7196 |
| AUROTHIOGLUCOSE | 50 MG | IM | J2910 |
| AUTOPLEX T | 1 IU | IV | J7198 |
| AVASTIN | 0.25 MG | IV | C9257 |
| AVASTIN | 10 MG | IV | J9035 |
| AVEED | 1 MG | IM | J3145 |
| AVELOX | 100 MG | IV | J2280 |
| AVONEX | 1 MCG | IM | Q3027 |
| AVONEX | 30 MCG | IM | J1826 |
| AVYCAZ | 0.5 G/0.125 G | IV | J0714 |
| AXUMIN | 1 MCI | IV | A9588 |
| AZACITIDINE | 1 MG | SC | J9025 |
| AZACTAM | 500 MG | IV | S0073 |
| AZASAN | 50 MG | ORAL | J7500 |
| AZATHIOPRINE | 100 MG | OTH | J7501 |
| AZATHIOPRINE | 50 MG | ORAL | J7500 |
| AZITHROMYCIN | 500 MG | IV | J0456 |
| AZITHROMYCIN | 1 G | ORAL | Q0144 |
| AZMACORT | PER MG | INH | J7684 |

| Drug Name | Unit Per | Route | Code |
|---|---|---|---|
| AZMACORT CONCENTRATED | PER MG | INH | J7683 |
| AZTREONAM | 500 MG | IV, IM | S0073 |
| BACLOFEN | 50 MCG | IT | J0476 |
| BACLOFEN | 10 MG | IT | J0475 |
| BACTOCILL | 250 MG | IM, IV | J2700 |
| BACTRIM IV | 10 ML | IV | S0039 |
| BAL | 100 MG | IM | J0470 |
| BASILIXIMAB | 20 MG | IV | J0480 |
| BCG INTRAVESICLE | VIAL | OTH | J9031 |
| BEBULIN VH | 1 IU | IV | J7194 |
| BECAPLERMIN GEL 0.01% | 0.5 G | OTH | S0157 |
| BECLOMETHASONE COMPOUNDED | 1 MG | INH | J7622 |
| BECLOVENT COMPOUNDED | 1 MG | INH | J7622 |
| BECONASE COMPOUNDED | 1 MG | INH | J7622 |
| BELATACEPT | 1 MG | IV | J0485 |
| BELEODAQ | 10 MG | IV | J9032 |
| BELIMUMAB | 10 MG | IV | J0490 |
| BELINOSTAT | 10 MG | IV | J9032 |
| BENA-D 10 | 50 MG | IV, IM | J1200 |
| BENA-D 50 | 50 MG | IV, IM | J1200 |
| BENADRYL | 50 MG | IV, IM | J1200 |
| BENAHIST 10 | 50 MG | IV, IM | J1200 |
| BENAHIST 50 | 50 MG | IV, IM | J1200 |
| BENDAMUSTINE HCL | 100 MG | IV | J9034 |
| BENDAMUSTINE HCL | 1 MG | IV | J9033 |
| BENDEKA | 100 MG | IV | J9034 |
| BENEFIX | 1 IU | IV | J7195 |
| BENLYSTA | 10 MG | IV | J0490 |
| BENOJECT-10 | 50 MG | IV, IM | J1200 |
| BENOJECT-50 | 50 MG | IV, IM | J1200 |
| BENTYL | 20 MG | IM | J0500 |
| BENZTROPINE MESYLATE | 1 MG | IM, IV | J0515 |
| BERINERT | 10 U | IV | J0597 |
| BERUBIGEN | 1,000 MCG | SC, IM | J3420 |
| BETA-2 | 1 MG | INH | J7648 |
| BETALIN 12 | 1,000 MCG | SC, IM | J3420 |
| BETAMETHASONE ACETATE AND BETAMETHASONE SODIUM PHOSPHATE | 3 MG, OF EACH | IM | J0702 |
| BETAMETHASONE COMPOUNDED, UNIT DOSE | 1 MG | INH | J7624 |
| BETASERON | 0.25 MG | SC | J1830 |
| BETHANECHOL CHLORIDE, MYOTONACHOL OR URECHOLINE | 5 MG | SC | J0520 |
| BEVACIZUMAB | 0.25 MG | IV | C9257 |
| BEVACIZUMAB | 10 MG | IV | J9035 |
| BEXXAR THERAPEUTIC | TX DOSE | IV | A9545 |
| BICILLIN CR | 100,000 UNITS | IM | J0558 |
| BICILLIN CR 900/300 | 100,000 UNITS | IM | J0558 |

| Drug Name | Unit Per | Route | Code |
|---|---|---|---|
| BICILLIN CR TUBEX | 100,000 UNITS | IM | J0558 |
| BICILLIN LA | 100,000 U | IM | J0561 |
| BICNU | 100 MG | IV | J9050 |
| BIO-CONNEKT | SQ CM | OTH | Q4161 |
| BIOCLATE | 1 IU | IV | J7192 |
| BIODEXCEL | SQ CM | OTH | Q4137 |
| BIODFENCE | SQ CM | OTH | Q4140 |
| BIODFENCE DRYFLEX | SQ CM | OTH | Q4138 |
| BIODMATRIX | 1 CC | OTH | Q4139 |
| BIORENEW | SQ CM | OTH | Q4163 |
| BIORENEW FLOW | 0.5 CC | OTH | Q4162 |
| BIOSKIN | SQ CM | OTH | Q4163 |
| BIOSKIN FLOW | 0.5 CC | OTH | Q4162 |
| BIOTROPIN | 1 MG | SC | J2941 |
| BIOVANCE | SQ CM | OTH | Q4154 |
| BIPERIDEN LACTATE | 5 MG | IM, IV | J0190 |
| BITOLTEROL MESYLATE, COMPOUNDED CONCENTRATED | PER MG | INH | J7628 |
| BITOLTEROL MESYLATE, COMPOUNDED UNIT DOSE | PER MG | INH | J7629 |
| BIVALIRUDIN | 1 MG | IV | J0583 |
| BIVIGAM | 500 MG | IV | J1556 |
| BLENOXANE | 15 U | IM, IV, SC | J9040 |
| BLEOMYCIN LYOPHILLIZED | 15 U | IM, IV, SC | J9040 |
| BLEOMYCIN SULFATE | 15 U | IM, IV, SC | J9040 |
| BLINATUMOMAB | 1 MCG | IV | J9039 |
| BLINCYTO | 1 MCG | IV | J9039 |
| BONIVA | 1 MG | IV | J1740 |
| BORTEZOMIB | 0.1 MG | IV | J9041 |
| BOTOX | 1 UNIT | IM, OTH | J0585 |
| BOTOX COSMETIC | 1 UNIT | IM, OTH | J0585 |
| BOTULINUM TOXIN TYPE A | 1 UNIT | IM, OTH | J0585 |
| BOTULINUM TOXIN TYPE B | 100 U | OTH | J0587 |
| BRAVELLE | 75 IU | SC, IM | J3355 |
| BRENTUXIMAB VENDOTIN | 1 MG | IV | J9042 |
| BRETHINE | PER MG | INH | J7681 |
| BRETHINE CONCENTRATED | PER MG | INH | J7680 |
| BRICANYL | PER MG | INH | J7681 |
| BRICANYL CONCENTRATED | PER MG | INH | J7680 |
| BROM-A-COT | 10 MG | IM, SC, IV | J0945 |
| BROMPHENIRAMINE MALEATE | 10 MG | IM, SC, IV | J0945 |
| BUDESONIDE COMPOUNDED, CONCETRATED | 0.25 MG | INH | J7634 |
| BUDESONIDE, COMPOUNDED, UNIT DOSE | 0.5 MG | INH | J7627 |
| BUDESONIDE, NONCOMPOUNDED, CONCENTRATED | 0.25 MG | INH | J7633 |
| BUDESONIDE, NONCOMPOUNDED, UNIT DOSE | 0.5 MG | INH | J7626 |
| BUMETANIDE | 0.5 MG | IM, IV | S0171 |
| BUNAVAIL | 2.1 MG | ORAL | J0572 |
| BUNAVAIL | 4.2 MG | ORAL | J0573 |

© 2016 Optum360, LLC

| Drug Name | Unit Per | Route | Code |
|---|---|---|---|
| BUNAVAIL | 6.3 MG | ORAL | J0574 |
| BUPIVACAINE HCL | 30 ML | VAR | S0020 |
| BUPIVACAINE LIPOSOME | 1 MG | VAR | C9290 |
| BUPRENEX | 0.1 MG | IM, IV | J0592 |
| BUPRENORPHIN/NALOXONE | UP TO 3 MG | ORAL | J0572 |
| BUPRENORPHIN/NALOXONE | > 10 MG | ORAL | J0575 |
| BUPRENORPHINE HCL | 0.1 MG | IM, IV | J0592 |
| BUPRENORPHINE IMPLANT | 74.2 MG | OTH | J0570 |
| BUPRENORPHINE ORAL | 1 MG | ORAL | J0571 |
| BUPRENORPHINE/NALOXONE | 3.1 TO 6 MG | ORAL | J0573 |
| BUPRENORPHINE/NALOXONE | 6.1 TO 10 MG | ORAL | J0574 |
| BUPROPION HCL | 150 MG | ORAL | S0106 |
| BUSULFAN | 2 MG | ORAL | J8510 |
| BUSULFAN | 1 MG | IV | J0594 |
| BUSULFEX | 2 MG | ORAL | J8510 |
| BUTORPHANOL TARTRATE | 2 MG | IM, IV | J0595 |
| BUTORPHANOL TARTRATE | 25 MG | OTH | S0012 |
| C 1 ESTERASE INHIBITOR (HUMAN) (BERINERT) | 10 UNITS | IV | J0597 |
| C1 ESTERASE INHIBITOR (HUMAN) (CINRYZE) | 10 UNITS | IV | J0598 |
| C1 ESTERASE INHIBITOR (RECOMBINANT) | 10 UNITS | IV | J0596 |
| CABAZITAXEL | 1 MG | IV | J9043 |
| CABERGOLINE | 0.25 MG | ORAL | J8515 |
| CAFCIT | 5 MG | IV | J0706 |
| CAFFEINE CITRATE | 5 MG | IV | J0706 |
| CALCIJEX | 0.1 MCG | IM | J0636 |
| CALCIJEX | 0.25 MCG | INJ | S0169 |
| CALCIMAR | UP TO 400 U | SC, IM | J0630 |
| CALCITONIN SALMON | 400 U | SC, IM | J0630 |
| CALCITRIOL | 0.1 MCG | IM | J0636 |
| CALCITROL | 0.25 MCG | IM | S0169 |
| CALCIUM DISODIUM VERSENATE | 1,000 MG | IV, SC, IM | J0600 |
| CALCIUM GLUCONATE | 10 ML | IV | J0610 |
| CALCIUM GLYCEROPHOSPHATE AND CALCIUM LACTATE | 10 ML | IM, SC | J0620 |
| CALDOLOR | 100 MG | IV | J1741 |
| CAMPTOSAR | 20 MG | IV | J9206 |
| CANAKINUMAB | 1 MG | SC | J0638 |
| CANCIDAS | 5 MG | IV | J0637 |
| CAPECITABINE | 150 MG | ORAL | J8520 |
| CAPROMAB PENDETIDE | STUDY DOSE UP TO 10 MCI | IV | A9507 |
| CAPSAICIN 8% PATCH | 1 SQ CM | OTH | J7336 |
| CARBIDOPA/LEVODOPA | 5 MG/20 MG | ORAL | J7340 |
| CARBOCAINE | 10 ML | VAR | J0670 |
| CARBOPLATIN | 50 MG | IV | J9045 |
| CARDIOGEN 82 | STUDY DOSE UP TO 60 MCI | IV | A9555 |
| CARDIOLITE | STUDY DOSE | IV | A9500 |
| CARFILZOMIB | 1 MG | IV | J9047 |

| Drug Name | Unit Per | Route | Code |
|---|---|---|---|
| CARIMUNE | 500 MG | IV | J1566 |
| CARMUSTINE | 100 MG | IV | J9050 |
| CARNITOR | 1 G | IV | J1955 |
| CARTICEL | | OTH | J7330 |
| CASPOFUNGIN ACETATE | 5 MG | IV | J0637 |
| CATAPRES | 1 MG | OTH | J0735 |
| CATHFLO | 1 MG | IV | J2997 |
| CAVERJECT | 1.25 MCG | VAR | J0270 |
| CEA SCAN | STUDY DOSE UP TO 45 MCI | IV | A9568 |
| CEENU | 10 MG | ORAL | S0178 |
| CEFAZOLIN SODIUM | 500 MG | IM, IV | J0690 |
| CEFEPIME HCL | 500 MG | IV | J0692 |
| CEFIZOX | 500 MG | IV, IM | J0715 |
| CEFOBID | 1 G | IV | S0021 |
| CEFOPERAZONE SODIUM | 1 G | IV | S0021 |
| CEFOTAN | 500 MG | IM, IV | S0074 |
| CEFOTAXIME SODIUM | 1 GM | IV, IM | J0698 |
| CEFOTETAN DISODIUM | 500 MG | IM. IV | S0074 |
| CEFOXITIN SODIUM | 1 GM | IV, IM | J0694 |
| CEFTAROLINE FOSAMIL | 10 MG | IV | J0712 |
| CEFTAZIDIME | 500 MG | IM, IV | J0713 |
| CEFTAZIDIME AND AVIBACTAM | 0.5 G/0.125 G | IV | J0714 |
| CEFTIZOXIME SODIUM | 500 MG | IV, IM | J0715 |
| CEFTOLOZANE AND TAZOBACTAM | 50 MG/25 MG | IV | J0695 |
| CEFTRIAXONE SODIUM | 250 MG | IV, IM | J0696 |
| CEFUROXIME | 750 MG | IM, IV | J0697 |
| CEFUROXIME SODIUM STERILE | 750 MG | IM, IV | J0697 |
| CELESTONE SOLUSPAN | 3 MG | IM | J0702 |
| CELLCEPT | 250 MG | ORAL | J7517 |
| CENACORT A-40 | 10 MG | IM | J3301 |
| CENACORT FORTE | 5 MG | IM | J3302 |
| CENTRUROIDES (SCORPION) IMMUNE F(AB)2 (EQUINE) | UP TO 120 MG | IV | J0716 |
| CEPHALOTHIN SODIUM | UP TO 1 G | INJ | J1890 |
| CEPHAPIRIN SODIUM | 1 G | IV | J0710 |
| CEPTAZ | 500 MG | IM, IV | J0713 |
| CEREBRYX | 50 MG | IM, IV | Q2009 |
| CEREBRYX | 750 MG | IM, IV | S0078 |
| CEREDASE | 10 U | IV | J0205 |
| CERETEC | STUDY DOSE UP TO 25 MCI | IV | A9521 |
| CEREZYME | 10 U | IV | J1786 |
| CERTOLIZUMAB PEGOL | 1 MG | SC | J0717 |
| CERUBIDINE | 10 MG | IV | J9150 |
| CESAMET | 1 MG | ORAL | J8650 |
| CETUXIMAB | 10 MG | IV | J9055 |
| CHEALAMIDE | 150 MG | IV | J3520 |
| CHLORAMBUCIL | 2 MG | ORAL | S0172 |

| Drug Name | Unit Per | Route | Code |
|---|---|---|---|
| CHLORAMPHENICOL SODIUM SUCCINATE | 1 G | IV | J0720 |
| CHLORDIAZEPOXIDE HCL | 100 MG | IM, IV | J1990 |
| CHLOROMYCETIN | 1 G | IV | J0720 |
| CHLOROPROCAINE HCL | 30 ML | VAR | J2400 |
| CHLOROQUINE HCL | UP TO 250 MG | IM, IV | J0390 |
| CHLOROTHIAZIDE SODIUM | 500 MG | IV | J1205 |
| CHLORPROMAZINE HCL | 50 MG | IM, IV | J3230 |
| CHLORPROMAZINE HCL | 5 MG | ORAL | Q0161 |
| CHOLETEC | STUDY DOSE UP TO 15 MCI | IV | A9537 |
| CHOLINE C 11, DIAGNOSTIC, PER STUDY DOSE | UP TO 20 MCI | IV | A9515 |
| ~~CHOLINE C 11, DIAGNOSTIC, PER STUDY DOSE~~ | ~~VAR~~ | ~~IV~~ | ~~C9461~~ |
| CHOREX | 1000 USP | IM | J0725 |
| CHORIONIC GONADOTROPIN | 1,000 USP U | IM | J0725 |
| CHROMIC PHOSPHATE P32 (THERAPEUTIC) | 1 MCI | IV | A9564 |
| CHROMITOPE SODIUM | STUDY DOSE UP TO 250 UCI | IV | A9553 |
| CHROMIUM CR-51 SODIUM IOTHALAMATE, DIAGNOSTIC | STUDY DOSE UP TO 250 UCI | IV | A9553 |
| CIDOFOVIR | 375 MG | IV | J0740 |
| CILASTATIN SODIUM | 250 MG | IV, IM | J0743 |
| CIMETIDINE HCL | 300 MG | IM, IV | S0023 |
| CIMZIA | 1 MG | SC | J0717 |
| ~~CINQUAIR~~ | ~~1 MG~~ | ~~IV~~ | ~~C9481~~ |
| CINQUAIR | 1 MG | IV | J2786 |
| CINRZYE | 10 UNITS | IV | J0598 |
| CIPRO | 200 MG | IV | J0744 |
| CIPROFLOXACIN FOR INTRAVENOUS INFUSION | 200 MG | IV | J0744 |
| CIPROFLOXACIN OTIC SUSPENSION | 6 MG | OTIC | J7342 |
| ~~CIPROFLOXACIN, OTIC SUSPENSION~~ | ~~6 MG~~ | ~~OTH~~ | ~~C9479~~ |
| CIS-MDP | STUDY DOSE UP TO 30 MCI | IV | A9503 |
| CIS-PYRO | STUDY DOSE UP TO 25 MCI | IV | A9538 |
| CISPLATIN | 10 MG | IV | J9060 |
| CLADRIBINE | 1 MG | IV | J9065 |
| CLAFORAN | 1 GM | IV, IM | J0698 |
| CLARIXFLO | 1 MG | OTH | Q4155 |
| CLEOCIN PHOSPHATE | 300 MG | IV | S0077 |
| CLEVIDIPINE BUTYRATE | 1 MG | IV | C9248 |
| CLEVIPREX | 1 MG | IV | C9248 |
| CLINDAMYCIN PHOSPHATE | 300 MG | IV | S0077 |
| CLOFARABINE | 1 MG | IV | J9027 |

| Drug Name | Unit Per | Route | Code |
|---|---|---|---|
| CLOLAR | 1 MG | IV | J9027 |
| CLONIDINE HCL | 1 MG | OTH | J0735 |
| CLOZAPINE | 25 MG | ORAL | S0136 |
| CLOZARIL | 25 MG | ORAL | S0136 |
| COAGADEX | 1 IU | IV | J7175 |
| COBAL | 1,000 MCG | IM, SC | J3420 |
| COBALT CO-57 CYNOCOBALAMIN, DIAGNOSTIC | STUDY DOSE UP TO 1 UCI | ORAL | A9559 |
| COBATOPE 57 | STUDY DOSE UP TO 1 UCI | ORAL | A9559 |
| COBEX | 1,000 MCG | SC, IM | J3420 |
| CODEINE PHOSPHATE | 30 MG | IM, IV, SC | J0745 |
| COGENTIN | 1 MG | IM, IV | J0515 |
| COGNEX | 10 MG | ORAL | S0014 |
| COLCHICINE | 1 MG | IV | J0760 |
| COLHIST | 10 MG | IM, SC, IV | J0945 |
| COLISTIMETHATE SODIUM | 150 MG | IM, IV | J0770 |
| COLISTIMETHATE SODIUM | 1 MG | INH | S0142 |
| COLLAGEN BASED WOUND FILLER DRY FOAM | 1 GM | OTH | A6010 |
| COLLAGEN BASED WOUND FILLER, GEL/PASTE | 1 GM | OTH | A6011 |
| COLLAGEN MATRIX NERVE WRAP | 0.5 CM | OTH | C9361 |
| COLLAGEN NERVE CUFF | 0.5 CM LENGTH | OTH | C9355 |
| COLLAGEN WOUND DRESSING | SQ CM | OTH | Q4164 |
| COLLAGENASE, CLOSTRIDIUM HISTOLYTICUM | 0.01 MG | OTH | J0775 |
| COLY-MYCIN M | 150 MG | IM, IV | J0770 |
| COMPAZINE | 10 MG | IM, IV | J0780 |
| COMPAZINE | 5 MG | ORAL | Q0164 |
| COMPAZINE | 5 MG | ORAL | S0183 |
| CONTRACEPTIVE SUPPLY, HORMONE CONTAINING PATCH | EACH | OTH | J7304 |
| CONTRAST FOR ECHOCARDIOGRAM | STUDY | IV | A9700 |
| COPAXONE | 20 MG | SC | J1595 |
| COPPER T MODEL TCU380A IUD COPPER WIRE/COPPER COLLAR | EA | OTH | J7300 |
| CORDARONE | 30 MG | IV | J0282 |
| CORIFACT | 1 IU | IV | J7180 |
| CORTASTAT | 1 MG | IM, IV, OTH | J1100 |
| CORTASTAT LA | 1 MG | IM | J1094 |
| CORTICORELIN OVINE TRIFLUTATE | 1 MCG | IV | J0795 |
| CORTICOTROPIN | 40 U | IV, IM, SC | J0800 |
| CORTIMED | 80 MG | IM | J1040 |
| CORTROSYN | 0.25 MG | IM, IV | J0834 |
| CORVERT | 1 MG | IV | J1742 |
| COSMEGEN | 0.5 MG | IV | J9120 |
| COSYNTROPIN | 0.25 MG | IM, IV | J0833 |
| COTOLONE | 5 MG | ORAL | J7510 |
| CRESEMBA | 1 MG | IV | J1833 |
| CROFAB | UP TO 1 GM | IV | J0840 |

| Drug Name | Unit Per | Route | Code |
|---|---|---|---|
| CROMOLYN SODIUM COMPOUNDED | PER 10 MG | INH | J7632 |
| CROMOLYN SODIUM NONCOMPOUNDED | 10 MG | INH | J7631 |
| CROTALIDAE POLYVALENT IMMUNE FAB (OVINE) | UP TO 1 GM | IV | J0840 |
| CRYSTAL B12 | 1,000 MCG | IM, SC | J3420 |
| CRYSTICILLIN 300 A.S. | 600,000 UNITS | IM, IV | J2510 |
| CRYSTICILLIN 600 A.S. | 600,000 UNITS | IM, IV | J2510 |
| CUBICIN | 1 MG | IV | J0878 |
| CYANO | 1,000 MCG | IM, SC | J3420 |
| CYANOCOBALAMIN | 1,000 MCG | IM, SC | J3420 |
| CYANOCOBALAMIN COBALT 57/58 | STUDY DOSE UP TO 1 UCI | IV | A9546 |
| CYANOCOBALAMIN COBALT CO-57 | STUDY DOSE UP TO 1 UCI | ORAL | A9559 |
| CYCLOPHOSPHAMIDE | 25 MG | ORAL | J8530 |
| CYCLOPHOSPHAMIDE | 100 MG | IV | J9070 |
| CYCLOSPORINE | 100 MG | ORAL | J7502 |
| CYCLOSPORINE | 25 MG | ORAL | J7515 |
| CYCLOSPORINE | 250 MG | IV | J7516 |
| CYGNUS | SQ CM | OTH | Q4170 |
| CYMETRA | 1 CC | INJ | Q4112 |
| CYRAMZA | 5 MG | IV | J9308 |
| CYSVIEW | STUDY DOSE | OTH | C9275 |
| CYTAL | SQ CM | OTH | Q4166 |
| CYTARABINE | 100 MG | SC, IV | J9100 |
| CYTARABINE LIPOSOME | 10 MG | IT | J9098 |
| CYTOGAM | VIAL | IV | J0850 |
| CYTOMEGALOVIRUS IMMUNE GLOB | VIAL | IV | J0850 |
| CYTOSAR-U | 100 MG | SC, IV | J9100 |
| CYTOTEC | 200 MCG | ORAL | S0191 |
| CYTOVENE | 500 MG | IV | J1570 |
| CYTOXAN | 100 MG | IV | J9070 |
| CYTOXAN | 25 MG | ORAL | J8530 |
| D.H.E. 45 | 1 MG | IM, IV | J1110 |
| DACARBAZINE | 100 MG | IV | J9130 |
| DACLIZUMAB | 25 MG | OTH | J7513 |
| DACOGEN | 1 MG | IV | J0894 |
| DACTINOMYCIN | 0.5 MG | IV | J9120 |
| DALALONE | 1 MG | IM, IV, OTH | J1100 |
| DALALONE LA | 1 MG | IM | J1094 |
| DALBAVANCIN | 5 MG | IV | J0875 |
| DALTEPARIN SODIUM | 2,500 IU | SC | J1645 |
| DALVANCE | 5 MG | IV | J0875 |
| DAPTOMYCIN | 1 MG | IV | J0878 |
| DARATUMUMAB | 10 MG | IV | J9145 |
| ~~DARATUMUMAB~~ | ~~10 MG~~ | ~~IV~~ | ~~C9476~~ |
| DARBEPOETIN ALFA, ESRD USE | 1 MCG | SC, IV | J0882 |
| DARBEPOETIN ALFA, NON-ESRD USE | 1 MCG | SC, IV | J0881 |

| Drug Name | Unit Per | Route | Code |
|---|---|---|---|
| ~~DARZALEX~~ | ~~10 MG~~ | ~~IV~~ | ~~C9476~~ |
| DARZALEX | 10 MG | IV | J9145 |
| DATSCAN | STUDY DOSE | IV | A9584 |
| DAUNORUBICIN | 10 MG | IV | J9150 |
| DAUNORUBICIN CITRATE, LIPOOSOMAL FORMULATION | 10 MG | IV | J9151 |
| DAUNOXOME | 10 MG | IV | J9151 |
| DDAVP | 1 MCG | IV, SC | J2597 |
| DECADRON | 0.25 MG | ORAL | J8540 |
| DECAJECT | 1 MG | IM, IV, OTH | J1100 |
| DECITABINE | 1 MG | IV | J0894 |
| DECOLONE-50 | 50 MG | IM | J2320 |
| DEFEROXAMINE MESYLATE | 500 MG | IM, SC, IV | J0895 |
| DEGARELIX | 1 MG | SC | J9155 |
| DELATESTRYL | 1 MG | IM | J3121 |
| DELESTROGEN | 10 MG | IM | J1380 |
| DELTA-CORTEF | 5 MG | ORAL | J7510 |
| DEMADEX | 10 MG | IV | J3265 |
| DEMEROL | 100 MG | IM, IV, SC | J2175 |
| DENILEUKIN DIFTITOX | 300 MCG | IV | J9160 |
| DENOSUMAB | 1 MG | SC | J0897 |
| DEPGYNOGEN | UP TO 5 MG | IM | J1000 |
| DEPHENACEN-50 | 50 MG | IM, IV | J1200 |
| DEPMEDALONE | 80 MG | IM | J1040 |
| DEPMEDALONE | 40 MG | IM | J1030 |
| DEPO-ESTRADIOL CYPIONATE | UP TO 5 MG | IM | J1000 |
| DEPO-MEDROL | 20 MG | IM, OTH | J1020 |
| DEPO-MEDROL | 40 MG | IM, OTH | J1030 |
| DEPO-MEDROL | 80 MG | IM, OTH | J1040 |
| DEPO-TESTOSTERONE | 1 MG | IM | J1071 |
| DEPOCYT | 10 MG | IT | J9098 |
| DEPODUR | 10 MG | OTH | J2274 |
| DEPODUR | UP TO 10 MG | IV | J2270 |
| DEPOGEN | UP TO 5 MG | IM | J1000 |
| DERMACELL | SQ CM | OTH | Q4122 |
| DERMAGRAFT | SQ CM | OTH | Q4106 |
| DERMAL SUBSTITUTE, NATIVE, NONDENATURED COLLAGEN, FETAL | 0.5 SQ CM | OTH | C9358 |
| DERMAL SUBSTITUTE, NATIVE, NONDENATURED COLLAGEN, NEONATAL | 0.5 SQ CM | OTH | C9360 |
| DERMAPURE | SQ CM | OTH | Q4152 |
| DERMAVEST AND PLURIVEST | SQ CM | OTH | Q4153 |
| DESFERAL | 500 MG | IM, SC, IV | J0895 |
| DESMOPRESSIN ACETATE | 1 MCG | IV, SC | J2597 |
| DEXAMETHASONE | 0.25 MG | ORAL | J8540 |
| DEXAMETHASONE ACETATE | 1 MG | IM | J1094 |
| DEXAMETHASONE ACETATE ANHYDROUS | 1 MG | IM | J1094 |
| DEXAMETHASONE INTRAVITREAL IMPLANT | 0.1 MG | OTH | J7312 |
| DEXAMETHASONE SODIUM PHOSPHATE | 1 MG | IM, IV, OTH | J1100 |

© 2016 Optum360, LLC

| Drug Name | Unit Per | Route | Code |
|---|---|---|---|
| DEXAMETHASONE, COMPOUNDED, CONCENTRATED | 1 MG | INH | J7637 |
| DEXAMETHASONE, COMPOUNDED, UNIT DOSE | 1 MG | INH | J7638 |
| DEXASONE | 1 MG | IM, IV, OTH | J1100 |
| DEXEDRINE | 5 MG | ORAL | S0160 |
| DEXIM | 1 MG | IM, IV, OTH | J1100 |
| DEXONE | 1 MG | IM, IV, OTH | J1100 |
| DEXONE | 0.25 MG | ORAL | J8540 |
| DEXONE LA | 1 MG | IM | J1094 |
| DEXRAZOXANE HCL | 250 MG | IV | J1190 |
| DEXTRAN 40 | 500 ML | IV | J7100 |
| DEXTROAMPHETAMINE SULFATE | 5 MG | ORAL | S0160 |
| DEXTROSE | 500 ML | IV | J7060 |
| DEXTROSE, STERILE WATER, AND/OR DEXTROSE DILUENT/FLUSH | 10 ML | VAR | A4216 |
| DEXTROSE/SODIUM CHLORIDE | 5% | VAR | J7042 |
| DEXTROSE/THEOPHYLLINE | 40 MG | IV | J2810 |
| DEXTROSTAT | 5 MG | ORAL | S0160 |
| DI-SPAZ | UP TO 20 MG | IM | J0500 |
| DIALYSIS/STRESS VITAMINS | 100 CAPS | ORAL | S0194 |
| DIAMOX | 500 MG | IM, IV | J1120 |
| DIASTAT | 5 MG | IV, IM | J3360 |
| DIAZEPAM | 5 MG | IV, IM | J3360 |
| DIAZOXIDE | 300 MG | IV | J1730 |
| DIBENT | UP TO 20 MG | IM | J0500 |
| DICLOFENAC SODIUM | 0.5 MG | OTH | J1130 |
| DICYCLOMINE HCL | 20 MG | IM | J0500 |
| DIDANOSINE (DDI) | 25 MG | ORAL | S0137 |
| DIDRONEL | 300 MG | IV | J1436 |
| DIETHYLSTILBESTROL DIPHOSPHATE | 250 MG | INJ | J9165 |
| DIFLUCAN | 200 MG | IV | J1450 |
| DIGIBIND | VIAL | IV | J1162 |
| DIGIFAB | VIAL | IV | J1162 |
| DIGOXIN | 0.5 MG | IM, IV | J1160 |
| DIGOXIN IMMUNE FAB | VIAL | IV | J1162 |
| DIHYDROERGOTAMINE MESYLATE | 1 MG | IM, IV | J1110 |
| DILANTIN | 50 MG | IM, IV | J1165 |
| DILAUDID | 250 MG | OTH | S0092 |
| DILAUDID | 4 MG | SC, IM, IV | J1170 |
| DIMENHYDRINATE | 50 MG | IM, IV | J1240 |
| DIMERCAPROL | 100 MG | IM | J0470 |
| DIMINE | 50 MG | IV, IM | J1200 |
| DINATE | 50 MG | IM, IV | J1240 |
| DIOVAL | 10 MG | IM | J1380 |
| DIOVAL 40 | 10 MG | IM | J1380 |
| DIOVAL XX | 10 MG | IM | J1380 |
| DIPHENHYDRAMINE HCL | 50 MG | ORAL | Q0163 |
| DIPHENHYDRAMINE HCL | 50 MG | IV, IM | J1200 |
| DIPRIVAN | 10 MG | IV | J2704 |
| DIPYRIDAMOLE | 10 MG | IV | J1245 |

| Drug Name | Unit Per | Route | Code |
|---|---|---|---|
| DISOTATE | 150 MG | IV | J3520 |
| DIURIL | 500 MG | IV | J1205 |
| DIURIL SODIUM | 500 MG | IV | J1205 |
| DIZAC | 5 MG | IV, IM | J3360 |
| DMSO, DIMETHYL SULFOXIDE | 50%, 50 ML | OTH | J1212 |
| DOBUTAMINE HCL | 250 MG | IV | J1250 |
| DOBUTREX | 250 MG | IV | J1250 |
| DOCETAXEL | 1 MG | IV | J9171 |
| DOLASETRON MESYLATE | 100 MG | ORAL | Q0180 |
| DOLASETRON MESYLATE | 10 MG | IV | J1260 |
| DOLASETRON MESYLATE | 50 MG | ORAL | S0174 |
| DOLOPHINE | 5 MG | ORAL | S0109 |
| DOLOPHINE HCL | 10 MG | IM, SC | J1230 |
| DOMMANATE | 50 MG | IM, IV | J1240 |
| DOPAMINE HCL | 40 MG | IV | J1265 |
| DORIBAX | 10 MG | IV | J1267 |
| DORIPENEM | 10 MG | IV | J1267 |
| DORNASE ALPHA, NONCOMPOUNDED, UNIT DOSE | 1 MG | INH | J7639 |
| DOSTINEX | 0.25 MG | ORAL | J8515 |
| DOTAREM | 0.1 ML | IV | A9575 |
| DOXERCALCIFEROL | 1 MG | IV | J1270 |
| DOXORUBICIN HCL | 10 MG | IV | J9000 |
| DOXORUBICIN HYDROCHLORIDE, LIPOSOMAL, IMPORTED LIPODOX | 10 MG | IV | Q2049 |
| DOXORUBICIN HYDROCHLORIDE, LIPOSOMAL, NOT OTHERWISE SPECIFIED, 10 MG | 10 MG | IV | Q2050 |
| DRAMAMINE | 50 MG | IM, IV | J1240 |
| DRAMANATE | 50 MG | IM, IV | J1240 |
| DRAMILIN | 50 MG | IM, IV | J1240 |
| DRAMOCEN | 50 MG | IM, IV | J1240 |
| DRAMOJECT | 50 MG | IM, IV | J1240 |
| DRAXIMAGE MDP-10 | STUDY DOSE UP TO 30 MCI | IV | A9503 |
| DRAXIMAGE MDP-25 | STUDY DOSE UP TO 30 MCI | IV | A9503 |
| DRONABINAL | 2.5 MG | ORAL | Q0167 |
| DROPERIDOL | 5 MG | IM, IV | J1790 |
| DROPERIDOL AND FENTANYL CITRATE | 2 ML | IM, IV | J1810 |
| DROXIA | 500 MG | ORAL | S0176 |
| DTIC-DOME | 100 MG | IV | J9130 |
| DTPA | STUDY DOSE UP TO 25 MCI | IV | A9539 |
| DTPA | STUDY DOSE UP TO 25 MCI | INH | A9567 |
| DUOPA | 5 MG/20 MG | ORAL | J7340 |
| DURACILLIN A.S. | 600,000 UNITS | IM, IV | J2510 |

© 2016 Optum360, LLC

| Drug Name | Unit Per | Route | Code |
|---|---|---|---|
| DURACLON | 1 MG | OTH | J0735 |
| DURAGEN-10 | 10 MG | IM | J1380 |
| DURAGEN-20 | 10 MG | IM | J1380 |
| DURAGEN-40 | 10 MG | IM | J1380 |
| DURAMORPH | 500 MG | OTH | S0093 |
| DURAMORPH PF | 10 MG | OTH | J2274 |
| DURO CORT | 80 MG | IM | J1040 |
| DYLOJECT | 0.5 MG | OTH | J1130 |
| DYMENATE | 50 MG | IM, IV | J1240 |
| DYPHYLLINE | 500 MG | IM | J1180 |
| DYSPORT | 5 UNITS | IM | J0586 |
| E.D.T.A. | 150 MG | IV | J3520 |
| ECALLANTIDE | 1 MG | SC | J1290 |
| ECHOCARDIOGRAM IMAGE ENHANCER OCTAFLUOROPROPANE | 1 ML | IV | Q9956 |
| ECHOCARDIOGRAM IMAGE ENHANCER PERFLEXANE | 1 ML | IV | Q9955 |
| ECULIZUMAB | 10 MG | IV | J1300 |
| EDETATE CALCIUM DISODIUM | 1,000 MG | IV, SC, IM | J0600 |
| EDETATE DISODIUM | 150 MG | IV | J3520 |
| EDEX | 1.25 MCG | VAR | J0270 |
| ELAPRASE | 1 MG | IV | J1743 |
| ELAVIL | 20 MG | IM | J1320 |
| ELELYSO | 10 U | IV | J3060 |
| ELIGARD | 7.5, 22.5, 30, 45 MG | SC | J9217 |
| ELITEK | 0.5 MG | IM | J2783 |
| ELLENCE | 2 MG | IV | J9178 |
| ELLIOTTS B SOLUTION | 1 ML | IV, IT | J9175 |
| ~~ELOCTATE~~ | ~~IU~~ | ~~IV~~ | ~~C9136~~ |
| ELOCTATE | IU | IV | J7205 |
| ELOSULFASE ALFA | 1 MG | IV | J1322 |
| ~~ELOTUZUMAB~~ | ~~1 MG~~ | ~~IV~~ | ~~C9477~~ |
| ELOTUZUMAB | 1 MG | IV | J9176 |
| ELOXATIN | 0.5 MG | IV | J9263 |
| ELSPAR | 1,000 IU | IM,IV, SC | J9019 |
| ELSPAR | 10,000 U | IM, IV, SC | J9020 |
| EMEND | 5 MG | ORAL | J8501 |
| EMEND | 1 MG | IV | J1453 |
| EMINASE | 30 U | IV | J0350 |
| ~~EMPLICITI~~ | ~~1 MG~~ | ~~IV~~ | ~~C9477~~ |
| EMPLICITI | 1 MG | IV | J9176 |
| ENBREL | 25 MG | IM, IV | J1438 |
| ENDOXAN-ASTA | 100 MG | IV | J9070 |
| ENDRATE | 150 MG | IV | J3520 |
| ENFUVIRTIDE | 1 MG | SC | J1324 |
| ENOXAPARIN SODIUM | 10 MG | SC | J1650 |
| ENTYVIO | 1 MG | IV | J3380 |
| ENVARSUS XR | 0.25 MG | ORAL | J7503 |
| EOVIST | 1 ML | IV | A9581 |
| EPIFIX, INJECTABLE | 1 MG | OTH | Q4145 |
| EPIFIX/EPICORD | PER SQ IN | OTH | Q4131 |

| Drug Name | Unit Per | Route | Code |
|---|---|---|---|
| EPINEPHRINE | 0.1 MG | VAR | J0171 |
| EPIRUBICIN HCL | 2 MG | IV | J9178 |
| EPOETIN ALFA FOR ESRD DIALYSIS | 100 U | INJ | Q4081 |
| EPOETIN ALFA, NON-ESRD USE | 1,000 U | SC, IV | J0885 |
| EPOETIN BETA FOR ESRD ON DIALYSIS | 1 MCG | IV | J0887 |
| EPOETIN BETA FOR NON-ESRD | 1 MCG | IV, SC | J0888 |
| EPOGEN/NON-ESRD | 1,000 U | SC, IV | J0885 |
| EPOPROSTENOL | 0.5 MG | IV | J1325 |
| EPOPROSTENOL STERILE DILUTANT | 50 ML | IV | S0155 |
| EPTIFIBATIDE | 5 MG | IM, IV | J1327 |
| ERAXIS | 1 MG | IV | J0348 |
| ERBITUX | 10 MG | IV | J9055 |
| ERGAMISOL | 50 MG | ORAL | S0177 |
| ERGONOVINE MALEATE | 0.2 MG | IM, IV | J1330 |
| ERIBULIN MESYLATE | 0.1 MG | IV | J9179 |
| ERTAPENEM SODIUM | 500 MG | IM, IV | J1335 |
| ERYTHROCIN LACTOBIONATE | 500 MG | IV | J1364 |
| ESTONE AQUEOUS | 1 MG | IM, IV | J1435 |
| ESTRA-L 20 | 10 MG | IM | J1380 |
| ESTRA-L 40 | 10 MG | IM | J1380 |
| ESTRADIOL CYPIONATE | UP TO 5 MG | IM | J1000 |
| ESTRADIOL L.A. | 10 MG | IM | J1380 |
| ESTRADIOL L.A. 20 | 10 MG | IM | J1380 |
| ESTRADIOL L.A. 40 | 10 MG | IM | J1380 |
| ESTRADIOL VALERATE | 10 MG | IM | J1380 |
| ESTRAGYN | 1 MG | IV, IM | J1435 |
| ESTRO-A | 1 MG | IV, IM | J1435 |
| ESTROGEN CONJUGATED | 25 MG | IV, IM | J1410 |
| ESTRONE | 1 MG | IV, IM | J1435 |
| ESTRONOL | 1 MG | IM, IV | J1435 |
| ETANERCEPT | 25 MG | IM, IV | J1438 |
| ETHAMOLIN | 100 MG | IV | J1430 |
| ETHANOLAMINE OLEATE | 100 MG | IV | J1430 |
| ETHYOL | 500 MG | IV | J0207 |
| ETIDRONATE DISODIUM | 300 MG | IV | J1436 |
| ETONOGESTREL | IMPLANT | OTH | J7307 |
| ETOPOSIDE | 50 MG | ORAL | J8560 |
| ETOPOSIDE | 10 MG | IV | J9181 |
| EUFLEXXA | DOSE | OTH | J7323 |
| EULEXIN | 125 MG | ORAL | S0175 |
| EVEROLIMUS | 0.25 MG | ORAL | J7527 |
| EXAMETAZIME LABELED AUTOLOGOUS WHITE BLOOD CELLS, TECHNETIUM TC-99M | STUDY DOSE | IV | A9569 |
| EXCELLAGEN | 0.1 CC | OTH | Q4149 |
| EXMESTANE | 25 MG | ORAL | S0156 |
| EXPAREL | 1 MG | VAR | C9290 |
| EZ-DERM | PER SQ CM | OTH | Q4136 |
| FABRAZYME | 1 MG | IV | J0180 |

| Drug Name | Unit Per | Route | Code |
|---|---|---|---|
| FACTOR IX (ANTIHEMOPHILIC FACTOR, RECOMBINANT), RIXIBUS, PER I.U. | IU | IV | J7200 |
| FACTOR IX NON-RECOMBINANT | 1 IU | IV | J7193 |
| FACTOR IX RECOMBINANT | 1 IU | IV | J7195 |
| FACTOR IX+ COMPLEX | 1 IU | IV | J7194 |
| FACTOR IX, ALBUMIN FUSION PROTEIN (RECOMBINANT) | 1 IU | IV | C9139 |
| FACTOR IX, ALBUMIN FUSION PROTEIN, (RECOMBINANT) | 1 IU | IV | J7202 |
| FACTOR IX, FC FUSION PROTEIN (ANTIHEMOPHILIC FACTOR, RECOMBINANT), ALPROLIX | IU | IV | J7201 |
| FACTOR VII FC FUSION PROTEIN, (RECOMBINANT) | IU | IV | C9136 |
| FACTOR VIIA RECOMBINANT | 1 MCG | IV | J7189 |
| FACTOR VIII (ANTIHEMOPHILIC FACTOR, RECOMBINANT) | IU | IV | C9138 |
| FACTOR VIII (ANTIHEMOPHILIC FACTOR, RECOMBINANT) | IU | IV | J7188 |
| FACTOR VIII (ANTIHEMOPHILIC FACTOR, RECOMBINANT) | 1 IU | IV | J7209 |
| FACTOR VIII (ANTIHEMOPHILIC FACTOR, RECOMBINANT) | 1 IU | IV | C9140 |
| FACTOR VIII (ANTIHEMOPHILIC FACTOR, RECOMBINANT) PEGYLATED | IU | IV | C9137 |
| FACTOR VIII (ANTIHEMOPHILIC FACTOR, RECOMBINANT) PEGYLATED | 1 IU | IV | J7207 |
| FACTOR VIII FC FUSION (RECOMBINANT) | IU | IV | J7205 |
| FACTOR VIII PORCINE | 1 IU | IV | J7191 |
| FACTOR VIII RECOMBINANT | 1 IU | IV | J7192 |
| FACTOR VIII, (ANTIHEMOPHILIC FACTOR, RECOMBINANT), (NOVOEIGHT), PER IU | IU | IV | J7182 |
| FACTOR VIII, HUMAN | 1 IU | IV | J7190 |
| FACTOR X (HUMAN) | 1 IU | IV | J7175 |
| FACTOR XIII (ANTIHEMOPHILIC FACTOR, HUMAN) | 1 IU | IV | J7180 |
| FACTOR XIII A-SUBUNIT (RECOMBINANT) | 10 IU | IV | J7181 |
| FACTREL | 100 MCG | SC, IV | J1620 |
| FAMOTIDINE | 20 MG | IV | S0028 |
| FASLODEX | 25 MG | IM | J9395 |
| FDG | STUDY DOSE UP TO 45 MCI | IV | A9552 |
| FEIBA-VH AICC | 1 IU | IV | J7198 |
| FENTANYL CITRATE | 0.1 MG | IM, IV | J3010 |
| FERAHEME (FOR ESRD) | 1 MG | IV | Q0139 |
| FERAHEME (NON-ESRD) | 1 MG | IV | Q0138 |
| FERIDEX IV | 1 ML | IV | Q9953 |
| FERRIC CARBOXYMALTOSE | 1 MG | IV | J1439 |
| FERRIC PYROPHOSPHATE CITRATE SOLUTION | 0.1 MG | IV | J1443 |

| Drug Name | Unit Per | Route | Code |
|---|---|---|---|
| FERRLECIT | 12.5 MG | IV | J2916 |
| FERTINEX | 75 IU | SC | J3355 |
| FERUMOXYTOL (FOR ESRD) | 1 MG | IV | Q0139 |
| FERUMOXYTOL (NON-ESRD) | 1 MG | IV | Q0138 |
| FIBRIN SEALANT (HUMAN) | 2 ML | OTH | C9250 |
| FILGRASTIM | 1 MCG | SC, IV | J1442 |
| FILGRASTIM (G-CSF), BIOSIMILAR | 1 MCG | SC, IV | Q5101 |
| FINASTERIDE | 5 MG | ORAL | S0138 |
| FIRAZYR | 1 MG | SC | J1744 |
| FIRMAGON | 1 MG | SC | J9155 |
| FLAGYL | 500 MG | IV | S0030 |
| FLEBOGAMMA | 500 MG | IV | J1572 |
| FLEXHD | SQ CM | OTH | Q4128 |
| FLEXON | 60 MG | IV, IM | J2360 |
| FLOLAN | 0.5 MG | IV | J1325 |
| FLORBETABEN F18 | PER STUDY DOSE | IV | C9458 |
| FLORBETABEN F18, DIAGNOSTIC | STUDY DOSE UP TO 8.1 MCI | IV | Q9983 |
| FLOWABLE WOUND MATRIX | 0.5 CC | OTH | Q4162 |
| FLOXIN IV | 400 MG | IV | S0034 |
| FLOXURIDINE | 500 MG | IV | J9200 |
| FLUCICLOVINE F-18, DIAGNOSTIC | 1 MCI | IV | A9588 |
| FLUCONAZOLE | 200 MG | IV | J1450 |
| FLUDARA | 50 MG | IV | J9185 |
| FLUDARABINE PHOSPHATE | 50 MG | IV | J9185 |
| FLUDARABINE PHOSPHATE | 10 MG | ORAL | J8562 |
| FLUDEOXYGLUCOSE F18 | STUDY DOSE UP TO 45 MCI | IV | A9552 |
| FLULAVAL | EA | IM | Q2036 |
| FLUMADINE (DEMONSTATION PROJECT) | 100 MG | ORAL | G9036 |
| FLUNISOLIDE, COMPOUNDED, UNIT DOSE | 1 MG | INH | J7641 |
| FLUOCINOLONE ACETONIDE INTRAVITREAL IMPLANT | IMPLANT | OTH | J7311 |
| FLUOCINOLONE ACETONIDE, INTRAVITREAL IMPLANT | 0.01 MG | OTH | J7313 |
| FLUORODEOXYGLUCOSE F-18 FDG, DIAGNOSTIC | STUDY DOSE UP TO 45 MCI | IV | A9552 |
| FLUOROURACIL | 500 MG | IV | J9190 |
| FLUPHENAZINE DECANOATE | 25 MG | SC, IM | J2680 |
| FLUTAMIDE | 125 MG | ORAL | S0175 |
| FLUTEMETAMOL F18 | PER STUDY DOSE | IV | C9459 |
| FLUTEMETAMOL F18, DIAGNOSTIC | STUDY DOSE UP TO 5 MCI | IV | Q9982 |
| FLUVIRIN | EA | IM | Q2037 |
| FLUZONE | EA | IM | Q2038 |
| FOLEX | 50 MG | IV, IM, IT, IA | J9260 |
| FOLEX | 5 MG | IV, IM, IT, IA | J9250 |

© 2016 Optum360, LLC

| Drug Name | Unit Per | Route | Code |
|---|---|---|---|
| FOLEX PFS | 50 MG | IV, IM, IT, IA | J9260 |
| FOLEX PFS | 5 MG | IV, IM, IT, IA | J9250 |
| FOLLISTIM | 75 IU | SC, IM | S0128 |
| FOLLITROPIN ALFA | 75 IU | SC | S0126 |
| FOLLITROPIN BETA | 75 IU | SC, IM | S0128 |
| FOLOTYN | 1 MG | IV | J9307 |
| FOMEPIZOLE | 15 MG | IV | J1451 |
| FOMIVIRSEN SODIUM | 1.65 MG | OTH | J1452 |
| FONDAPARINUX SODIUM | 0.5 MG | SC | J1652 |
| FORMOTEROL FUMERATE NONCOMPOUNDED UNIT DOSE FORM | 20 MCG | INH | J7606 |
| FORMOTEROL, COMPOUNDED, UNIT DOSE | 12 MCG | INH | J7640 |
| FORTAZ | 500 MG | IM, IV | J0713 |
| FORTEO | 10 MCG | SC | J3110 |
| FORTOVASE | 200 MG | ORAL | S0140 |
| FOSAPREPITANT | 1 MG | IV | J1453 |
| FOSCARNET SODIUM | 1,000 MG | IV | J1455 |
| FOSCAVIR | 1,000 MG | IV | J1455 |
| FOSPHENYTOIN | 50 MG | IM, IV | Q2009 |
| FOSPHENYTOIN SODIUM | 750 MG | IM, IV | S0078 |
| FRAGMIN | 2,500 IU | SC | J1645 |
| FUDR | 500 MG | IV | J9200 |
| FULVESTRANT | 25 MG | IM | J9395 |
| FUNGIZONE | 50 MG | IV | J0285 |
| FUROSEMIDE | 20 MG | IM, IV | J1940 |
| FUSILEV | 0.5 MG | IV | J0641 |
| FUZEON | 1 MG | SC | J1324 |
| GABLOFEN | 50 MCG | IT | J0476 |
| GABLOFEN | 10 MG | IT | J0475 |
| GADAVIST | 0.1 ML | IV | A9585 |
| GADOBENATE DIMEGLUMINE (MULTIHANCE MULTIPACK) | 1 ML | IV | A9577 |
| GADOBUTROL | 0.1 ML | IV | A9585 |
| GADOFOSVESET TRISODIUM | 1 ML | IV | A9583 |
| GADOLINIUM -BASED CONTRAST NOS | 1 ML | IV | A9579 |
| GADOTERATE MEGLUMINE | 0.1 ML | IV | A9575 |
| GADOTERIDOL (PROHANCE MULTIPACK) | 1 ML | IV | A9576 |
| GADOXETATE DISODIUM | 1 ML | IV | A9581 |
| GALLIUM GA-67 | 1 MCI | IV | A9556 |
| GALLIUM GA-68, DOTATATE, DIAGNOSTIC | 0.1 MCI | IV | A9587 |
| GALLIUM NITRATE | 1 MG | IV | J1457 |
| GALSULFASE | 1 MG | IV | J1458 |
| GAMASTAN | 1 CC | IM | J1460 |
| GAMASTAN | OVER 10 CC | IM | J1560 |
| GAMASTAN SD | OVER 10 CC | IM | J1560 |
| GAMASTAN SD | 1 CC | IM | J1460 |
| GAMMA GLOBULIN | OVER 10 CC | IM | J1560 |
| GAMMA GLOBULIN | 1 CC | IM | J1460 |
| GAMMAGARD | 500 MG | IV | J1569 |

| Drug Name | Unit Per | Route | Code |
|---|---|---|---|
| GAMMAGRAFT | SQ CM | OTH | Q4111 |
| GAMMAKED | 500 MG | IV, SC | J1561 |
| GAMMAPLEX | 500 MG | IV | J1557 |
| GAMUNEX | 500 MG | IV, SQ | J1561 |
| GAMUNEX-C | 500 MG | IV, SC | J1561 |
| GANCICLOVIR | 4.5 MG | OTH | J7310 |
| GANCICLOVIR SODIUM | 500 MG | IV | J1570 |
| GANIRELIX ACETATE | 250 MCG | SC | S0132 |
| GANITE | 1 MG | IV | J1457 |
| GARAMYCIN | 80 MG | IM, IV | J1580 |
| GASTROCROM | 10 MG | INH | J7631 |
| GASTROMARK | 1 ML | ORAL | Q9954 |
| GATIFLOXACIN | 10 MG | IV | J1590 |
| GAZYVA | 10 MG | IV | J9301 |
| GEFITINIB | 250 MG | ORAL | J8565 |
| GEL-ONE | DOSE | OTH | J7326 |
| GEL-SYN | 0.1 MG | INJ | J7328 |
| GEMCITABINE HCL | 200 MG | IV | J9201 |
| GEMTUZUMAB OZOGAMICIN | 5 MG | IV | J9300 |
| GEMZAR | 200 MG | IV | J9201 |
| GENGRAF | 100 MG | ORAL | J7502 |
| GENGRAF | 25 MG | ORAL | J7515 |
| GENOTROPIN | 1 MG | SC | J2941 |
| GENOTROPIN MINIQUICK | 1 MG | SC | J2941 |
| GENOTROPIN NUTROPIN | 1 MG | SC | J2941 |
| GENTAMICIN | 80 MG | IM, IV | J1580 |
| GENTRAN | 500 ML | IV | J7100 |
| GENTRAN 75 | 500 ML | IV | J7110 |
| GENVISC | 1 MG | INJ | Q9980 |
| GENVISC 850 | 1 MG | OTH | J7320 |
| GEODON | 10 MG | IM | J3486 |
| GEREF | 1MCG | SC | Q0515 |
| GLASSIA | 10 MG | IV | J0257 |
| GLATIRAMER ACETATE | 20 MG | SC | J1595 |
| GLEEVEC | 100 MG | ORAL | S0088 |
| GLOFIL-125 | STUDY DOSE UP TO 10 UCI | IV | A9554 |
| GLUCAGEN | 1 MG | SC, IM, IV | J1610 |
| GLUCAGON | 1 MG | SC, IM, IV | J1610 |
| GLUCOTOPE | STUDY DOSE UP TO 45 MCI | IV | A9552 |
| GLYCOPYRROLATE, COMPOUNDED CONCENTRATED | PER MG | INH | J7642 |
| GLYCOPYRROLATE, COMPOUNDED, UNIT DOSE | 1 MG | INH | J7643 |
| GOLD SODIUM THIOMALATE | 50 MG | IM | J1600 |
| GOLIMUMAB | 1 MG | IV | J1602 |
| GONADORELIN HCL | 100 MCG | SC, IV | J1620 |
| GONAL-F | 75 IU | SC | S0126 |
| GOSERELIN ACETATE | 3.6 MG | SC | J9202 |
| GRAFIX CORE | SQ CM | OTH | Q4132 |
| GRAFIX PRIME | SQ CM | OTH | Q4133 |

*Appendix 1 — Table of Drugs and Biologicals*

| Drug Name | Unit Per | Route | Code |
|---|---|---|---|
| GRAFTJACKET | SQ CM | OTH | Q4107 |
| GRAFTJACKET EXPRESS | 1 CC | INJ | Q4113 |
| GRANISETRON HCL | 100 MCG | IV | J1626 |
| GRANISETRON HCL | 1 MG | IV | S0091 |
| GRANISETRON HCL | 1 MG | ORAL | Q0166 |
| GRANIX | 1 MCG | IV | J1447 |
| GUARDIAN | SQ CM | OTH | Q4151 |
| GYNOGEN L.A. 10 | 10 MG | IM | J1380 |
| GYNOGEN L.A. 20 | 10 MG | IM | J1380 |
| GYNOGEN L.A. 40 | 10 MG | IM | J1380 |
| H.P. ACTHAR GEL | UP TO 40 UNITS | OTH | J0800 |
| HALAVEN | 0.1 MG | IV | J9179 |
| HALDOL | 5 MG | IM, IV | J1630 |
| HALDOL DECANOATE | 50 MG | IM | J1631 |
| HALOPERIDOL | 5 MG | IM, IV | J1630 |
| HECTOROL | 1 MG | IV | J1270 |
| HELICOLL | SQ CM | OTH | Q4164 |
| HELIXATE FS | 1 IU | IV | J7192 |
| HEMIN | 1 MG | IV | J1640 |
| HEMOFIL | 1 IU | IV | J7192 |
| HEMOFIL-M | 1 IU | IV | J7190 |
| HEMOPHILIA CLOTTING FACTOR, NOC | VAR | INJ | J7199 |
| HEP LOCK | 10 U | IV | J1642 |
| HEP-PAK | 10 UNITS | IV | J1642 |
| HEPAGAM B | 0.5 ML | IV | J1573 |
| HEPAGAM B | 0.5 ML | IM | J1571 |
| HEPARIN SODIUM | 1,000 U | IV, SC | J1644 |
| HEPARIN SODIUM | 10 U | IV | J1642 |
| HEPATITIS B IMMUNE GLOBULIN | 0.5 ML | IV | J1573 |
| HEPATOLITE | STUDY DOSE UP TO 15 MCI | IV | A9510 |
| HERCEPTIN | 10 MG | IV | J9355 |
| HEXADROL | 0.25 MG | ORAL | J8540 |
| HEXAMINOLEVULINATE | STUDY DOSE | OTH | C9275 |
| HIGH OSMOLAR CONTRAST MATERIAL, UP TO 149 MG/ML IODINE CONCENTRATION | 1 ML | IV | Q9958 |
| HIGH OSMOLAR CONTRAST MATERIAL, UP TO 150-199 MG/ML IODINE CONCENTRATION | 1 ML | IV | Q9959 |
| HIGH OSMOLAR CONTRAST MATERIAL, UP TO 200-249 MG/ML IODINE CONCENTRATION | 1 ML | IV | Q9960 |
| HIGH OSMOLAR CONTRAST MATERIAL, UP TO 250-299 MG/ML IODINE CONCENTRATION | 1 ML | IV | Q9961 |
| HIGH OSMOLAR CONTRAST MATERIAL, UP TO 300-349 MG/ML IODINE CONCENTRATION | 1 ML | IV | Q9962 |
| HIGH OSMOLAR CONTRAST MATERIAL, UP TO 350-399 MG/ML IODINE CONCENTRATION | 1 ML | IV | Q9963 |
| HIGH OSMOLAR CONTRAST MATERIAL, UP TO 400 OR GREATER MG/ML IODINE CONCENTRATION | 1 ML | IV | Q9964 |
| HISTERLIN IMPLANT (VANTAS) | 50 MG | OTH | J9225 |
| HISTRELIN ACETATE | 10 MG | INJ | J1675 |
| HISTRELIN IMPLANT (SUPPRELIN LA) | 50 MG | OTH | J9226 |
| HIZENTRA | 100 MG | SC | J1559 |
| HMATRIX | PER SQ CM | OTH | Q4134 |
| HUMALOG | 5 U | SC | J1815 |
| HUMALOG | 50 U | SC | J1817 |
| HUMAN AMNIOTIC TISSUE ALLOGRAFT | SQ CM | OTH | Q4163 |
| HUMAN FIGRINOGEN CONCENTRATE | 1 MG | IV | J7178 |
| HUMATE-P | 1 IU | IV | J7187 |
| HUMATROPE | 1 MG | SC | J2941 |
| HUMIRA | 20 MG | SC | J0135 |
| HUMULIN | 50 U | SC | J1817 |
| HUMULIN | 5 U | SC | J1815 |
| HUMULIN R | 5 U | SC | J1815 |
| HUMULIN R U-500 | 5 U | SC | J1815 |
| HYALGAN | DOSE | OTH | J7321 |
| HYALOMATRIX | SQ CM | OTH | Q4117 |
| HYALURONAN OR DERITIVE, GEL-ONE | DOSE | OTH | J7326 |
| HYALURONAN OR DERIVATIVE, FOR INTRA-ARTICULAR INJECTION | 0.1 MG | INJ | J7328 |
| ~~HYALURONAN OR DERIVATIVE, FOR INTRA-ARTICULAR INJECTION~~ | ~~1 MG~~ | ~~INJ~~ | ~~Q9980~~ |
| ~~HYALURONAN OR DERIVATIVE, HYMOVIS, FOR INTRA-ARTICULAR INJECTION~~ | ~~MG~~ | ~~INJ~~ | ~~C9471~~ |
| HYALURONAN OR DERIVATIVE, MONOVISC | DOSE | OTH | J7327 |
| HYALURONAN OR DERIVITIVE FOR INTRA-ARTICULAR INJECTION | 1 MG | OTH | J7322 |
| HYALURONAN OR DERIVITIVE FOR INTRA-ARTICULAR INJECTION | 1 MG | OTH | J7320 |
| HYALURONAN, EUFLEXXA | DOSE | OTH | J7323 |
| HYALURONAN, HYALGAN OR SUPARTZ | DOSE | OTH | J7321 |
| HYALURONAN, ORTHOVISC | DOSE | OTH | J7324 |
| HYALURONAN, SYNVISC/SYNVISC-ONE | 1 MG | OTH | J7325 |
| HYALURONIDASE | 150 UNITS | VAR | J3470 |
| HYALURONIDASE RECOMBINANT | 1 USP UNIT | SC | J3473 |
| HYALURONIDASE, OVINE, PRESERVATIVE FREE | 1000 USP | OTH | J3472 |
| HYALURONIDASE, OVINE, PRESERVATIVE FREE | 1 USP | OTH | J3471 |

 © 2016 Optum360, LLC

| Drug Name | Unit Per | Route | Code |
|---|---|---|---|
| HYCAMTIN | 0.25 MG | ORAL | J8705 |
| HYCAMTIN | 0.1 MG | IV | J9351 |
| HYDRALAZINE HCL | 20 MG | IV, IM | J0360 |
| HYDRATE | 50 MG | IM, IV | J1240 |
| HYDREA | 500 MG | ORAL | S0176 |
| HYDROCORTISONE ACETATE | 25 MG | IV, IM, SC | J1700 |
| HYDROCORTISONE SODIUM PHOSPHATE | 50 MG | IV, IM, SC | J1710 |
| HYDROCORTISONE SODIUM SUCCINATE | 100 MG | IV, IM, SC | J1720 |
| HYDROCORTONE PHOSPHATE | 50 MG | SC, IM, IV | J1710 |
| HYDROMORPHONE HCL | 250 MG | OTH | S0092 |
| HYDROMORPHONE HCL | 4 MG | SC, IM, IV | J1170 |
| HYDROXOCOBALAMIN | 1,000 MCG | IM, SC | J3420 |
| HYDROXYCOBAL | 1,000 MCG | IM, SC | J3420 |
| HYDROXYPROGESTERONE CAPROATE | 1 MG | IM | J1725 |
| HYDROXYUREA | 500 MG | ORAL | S0176 |
| HYDROXYZINE HCL | 25 MG | IM | J3410 |
| HYDROXYZINE PAMOATE | 25 MG | ORAL | Q0177 |
| HYMOVIS | 1 MG | OTH | J7322 |
| HYMOVIS | MG | INJ | C9471 |
| HYOSCYAMINE SULFATE | 0.25 MG | SC, IM, IV | J1980 |
| HYPERRHO S/D | 300 MCG | IV | J2790 |
| HYPERTET SD | UP TO 250 MG | IM | J1670 |
| HYPERTONIC SALINE SOLUTION | 1 ML | VAR | J7131 |
| HYQVIA | 100 MG | IV | J1575 |
| HYREXIN | 50 MG | IV, IM | J1200 |
| HYZINE | 25 MG | IM | J3410 |
| HYZINE-50 | 25 MG | IM | J3410 |
| I-131 TOSITUMOMAB DIAGNOSTIC | STUDY DOSE | IV | A9544 |
| I-131 TOSITUMOMAB THERAPEUTIC | TX DOSE | IV | A9545 |
| IBANDRONATE SODIUM | 1 MG | IV | J1740 |
| IBRITUMOMAB TUXETAN | STUDY DOSE UP TO 5 MCI | IV | A9542 |
| IBUPROFEN | 100 MG | IV | J1741 |
| IBUTILIDE FUMARATE | 1 MG | IV | J1742 |
| ICATIBANT | 1 MG | SC | J1744 |
| IDAMYCIN | 5 MG | IV | J9211 |
| IDAMYCIN PFS | 5 MG | IV | J9211 |
| IDARUBICIN HCL | 5 MG | IV | J9211 |
| IDELVION | 1 IU | IV | C9139 |
| IDELVION | 1 IU | IV | J7202 |
| IDURSULFASE | 1 MG | IV | J1743 |
| IFEX | 1 G | IV | J9208 |
| IFOSFAMIDE | 1 G | IV | J9208 |
| IL-2 | 1 VIAL | IV | J9015 |
| ILARIS | 1 MG | SC | J0638 |
| ILETIN | 5 UNITS | SC | J1815 |
| ILETIN II NPH PORK | 50 U | SC | J1817 |
| ILETIN II REGULAR PORK | 5 U | SC | J1815 |

| Drug Name | Unit Per | Route | Code |
|---|---|---|---|
| ILOPROST INHALATION SOLUTION | PER DOSE UP TO 20 MCG | INH | Q4074 |
| ILUVIEN | 0.01 MG | OTH | J7313 |
| IMAGENT | 1 ML | IV | Q9955 |
| IMATINIB | 100 MG | ORAL | S0088 |
| IMIGLUCERASE | 10 U | IV | J1786 |
| IMITREX | 6 MG | SC | J3030 |
| IMLYGIC | 1 MILLION | INTRALESIONAL | J9325 |
| IMLYGIC | PFU | INJ | C9472 |
| IMMUNE GLOBULIN (BIVIGAM) | 500 MG | IV | J1556 |
| IMMUNE GLOBULIN (FLEBOGAMMA, FLEBOGAMMA DIF) | 500 MG | IV | J1572 |
| IMMUNE GLOBULIN (GAMMAGARD LIQUID) | 500 MG | IV | J1569 |
| IMMUNE GLOBULIN (GAMMAPLEX) | 500 MG | IV | J1557 |
| IMMUNE GLOBULIN (GAMUNEX) | 500 MG | IV | J1561 |
| IMMUNE GLOBULIN (HIZENTRA) | 100 MG | SC | J1559 |
| IMMUNE GLOBULIN (OCTAGAM) | 500 MG | IV | J1568 |
| IMMUNE GLOBULIN (PRIVIGEN) NONLYOPHILIZED | 500 MG | IV | J1459 |
| IMMUNE GLOBULIN (RHOPHYLAC) | 100 IU | IM, IV | J2791 |
| IMMUNE GLOBULIN LYOPHILIZED | 500 MG | IV | J1566 |
| IMMUNE GLOBULIN SUBCUTANEOUS | 100 MG | SC | J1562 |
| IMMUNE GLOBULIN, NONLYOPHILIZED (NOS) | 500 MG | IV | J1599 |
| IMMUNE GLOBULIN/HYALURONIDASE | 100 MG | IV | J1575 |
| IMPLANON | IMPLANT | OTH | J7307 |
| IMURAN | 50 MG | ORAL | J7500 |
| IN-111 SATUMOMAB PENDETIDE | STUDY DOSE UP TO MCI | IV | A4642 |
| INAPSINE | 5 MG | IM, IV | J1790 |
| INCOBUTULINUMTOXINA | 1 UNIT | IM | J0588 |
| INDERAL | 1 MG | IV | J1800 |
| INDIUM IN-111 IBRITUMOMAB TIUXETAN, DIAGNOSTIC | STUDY DOSE UP TO 5 MCI | IV | A9542 |
| INDIUM IN-111 LABELED AUTOLOGOUS PLATELETS | STUDY DOSAGE | IV | A9571 |
| INDIUM IN-111 LABELED AUTOLOGOUS WHITE BLOOD CELLS | STUDY DOSE | IV | A9570 |
| INDIUM IN-111 OXYQUINOLINE | 0.5 MCI | IV | A9547 |
| INDIUM IN-111 PENTETREOTIDE | STUDY DOSE UP TO 6 MCI | IV | A9572 |
| INDURSALFASE | 1 MG | IV | J1743 |
| INFED | 50 MG | IM, IV | J1750 |
| INFERGEN | 1 MCG | SC | J9212 |
| INFLECTRA | 10 MG | IV | Q5102 |
| INFLIXIMAB | 10 MG | IV | J1745 |
| INFLIXIMAB, BIOSIMILAR | 10 MG | IV | Q5102 |

| Drug Name | Unit Per | Route | Code | Drug Name | Unit Per | Route | Code |
|---|---|---|---|---|---|---|---|
| INFLUENZA VACCINE, AGRIFLU | UNKNOWN | IM | Q2034 | INTRON A | 1,000,000 U | SC, IM | J9214 |
| INFLUENZA VIRUS VACCINE (AFLURIA) | EA | IM | Q2035 | INVANZ | 500 MG | IM, IV | J1335 |
| INFLUENZA VIRUS VACCINE (FLULAVAL) | EA | IM | Q2036 | INVEGA SUSTENNA | 1 MG | IM | J2426 |
| | | | | INVIRASE | 200 MG | ORAL | S0140 |
| INFLUENZA VIRUS VACCINE (FLUVIRIN) | EA | IM | Q2037 | IOBENGUANE SULFATE I-131 | 0.5 MCI | IV | A9508 |
| INFLUENZA VIRUS VACCINE (FLUZONE) | EA | IM | Q2038 | IOBENGUANE, I-123, DIAGNOSTIC | PER STUDY DOSE UP TO 15 MCI | IV | A9582 |
| INFLUENZA VIRUS VACCINE, NOT OTHERWISE SPECIFIED | EA | IM | Q2039 | IODINE I-123 IOBENGUANE, DIAGNOSTIC | 15 MCI | IV | A9582 |
| INFUMORPH | 10 MG | IM, IV, SC | J2270 | IODINE I-123 IOFLUPANE | STUDY DOSE UP TO 5 MCI | IV | A9584 |
| INJECTAFER | 1 MG | IV | J1439 | IODINE I-123 SODIUM IODIDE CAPSULE(S), DIAGNOSTIC | 100-9999 UCI | ORAL | A9516 |
| INNOHEP | 1,000 IU | SC | J1655 | IODINE I-123 SODIUM IODIDE, DIAGNOSTIC | 1 MCI | IV | A9509 |
| INSULIN | 50 U | SC | J1817 | IODINE I-125 SERUM ALBUMIN, DIAGNOSTIC | 5 UCI | IV | A9532 |
| INSULIN | 5 U | SC | J1815 | IODINE I-125 SODIUM IOTHALAMATE, DIAGNOSTIC | STUDY DOSE UP TO 10 UCI | IV | A9554 |
| INSULIN LISPRO | 5 U | SC | S5551 | IODINE I-125, SODIUM IODIDE SOLUTION, THERAPEUTIC | 1 MCI | ORAL | A9527 |
| INSULIN LISPRO | 5 U | SC | J1815 | IODINE I-131 IOBENGUANE SULFATE, DIAGNOSTIC | 0.5 MCI | IV | A9508 |
| INSULIN PURIFIED REGULAR PORK | 5 U | SC | J1815 | IODINE I-131 IODINATED SERUM ALBUMIN, DIAGNOSTIC | PER 5 UCI | IV | A9524 |
| INTAL | 10 MG | INH | J7631 | IODINE I-131 SODIUM IODIDE CAPSULE(S), DIAGNOSTIC | 1 MCI | ORAL | A9528 |
| INTEGRA BILAYER MATRIX DRESSING | SQ CM | OTH | Q4104 | IODINE I-131 SODIUM IODIDE CAPSULE(S), THERAPEUTIC | 1 MCI | ORAL | A9517 |
| INTEGRA DERMAL REGENERATION TEMPLATE | SQ CM | OTH | Q4105 | IODINE I-131 SODIUM IODIDE SOLUTION, DIAGNOSTIC | 1 MCI | ORAL | A9529 |
| INTEGRA FLOWABLE WOUND MATRIX | 1 CC | INJ | Q4114 | IODINE I-131 SODIUM IODIDE SOLUTION, THERAPEUTIC | 1 MCI | ORAL | A9530 |
| INTEGRA MATRIX | SQ CM | OTH | Q4108 | ~~IODINE I-131 SODIUM IODIDE, DIAGNOSTIC~~ | ~~PER UCI UP TO 100 UCI~~ | ~~IV~~ | ~~A9531~~ |
| INTEGRA MOZAIK OSTEOCONDUCTIVE SCAFFOLD PUTTY | 0.5 CC | OTH | C9359 | ~~IODINE I-131 TOSITUMOMAB, DIAGNOSTIC~~ | ~~STUDY DOSE~~ | ~~IV~~ | ~~A9544~~ |
| INTEGRA MOZAIK OSTEOCONDUCTIVE SCAFFOLD STRIP | 0.5 CC | OTH | C9362 | ~~IODINE I-131 TOSITUMOMAB, THERAPEUTIC~~ | ~~TX DOSE~~ | ~~IV~~ | ~~A9545~~ |
| INTEGRA OMNIGRAFT DERMAL REGENERATION MATRIX | SQ CM | OTH | Q4105 | IODOTOPE THERAPEUTIC CAPSULE(S) | 1 MCI | ORAL | A9517 |
| INTEGRA OS OSTEOCONDUCTIVE SCAFFOLD PUTTY | 0.5 CC | OTH | C9359 | IODOTOPE THERAPEUTIC SOLUTION | 1 MCI | ORAL | A9530 |
| INTEGRILIN | 5 MG | IM, IV | J1327 | IOFLUPANE | STUDY DOSE UP TO 5 MCI | IV | A9584 |
| INTERFERON ALFA-2A | 3,000,000 U | SC, IM | J9213 | | | | |
| INTERFERON ALFA-2B | 1,000,000 U | SC, IM | J9214 | ION-BASED MAGNETIC RESONANCE CONTRAST AGENT | 1 ML | IV | Q9953 |
| INTERFERON ALFA-N3 | 250,000 IU | IM | J9215 | IOTHALAMATE SODIUM I-125 | STUDY DOSE UP TO 10 UCI | IV | A9554 |
| INTERFERON ALFACON-1 | 1 MCG | SC | J9212 | | | | |
| INTERFERON BETA-1A | 1 MCG | IM | Q3027 | IPILIMUMAB | 1 MG | IV | J9228 |
| INTERFERON BETA-1A | 1 MCG | SC | Q3028 | IPLEX | 1 MG | SC | J2170 |
| INTERFERON BETA-1A | 30 MCG | IM, SC | J1826 | IPRATROPIUM BROMIDE, NONCOMPOUNDED, UNIT DOSE | 1 MG | INH | J7644 |
| INTERFERON BETA-1B | 0.25 MG | SC | J1830 | IPTRATROPIUM BROMIDE COMPOUNDED, UNIT DOSE | 1 MG | INH | J7645 |
| INTERFERON, ALFA-2A, RECOMBINANT | 3,000,000 U | SC, IM | J9213 | IRESSA | 250 MG | ORAL | J8565 |
| INTERFERON, ALFA-2B, RECOMBINANT | 1,000,000 U | SC, IM | J9214 | IRINOTECAN | 20 MG | IV | J9206 |
| INTERFERON, ALFA-N3, (HUMAN LEUKOCYTE DERIVED) | 250,000 IU | IM | J9215 | | | | |
| INTERFERON, GAMMA 1-B | 3,000,000 U | SC | J9216 | | | | |
| INTERFYL | 1 MG | OTH | Q4171 | | | | |
| INTERLUEKIN | 1 VIAL | IV | J9015 | | | | |

                                                      © 2016 Optum360, LLC

| Drug Name | Unit Per | Route | Code |
|---|---|---|---|
| IRINOTECAN LIPOSOME | 1 MG | IV | J9205 |
| IRINOTECAN LIPOSOME | ~~MG~~ | ~~IV~~ | C9474 |
| IRON DEXTRAN, 50 MG | 50 MG | IM, IV | J1750 |
| IRON SUCROSE | 1 MG | IV | J1756 |
| ISAVUCONAZONIUM | 1 MG | IV | J1833 |
| ISOCAINE | 10 ML | VAR | J0670 |
| ISOETHARINE HCL COMPOUNDED, CONCENTRATED | 1 MG | INH | J7647 |
| ISOETHARINE HCL COMPOUNDED, UNIT DOSE | 1 MG | INH | J7650 |
| ISOETHARINE HCL, NONCOMPOUNDED CONCENTRATED | PER MG | INH | J7648 |
| ISOETHARINE HCL, NONCOMPOUNDED, UNIT DOSE | 1 MG | INH | J7649 |
| ISOJEX | 5 UCI | IV | A9532 |
| ISOPROTERENOL HCL COMPOUNDED, CONCENTRATED | 1 MG | INH | J7657 |
| ISOPROTERENOL HCL COMPOUNDED, UNIT DOSE | 1 MG | INH | J7660 |
| ISOPROTERENOL HCL, NONCOMPOUNDED CONCENTRATED | 1 MG | INH | J7658 |
| ISOPROTERNOL HCL, NONCOMPOUNDED, UNIT DOSE | 1MG | INH | J7659 |
| ISOSULFAN BLUE | 1 MG | SC | Q9968 |
| ISTODAX | 1 MG | IV | J9315 |
| ISUPREL | 1 MG | INH | J7658 |
| ISUPREL | 1 MG | INH | J7659 |
| ITRACONAZOLE | 50 MG | IV | J1835 |
| IVEEGAM | 500 MG | IV | J1566 |
| IXABEPILONE | 1 MG | IV | J9207 |
| IXEMPRA | 1 MG | IV | J9207 |
| JETREA | 0.125 MG | OTH | J7316 |
| JEVTANA | 1 MG | IV | J9043 |
| KADCYLA | 1 MG | IV | J9354 |
| KALBITOR | 1 MG | SC | J1290 |
| KANAMYCIN | 75 MG | IM, IV | J1850 |
| KANAMYCIN | 500 MG | IM, IV | J1840 |
| KANTREX | 75 MG | IM, IV | J1850 |
| KANTREX | 500 MG | IM, IV | J1840 |
| KANUMA | ~~1 MG~~ | ~~IV~~ | C9478 |
| KANUMA | 1 MG | IV | J2840 |
| KCENTRA | PER I.U. | IV | C9132 |
| KEFZOL | 500 MG | IM, IV | J0690 |
| KENAJECT-40 | 10 MG | IM | J3301 |
| KENALOG-10 | 10 MG | IM | J3301 |
| KEPIVANCE | 50 MCG | IV | J2425 |
| KEPPRA | 10 MG | IV | J1953 |
| KERAMATRIX | SQ CM | OTH | Q4165 |
| KESTRONE | 1 MG | IV, IM | J1435 |
| KETOROLAC TROMETHAMINE | 15 MG | IM, IV | J1885 |
| KEYTRUDA | 1 MG | IV | J9271 |
| KINEVAC | 5 MCG | IV | J2805 |

| Drug Name | Unit Per | Route | Code |
|---|---|---|---|
| KOATE-DVI | 1 IU | IV | J7190 |
| KOGENATE FS | 1 IU | IV | J7192 |
| KONAKION | 1 MG | SC, IM, IV | J3430 |
| KONYNE 80 | 1 IU | IV | J7194 |
| KRYSTEXXA | 1 MG | IV | J2507 |
| KYPROLIS | 1 MG | IV | J9047 |
| KYTRIL | 100 MCG | IV | J1626 |
| KYTRIL | 1 MG | IV | S0091 |
| KYTRIL | 1 MG | ORAL | Q0166 |
| L-PHENYLALANINE MUSTARD | 50 MG | IV | J9245 |
| L.A.E. 20 | 10 MG | IM | J1380 |
| LACOSAMIDE | 1 MG | IV | C9254 |
| LAETRILE | VAR | INJ | J3570 |
| LANOXIN | 0.5 MG | IM, IV | J1160 |
| LANREOTIDE | 1 MG | SC | J1930 |
| LANTUS | 5 U | SC | J1815 |
| LARONIDASE | 0.1 MG | IV | J1931 |
| LASIX | 20 MG | IM, IV | J1940 |
| LEMTRADA | 1 MG | IV | J0202 |
| LENTE ILETIN I | 5 U | SC | J1815 |
| LEPIRUDIN | 50 MG | IV | J1945 |
| LEUCOVORIN CALCIUM | 50 MG | IM, IV | J0640 |
| LEUKERAN | 2 MG | ORAL | S0172 |
| LEUKINE | 50 MCG | IV | J2820 |
| LEUPROLIDE ACETATE | 1 MG | IM | J9218 |
| LEUPROLIDE ACETATE | 7.5, 22.5, 30, 45 MG | SC | J9217 |
| LEUPROLIDE ACETATE (FOR DEPOT SUSPENSION) | 3.75 MG | IM | J1950 |
| LEUPROLIDE ACETATE DEPOT | 7.5, 22.5, 30, 45 MG | SC | J9217 |
| LEUPROLIDE ACETATE IMPLANT | 65 MG | OTH | J9219 |
| LEUSTATIN | 1 MG | IV | J9065 |
| LEVABUTEROL COMPOUNDED, UNIT DOSE | 1 MG | INH | J7615 |
| LEVABUTEROL, COMPOUNDED, CONCENTRATED | 0.5 MG | INH | J7607 |
| LEVALBUTEROL NONCOMPOUNDED, CONCENTRATED FORM | 0.5 MG | INH | J7612 |
| LEVALBUTEROL, NONCOMPOUNDED, UNIT DOSE | 0.5 MG | INH | J7614 |
| LEVAMISOLE HCL | 50 MG | ORAL | S0177 |
| LEVAQUIN | 250 MG | IV | J1956 |
| LEVEMIR | 5 U | SC | J1815 |
| LEVETIRACETAM | 10 MG | IV | J1953 |
| LEVO-DROMORAN | UP TO 2 MG | IV, IM | J1960 |
| LEVOCARNITINE | 1 G | IV | J1955 |
| LEVOFLOXACIN | 250 MG | IV | J1956 |
| LEVOLEUCOVORIN CALCIUM | 0.5 MG | IV | J0641 |
| LEVONORGESTREL IMPLANT | IMPLANT | OTH | J7306 |
| LEVONORGESTREL-RELEASING INTRAUTERINE CONTRACEPTIVE (LILETTA) | 52 MG | OTH | J7298 |

© 2016 Optum360, LLC

| Drug Name | Unit Per | Route | Code |
|---|---|---|---|
| LEVONORGESTREL-RELEASING INTRAUTERINE CONTRACEPTIVE (MIRENA) | 52 MG | OTH | J7297 |
| LEVONORGESTREL-RELEASING INTRAUTERINE CONTRACEPTIVE SYSTEM (SKYLA) | 13.5 MG | OTH | J7301 |
| LEVORPHANOL TARTRATE | 2 MG | SC, IV, IM | J1960 |
| LEVSIN | 0.25 MG | SC, IM, IV | J1980 |
| LEVULAN KERASTICK | 354 MG | OTH | J7308 |
| LEXISCAN | 0.1 MG | IV | J2785 |
| LIBRIUM | 100 MG | IM, IV | J1990 |
| LIDOCAINE 70 MG/TETRACAINE 70 MG | PATCH | OTH | C9285 |
| LIDOCAINE HCL | 10 MG | IV | J2001 |
| LILETTA | 52 MG | OTH | J7297 |
| LINCOCIN HCL | 300 MG | IV | J2010 |
| LINCOMYCIN HCL | 300 MG | IM, IV | J2010 |
| LINEZOLID | 200 MG | IV | J2020 |
| LIORESAL | 10 MG | IT | J0475 |
| LIORESAL INTRATHECAL REFILL | 50 MCG | IT | J0476 |
| LIPODOX | 10 MG | IV | Q2049 |
| LIQUAEMIN SODIUM | 1,000 UNITS | SC, IV | J1644 |
| LISPRO-PFC | 50 U | SC | J1817 |
| LOK-PAK | 10 UNITS | IV | J1642 |
| LOMUSTINE | 10 MG | ORAL | S0178 |
| LORAZEPAM | 2 MG | IM, IV | J2060 |
| LOVENOX | 10 MG | SC | J1650 |
| LOW OSMOLAR CONTRAST MATERIAL, 100-199 MG/ML IODINE CONCENTRATIONS | 1 ML | IV | Q9965 |
| LOW OSMOLAR CONTRAST MATERIAL, 200-299 MG/ML IODINE CONCENTRATION | 1 ML | IV | Q9966 |
| LOW OSMOLAR CONTRAST MATERIAL, 300-399 MG/ML IODINE CONCENTRATION | 1 ML | IV | Q9967 |
| LOW OSMOLAR CONTRAST MATERIAL, 400 OR GREATER MG/ML IODINE CONCENTRATION | 1 ML | IV | Q9951 |
| LOXAPINE, INHALATION POWDER | 10 MG | OTH | C9497 |
| LUCENTIS | 0.1 MG | IV | J2778 |
| LUMASON | 1 ML | IV | Q9950 |
| LUMIZYME | 10 MG | IV | J0221 |
| LUPRON | 1 MG | SC | J9218 |
| LUPRON DEPOT | 7.5, 22.5, 30, 45 MG | SC | J9217 |
| LUPRON DEPOT | PER 3.75 MG | IM | J1950 |
| LUPRON IMPLANT | 65 MG | OTH | J9219 |
| LUTREPULSE | 100 MCG | SC, IV | J1620 |
| LYMPHAZURIN | 1 MG | SC | Q9968 |
| LYMPHOCYTE IMMUNE GLOBULIN, ANTITHYMOCYTE GLOBULIN, EQUINE | 250 MG | OTH | J7504 |
| LYMPHOCYTE IMMUNE GLOBULIN, ANTITHYMOCYTE GLOBULIN, RABBIT | 25 MG | OTH | J7511 |

| Drug Name | Unit Per | Route | Code |
|---|---|---|---|
| LYMPHOSEEK | 0.5 MCI | SC, OTH | A9520 |
| MACUGEN | 0.3 MG | OTH | J2503 |
| MAGNESIUM SULFATE | 500 MG | IV | J3475 |
| MAGNETIC RESONANCE CONTRAST AGENT | 1 ML | ORAL | Q9954 |
| MAGNEVIST | 1 ML | IV | A9579 |
| MAGROTEC | STUDY DOSE UP TO 10 MCI | IV | A9540 |
| MAKENA | 1 MG | IM | J1725 |
| MANNITOL | 25% IN 50 ML | IV | J2150 |
| MANNITOL | 5 MG | INH | J7665 |
| MARCAINE HCL | 30 ML | VAR | S0020 |
| MARIGEN | SQ CM | OTH | Q4158 |
| MARINOL | 2.5 MG | ORAL | Q0167 |
| MARMINE | 50 MG | IM, IV | J1240 |
| MARQIBO KIT | 5 MG | IV | J9371 |
| MATRISTEM BURN MATRIX | SQ CM | OTH | Q4120 |
| MATRISTEM MICROMATRIX | 1 MG | OTH | Q4118 |
| MATRISTEM WOUND MATRIX | SQ CM | OTH | Q4119 |
| MATULANE | 50 MG | ORAL | S0182 |
| MAXIPIME | 500 MG | IV | J0692 |
| MDP-BRACCO | STUDY DOSE UP TO 30 MCI | IV | A9503 |
| MECASERMIN | 1 MG | SC | J2170 |
| MECHLORETHAMINE HCL (NITROGEN MUSTARD) | 10 MG | IV | J9230 |
| MEDIDEX | 1 MG | IM, IV, OTH | J1100 |
| MEDISKIN | PER SQ CM | OTH | Q4135 |
| MEDROL | 4 MG | ORAL | J7509 |
| MEDROXYPROGESTERONE ACETATE | 1 MG | IM | J1050 |
| MEFOXIN | 1 G | IV | J0694 |
| MEGACE | 20 MG | ORAL | S0179 |
| MEGESTROL ACETATE | 20 MG | ORAL | S0179 |
| MELPHALAN HCL | 2 MG | ORAL | J8600 |
| MELPHALAN HCL | 50 MG | IV | J9245 |
| MEMETASONE SINUS IMPLANT | 370 MCG | OTH | S1090 |
| MEMODERM | SQ CM | OTH | Q4126 |
| MENADIONE | 1 MG | IM, SC, IV | J3430 |
| MENOTROPINS | 75 IU | SC, IM, IV | S0122 |
| MEPERGAN | 50 MG | IM, IV | J2180 |
| MEPERIDINE AND PROMETHAZINE HCL | 50 MG | IM, IV | J2180 |
| MEPERIDINE HCL | 100 MG | IM, IV, SC | J2175 |
| MEPIVACAINE HCL | 10 ML | VAR | J0670 |
| MEPOLIZUMAB | 100 MG | SQ | J2182 |
| MEPOLIZUMAB | MG | SQ | C9473 |
| MERCAPTOPURINE | 50 MG | ORAL | S0108 |
| MERITATE | 150 MG | IV | J3520 |
| MEROPENEM | 100 MG | IV | J2185 |
| MERREM | 100 MG | IV | J2185 |

© 2016 Optum360, LLC

| Drug Name | Unit Per | Route | Code |
|---|---|---|---|
| MESNA | 200 MG | IV | J9209 |
| MESNEX | 200 MG | IV | J9209 |
| METAPROTERENOL SULFATE COMPOUNDED, UNIT DOSE | 10 MG | INH | J7670 |
| METAPROTERENOL SULFATE, NONCOMPOUNDED, CONCENTRATED | 10 MG | INH | J7668 |
| METAPROTERENOL SULFATE, NONCOMPOUNDED, UNIT DOSE | 10 MG | INH | J7669 |
| METARAMINOL BITARTRATE | 10 MG | IV, IM, SC | J0380 |
| METASTRON STRONTIUM 89 CHLORIDE | 1 MCI | IV | A9600 |
| METATRACE | STUDY DOSE UP TO 45 MCI | IV | A9552 |
| METHACHOLINE CHLORIDE | 1 MG | INH | J7674 |
| METHADONE | 5 MG | ORAL | S0109 |
| METHADONE HCL | 10 MG | IM, SC | J1230 |
| METHAPREL, COMPOUNDED, UNIT DOSE | 10 MG | INH | J7670 |
| METHAPREL, NONCOMPOUNDED, CONCENTRATED | 10 MG | INH | J7668 |
| METHAPREL, NONCOMPOUNDED, UNIT DOSE | 10 MG | INH | J7669 |
| METHERGINE | 0.2 MG | IM, IV | J2210 |
| METHOTREXATE | 2.5 MG | ORAL | J8610 |
| METHOTREXATE | 50 MG | IV, IM, IT, IA | J9260 |
| METHOTREXATE | 5 MG | IV, IM, IT, IA | J9250 |
| METHOTREXATE LPF | 50 MG | IV, IM, IT, IA | J9260 |
| METHOTREXATE LPF | 5 MG | IV, IM, IT, IA | J9250 |
| METHYL AMINOLEVULINATE 16.8% | 1 G | OTH | J7309 |
| METHYLCOTOLONE | 80 MG | IM | J1040 |
| METHYLDOPA HCL | UP TO 250 MG | IV | J0210 |
| METHYLDOPATE HCL | UP TO 250 MG | IV | J0210 |
| METHYLENE BLUE | 1 MG | SC | Q9968 |
| METHYLERGONOVINE MALEATE | 0.2 MG | IM, IV | J2210 |
| METHYLNALTREXONE | 0.1 MG | SC | J2212 |
| METHYLPRED | 4 MG | ORAL | J7509 |
| METHYLPREDNISOLONE | 4 MG | ORAL | J7509 |
| METHYLPREDNISOLONE | UP TO 40 MG | IM, IV | J2920 |
| METHYLPREDNISOLONE | 125 MG | IM, IV | J2930 |
| METHYLPREDNISOLONE ACETATE | 40 MG | IM | J1030 |
| METHYLPREDNISOLONE ACETATE | 80 MG | IM | J1040 |
| METHYLPREDNISOLONE ACETATE | 20 MG | IM | J1020 |
| METOCLOPRAMIDE | 10 MG | IV | J2765 |
| METRONIDAZOLE | 500 MG | IV | S0030 |
| METVIXIA 16.8% | 1 G | OTH | J7309 |
| MIACALCIN | 400 U | SC, IM | J0630 |
| MIBG | 0.5 MCI | IV | A9508 |

| Drug Name | Unit Per | Route | Code |
|---|---|---|---|
| MICAFUNGIN SODIUM | 1 MG | IV | J2248 |
| MICRHOGAM | 50 MCG | IV | J2788 |
| MICROPOROUS COLLAGEN IMPLANTABLE SLIT TUBE | 1 CM LENGTH | OTH | C9353 |
| MICROPOROUS COLLAGEN IMPLANTABLE TUBE | 1 CM LENGTH | OTH | C9352 |
| MIDAZOLAM HCI | 1 MG | IM, IV | J2250 |
| MIFEPRISTONE | 200 MG | ORAL | S0190 |
| MILRINONE LACTATE | 5 MG | IV | J2260 |
| MINOCIN | 1 MG | IV | J2265 |
| MINOCYCLINE HCL | 1 MG | IV | J2265 |
| MINOXIDIL | 10 MG | ORAL | S0139 |
| MIRCERA | 1 MCG | IV | J0887 |
| MIRCERA | 1 MCG | SC | J0888 |
| MIRENA | 52 MG | OTH | J7298 |
| MIRODERM | SQ CM | OTH | Q4175 |
| MISOPROSTOL | 200 MG | ORAL | S0191 |
| MITHRACIN | 2.5 MG | IV | J9270 |
| MITOMYCIN | 0.2 MG | OTH | J7315 |
| MITOMYCIN | 5 MG | IV | J9280 |
| MITOSOL | 0.2 MG | OTH | J7315 |
| MITOXANA | 1 G | IV | J9208 |
| MITOXANTRONE HCL | 5 MG | IV | J9293 |
| MONARC-M | 1 IU | IV | J7190 |
| MONOCLATE-P | 1 IU | IV | J7190 |
| MONONINE | 1 IU | IV | J7193 |
| MONOPUR | 75 IU | SC, IM | S0122 |
| MONOVISC | DOSE | OTH | J7327 |
| MORPHINE SULFATE | 10 MG | IM, IV, SC | J2270 |
| MORPHINE SULFATE | 500 MG | OTH | S0093 |
| MORPHINE SULFATE, PRESERVATIVE-FREE FOR EPIDURAL OR INTRATHECAL USE | 10 MG | OTH | J2274 |
| MOXIFLOXACIN | 100 MG | IV | J2280 |
| MOZOBIL | 1 MG | SC | J2562 |
| MPI INDIUM DTPA | 0.5 MCI | IV | A9548 |
| MS CONTIN | 500 MG | OTH | S0093 |
| MUCOMYST | 1 G | INH | J7608 |
| MUCOSIL | 1 G | INH | J7608 |
| MULTIHANCE | 1 ML | IV | A9577 |
| MULTIHANCE MULTIPACK | 1 ML | IV | A9578 |
| MUROMONAB-CD3 | 5 MG | OTH | J7505 |
| MUSE | EA | OTH | J0275 |
| MUSTARGEN | 10 MG | IV | J9230 |
| MUTAMYCIN | 5 MG | IV | J9280 |
| MYCAMINE | 1 MG | IV | J2248 |
| MYCOPHENOLATE MOFETIL | 250 MG | ORAL | J7517 |
| MYCOPHENOLIC ACID | 180 MG | ORAL | J7518 |
| MYFORTIC DELAYED RELEASE | 180 MG | ORAL | J7518 |
| MYLERAN | 2 MG | ORAL | J8510 |
| MYLOCEL | 500 MG | ORAL | S0176 |
| MYOBLOC | 100 U | IM | J0587 |
| MYOCHRYSINE | 50 MG | IM | J1600 |

© 2016 Optum360, LLC

| Drug Name | Unit Per | Route | Code |
|---|---|---|---|
| MYOZYME | 10 MG | IV | J0220 |
| NABILONE | 1 MG | ORAL | J8650 |
| NAFCILLIN SODIUM | 2 GM | IM, IV | S0032 |
| NAGLAZYME | 1 MG | IV | J1458 |
| NALBUPHINE HCL | 10 MG | IM, IV, SC | J2300 |
| NALLPEN | 2 GM | IM, IV | S0032 |
| NALOXONE HCL | 1 MG | IM, IV, SC | J2310 |
| NALTREXONE, DEPOT FORM | 1 MG | IM | J2315 |
| NANDROLONE DECANOATE | 50 MG | IM | J2320 |
| NARCAN | 1 MG | IM, IV, SC | J2310 |
| NAROPIN | 1 MG | VAR | J2795 |
| NASALCROM | 10 MG | INH | J7631 |
| NATALIZUMAB | 1 MG | IV | J2323 |
| NATRECOR | 0.1 MG | IV | J2325 |
| NATURAL ESTROGENIC SUBSTANCE | 1 MG | IM, IV | J1410 |
| NAVELBINE | 10 MG | IV | J9390 |
| ND-STAT | 10 MG | IM, SC, IV | J0945 |
| NEBCIN | 80 MG | IM, IV | J3260 |
| NEBUPENT | 300 MG | INH | J2545 |
| NEBUPENT | 300 MG | IM, IV | S0080 |
| NECITUMUMAB | 1 MG | IV | J9295 |
| ~~NECITUMUMAB~~ | ~~MG~~ | ~~IV~~ | ~~C9475~~ |
| NELARABINE | 50 MG | IV | J9261 |
| NEMBUTAL SODIUM | 50 MG | IM, IV, OTH | J2515 |
| NEORAL | 250 MG | ORAL | J7516 |
| NEORAL | 25 MG | ORAL | J7515 |
| NEOSAR | 100 MG | IV | J9070 |
| NEOSCAN | 1 MCI | IV | A9556 |
| NEOSTIGMINE METHYLSULFATE | 0.5 MG | IM, IV | J2710 |
| NEOTECT | STUDY DOSE UP TO 35 MCI | IV | A9536 |
| NEOX 100 | SQ CM | OTH | Q4156 |
| NEOX 1K | SQ CM | OTH | Q4148 |
| NEOXFLO | 1 MG | OTH | Q4155 |
| NESACAINE | 30 ML | VAR | J2400 |
| NESACAINE-MPF | 30 ML | VAR | J2400 |
| NESIRITIDE | 0.1 MG | IV | J2325 |
| NETSPOT | 0.1 MCI | IV | A9587 |
| NETUPITANT AND PALONOSETRON | 300 MG/0.5 MG | ORAL | J8655 |
| ~~NETUPITANT AND PALONOSETRON~~ | ~~300 MG/0.5 MG~~ | ~~ORAL~~ | ~~C9448~~ |
| NEULASTA | 6 MG | SC, SQ | J2505 |
| NEUMEGA | 5 MG | SC | J2355 |
| NEUPOGEN | 1 MCG | SC, IV | J1442 |
| NEURAGEN NERVE GUIDE | 1 CM LENGTH | OTH | C9352 |
| NEUROLITE | STUDY DOSE UP TO 25 MCI | IV | A9557 |
| NEUROMATRIX | 0.5 CM LENGTH | OTH | C9355 |

| Drug Name | Unit Per | Route | Code |
|---|---|---|---|
| NEUROMEND NERVE WRAP | 0.5 CM | OTH | C9361 |
| NEUROWRAP NERVE PROTECTOR | 1 CM LENGTH | OTH | C9353 |
| NEUTREXIN | 25 MG | IV | J3305 |
| NEUTROSPEC | STUDY DOSE UP TO 25 MCI | IV | A9566 |
| NEXPLANON | IMPLANT | OTH | J7307 |
| NIPENT | 10 MG | IV | J9268 |
| NITROGEN MUSTARD | 10 MG | IV | J9230 |
| NITROGEN N-13 AMMONIA, DIAGNOSTIC | STUDY DOSE UP TO 40 MCI | INJ | A9526 |
| NIVOLUMAB | 1 MG | IV | J9299 |
| NOC DRUGS, INHALATION SOLUTION ADMINISTERED THROUGH DME | 1 EA | | J7699 |
| NOLVADEX | 10 MG | ORAL | S0187 |
| NORDITROPIN | 1 MG | SC | J2941 |
| NORDYL | 50 MG | IV, IM | J1200 |
| NORFLEX | 60 MG | IV, IM | J2360 |
| NORMAL SALINE SOLUTION | 500 ML | IV | J7040 |
| NORMAL SALINE SOLUTION | 1000 CC | IV | J7030 |
| NORMAL SALINE SOLUTION | 250 CC | IV | J7050 |
| NOT OTHERWISE CLASSIFIED, ANTINEOPLASTIC DRUGS | | | J9999 |
| NOVANTRONE | 5 MG | IV | J9293 |
| NOVAREL | 1,000 USP U | IM | J0725 |
| ~~NOVASTAN~~ | ~~5 MG~~ | ~~IV~~ | ~~C9121~~ |
| NOVOEIGHT | IU | IV | J7182 |
| NOVOLIN | 50 U | SC | J1817 |
| NOVOLIN R | 5 U | SC | J1815 |
| NOVOLOG | 50 U | SC | J1817 |
| NOVOSEVEN | 1 MCG | IV | J7189 |
| NPH | 5 UNITS | SC | J1815 |
| NPLATE | 10 MCG | SC | J2796 |
| NUBAIN | 10 MG | IM, IV, SC | J2300 |
| ~~NUCALA~~ | ~~MG~~ | ~~SQ~~ | ~~C9473~~ |
| NUCALA | 100 MG | SQ | J2182 |
| NULOJIX | 1 MG | IV | J0485 |
| NUMORPHAN | 1 MG | IV, SC, IM | J2410 |
| NUSHIELD | SQ CM | OTH | Q4160 |
| NUTRI-TWELVE | 1,000 MCG | IM, SC | J3420 |
| NUTROPIN | 1 MG | SC | J2941 |
| NUTROPIN A.Q. | 1 MG | SC | J2941 |
| NUVARING VAGINAL RING | EACH | OTH | J7303 |
| NUWIQ | 1 IU | IV | J7209 |
| ~~NUWIQ~~ | ~~IU~~ | ~~IV~~ | ~~C9138~~ |
| OASIS BURN MATRIX | SQ CM | OTH | Q4103 |
| OASIS ULTRA TRI-LAYER WOUND MATRIX | SQ CM | OTH | Q4124 |
| OASIS WOUND MATRIX | SQ CM | OTH | Q4102 |
| OBINUTUZUMAB | 10 MG | IV | J9301 |
| OBIZUR | IU | IV | J7188 |

© 2016 Optum360, LLC

| Drug Name | Unit Per | Route | Code | Drug Name | Unit Per | Route | Code |
|---|---|---|---|---|---|---|---|
| OCRIPLASMIN | 0.125 MG | OTH | J7316 | ORTHOCLONE OKT3 | 5 MG | OTH | J7505 |
| OCTAFLUOROPROPANE UCISPHERES | 1 ML | IV | Q9956 | ORTHOVISC | DOSE | OTH | J7324 |
| OCTAGAM | 500 MG | IV | J1568 | OSELTAMIVIR PHOSPHATE (BRAND NAME) (DEMONSTRATION PROJECT) | 75 MG | ORAL | G9035 |
| OCTREOSCAN | STUDY DOSE UP TO 6 MCI | IV | A9572 | OSELTAMIVIR PHOSPHATE (GENERIC) (DEMONSTRATION PROJECT) | 75 MG | ORAL | G9019 |
| OCTREOTIDE ACETATE DEPOT | 1 MG | IM | J2353 | OSMITROL | 25% IN 50 ML | IV | J2150 |
| OCTREOTIDE, NON-DEPOT FORM | 25 MCG | SC, IV | J2354 | | | | |
| OFATUMUMAB | 10 MG | IV | J9302 | OTIPRIO | 6 MG | OTIC | J7342 |
| OFIRMEV | 10 MG | IV | J0131 | OXACILLIN SODIUM | 250 MG | IM, IV | J2700 |
| OFLOXACIN | 400 MG | IV | S0034 | OXALIPLATIN | 0.5 MG | IV | J9263 |
| OFORTA | 10 MG | ORAL | J8562 | OXILAN 300 | PER ML | IV | Q9967 |
| OLANZAPINE | 2.5 MG | IM | S0166 | OXILAN 350 | PER ML | IV | Q9967 |
| OLANZAPINE LONG ACTING | 1 MG | IM | J2358 | OXYMORPHONE HCL | 1 MG | IV, SC, IM | J2410 |
| OMACETAXINE MEPESUCCINATE | 0.01 MG | SC | J9262 | OXYTETRACYCLINE HCL | 50 MG | IM | J2460 |
| OMALIZUMAB | 5 MG | SC | J2357 | OXYTOCIN | 10 U | IV, IM | J2590 |
| OMIDRIA | 4 ML | IRR | C9447 | OZURDEX | 0.1 MG | OTH | J7312 |
| OMNIPAQUE 140 | PER ML | IV | Q9965 | PACIS BCG | VIAL | OTH | J9031 |
| OMNIPAQUE 180 | PER ML | IV | Q9965 | PACLITAXEL | 1 MG | IV | J9267 |
| OMNIPAQUE 240 | PER ML | IV | Q9966 | PACLITAXEL PROTEIN-BOUND PARTICLES | 1 MG | IV | J9264 |
| OMNIPAQUE 300 | PER ML | IV | Q9967 | PALIFERMIN | 50 MCG | IV | J2425 |
| ~~OMNIPAQUE 300~~ | ~~PER ML~~ | ~~IV~~ | ~~Q9966~~ | PALINGEN OR PALINGEN XPLU | SQ CM | OTH | Q4173 |
| OMNIPAQUE 350 | PER ML | IV | Q9967 | PALINGEN OR PROMATRX | 0.36 MG/0.25 CC | OTH | Q4174 |
| OMNISCAN | 1 ML | IV | A9579 | PALIPERIDONE PALMITATE EXTENDED RELEASED | 1 MG | IM | J2426 |
| OMONTYS (FOR ESRD ON DIALYSIS) | 0.1 MG | SC, IV | J0890 | PALONOSETRON HCL | 25 MCG | IV | J2469 |
| ONABOTULINUMTOXINA | 1 UNIT | IM, OTH | J0585 | PAMIDRONATE DISODIUM | 30 MG | IV | J2430 |
| ONCASPAR | VIAL | IM, IV | J9266 | PANHEMATIN | 1 MG | IV | J1640 |
| ONCOSCINT | STUDY DOSE, UP TO 6 MCI | IV | A4642 | PANITUMUMAB | 10 MG | IV | J9303 |
| ONDANSETRON | 4 MG | ORAL | S0119 | PANTOPRAZOLE SODIUM | VIAL | IV | C9113 |
| ONDANSETRON | 1 MG | ORAL | Q0162 | PANTOPRAZOLE SODIUM | 40 MG | IV | S0164 |
| ONDANSETRON HYDROCHLORIDE | 1 MG | IV | J2405 | PAPAVERINE HCL | 60 MG | IV, IM | J2440 |
| ONIVYDE | 1 MG | IV | J9205 | PARAGARD T380A | EA | OTH | J7300 |
| ~~ONIVYDE~~ | ~~MG~~ | ~~IV~~ | ~~C9474~~ | PARAPLANTIN | 50 MG | IV | J9045 |
| ONTAK | 300 MCG | IV | J9160 | PARICALCITOL | 1 MCG | IV, IM | J2501 |
| OPDIVO | 1 MG | IV | J9299 | PASIREOTIDE LONG ACTING | 1 MG | IV | J2502 |
| OPRELVEKIN | 5 MG | SC | J2355 | PEDIAPRED | 5 MG | ORAL | J7510 |
| ~~OPTIPRIO~~ | ~~6 MG~~ | ~~OTH~~ | ~~C9479~~ | PEG-INTRON | 180 MCG | SC | S0145 |
| OPTIRAY | PER ML | IV | Q9967 | PEGADEMASE BOVINE | 25 IU | IM | J2504 |
| OPTIRAY 160 | PER ML | IV | Q9965 | PEGAPTANIB SODIUM | 0.3 MG | OTH | J2503 |
| OPTIRAY 240 | PER ML | IV | Q9966 | PEGASPARGASE | VIAL | IM, IV | J9266 |
| OPTIRAY 300 | PER ML | IV | Q9967 | PEGFILGRASTIM | 6 MG | SC | J2505 |
| OPTIRAY 320 | PER ML | IV | Q9967 | PEGINESATIDE (FOR ESRD ON DIALYSIS) | 0.1 MG | SC, IV | J0890 |
| OPTISON | 1 ML | IV | Q9956 | PEGINTERFERON ALFA-2A | 180 MCG | SC | S0145 |
| ORAL MAGNETIC RESONANCE CONTRAST AGENT, PER 100 ML | 100 ML | ORAL | Q9954 | PEGLOTICASE | 1 MG | IV | J2507 |
| ORBACTIV | 10 MG | IV | J2407 | PEGYLATED INTERFERON ALFA-2A | 180 MCG | SC | S0145 |
| ORENCIA | 10 MG | IV | J0129 | | | | |
| ORITAVANCIN | 10 MG | IV | J2407 | PEGYLATED INTERFERON ALFA-2B | 10 MCG | SC | S0148 |
| ORPHENADRINE CITRATE | 60 MG | IV, IM | J2360 | | | | |
| ORTHADAPT BIOIMPLANT | SQ CM | OTH | C1781 | PEMBROLIZUMAB | 1 MG | IV | J9271 |

| Drug Name | Unit Per | Route | Code |
|---|---|---|---|
| PEMETREXED | 10 MG | IV | J9305 |
| PENICILLIN G BENZATHINE | 100,000 U | IM | J0561 |
| PENICILLIN G BENZATHINE AND PENICILLIN G PROCAINE | 100,000 UNITS | IM | J0558 |
| PENICILLIN G POTASSIUM | 600,000 U | IM, IV | J2540 |
| PENICILLIN G PROCAINE | 600,000 U | IM, IV | J2510 |
| PENTACARINAT | 300 MG | INH | S0080 |
| PENTAM | 300 MG | IM, IV | J2545 |
| PENTAM 300 | 300 MG | IM, IV | S0080 |
| PENTAMIDINE ISETHIONATE | 300 MG | IM, IV | S0080 |
| PENTAMIDINE ISETHIONATE COMPOUNDED | PER 300 MG | INH | J7676 |
| PENTAMIDINE ISETHIONATE NONCOMPOUNDED | 300 MG | INH | J2545 |
| PENTASPAN | 100 ML | IV | J2513 |
| PENTASTARCH 10% SOLUTION | 100 ML | IV | J2513 |
| PENTATE CALCIUM TRISODIUM | STUDY DOSE UP TO 25 MCI | IV | A9539 |
| PENTATE CALCIUM TRISODIUM | STUDY DOSE UP TO 75 MCI | INH | A9567 |
| PENTATE ZINC TRISODIUM | STUDY DOSE UP TO 75 MCI | INH | A9567 |
| PENTATE ZINC TRISODIUM | STUDY DOSE UP TO 25 MCI | IV | A9539 |
| PENTAZOCINE | 30 MG | IM, SC, IV | J3070 |
| PENTOBARBITAL SODIUM | 50 MG | IM, IV, OTH | J2515 |
| PENTOSTATIN | 10 MG | IV | J9268 |
| PEPCID | 20 MG | IV | S0028 |
| PERAMIVIR | 1 MG | IV | J2547 |
| PERFLEXANE LIPID MICROSPHERE | 1 ML | IV | Q9955 |
| PERFLUTREN LIPID MICROSPHERE | 1 ML | IV | Q9957 |
| PERFOROMIST | 20 MCG | INH | J7606 |
| PERJETA | 1 MG | IV | J9306 |
| PERMACOL | SQ CM | OTH | C9364 |
| PERPHENAZINE | 4 MG | ORAL | Q0175 |
| PERPHENAZINE | 5 MG | IM, IV | J3310 |
| PERSANTINE | 10 MG | IV | J1245 |
| PERTUZUMAB | 1 MG | IV | J9306 |
| PFIZERPEN A.S. | 600,000 U | IM, IV | J2510 |
| PHENERGAN | 50 MG | IM, IV | J2550 |
| PHENERGAN | 12.5 MG | ORAL | Q0169 |
| PHENOBARBITAL SODIUM | 120 MG | IM, IV | J2560 |
| PHENTOLAMINE MESYLATE | 5 MG | IM, IV | J2760 |
| PHENYLEPHRINE HCL | 1 ML | SC, IM, IV | J2370 |
| PHENYLEPHRINE KETOROLAC | 4 ML | IRR | C9447 |
| PHENYTOIN SODIUM | 50 MG | IM, IV | J1165 |
| PHOSPHOCOL | 1 MCI | IV | A9563 |
| PHOSPHOTEC | STUDY DOSE UP TO 25 MCI | IV | A9538 |

| Drug Name | Unit Per | Route | Code |
|---|---|---|---|
| PHOTOFRIN | 75 MG | IV | J9600 |
| PHYTONADIONE | 1 MG | IM, SC, IV | J3430 |
| PIPERACILLIN SODIUM | 500 MG | IM, IV | S0081 |
| PIPERACILLIN SODIUM/TAZOBACTAM SODIUM | 1 G/1.125 GM | IV | J2543 |
| PITOCIN | 10 U | IV, IM | J2590 |
| PLATINOL AQ | 10 MG | IV | J9060 |
| PLERIXAFOR | 1 MG | SC | J2562 |
| PLICAMYCIN | 2.5 MG | IV | J9270 |
| PNEUMOCOCCAL CONJUGATE | EA | IM | S0195 |
| PNEUMOVAX II | EA | IM | S0195 |
| POLOCAINE | 10 ML | VAR | J0670 |
| POLYGAM | 500 MG | IV | J1566 |
| POLYGAM S/D | 500 MG | IV | J1566 |
| PORCINE IMPLANT, PERMACOL | SQ CM | OTH | C9364 |
| PORFIMER SODIUM | 75 MG | IV | J9600 |
| PORK INSULIN | 5 U | SC | J1815 |
| POROUS PURIFIED COLLAGEN MATRIX BONE VOID FILLER | 0.5 CC | OTH | C9362 |
| POROUS PURIFIED COLLAGEN MATRIX BONE VOID FILLER, PUTTY | 0.5 CC | OTH | C9359 |
| ~~PORTRAZZA~~ | ~~MG~~ | ~~IV~~ | ~~C9475~~ |
| PORTRAZZA. | 1 MG | IV | J9295 |
| POTASSIUM CHLORIDE | 2 MEQ | IV | J3480 |
| PRALATREXATE | 1 MG | IV | J9307 |
| PRALIDOXIME CHLORIDE | 1 MG | IV, IM, SC | J2730 |
| PREDNISOLONE | 5 MG | ORAL | J7510 |
| PREDNISOLONE ACETATE | 1 ML | IM | J2650 |
| PREDNISONE, IMMEDIATE RELEASE OR DELAYED RELEASE | 1 MG | ORAL | J7512 |
| PREDNORAL | 5 MG | ORAL | J7510 |
| PREGNYL | 1,000 USP U | IM | J0725 |
| PRELONE | 5 MG | ORAL | J7510 |
| PREMARIN | 25 MG | IV, IM | J1410 |
| PRENATAL VITAMINS | 30 TABS | ORAL | S0197 |
| PRI-METHYLATE | 80 MG | IM | J1040 |
| PRIALT | 1 MCG | OTH | J2278 |
| PRIMACOR | 5 MG | IV | J2260 |
| PRIMATRIX | SQ CM | OTH | Q4110 |
| PRIMAXIN | 250 MG | IV, IM | J0743 |
| PRIMESTRIN AQUEOUS | 1 MG | IM, IV | J1410 |
| PRIMETHASONE | 1 MG | IM, IV, OTH | J1100 |
| PRIVIGEN | 500 MG | IV | J1459 |
| PROBUPHINE IMPLANT | 74.2 MG | OTH | J0570 |
| PROCAINAMIDE HCL | 1 G | IM, IV | J2690 |
| PROCARBAZINE HCL | 50 MG | ORAL | S0182 |
| PROCHLOPERAZINE MALEATE | 5 MG | ORAL | S0183 |
| PROCHLORPERAZINE | 10 MG | IM, IV | J0780 |
| PROCHLORPERAZINE MALEATE | 5 MG | ORAL | Q0164 |
| PROCRIT, NON-ESRD USE | 1,000 U | SC, IV | J0885 |
| PROFILNINE HEAT-TREATED | 1 IU | IV | J7194 |
| PROFILNINE SD | 1 IU | IV | J7194 |

© 2016 Optum360, LLC

| Drug Name | Unit Per | Route | Code |
|---|---|---|---|
| PROFONIX | VIAL | INJ | C9113 |
| PROGESTERONE | 50 MG | IM | J2675 |
| PROGRAF | 1 MG | ORAL | J7507 |
| PROGRAF | 5 MG | OTH | J7525 |
| PROLASTIN | 10 MG | IV | J0256 |
| PROLEUKIN | 1 VIAL | VAR | J9015 |
| PROLIA | 1 MG | SC | J0897 |
| PROLIXIN DECANOATE | 25 MG | SC, IM | J2680 |
| PROMAZINE HCL | 25 MG | IM | J2950 |
| PROMETHAZINE HCL | 50 MG | IM, IV | J2550 |
| PROMETHAZINE HCL | 12.5 MG | ORAL | Q0169 |
| PRONESTYL | 1 G | IM, IV | J2690 |
| PROPECIA | 5 MG | ORAL | S0138 |
| PROPLEX SX-T | 1 IU | IV | J7194 |
| PROPLEX T | 1 IU | IV | J7194 |
| PROPOFOL | 10 MG | IV | J2704 |
| PROPRANOLOL HCL | 1 MG | IV | J1800 |
| PROREX | 50 MG | IM, IV | J2550 |
| PROSCAR | 5 MG | ORAL | S0138 |
| PROSTASCINT | STUDY DOSE UP TO 10 MCI | IV | A9507 |
| PROSTIGMIN | 0.5 MG | IM, IV | J2710 |
| PROSTIN VR | 1.25 MCG | INJ | J0270 |
| PROTAMINE SULFATE | 10 MG | IV | J2720 |
| PROTEIN C CONCENTRATE | 10 IU | IV | J2724 |
| PROTEINASE INHIBITOR (HUMAN) | 10 MG | IV | J0256 |
| PROTIRELIN | 250 MCG | IV | J2725 |
| PROTONIX IV | 40 MG | IV | S0164 |
| PROTONIX IV | VIAL | IV | C9113 |
| PROTOPAM CHLORIDE | 1 G | SC, IM, IV | J2730 |
| PROTROPIN | 1 MG | SC, IM | J2940 |
| PROVENGE | INFUSION | IV | Q2043 |
| PROVENTIL NONCOMPOUNDED, CONCENTRATED | 1 MG | INH | J7611 |
| PROVENTIL NONCOMPOUNDED, UNIT DOSE | 1 MG | INH | J7613 |
| PROVOCHOLINE POWDER | 1 MG | INH | J7674 |
| PROZINE-50 | 25 MG | IM | J2950 |
| PULMICORT | 0.25 MG | INH | J7633 |
| PULMICORT RESPULES | 0.5 MG | INH | J7627 |
| PULMICORT RESPULES NONCOMPOUNDED, CONCETRATED | 0.25 MG | INH | J7626 |
| PULMOZYME | 1 MG | INH | J7639 |
| PURAPLY AND PURAPLY ANTIMICROBIAL | SQ CM | OTH | C9349 |
| PURAPLY OR PURAPLY AM | SQ CM | OTH | Q4172 |
| PURINETHOL | 50 MG | ORAL | S0108 |
| PYRIDOXINE HCL | 100 MG | IM, IV | J3415 |
| QUADRAMET | PER DOSE UP TO 150 MCI | IV | A9604 |
| QUELICIN | 20 MG | IM, IV | J0330 |

| Drug Name | Unit Per | Route | Code |
|---|---|---|---|
| QUINUPRISTIN/DALFOPRISTIN | 500 MG | IV | J2770 |
| QUTENZA | 1 SQ CM | OTH | J7336 |
| RADIESSE | 0.1 ML | OTH | Q2026 |
| RADIUM (RA) 223 DICHLORIDE THERAPEUTIC | PER MICROCURIE | IV | A9606 |
| RAMUCIRUMAB | 5 MG | IV | J9308 |
| RANIBIZUMAB | 0.1 MG | OTH | J2778 |
| RANITIDINE HCL | 25 MG | INJ | J2780 |
| RAPAMUNE | 1 MG | ORAL | J7520 |
| RAPIVAB | 1 MG | IV | J2547 |
| RASBURICASE | 0.5 MG | IM | J2783 |
| REBETRON KIT | 1,000,000 U | SC, IM | J9214 |
| REBIF | 1 MCG | SC | Q3028 |
| REBIF | 30 MCG | SC | J1826 |
| RECLAST | 1 MG | IV | J3489 |
| RECOMBINATE | 1 IU | IV | J7192 |
| REDISOL | 1,000 MCG | SC. IM | J3420 |
| REFACTO | 1 IU | IV | J7192 |
| REFLUDAN | 50 MG | IM, IV | J1945 |
| REGADENOSON | 0.1 MG | IV | J2785 |
| REGITINE | 5 MG | IM, IV | J2760 |
| REGLAN | 10 MG | IV | J2765 |
| REGRANEX GEL | 0.5 G | OTH | S0157 |
| REGULAR INSULIN | 5 UNITS | SC | J1815 |
| RELAXIN | 10 ML | IV, IM | J2800 |
| RELENZA (DEMONSTRATION PROJECT) | 10 MG | INH | G9034 |
| RELION | 5 U | SC | J1815 |
| RELION NOVOLIN | 50 U | SC | J1817 |
| RELISTOR | 0.1 MG | SC | J2212 |
| REMICADE | 10 MG | IV | J1745 |
| REMODULIN | 1 MG | SC | J3285 |
| REODULIN | 1 MG | SC | J3285 |
| REOPRO | 10 MG | IV | J0130 |
| REPRIZA | SQ CM | OTH | Q4143 |
| REPRONEX | 75 IU | SC, IM, IV | S0122 |
| RESLIZUMAB | 1 MG | IV | J2786 |
| RESLIZUMAB | 1 MG | IV | C9481 |
| RESPIROL NONCOMPOUNDED, CONCENTRATED | 1 MG | INH | J7611 |
| RESPIROL NONCOMPOUNDED, UNIT DOSE | 1 MG | INH | J7613 |
| RETAVASE | 18.1 MG | IV | J2993 |
| RETEPLASE | 18.1 MG | IV | J2993 |
| RETISERT | IMPLANT | OTH | J7311 |
| RETROVIR | 10 MG | IV | J3485 |
| RETROVIR | 100 MG | ORAL | S0104 |
| REVITALON | SQ CM | OTH | Q4157 |
| RHEOMACRODEX | 500 ML | IV | J7100 |
| RHEUMATREX | 2.5 MG | ORAL | J8610 |
| RHEUMATREX DOSE PACK | 2.5 MG | ORAL | J8610 |
| RHO D IMMUNE GLOBULIN | 300 MCG | IV | J2790 |

© 2016 Optum360, LLC

| Drug Name | Unit Per | Route | Code |
|---|---|---|---|
| RHO D IMMUNE GLOBULIN (RHOPHYLAC) | 100 IU | IM, IV | J2791 |
| RHO D IMMUNE GLOBULIN MINIDOSE | 50 MCG | IM | J2788 |
| RHO D IMMUNE GLOBULIN SOLVENT DETERGENT | 100 IU | IV | J2792 |
| RHOGAM | 300 MCG | IM | J2790 |
| RHOGAM | 50 MCG | IM | J2788 |
| RHOPHYLAC | 100 IU | IM, IV | J2791 |
| RILONACEPT | 1 MG | SC | J2793 |
| RIMANTADINE HCL (DEMONSTRATION PROJECT) | 100 MG | ORAL | G9036 |
| RIMANTADINE HCL (DEMONSTRATION PROJECT) | 100 MG | ORAL | G9020 |
| RIMSO 50 | 50 ML | IV | J1212 |
| RINGERS LACTATE INFUSION | UP TO 1000 CC | IV | J7120 |
| RISPERDAL COSTA LONG ACTING | 0.5 MG | IM | J2794 |
| RISPERIDONE, LONG ACTING | 0.5 MG | IM | J2794 |
| RITUXAN | 100 MG | IV | J9310 |
| RITUXIMAB | 100 MG | IV | J9310 |
| RIXUBIS | IU | IV | J7200 |
| ROBAXIN | 10 ML | IV, IM | J2800 |
| ROCEPHIN | 250 MG | IV, IM | J0696 |
| ROFERON-A | 3,000,000 U | SC, IM | J9213 |
| ROLAPITANT | 1 MG | ORAL | J8670 |
| ROLAPITANT | ~~1 MG~~ | ~~ORAL~~ | ~~Q9981~~ |
| ROMIDEPSIN | 1 MG | IV | J9315 |
| ROMIPLOSTIM | 10 MCG | SC | J2796 |
| ROPIVACAINE HYDROCHLORIDE | 1 MG | VAR | J2795 |
| RUBEX | 10 MG | IV | J9000 |
| RUBIDIUM RB-82 | STUDY DOSE UP TO 60 MCI | IV | A9555 |
| RUBRAMIN PC | 1,000 MCG | SC, IM | J3420 |
| RUBRATOPE 57 | STUDY DOSE UP TO 1 UCI | ORAL | A9559 |
| RUCONEST | 10 UNITS | IV | J0596 |
| SAIZEN | 1 MG | SC | J2941 |
| SAIZEN SOMATROPIN RDNA ORIGIN | 1 MG | SC | J2941 |
| SALINE OR STERILE WATER, METERED DOSE DISPENSER | 10 ML | INH | A4218 |
| SALINE, STERILE WATER, AND/OR DEXTROSE DILUENT/FLUSH | 10 ML | VAR | A4216 |
| SALINE/STERILE WATER | 500 ML | VAR | A4217 |
| SAMARIUM LEXIDRONAM | PER DOSE UP TO 150 MCI | IV | A9604 |
| SANDIMMUNE | 100 MG | ORAL | J7502 |
| SANDIMMUNE | 250 MG | IV | J7516 |
| SANDIMMUNE | 25 MG | ORAL | J7515 |
| SANDOSTATIN | 25 MCG | SC, IV | J2354 |
| SANDOSTATIN LAR | 1 MG | IM | J2353 |
| SANGCYA | 100 MG | ORAL | J7502 |

| Drug Name | Unit Per | Route | Code |
|---|---|---|---|
| SANO-DROL | 40 MG | IM | J1030 |
| SANO-DROL | 80 MG | IM | J1040 |
| SAQUINAVIR | 200 MG | ORAL | S0140 |
| SARGRAMOSTIM (GM-CSF) | 50 MCG | IV | J2820 |
| SCANDONEST | PER 10 ML | IV | J0670 |
| SCULPTRA | 0.5 ML | OTH | Q2028 |
| ~~SEBELIPASE ALFA~~ | ~~1 MG~~ | ~~IV~~ | ~~C9478~~ |
| SEBELIPASE ALFA | 1 MG | IV | J2840 |
| SECREFLO | 1 MCG | IV | J2850 |
| SECRETIN, SYNTHETIC, HUMAN | 1 MCG | IV | J2850 |
| SENSORCAINE | 30 ML | VAR | S0020 |
| SEPTRA IV | 10 ML | IV | S0039 |
| SERMORELIN ACETATE | 1 MCG | IV | Q0515 |
| SEROSTIM | 1 MG | SC | J2941 |
| SEROSTIM RDNA ORIGIN | 1 MG | SC | J2941 |
| SIGNIFOR LAR | 1 MG | IV | J2502 |
| SILDENAFIL CITRATE | 25 MG | ORAL | S0090 |
| SILTUXIMAB | 10 MG | IV | J2860 |
| SIMPONI | 1 MG | IV | J1602 |
| SIMULECT | 20 MG | IV | J0480 |
| SINCALIDE | 5 MCG | IV | J2805 |
| SIPULEUCEL-T | INFUSION | IV | Q2043 |
| SIROLIMUS | 1 MG | ORAL | J7520 |
| SIVEXTRO | 1 MG | IV | J3090 |
| SKIN SUBSTITUTE, ALLODERM | SQ CM | OTH | Q4116 |
| SKIN SUBSTITUTE, ALLOSKIN | SQ CM | OTH | Q4115 |
| SKIN SUBSTITUTE, APLIGRAF | SQ CM | OTH | Q4101 |
| SKIN SUBSTITUTE, DERMAGRAFT | SQ CM | OTH | Q4106 |
| SKIN SUBSTITUTE, GAMMAGRAFT | SQ CM | OTH | Q4111 |
| SKIN SUBSTITUTE, GRAFTJACKET | SQ CM | OTH | Q4107 |
| SKIN SUBSTITUTE, INTEGRA BILAYER MATRIX WOUND DRESSING | SQ CM | OTH | Q4104 |
| SKIN SUBSTITUTE, INTEGRA DERMAL REGENERATION TEMPLATE | SQ CM | OTH | Q4105 |
| SKIN SUBSTITUTE, INTEGRA MATRIX | SQ CM | OTH | Q4108 |
| SKIN SUBSTITUTE, INTEGRA MESHED BILAYER WOUND MATRIX | SQ CM | OTH | C9363 |
| SKIN SUBSTITUTE, KERAMATRIX | SQ CM | OTH | Q4165 |
| SKIN SUBSTITUTE, OASIS BURN MATRIX | SQ CM | OTH | Q4103 |
| SKIN SUBSTITUTE, OASIS WOUND MATRIX | SQ CM | OTH | Q4102 |
| SKIN SUBSTITUTE, PRIMATRIX | SQ CM | OTH | Q4110 |
| SKYLA | 13.5 MG | OTH | J7301 |
| SMZ-TMP | 10 ML | IV | S0039 |
| SODIUM FERRIC GLUCONATE COMPLEX IN SUCROSE | 12.5 MG | IV | J2916 |

© 2016 Optum360, LLC

| Drug Name | Unit Per | Route | Code |
|---|---|---|---|
| SODIUM FLUORIDE F-18, DIAGNOSTIC | STUDY DOSE UP TO 30 MCI | IV | A9580 |
| SODIUM IODIDE I-131 CAPSULE DIAGNOSTIC | 1 MCI | ORAL | A9528 |
| SODIUM IODIDE I-131 CAPSULE THERAPEUTIC | 1 MCI | ORAL | A9517 |
| SODIUM IODIDE I-131 SOLUTION THERAPEUTIC | 1 MCI | ORAL | A9530 |
| SODIUM PHOSPHATE P32 | 1 MCI | IV | A9563 |
| SOLGANAL | 50 MG | IM | J2910 |
| SOLIRIS | 10 MG | IV | J1300 |
| SOLTAMOX | 10 MG | ORAL | S0187 |
| SOLU-CORTEF | 100 MG | IV, IM, SC | J1720 |
| SOLU-MEDROL | 40 MG | IM, IV | J2920 |
| SOLU-MEDROL | 125 MG | IM, IV | J2930 |
| SOLUREX | 1 MG | IM, IV, OTH | J1100 |
| SOMATREM | 1 MG | SC, IM | J2940 |
| SOMATROPIN | 1 MG | SC | J2941 |
| SOMATULINE | 1 MG | SC | J1930 |
| SOTALOL HYDROCHLORIDE | 1 MG | IV | C9482 |
| SPECTINOMYCIN DIHYDROCHLORIDE | 2 G | IM | J3320 |
| SPECTRO-DEX | 1 MG | IM, IV, OTH | J1100 |
| SPORANOX | 50 MG | IV | J1835 |
| STADOL | 1 MG | IM, IV | J0595 |
| STADOL NS | 25 MG | OTH | S0012 |
| STELARA | 1 MG | SC | J3357 |
| STERILE WATER OR SALINE, METERED DOSE DISPENSER | 10 ML | INH | A4218 |
| STERILE WATER, SALINE, AND/OR DEXTROSE DILUENT/FLUSH | 10 ML | VAR | A4216 |
| STERILE WATER/SALINE | 500 ML | VAR | A4217 |
| STRATTICE TM | SQ CM | OTH | Q4130 |
| STREPTASE | 250,000 IU | IV | J2995 |
| STREPTOKINASE | 250,000 IU | IV | J2995 |
| STREPTOMYCIN | 1 G | IM | J3000 |
| STREPTOZOCIN | 1 G | IV | J9320 |
| STRONTIUM 89 CHLORIDE | 1 MCI | IV | A9600 |
| SUBLIMAZE | 0.1 MG | IM, IV | J3010 |
| SUBOXONE | 12 MG | ORAL | J0575 |
| SUBOXONE | 2 MG | ORAL | J0572 |
| SUBOXONE | 8 MG | ORAL | J0574 |
| SUBOXONE | 4 MG | ORAL | J0573 |
| SUBUTEX | 1 MG | ORAL | J0571 |
| SUCCINYLCHOLINE CHLORIDE | 20 MG | IM, IV | J0330 |
| SULFAMETHOXAZOLE AND TRIMETHOPRIM | 10 ML | IV | S0039 |
| SULFUR HEXAFLUORIDE LIPID MICROSPHERES | 1 ML | IV | Q9950 |
| SULFUTRIM | 10 ML | IV | S0039 |
| SUMATRIPTAN SUCCINATE | 6 MG | SC | J3030 |
| SUPARTZ | DOSE | OTH | J7321 |
| SUPPRELIN LA | 10 MCG | OTH | J1675 |

| Drug Name | Unit Per | Route | Code |
|---|---|---|---|
| SURGIMEND COLLAGEN MATRIX, FETAL | 0.5 SQ CM | OTH | C9358 |
| SURGIMEND COLLAGEN MATRIX, NEONATAL | 0.5 SQ CM | OTH | C9360 |
| SYLVANT | 10 MG | IV | J2860 |
| SYMMETREL (DEMONSTRATION PROJECT) | 100 MG | ORAL | G9033 |
| SYNERA | 70 MG/70 MG | OTH | C9285 |
| SYNERCID | 500 MG | IV | J2770 |
| SYNRIBO | 0.01 MG | SC | J9262 |
| SYNTOCINON | 10 UNITS | IV | J2590 |
| SYNVISC/SYNVISC-ONE | 1 MG | OTH | J7325 |
| SYTOBEX | 1,000 MCG | SC, IM | J3420 |
| T-GEN | 250 MG | ORAL | Q0173 |
| TACRINE HCL | 10 MG | ORAL | S0014 |
| TACROLIMUS | 1 MG | ORAL | J7507 |
| TACROLIMUS | 5 MG | OTH | J7525 |
| TACROLIMUS, EXTENDED RELEASE | 0.1 MG | ORAL | J7508 |
| TACROLIMUS, EXTENDED RELEASE | 0.25 MG | ORAL | J7503 |
| TAGAMET HCL | 300 MG | IM, IV | S0023 |
| TALIGLUCERASE ALFA | 10 U | IV | J3060 |
| TALIMOGENE LAHERPAREPVEC | 1 MILLION | INTRALESIONAL | J9325 |
| ~~TALIMOGENE LAHERPAREPVEC, 1 MILLION PLAQUE FORMING UNITS~~ | ~~PFU~~ | ~~INJ~~ | ~~C9472~~ |
| TALWIN | 30 MG | IM, SC, IV | J3070 |
| TALYMED | SQ CM | OTH | Q4127 |
| TAMIFLU (DEMONSTRATION PROJECT) | 75 MG | ORAL | G9019 |
| TAMIFLU (DEMONSTRATION PROJECT) | 75 MG | ORAL | G9035 |
| TAMOXIFEN CITRATE | 10 MG | ORAL | S0187 |
| TAXOL | 1 MG | IV | J9267 |
| TAXOTERE | 1 MG | IV | J9171 |
| TAZICEF | 500 MG | IM, IV | J0713 |
| TBO-FILGRASTIM | 1 MCG | IV | J1447 |
| TC 99M TILOMANOCEPT | 0.5 MCI | SC, OTH | A9520 |
| TEBAMIDE | 250 MG | ORAL | Q0173 |
| TEBOROXIME TECHNETIUM TC 99M | STUDY DOSE | IV | A9501 |
| TEBOROXIME, TECHNETIUM | STUDY DOSE | IV | A9501 |
| TECENTRIQ | 10 MG | IV | C9483 |
| TECHNEPLEX | STUDY DOSE UP TO 25 MCI | IV | A9539 |
| TECHNESCAN | STUDY DOSE UP TO 30 MCI | IV | A9561 |
| TECHNESCAN FANOLESOMAB | STUDY DOSE UP TO 25 MCI | IV | A9566 |

| Drug Name | Unit Per | Route | Code |
|---|---|---|---|
| TECHNESCAN MAA | STUDY DOSE UP TO 10 MCI | IV | A9540 |
| TECHNESCAN MAG3 | STUDY DOSE UP TO 15 MCI | IV | A9562 |
| TECHNESCAN PYP | STUDY DOSE UP TO 25 MCI | IV | A9538 |
| TECHNESCAN PYP KIT | STUDY DOSE UP TO 25 MCI | IV | A9538 |
| TECHNETIUM SESTAMBI | STUDY DOSE | IV | A9500 |
| TECHNETIUM TC 99M APCITIDE | STUDY DOSE UP TO 20 MCI | IV | A9504 |
| TECHNETIUM TC 99M ARCITUMOMAB, DIAGNOSTIC | STUDY DOSE UP TO 45 MCI | IV | A9568 |
| TECHNETIUM TC 99M BICISATE | STUDY DOSE UP TO 25 MCI | IV | A9557 |
| TECHNETIUM TC 99M DEPREOTIDE | STUDY DOSE UP TO 35 MCI | IV | A9536 |
| TECHNETIUM TC 99M EXAMETAZIME | STUDY DOSE UP TO 25 MCI | IV | A9521 |
| TECHNETIUM TC 99M FANOLESOMAB | STUDY DOSE UP TO 25 MCI | IV | A9566 |
| TECHNETIUM TC 99M LABELED RED BLOOD CELLS | STUDY DOSE UP TO 30 MCI | IV | A9560 |
| TECHNETIUM TC 99M MACROAGGREGATED ALBUMIN | STUDY DOSE UP TO 10 MCI | IV | A9540 |
| TECHNETIUM TC 99M MDI-MDP | STUDY DOSE UP TO 30 MCI | IV | A9503 |
| TECHNETIUM TC 99M MEBROFENIN | STUDY DOSE UP TO 15 MCI | IV | A9537 |
| TECHNETIUM TC 99M MEDRONATE | STUDY DOSE UP TO 30 MCI | IV | A9503 |
| TECHNETIUM TC 99M MERTIATIDE | STUDY DOSE UP TO 15 MCI | IV | A9562 |
| TECHNETIUM TC 99M OXIDRONATE | STUDY DOSE UP TO 30 MCI | IV | A9561 |
| TECHNETIUM TC 99M PENTETATE | STUDY DOSE UP TO 25 MCI | IV | A9539 |
| TECHNETIUM TC 99M PYROPHOSPHATE | STUDY DOSE UP TO 25 MCI | IV | A9538 |
| TECHNETIUM TC 99M SODIUM GLUCEPATATE | STUDY DOSE UP TO 25 MCI | IV | A9550 |

| Drug Name | Unit Per | Route | Code |
|---|---|---|---|
| TECHNETIUM TC 99M SUCCIMER | STUDY DOSE UP TO 10 MCI | IV | A9551 |
| TECHNETIUM TC 99M SULFUR COLLOID | STUDY DOSE UP TO 20 MCI | IV | A9541 |
| TECHNETIUM TC 99M TETROFOSMIN, DIAGNOSTIC | STUDY DOSE | IV | A9502 |
| TECHNETIUM TC-99M EXAMETAZIME LABELED AUTOLOGOUS WHITE BLOOD CELLS | STUDY DOSE | IV | A9569 |
| TECHNETIUM TC-99M TEBOROXIME | STUDY DOSE | IV | A9501 |
| TECHNILITE | 1 MCI | IV | A9512 |
| TEDIZOLID PHOSPHATE | 1 MG | IV | J3090 |
| TEFLARO | 10 MG | IV | J0712 |
| TELAVANCIN | 10 MG | IV | J3095 |
| TEMODAR | 5 MG | ORAL | J8700 |
| TEMODAR | 1 MG | IV | J9328 |
| TEMOZOLOMIDE | 5 MG | ORAL | J8700 |
| TEMOZOLOMIDE | 1 MG | IV | J9328 |
| TEMSIROLIMUS | 1 MG | IV | J9330 |
| TENDON, POROUS MATRIX | SQ CM | OTH | C9356 |
| TENDON, POROUS MATRIX CROSS-LINKED AND GLYCOSAMINOGLYCAN MATRIX | SQ CM | OTH | C9356 |
| TENECTEPLASE | 1 MG | IV | J3101 |
| TENIPOSIDE | 50 MG | IV | Q2017 |
| TENOGLIDE TENDON PROTECTOR | SQ CM | OTH | C9356 |
| TENOGLIDE TENDON PROTECTOR SHEET | SQ CM | OTH | C9356 |
| TENSIX | SQ CM | OTH | Q4146 |
| TEQUIN | 10 MG | IV | J1590 |
| TERBUTALINE SULFATE | 1 MG | SC, IV | J3105 |
| TERBUTALINE SULFATE, COMPOUNDED, CONCENTRATED | 1 MG | INH | J7680 |
| TERBUTALINE SULFATE, COMPOUNDED, UNIT DOSE | 1 MG | INH | J7681 |
| TERIPARATIDE | 10 MCG | SC | J3110 |
| TERRAMYCIN | 50 MG | IM | J2460 |
| TESTOSTERONE CYPIONATE | 1 MG | IM | J1071 |
| TESTOSTERONE ENANTHATE | 1 MG | IM | J3121 |
| TESTOSTERONE PELLET | 75 MG | OTH | S0189 |
| TESTOSTERONE UNDECANOATE | 1 MG | IM | J3145 |
| TETANUS IMMUNE GLOBULIN | 250 U | IM | J1670 |
| TETRACYCLINE HCL | 250 MG | IV | J0120 |
| THALLOUS CHLORIDE | 1 MCI | IV | A9505 |
| THALLOUS CHLORIDE TL-201 | 1 MCI | IV | A9505 |
| THALLOUS CHLORIDE USP | 1 MCI | IV | A9505 |
| THEELIN AQUEOUS | 1 MG | IM, IV | J1435 |
| THEOPHYLLINE | 40 MG | IV | J2810 |
| THERACYS | VIAL | OTH | J9031 |
| THERASKIN | SQ CM | OTH | Q4121 |
| THIAMINE HCL | 100 MG | INJ | J3411 |

© 2016 Optum360, LLC

| Drug Name | Unit Per | Route | Code |
|---|---|---|---|
| THIETHYLPERAZINE MALEATE | 10 MG | ORAL | Q0174 |
| THIETHYLPERAZINE MALEATE | 10 MG | IM | J3280 |
| THIMAZIDE | 250 MG | ORAL | Q0173 |
| THIOTEPA | 15 MG | IV | J9340 |
| THORAZINE | 50 MG | IM, IV | J3230 |
| THROMBATE III | 1 IU | IV | J7197 |
| THYMOGLOBULIN | 25 MG | OTH | J7511 |
| THYROGEN | 0.9 MG | IM, SC | J3240 |
| THYROTROPIN ALPHA | 0.9 MG | IM, SC | J3240 |
| TICARCILLIN DISODIUM AND CLAVULANATE | 3.1 G | IV | S0040 |
| TICE BCG | VIAL | OTH | J9031 |
| TICON | 250 MG | IM | Q0173 |
| TIGAN | 200 MG | IM | J3250 |
| TIGECYCLINE | 1 MG | IV | J3243 |
| TIJECT-20 | 200 MG | IM | J3250 |
| TIMENTIN | 3.1 G | IV | S0040 |
| TINZAPARIN | 1,000 IU | SC | J1655 |
| TIROFIBAN HCL | 0.25 MG | IM, IV | J3246 |
| TNKASE | 1 MG | IV | J3101 |
| TOBI | 300 MG | INH | J7682 |
| TOBRAMYCIN COMPOUNDED, UNIT DOSE | 300 MG | INH | J7685 |
| TOBRAMYCIN SULFATE | 80 MG | IM, IV | J3260 |
| TOBRAMYCIN, NONCOMPOUNDED, UNIT DOSE | 300 MG | INH | J7682 |
| TOCILIZUMAB | 1 MG | IV | J3262 |
| TOLAZOLINE HCL | 25 MG | IV | J2670 |
| TOPOSAR | 10 MG | IV | J9181 |
| TOPOTECAN | 0.1 MG | IV | J9351 |
| TOPOTECAN | 0.25 MG | ORAL | J8705 |
| TORADOL | 15 MG | IV | J1885 |
| TORISEL | 1 MG | IV | J9330 |
| TORNALATE | PER MG | INH | J7629 |
| TORNALATE CONCENTRATE | PER MG | INH | J7628 |
| TORSEMIDE | 10 MG | IV | J3265 |
| TOSITUMOMAB | 450 MG | IV | G3001 |
| ~~TOSITUMOMAB I-131 DIAGNOSTIC~~ | ~~STUDY DOSE~~ | ~~IV~~ | ~~A9544~~ |
| ~~TOSITUMOMAB I-131 THERAPEUTIC~~ | ~~TX DOSE~~ | ~~IV~~ | ~~A9545~~ |
| TOTECT | PER 250 MG | IV | J1190 |
| ~~TRABECTEDIN~~ | ~~0.1 MG~~ | ~~INJ, IV~~ | ~~C9480~~ |
| TRABECTEDIN | 0.1 MG | IV | J9352 |
| TRASTUZUMAB | 10 MG | IV | J9355 |
| TRASYLOL | 10,000 KIU | IV | J0365 |
| TREANDA | 1 MG | IV | J9033 |
| TRELSTAR DEPOT | 3.75 MG | IM | J3315 |
| TRELSTAR DEPOT PLUS DEBIOCLIP KIT | 3.75 MG | IM | J3315 |
| TRELSTAR LA | 3.75 MG | IM | J3315 |
| TREPROSTINIL | 1 MG | SC | J3285 |
| TREPROSTINIL, INHALATION SOLUTION | 1.74 MG | INH | J7686 |

| Drug Name | Unit Per | Route | Code |
|---|---|---|---|
| TRETINOIN | 5 G | OTH | S0117 |
| TRETTEN | 10 IU | IV | J7181 |
| TRI-KORT | 10 MG | IM | J3301 |
| TRIAM-A | 10 MG | IM | J3301 |
| TRIAMCINOLONE ACETONIDE | 10 MG | IM | J3301 |
| TRIAMCINOLONE ACETONIDE, PRESERVATIVE FREE | 1 MG | INJ | J3300 |
| TRIAMCINOLONE DIACETATE | 5 MG | IM | J3302 |
| TRIAMCINOLONE HEXACETONIDE | 5 MG | VAR | J3303 |
| TRIAMCINOLONE, COMPOUNDED, CONCENTRATED | 1 MG | INH | J7683 |
| TRIAMCINOLONE, COMPOUNDED, UNIT DOSE | 1 MG | INH | J7684 |
| TRIBAN | 250 MG | ORAL | Q0173 |
| TRIESENCE | 1 MG | OTH | J3300 |
| TRIFERIC | 0.1 MG | IV | J1443 |
| TRIFLUPROMAZINE HCL | UP TO 20 MG | INJ | J3400 |
| TRILIFON | 4 MG | ORAL | Q0175 |
| TRILOG | 10 MG | IM | J3301 |
| TRILONE | 5 MG | IM | J3302 |
| TRIMETHOBENZAMIDE HCL | 250 MG | ORAL | Q0173 |
| TRIMETHOBENZAMIDE HCL | 200 MG | IM | J3250 |
| TRIMETREXATE GLUCURONATE | 25 MG | IV | J3305 |
| TRIPTORELIN PAMOATE | 3.75 MG | IM | J3315 |
| TRISENOX | 1 MG | IV | J9017 |
| TRIVARIS | 1 MG | VAR | J3300 |
| TROBICIN | 2 G | IM | J3320 |
| TRUSKIN | SQ CM | OTH | Q4167 |
| TRUXADRYL | 50 MG | IV, IM | J1200 |
| TYGACIL | 1 MG | IV | J3243 |
| TYPE A BOTOX | 1 UNIT | IM, OTH | J0585 |
| TYSABRI | 1 MG | IV | J2323 |
| TYVASO | 1.74 MG | INH | J7686 |
| ULTRA-TECHNEKOW | 1 MCI | IV | A9512 |
| ULTRALENTE | 5 U | SC | J1815 |
| ULTRATAG | STUDY DOSE UP TO 30 MCI | IV | A9560 |
| ULTRAVIST 150 | 1 ML | IV | Q9965 |
| ULTRAVIST 240 | 1 ML | IV | Q9966 |
| ULTRAVIST 300 | 1 ML | IV | Q9967 |
| ULTRAVIST 370 | 1 ML | IV | Q9967 |
| UNASYN | 1.5 G | IM, IV | J0295 |
| UNCLASSIFIED BIOLOGICS | | | J3590 |
| UNCLASSIFIED DRUGS OR BIOLOGICALS | VAR | VAR | C9399 |
| ~~UNITE BIOMATRIX~~ | ~~SQ CM~~ | ~~OTH~~ | ~~Q4129~~ |
| UREA | 40 G | IV | J3350 |
| URECHOLINE | UP TO 5 MG | SC | J0520 |
| UROFOLLITROPIN | 75 IU | SC, IM | J3355 |
| UROKINASE | 250,000 IU | IV | J3365 |
| UROKINASE | 5,000 IU | IV | J3364 |
| USTEKINUMAB | 1 MG | SC | J3357 |

© 2016 Optum360, LLC

| Drug Name | Unit Per | Route | Code | Drug Name | Unit Per | Route | Code |
|---|---|---|---|---|---|---|---|
| VALERGEN | 10 MG | IM | J1380 | VIVITROL | 1 MG | IM | J2315 |
| VALIUM | 5 MG | IV, IM | J3360 | VON WILLEBRAND FACTOR (RECOMBINANT) | 1 IU | IV | J7179 |
| VALRUBICIN INTRAVESICAL | 200 MG | OTH | J9357 | VON WILLEBRAND FACTOR COMPLEX (HUMAN) (WILATE) | 1 IU | IV | J7183 |
| VALSTAR | 200 MG | OTH | J9357 | VON WILLEBRAND FACTOR COMPLEX, HUMATE-P | 1 IU | IV | J7187 |
| VANCOCIN | 500 MG | IM, IV | J3370 | VON WILLEBRAND FACTOR VIII COMPLEX, HUMAN | PER FACTOR VIII IU | IV | J7186 |
| VANCOMYCIN HCL | 500 MG | IV, IM | J3370 | VONVENDI | 1 IU | IV | J7179 |
| VANTAS | 50 MG | OTH | J9225 | VORAXAZE | 10 UNITS | IV | C9293 |
| VARUBI | 1 MG | ORAL | J8670 | VORICONAZOLE | 200 MG | IV | J3465 |
| ~~VARUBI~~ | ~~1 MG~~ | ~~ORAL~~ | ~~Q9981~~ | VPRIV | 100 U | IV | J3385 |
| VECTIBIX | 10 MG | IV | J9303 | VUMON | 50 MG | IV | Q2017 |
| VEDOLIZUMAB | 1 MG | IV | J3380 | WEHAMINE | 50 MG | IM, IV | J1240 |
| VELAGLUCERASE ALFA | 100 U | IV | J3385 | WEHDRYL | 50 MG | IM, IV | J1200 |
| VELBAN | I MG | IV | J9360 | WELBUTRIN SR | 150 MG | ORAL | S0106 |
| VELCADE | 0.1 MG | IV | J9041 | WILATE | 1 IU | IV | J7183 |
| VELETRI | 0.5 MG | IV | J1325 | WINRHO SDF | 100 IU | IV | J2792 |
| VELOSULIN | 5 U | SC | J1815 | WOUNDEX | SQ CM | OTH | Q4163 |
| VELOSULIN BR | 5 U | SC | J1815 | WOUNDEX FLOW | 0.5 CC | OTH | Q4162 |
| VENOFER | 1 MG | IV | J1756 | WYCILLIN | 600,000 U | IM, IV | J2510 |
| VENTOLIN NONCOMPOUNDED, CONCENTRATED | 1 MG | INH | J7611 | XCM BIOLOGIC TISSUE MATRIX | SQ CM | OTH | Q4142 |
| VENTOLIN NONCOMPOUNDED, UNIT DOSE | 1 MG | INH | J7613 | XELODA | 500 MG | ORAL | J8521 |
| VEPESID | 50 MG | ORAL | J8560 | XELODA | 150 MG | ORAL | J8520 |
| VEPESID | 10 MG | IV | J9181 | XENON XE-133 | 10 MCI | INH | A9558 |
| VERITAS | SQ CM | OTH | C9354 | XEOMIN | 1 UNIT | IM | J0588 |
| VERSED | 1 MG | IM, IV | J2250 | XGEVA | 1 MG | SC | J0897 |
| VERTEPORFIN | 0.1 MG | IV | J3396 | XIAFLEX | 0.01 MG | OTH | J0775 |
| VFEND | 200 MG | IV | J3465 | XOFIGO | PER MICROCURIE | IV | A9606 |
| VIAGRA | 25 MG | ORAL | S0090 | XOLAIR | 5 MG | SC | J2357 |
| VIBATIV | 10 MG | IV | J3095 | XYLOCAINE | 10 MG | IV | J2001 |
| VIDAZA | 1 MG | SC | J9025 | XYNTHA | 1 IU | IV | J7185 |
| VIDEX | 25 MG | ORAL | S0137 | YERVOY | 1 MG | IV | J9228 |
| VIMIZIM | 1 MG | IV | J1322 | YONDELIS | 0.1 MG | IV | J9352 |
| VIMPAT | 1 MG | IV, ORAL | C9254 | ~~YONDELIS~~ | ~~0.1 MG~~ | ~~INJ, IV~~ | ~~C9480~~ |
| VINBLASTINE SULFATE | 1 MG | IV | J9360 | YTTRIUM 90 IBRITUMOMAB TIUXETAN | TX DOSE UP TO 40 MCI | IV | A9543 |
| VINCASCAR | 1 MG | IV | J9370 | ZALTRAP | 1 MG | IV | J9400 |
| VINCRISTINE SULFATE | 1 MG | IV | J9370 | ZANAMIVIR (BRAND) (DEMONSTRATION PROJECT) | 10 MG | INH | G9034 |
| VINCRISTINE SULFATE LIPOSOME | 5 MG | IV | J9371 | ZANAMIVIR (GENERIC) (DEMONSTRATION PROJECT) | 10 MG | INH | G9018 |
| VINORELBINE TARTRATE | 10 MG | IV | J9390 | ZANOSAR | 1 GM | IV | J9320 |
| VIRILON | 1 CC, 200 MG | IM | J1080 | ZANTAC | 25 MG | INJ | J2780 |
| VISTAJECT-25 | 25 MG | IM | J3410 | ZARXIO | 1 MCG | SC, IV | Q5101 |
| VISTARIL | 25 MG | IM | J3410 | ZEMAIRA | 10 MG | IV | J0256 |
| VISTARIL | 25 MG | ORAL | Q0177 | ZEMPLAR | 1 MCG | IV, IM | J2501 |
| VISTIDE | 375 MG | IV | J0740 | ZENAPAX | 25 MG | OTH | J7513 |
| VISUDYNE | 0.1 MG | IV | J3396 | ZERBAXA | 50 MG/25 MG | IV | J0695 |
| VITAMIN B-12 CYANOCOBALAMIN | 1,000 MCG | IM, SC | J3420 | ZEVALIN | STUDY DOSE UP TO 5 MCI | IV | A9542 |
| VITAMIN B-17 | VAR | INJ | J3570 | | | | |
| VITRASE | 1 USP | OTH | J3471 | | | | |
| VITRASE | 1,000 USP | OTH | J3472 | | | | |
| VITRASERT | 4.5 MG | OTH | J7310 | | | | |
| VITRAVENE | 1.65 MG | OTH | J1452 | | | | |

© 2016 Optum360, LLC

| Drug Name | Unit Per | Route | Code |
|---|---|---|---|
| ZEVALIN DIAGNOSTIC | STUDY DOSE UP TO 5 MCI | IV | A9542 |
| ZEVALIN THERAPEUTIC | TX DOSE UP TO 40 MCI | IV | A9543 |
| ZICONOTIDE | 1 MCG | IT | J2278 |
| ZIDOVUDINE | 100 MG | ORAL | S0104 |
| ZIDOVUDINE | 10 MG | IV | J3485 |
| ZINACEFT | PER 750 MG | IM, IV | J0697 |
| ZINECARD | 250 MG | IV | J1190 |
| ZIPRASIDONE MESYLATE | 10 MG | IM | J3486 |
| ZITHROMAX | 500 MG | IV | J0456 |
| ZITHROMAX | 1 G | ORAL | Q0144 |
| ZIV-AFLIBERCEPT | 1 MG | IV | J9400 |
| ZOFRAN | 4 MG | ORAL | S0119 |
| ZOFRAN | 1 MG | ORAL | Q0162 |
| ZOFRAN | 1 MG | IV | J2405 |
| ZOLADEX | 3.6 MG | SC | J9202 |
| ZOLEDRONIC ACID | 1 MG | IV | J3489 |
| ZOMETA | 1 MG | IV | J3489 |
| ZORBTIVE | 1 MG | SC | J2941 |
| ZORTRESS | 0.25 MG | ORAL | J7527 |
| ZOSYN | 1 G/1.125 GM | IV | J2543 |
| ZOVIRAX | 5 MG | IV | J0133 |
| ZUBSOLV | 1.4 MG | ORAL | J0572 |
| ZUBSOLV | 5.7 MG | ORAL | J0573 |
| ZUPLENZ | 1 MG | ORAL | Q0162 |
| ZUPLENZ | 4 MG | ORAL | S0119 |
| ZYPREXA | 2.5 MG | IM | S0166 |
| ZYPREXA RELPREVV | 1 MG | IM | J2358 |
| ZYVOX | 200 MG | IV | J2020 |

## NOT OTHERWISE CLASSIFIED DRUGS

| Drug Name | Unit Per | Route | Code |
|---|---|---|---|
| ALFENTANIL | 500 MCG | IV | J3490 |
| ALLOPURINOL SODIUM | 500 MG | IV | J3490 |
| AMINOCAPROIC ACID | 250 MG | IV | J3490 |
| AZTREONAM | 500 MG | IM, IV | J3490 |
| BUMETANIDE | 0.25 MG | IM, IV | J3490 |
| BUPIVACAINE, 0.25% | 1 ML | OTH | J3490 |
| BUPIVACAINE, 0.50% | 1 ML | OTH | J3490 |
| BUPIVACAINE, 0.75% | 1 ML | OTH | J3490 |
| CALCIUM CHLORIDE | 100 MG | IV | J3490 |
| CLAVULANTE POTASSIUM/TICARCILLIN DISODIUM | 0.1-3 GM | IV | J3490 |
| CLEVIDIPINE BUTYRATE | 1 MG | IV | J3490 |
| CLINDAMYCIN PHOSPHATE | 150 MG | IV | J3490 |
| COMPOUNDED DRUG, NOT OTHERWISE CLASSIFIED | VAR | VAR | J7999 |
| COPPER SULFATE | 0.4 MG | INJ | J3490 |

| Drug Name | Unit Per | Route | Code |
|---|---|---|---|
| DIAGNOSTIC RADIOPHARMACEUTICAL FOR BETA-AMYLOID PET | STUDY DOSE | IV | A9599 |
| DILTIAZEM HCL | 5 MG | IV | J3490 |
| DOXAPRAM HCL | 20 MG | IV | J3490 |
| DOXYCYCLINE HYCLATE | 100 MG | INJ | J3490 |
| ENALAPRILAT | 1.25 MG | IV | J3490 |
| ESMOLOL HYDROCHLORIDE | 10 MG | IV | J3490 |
| ESOMEPRAZOLE SODIUM | 20 MG | IV | J3490 |
| ETOMIDATE | 2 MG | IV | J3490 |
| FAMOTIDINE | 10 MG | IV | J3490 |
| FLUMAZENIL | 0.1 MG | IV | J3490 |
| FOLIC ACID | 5 MG | SC, IM, IV | J3490 |
| FOSPROPOFOL DISODIUM | 35 MG | IV | J3490 |
| GLUCARPIDASE | 10 U | IV | J3490 |
| GLYCOPYRROLATE | 0.2 MG | IM, IV | J3490 |
| HEXAMINOLEVULINATE HCL | 100 MG PER STUDY DOSE | IV | J3490 |
| INTEGRA MESHED BILAYER WOUND MATRIX | SQ CM | OTH | C9363 |
| LABETALOL HCL | 5 MG | INJ | J3490 |
| METOPROLOL TARTRATE | 1 MG | IV | J3490 |
| METRONIDAZOLE INJ | 500 MG | IV | J3490 |
| MORRHUATE SODIUM | 50 MG | OTH | J3490 |
| NITROGLYCERIN | 5 MG | IV | J3490 |
| OLANZAPINE SHORT ACTING INTRAMUSCULAR INJECTION | 0.5 MG | IM | J3490 |
| PHENYLEPHRINE KETOROLAC | 4 ML | IRR | J3490 |
| RIFAMPIN | 600 MG | IV | J3490 |
| SODIUM ACETATE | 2 MEQ | IV | J3490 |
| SODIUM CHLORIDE, HYPERTONIC (3%-5% INFUSION) | 250 CC | IV | J3490 |
| SULFAMETHOXAZOLE-TRIMETHOPRIM | 80 MG/16 MG | IV | J3490 |
| SURGIMEND | 0.5 SQ CM | OTH | J3490 |
| VASOPRESSIN | 20 UNITS | SC, IM | J3490 |
| VECURONIUM BROMIDE | 1 MG | IV | J3490 |

© 2016 Optum360, LLC

# Appendix 2 — Modifiers

A modifier is a two-position code that is added to the end of a code to clarify the services being billed. Modifiers provide a means by which a service can be altered without changing the procedure code. They add more information, such as the anatomical site, to the code. In addition, they help to eliminate the appearance of duplicate billing and unbundling. Modifiers are used to increase accuracy in reimbursement, coding consistency, editing, and to capture payment data.

| | |
|---|---|
| A1 | Dressing for one wound |
| A2 | Dressing for 2 wounds |
| A3 | Dressing for 3 wounds |
| A4 | Dressing for 4 wounds |
| A5 | Dressing for 5 wounds |
| A6 | Dressing for 6 wounds |
| A7 | Dressing for 7 wounds |
| A8 | Dressing for 8 wounds |
| A9 | Dressing for 9 or more wounds |
| AA | Anesthesia services performed personally by anesthesiologist |
| AD | Medical supervision by a physician: more than 4 concurrent anesthesia procedures |
| AE | Registered dietician |
| AF | Specialty physician |
| AG | Primary physician |
| AH | Clinical psychologist |
| AI | Principal physician of record |
| AJ | Clinical social worker |
| AK | Nonparticipating physician |
| AM | Physician, team member service |
| AO | Alternate payment method declined by provider of service |
| AP | Determination of refractive state was not performed in the course of diagnostic ophthalmological examination |
| AQ | Physician providing a service in an unlisted health professional shortage area (HPSA) |
| AR | Physician provider services in a physician scarcity area |
| AS | Physician assistant, nurse practitioner, or clinical nurse specialist services for assistant at surgery |
| AT | Acute treatment (this modifier should be used when reporting service 98940, 98941, 98942) |
| AU | Item furnished in conjunction with a urological, ostomy, or tracheostomy supply |
| AV | Item furnished in conjunction with a prosthetic device, prosthetic or orthotic |
| AW | Item furnished in conjunction with a surgical dressing |
| AX | Item furnished in conjunction with dialysis services |
| AY | Item or service furnished to an ESRD patient that is not for the treatment of ESRD |
| AZ | Physician providing a service in a dental health professional shortage area for the purpose of an electronic health record incentive payment |
| BA | Item furnished in conjunction with parenteral enteral nutrition (PEN) services |
| BL | Special acquisition of blood and blood products |
| BO | Orally administered nutrition, not by feeding tube |
| BP | The beneficiary has been informed of the purchase and rental options and has elected to purchase the item |
| BR | The beneficiary has been informed of the purchase and rental options and has elected to rent the item |
| BU | The beneficiary has been informed of the purchase and rental options and after 30 days has not informed the supplier of his/her decision |
| CA | Procedure payable only in the inpatient setting when performed emergently on an outpatient who expires prior to admission |
| CB | Service ordered by a renal dialysis facility (RDF) physician as part of the ESRD beneficiary's dialysis benefit, is not part of the composite rate, and is separately reimbursable |
| CC | Procedure code change (use CC when the procedure code submitted was changed either for administrative reasons or because an incorrect code was filed) |
| CD | AMCC test has been ordered by an ESRD facility or MCP physician that is part of the composite rate and is not separately billable |
| CE | AMCC test has been ordered by an ESRD facility or MCP physician that is a composite rate test but is beyond the normal frequency covered under the rate and is separately reimbursable based on medical necessity |
| CF | AMCC test has been ordered by an ESRD facility or MCP physician that is not part of the composite rate and is separately billable |
| CG | Policy criteria applied |
| CH | 0 percent impaired, limited or restricted |
| CI | At least 1 percent but less than 20 percent impaired, limited or restricted |
| CJ | At least 20 percent but less than 40 percent impaired, limited or restricted |
| CK | At least 40 percent but less than 60 percent impaired, limited or restricted |
| CL | At least 60 percent but less than 80 percent impaired, limited or restricted |
| CM | At least 80 percent but less than 100 percent impaired, limited or restricted |
| CN | 100 percent impaired, limited or restricted |
| CP | Adjunctive service related to a procedure assigned to a comprehensive ambulatory payment classification (C-APC) procedure, but reported on a different claim |
| CR | Catastrophe/Disaster related |
| CS | Item or service related, in whole or in part, to an illness, injury, or condition that was caused by or exacerbated by the effects, direct or indirect, of the 2010 oil spill in the gulf of Mexico, including but not limited to subsequent clean up activities |
| CT | Computed tomography services furnished using equipment that does not meet each of the attributes of the national electrical manufacturers association (NEMA) XR-29-2013 standard |
| DA | Oral health assessment by a licensed health professional other than a dentist |
| E1 | Upper left, eyelid |
| E2 | Lower left, eyelid |
| E3 | Upper right, eyelid |
| E4 | Lower right, eyelid |

| | |
|---|---|
| **EA** | Erythropoetic stimulating agent (ESA) administered to treat anemia due to anticancer chemotherapy |
| **EB** | Erythropoetic stimulating agent (ESA) administered to treat anemia due to anticancer radiotherapy |
| **EC** | Erythropoetic stimulating agent (ESA) administered to treat anemia not due to anticancer radiotherapy or anticancer chemotherapy |
| **ED** | Hematocrit level has exceeded 39% (or hemoglobin level has exceeded 13.0 G/dl) for 3 or more consecutive billing cycles immediately prior to and including the current cycle |
| **EE** | Hematocrit level has not exceeded 39% (or hemoglobin level has not exceeded 13.0 G/dl) for 3 or more consecutive billing cycles immediately prior to and including the current cycle |
| **EJ** | Subsequent claims for a defined course of therapy, e.g., EPO, sodium hyaluronate, infliximab |
| **EM** | Emergency reserve supply (for ESRD benefit only) |
| **EP** | Service provided as part of Medicaid early periodic screening diagnosis and treatment (EPSDT) program |
| **ET** | Emergency services |
| **EX** | Expatriate beneficiary |
| **EY** | No physician or other licensed health care provider order for this item or service |
| **F1** | Left hand, 2nd digit |
| **F2** | Left hand, third digit |
| **F3** | Left hand, 4th digit |
| **F4** | Left hand, fifth digit |
| **F5** | Right hand, thumb |
| **F6** | Right hand, 2nd digit |
| **F7** | Right hand, third digit |
| **F8** | Right hand, 4th digit |
| **F9** | Right hand, 5th digit |
| **FA** | Left hand, thumb |
| **FB** | Item provided without cost to provider, supplier or practitioner, or full credit received for replaced device (examples, but not limited to, covered under warranty, replaced due to defect, free samples) |
| **FC** | Partial credit received for replaced device |
| **FP** | Service provided as part of family planning program |
| ● **FX** | X-ray taken using film |
| **G1** | Most recent URR reading of less than 60 |
| **G2** | Most recent URR reading of 60 to 64.9 |
| **G3** | Most recent URR reading of 65 to 69.9 |
| **G4** | Most recent URR reading of 70 to 74.9 |
| **G5** | Most recent URR reading of 75 or greater |
| **G6** | ESRD patient for whom less than 6 dialysis sessions have been provided in a month |
| **G7** | Pregnancy resulted from rape or incest or pregnancy certified by physician as life threatening |
| **G8** | Monitored anesthesia care (MAC) for deep complex, complicated, or markedly invasive surgical procedure |
| **G9** | Monitored anesthesia care for patient who has history of severe cardiopulmonary condition |
| **GA** | Waiver of liability statement issued as required by payer policy, individual case |
| **GB** | Claim being resubmitted for payment because it is no longer covered under a global payment demonstration |
| **GC** | This service has been performed in part by a resident under the direction of a teaching physician |
| **GD** | Units of service exceeds medically unlikely edit value and represents reasonable and necessary services |
| **GE** | This service has been performed by a resident without the presence of a teaching physician under the primary care exception |
| **GF** | Nonphysician (e.g., nurse practitioner (NP), certified registered nurse anesthetist (CRNA), certified registered nurse (CRN), clinical nurse specialist (CNS), physician assistant (PA)) services in a critical access hospital |
| **GG** | Performance and payment of a screening mammogram and diagnostic mammogram on the same patient, same day |
| **GH** | Diagnostic mammogram converted from screening mammogram on same day |
| **GJ** | "Opt out" physician or practitioner emergency or urgent service |
| **GK** | Reasonable and necessary item/service associated with GA or GZ modifier |
| **GL** | Medically unnecessary upgrade provided instead of nonupgraded item, no charge, no advance beneficiary notice (ABN) |
| **GM** | Multiple patients on one ambulance trip |
| **GN** | Services delivered under an outpatient speech language pathology plan of care |
| **GO** | Services delivered under an outpatient occupational therapy plan of care |
| **GP** | Services delivered under an outpatient physical therapy plan of care |
| **GQ** | Via asynchronous telecommunications system |
| **GR** | This service was performed in whole or in part by a resident in a department of veterans affairs medical center or clinic, supervised in accordance with VA policy |
| **GS** | Dosage of erythropoietin stimulating agent has been reduced and maintained in response to hematocrit or hemoglobin level |
| **GT** | Via interactive audio and video telecommunication systems |
| **GU** | Waiver of liability statement issued as required by payer policy, routine notice |
| **GV** | Attending physician not employed or paid under arrangement by the patient's hospice provider |
| **GW** | Service not related to the hospice patient's terminal condition |
| **GX** | Notice of liability issued, voluntary under payer policy |
| **GY** | Item or service statutorily excluded, does not meet the definition of any Medicare benefit or for non-Medicare insurers, is not a contract benefit |
| **GZ** | Item or service expected to be denied as not reasonable and necessary |
| **H9** | Court-ordered |
| **HA** | Child/adolescent program |
| **HB** | Adult program, nongeriatric |
| **HC** | Adult program, geriatric |
| **HD** | Pregnant/parenting women's program |
| **HE** | Mental health program |
| **HF** | Substance abuse program |
| **HG** | Opioid addiction treatment program |
| **HH** | Integrated mental health/substance abuse program |
| **HI** | Integrated mental health and intellectual disability/developmental disabilities program |
| **HJ** | Employee assistance program |
| **HK** | Specialized mental health programs for high-risk populations |
| **HL** | Intern |

| | |
|---|---|
| HM | Less than bachelor degree level |
| HN | Bachelors degree level |
| HO | Masters degree level |
| HP | Doctoral level |
| HQ | Group setting |
| HR | Family/couple with client present |
| HS | Family/couple without client present |
| HT | Multi-disciplinary team |
| HU | Funded by child welfare agency |
| HV | Funded state addictions agency |
| HW | Funded by state mental health agency |
| HX | Funded by county/local agency |
| HY | Funded by juvenile justice agency |
| HZ | Funded by criminal justice agency |
| J1 | Competitive acquisition program no-pay submission for a prescription number |
| J2 | Competitive acquisition program, restocking of emergency drugs after emergency administration |
| J3 | Competitive acquisition program (CAP), drug not available through CAP as written, reimbursed under average sales price methodology |
| J4 | DMEPOS item subject to DMEPOS competitive bidding program that is furnished by a hospital upon discharge |
| JA | Administered intravenously |
| JB | Administered subcutaneously |
| JC | Skin substitute used as a graft |
| JD | Skin substitute not used as a graft |
| JE | Administered via dialysate |
| JW | Drug amount discarded/not administered to any patient |
| K0 | Lower extremity prosthesis functional level 0 - does not have the ability or potential to ambulate or transfer safely with or without assistance and a prosthesis does not enhance their quality of life or mobility |
| K1 | Lower extremity prosthesis functional level 1 - has the ability or potential to use a prosthesis for transfers or ambulation on level surfaces at fixed cadence, typical of the limited and unlimited household ambulator. |
| K2 | Lower extremity prosthesis functional level 2 - has the ability or potential for ambulation with the ability to traverse low level environmental barriers such as curbs, stairs or uneven surfaces. typical of the limited community ambulator. |
| K3 | Lower extremity prosthesis functional level 3 - has the ability or potential for ambulation with variable cadence, typical of the community ambulator who has the ability to traverse most environmental barriers and may have vocational, therapeutic, or exercise activity that demands prosthetic utilization beyond simple locomotion |
| K4 | Lower extremity prosthesis functional level 4 - has the ability or potential for prosthetic ambulation that exceeds the basic ambulation skills, exhibiting high impact, stress, or energy levels, typical of the prosthetic demands of the child, active adult, or athlete. |
| KA | Add on option/accessory for wheelchair |
| KB | Beneficiary requested upgrade for ABN, more than 4 modifiers identified on claim |
| KC | Replacement of special power wheelchair interface |
| KD | Drug or biological infused through DME |
| KE | Bid under round one of the DMEPOS competitive bidding program for use with noncompetitive bid base equipment |
| KF | Item designated by FDA as class III device |

| | |
|---|---|
| KG | DMEPOS item subject to DMEPOS competitive bidding program number 1 |
| KH | DMEPOS item, initial claim, purchase or first month rental |
| KI | DMEPOS item, 2nd or 3rd month rental |
| KJ | DMEPOS item, parenteral enteral nutrition (PEN) pump or capped rental, months 4 to 15 |
| KK | DMEPOS item subject to DMEPOS competitive bidding program number 2 |
| KL | DMEPOS item delivered via mail |
| KM | Replacement of facial prosthesis including new impression/moulage |
| KN | Replacement of facial prosthesis using previous master model |
| KO | Single drug unit dose formulation |
| KP | First drug of a multiple drug unit dose formulation |
| KQ | Second or subsequent drug of a multiple drug unit dose formulation |
| KR | Rental item, billing for partial month |
| KS | Glucose monitor supply for diabetic beneficiary not treated with insulin |
| KT | Beneficiary resides in a competitive bidding area and travels outside that competitive bidding area and receives a competitive bid item. |
| KU | DMEPOS item subject to DMEPOS competitive bidding program number 3 |
| KV | DMEPOS item subject to DMEPOS competitive bidding program that is furnished as part of a professional service |
| KW | DMEPOS item subject to DMEPOS competitive bidding program number 4 |
| KX | Requirements specified in the medical policy have been met |
| KY | DMEPOS item subject to DMEPOS competitive bidding program number 5 |
| KZ | New coverage not implemented by managed care |
| L1 | ~~Provider attestation that the hospital laboratory test(s) is not packaged under the hospital OPPS~~ |
| LC | Left circumflex coronary artery |
| LD | Left anterior descending coronary artery |
| LL | Lease/rental (use the LL modifier when DME equipment rental is to be applied against the purchase price) |
| LM | Left main coronary artery |
| LR | Laboratory round trip |
| LS | FDA-monitored intraocular lens implant |
| LT | Left side (used to identify procedures performed on the left side of the body) |
| M2 | Medicare secondary payer (MSP) |
| MS | Six month maintenance and servicing fee for reasonable and necessary parts and labor which are not covered under any manufacturer or supplier warranty |
| NB | Nebulizer system, any type, FDA-cleared for use with specific drug |
| NR | New when rented (use the NR modifier when DME which was new at the time of rental is subsequently purchased) |
| NU | New equipment |
| P1 | A normal healthy patient |
| P2 | A patient with mild systemic disease |
| P3 | A patient with severe systemic disease |
| P4 | A patient with severe systemic disease that is a constant threat to life |

| | | |
|---|---|---|
| P5 | A moribund patient who is not expected to survive without the operation |
| P6 | A declared brain-dead patient whose organs are being removed for donor purposes |
| PA | Surgical or other invasive procedure on wrong body part |
| PB | Surgical or other invasive procedure on wrong patient |
| PC | Wrong surgery or other invasive procedure on patient |
| PD | Diagnostic or related non diagnostic item or service provided in a wholly owned or operated entity to a patient who is admitted as an inpatient within 3 days |
| PI | Positron emission tomography (PET) or PET/computed tomography (CT) to inform the initial treatment strategy of tumors that are biopsy proven or strongly suspected of being cancerous based on other diagnostic testing |
| PL | Progressive addition lenses |
| PM | Post mortem |
| ● PN | Non-excepted service provided at an off-campus, outpatient, provider-based department of a hospital |
| ▲ PO | Excepted service provided at an off-campus, outpatient, provider-based department of a hospital |
| PS | Positron emission tomography (PET) or PET/computed tomography (CT) to inform the subsequent treatment strategy of cancerous tumors when the beneficiary's treating physician determines that the PET study is needed to inform subsequent anti-tumor strategy |
| PT | Colorectal cancer screening test; converted to diagnostic test or other procedure |
| Q0 | Investigational clinical service provided in a clinical research study that is in an approved clinical research study |
| Q1 | Routine clinical service provided in a clinical research study that is in an approved clinical research study |
| ▲ Q2 | Demonstration procedure/service |
| Q3 | Live kidney donor surgery and related services |
| Q4 | Service for ordering/referring physician qualifies as a service exemption |
| Q5 | Service furnished by a substitute physician under a reciprocal billing arrangement |
| Q6 | Service furnished by a locum tenens physician |
| Q7 | One Class A finding |
| Q8 | Two Class B findings |
| Q9 | One class B and 2 class C findings |
| QC | Single channel monitoring |
| QD | Recording and storage in solid state memory by a digital recorder |
| QE | Prescribed amount of oxygen is less than 1 liter per minute (LPM) |
| QF | Prescribed amount of oxygen exceeds 4 liters per minute (LPM) and portable oxygen is prescribed |
| QG | Prescribed amount of oxygen is greater than 4 liters per minute (LPM) |
| QH | Oxygen conserving device is being used with an oxygen delivery system |
| QJ | Services/items provided to a prisoner or patient in state or local custody, however the state or local government, as applicable, meets the requirements in 42 CFR 411.4(B) |
| QK | Medical direction of 2, 3, or 4 concurrent anesthesia procedures involving qualified individuals |
| QL | Patient pronounced dead after ambulance called |
| QM | Ambulance service provided under arrangement by a provider of services |
| QN | Ambulance service furnished directly by a provider of services |
| QP | Documentation is on file showing that the laboratory test(s) was ordered individually or ordered as a CPT-recognized panel other than automated profile codes 80002-80019, G0058, G0059, and G0060 |
| QS | Monitored anesthesiology care services (can be billed by a qualified nonphysician anesthetist or a physician) |
| QT | Recording and storage on tape by an analog tape recorder |
| QW | CLIA waived test |
| QX | Qualified nonphysician anesthetist with medical direction by a physician |
| QY | Medical direction of one qualified nonphysician anesthetist by an anesthesiologist |
| QZ | CRNA without medical direction by a physician. |
| RA | Replacement of a DME, orthotic or prosthetic item |
| RB | Replacement of a part of a DME, orthotic or prosthetic item furnished as part of a repair |
| RC | Right coronary artery |
| RD | Drug provided to beneficiary, but not administered "incident-to" |
| RE | Furnished in full compliance with FDA-mandated risk evaluation and mitigation strategy (REMS) |
| RI | Ramus intermedius coronary artery |
| RR | Rental (use the RR modifier when DME is to be rented) |
| RT | Right side (used to identify procedures performed on the right side of the body) |
| SA | Nurse practitioner rendering service in collaboration with a physician |
| SB | Nurse midwife |
| SC | Medically necessary service or supply |
| SD | Services provided by registered nurse with specialized, highly technical home infusion training |
| SE | State and/or federally-funded programs/services |
| SF | Second opinion ordered by a professional review organization (PRO) per section 9401, p.l. 99-272 (100% reimbursement - no Medicare deductible or coinsurance) |
| SG | Ambulatory surgical center (ASC) facility service |
| SH | Second concurrently administered infusion therapy |
| SJ | Third or more concurrently administered infusion therapy |
| SK | Member of high risk population (use only with codes for immunization) |
| SL | State supplied vaccine |
| SM | Second surgical opinion |
| SN | Third surgical opinion |
| SQ | Item ordered by home health |
| SS | Home infusion services provided in the infusion suite of the IV therapy provider |
| ST | Related to trauma or injury |
| SU | Procedure performed in physician's office (to denote use of facility and equipment) |
| SV | Pharmaceuticals delivered to patient's home but not utilized |
| SW | Services provided by a certified diabetic educator |
| SY | Persons who are in close contact with member of high-risk population (use only with codes for immunization) |
| SZ | Habilitative services |
| T1 | Left foot, 2nd digit |
| T2 | Left foot, 3rd digit |
| T3 | Left foot, 4th digit |
| T4 | Left foot, 5th digit |

© 2016 Optum360, LLC

| | |
|---|---|
| **T5** | Right foot, great toe |
| **T6** | Right foot, 2nd digit |
| **T7** | Right foot, 3rd digit |
| **T8** | Right foot, 4th digit |
| **T9** | Right foot, 5th digit |
| **TA** | Left foot, great toe |
| **TC** | Technical component. Under certain circumstances, a charge may be made for the technical component alone. Under those circumstances the technical component charge is identified by adding modifier 'TC' to the usual procedure number. Technical component charges are institutional charges and not billed separately by physicians. However, portable x-ray suppliers only bill for technical component and should utilize modifier TC. The charge data from portable x-ray suppliers will then be used to build customary and prevailing profiles. |
| **TD** | RN |
| **TE** | LPN/LVN |
| **TF** | Intermediate level of care |
| **TG** | Complex/high tech level of care |
| **TH** | Obstetrical treatment/services, prenatal or postpartum |
| **TJ** | Program group, child and/or adolescent |
| **TK** | Extra patient or passenger, nonambulance |
| **TL** | Early intervention/individualized family service plan (IFSP) |
| **TM** | Individualized education program (IEP) |
| **TN** | Rural/outside providers' customary service area |
| **TP** | Medical transport, unloaded vehicle |
| **TQ** | Basic life support transport by a volunteer ambulance provider |
| **TR** | School-based individualized education program (IEP) services provided outside the public school district responsible for the student |
| **TS** | Follow-up service |
| **TT** | Individualized service provided to more than one patient in same setting |
| **TU** | Special payment rate, overtime |
| **TV** | Special payment rates, holidays/weekends |
| **TW** | Back-up equipment |
| **U1** | Medicaid level of care 1, as defined by each state |
| **U2** | Medicaid level of care 2, as defined by each state |
| **U3** | Medicaid level of care 3, as defined by each state |
| **U4** | Medicaid level of care 4, as defined by each state |
| **U5** | Medicaid level of care 5, as defined by each state |

| | |
|---|---|
| **U6** | Medicaid level of care 6, as defined by each state |
| **U7** | Medicaid level of care 7, as defined by each state |
| **U8** | Medicaid level of care 8, as defined by each state |
| **U9** | Medicaid level of care 9, as defined by each state |
| **UA** | Medicaid level of care 10, as defined by each state |
| **UB** | Medicaid level of care 11, as defined by each state |
| **UC** | Medicaid level of care 12, as defined by each state |
| **UD** | Medicaid level of care 13, as defined by each state |
| **UE** | Used durable medical equipment |
| **UF** | Services provided in the morning |
| **UG** | Services provided in the afternoon |
| **UH** | Services provided in the evening |
| **UJ** | Services provided at night |
| **UK** | Services provided on behalf of the client to someone other than the client (collateral relationship) |
| **UN** | 2 patients served |
| **UP** | 3 patients served |
| **UQ** | 4 patients served |
| **UR** | 5 patients served |
| **US** | 6 or more patients served |
| ● **V1** | Demonstration modifier 1 |
| ● **V2** | Demonstration modifier 2 |
| ● **V3** | Demonstration modifier 3 |
| **V5** | Vascular catheter (alone or with any other vascular access) |
| **V6** | Arteriovenous graft (or other vascular access not including a vascular catheter) |
| **V7** | Arteriovenous fistula only (in use with 2 needles) |
| **VP** | Aphakic patient |
| **XE** | Separate encounter, a service that is distinct because it occurred during a separate encounter |
| **XP** | Separate practitioner, a service that is distinct because it was performed by a different practitioner |
| **XS** | Separate structure, a service that is distinct because it was performed on a separate organ/structure |
| **XU** | Unusual non-overlapping service, the use of a service that is distinct because it does not overlap usual components of the main service |
| **ZA** | Novartis/Sandoz |
| ● **ZB** | Pfizer/Hospira |

# Appendix 3 — Abbreviations and Acronyms

## HCPCS Abbreviations and Acronyms

The following abbreviations and acronyms are used in the HCPCS descriptions:

| | |
|---|---|
| / | or |
| < | less than |
| <= | less than equal to |
| > | greater than |
| >= | greater than equal to |
| AC | alternating current |
| AFO | ankle-foot orthosis |
| AICC | anti-inhibitor coagulant complex |
| AK | above the knee |
| AKA | above knee amputation |
| ALS | advanced life support |
| AMP | ampule |
| ART | artery |
| ART | Arterial |
| ASC | ambulatory surgery center |
| ATT | attached |
| A-V | Arteriovenous |
| AVF | arteriovenous fistula |
| BICROS | bilateral routing of signals |
| BK | below the knee |
| BLS | basic life support |
| BMI | body mass index |
| BP | blood pressure |
| BTE | behind the ear (hearing aid) |
| CAPD | continuous ambulatory peritoneal dialysis |
| Carb | carbohydrate |
| CBC | complete blood count |
| cc | cubic centimeter |
| CCPD | continuous cycling peritoneal analysis |
| CHF | congestive heart failure |
| CIC | completely in the canal (hearing aid) |
| CIM | Coverage Issue Manual |
| Clsd | closed |
| cm | centimeter |
| CMN | certificate of medical necessity |
| CMS | Centers for Medicare and Medicaid Services |
| CMV | Cytomegalovirus |
| Conc | concentrate |
| Conc | concentrated |
| Cont | continuous |
| CP | clinical psychologist |
| CPAP | continuous positive airway pressure |
| CPT | Current Procedural Terminology |
| CRF | chronic renal failure |
| CRNA | certified registered nurse anesthetist |
| CROS | contralateral routing of signals |
| CSW | clinical social worker |
| CT | computed tomography |
| CTLSO | cervical-thoracic-lumbar-sacral orthosis |
| cu | cubic |

| | |
|---|---|
| DC | direct current |
| DI | diurnal rhythm |
| Dx | diagnosis |
| DLI | donor leukocyte infusion |
| DME | durable medical equipment |
| DME MAC | durable medical equipment Medicare administrative contractor |
| DMEPOS | Durable Medical Equipment, Prosthestics, Orthotics and Other Supplies |
| DMERC | durable medical equipment regional carrier |
| DR | diagnostic radiology |
| DX | diagnostic |
| e.g. | for example |
| Ea | each |
| ECF | extended care facility |
| EEG | electroencephalogram |
| EKG | electrocardiogram |
| EMG | electromyography |
| EO | elbow orthosis |
| EP | electrophysiologic |
| EPO | epoetin alfa |
| EPSDT | early periodic screening, diagnosis and treatment |
| ESRD | end-stage renal disease |
| Ex | extended |
| Exper | experimental |
| Ext | external |
| F | french |
| FDA | Food and Drug Administration |
| FDG-PET | Positron emission with tomography with 18 fluorodeoxyglucose |
| Fem | female |
| FO | finger orthosis |
| FPD | fixed partial denture |
| Fr | french |
| ft | foot |
| G-CSF | filgrastim (granulocyte colony-stimulating factor) |
| gm | gram (g) |
| H2O | water |
| HCl | hydrochloric acid, hydrochloride |
| HCPCS | Healthcare Common Procedural Coding System |
| HCT | hematocrit |
| HFO | hand-finger orthosis |
| HHA | home health agency |
| HI | high |
| HI-LO | high-low |
| HIT | home infusion therapy |
| HKAFO | hip-knee-ankle foot orthosis |
| HLA | human leukocyte antigen |
| HMES | heat and moisture exchange system |
| HNPCC | hereditary non-polyposis colorectal cancer |
| HO | hip orthosis |
| HPSA | health professional shortage area |
| HST | home sleep test |
| IA | intra-arterial administration |
| ip | interphalangeal |

| | | | | |
|---|---|---|---|---|
| I-131 | Iodine 131 | | OSA | obstructive sleep apnea |
| ICF | intermediate care facility | | Ost | ostomy |
| ICU | intensive care unit | | OTH | other routes of administration |
| IM | intramuscular | | oz | ounce |
| in | inch | | PA | physician's assistant |
| INF | infusion | | PAR | parenteral |
| INH | inhalation solution | | PCA | patient controlled analgesia |
| INJ | injection | | PCH | pouch |
| IOL | intraocular lens | | PEN | parenteral and enteral nutrition |
| IPD | intermittent peritoneal dialysis | | PENS | percutaneous electrical nerve stimulation |
| IPPB | intermittent positive pressure breathing | | PET | positron emission tomography |
| IT | intrathecal administration | | PHP | pre-paid health plan |
| ITC | in the canal (hearing aid) | | PHP | physician hospital plan |
| ITE | in the ear (hearing aid) | | PI | paramedic intercept |
| IU | international units | | PICC | peripherally inserted central venous catheter |
| IV | intravenous | | PKR | photorefractive keratotomy |
| IVF | in vitro fertilization | | Pow | powder |
| KAFO | knee-ankle-foot orthosis | | PQRS | Physician Quality Reporting System |
| KO | knee orthosis | | PRK | photoreactive keratectomy |
| KOH | potassium hydroxide | | PRO | peer review organization |
| L | left | | PSA | prostate specific antigen |
| LASIK | laser in situ keratomileusis | | PTB | patellar tendon bearing |
| LAUP | laser assisted uvulopalatoplasty | | PTK | phototherapeutic keratectomy |
| lbs | pounds | | PVC | polyvinyl chloride |
| LDL | low density lipoprotein | | R | right |
| LDS | lipodystrophy syndrome | | Repl | replace |
| Lo | low | | RN | registered nurse |
| LPM | liters per minute | | RP | retrograde pyelogram |
| LPN/LVN | Licensed Practical Nurse/Licensed Vocational Nurse | | Rx | prescription |
| LSO | lumbar-sacral orthosis | | SACH | solid ankle, cushion heel |
| MAC | Medicare administrative contractor | | SC | subcutaneous |
| mp | metacarpophalangeal | | SCT | specialty care transport |
| mcg | microgram | | SEO | shoulder-elbow orthosis |
| mCi | millicurie | | SEWHO | shoulder-elbow-wrist-hand orthosis |
| MCM | Medicare Carriers Manual | | SEXA | single energy x-ray absorptiometry |
| MCP | metacarparpophalangeal joint | | SGD | speech generating device |
| MCP | monthly capitation payment | | SGD | sinus rhythm |
| mEq | milliequivalent | | SM | samarium |
| MESA | microsurgical epididymal sperm aspiration | | SNCT | sensory nerve conduction test |
| mg | milligram | | SNF | skilled nursing facility |
| mgs | milligrams | | SO | sacroilliac othrosis |
| MHT | megahertz | | SO | shoulder orthosis |
| ml | milliliter | | Sol | solution |
| mm | millimeter | | SQ | square |
| mmHg | millimeters of Mercury | | SR | screen |
| MRA | magnetic resonance angiography | | ST | standard |
| MRI | magnetic resonance imaging | | ST | sustained release |
| NA | sodium | | Syr | syrup |
| NCI | National Cancer Institute | | TABS | tablets |
| NEC | not elsewhere classified | | Tc | Technetium |
| NG | nasogastric | | Tc 99m | technetium isotope |
| NH | nursing home | | TENS | transcutaneous electrical nerve stimulator |
| NMES | neuromuscular electrical stimulation | | THKAO | thoracic-hip-knee-ankle orthosis |
| NOC | not otherwise classified | | TLSO | thoracic-lumbar-sacral-orthosis |
| NOS | not otherwise specified | | TM | temporomandibular |
| O2 | oxygen | | TMJ | temporomandibular joint |
| OBRA | Omnibus Budget Reconciliation Act | | TPN | total parenteral nutrition |
| OMT | osteopathic manipulation therapy | | U | unit |
| OPPS | outpatient prospective payment system | | uCi | microcurie |
| ORAL | oral administration | | VAR | various routes of administration |

© 2016 Optum360, LLC

| | |
|---|---|
| w | with |
| w/ | with |
| w/o | without |
| WAK | wearable artificial kidney |
| wc | wheelchair |
| WHFO | wrist-hand-finger orthotic |
| Wk | week |
| w/o | without |
| Xe | xenon (isotope mass of xenon 133) |

# Appendix 4 — Internet-only Manuals (IOMs)

The Centers for Medicare and Medicaid Services restructured its paper-based manual system as a web-based system on October 1, 2003. Called the online CMS manual system, it combines all of the various program instructions into Internet-only Manuals (IOMs), which are used by all CMS programs and contractors. In many instances, the references from the online manuals in appendix 4 contain a mention of the old paper manuals from which the current information was obtained when the manuals were converted. This information is shown in the header of the text, in the following format, when applicable, as A3-3101, HO-210, and B3-2049. Complete versions of all of the manuals can be found at http://www.cms.gov/manuals.

Effective with implementation of the IOMs, the former method of publishing program memoranda (PMs) to communicate program instructions was replaced by the following four templates:

*   One-time notification
*   Manual revisions
*   Business requirements
*   Confidential requirements

The web-based system has been organized by functional area (e.g., eligibility, entitlement, claims processing, benefit policy, program integrity) in an effort to eliminate redundancy within the manuals, simplify updating, and make CMS program instructions available more quickly. The web-based system contains the functional areas included below:

| | |
|---|---|
| Pub. 100 | Introduction |
| Pub. 100-01 | Medicare General Information, Eligibility, and Entitlement Manual |
| Pub. 100-02 | Medicare Benefit Policy Manual |
| Pub. 100-03 | Medicare National Coverage Determinations (NCD) Manual |
| Pub. 100-04 | Medicare Claims Processing Manual |
| Pub. 100-05 | Medicare Secondary Payer Manual |
| Pub. 100-06 | Medicare Financial Management Manual |
| Pub. 100-07 | State Operations Manual |
| Pub. 100-08 | Medicare Program Integrity Manual |
| Pub. 100-09 | Medicare Contractor Beneficiary and Provider Communications Manual |
| Pub. 100-10 | Quality Improvement Organization Manual |
| Pub. 100-11 | Programs of All-Inclusive Care for the Elderly (PACE) Manual |
| Pub. 100-12 | State Medicaid Manual (under development) |
| Pub. 100-13 | Medicaid State Children's Health Insurance Program (under development) |
| Pub. 100-14 | Medicare ESRD Network Organizations Manual |
| Pub. 100-15 | Medicaid Integrity Program (MIP) |
| Pub. 100-16 | Medicare Managed Care Manual |
| Pub. 100-17 | CMS/Business Partners Systems Security Manual |
| Pub. 100-18 | Medicare Prescription Drug Benefit Manual |
| Pub. 100-19 | Demonstrations |
| Pub. 100-20 | One-Time Notification |
| Pub. 100-21 | Recurring Update Notification |
| Pub. 100-22 | Medicare Quality Reporting Incentive Programs Manual |
| Pub. 100-24 | State Buy-In Manual |
| Pub. 100-25 | Information Security Acceptable Risk Safeguards Manual |

A brief description of the Medicare manuals primarily used for *CPC Expert* follows:

The *National Coverage Determinations Manual* (NCD), is organized according to categories such as diagnostic services, supplies, and medical procedures.

The table of contents lists each category and subject within that category. Revision transmittals identify any new or background material, recap the changes, and provide an effective date for the change.

When complete, the manual will contain two chapters. Chapter 1 currently includes a description of CMS's national coverage determinations. When available, chapter 2 will contain a list of HCPCS codes related to each coverage determination. The manual is organized in accordance with CPT category sequences.

The *Medicare Benefit Policy Manual* contains Medicare general coverage instructions that are not national coverage determinations. As a general rule, in the past these instructions have been found in chapter II of the *Medicare Carriers Manual*, the *Medicare Intermediary Manual*, other provider manuals, and program memoranda.

The *Medicare Claims Processing Manual* contains instructions for processing claims for contractors and providers.

The *Medicare Program Integrity Manual* communicates the priorities and standards for the Medicare integrity programs.

## 100-01, 3, 20.5

### Blood Deductibles (Part A and Part B)
Program payment may not be made for the first 3 pints of whole blood or equivalent units of packed red cells received under Part A and Part B combined in a calendar year. However, blood processing (e.g., administration, storage) is not subject to the deductible.

The blood deductibles are in addition to any other applicable deductible and coinsurance amounts for which the patient is responsible.

The deductible applies only to the first 3 pints of blood furnished in a calendar year, even if more than one provider furnished blood.

## 100-01, 3, 20.5.2

### Part B Blood Deductible
Blood is furnished on an outpatient basis or is subject to the Part B blood deductible and is counted toward the combined limit. It should be noted that payment for blood may be made to the hospital under Part B only for blood furnished in an outpatient setting. Blood is not covered for inpatient Part B services.

## 100-01, 3, 20.5.3

### Items Subject to Blood Deductibles
The blood deductibles apply only to whole blood and packed red cells. The term whole blood means human blood from which none of the liquid or cellular components have been removed. Where packed red cells are furnished, a unit of packed red cells is considered equivalent to a pint of whole blood. Other components of blood such as platelets, fibrinogen, plasma, gamma globulin, and serum albumin are not subject to the blood deductible. However, these components of blood are covered as biologicals.

Refer to Pub. 100-04, Medicare Claims Processing Manual, chapter 4, Sec.231 regarding billing for blood and blood products under the Hospital Outpatient Prospective Payment System (OPPS).

## 100-01, 3, 30

### Outpatient Mental Health Treatment Limitation
Regardless of the actual expenses a beneficiary incurs in connection with the treatment of mental, psychoneurotic, and personality disorders while the beneficiary is not an inpatient of a hospital at the time such expenses are incurred, the amount of those expenses that may be recognized for Part B deductible and payment purposes is limited to 62.5 percent of the Medicare approved amount for those services. The limitation is called the outpatient mental health treatment limitation (the limitation). The 62.5 percent limitation has been in place since the inception of the Medicare Part B program and it will remain effective at this percentage amount until January 1, 2010. However, effective January 1, 2010, through January 1, 2014, the limitation will be phased out as follows:

- January 1, 2010–December 31, 2011, the limitation percentage is 68.75%. (Medicare pays 55% and the patient pays 45%).

- January 1, 2012–December 31, 2012, the limitation percentage is 75%. (Medicare pays 60% and the patient pays 40%).

- January 1, 2013–December 31, 2013, the limitation percentage is 81.25%. (Medicare pays 65% and the patient pays 35%).

- January 1, 2014–onward, the limitation percentage is 100%. (Medicare pays 80% and the patient pays 20%).

For additional details concerning the outpatient mental health treatment limitation, please see the Medicare Claims Processing Manual, Publication 100-04, chapter 9, section 60 and chapter 12, section 210.

## 100-01, 3, 30.3

### Diagnostic Services

The mental health limitation does not apply to tests and evaluations performed to establish or confirm the patient's diagnosis. Diagnostic services include psychiatric or psychological tests and interpretations, diagnostic consultations, and initial evaluations. However, testing services performed to evaluate a patient's progress during treatment are considered part of treatment and are subject to the limitation.

## 100-02, 1, 10

### Covered Inpatient Hospital Services Covered Under Part A

A3-3101, HO-210

Patients covered under hospital insurance are entitled to have payment made on their behalf for inpatient hospital services. (Inpatient hospital services do not include extended care services provided by hospitals pursuant to swing bed approvals. See Pub. 100-01, Chapter 8, Sec.10.1, "Hospital Providers of Extended Care Services."). However, both inpatient hospital and inpatient SNF benefits are provided under Part A - Hospital Insurance Benefits for the Aged and Disabled, of Title XVIII).

Additional information concerning the following topics can be found in the following manual chapters:

- Benefit periods is found in Chapter 3, "Duration of Covered Inpatient Services";
- Copayment days is found in Chapter 2, "Duration of Covered Inpatient Services";
- Lifetime reserve days is found in Chapter 5, "Lifetime Reserve Days";
- Related payment information is housed in the Provider Reimbursement Manual.

Blood must be furnished on a day which counts as a day of inpatient hospital services to be covered as a Part A service and to count toward the blood deductible. Thus, blood is not covered under Part A and does not count toward the Part A blood deductible when furnished to an inpatient after the inpatient has exhausted all benefit days in a benefit period, or where the individual has elected not to use lifetime reserve days. However, where the patient is discharged on their first day of entitlement or on the hospital's first day of participation, the hospital is permitted to submit a billing form with no accommodation charge, but with ancillary charges including blood.

The records for all Medicare hospital inpatient discharges are maintained in CMS for statistical analysis and use in determining future PPS DRG classifications and rates.

Non-PPS hospitals do not pay for noncovered services generally excluded from coverage in the Medicare Program. This may result in denial of a part of the billed charges or in denial of the entire admission, depending upon circumstance. In PPS hospitals, the following are also possible:

1. In appropriately admitted cases where a noncovered procedure was performed, denied services may result in payment of a different DRG (i.e., one which excludes payment for the noncovered procedure); or

2. In appropriately admitted cases that become cost outlier cases, denied services may lead to denial of some or all of an outlier payment.

The following examples illustrate this principle. If care is noncovered because a patient does not need to be hospitalized, the intermediary denies the admission and makes no Part A (i.e., PPS) payment unless paid under limitation on liability. Under limitation on liability, Medicare payment may be made when the provider and the beneficiary were not aware the services were not necessary and could not reasonably be expected to know that he services were not necessary. For detailed instructions, see the Medicare Claims Processing Manual, Chapter 30,"Limitation on Liability." If a patient is appropriately hospitalized but receives (beyond routine services) only noncovered care, the admission is denied.

NOTE: The intermediary does not deny an admission that includes covered care, even if noncovered care was also rendered. Under PPS, Medicare assumes that it is paying for only the covered care rendered whenever covered services needed to treat and/or diagnose the illness were in fact provided.

If a noncovered procedure is provided along with covered nonroutine care, a DRG change rather than an admission denial might occur. If noncovered procedures are elevating costs into the cost outlier category, outlier payment is denied in whole or in part.

When the hospital is included in PPS, most of the subsequent discussion regarding coverage of inpatient hospital services is relevant only in the context of determining the appropriateness of admissions, which DRG, if any, to pay, and the appropriateness of payment for any outlier cases.

If a patient receives items or services in excess of, or more expensive than, those for which payment can be made, payment is made only for the covered items or services or for only the appropriate prospective payment amount. This provision applies not only to inpatient services, but also to all hospital services under Parts A and B of the program. If the items or services were requested by the patient, the hospital may charge him the difference between the amount customarily charged for the services requested and the amount customarily charged for covered services.

An inpatient is a person who has been admitted to a hospital for bed occupancy for purposes of receiving inpatient hospital services. Generally, a patient is considered an inpatient if formally admitted as inpatient with the expectation that he or she will remain at least overnight and occupy a bed even though it later develops that the patient can be discharged or transferred to another hospital and not actually use a hospital bed overnight.

The physician or other practitioner responsible for a patient's care at the hospital is also responsible for deciding whether the patient should be admitted as an inpatient. Physicians should use a 24-hour period as a benchmark, i.e., they should order admission for patients who are expected to need hospital care for 24 hours or more, and treat other patients on an outpatient basis. However, the decision to admit a patient is a complex medical judgment which can be made only after the physician has considered a number of factors, including the patient's medical history and current medical needs, the types of facilities available to inpatients and to outpatients, the hospital's by-laws and admissions policies, and the relative appropriateness of treatment in each setting. Factors to be considered when making the decision to admit include such things as:

The severity of the signs and symptoms exhibited by the patient;

The medical predictability of something adverse happening to the patient;

The need for diagnostic studies that appropriately are outpatient services (i.e., their performance does not ordinarily require the patient to remain at the hospital for 24 hours or more) to assist in assessing whether the patient should be admitted; and

The availability of diagnostic procedures at the time when and at the location where the patient presents.

Admissions of particular patients are not covered or noncovered solely on the basis of the length of time the patient actually spends in the hospital. In certain specific situations coverage of services on an inpatient or outpatient basis is determined by the following rules:

Minor Surgery or Other Treatment - When patients with known diagnoses enter a hospital for a specific minor surgical procedure or other treatment that is expected to keep them in the hospital for only a few hours (less than 24), they are considered outpatients for coverage purposes regardless of: the hour they came to the hospital, whether they used a bed, and whether they remained in the hospital past midnight.

Renal Dialysis - Renal dialysis treatments are usually covered only as outpatient services but may under certain circumstances be covered as inpatient services depending on the patient's condition. Patients staying at home, who are ambulatory, whose conditions are stable and who come to the hospital for routine chronic dialysis treatments, and not for a diagnostic workup or a change in therapy, are considered outpatients. On the other hand, patients undergoing short-term dialysis until their kidneys recover from an acute illness (acute dialysis), or persons with borderline renal failure who develop acute renal failure every time they have an illness and require dialysis (episodic dialysis) are usually inpatients. A patient may begin dialysis as an inpatient and then progress to an outpatient status.

Under original Medicare, the Quality Improvement Organization (QIO), for each hospital is responsible for deciding, during review of inpatient admissions on a case-by-case basis, whether the admission was medically necessary. Medicare law authorizes the QIO to make these judgments, and the judgments are binding for purposes of Medicare coverage. In making these judgments, however, QIOs consider only the medical evidence which was available to the physician at the time an admission decision had to be made. They do not take into account other information (e.g., test results) which became available only after admission, except in cases where considering the post-admission information would support a finding that an admission was medically necessary.

Refer to Parts 4 and 7 of the QIO Manual with regard to initial determinations for these services. The QIO will review the swing bed services in these PPS hospitals as well.

NOTE: When patients requiring extended care services are admitted to beds in a hospital, they are considered inpatients of the hospital. In such cases, the services furnished in the hospital will not be considered extended care services, and payment may not be made under the program for such services unless the services are extended care services furnished pursuant to a swing bed agreement granted to the hospital by the Secretary of Health and Human Services.

## 100-02, 1, 10.1.4

### Charges for Deluxe Private Room
A3-3101.1.D, HO-210.1.D

Beneficiaries found to need a private room (either because they need isolation for medical reasons or because they need immediate admission when no other accommodations are available) may be assigned to any of the provider's private rooms. They do not have the right to insist on the private room of their choice, but their preferences should be given the same consideration as if they were paying all provider charges themselves. The program does not, under any circumstances, pay for personal comfort items. Thus, the program does not pay for deluxe accommodations and/or services. These would include a suite, or a room substantially more spacious than is required for treatment, or specially equipped or decorated, or serviced for the comfort and convenience of persons willing to pay a differential for such amenities. If the beneficiary (or representative) requests such deluxe accommodations, the provider should advise that there will be a charge, not covered by Medicare, of a specified amount per day (not exceeding the differential defined in the next sentence); and may charge the beneficiary that amount for each day he/she occupies the deluxe accommodations. The maximum amount the provider may charge the beneficiary for such accommodations is the differential between the most prevalent private room rate at the time of admission and the customary charge for the room occupied. Beneficiaries may not be charged this differential if they (or their representative) do not request the deluxe accommodations.

The beneficiary may not be charged such a differential in private room rates if that differential is based on factors other than personal comfort items. Such factors might include differences between older and newer wings, proximity to lounge, elevators or nursing stations, desirable view, etc. Such rooms are standard 1-bed units and not deluxe rooms for purposes of these instructions, even though the provider may call them deluxe and have a higher customary charge for them. No additional charge may be imposed upon the beneficiary who is assigned to a room that may be somewhat more desirable because of these factors.

## 100-02, 6, 20.6

### Outpatient Observation Services

#### A. Outpatient Observation Services Defined
Observation care is a well-defined set of specific, clinically appropriate services, which include ongoing short term treatment, assessment, and reassessment before a decision can be made regarding whether patients will require further treatment as hospital inpatients or if they are able to be discharged from the hospital. Observation services are commonly ordered for patients who present to the emergency department and who then require a significant period of treatment or monitoring in order to make a decision concerning their admission or discharge.

Observation services are covered only when provided by the order of a physician or another individual authorized by State licensure law and hospital staff bylaws to admit patients to the hospital or to order outpatient tests. In the majority of cases, the decision whether to discharge a patient from the hospital following resolution of the reason for the observation care or to admit the patient as an inpatient can be made in less than 48 hours, usually in less than 24 hours. In only rare and exceptional cases do reasonable and necessary outpatient observation services span more than 48 hours.

Hospitals may bill for patients who are directly referred to the hospital for outpatient observation services. A direct referral occurs when a physician in the community refers a patient to the hospital for outpatient observation, bypassing the clinic or emergency department (ED) visit. Effective for services furnished on or after January 1, 2003, hospitals may bill for patients directly referred for observation services.

See Pub. 100-04, *Medicare Claims Processing Manual*, chapter 4, section 290, at http://www.cms.hhs.gov/manuals/downloads/clm104c04.pdf for billing and payment instructions for outpatient observation services.

Future updates will be issued in a Recurring Update Notification.

#### B. Coverage of Outpatient Observation Services
When a physician orders that a patient receive observation care, the patient's status is that of an outpatient. The purpose of observation is to determine the need for further treatment or for inpatient admission. Thus, a patient receiving observation services may improve and be released, or be admitted as an inpatient (see Pub. 100-02, *Medicare Benefit Policy Manual*, Chapter 1, Section 10 "Covered Inpatient Hospital Services Covered Under Part A" at http://www.cms.hhs.gov/manuals/Downloads/bp102c01.pdf). For more information on correct reporting of observation services, see Pub. 100-04, *Medicare Claims Processing Manual*, chapter 4, section 290.2.2.)

All hospital observation services, regardless of the duration of the observation care, that are medically reasonable and necessary are covered by Medicare.

Observation services are reported using HCPCS code G0378 (Hospital observation service, per hour). Beginning January 1, 2008, HCPCS code G0378 for hourly observation services is assigned status indicator N, signifying that its payment is always packaged. No separate payment is made for observation services reported with HCPCS code G0378. In most circumstances, observation services are supportive and ancillary to the other separately payable services provided to a patient. In certain circumstances when observation care is billed in conjunction with a high level clinic visit (Level 5), high level Type A emergency department visit (Level 4 or 5), high level Type B emergency department visit (Level 5), critical care services, or direct referral for observation services as an integral part of a patient's extended encounter of care, payment may be made for the entire extended care encounter through one of two composite APCs when certain criteria are met. For information about billing and payment methodology for observation services in years prior to CY 2008, see Pub. 100-04, *Medicare Claims Processing Manual*, Chapter 4, Sec.Sec.290.3-290.4. For information about payment for extended assessment and management under composite APCs, see Sec.290.5.

Payment for all reasonable and necessary observation services is packaged into the payments for other separately payable services provided to the patient in the same encounter. Observation services packaged through assignment of status indicator N are covered OPPS services. Since the payment for these services is included in the APC payment for other separately payable services on the claim, hospitals must not bill Medicare beneficiaries directly for the packaged services.

#### C. Services Not Covered by Medicare and Notification to the Beneficiary
In making the determination whether an ABN can be used to shift liability to a beneficiary for the cost of non-covered items or services related to an encounter that includes observation care, the provider should follow a two step process. First, the provider must decide whether the item or service meets either the definition of observation care or would be otherwise covered. If the item or service does not meet the definitional requirements of any Medicare-covered benefit under Part B, then the item or service is not covered by Medicare and an ABN is not required to shift the liability to the beneficiary. However, the provider may choose to provide voluntary notification for these items or services.

Second, if the item or service meets the definition of observation services or would be otherwise covered, then the provider must decide whether the item or service is "reasonable and necessary" for the beneficiary on the occasion in question, or if the item or service exceeds any frequency limitation for the particular benefit or falls outside of a timeframe for receipt of a particular benefit. In these cases, the ABN would be used to shift the liability to the beneficiary (see Pub. 100-04, *Medicare Claims Processing Manual*; Chapter 30, "Financial Liability Protections," Section 20, at http://www.cms.hhs.gov/manuals/downloads/clm104c30.pdf for information regarding Limitation On Liability (LOL) Under Sec.1879 Where Medicare Claims Are Disallowed).

If an ABN is not issued to the beneficiary, the provider may be held liable for the cost of the item or service unless the provider/supplier is able to demonstrate that they did not know and could not have reasonably been expected to know that Medicare would not pay for the item or service.

## 100-02, 10, 10.1

### The Vehicle
Any vehicle used as an ambulance must be designed and equipped to respond to medical emergencies and, in nonemergency situations, be capable of transporting beneficiaries with acute medical conditions. The vehicle must comply with State or local laws governing the licensing and certification of an emergency medical transportation vehicle. At a minimum, the ambulance must contain a stretcher, linens, emergency medical supplies, oxygen equipment, and other lifesaving emergency medical equipment and be equipped with emergency warning lights, sirens, and telecommunications equipment as required by State or local law. This should include, at a minimum, one 2-way voice radio or wireless telephone.

## 100-02, 10, 10.2.2

### Reasonableness of the Ambulance Trip

Under the FS payment is made according to the level of medically necessary services actually furnished. That is, payment is based on the level of service furnished (provided they were medically necessary), not simply on the vehicle used. Even if a local government requires an ALS response for all calls, payment under the FS is made only for the level of service furnished, and then only when the service is medically necessary.

## 100-02, 10, 10.3.3

### Separately Payable Ambulance Transport Under Part B versus Patient Transportation that is Covered Under a Packaged Hospital Service

Transportation of a beneficiary from his or her home, an accident scene, or any other point of origin is covered under Part B as an ambulance service only to the nearest hospital, critical access hospital (CAH), or skilled nursing facility (SNF) that is capable of furnishing the required level and type of care for the beneficiary's illness or injury and only if medical necessity and other program coverage criteria are met.

Medicare-covered ambulance services are paid either as separately billed services, in which case the entity furnishing the ambulance service bills Part B of the program, or as a packaged service, in which case the entity furnishing the ambulance service must seek payment from the provider who is responsible for the beneficiary's care. If either the origin or the destination of the ambulance transport is the beneficiary's home, then the ambulance transport is paid separately by Medicare Part B, and the entity that furnishes the ambulance transport may bill its Medicare carrier or intermediary directly. If both the origin and destination of the ambulance transport are providers, e.g., a hospital, critical access hospital (CAH), skilled nursing facility (SNF), then responsibility for payment for the ambulance transport is determined in accordance with the following sequential criteria.

NOTE: These criteria must be applied in sequence as a flow chart and not independently of one another.

1. Provider Numbers:

   If the Medicare-assigned provider numbers of the two providers are different, then the ambulance service is separately billable to the program. If the provider number of both providers is the same, then consider criterion 2, "campus".

2. Campus:

   Following criterion 1, if the campuses of the two providers (sharing the same provider numbers) are the same, then the transport is not separately billable to the program. In this case the provider is responsible for payment. If the campuses of the two providers are different, then consider criterion 3, "patient status." "Campus" means the physical area immediately adjacent to the provider's main buildings, other areas and structures that are not strictly contiguous to the main buildings, but are located within 250 yards of the main buildings, and any of the other areas determined on an individual case basis by the CMS regional office to be part of the provider's campus.

3. Patient Status: Inpatient vs. Outpatient

   Following criteria 1 and 2, if the patient is an inpatient at both providers (i.e., inpatient status both at the origin and at the destination, providers sharing the same provider number but located on different campuses), then the transport is not separately billable. In this case the provider is responsible for payment. All other combinations (i.e., outpatient-to-inpatient, inpatient-to-outpatient, outpatient-to-outpatient) are separately billable to the program.

In the case where the point of origin is not a provider, Part A coverage is not available because, at the time the beneficiary is being transported, the beneficiary is not an inpatient of any provider paid under Part A of the program and ambulance services are excluded from the 3-day preadmission payment window.

The transfer, i.e., the discharge of a beneficiary from one provider with a subsequent admission to another provider, is also payable as a Part B ambulance transport, provided all program coverage criteria are met, because, at the time that the beneficiary is in transit, the beneficiary is not a patient of either provider and not subject to either the inpatient preadmission payment window or outpatient payment packaging requirements. This includes an outpatient transfer from a remote, off-campus emergency department (ER) to becoming an inpatient or outpatient at the main campus hospital, even if the ER is owned and operated by the hospital.

Once a beneficiary is admitted to a hospital, CAH, or SNF, it may be necessary to transport the beneficiary to another hospital or other site temporarily for specialized care while the beneficiary maintains inpatient status with the original provider. This movement of the patient is considered "patient transportation" and is covered as an inpatient hospital or CAH service and as a SNF service when the SNF is furnishing it as a covered SNF service and payment is made under Part A for that service. (If the beneficiary is a resident of a SNF and must be transported by ambulance to receive dialysis or certain other high-end outpatient hospital services, the ambulance transport may be separately payable under Part B.) Because the service is covered and payable as a beneficiary transportation service under Part A, the service cannot be classified and paid for as an ambulance service under Part B. This includes intra-campus transfers between different departments of the same hospital, even where the departments are located in separate buildings. Such intra-campus transfers are not separately payable under the Part B ambulance benefit. Such costs are accounted for in the same manner as the costs of such a transfer within a single building.

## 100-02, 10, 20

### Coverage Guidelines for Ambulance Service Claims.

Payment may be made for expenses incurred by a patient for ambulance service provided conditions l, 2, and 3 in the left-hand column have been met. The right-hand column indicates the documentation needed to establish that the condition has been met

| Conditions | Review Action |
|---|---|
| 1. Patient was transported by an approved supplier of ambulance services. | 1. Ambulance suppliers are explained in greater detail in §10.1.3 |
| 2. The patient was suffering from an illness or injury, which contraindicated transportation by other means. (§10.2) | 2. (a) The contractor presumes the requirement was met if the submitted documentation indicates that the patient:<br><br>• Was transported in an emergency situation, e.g., as a result of an accident, injury or acute illness, or<br>• Needed to be restrained to prevent injury to the beneficiary or others; or<br>• Was unconscious or in shock; or<br>• Required oxygen or other emergency treatment during transport to the nearest appropriate facility; or<br>• Exhibits signs and symptoms of acute respiratory distress or cardiac distress such as shortness of breath or chest pain; or<br>• Exhibits signs and symptoms that indicate the possibility of acute stroke; or<br>• Had to remain immobile because of a fracture that had not been set or the possibility of a fracture; or<br>• Was experiencing severe hemorrhage; or<br>• Could be moved only by stretcher; or<br>• Was bed-confined before and after the ambulance trip. |
| 2. The patient was suffering from an illness or injury, which contraindicated transportation by other means. (§10.2) (Continued) | (b)<br><br>In the absence of any of the conditions listed in (a) above additional documentation should be obtained to establish medical need where the evidence indicates the existence of the circumstances listed below:<br><br>(i) Patient's condition would not ordinarily require movement by stretcher, or<br><br>(ii) The individual was not admitted as a hospital inpatient (except in accident cases), or<br><br>(iii) The ambulance was used solely because other means of transportation were unavailable, or<br><br>(iv) The individual merely needed assistance in getting from his room or home to a vehicle.<br><br>(c) Where the information indicates a situation not listed in 2(a) or 2(b) above, refer the case to your supervisor. |

| Conditions | Review Action |
|---|---|
| 3. The patient was transported from and to points listed below. | 3. Claims should show the ZIP Code of the point of pickup. |
| (a) From patient's residence (or other place where need arose) to hospital or skilled nursing facility. | (a)<br><br>   i. Condition met if trip began within the institution's service area as shown in the carrier's locality guide.<br><br>   ii. Condition met where the trip began outside the institution's service area if the institution was the nearest one with appropriate facilities. |

NOTE: A Patient'sresidence is the place where he or she makes his/her home and dwells permanently, or for an extended period of time. A skilled nursing facility is one, which is listed in the Directory of Medical Facilities as a participating SNF or as an institution which meets §1861(j)(1) of the Act.

NOTE: A claim for ambulance service to a participating hospital or skilled nursing facility should not be denied on the grounds that there is a nearer nonparticipating institution having appropriate facilities.

| | |
|---|---|
| (b) Skilled nursing facility to a hospital or hospital to a skilled nursing facility. | (b)<br><br>   (i) Condition met if the ZIP Code of the pickup point is within the service area of the destination as shown in the carrier's locality guide.<br><br>   (ii) Condition met where the ZIP Code of the pickup point is outside the service area of the destination if the destination institution was the nearest appropriate facility. |
| (c) Hospital to hospital or skilled nursing facility to skilled nursing facility. | (c) Condition met if the discharging institution was not an appropriate facility and the admitting institution was the nearest appropriate facility. |
| (d) From a hospital or skilled nursing facility to patient's residence. | (d)<br><br>   (i) Condition met if patient's residence is within the institution's service area as shown in the carrier's locality guide.<br><br>   (ii) Condition met where the patient's residence is outside the institution's service area if the institution was the nearest appropriate facility. |
| (e) Round trip for hospital or participating skilled nursing facility inpatients to the nearest hospital or nonhospital treatment facility. | (e) Condition met if the reasonable and necessary diagnostic or therapeutic service required by patient's condition is not available at the institution where the beneficiary is an inpatient. |

NOTE: Ambulance service to a physician's office or a physician-directed clinic is not covered. See §10.3.8 above, where a stop is made at a physician's office en route to a hospital and §10.3.3 for additional exceptions.)

| | |
|---|---|
| 4. Ambulance services involving hospital admissions in Canada or Mexico are covered (Medicare Claims Processing Manual, Chapter 1, "General Billing Requirements, "§10.1.3.) if the following conditions are met: | 4.<br><br>(a) The foreign hospitalization has been determined to be covered; and<br><br>(b) The ambulance service meets the coverage requirements set forth in §§10-10.3. If the foreign hospitalization has been determined to be covered on the basis of emergency services (See the Medicare Claims Processing Manual, Chapter 1, "General Billing Requirements," §10.1.3), the necessity requirement (§10.2) and the destination requirement (§10.3) are considered met. |

| | |
|---|---|
| 5. The carrier will make partial payment for otherwise covered ambulance service, which exceeded limits defined in item | 5 & 6 (a) From the pickup point to the nearest appropriate facility, or 5 & 6 (b) From the nearest appropriate facility to the beneficiary's residence where he or she is being returned home from a distant institution. |
| 6. The carrier will base the payment on the amount payable had the patient been transported: | |

## 100-02, 10, 30.1.1

### Ground Ambulance Services:

**Basic Life Support (BLS)**

Definition: Basic life support (BLS) is transportation by ground ambulance vehicle and the provision of medically necessary supplies and services, including BLS ambulance services as defined by the State. The ambulance must be staffed by an individual who is qualified in accordance with State and local laws as an emergency medical technician-basic (EMT-Basic). These laws may vary from State to State or within a State. For example, only in some jurisdictions is an EMT-Basic permitted to operate limited equipment onboard the vehicle, assist more qualified personnel in performing assessments and interventions, and establish a peripheral intravenous (IV) line.

**Basic Life Support (BLS) - Emergency**

Definition: When medically necessary, the provision of BLS services, as specified above, in the context of an emergency response. An emergency response is one that, at the time the ambulance provider or supplier is called, it responds immediately. An immediate response is one in which the ambulance provider/supplier begins as quickly as possible to take the steps necessary to respond to the call.

Application: The determination to respond emergently with a BLS ambulance must be in accord with the local 911 or equivalent service dispatch protocol. If the call came in directly to the ambulance provider/supplier, then the provider's/supplier's dispatch protocol must meet, at a minimum, the standards of the dispatch protocol of the local 911 or equivalent service. In areas that do not have a local 911 or equivalent service, then the protocol must meet, at a minimum, the standards of a dispatch protocol in another similar jurisdiction within the State or, if there is no similar jurisdiction within the State, then the standards of any other dispatch protocol within the State. Where the dispatch was inconsistent with this standard of protocol, including where no protocol was used, the beneficiary's condition (for example, symptoms) at the scene determines the appropriate level of payment.

**Advanced Life Support, Level 1 (ALS1)**

Definition: Advanced life support, level 1 (ALS1) is the transportation by ground ambulance vehicle and the provision of medically necessary supplies and services including the provision of an ALS assessment or at least one ALS intervention.

**Advanced Life Support Assessment**

Definition: An advanced life support (ALS) assessment is an assessment performed by an ALS crew as part of an emergency response that was necessary because the patient's reported condition at the time of dispatch was such that only an ALS crew was qualified to perform the assessment. An ALS assessment does not necessarily result in a determination that the patient requires an ALS level of service.

Application: The determination to respond emergently with an ALS ambulance must be in accord with the local 911 or equivalent service dispatch protocol. If the call came in directly to the ambulance provider/supplier, then the provider's/supplier's dispatch protocol must meet, at a minimum, the standards of the dispatch protocol of the local 911 or equivalent service. In areas that do not have a local 911 or equivalent service, then the protocol must meet, at a minimum, the standards of a dispatch protocol in another similar jurisdiction within the State or, if there is no similar jurisdiction within the State, then the standards of any other dispatch protocol within the State. Where the dispatch was inconsistent with this standard of protocol, including where no protocol was used, the beneficiary's condition (for example, symptoms) at the scene determines the appropriate level of payment.

**Advanced Life Support Intervention**

Definition: An advanced life support (ALS) intervention is a procedure that is in accordance with State and local laws, required to be done by an emergency medical technician-intermediate (EMT-Intermediate) or EMT-Paramedic.

Application: An ALS intervention must be medically necessary to qualify as an intervention for payment for an ALS level of service. An ALS intervention applies only to ground transports.

**Advanced Life Support, Level 1 (ALS1) - Emergency**

Definition: When medically necessary, the provision of ALS1 services, as specified above, in the context of an emergency response. An emergency response is one that, at the time the ambulance provider or supplier is called, it responds immediately. An immediate response is one in which the ambulance provider/supplier begins as quickly as possible to take the steps necessary to respond to the call.

Application: The determination to respond emergently with an ALS ambulance must be in accord with the local 911 or equivalent service dispatch protocol. If the call came in directly to the ambulance provider/supplier, then the provider's/supplier's dispatch protocol must meet, at a minimum, the standards of the dispatch protocol of the local 911 or equivalent service. In areas that do not have a local 911 or equivalent service, then the protocol must meet, at a minimum, the standards of a dispatch protocol in another similar jurisdiction within the State or, if there is no similar jurisdiction within the State, then the standards of any other dispatch protocol within the State. Where the dispatch was inconsistent with this standard of protocol, including where no protocol was used, the beneficiary's condition (for example, symptoms) at the scene determines the appropriate level of payment.

**Advanced Life Support, Level 2 (ALS2)**
Definition: Advanced life support, level 2 (ALS2) is the transportation by ground ambulance vehicle and the provision of medically necessary supplies and services including (1) at least three separate administrations of one or more medications by intravenous push/bolus or by continuous

infusion (excluding crystalloid fluids) or (2) ground ambulance transport, medically necessary supplies and services, and the provision of at least one of the ALS2 procedures listed below:

a. Manual defibrillation/cardioversion;

b. Endotracheal intubation;

c. Central venous line;

d. Cardiac pacing;

e. Chest decompression;

f. Surgical airway; or

g. Intraosseous line.

Application: Crystalloid fluids include fluids such as 5 percent Dextrose in water, Saline and Lactated Ringer's. Medications that are administered by other means, for example: intramuscular/subcutaneous injection, oral, sublingually or nebulized, do not qualify to determine whether the ALS2 level rate is payable. However, this is not an all-inclusive list. Likewise, a single dose of medication administered fractionally (i.e., one-third of a single dose quantity) on three separate occasions does not qualify for the ALS2 payment rate. The criterion of multiple administrations of the same drug requires a suitable quantity and amount of time between administrations that is in accordance with standard medical practice guidelines. The fractional administration of a single dose (for this purpose meaning a standard or protocol dose) on three separate occasions does not qualify for ALS2 payment.

In other words, the administration of 1/3 of a qualifying dose 3 times does not equate to three qualifying doses for purposes of indicating ALS2 care. One-third of X given 3 times might = X (where X is a standard/protocol drug amount), but the same sequence does not equal 3 times X. Thus, if 3 administrations of the same drug are required to show that ALS2 care was given, each of those administrations must be in accord with local protocols. The run will not qualify on the basis of drug administration if that administration was not according to protocol.

An example of a single dose of medication administered fractionally on three separate occasions that would not qualify for the ALS2 payment rate would be the use of Intravenous (IV) Epinephrine in the treatment of pulseless Ventricular Tachycardia/Ventricular Fibrillation (VF/VT) in the adult patient. Administering this medication in increments of 0.25 mg, 0.25 mg, and 0.50 mg would not qualify for the ALS2 level of payment. This medication, according to the American Heart Association (AHA), Advanced Cardiac Life Support (ACLS) protocol, calls for Epinephrine to be administered in 1 mg increments every 3 to 5 minutes. Therefore, in order to receive payment for an ALS2 level of service, based in part on the administration of Epinephrine, three separate administrations of Epinephrine in 1 mg increments must be administered for the treatment of pulseless VF/VT.

A second example that would not qualify for the ALS2 payment level is the use of Adenosine in increments of 2 mg, 2 mg, and 2 mg for a total of 6 mg in the treatment of an adult patient with Paroxysmal Supraventricular Tachycardia (PSVT). According to ACLS guidelines, 6 mg of Adenosine should be given by rapid intravenous push (IVP) over 1 to 2 seconds. If the first dose does not result in the elimination of the supraventricular tachycardia within 1 to 2 minutes, 12 mg of Adenosine should be administered IVP. If the supraventricular tachycardia persists, a second 12 mg dose of Adenosine can be administered for a total of 30 mg of Adenosine. Three separate administrations of the drug Adenosine in the dosage amounts outlined in the later case would qualify for ALS2 payment.

Endotracheal intubation is one of the services that qualifies for the ALS2 level of payment; therefore, it is not necessary to consider medications administered by endotracheal intubation for the purpose of determining whether the ALS2 rate is payable. The monitoring and maintenance of an endotracheal tube that was previously inserted prior to transport also qualifies as an ALS2 procedure.

**Advanced Life Support (ALS) Personnel**
Definition: ALS personnel are individuals trained to the level of the emergency medical technician-intermediate (EMT-Intermediate) or paramedic.

**Specialty Care Transport (SCT)**
Definition: Specialty care transport (SCT) is the interfacility transportation of a critically injured or ill beneficiary by a ground ambulance vehicle, including the provision of medically necessary supplies and services, at a level of service beyond the scope of the EMT-Paramedic. SCT is necessary when a beneficiary's condition requires ongoing care that must be furnished by one or more health professionals in an appropriate specialty area, for example, emergency or critical care nursing, emergency medicine, respiratory care, cardiovascular care, or a paramedic with additional training.

Application: The EMT-Paramedic level of care is set by each State. SCT is necessary when a beneficiary's condition requires ongoing care that must be furnished by one or more health professionals in an appropriate specialty area. Care above that level that is medically necessary and that is furnished at a level of service above the EMT-Paramedic level of care is considered SCT. That is to say, if EMT-Paramedics - without specialty care certification or qualification - are permitted to furnish a given service in a State, then that service does not qualify for SCT. The phrase "EMT-Paramedic with additional training" recognizes that a State may permit a person who is not only certified as an EMT-Paramedic, but who also has successfully completed additional education as determined by the State in furnishing higher level medical services required by critically ill or critically injured patients, to furnish a level of service that otherwise would require a health professional in an appropriate specialty care area (for example, a nurse) to provide. "Additional training" means the specific additional training that a State requires a paramedic to complete in order to qualify to furnish specialty care to a critically ill or injured patient during an SCT.

**Paramedic Intercept (PI)**
Definition: Paramedic Intercept services are ALS services provided by an entity that does not provide the ambulance transport. This type of service is most often provided for an emergency ambulance transport in which a local volunteer ambulance that can provide only basic life support (BLS) level of service is dispatched to transport a patient. If the patient needs ALS services such as EKG monitoring, chest decompression, or I.V. therapy, another entity dispatches a paramedic to meet the BLS ambulance at the scene or once the ambulance is on the way to the hospital. The ALS paramedics then provide services to the patient.

This tiered approach to life saving is cost effective in many areas because most volunteer ambulances do not charge for their services and one paramedic service can cover many communities. Prior to March 1, 1999, Medicare payment could be made for these services, but only when the claim was submitted by the entity that actually furnished the ambulance transport. Payment could not be made directly to the intercept service provider. In those areas where State laws prohibit volunteer ambulances from billing Medicare and other health insurance, the intercept service could not receive payment for treating a Medicare beneficiary and was forced to bill the beneficiary for the entire service.

Paramedic intercept services furnished on or after March 1, 1999, may be payable separate from the ambulance transport, subject to the requirements specified below.

The intercept service(s) is:

- Furnished in a rural area;
- Furnished under a contract with one or more volunteer ambulance services; and,
- Medically necessary based on the condition of the beneficiary receiving the ambulance service.
- In addition, the volunteer ambulance service involved must:
- Meet the program's certification requirements for furnishing ambulance services;
- Furnish services only at the BLS level at the time of the intercept; and,
- Be prohibited by State law from billing anyone for any service.

Finally, the entity furnishing the ALS paramedic intercept service must:

- Meet the program's certification requirements for furnishing ALS services, and,
- Bill all recipients who receive ALS paramedic intercept services from the entity, regardless of whether or not those recipients are Medicare beneficiaries.

For purposes of the paramedic intercept benefit, a rural area is an area that is designated as rural by a State law or regulation or any area outside of a Metropolitan Statistical Area or in New England, outside a New England County Metropolitan Area as defined by the Office of Management and Budget. The current list of these areas is periodically published in the Federal Register.

See the Medicare Claims Processing Manual, Chapter 15, "Ambulance," Sec.20.1.4 for payment of paramedic intercept services.

### Services in a Rural Area

Definition: Services in a rural area are services that are furnished (1) in an area outside a Metropolitan Statistical Area (MSA); or, (2) in New England, outside a New England County Metropolitan Area (NECMA); or, (3) an area identified as rural using the Goldsmith modification even though the area is within an MSA.

### Emergency Response

Definition: Emergency response is a BLS or ALS1 level of service that has been provided in immediate response to a 911 call or the equivalent. An immediate response is one in which the ambulance provider/supplier begins as quickly as possible to take the steps necessary to respond to the call.

Application: The phrase "911 call or equivalent" is intended to establish the standard that the nature of the call at the time of dispatch is the determining factor. Regardless of the medium by which the call is made (e.g., a radio call could be appropriate) the call is of an emergent nature when, based on the information available to the dispatcher at the time of the call, it is reasonable for the dispatcher to issue an emergency dispatch in light of accepted, standard dispatch protocol. An emergency call need not come through 911 even in areas where a 911 call system exists. However, the determination to respond emergently must be in accord with the local 911 or equivalent service dispatch protocol. If the call came in directly to the ambulance provider/supplier, then the provider's/supplier's dispatch protocol and the dispatcher's actions must meet, at a minimum, the standards of the dispatch protocol of the local 911 or equivalent service. In areas that do not have a local 911 or equivalent service, then both the protocol and the dispatcher's actions must meet, at a minimum, the standards of the dispatch protocol in another similar jurisdiction within the State, or if there is no similar jurisdiction, then the standards of any other dispatch protocol within the State. Where the dispatch was inconsistent with this standard of protocol, including where no protocol was used, the beneficiary's condition (for example, symptoms) at the scene determines the appropriate level of payment.

### EMT-Intermediate

Definition: EMT-Intermediate is an individual who is qualified, in accordance with State and local laws, as an EMT-Basic and who is also certified in accordance with State and local laws to perform essential advanced techniques and to administer a limited number of medications.

### EMT-Paramedic

Definition: EMT-Paramedic possesses the qualifications of the EMT-Intermediate and, in accordance with State and local laws, has enhanced skills that include being able to administer additional interventions and medications.

### Relative Value Units

Definition: Relative value units (RVUs) measure the value of ambulance services relative to the value of a base level ambulance service.

Application: The RVUs for the ambulance fee schedule are as follows:

Service Level RVUs

- BLS 1.00
- BLS - Emergency 1.60
- ALS1 1.20
- ALS1 - Emergency 1.90
- ALS2 2.75
- SCT 3.25
- PI 1.75
- RVUs are not applicable to FW and RW services

## 100-02, 11, 20.2

(Rev. 224, Issued: 06-03-16, Effective: 01-01-16, Implementation: 09-06-16)

All laboratory services furnished to individuals for the treatment of ESRD are included in the ESRD PPS as Part B services and are not paid separately as of January 1, 2011. The laboratory services include but are not limited to:

- Laboratory tests included under the composite rate as of December 31, 2010 (discussed below); and
- Former separately billable Part B laboratory tests that were billed by ESRD facilities and independent laboratories for ESRD patients.

Composite rate laboratory tests are listed in §20.2.E of this chapter. More information regarding composite rate laboratory tests can be found in Pub. 100-04, Medicare Claims Processing Manual, chapter 8, §50.1, §60.1, and §80. As discussed below, composite rate laboratory services should not be reported on claims.

*To the extent a laboratory test is performed to monitor the levels or effects of any of the drugs that were specifically excluded from the ESRD PPS, these tests would be separately billable. The following table lists the drug categories that were excluded from the ESRD PPS and the rationale for their exclusion. Laboratory services furnished to monitor the medication levels or effects of drugs and biologicals that fall in those categories would not be considered to be furnished for the treatment of ESRD.*

DRUG CATEGORIES EXCLUDED FROM THE ESRD PPS BASE RATE FOR THE PURPOSE OF REPORTING LABS

| Drug Category | Rationale for Exclusion |
|---|---|
| Anticoagulant | Drugs labeled for non-renal dialysis conditions and not for vascular access. |
| Antidiuretic | Used to prevent fluid loss. |
| Antiepileptic | Used to prevent seizures. |
| Anti-inflammatory | May be used to treat kidney disease (glomerulonephritis) and other inflammatory conditions. |
| Antipsychotic | Used to treat psychosis. |
| Antiviral | Used to treat viral conditions such as shingles. |
| Cancer management | Includes oral, parenteral and infusions. Cancer drugs are covered under a separate benefit category. |
| Cardiac management | Drugs that manage blood pressure and cardiac conditions. |
| Cartilage | Used to replace synovial fluid in a joint space. |
| Coagulants | Drugs that cause blood to clot after anti-coagulant overdose or factor VII deficiency. |
| Cytoprotective agents | Used after chemotherapy treatment. |
| Endocrine/metabolic management | Used for endocrine/metabolic disorders such as thyroid or endocrine deficiency, hypoglycemia, and hyperglycemia. |
| Erectile dysfunction management | Androgens were used prior to the development of ESAs for anemia management and currently are not recommended practice. Also used for hypogonadism and erectile dysfunction. |
| Gastrointestinal management | Used to treat gastrointestinal conditions such as ulcers and gallbladder disease. |
| Immune system management | Anti-rejection drugs covered under a separate benefit category. |
| Migraine management | Used to treat migraine headaches and symptoms. |
| Musculoskeletal management | Used to treat muscular disorders such as prevent muscle spasms, relax muscles, improve muscle tone as in myasthenia gravis, relax muscles for intubation and induce uterine contractions. |
| Pharmacy handling for oral anti-cancer, anti-emetics and immunosuppressant drugs | Not a function performed by an ESRD facility. |
| Pulmonary system management | Used for respiratory/lung conditions such as opening airways and newborn apnea. |
| Radiopharmaceutical procedures | Includes contrasts and procedure preparation. |
| Unclassified drugs | Should only be used for drugs that do not have a HCPCS code and therefore cannot be identified. |
| Vaccines | Covered under a separate benefit category. |

The distinction of what is considered to be a renal dialysis laboratory test is a clinical decision determined by the ESRD patient's ordering practitioner. If a laboratory test is ordered for the treatment of ESRD, then the laboratory test is not paid separately.

Payment for all renal dialysis laboratory tests furnished under the ESRD PPS is made directly to the ESRD facility responsible for the patient's care. The ESRD facility must furnish the laboratory tests directly or under arrangement and report renal dialysis laboratory tests on the ESRD facility claim (with the exception of composite rate laboratory services).

An ESRD facility must report renal dialysis laboratory services on its claims in order for the laboratory tests to be included in the outlier payment calculation. Renal dialysis laboratory services that were or would have been paid separately under Medicare Part B prior to January 1, 2011, are priced for the outlier payment calculation using the Clinical Laboratory Fee Schedule. Further information regarding the outlier policy can be found in §60.D of this chapter.

Certain laboratory services will be subject to Part B consolidated billing requirements and will no longer be separately payable when provided to ESRD beneficiaries by providers other than the ESRD facility. The list below includes the renal dialysis laboratory tests that are routinely performed for the treatment of ESRD. Payment for the laboratory tests identified on this list is included in the ESRD PPS. The laboratory tests listed in the table are used to enforce consolidated billing edits to ensure that payment is not made for renal dialysis laboratory tests outside of the ESRD PPS. The list of renal dialysis laboratory tests is not an all-inclusive list. If any laboratory test is ordered for the treatment of ESRD, then the laboratory test is considered to be included in the ESRD PPS and is the responsibility of the ESRD facility. Additional renal dialysis laboratory tests may be added through administrative issuances in the future.

LABS SUBJECT TO ESRD CONSOLIDATED BILLING

| CPT/ HCPCS | Short Description |
|---|---|
| 80047 | Basic Metabolic Panel (Calcium, ionized) |
| 80048 | Basic Metabolic Panel (Calcium, total) |
| 80051 | Electrolyte Panel |
| 80053 | Comprehensive Metabolic Panel |
| 80061* | Lipid Panel* |
| 80069 | Renal Function Panel |
| 80076 | Hepatic Function Panel |
| 82040 | Assay of serum albumin |
| 82108 | Assay of aluminum |
| 82306 | Vitamin d, 25 hydroxy |
| 82310 | Assay of calcium |
| 82330 | Assay of calcium, Ionized |
| 82374 | Assay, blood carbon dioxide |
| 82379 | Assay of carnitine |
| 82435 | Assay of blood chloride |
| 82565 | Assay of creatinine |
| 82570 | Assay of urine creatinine |
| 82575 | Creatinine clearance test |
| 82607 | Vitamin B-12 |
| 82652 | Vit d 1, 25-dihydroxy |
| 82668 | Assay of erythropoietin |
| 82728 | Assay of ferritin |
| 82746 | Blood folic acid serum |
| 83540 | Assay of iron |
| 83550 | Iron binding test |
| 83735 | Assay of magnesium |
| 83970 | Assay of parathormone |
| 84075 | Assay alkaline phosphatase |
| 84100 | Assay of phosphorus |
| 84132 | Assay of serum potassium |
| 84134 | Assay of prealbumin |
| 84155 | Assay of protein, serum |
| 84157 | Assay of protein by other source |
| 84295 | Assay of serum sodium |
| 84466 | Assay of transferrin |
| 84520 | Assay of urea nitrogen |
| 84540 | Assay of urine/urea-n |
| 84545 | Urea-N clearance test |
| 85014 | Hematocrit |

| CPT/ HCPCS | Short Description |
|---|---|
| 85018 | Hemoglobin |
| 85025 | Complete (cbc), automated (HgB, Hct, RBC, WBC, and Platelet count) and automated differential WBC count. |
| 85027 | Complete (cbc), automated (HgB, Hct, RBC, WBC, and Platelet count) |
| 85041 | Automated rbc count |
| 85044 | Manual reticulocyte count |
| 85045 | Automated reticulocyte count |
| 85046 | Reticyte/hgb concentrate |
| 85048 | Automated leukocyte count |
| 86704 | Hep b core antibody, total |
| 86705 | Hep b core antibody, igm |
| 86706 | Hep b surface antibody |
| 87040 | Blood culture for bacteria |
| 87070 | Culture, bacteria, other |
| 87071 | Culture bacteri aerobic othr |
| 87073 | Culture bacteria anaerobic |
| 87075 | Cultr bacteria, except blood |
| 87076 | Culture anaerobe ident, each |
| 87077 | Culture aerobic identify |
| 87081 | Culture screen only |
| 87340 | Hepatitis b surface ag, eia |
| G0306 | CBC/diff wbc w/o platelet |
| G0307 | CBC without platelet |

\* Effective January 1, 2016, the lipid panel is no longer considered to be a renal dialysis service. However, if the panel is furnished for the treatment of ESRD it is the responsibility of the ESRD facility and should be reported on the facility's claim.

**A. Automated Multi-Channel Chemistry (AMCC) Tests**
During the ESRD PPS transition period (see §70 of this chapter) ESRD facilities are required to report the renal dialysis AMCC tests with the appropriate modifiers (CD, CE, or CF) on their claims for purposes of applying the 50/50 rule under the composite rate portion of the blended payment. Refer to §70.B of this chapter for additional information regarding the composite rate portion of the blended payment during the transition.

The 50/50 rule is necessary for those ESRD facilities that chose to go through the transition period. If the 50/50 rule allows for separate payment, then the laboratory tests are priced using the clinical laboratory fee schedule. Information regarding the 50/50 rule can be found in §20.2.E of this chapter and in Pub. 100-04, Medicare Claims Processing Manual, chapter 16, §40.6.

NOTE: An ESRD facility billing a renal dialysis AMCC test must use the CF modifier when the AMCC is not in the composite rate but is a renal dialysis service. AMCC tests that are furnished to individuals for reasons other than for the treatment of ESRD should be billed with the AY modifier to Medicare directly by the entity furnishing the service with the AY modifier.

**B. Laboratory Services Furnished for Reasons Other Than for the Treatment of ESRD**
1. Independent Laboratory

   A patient's physician or practitioner may order a laboratory test that is included on the list of items and services subject to consolidated billing edits for reasons other than for the treatment of ESRD. When this occurs, the patient's physician or practitioner should notify the independent laboratory or the ESRD facility (with the appropriate clinical laboratory certification in accordance with the Clinical Laboratory Improvement Act) that furnished the laboratory service that the test is not a renal dialysis service and that entity may bill Medicare separately using the AY modifier. The AY modifier serves as an attestation that the item or service is medically necessary for the patient but is not being used for the treatment of ESRD.

2. Hospital-Based Laboratory

   Hospital outpatient clinical laboratories furnishing renal dialysis laboratory tests to ESRD patients for reasons other than for the treatment of ESRD may submit a claim for separate payment using the AY modifier. The AY modifier serves as an attestation that the item or service is medically necessary for the patient but is not being used for the treatment of ESRD.

### C. Laboratory Services Performed in Emergency Rooms or Emergency Departments

In an emergency room or emergency department, the ordering physician or practitioner may not know at the time the laboratory test is being ordered, if it is being ordered as a renal dialysis service. Consequently, emergency rooms or emergency departments are not required to append an AY modifier to these laboratory tests when submitting claims with dates of service on or after January 1, 2012.

When a renal dialysis laboratory service is furnished to an ESRD patient in an emergency room or emergency department on a different date of service, hospitals can append an ET modifier to the laboratory tests furnished to ESRD patients to indicate that the laboratory test was furnished in conjunction with the emergency visit. Appending the ET modifier indicates that the laboratory service being furnished on a day other than the emergency visit is related to the emergency visit and at the time the ordering physician was unable to determine if the test was ordered for reasons of treating the patient's ESRD.

Allowing laboratory testing to bypass consolidated billing edits in the emergency room or department does not mean that ESRD facilities should send patients to other settings for routine laboratory testing for the purpose of not assuming financial responsibility of renal dialysis items and services. For additional information regarding laboratory services furnished in a variety of settings, see Pub. 100-04, Medicare Claims Processing Manual, chapter 16, §30.3 and §40.6.

### D. Hepatitis B Laboratory Services for Transient Patients

Laboratory testing for hepatitis B is a renal dialysis service. Effective January 1, 2011, hepatitis B testing is included in the ESRD PPS and therefore cannot be billed separately to Medicare.

The Conditions for Coverage for ESRD facilities require routine hepatitis B testing (42 CFR §494.30(a)(1)). The ESRD facility is responsible for the payment of the laboratory test, regardless of frequency. If an ESRD patient wishes to travel, the patient's home ESRD facility should have systems in place for communicating hepatitis B test results to the destination ESRD facility.

### E. Laboratory Services Included Under Composite Rate

Prior to the implementation of the ESRD PPS, the costs of certain ESRD laboratory services furnished for outpatient maintenance dialysis by either the ESRD facility's staff or an independent laboratory, were included in the composite rate calculations. Therefore, payment for all of these laboratory tests was included in the ESRD facility's composite rate and the tests could not have been billed separately to the Medicare program.

All laboratory services that were included under the composite rate are included under the ESRD PPS unless otherwise specified. Payments for these laboratory tests are included in the ESRD PPS and are not paid separately under the composite rate portion of the blended payment and are not eligible for outlier payments. Therefore, composite rate laboratory services should not be reported on the claim. Laboratory tests included in the composite payment rate are identified below.

1. Routinely Covered Tests Paid Under Composite Rate

    The tests listed below are usually performed for dialysis patients and were routinely covered at the frequency specified in the absence of indications to the contrary, (i.e., no documentation of medical necessity was required other than knowledge of the patient's status as an ESRD beneficiary). When any of these tests were performed at a frequency greater than that specified, the additional tests were separately billable and were covered only if they were medically justified by accompanying documentation. A diagnosis of ESRD alone was not sufficient medical evidence to warrant coverage of the additional tests. The nature of the illness or injury (diagnosis, complaint, or symptom) requiring the performance of the test(s) must have been present, along with ICD diagnosis coding, on the claim for payment.

    a. Hemodialysis, IPD, CCPD, and Hemofiltration

    – Per Treatment - All hematocrit, hemoglobin, and clotting time tests furnished incident to dialysis treatments;

    – Weekly - Prothrombin time for patients on anticoagulant therapy and Serum Creatinine;

    – Weekly or Thirteen Per Quarter - BUN;

    – Monthly - Serum Calcium, Serum Potassium, Serum Chloride, CBC, Serum Bicarbonate, Serum Phosphorous, Total Protein, Serum Albumin, Alkaline Phosphatase, aspartate amino transferase (AST) (SGOT) and LDH; and

    – Automated Multi-Channel Chemistry (AMCC) - If an automated battery of tests, such as the SMA-12, is performed and contains most of the tests listed in one of the weekly or monthly categories, it is not necessary to separately identify any tests in the battery that are not listed. Further information concerning automated tests and the "50 percent rule" can be found below

and in Pub. 100-04, Medicare Claims Processing Manual, chapter 16, §40.6.1.

    b. CAPD

    – Monthly – BUN, Creatinine, Sodium, Potassium, $CO_2$, Calcium, Magnesium, Phosphate, Total Protein, Albumin, Alkaline Phosphatase, LDH, AST, SGOT, HCT, Hbg, and Dialysate Protein.

Under the ESRD PPS, frequency requirements do not apply for the purpose of payment. However, laboratory tests should be ordered as necessary and should not be restricted because of financial reasons.

2. Separately Billable Tests Under the Composite Rate

    The following list identifies certain separately billable laboratory tests that were covered routinely and without documentation of medical necessity other than knowledge of the patient's status as an ESRD beneficiary, when furnished at specified frequencies. If they were performed at a frequency greater than that specified, they were covered only if accompanied by medical documentation. A diagnosis of ESRD alone was not sufficient documentation. The medical necessity of the test(s), the nature of the illness or injury (diagnosis, complaint or symptom) requiring the performance of the test(s) must have been furnished on claims using the ICD diagnosis coding system.

    • Separately Billable Tests for Hemodialysis, IPD, CCPD, and Hemofiltration

      Serum Aluminum - one every 3 months

      Serum Ferritin - one every 3 months

    • Separately Billable Tests for CAPD

      WBC, RBC, and Platelet count – One every 3 months

      Residual renal function and 24 hour urine volume – One every 6 months

Under the ESRD PPS frequency requirements do not apply for the purpose of payment. However, laboratory tests should be ordered as necessary and should not be restricted because of financial reasons.

3. Automated Multi-Channel Chemistry (AMCC) Tests Under the Composite Rate

    Clinical diagnostic laboratory tests that comprise the AMCC (listed in Appendix A and B) could be considered to be composite rate and non-composite rate laboratory services. Composite rate payment was paid by the A/B MAC (A). To determine if separate payment was allowed for non-composite rate tests for a particular date of service, 50 percent or more of the covered tests must be non-composite rate tests. This policy also applies to the composite rate portion of the blended payment during the transition. Beginning January 1, 2014, the 50 percent rule will no longer apply and no separate payment will be made under the composite rate portion of the blended payment.

    Medicare applied the following to AMCC tests for ESRD beneficiaries:

    • Payment was the lowest rate for services performed by the same provider, for the same beneficiary, for the same date of service.

    • The A/B MAC identified, for a particular date of service, the AMCC tests ordered that were included in the composite rate and those that were not included. The composite rate tests were defined for Hemodialysis, IPD, CCPD, and Hemofiltration (see Appendix A) and for CAPD (see Appendix B).

    • If 50 percent or more of the covered tests were included under the composite rate payment, then all submitted tests were included within the composite payment. In this case, no separate payment in addition to the composite rate was made for any of the separately billable tests.

    • If less than 50 percent of the covered tests were composite rate tests, all AMCC tests submitted for that Date of Service (DOS) were separately payable.

    • A non-composite rate test was defined as any test separately payable outside of the composite rate or beyond the normal frequency covered under the composite rate that was reasonable and necessary.

    Three pricing modifiers identify the different payment situations for ESRD AMCC tests. The physician who ordered the tests was responsible for identifying the appropriate modifier when ordering the tests.

    • CD - AMCC test had been ordered by an ESRD facility or Medicare capitation payment (MCP) physician that was part of the composite rate and was not separately billable

    • CE - AMCC test had been ordered by an ESRD facility or MCP physician that was a composite rate test but was beyond the normal frequency covered under the rate and was separately reimbursable based on medical necessity

    • CF - AMCC test had been ordered by an ESRD facility or MCP physician that was not part of the composite rate and was separately billable

The ESRD clinical diagnostic laboratory tests identified with modifiers "CD", "CE" or "CF" may not have been billed as organ or disease panels. Effective October 1, 2003, all ESRD clinical diagnostic laboratory tests must be billed individually. See Pub. 100-04, Medicare Claims Processing Manual, chapter 16, §40.6.1, for additional billing and payment instructions as well as examples of the 50/50 rule.

For ESRD dialysis patients, CPT code 82330 Calcium; ionized shall be included in the calculation for the 50/50 rule (Pub. 100-04, Medicare Claims Processing Manual, chapter 16, §40.6.1). When CPT code 82330 is billed as a substitute for CPT code 82310, Calcium; total, it shall be billed with modifier CD or CE. When CPT code 82330 is billed in addition to CPT 82310, it shall be billed with CF modifier.

## 100-02, 12, 30.1

### Rules for Payment of CORF Services
The payment basis for CORF services is 80 percent of the lesser of: (1) the actual charge for the service or (2) the physician fee schedule amount for the service when the physician fee schedule establishes a payment amount for such service. Payment for CORF services under the physician fee schedule is made for physical therapy, occupational therapy, speech-language pathology and respiratory therapy services, as well as the nursing and social and/or psychological services, which are a part of, or directly relate to, the rehabilitation plan of treatment.

Payment for covered durable medical equipment, orthotic and prosthetic (DMEPOS) devices and supplies provided by a CORF is based upon: the lesser of 80 percent of actual charges or the payment amount established under the DMEPOS fee schedule; or, the single payment amount established under the DMEPOS competitive bidding program, provided that payment for such an item is not included in the payment amount for other CORF services.

If there is no fee schedule amount for a covered CORF item or service, payment should be based on the lesser of 80 percent of the actual charge for the service provided or an amount determined by the local Medicare contractor.

Payment for CORF social and/or psychological services is made under the physician fee schedule only for HCPCS code G0409, as appropriate, and only when billed using revenue codes 0560, 0569, 0910, 0911, 0914 and 0919.

Payment for CORF respiratory therapy services is made under the physician fee schedule when provided by a respiratory therapist as defined at 42CFR485.70(j) and, only to the extent that these services support or are an adjunct to the rehabilitation plan of treatment, when billed using revenue codes 0410, 0412 and 0419. Separate payment is not made for diagnostic tests or for services related to physiologic monitoring services which are bundled into other respiratory therapy services appropriately performed by a respiratory therapist, such as Healthcare Common Procedure Coding System (HCPCS) codes G0237, G0238 and G0239.

Payment for CORF nursing services is made under the physician fee schedule only when provided by a registered nurse as defined at 42CFR485.70(h) for nursing services only to the extent that these services support or are an adjunct to the rehabilitation plan of treatment. In addition, payment for CORF nursing services is made only when provided by a registered nurse. HCPCS code G0128 is used to bill for these services and only with revenue codes 0550 and 0559.

For specific payment requirements for CORF, items and services see Pub. 100-04, Medicare Claims Processing Manual, Chapter 5, Part B Outpatient Rehabilitation and CORF/OPT Services.

## 100-02, 12, 40.5

### Respiratory Therapy Services
A respiratory therapy plan of treatment is wholly established and signed by the referring physician before the respiratory therapist initiates the actual treatment.

### A. Definition
Respiratory therapy services include only those services that can be appropriately provided to CORF patients by a qualified respiratory therapist, as defined at 42CFR485.70(j), under a physician-established respiratory therapy plan of treatment. The facility physician must be present in the facility for a sufficient time to provide, in accordance with accepted principles of medical practice, medical direction, medical care services and consultation. Respiratory therapy services include the physiological monitoring necessary to furnish these services. Payment for these services is bundled into the payment for respiratory therapy services and is not payable separately. Diagnostic and other medical services provided in the CORF setting are not considered CORF services, and therefore may not be included in a respiratory therapy plan of treatment because these are covered under separate benefit categories.

The respiratory therapist assesses the patient to determine the appropriateness of pursed lip breathing activity and may check the patient's oxygen saturation level (via pulse oximetry). If appropriate, the respiratory therapist then provides the initial training in order to ensure that the patient can accurately perform the activity. The respiratory therapist may again check the patient's oxygen saturation level, or perform peak respiratory flow, or check other respiratory parameters. These types of services are considered "physiological monitoring" and are bundled into the payment

for HCPCS codes G0237, G0238 and G0239. Physiological monitoring also includes the provision of a 6-minute walk test that is typically conducted before the start of the patient's respiratory therapy activities. The time to provide this walk "test" assessment is included as part of the HCPCS code G0238. When provided as part of a CORF respiratory therapy plan of treatment, payment for these monitoring activities is bundled into the payment for other services provided by the respiratory therapist, such as the three respiratory therapy specific G-codes.

### B. Guidelines for Applying Coverage Criteria
There are some conditions for which respiratory therapy services may be indicated. However, respiratory therapy performed as part of a standard protocol without regard to the individual patient's actual condition, capacity for improving, and the need for such services as established, is not reasonable and medically necessary. All respiratory therapy services must meet the test of being "reasonable and medically necessary" pursuant to Sec.1862(a)(1)(A) of the Act. Determinations of medical necessity are made based on local contractor decisions on a claim-by-claim basis.

The three HCPCS codes G0237, G0238, and G0239 are specific to services provided under the respiratory therapy plan of treatment and, as such, are not designated as subject to the therapy caps.

### C. Patient Education Programs
Instructing a patient in the use of equipment, breathing exercises, etc. may be considered reasonable and necessary to the patient's respiratory therapy plan of treatment and can usually be given to a patient during the course of treatment by the respiratory therapist. These educational instructions are bundled into the covered service and separate payment is not made.

## 100-02, 12, 40.8

### Nursing Services
CORF nursing services may only be provided by an individual meeting the qualifications of a registered nurse, as defined at 42CFR485.70(h). They must relate to, or be a part of, the rehabilitation plan of treatment.

CORF nursing services must be reasonable and medically necessary and are provided as an adjunct to the rehabilitation plan of treatment. For example, a registered nurse may perform or instruct a patient, as appropriate, in the proper procedure of "in and out" urethral catheterization, tracheostomy tube suctioning, or the cleaning for ileostomy or colostomy bags.

Nursing services may not substitute for or supplant the services of physical therapists, occupational therapists, speech-language pathologists and respiratory therapists, but instead must support or further the services and goals provided in the rehabilitation plan of treatment.

CORF nursing services must be provided by a registered nurse and may only be coded as HCPCS code G0128 indicating that CORF "nursing services" were provided.

## 100-02, 12, 40.11

### Vaccines
A CORF may provide pneumococcal pneumonia, influenza virus, and hepatitis B vaccines to its patients. While not included as a service under the CORF benefit, Medicare will make payment to the CORF for certain vaccines and their administration provided to CORF patients (CY 2008 PFS Rule 72 FR 66293).

The following three vaccinations are covered in a CORF if a physician who is a doctor of medicine or osteopathy orders it for a CORF patient:

   Pneumococcal pneumonia vaccine and its administration;

   Hepatitis B vaccine and its administration furnished to a beneficiary who is at high or intermediate risk of contracting hepatitis B; and

   Influenza virus vaccine and its administration

Payment for covered pneumococcal pneumonia, influenza virus, and hepatitis B vaccines provided in the CORF setting is based on 95 percent of the average wholesale price. The CORF registered nurse provides administration of any of these vaccines using HCPCS codes G0008, G0009 or G0010 with payment based on CPT code 90471.

## 100-02, 15, 50.4.4.2

### Immunizations
Vaccinations or inoculations are excluded as immunizations unless they are directly related to the treatment of an injury or direct exposure to a disease or condition, such as anti-rabies treatment, tetanus antitoxin or booster vaccine, botulin antitoxin, antivenin sera, or immune globulin. In the absence of injury or direct exposure, preventive immunization (vaccination or inoculation) against such diseases as smallpox, polio, diphtheria, etc., is not covered. However, pneumococcal, hepatitis B, and influenza virus vaccines are exceptions to this rule. (See items A, B, and C below.)

© 2016 Optum360, LLC

In cases where a vaccination or inoculation is excluded from coverage, related charges are also not covered.

### A. Pneumococcal Pneumonia Vaccinations

Effective for services furnished on or after May 1, 1981, the Medicare Part B program covers pneumococcal pneumonia vaccine and its administration when furnished in compliance with any applicable State law by any provider of services or any entity or individual with a supplier number. This includes revaccination of patients at highest risk of pneumococcal infection. Typically, these vaccines are administered once in a lifetime except for persons at highest risk. Effective July 1, 2000, Medicare does not require for coverage purposes that a doctor of medicine or osteopathy order the vaccine. Therefore, the beneficiary may receive the vaccine upon request without a physician's order and without physician supervision.

An initial vaccine may be administered only to persons at high risk (see below) of pneumococcal disease. Revaccination may be administered only to persons at highest risk of serious pneumococcal infection and those likely to have a rapid decline in pneumococcal antibody levels, provided that at least 5 years have [passed since the previous dose of pneumococcal vaccine.

Persons at high risk for whom an initial vaccine may be administered include all people age 65 and older; immunocompetent adults who are at increased risk of pneumococcal disease or its complications because of chronic illness (e.g., cardiovascular disease, pulmonary disease, diabetes mellitus, alcoholism, cirrhosis, or cerebrospinal fluid leaks); and individuals with compromised immune

(e.g., splenic dysfunction or anatomic asplenia, Hodgkin's disease, lymphoma, multiple myeloma, chronic renal failure, HIV infection, nephrotic syndrome, sickle cell disease, or organ transplantation).

Persons at highest risk and those most likely to have rapid declines in antibody levels are those for whom revaccination may be appropriate. This group includes persons with functional or anatomic asplenia (e.g., sickle cell disease, splenectomy), HIV infection, leukemia, lymphoma, Hodgkin's disease, multiple myeloma, generalized malignancy, chronic renal failure, nephrotic syndrome, or other conditions associated with immunosuppression such as organ or bone marrow transplantation, and those receiving immunosuppressive chemotherapy. It is not appropriate for routine revaccination of people age 65 or older that are not at highest risk.

Those administering the vaccine should not require the patient to present an immunization record prior to administering the pneumococcal vaccine, nor should they feel compelled to review the patient's complete medical record if it is not available. Instead, provided that the patient is competent, it is acceptable to rely on the patient's verbal history to determine prior vaccination status. If the patient is uncertain about his or her vaccination history in the past 5 years, the vaccine should be given. However, if the patient is certain he/she was were vaccinated in the last 5 years, the vaccine should not be given. If the patient is certain that the vaccine was given more than 5 years ago, revaccination is covered only if the patient is at high risk.

### B. Hepatitis B Vaccine

Effective for services furnished on or after September 1, 1984, P.L. 98-369 provides coverage under Part B for hepatitis B vaccine and its administration, furnished to a Medicare beneficiary who is at high or intermediate risk of contracting hepatitis B. This coverage is effective for services furnished on or after September 1, 1984. High-risk groups currently identified include (see exception below):

- ESRD patients;
- Hemophiliacs who receive Factor VIII or IX concentrates;
- Clients of institutions for the mentally retarded;
- Persons who live in the same household as a Hepatitis B Virus (HBV) carrier;
- Homosexual men; and
- Illicit injectable drug abusers; and
- Persons diagnosed with diabetes mellitus.

Intermediate risk groups currently identified include:

- Staff in institutions for the mentally retarded; and
- Workers in health care professions who have frequent contact with blood or blood-derived body fluids during routine work.

EXCEPTION: Persons in both of the above-listed groups in paragraph B, would not be considered at high or intermediate risk of contracting hepatitis B, however, if there were laboratory evidence positive for antibodies to hepatitis B. (ESRD patients are routinely tested for hepatitis B antibodies as part of their continuing monitoring and therapy.)

For Medicare program purposes, the vaccine may be administered upon the order of a doctor of medicine or osteopathy, by a doctor of medicine or osteopathy, or by home health agencies, skilled nursing facilities, ESRD facilities, hospital outpatient

departments, and persons recognized under the incident to physicians' services provision of law.

A charge separate from the ESRD composite rate will be recognized and paid for administration of the vaccine to ESRD patients.

### C. Influenza Virus Vaccine

Effective for services furnished on or after May 1, 1993, the Medicare Part B program covers influenza virus vaccine and its administration when furnished in compliance with any applicable State law by any provider of services or any entity or individual with a supplier number. Typically, these vaccines are administered once a flu season. Medicare does not require, for coverage purposes, that a doctor of medicine or osteopathy order the vaccine. Therefore, the beneficiary may receive the vaccine upon request without a physician's order and without physician supervision

## 100-02, 15, 50.5

### Self-Administered Drugs and Biologicals

B3-2049.5 Medicare Part B does not cover drugs that are usually self-administered by the patient unless the statute provides for such coverage. The statute explicitly provides coverage, for blood clotting factors, drugs used in immunosuppressive therapy, erythropoietin for dialysis patients, certain oral anti-cancer drugs and anti-emetics used in certain situations.

## 100-02, 15, 50.5.4

### Oral Anti-Nausea (Anti-Emetic) Drugs

Effective January 1, 1998, Medicare also covers self-administered anti-emetics, which are necessary for the administration and absorption of the anti-neoplastic chemotherapeutic agents when a high likelihood of vomiting exists. The anti-emetic drug is covered as a necessary means for administration of the anti-neoplastic chemotherapeutic agents. Oral drugs prescribed for use with the primary drug, which enhance the anti-neoplastic effect of the primary drug or permit the patient to tolerate the primary anti-neoplastic drug in higher doses for longer periods, are not covered. Self-administered anti-emetics to reduce the side effects of nausea and vomiting brought on by the primary drug are not included beyond the administration necessary to achieve drug absorption.

Section 1861(s)(2) of the Social Security Act extends coverage to oral anti-emetic drugs that are used as full replacement for intravenous dosage forms of a cancer regimen under the following conditions:

- Coverage is provided only for oral drugs approved by the Food and Drug Administration (FDA) for use as anti-emetics;
- The oral anti-emetic must either be administered by the treating physician or in accordance with a written order from the physician as part of a cancer chemotherapy regimen;
- Oral anti-emetic drugs administered with a particular chemotherapy treatment must be initiated within two hours of the administration of the chemotherapeutic agent and may be continued for a period not to exceed 48 hours from that time;
- The oral anti-emetic drugs provided must be used as a full therapeutic replacement for the intravenous anti-emetic drugs that would have otherwise been administered at the time of the chemotherapy treatment.

Only drugs pursuant to a physician's order at the time of the chemotherapy treatment qualify for this benefit. The dispensed number of dosage units may not exceed a loading dose administered within two hours of the treatment, plus a supply of additional dosage units not to exceed 48 hours of therapy.

Oral drugs that are not approved by the FDA for use as anti-emetics and which are used by treating physicians adjunctively in a manner incidental to cancer chemotherapy are not covered by this benefit and are not reimbursable within the scope of this benefit.

It is recognized that a limited number of patients will fail on oral anti-emetic drugs. Intravenous anti-emetics may be covered (subject to the rules of medical necessity) when furnished to patients who fail on oral anti-emetic therapy.

More than one oral anti emetic drug may be prescribed and may be covered for concurrent use if needed to fully replace the intravenous drugs that otherwise would be given. See the Medicare National Coverage Determinations Manual, Publication 100-04, Chapter 1, Section 110.18, for detailed coverage criteria.

## 100-02, 15, 50.6

### Coverage of Intravenous Immune Globulin for Treatment of Primary Immune Deficiency Diseases in the Home

Beginning for dates of service on or after January 1, 2004, The Medicare Prescription Drug, Improvement, and Modernization Act of 2003 provides coverage of intravenous immune globulin (IVIG) for the treatment of primary immune deficiency diseases in the home (ICD-9 diagnosis codes 279.04, 279.05, 279.06, 279.12, and 279.2 or ICD-10-

CM codes D80.0, D80.5, D81.0, D81.1, D81.2, D81.6, D81.7, D81.89, D81.9, D82.0, D83.0, D83.2, D83.8, or D83.9 if only an unspecified diagnosis is necessary). The Act defines "intravenous immune globulin" as an approved pooled plasma derivative for the treatment of primary immune deficiency disease. It is covered under this benefit when the patient has a diagnosed primary immune deficiency disease, it is administered in the home of a patient with a diagnosed primary immune deficiency disease, and the physician determines that administration of the derivative in the patient's home is medically appropriate. The benefit does not include coverage for items or services related to the administration of the derivative. For coverage of IVIG under this benefit, it is not necessary for the derivative to be administered through a piece of durable medical equipment.

## 100-02, 15, 110

### Durable Medical Equipment - General

B3-2100, A3-3113, HO-235, HHA-220

Expenses incurred by a beneficiary for the rental or purchases of durable medical equipment (DME) are reimbursable if the following three requirements are met:

- The equipment meets the definition of DME (Sec.110.1);
- The equipment is necessary and reasonable for the treatment of the patient's illness or injury or to improve the functioning of his or her malformed body member (Sec.110.1); and
- The equipment is used in the patient's home. The decision whether to rent or purchase an item of equipment generally resides with the beneficiary, but the decision on how to pay rests with CMS. For some DME, program payment policy calls for lump sum payments and in others for periodic payment. Where covered DME is furnished to a beneficiary by a supplier of services other than a provider of services, the DMERC makes the reimbursement. If a provider of services furnishes the equipment, the intermediary makes the reimbursement. The payment method is identified in the annual fee schedule update furnished by CMS. The CMS issues quarterly updates to a fee schedule file that contains rates by HCPCS code and also identifies the classification of the HCPCS code within the following categories. Category Code Definition IN Inexpensive and Other Routinely Purchased Items FS Frequently Serviced Items CR Capped Rental Items OX Oxygen and Oxygen Equipment OS Ostomy, Tracheostomy & Urological Items SD Surgical Dressings PO Prosthetics & Orthotics SU Supplies TE Transcutaneous Electrical Nerve Stimulators The DMERCs, carriers, and intermediaries, where appropriate, use the CMS files to determine payment rules. See the Medicare Claims Processing Manual, Chapter 20, "Durable Medical Equipment, Surgical Dressings and Casts, Orthotics and Artificial Limbs, and Prosthetic Devices," for a detailed description of payment rules for each classification. Payment may also be made for repairs, maintenance, and delivery of equipment and for expendable and nonreusable items essential to the effective use of the equipment subject to the conditions in Sec.110.2. See the Medicare Benefit Policy Manual, Chapter 11, "End Stage Renal Disease," for hemodialysis equipment and supplies.

## 100-02, 15, 140

### Therapeutic Shoes for Individuals with Diabetes

B3-2134 Coverage of therapeutic shoes (depth or custom-molded) along with inserts for individuals with diabetes is available as of May 1, 1993. These diabetic shoes are covered if the requirements as specified in this section concerning certification and prescription are fulfilled. In addition, this benefit provides for a pair of diabetic shoes even if only one foot suffers from diabetic foot disease. Each shoe is equally equipped so that the affected limb, as well as the remaining limb, is protected. Claims for therapeutic shoes for diabetics are processed by the Durable Medical Equipment Regional Carriers (DMERCs). Therapeutic shoes for diabetics are not DME and are not considered DME nor orthotics, but a separate category of coverage under Medicare Part B. (See Sec.1861(s)(12) and Sec.1833(o) of the Act.)

### A. Definitions

The following items may be covered under the diabetic shoe benefit:

1. Custom-Molded ShoesCustom-molded shoes are shoes that:
   - Are constructed over a positive model of the patient's foot;
   - Are made from leather or other suitable material of equal quality;
   - Have removable inserts that can be altered or replaced as the patient's condition warrants; and
   - Have some form of shoe closure.
2. Depth Shoes

Depth shoes are shoes that:

- Have a full length, heel-to-toe filler that, when removed, provides a minimum of 3/16 inch of additional depth used to accommodate custom-molded or customized inserts;
- Are made from leather or other suitable material of equal quality;
- Have some form of shoe closure; and
- Are available in full and half sizes with a minimum of three widths so that the sole is graded to the size and width of the upper portions of the shoes according to the American standard last sizing schedule or its equivalent. (The American standard last sizing schedule is the numerical shoe sizing system used for shoes sold in the United States.)

3. Inserts

Inserts are total contact, multiple density, removable inlays that are directly molded to the patient's foot or a model of the patient's foot and that are made of a suitable material with regard to the patient's condition.

### B. Coverage

1. Limitations For each individual, coverage of the footwear and inserts is limited to one of the following within one calendar year:
   - No more than one pair of custom-molded shoes (including inserts provided with such shoes) and two additional pairs of inserts; or
   - No more than one pair of depth shoes and three pairs of inserts (not including the noncustomized removable inserts provided with such shoes).

2. Coverage of Diabetic Shoes and Brace
   Orthopedic shoes, as stated in the Medicare Claims Processing Manual, Chapter 20, "Durable Medical Equipment, Surgical Dressings and Casts, Orthotics and Artificial Limbs, and Prosthetic Devices," generally are not covered. This exclusion does not apply to orthopedic shoes that are an integral part of a leg brace. In situations in which an individual qualifies for both diabetic shoes and a leg brace, these items are covered separately. Thus, the diabetic shoes may be covered if the requirements for this section are met, while the brace may be covered if the requirements of Sec.130 are met.

3. Substitution of Modifications for Inserts
   An individual may substitute modification(s) of custom-molded or depth shoes instead of obtaining a pair(s) of inserts in any combination. Payment for the modification(s) may not exceed the limit set for the inserts for which the individual is entitled. The following is a list of the most common shoe modifications available, but it is not meant as an exhaustive list of the modifications available for diabetic shoes:
   - Rigid Rocker Bottoms - These are exterior elevations with apex positions for 51 percent to 75 percent distance measured from the back end of the heel. The apex is a narrowed or pointed end of an anatomical structure. The apex must be positioned behind the metatarsal heads and tapered off sharply to the front tip of the sole. Apex height helps to eliminate pressure at the metatarsal heads. Rigidity is ensured by the steel in the shoe. The heel of the shoe tapers off in the back in order to cause the heel to strike in the middle of the heel;
   - Roller Bottoms (Sole or Bar) - These are the same as rocker bottoms, but the heel is tapered from the apex to the front tip of the sole;
   - Metatarsal Bars- An exterior bar is placed behind the metatarsal heads in order to remove pressure from the metatarsal heads. The bars are of various shapes, heights, and construction depending on the exact purpose;
   - Wedges (Posting) - Wedges are either of hind foot, fore foot, or both and may be in the middle or to the side. The function is to shift or transfer weight bearing upon standing or during ambulation to the opposite side for added support, stabilization, equalized weight distribution, or balance; and
   - Offset Heels- This is a heel flanged at its base either in the middle, to the side, or a combination, that is then extended upward to the shoe in order to stabilize extreme positions of the hind foot. Other modifications to diabetic shoes include, but are not limited to flared heels, Velcro closures, and inserts for missing toes.

4. Separate Inserts
   Inserts may be covered and dispensed independently of diabetic shoes if the supplier of the shoes verifies in writing that the patient has appropriate footwear into which the insert can be placed. This footwear must meet the definitions found above for depth shoes and custom-molded shoes.

### C. Certification

The need for diabetic shoes must be certified by a physician who is a doctor of medicine or a doctor of osteopathy and who is responsible for diagnosing and treating the patient's diabetic systemic condition through a comprehensive plan of care. This managing physician must:

- Document in the patient's medical record that the patient has diabetes;

- Certify that the patient is being treated under a comprehensive plan of care for diabetes, and that the patient needs diabetic shoes; and
- Document in the patient's record that the patient has one or more of the following conditions:
  - Peripheral neuropathy with evidence of callus formation;
  - History of pre-ulcerative calluses;
  - History of previous ulceration;
  - Foot deformity;
  - Previous amputation of the foot or part of the foot; or
  - Poor circulation.

### D. Prescription

Following certification by the physician managing the patient's systemic diabetic condition, a podiatrist or other qualified physician who is knowledgeable in the fitting of diabetic shoes and inserts may prescribe the particular type of footwear necessary.

### E. Furnishing Footwear

The footwear must be fitted and furnished by a podiatrist or other qualified individual such as a pedorthist, an orthotist, or a prosthetist. The certifying physician may not furnish the diabetic shoes unless the certifying physician is the only qualified individual in the area. It is left to the discretion of each carrier to determine the meaning of "in the area."

## 100-02, 15, 200

### Nurse Practitioner (NP) Services

Effective for services rendered after January 1, 1998, any individual who is participating under the Medicare program as a nurse practitioner (NP) for the first time ever, may have his or her professional services covered if he or she meets the qualifications listed below, and he or she is legally authorized to furnish NP services in the State where the services are performed. NPs who were issued billing provider numbers prior to January 1, 1998, may continue to furnish services under the NP benefit.

Payment for NP services is effective on the date of service, that is, on or after January 1, 1998, and payment is made on an assignment-related basis only.

### A. Qualifications for NPs

In order to furnish covered NP services, an NP must meet the conditions as follows:

- Be a registered professional nurse who is authorized by the State in which the services are furnished to practice as a nurse practitioner in accordance with State law; and be certified as a nurse practitioner by a recognized national certifying body that has established standards for nurse practitioners; or
- Be a registered professional nurse who is authorized by the State in which the services are furnished to practice as a nurse practitioner by December 31, 2000.

The following organizations are recognized national certifying bodies for NPs at the advanced practice level:

- American Academy of Nurse Practitioners;
- American Nurses Credentialing Center;
- National Certification Corporation for Obstetric, Gynecologic and Neonatal Nursing Specialties;
- Pediatric Nursing Certification Board (previously named the National Certification Board of Pediatric Nurse Practitioners and Nurses);
- Oncology Nurses Certification Corporation;
- AACN Certification Corporation; and
- National Board on Certification of Hospice and Palliative Nurses.

The NPs applying for a Medicare billing number for the first time on or after January 1, 2001, must meet the requirements as follows:

- Be a registered professional nurse who is authorized by the State in which the services are furnished to practice as a nurse practitioner in accordance with State law; and
- Be certified as a nurse practitioner by a recognized national certifying body that has established standards for nurse practitioners.

The NPs applying for a Medicare billing number for the first time on or after January 1, 2003, must meet the requirements as follows:

- Be a registered professional nurse who is authorized by the State in which the services are furnished to practice as a nurse practitioner in accordance with State law;
- Be certified as a nurse practitioner by a recognized national certifying body that has established standards for nurse practitioners; and
- Possess a master's degree in nursing.

### B. Covered Services

Coverage is limited to the services an NP is legally authorized to perform in accordance with State law (or State regulatory mechanism established by State law).

#### 1. General

The services of an NP may be covered under Part B if all of the following conditions are met:

- They are the type that are considered physician's services if furnished by a doctor of medicine or osteopathy (MD/DO);
- They are performed by a person who meets the definition of an NP (see subsection A);
- The NP is legally authorized to perform the services in the State in which they are performed;
- They are performed in collaboration with an MD/DO (see subsection D); and
- They are not otherwise precluded from coverage because of one of the statutory exclusions. (See subsection C.2.)

#### 2. Incident To

If covered NP services are furnished, services and supplies furnished incident to the services of the NP may also be covered if they would have been covered when furnished incident to the services of an MD/DO as described in §60.

### C. Application of Coverage Rules
#### 1. Types of NP Services That May Be Covered

State law or regulation governing an NP's scope of practice in the State in which the services are performed applies. Consider developing a list of covered services based on the State scope of practice. Examples of the types of services that NP's may include services that traditionally have been reserved to physicians, such as physical examinations, minor surgery, setting casts for simple fractures, interpreting x-rays, and other activities that involve an independent evaluation or treatment of the patient's condition. Also, if authorized under the scope of their State license, NPs may furnish services billed under all levels of evaluation and management codes and diagnostic tests if furnished in collaboration with a physician.

See §60.2 for coverage of services performed by NPs incident to the services of physicians.

#### 2. Services Otherwise Excluded From Coverage

The NP services may not be covered if they are otherwise excluded from coverage even though an NP may be authorized by State law to perform them. For example, the Medicare law excludes from coverage routine foot care, routine physical checkups, and services that are not reasonable and necessary for the diagnosis or treatment of an illness or injury or to improve the functioning of a malformed body member. Therefore, these services are precluded from coverage even though they may be within an NP's scope of practice under State law.

### D. Collaboration

Collaboration is a process in which an NP works with one or more physicians (MD/DO) to deliver health care services, with medical direction and appropriate supervision as required by the law of the State in which the services are furnished. In the absence of State law governing collaboration, collaboration is to be evidenced by NPs documenting their scope of practice and indicating the relationships that they have with physicians to deal with issues outside their scope of practice.

The collaborating physician does not need to be present with the NP when the services are furnished or to make an independent evaluation of each patient who is seen by the NP.

### E. Direct Billing and Payment

Direct billing and payment for NP services may be made to the NP.

### F. Assignment

Assignment is mandatory.

## 100-02, 15, 232

### Cardiac Rehabilitation (CR) and Intensive Cardiac Rehabilitation (ICR) Services Furnished On or After January 1, 2010

Cardiac rehabilitation (CR) services mean a physician-supervised program that furnishes physician prescribed exercise, cardiac risk factor modification, including education, counseling, and behavioral intervention; psychosocial assessment, outcomes assessment, and other items/services as determined by the Secretary under certain conditions. Intensive cardiac rehabilitation (ICR) services mean a physician-supervised program that furnishes the same items/services under the same conditions as a CR program but must also demonstrate, as shown in peer-reviewed published research, that it improves patients' cardiovascular disease through specific outcome measurements described in 42 CFR 410.49(c). Effective

January 1, 2010, Medicare Part B pays for CR/ICR programs and related items/services if specific criteria is met by the Medicare beneficiary, the CR/ICR program itself, the setting in which is it administered, and the physician administering the program, as outlined below:

CR/ICR Program Beneficiary Requirements:

- Medicare covers CR/ICR program services for beneficiaries who have experienced one or more of the following:
- Acute myocardial infarction within the preceding 12 months;
- Coronary artery bypass surgery;
- Current stable angina pectoris;
- Heart valve repair or replacement;
- Percutaneous transluminal coronary angioplasty (PTCA) or coronary stenting;
- Heart or heart-lung transplant.

For cardiac rehabilitation only: Stable, chronic heart failure defined as patients with left ventricular ejection fraction of 35% or less and New York Heart Association (NYHA) class II to IV symptoms despite being on optimal heart failure therapy for at least 6 weeks. (Effective February 18, 2014.)

**CR/ICR Program Component Requirements:**
Physician-prescribed exercise. This physical activity includes aerobic exercise combined with other types of exercise (i.e., strengthening, stretching) as determined to be appropriate for individual patients by a physician each day CR/ICR items/services are furnished.

Cardiac risk factor modification. This includes education, counseling, and behavioral intervention, tailored to the patients' individual needs.

Psychosocial assessment. This assessment means an evaluation of an individual's mental and emotional functioning as it relates to the individual's rehabilitation. It should include: (1) an assessment of those aspects of the individual's family and home situation that affects the individual's rehabilitation treatment, and, (2) a psychosocial evaluation of the individual's response to, and rate of progress under, the treatment plan.

Outcomes assessment. These should include: (i) minimally, assessments from the commencement and conclusion of CR/ICR, based on patient-centered outcomes which must be measured by the physician immediately at the beginning and end of the program, and, (ii) objective clinical measures of the effectiveness of the CR/ICR program for the individual patient, including exercise performance and self-reported measures of exertion and behavior.

Individualized treatment plan. This plan should be written and tailored to each individual patient and include (i) a description of the individual's diagnosis; (ii) the type, amount, frequency, and duration of the CR/ICR items/services furnished; and (iii) the goals set for the individual under the plan. The individualized treatment plan must be established, reviewed, and signed by a physician every 30 days.

As specified at 42 CFR 410.49(f)(1), CR sessions are limited to a maximum of 2 1-hour sessions per day for up to 36 sessions over up to 36 weeks with the option for an additional 36 sessions over an extended period of time if approved by the contractor under section 1862(a)(1)(A) of the Act. ICR sessions are limited to 72 1-hour sessions (as defined in section 1848(b)(5) of the Act), up to 6 sessions per day, over a period of up to 18 weeks.

**CR/ICR Program Setting Requirements:**
CR/ICR services must be furnished in a physician's office or a hospital outpatient setting (for ICR, the hospital outpatient setting must provide ICR using an approved ICR program). All settings must have a physician immediately available and accessible for medical consultations and emergencies at all times when items/services are being furnished under the program. This provision is satisfied if the physician meets the requirements for direct supervision of physician office services as specified at 42 CFR 410.26, and for hospital outpatient services as specified at 42 CFR 410.27.

**ICR Program Approval Requirements:**
All prospective ICR programs must be approved through the national coverage determination (NCD) process. To be approved as an ICR program, it must demonstrate through peer-reviewed, published research that it has accomplished one or more of the following for its patients: (i) positively affected the progression of coronary heart disease, (ii) reduced the need for coronary bypass surgery, or, (iii) reduced the need for percutaneous coronary interventions.

An ICR program must also demonstrate through peer-reviewed, published research that it accomplished a statistically significant reduction in five or more of the following measures for patients from their levels before CR services to after CR services: (i) low density lipoprotein, (ii) triglycerides, (iii) body mass index, (iv) systolic blood pressure, (v) diastolic blood pressure, and (vi) the need for cholesterol, blood pressure, and diabetes medications.

A list of approved ICR programs, identified through the NCD process, will be posted to the CMS Web site and listed in the Federal Register.

Once an ICR program is approved through the NCD process, all prospective ICR sites wishing to furnish ICR items/services via an approved ICR program may enroll with their local contractor to become an ICR program supplier using the designated forms as specified at 42 CFR 424.510, and report specialty code 31 to be identified as an enrolled ICR supplier. For purposes of appealing an adverse determination concerning site approval, an ICR site is considered a supplier (or prospective supplier) as defined in 42 CFR 498.2.

**CR/ICR Program Physician Requirements:**
Physicians responsible for CR/ICR programs are identified as medical directors who oversee or supervise the CR/ICR program at a particular site. The medical director, in consultation with staff, is involved in directing the progress of individuals in the program. The medical director, as well as physicians acting as the supervising physician, must possess all of the following: (1) expertise in the management of individuals with cardiac pathophysiology, (2) cardiopulmonary training in basic life support or advanced cardiac life support, and (3) licensed to practice medicine in the state in which the CR/ICR program is offered. Direct physician supervision may be provided by a supervising physician or the medical director.

(See Pub. 100-03, Medicare National Coverage Determinations Manual, Chapter 1, Part 1, section 20.10.1, Pub. 100-04, Medicare Claims Processing Manual, Chapter 32, section 140, Pub. 100-08, Medicare Program Integrity Manual, Chapter 15, section 15.4.2.8, for specific claims processing, coding, and billing requirements for CR/ICR program services.)

## 100-02, 15, 270.2

**List of Medicare Telehealth Services**
The use of a telecommunications system may substitute for an in-person encounter for professional consultations, office visits, office psychiatry services, and a limited number of other physician fee schedule (PFS) services. These services are listed below.

- Consultations (Effective October 1, 2001- December 31, 2009)
- Telehealth consultations, emergency department or initial inpatient (Effective January 1, 2010)
- Follow-up inpatient telehealth consultations (Effective January 1, 2009)
- Office or other outpatient visits
- Subsequent hospital care services (with the limitation of one telehealth visit every 3 days) (Effective January 1, 2011)
- Subsequent nursing facility care services (with the limitation of one telehealth visit every 30 days) (Effective January 1, 2011)
- Individual psychotherapy
- Pharmacologic management (Effective March 1, 2003 – December 31, 2012)
- Psychiatric diagnostic interview examination (Effective March 1, 2003)
- End stage renal disease related services (Effective January 1, 2005)
- Individual and group medical nutrition therapy (Individual effective January 1, 2006; group effective January 1, 2011)
- Neurobehavioral status exam (Effective January 1, 2008)
- Individual and group health and behavior assessment and intervention (Individual effective January 1, 2010; group effective January 1, 2011)
- Individual and group kidney disease education (KDE) services (Effective January 1, 2011)
- Individual and group diabetes self-management training (DSMT) services (with a minimum of 1 hour of in-person instruction to be furnished in the initial year training period to ensure effective injection training) (Effective January 1, 2011)
- Smoking Cessation Services (Effective January 1, 2012)
- Alcohol and/or substance (other than tobacco) abuse structured assessment and intervention services (Effective January 1, 2013)
- Annual alcohol misuse screening (Effective January 1, 2013)
- Brief face-to-face behavioral counseling for alcohol misuse (Effective January 1, 2013).
- Annual Depression Screening (Effective January 1, 2013)
- High-intensity behavioral counseling to prevent sexually transmitted infections (Effective January 1, 2013)
- Annual, face-to-face Intensive behavioral therapy for cardiovascular disease (Effective January 1, 2013)
- Face-to-face behavioral counseling for obesity (Effective January 1, 2013)

- Transitional Care Management Services (Effective January 1, 2014)

NOTE: Beginning January 1, 2010, CMS eliminated the use of all consultation codes, except for inpatient telehealth consultation G-codes. CMS no longer recognizes office/outpatient or inpatient consultation CPT codes for payment of office/outpatient or inpatient visits. Instead, physicians and practitioners are instructed to bill a new or established patient office/outpatient visit CPT code or appropriate hospital or nursing facility care code, as appropriate to the particular patient, for all office/outpatient or inpatient visits. For detailed instructions regarding reporting these and other telehealth services, see Pub. 100-04, Medicare Claims Processing Manual, chapter 12, section 190.3.

The conditions of payment for Medicare telehealth services, including qualifying originating sites and the types of telecommunications systems recognized by Medicare, are subject to the provisions of 42 CFR 410.78. Payment for these services is subject to the provisions of 42 CFR 414.65.

## 100-02, 15, 270.4

### Payment - Physician/Practitioner at a Distant Site

The term "distant site" means the site where the physician or practitioner providing the professional service is located at the time the service is provided via a telecommunications system.

The payment amount for the professional service provided via a telecommunications system by the physician or practitioner at the distant site is equal to the current physician fee schedule amount for the service. Payment for telehealth services (see section 270.2 of this chapter) should be made at the same amount as when these services are furnished without the use of a telecommunications system. For Medicare payment to occur, the service must be within a practitioner's scope of practice under State law. The beneficiary is responsible for any unmet deductible amount and applicable coinsurance.

### Medicare Practitioners Who May Receive Payment at the Distant Site (i.e., at a Site Other Than Where the Beneficiary is Located)

As a condition of Medicare Part B payment for telehealth services, the physician or practitioner at the distant site must be licensed to provide the service under State law. When the physician or practitioner at the distant site is licensed under State law to provide a covered telehealth service (see section 270.2 of this chapter) then he or she may bill for and receive payment for this service when delivered via a telecommunications system.

Medicare practitioners who may bill for a covered telehealth service are listed below (subject to State law):

- Physician;
- Nurse practitioner;
- Physician assistant;
- Nurse midwife;
- Clinical nurse specialist;
- Clinical psychologist;
- Clinical social worker; and
- Registered dietitian or nutrition professional.

\* Clinical psychologists and clinical social workers cannot bill for psychotherapy services that include medical evaluation and management services under Medicare. These practitioners may not bill or receive payment for the following CPT codes: 90805, 90807, and 90809.

## 100-02, 15, 280.1

### Glaucoma Screening

#### A. Conditions of Coverage

The regulations implementing the Benefits Improvements and Protection Act of 2000, Sec.102, provide for annual coverage for glaucoma screening for beneficiaries in the following high risk categories:

- Individuals with diabetes mellitus;
- Individuals with a family history of glaucoma; or
- African-Americans age 50 and over.

In addition, beginning with dates of service on or after January 1, 2006, 42 CFR 410.23(a)(2), revised, the definition of an eligible beneficiary in a high-risk category is expanded to include:

- Hispanic-Americans age 65 and over.

Medicare will pay for glaucoma screening examinations where they are furnished by or under the direct supervision in the office setting of an ophthalmologist or optometrist, who is legally authorized to perform the services under State law. Screening for glaucoma is defined to include:

- A dilated eye examination with an intraocular pressure measurement; and
- A direct ophthalmoscopy examination, or a slit-lamp biomicroscopic examination.

Payment may be made for a glaucoma screening examination that is performed on an eligible beneficiary after at least 11 months have passed following the month in which the last covered glaucoma screening examination was performed.

The following HCPCS codes apply for glaucoma screening:

G0117   Glaucoma screening for high-risk patients furnished by an optometrist or ophthalmologist; and

G0118   Glaucoma screening for high-risk patients furnished under the direct supervision of an optometrist or ophthalmologist.

The type of service for the above G codes is: TOS Q.

For providers who bill intermediaries, applicable types of bill for screening glaucoma services are 13X, 22X, 23X, 71X, 73X, 75X, and 85X. The following revenue codes should be reported when billing for screening glaucoma services:

- Comprehensive outpatient rehabilitation facilities (CORFs), critical access hospitals (CAHs), skilled nursing facilities (SNFs), independent and provider-based RHCs and free standing and provider-based FQHCs bill for this service under revenue code 770. CAHs electing the optional method of payment for outpatient services report this service under revenue codes 96X, 97X, or 98X.
- Hospital outpatient departments bill for this service under any valid/appropriate revenue code. They are not required to report revenue code 770.

#### B. Calculating the Frequency

Once a beneficiary has received a covered glaucoma screening procedure, the beneficiary may receive another procedure after 11 full months have passed. To determine the 11-month period, start the count beginning with the month after the month in which the previous covered screening procedure was performed.

#### C. Diagnosis Coding Requirements

Providers bill glaucoma screening using screening ("V") code V80.1 (Special Screening for Neurological, Eye, and Ear Diseases, Glaucoma). Claims submitted without a screening diagnosis code may be returned to the provider as unprocessable.

#### D. Payment Methodology

1. Carriers

   Contractors pay for glaucoma screening based on the Medicare physician fee schedule. Deductible and coinsurance apply. Claims from physicians or other providers where assignment was not taken are subject to the Medicare limiting charge (refer to the Medicare Claims Processing Manual, Chapter 12, "Physician/Non-physician Practitioners," for more information about the Medicare limiting charge).

2. Intermediaries

   Payment is made for the facility expense as follows:

   - Independent and provider-based RHC/free standing and provider-based FQHC - payment is made under the all inclusive rate for the screening glaucoma service based on the visit furnished to the RHC/FQHC patient;
   - CAH - payment is made on a reasonable cost basis unless the CAH has elected the optional method of payment for outpatient services in which case, procedures outlined in the Medicare Claims Processing Manual, Chapter 3, Sec.30.1.1, should be followed;
   - CORF - payment is made under the Medicare physician fee schedule;
   - Hospital outpatient department - payment is made under outpatient prospective payment system (OPPS);
   - Hospital inpatient Part B - payment is made under OPPS;
   - SNF outpatient - payment is made under the Medicare physician fee schedule (MPFS); and
   - SNF inpatient Part B - payment is made under MPFS.

   Deductible and coinsurance apply.

#### E. Special Billing Instructions for RHCs and FQHCs

Screening glaucoma services are considered RHC/FQHC services. RHCs and FQHCs bill the contractor under bill type 71X or 73X along with revenue code 770 and HCPCS codes G0117 or G0118 and RHC/FQHC revenue code 520 or 521 to report the related visit. Reporting of revenue code 770 and HCPCS codes G0117 and G0118 in addition to revenue code 520 or 521 is required for this service in order for CWF to perform frequency editing.

Payment should not be made for a screening glaucoma service unless the claim also contains a visit code for the service. Therefore, the contractor installs an edit in its

**Appendix 4 — Internet-only Manuals (IOMs)**

system to assure payment is not made for revenue code 770 unless the claim also contains a visit revenue code (520 or 521).

## 100-02, 15, 280.2.2

### Coverage Criteria

(Rev. 196, Issued: 10-17-14, Effective: 01-27-14, Implementation: 11-18-14)

The following are the coverage criteria for these screenings:

### A. Screening Fecal-Occult Blood Tests (FOBT) (Codes G0107 & G0328)

Effective for services furnished on or after January 1, 2004, one screening FOBT (code G0107 or G0328) is covered for beneficiaries who have attained age 50, at a frequency of once every 12 months (i.e., at least 11 months have passed following the month in which the last covered screening FOBT was done). Screening FOBT means: (1) a guaiac-based test for peroxidase activity in which the beneficiary completes it by taking samples from two different sites of three consecutive stools or, (2) an immunoassay (or immunochemical) test for antibody activity in which the beneficiary completes the test by taking the appropriate number of samples according to the specific manufacturer's

instructions. This expanded coverage is in accordance with revised regulations at 42 CFR 410.37(a)(2) that includes " other tests determined by the Secretary through a national coverage determination." This screening requires a written order from the beneficiary's attending physician or for claims with dates of service on or after January 27, 2014, from the beneficiary's attending physician assistant, nurse practitioner, or clinical nurse specialist. (The term "attending physician" is defined to mean a doctor of medicine or osteopathy (as defined in §1861(r)(1) of the Act) who is fully knowledgeable about the beneficiary's medical condition, and who would be responsible for using the results of any examination performed in the overall management of the beneficiary's specific medical problem.)

NOTE: For claims with dates of service prior to January 1, 2007, physicians, suppliers, and providers report HCPCS code G0107. Effective January 1, 2007, code G0107, is discontinued and replaced with CPT code 82270. For complete claims processing information refer to Pub. 100-04, Medicare Claims Processing Manual, chapter 18, section 60.

### B. Screening Flexible Sigmoidoscopies (code G0104)

For claims with dates of service on or after January 1, 2002, A/B MACs (B) pay for screening flexible sigmoidoscopies (Code G0104) for beneficiaries who have attained age 50 when these services were performed by a doctor of medicine or osteopathy, or by a physician assistant, nurse practitioner, or clinical nurse specialist (as defined in §1861(aa)(5) of the Act and at 42 CFR 410.74, 410.75, and 410.76) at the frequencies noted below. For claims with dates of service prior to January 1, 2002, pay for these services under the conditions noted only when they are performed by a doctor of medicine or osteopathy.

#### For services furnished from January 1, 1998, through June 30, 2001, inclusive

Once every 48 months (i.e., at least 47 months have passed following the month in which the last covered screening flexible sigmoidoscopy was done).

#### For services furnished on or after July 1, 2001

Once every 48 months as calculated above unless the beneficiary does not meet the criteria for high risk of developing colorectal cancer (refer to §280.2.3) and the beneficiary has had a screening colonoscopy (code G0121) within the preceding 10 years. If such a beneficiary has had a screening colonoscopy within the preceding 10 years, then he or she can have covered a screening flexible sigmoidoscopy only after at least 119 months have passed following the month that he/she received the screening colonoscopy (code G0121).

NOTE: If during the course of a screening flexible sigmoidoscopy a lesion or growth is detected which results in a biopsy or removal of the growth, the appropriate diagnostic

procedure classified as a flexible sigmoidoscopy with biopsy or removal should be billed and paid rather than code G0104.

### C. Screening Colonoscopies for Beneficiaries at High Risk of Developing Colorectal Cancer (Code G0105)

The A/B MAC (B) must pay for screening colonoscopies (code G0105) when performed by a doctor of medicine or osteopathy at a frequency of once every 24 months for beneficiaries at high risk for developing colorectal cancer (i.e., at least 23 months have passed following the month in which the last covered G0105 screening colonoscopy was performed). Refer to §280.2.3 for the criteria to use in determining whether or not an individual is at high risk for developing colorectal cancer.

NOTE: If during the course of the screening colonoscopy, a lesion or growth is detected which results in a biopsy or removal of the growth, the appropriate diagnostic procedure classified as a colonoscopy with biopsy or removal should be billed and paid rather than code G0105.

### D. Screening Colonoscopies Performed on Individuals Not Meeting the Criteria for Being at High-Risk for Developing Colorectal Cancer (Code G0121)

Effective for services furnished on or after July 1, 2001, screening colonoscopies (code G0121) are covered when performed under the following conditions:

1. On individuals not meeting the criteria for being at high risk for developing colorectal cancer (refer to §280.2.3);

2. At a frequency of once every 10 years (i.e., at least 119 months have passed following the month in which the last covered G0121 screening colonoscopy was performed); and

3. If the individual would otherwise qualify to have covered a G0121 screening colonoscopy based on the above (see §§280.2.2.D.1 and 2) but has had a covered screening flexible sigmoidoscopy (code G0104), then the individual may have a covered G0121 screening colonoscopy only after at least 47 months have passed following the month in which the last covered G0104 flexible sigmoidoscopy was performed.

NOTE: I f during the course of the screening colonoscopy, a lesion or growth is detected which results in a biopsy or removal of the growth, the appropriate diagnostic procedure classified as a colonoscopy with biopsy or removal should be billed and paid rather than code G0121.

### E. Screening Barium Enema Examinations (codes G0106 and G0120)

Screening barium enema examinations are covered as an alternative to either a screening sigmoidoscopy (code G0104) or a screening colonoscopy (code G0105) examination. The same frequency parameters for screening sigmoidoscopies and screening colonoscopies above apply.

In the case of an individual aged 50 or over, payment may be made for a screening barium enema examination (code G0106) performed after at least 47 months have passed following the month in which the last screening barium enema or screening flexible sigmoidoscopy was performed. For example, the beneficiary received a screening barium enema examination as an alternative to a screening flexible sigmoidoscopy in January 1999. The count starts beginning February 1999. The beneficiary is eligible for another screening barium enema in January 2003.

In the case of an individual who is at high risk for colorectal cancer, payment may be made for a screening barium enema examination (code G0120) performed after at least 23 months have passed following the month in which the last screening barium enema or the last screening colonoscopy was performed. For example, a beneficiary at high risk for developing colorectal cancer received a screening barium enema examination (code G0120) as an alternative to a screening colonoscopy (code G0105) in January 2000. The count starts beginning February 2000. The beneficiary is eligible for another screening barium enema examination (code G0120) in January 2002.

The screening barium enema must be ordered in writing after a determination that the test is the appropriate screening test. Generally, it is expected that this will be a screening double contrast enema unless the individual is unable to withstand such an exam. This means that in the case of a particular individual, the attending physician must determine that the estimated screening potential for the barium enema is equal to or greater than the screening potential that has been estimated for a screening flexible sigmoidoscopy, or for a screening colonoscopy, as appropriate, for the same individual. The screening single contrast barium enema also requires a written order from the beneficiary's attending physician in the same manner as described above for the screening double contrast barium enema examination.

## 100-02, 15, 280.4

### Screening Pap Smears

Effective, January 1, 1998, §4102 of the Balanced Budget Act (BBA) of 1997 (P.L. 105-33) amended §1861(nn) of the Act (42 USC 1395X(nn)) to include coverage every 3 years for a screening Pap smear or more frequent coverage for women:

1. At high risk for cervical or vaginal cancer; or

2. Of childbearing age who have had a Pap smear during any of the preceding 3 years indicating the presence of cervical or vaginal cancer or other abnormality.

Effective July 1, 2001, the Consolidated Appropriations Act of 2001 (P.L. 106-554) modifies §1861(nn) to provide Medicare coverage for biennial screening Pap smears. Specifications for frequency limitations are defined below.

For claims with dates of service from January 1, 1998, through June 30, 2001, screening Pap smears are covered when ordered and collected by a doctor of medicine or osteopathy (as defined in §1861(r)(1) of the Act), or other authorized practitioner (e.g., a certified nurse midwife, physician assistant, nurse practitioner, or clinical nurse specialist, who is authorized under State law to perform the examination) under one of the following conditions:

The beneficiary has not had a screening Pap smear test during the preceding 3 years (i.e., 35 months have passed following the month that the woman had the last

© 2016 Optum360, LLC

covered Pap smear – ICD-9-CM code V76.2 or ICD-10 code Z112.4 is used to indicate special screening for malignant neoplasm, cervix); or

There is evidence (on the basis of her medical history or other findings) that she is of childbearing age and has had an examination that indicated the presence of cervical or vaginal cancer or other abnormalities during any of the preceding 3 years; and at least 11 months have passed following the month that the last covered Pap smear was performed; or

She is at high risk of developing cervical or vaginal cancer – ICD-9-CM code V15.89, other specified personal history presenting hazards to health) or as applicable, ICD-10 code Z77.21, Z77.22, Z77.9, Z91.89, OR Z92.89 and at least 11 months have passed following the month that the last covered screening Pap smear was performed. The high risk factors for cervical and vaginal cancer are:

#### Cervical Cancer High Risk Factors
- Early onset of sexual activity (under 16 years of age);
- Multiple sexual partners (five or more in a lifetime);
- History of a sexually transmitted disease (including HIV infection); and
- Fewer than three negative or any Pap smears within the previous 7 years.

#### Vaginal Cancer High Risk Factors
- The DES (diethylstilbestrol) - exposed daughters of women who took DES during pregnancy.

The term "woman of childbearing age" means a woman who is premenopausal, and has been determined by a physician, or qualified practitioner, to be of childbearing age, based on her medical history or other findings. Payment is not made for a screening Pap smear for women at high risk or who qualify for coverage under the childbearing provision more frequently than once every 11 months after the month that the last screening Pap smear covered by Medicare was performed.

#### B. For Claims with Dates of Service on or After July 1, 2001
When the beneficiary does not qualify for a more frequently performed screening Pap smear as noted in items 1 and 2 above, contractors pay for the screening Pap smear only after at least 23 months have passed following the month during which the beneficiary received her last covered screening Pap smear. All other coverage and payment requirements remain the same.

See the Medicare Claims Processing Manual, Chapter 18, "Preventive and Screening Services," for billing procedures.

### 100-02, 15, 280.5

#### Annual Wellness Visit (AWV) Providing Personalized Prevention Plan Services (PPPS)

#### A. General
Pursuant to section 4103 of the Affordable Care Act of 2010 (the ACA), the Centers for Medicare & Medicaid Services (CMS) amended section 411.15(a)(1) and 411.15(k)(15) of the Code of Federal Regulations (CFR)(list of examples of routine physical examinations excluded from coverage), effective for services furnished on or after January 1, 2011. This expanded coverage, as established at 42 CFR 410.15, is subject to certain eligibility and other limitations that allow payment for an annual wellness visit (AWV), providing personalized prevention plan services (PPPS), for an individual who is no longer within 12 months after the effective date of his/her first Medicare Part B coverage period, and has not received either an initial preventive physical examination (IPPE) or an AWV within the past 12 months. Medicare coinsurance and Part B deductibles do not apply.

The AWV will include the establishment of, or update to, the individual's medical/family history, measurement of his/her height, weight, body-mass index (BMI) or waist circumference, and blood pressure (BP), with the goal of health promotion and disease detection and encouraging patients to obtain the screening and preventive services that may already be covered and paid for under Medicare Part B. Definitions relative to the AWV are included below.

Coverage is available for an AWV that meets the following requirements:

1. It is performed by a health professional; and,
2. It is furnished to an eligible beneficiary who is no longer within 12 months after the effective date of his/her first Medicare Part B coverage period, and he/she has not received either an IPPE or an AWV providing PPPS within the past 12 months.

Sections 4103 and 4104 of the ACA also provide for a waiver of the Medicare coinsurance and Part B deductible requirements for an AWV effective for services furnished on or after January 1, 2011.

#### B. Definitions Relative to the AWV:
Detection of any cognitive impairment: The assessment of an individual's cognitive function by direct observation, with due consideration of information obtained by way of patient reports, concerns raised by family members, friends, caretakers, or others.

Eligible beneficiary: An individual who is no longer within 12 months after the effective date of his/her first Medicare Part B coverage period and who has not received either an IPPE or an AWV providing PPPS within the past 12 months.

Establishment of, or an update to, the individual's medical/family history: At a minimum, the collection and documentation of the following:

a. Past medical and surgical history, including experiences with illnesses, hospital stays, operations, allergies, injuries, and treatments.

b. Use or exposure to medications and supplements, including calcium and vitamins.

c. Medical events in the beneficiary's parents and any siblings and children, including diseases that may be hereditary or place the individual at increased risk.

First AWV providing PPPS: The provision of the following services to an eligible beneficiary by a health professional that include, and take into account the results of, a health risk assessment as those terms are defined in this section:

a. Review (and administration if needed) of a health risk assessment (as defined in this section).

b. Establishment of an individual's medical/family history.

c. Establishment of a list of current providers and suppliers that are regularly involved in providing medical care to the individual.

d. Measurement of an individual's height, weight, BMI (or waist circumference, if appropriate), BP, and other routine measurements as deemed appropriate, based on the beneficiary's medical/family history.

e. Detection of any cognitive impairment that the individual may have as defined in this section.

f. Review of the individual's potential (risk factors) for depression, including current or past experiences with depression or other mood disorders, based on the use of an appropriate screening instrument for persons without a current diagnosis of depression, which the health professional may select from various available standardized screening tests designed for this purpose and recognized by national medical professional organizations.

g. Review of the individual's functional ability and level of safety based on direct observation, or the use of appropriate screening questions or a screening questionnaire, which the health professional may select from various available screening questions or standardized questionnaires designed for this purpose and recognized by national professional medical organizations.

h. Establishment of the following:

(1) A written screening schedule for the individual, such as a checklist for the next 5 to 10 years, as appropriate, based on recommendations of the United States Preventive Services Task Force (USPSTF) and the Advisory Committee on Immunization Practices (ACIP), and the individual's health risk assessment (as that term is defined in this section), the individual's health status, screening history, and age-appropriate preventive services covered by Medicare.

(2) A list of risk factors and conditions for which primary, secondary, or tertiary interventions are recommended or are underway for the individual, including any mental health conditions or any such risk factors or conditions that have been identified through an IPPE, and a list of treatment options and their associated risks and benefits.

i. Furnishing of personalized health advice to the individual and a referral, as appropriate, to health education or preventive counseling services or programs aimed at reducing identified risk factors and improving self-management, or community-based lifestyle interventions to reduce health risks and promote self-management and wellness, including weight loss, physical activity, smoking cessation, fall prevention, and nutrition.

j. Any other element determined appropriate through the National Coverage Determination (NCD) process.

Health professional:

a. A physician who is a doctor of medicine or osteopathy (as defined in section 1861(r)(1) of the Social Security Act (the Act); or,

b. A physician assistant, nurse practitioner, or clinical nurse specialist (as defined in section 1861(aa)(5) of the Act); or,

c. A medical professional (including a health educator, registered dietitian, or nutrition professional or other licensed practitioner) or a team of such medical professionals, working under the direct supervision (as defined in 42CFR 410.32(b)(3)(ii)) of a physician as defined in this section.

Health Risk Assessment means, for the purposes of the annual wellness visit, an evaluation tool that meets the following criteria:

a. collects self-reported information about the beneficiary.

b. can be administered independently by the beneficiary or administered by a health professional prior to or as part of the AWV encounter.

c. is appropriately tailored to and takes into account the communication needs of underserved populations, persons with limited English proficiency, and persons with health literacy needs.

d. takes no more than 20 minutes to complete.

e. addresses, at a minimum, the following topics:

1. demographic data, including but not limited to age, gender, race, and ethnicity.

2. self assessment of health status, frailty, and physical functioning.

3. psychosocial risks, including but not limited to, depression/life satisfaction, stress, anger, loneliness/social isolation, pain, and fatigue.

4. Behavioral risks, including but not limited to, tobacco use, physical activity, nutrition and oral health, alcohol consumption, sexual health, motor vehicle safety (seat belt use), and home safety.

5. Activities of daily living (ADLs), including but not limited to, dressing, feeding, toileting, grooming, physical ambulation (including balance/risk of falls), and bathing.

6. Instrumental activities of daily living (IADLs), including but not limited to, shopping, food preparation, using the telephone, housekeeping, laundry, mode of transportation, responsibility for own medications, and ability to handle finances.

Review of the individual's functional ability and level of safety: At a minimum, includes assessment of the following topics:

a. Hearing impairment,

b. Ability to successfully perform activities of daily living,

c. Fall risk, and, d. Home safety.

Subsequent AWV providing PPPS: The provision of the following services to an eligible beneficiary by a health professional that include, and take into account the results of an updated health risk assessment, as those terms are defined in this section:

a. Review (and administration if needed) of an updated health risk assessment (as defined in this section).

b. An update of the individual's medical/family history.

c. An update of the list of current providers and suppliers that are regularly involved in providing medical care to the individual, as that list was developed for the first AWV providing PPPS or the previous subsequent AWV providing PPPS.

d. Measurement of an individual's weight (or waist circumference), BP, and other routine measurements as deemed appropriate, based on the individual's medical/family history.

e. Detection of any cognitive impairment that the individual may have as defined in this section.

f. An update to the following:

(1) The written screening schedule for the individual as that schedule is defined in this section, that was developed at the first AWV providing PPPS, and,

(2) The list of risk factors and conditions for which primary, secondary, or tertiary interventions are recommended or are under way for the individual, as that list was developed at the first AWV providing PPPS or the previous subsequent AWV providing PPPS.

g. Furnishing of personalized health advice to the individual and a referral, as appropriate, to health education or preventive counseling services or programs as that advice and related services are defined for the first AWV providing PPPS.

h. Any other element determined appropriate by the Secretary through the NCD process.

See Pub. 100-04, Medicare Claims Processing Manual, chapter 18, section 140, for detailed claims processing and billing instructions.

## 100-02, 15, 290
### Foot Care

#### A. Treatment of Subluxation of Foot
Subluxations of the foot are defined as partial dislocations or displacements of joint surfaces, tendons ligaments, or muscles of the foot. Surgical or nonsurgical treatments undertaken for the sole purpose of correcting a subluxated structure in the foot as an isolated entity are not covered.

However, medical or surgical treatment of subluxation of the ankle joint (talo-crural joint) is covered. In addition, reasonable and necessary medical or surgical services, diagnosis, or treatment for medical conditions that have resulted from or are associated with partial displacement of structures is covered. For example, if a patient has osteoarthritis that has resulted in a partial displacement of joints in the foot, and the primary treatment is for the osteoarthritis, coverage is provided.

#### B. Exclusions from Coverage
The following foot care services are generally excluded from coverage under both Part A and Part B. (See Sec.290.F and Sec.290.G for instructions on applying foot care exclusions.)

1. Treatment of Flat Foot
The term "flat foot" is defined as a condition in which one or more arches of the foot have flattened out. Services or devices directed toward the care or correction of such conditions, including the prescription of supportive devices, are not covered.

2. Routine Foot Care
Except as provided above, routine foot care is excluded from coverage. Services that normally are considered routine and not covered by Medicare include the following:

- The cutting or removal of corns and calluses;
- The trimming, cutting, clipping, or debriding of nails; and
- Other hygienic and preventive maintenance care, such as cleaning and soaking the feet, the use of skin creams to maintain skin tone of either ambulatory or bedfast patients, and any other service performed in the absence of localized illness, injury, or symptoms involving the foot.

3. Supportive Devices for Feet
Orthopedic shoes and other supportive devices for the feet generally are not covered. However, this exclusion does not apply to such a shoe if it is an integral part of a leg brace, and its expense is included as part of the cost of the brace. Also, this exclusion does not apply to therapeutic shoes furnished to diabetics.

#### C. Exceptions to Routine Foot Care Exclusion
1. Necessary and Integral Part of Otherwise Covered Services
In certain circumstances, services ordinarily considered to be routine may be covered if they are performed as a necessary and integral part of otherwise covered services, such as diagnosis and treatment of ulcers, wounds, or infections.

2. Treatment of Warts on Foot
The treatment of warts (including plantar warts) on the foot is covered to the same extent as services provided for the treatment of warts located elsewhere on the body.

3. Presence of Systemic Condition
The presence of a systemic condition such as metabolic, neurologic, or peripheral vascular disease may require scrupulous foot care by a professional that in the absence of such condition(s) would be considered routine (and, therefore, excluded from coverage). Accordingly, foot care that would otherwise be considered routine may be covered when systemic condition(s) result in severe circulatory embarrassment or areas of diminished sensation in the individual's legs or feet. (See subsection A.)

In these instances, certain foot care procedures that otherwise are considered routine (e.g., cutting or removing corns and calluses, or trimming, cutting, clipping, or debriding nails) may pose a hazard when performed by a nonprofessional person on patients with such systemic conditions. (See Sec.290.G for procedural instructions.)

4. Mycotic Nails
In the absence of a systemic condition, treatment of mycotic nails may be covered.
The treatment of mycotic nails for an ambulatory patient is covered only when the physician attending the patient's mycotic condition documents that (1) there is clinical evidence of mycosis of the toenail, and (2) the patient has marked limitation of ambulation, pain, or secondary infection resulting from the thickening and dystrophy of the infected toenail plate.

© 2016 Optum360, LLC

The treatment of mycotic nails for a nonambulatory patient is covered only when the physician attending the patient's mycotic condition documents that (1) there is clinical evidence of mycosis of the toenail, and (2) the patient suffers from pain or secondary infection resulting from the thickening and dystrophy of the infected toenail plate.

For the purpose of these requirements, documentation means any written information that is required by the carrier in order for services to be covered. Thus, the information submitted with claims must be substantiated by information found in the patient's medical record. Any information, including that contained in a form letter, used for documentation purposes is subject to carrier verification in order to ensure that the information adequately justifies coverage of the treatment of mycotic nails.

## D. Systemic Conditions That Might Justify Coverage

Although not intended as a comprehensive list, the following metabolic, neurologic, and peripheral vascular diseases (with synonyms in parentheses) most commonly represent the underlying conditions that might justify coverage for routine foot care.

- Diabetes mellitus *
- Arteriosclerosis obliterans (A.S.O., arteriosclerosis of the extremities, occlusive peripheral arteriosclerosis)
- Buerger's disease (thromboangiitis obliterans)
- Chronic thrombophlebitis *
- Peripheral neuropathies involving the feet -
- Associated with malnutrition and vitamin deficiency *
  – Malnutrition (general, pellagra)
  – Alcoholism
  – Malabsorption (celiac disease, tropical sprue)
  – Pernicious anemia
- Associated with carcinoma *
- Associated with diabetes mellitus *
- Associated with drugs and toxins *
- Associated with multiple sclerosis *
- Associated with uremia (chronic renal disease) *
- Associated with traumatic injury
- Associated with leprosy or neurosyphilis
- Associated with hereditary disorders
- Hereditary sensory radicular neuropathy
- Angiokeratoma corporis diffusum (Fabry's)
- Amyloid neuropathy

When the patient's condition is one of those designated by an asterisk (*), routine procedures are covered only if the patient is under the active care of a doctor of medicine or osteopathy who documents the condition.

## E. Supportive Devices for Feet

Orthopedic shoes and other supportive devices for the feet generally are not covered. However, this exclusion does not apply to such a shoe if it is an integral part of a leg brace, and its expense is included as part of the cost of the brace. Also, this exclusion does not apply to therapeutic shoes furnished to diabetics.

## F. Presumption of Coverage

In evaluating whether the routine services can be reimbursed, a presumption of coverage may be made where the evidence available discloses certain physical and/or clinical findings consistent with the diagnosis and indicative of severe peripheral involvement. For purposes of applying this presumption the following findings are pertinent:

Class A Findings
Nontraumatic amputation of foot or integral skeletal portion thereof.

Class B Findings
Absent posterior tibial pulse;

Advanced trophic changes as: hair growth (decrease or absence) nail changes (thickening) pigmentary changes (discoloration) skin texture (thin, shiny) skin color (rubor or redness) (Three required); and

Absent dorsalis pedis pulse.

Class C Findings
Claudication;

Temperature changes (e.g., cold feet);

Edema;

Paresthesias (abnormal spontaneous sensations in the feet); and

Burning.

The presumption of coverage may be applied when the physician rendering the routine foot care has identified:

1. A Class A finding;
2. Two of the Class B findings; or
3. One Class B and two Class C findings.

Cases evidencing findings falling short of these alternatives may involve podiatric treatment that may constitute covered care and should be reviewed by the intermediary's medical staff and developed as necessary.

For purposes of applying the coverage presumption where the routine services have been rendered by a podiatrist, the contractor may deem the active care requirement met if the claim or other evidence available discloses that the patient has seen an M.D. or D.O. for treatment and/or evaluation of the complicating disease process during the 6-month period prior to the rendition of the routine-type services. The intermediary may also accept the podiatrist's statement that the diagnosing and treating M.D. or D.O. also concurs with the podiatrist's findings as to the severity of the peripheral involvement indicated.

Services ordinarily considered routine might also be covered if they are performed as a necessary and integral part of otherwise covered services, such as diagnosis and treatment of diabetic ulcers, wounds, and infections.

## G. Application of Foot Care Exclusions to Physician's Services

The exclusion of foot care is determined by the nature of the service. Thus, payment for an excluded service should be denied whether performed by a podiatrist, osteopath, or a doctor of medicine, and without regard to the difficulty or complexity of the procedure.

When an itemized bill shows both covered services and noncovered services not integrally related to the covered service, the portion of charges attributable to the noncovered services should be denied. (For example, if an itemized bill shows surgery for an ingrown toenail and also removal of calluses not necessary for the performance of toe surgery, any additional charge attributable to removal of the calluses should be denied.)

In reviewing claims involving foot care, the carrier should be alert to the following exceptional situations:

1. Payment may be made for incidental noncovered services performed as a necessary and integral part of, and secondary to, a covered procedure. For example, if trimming of toenails is required for application of a cast to a fractured foot, the carrier need not allocate and deny a portion of the charge for the trimming of the nails. However, a separately itemized charge for such excluded service should be disallowed. When the primary procedure is covered the administration of anesthesia necessary for the performance of such procedure is also covered.

2. Payment may be made for initial diagnostic services performed in connection with a specific symptom or complaint if it seems likely that its treatment would be covered even though the resulting diagnosis may be one requiring only noncovered care.

The name of the M.D. or D.O. who diagnosed the complicating condition must be submitted with the claim. In those cases, where active care is required, the approximate date the beneficiary was last seen by such physician must also be indicated.

NOTE: Section 939 of P.L. 96-499 removed "warts" from the routine foot care exclusion effective July 1, 1981.

Relatively few claims for routine-type care are anticipated considering the severity of conditions contemplated as the basis for this exception. Claims for this type of foot care should not be paid in the absence of convincing evidence that nonprofessional performance of the service would have been hazardous for the beneficiary because of an underlying systemic disease. The mere statement of a diagnosis such as those mentioned in Sec.D above does not of itself indicate the severity of the condition. Where development is indicated to verify diagnosis and/or severity the carrier should follow existing claims processing practices which may include review of carrier's history and medical consultation as well as physician contacts.

The rules in Sec.290.F concerning presumption of coverage also apply.

Codes and policies for routine foot care and supportive devices for the feet are not exclusively for the use of podiatrists. These codes must be used to report foot care services regardless of the specialty of the physician who furnishes the services. Carriers must instruct physicians to use the most appropriate code available when billing for routine foot care.

## 100-02, 15, 300

### Diabetes Self-Management Training Services

Section 4105 of the Balanced Budget Act of 1997 permits Medicare coverage of diabetes self-management training (DSMT) services when these services are furnished by a certified provider who meets certain quality standards. This program is intended to educate beneficiaries in the successful self-management of diabetes. The program includes instructions in self-monitoring of blood glucose; education about diet and exercise; an insulin treatment plan developed specifically for the patient who is insulin-dependent; and motivation for patients to use the skills for self-management.

Diabetes self-management training services may be covered by Medicare only if the treating physician or treating qualified non-physician practitioner who is managing the beneficiary's diabetic condition certifies that such services are needed. The referring physician or qualified non-physician practitioner must maintain the plan of care in the beneficiary's medical record and documentation substantiating the need for training on an individual basis when group training is typically covered, if so ordered. The order must also include a statement signed by the physician that the service is needed as well as the following:

- The number of initial or follow-up hours ordered (the physician can order less than 10 hours of training);
- The topics to be covered in training (initial training hours can be used for the full initial training program or specific areas such as nutrition or insulin training); and
- A determination that the beneficiary should receive individual or group training.

The provider of the service must maintain documentation in a file that includes the original order from the physician and any special conditions noted by the physician.

When the training under the order is changed, the training order/referral must be signed by the physician or qualified non-physician practitioner treating the beneficiary and maintained in the beneficiary's file in the DSMT's program records.

NOTE: All entities billing for DSMT under the fee-for-service payment system or other payment systems must meet all national coverage requirements.

## 100-02, 15, 300.2

### Certified Providers

A designated certified provider bills for DSMT provided by an accredited DSMT program. Certified providers must submit a copy of their accreditation certificate to the contractor. The statute states that a "certified provider" is a physician or other individual or entity designated by the Secretary that, in addition to providing outpatient self-management training services, provides other items and services for which payment may be made under title XVIII, and meets certain quality standards. The CMS is designating all providers and suppliers that bill Medicare for other individual services such as hospital outpatient departments, renal dialysis facilities, physicians and durable medical equipment suppliers as certified. All suppliers/providers who may bill for other Medicare services or items and who represent a DSMT program that is accredited as meeting quality standards can bill and receive payment for the entire DSMT program. Registered dietitians are eligible to bill on behalf of an entire DSMT program on or after January 1, 2002, as long as the provider has obtained a Medicare provider number. A dietitian may not be the sole provider of the DSMT service. There is an exception for rural areas. In a rural area, an individual who is qualified as a registered dietitian and as a certified diabetic educator who is currently certified by an organization approved by CMS may furnish training and is deemed to meet the multidisciplinary team requirement.

The CMS will not reimburse services on a fee-for-service basis rendered to a beneficiary under Part A.

NOTE: While separate payment is not made for this service to Rural Health Clinics (RHCs), the service is covered but is considered included in the all-inclusive encounter rate. Effective January 1, 2006, payment for DSMT provided in a Federally Qualified Health Clinic (FQHC) that meets all of the requirements identified in Pub. 100-04, chapter 18, section 120 may be made in addition to one other visit the beneficiary had during the same day.

All DSMT programs must be accredited as meeting quality standards by a CMS approved national accreditation organization. Currently, CMS recognizes the American Diabetes Association, American Association of Diabetes Educators and the Indian Health Service as approved national accreditation organizations. Programs without accreditation by a CMS-approved national accreditation organization are not covered. Certified providers may be asked to submit updated accreditation documents at any time or to submit outcome data to an organization designated by CMS.

### Enrollment of DMEPOS Suppliers

The DMEPOS suppliers are reimbursed for diabetes training through local carriers. In order to file claims for DSMT, a DMEPOS supplier must be enrolled in the Medicare program with the National Supplier Clearinghouse (NSC). The supplier must also meet the quality standards of a CMS-approved national accreditation organization as stated above. DMEPOS suppliers must obtain a provider number from the local carrier in order to bill for DSMT.

The carrier requires a completed Form CMS-855, along with an accreditation certificate as part of the provider application process. After it has been determined that the quality standards are met, a billing number is assigned to the supplier. Once a supplier has received a provider identification (PIN) number, the supplier can begin receiving reimbursement for this service.

Carriers should contact the National Supplier Clearinghouse (NSC) according to the instruction in Pub 100-08, the Medicare Program Integrity Manual, Chapter 10, "Healthcare Provider/Supplier Enrollment," to verify an applicant is currently enrolled and eligible to receive direct payment from the Medicare program.

The applicant is assigned specialty 87.

Any DMEPOS supplier that has its billing privileges deactivated or revoked by the NSC will also have the billing number deactivated by the carrier.

## 100-02, 15, 300.3

### Frequency of Training

#### A - Initial Training

The initial year for DSMT is the 12 month period following the initial date.

Medicare will cover initial training that meets the following conditions:

- Is furnished to a beneficiary who has not previously received initial or follow-up training under HCPCS codes G0108 or G0109;
- Is furnished within a continuous 12-month period;
- Does not exceed a total of 10 hours* (the 10 hours of training can be done in any combination of 1/2 hour increments);
- With the exception of 1 hour of individual training, training is usually furnished in a group setting, which can contain other patients besides Medicare beneficiaries, and;
- One hour of individual training may be used for any part of the training including insulin training.

* When a claim contains a DSMT HCPCS code and the associated units cause the total time for the DSMT initial year to exceed '10' hours, a CWF error will set.

#### B - Follow-Up Training

Medicare covers follow-up training under the following conditions:

- No more than 2 hours individual or group training per beneficiary per year;
- Group training consists of 2 to 20 individuals who need not all be Medicare beneficiaries;
- Follow-up training for subsequent years is based on a 12 month calendar after completion of the full 10 hours of initial training;
- Follow-up training is furnished in increments of no less than one-half hour*; and
- The physician (or qualified non-physician practitioner) treating the beneficiary must document in the beneficiary's medical record that the beneficiary is a diabetic.

*When a claim contains a DSMT HCPCS code and the associated units cause the total time for any follow-up year to exceed 2 hours, a CWF error will set.

## 100-02, 15, 300.4

### Coverage Requirements for Individual Training

Medicare covers training on an individual basis for a Medicare beneficiary under any of the following conditions:

- No group session is available within 2 months of the date the training is ordered;
- The beneficiary's physician (or qualified non-physician practitioner) documents in the beneficiary's medical record that the beneficiary has special needs resulting from conditions, such as severe vision, hearing or language limitations or other such special conditions as identified by the treating physician or non-physician practitioner, that will hinder effective participation in a group training session; or
- The physician orders additional insulin training.

The need for individual training must be identified by the physician or non-physician practitioner in the referral.

NOTE: If individual training has been provided to a Medicare beneficiary and subsequently the carrier or intermediary determines that training should have been provided in a group, carriers and intermediaries down-code the reimbursement from individual to the group level and provider education would be the appropriate actions instead of denying the service as billed.

## 100-02, 15, 310

### Kidney Disease Patient Education Services

By definition, chronic kidney disease (CKD) is kidney damage for 3 months or longer, regardless of the cause of kidney damage. CKD typically evolves over a long period of time and patients may not have symptoms until significant, possibly irreversible, damage has been done. Complications can develop from kidneys that do not function properly, such as high blood pressure, anemia, and weak bones. When CKD progresses, it may lead to kidney failure, which requires artificial means to perform kidney functions (dialysis) or a kidney transplant to maintain life.

Patients can be classified into 5 stages based on their glomerular filtration rate (GFR, how quickly blood is filtered through the kidneys), with stage I having kidney damage with normal or increased GFR to stage V with kidney failure, also called end-stage renal disease (ESRD). Once patients with CKD are identified, treatment is available to help prevent complications of decreased kidney function, slow the progression of kidney disease, and reduce the risk of other diseases such as heart disease.

Beneficiaries with CKD may benefit from kidney disease education (KDE) interventions due to the large amount of medical information that could affect patient outcomes, including the increasing emphasis on self-care and patients' desire for informed, autonomous decision-making. Pre-dialysis education can help patients achieve better understanding of their illness, dialysis modality options, and may help delay the need for dialysis. Education interventions should be patient-centered, encourage collaboration, offer support to the patient, and be delivered consistently.

Effective for claims with dates of service on and after January 1, 2010, Section 152(b) of the Medicare Improvements for Patients and Providers Act of 2008 (MIPPA) covers KDE services under Medicare Part B. KDE services are designed to provide beneficiaries with Stage IV CKD comprehensive information regarding: the management of comorbidities, including delaying the need for dialysis; prevention of uremic complications; all therapeutic options (each option for renal replacement therapy, dialysis access options, and transplantation); ensuring that the beneficiary has opportunities to actively participate in his/her choice of therapy; and that the services be tailored to meet the beneficiary's needs.

Regulations for KDE services were established at 42 CFR 410.48. Claims processing instructions and billing requirements can be found in Pub. 100-04, Medicare Claims Processing Manual, Chapter 32 - Billing Requirements for Special Services, Section 20.

## 100-02, 15, 310.1

### Beneficiaries Eligible for Coverage

Medicare Part B covers outpatient, face-to-face KDE services for a beneficiary that:

- is diagnosed with Stage IV CKD, using the Modification of Diet in Renal Disease (MDRD) Study formula (severe decrease in GFR, GFR value of 15-29 mL/min/1.73 m2), and
- obtains a referral from the physician managing the beneficiary's kidney condition. The referral should be documented in the beneficiary's medical records.

## 100-02, 15, 310.2

### Qualified Person

Medicare Part B covers KDE services provided by a ,Àòqualified person,' meaning a: physician (as defined in section 30 of this chapter), physician assistant, nurse practitioner, or clinical nurse specialist (as defined in sections 190, 200, and 210 of this chapter), hospital, critical access hospital (CAH), skilled nursing facility (SNF), comprehensive outpatient rehabilitation facility (CORF), home health agency (HHA), or hospice, if the KDE services are provided in a rural area (using the actual geographic location core based statistical area (CBSA) to identify facilities located in rural areas), or hospital or CAH that is treated as being rural (was reclassified from urban to rural status per 42 CFR 412.103).

NOTE: The "incident to" requirements at section 1861(s)(2)(A) of the Social Security Act (the Act) do not apply to KDE services.

The following providers are not ,Àòqualified persons' and are excluded from furnishing KDE services:

- A hospital, CAH, SNF, CORF, HHA, or hospice located outside of a rural area (using the actual geographic location CBSA to identify facilities located outside of a rural area), unless the services are furnished by a hospital or CAH that is treated as being in a rural area; and

- Renal dialysis facilities.

## 100-02, 15, 310.4

### Standards for Content

Medicare Part B covers KDE services, provided by a qualified person, which provide comprehensive information regarding:

A. The management of comorbidities, including delaying the need for dialysis, which includes, but is not limited to, the following topics:

- Prevention and treatment of cardiovascular disease,
- Prevention and treatment of diabetes,
- Hypertension management,
- Anemia management,
- Bone disease and disorders of calcium and phosphorus metabolism management,
- Symptomatic neuropathy management, and
- Impairments in functioning and well-being.

B. Prevention of uremic complications, which includes, but is not limited to, the following topics:

- Information on how the kidneys work and what happens when the kidneys fail,
- Understanding if remaining kidney function can be protected, preventing disease
  progression, and realistic chances of survival,
- Diet and fluid restrictions, and
- Medication review, including how each medication works, possible side effects and minimization of side effects, the importance of compliance, and informed decision making if the patient decides not to take a specific drug.

C. Therapeutic options, treatment modalities and settings, advantages and disadvantages of each treatment option, and how the treatments replace the kidney, including, but not limited to, the following topics: Hemodialysis, both at home and in-facility;

- Peritoneal dialysis (PD), including intermittent PD, continuous ambulatory PD, and continuous cycling PD, both at home and in-facility;
- All dialysis access options for hemodialysis and peritoneal dialysis; and
- Transplantation.

D. Opportunities for beneficiaries to actively participate in the choice of therapy and be tailored to meet the needs of the individual beneficiary involved, which includes, but is not limited to, the following topics: Physical symptoms,

- Impact on family and social life,
- Exercise,
- The right to refuse treatment,
- Impact on work and finances,
- The meaning of test results, and
- Psychological impact.

## 100-02, 15, 310.5

### Outcomes Assessment

Qualified persons that provide KDE services must develop outcomes assessments that are designed to measure beneficiary knowledge about CKD and its treatment. The assessment must be administered to the beneficiary during a KDE session, and be made available to the Centers for Medicare & Medicaid Services (CMS) upon request. The outcomes assessments serve to assist KDE educators and CMS in improving subsequent KDE programs, patient understanding, and assess program effectiveness of:

Preparing the beneficiary to make informed decisions about their healthcare options related to CKD, and

Meeting the communication needs of underserved populations, including persons with disabilities, persons with limited English proficiency, and persons with health literacy needs.

## 100-02, 32, 20.2

### Healthcare Common Procedure Coding System (HCPCS) Procedure Codes and Applicable Diagnosis Codes

Effective for services performed on and after January 1, 2010, the following new HCPCS codes have been created for KDE services when provided to patients with stage IV CKD.

G0420:  Face-to-face educational services related to the care of chronic kidney disease; individual, per session, per one hour

G0421:    Face-to-face educational services related to the care of chronic kidney disease; group, per session, per one hour

The following diagnosis code should be reported when billing for KDE services:

585.4    (chronic kidney disease, Stage IV (severe)).

NOTE: Claims with HCPCS codes G0420 or G0421 and ICD-9 code 585.4 that are billed for KDE services are not allowed on a professional and institutional claim on the same service date.

## 100-03, 10.2

### NCD for Transcutaneous Electrical Nerve Stimulation (TENS) for Acute Post-Operative Pain (10.2)

NCD for Transcutaneous Electrical Nerve Stimulation (TENS) for Acute Post-Operative Pain (10.2)

#### Indications and Limitations of Coverage

The use of Transcutaneous Electrical Nerve Stimulation (TENS) for the relief of acute post-operative pain is covered under Medicare. TENS may be covered whether used as an adjunct to the use of drugs, or as an alternative to drugs, in the treatment of acute pain resulting from surgery.

TENS devices, whether durable or disposable, may be used in furnishing this service. When used for the purpose of treating acute post-operative pain, TENS devices are considered supplies. As such they may be hospital supplies furnished inpatients covered under Part A, or supplies incident to a physician's service when furnished in connection with surgery done on an outpatient basis, and covered under Part B.

It is expected that TENS, when used for acute post-operative pain, will be necessary for relatively short periods of time, usually 30 days or less. In cases when TENS is used for longer periods, Medicare Administrative Contractors should attempt to ascertain whether TENS is no longer being used for acute pain but rather for chronic pain, in which case the TENS device may be covered as durable medical equipment as described in §160.27.

#### Cross-references:

Medicare Benefit Policy Manual, Chapter 1, "Inpatient Hospital Services," §40;

Medicare Benefit Policy Manual, Chapter 2, "Hospital Services Covered Under Part B," §§20, 20.4, and 80; Medicare Benefit Policy Manual, Chapter 15, "Covered Medical and other Health Services, §110."

## 100-03, 20.21

### NCD for Chelation Therapy for Treatment of Atherosclerosis (20.21)

The application of chelation therapy using ethylenediamine-tetra-acetic acid (EDTA) for the treatment and prevention of atherosclerosis is controversial. There is no widely accepted rationale to explain the beneficial effects attributed to this therapy. Its safety is questioned and its clinical effectiveness has never been established by well designed, controlled clinical trials. It is not widely accepted and practiced by American physicians. EDTA chelation therapy for atherosclerosis is considered experimental. For these reasons, EDTA chelation therapy for the treatment or prevention of atherosclerosis is not covered.

Some practitioners refer to this therapy as chemoendarterectomy and may also show a diagnosis other than atherosclerosis, such as arteriosclerosis or calcinosis. Claims employing such variant terms should also be denied under this section.

## 100-03, 20.22

### NCD for Ethylenediamine-Tetra-Acetic (EDTA) Chelation Therapy for Treatment of Atherosclerosis (20.22)

The use of EDTA as a chelating agent to treat atherosclerosis, arteriosclerosis, calcinosis, or similar generalized condition not listed by the FDA as an approved use is not covered. Any such use of EDTA is considered experimental.

## 100-03, 40.7

### NCD for Outpatient Intravenous Insulin Treatment (40.7) (Effective December 23, 2009)

#### Indications and Limitations of Coverage

#### B. Nationally Covered Indications
N/A

#### C. Nationally Non-Covered Indications
Effective for claims with dates of service on and after December 23, 2009, the Centers for Medicare and Medicaid Services (CMS) determines that the evidence is adequate to conclude that OIVIT does not improve health outcomes in Medicare beneficiaries. Therefore, CMS determines that OIVIT is not reasonable and necessary for any indication under section 1862(a)(1)(A) of the Social Security Act. Services comprising an Outpatient Intravenous Insulin Therapy regimen are nationally non-covered under Medicare when furnished pursuant to an OIVIT regimen (see subsection A. above).

#### D. Other
Individual components of OIVIT may have medical uses in conventional treatment regimens for diabetes and other conditions. Coverage for such other uses may be determined by other local or national Medicare determinations, and do not pertain to OIVIT. For example, see Pub. 100-03, NCD Manual, Section 40.2, Home Blood Glucose Monitors, Section 40.3, Closed-loop Blood Glucose Control Devices (CBGCD), Section 190.20, Blood Glucose Testing, and Section 280.14, Infusion Pumps, as well as Pub. 100-04, Claims Processing Manual, Chapter 18, Section 90, Diabetics Screening.

(This NCD last reviewed December 2009.)

## 100-03, 70.2.1

### Services Provided for the Diagnosis and Treatment of Diabetic Sensory Neuropathy with Loss of Protective Sensation (aka Diabetic Peripheral Neuropathy)
(Rev. 1, 10-03-03)

CIM 50-8.1

Presently, peripheral neuropathy, or diabetic sensory neuropathy, is the most common factor leading to amputation in people with diabetes. In diabetes, sensory neuropathy is an anatomically diffuse process primarily affecting sensory and autonomic fibers; however, distal motor findings may be present in advanced cases. Long nerves are affected first, with symptoms typically beginning insidiously in the toes and then advancing proximally. This leads to loss of protective sensation (LOPS), whereby a person is unable to feel minor trauma from mechanical, thermal, or chemical sources. When foot lesions are present, the reduction in autonomic nerve functions may also inhibit wound healing.

Diabetic sensory neuropathy with LOPS is a localized illness of the feet and falls within the regulation's exception to the general exclusionary rule (see 42 CFR 411.15(l)(1)(i)). Foot exams for people with diabetic sensory neuropathy with LOPS are reasonable and necessary to allow for early intervention in serious complications that typically afflict diabetics with the disease.

Effective for services furnished on or after July 1, 2002, Medicare covers, as a physician service, an evaluation (examination and treatment) of the feet no more often than every six months for individuals with a documented diagnosis of diabetic sensory neuropathy and LOPS, as long as the beneficiary has not seen a foot care specialist for some other reason in the interim. LOPS shall be diagnosed through sensory testing with the 5.07 monofilament using established guidelines, such as those developed by the National Institute of Diabetes and Digestive and Kidney Diseases guidelines. Five sites should be tested on the plantar surface of each foot, according to the National Institute of Diabetes and Digestive and Kidney Diseases guidelines. The areas must be tested randomly since the loss of protective sensation may be patchy in distribution, and the patient may get clues if the test is done rhythmically. Heavily callused areas should be avoided. As suggested by the American Podiatric Medicine Association, an absence of sensation at two or more sites out of 5 tested on either foot when tested with the 5.07 Semmes-Weinstein monofilament must be present and documented to diagnose peripheral neuropathy with loss of protective sensation.

The examination includes:

1. A patient history, and
2. A physical examination that must consist of at least the following elements:
   – Visual inspection of forefoot and hindfoot (including toe web spaces);
   – Evaluation of protective sensation;
   – Evaluation of foot structure and biomechanics;
   – Evaluation of vascular status and skin integrity;
   – Evaluation of the need for special footwear; and
3. Patient education.

#### A. Treatment includes, but is not limited to:
- Local care of superficial wounds;
- Debridement of corns and calluses; and
- Trimming and debridement of nails.

The diagnosis of diabetic sensory neuropathy with LOPS should be established and documented prior to coverage of foot care. Other causes of peripheral neuropathy should be considered and investigated by the primary care physician prior to initiating or referring for foot care for persons with LOPS.

© 2016 Optum360, LLC

## 100-03, 80.2

### Photodynamic Therapy

Photodynamic therapy is a medical procedure which involves the infusion of a photosensitive (light-activated) drug with a very specific absorption peak. This drug is chemically designed to have a unique affinity for the diseased tissue intended for treatment. Once introduced to the body, the drug accumulates and is retained in diseased tissue to a greater degree than in normal tissue. Infusion is followed by the targeted irradiation of this tissue with a non-thermal laser, calibrated to emit light at a wavelength that corresponds to the drug? absorption peak. The drug then becomes active and locally treats the diseased tissue.

### Ocular Photodynamic Therapy (OPT)

Ocular Photodynamic Therapy (OPT) is used in the treatment of ophthalmologic diseases. OPT is only covered when used in conjunction with verteporfin (see section 80.3, "Photosensitive Drugs").

- Classic Subfoveal Choroidal Neovascular (CNV) Lesions - OPT is covered with a diagnosis of neovascular age-related macular degeneration (AMD) with predominately classic subfoveal choroidal neovascular (CNV) lesions (where the area of classic CNV occupies = 50 percent of the area of the entire lesion) at the initial visit as determined by a fluorescein angiogram. Subsequent follow-up visits will require either an optical coherence tomography (OCT) or a fluorescein angiogram (FA) to access treatment response. There are no requirements regarding visual acuity, lesion size, and number of re-treatments.

- Occult Subfoveal Choroidal Neovascular (CNV) Lesions - OPT is noncovered for patients with a diagnosis of age-related macular degeneration (AMD) with occult and no classic CNV lesions.

- Other Conditions - Use of OPT with verteporfin for other types of AMD (e.g., patients with minimally classic CNV lesions, atrophic, or dry AMD) is noncovered. OPT with verteporfin for other ocular indications such as pathologic myopia or presumed ocular histoplasmosis syndrome, is eligible for coverage through individual contractor discretion.

## 100-03, 80.2.1

### Ocular Photodynamic Therapy (OPT)- Effective April 3, 2013

#### A. General

Ocular Photodynamic Therapy (OPT) is used in the treatment of ophthalmologic diseases; specifically, for age-related macular degeneration (AMD), a common eye disease among the elderly. OPT involves the infusion of an intravenous photosensitizing drug called verteporfin followed by exposure to a laser. OPT is only covered when used in conjunction with verteporfin.

Effective July 1, 2001, OPT with verteporfin was approved for a diagnosis of neovascular AMD with predominately classic subfoveal choroidal neovascularization (CNV) lesions (where the area of classic CNV occupies = 50% of the area of the entire lesion) at the initial visit as determined by a fluorescein angiogram (FA).

On October 17, 2001, the Centers for Medicare & Medicaid Services (CMS) announced its "intent to cover" OPT with verteporfin for AMD patients with occult and no classic subfoveal CNV as determined by an FA. The October 17, 2001, decision was never implemented.

On March 28, 2002, after thorough review and reconsideration of the October 17, 2001, intent to cover policy, CMS determined that the current non-coverage policy for OPT for verteporfin for AMD patients with occult and no classic subfoveal CNV as determined by an FA should remain in effect.

Effective August 20, 2002, CMS issued a non-covered instruction for OPT with verteporfin for AMD patients with occult and no classic subfoveal CNV as determined by an FA.

#### B. Nationally Covered Indications

Effective April 1, 2004, OPT with verteporfin continues to be approved for a diagnosis of neovascular AMD with predominately classic subfoveal CNV lesions (where the area of classic CNV occupies = 50% of the area of the entire lesion) at the initial visit as determined by an FA. (CNV lesions are comprised of classic and/or occult components.) Subsequent follow-up visits require either an optical coherence tomography (OCT) (effective April 3. 2013) or an FA (effective April 1, 2004) to access treatment response. There are no requirements regarding visual acuity, lesion size, and number of re-treatments when treating predominantly classic lesions.

In addition, after thorough review and reconsideration of the August 20, 2002, non-coverage policy, CMS determines that the evidence is adequate to conclude that OPT with verteporfin is reasonable and necessary for treating:

1. Subfoveal occult with no classic CNV associated with AMD; and,

2. Subfoveal minimally classic CNV (where the area of classic CNV occupies <50% of the area of the entire lesion) associated with AMD.

The above 2 indications are considered reasonable and necessary only when:

1. The lesions are small (4 disk areas or less in size) at the time of initial treatment or within the 3 months prior to initial treatment; and,

2. The lesions have shown evidence of progression within the 3 months prior to initial treatment. Evidence of progression must be documented by deterioration of visual acuity (at least 5 letters on a standard eye examination chart), lesion growth (an increase in at least 1 disk area), or the appearance of blood associated with the lesion.

#### C. Nationally Non-Covered Indications

Other uses of OPT with verteporfin to treat AMD not already addressed by CMS will continue to be non-covered. These include, but are not limited to, the following AMD indications:

- Juxtafoveal or extrafoveal CNV lesions (lesions outside the fovea),
- Inability to obtain a fluorescein angiogram,
- Atrophic or "dry" AMD.

#### D. Other

The OPT with verteporfin for other ocular indications, such as pathologic myopia or presumed ocular histoplasmosis syndrome, continue to be eligible for local coverage determinations through individual contractor discretion.

## 100-03, 80.3

### (NCD) for Photosensitive Drugs (80.3)

Photosensitive drugs are the light-sensitive agents used in photodynamic therapy. Once introduced into the body, these drugs selectively identify and adhere to diseased tissue. The drugs remain inactive until they are exposed to a specific wavelength of light, by means of a laser, that corresponds to their absorption peak. The activation of a photosensitive drug results in a photochemical reaction which treats the diseased tissue without affecting surrounding normal tissue.

### Verteporfin

Verteporfin, a benzoporphyrin derivative, is an intravenous lipophilic photosensitive drug with an absorption peak of 690 nm. This drug was first approved by the Food and Drug Administration (FDA) on April 12, 2000, and subsequently, approved for inclusion in the United States Pharmacopoeia on July 18, 2000, meeting Medicare's definition of a drug when used in conjunction with ocular photodynamic therapy (OPT) (see section 80.2, "Photodynamic Therapy") when furnished intravenously incident to a physician? service. For patients with age-related macular degeneration (AMD), Verteporfin is only covered with a diagnosis of neovascular age-related macular degeneration with predominately classic subfoveal choroidal neovascular (CNV) lesions (where the area of classic CNV occupies = 50 percent of the area of the entire lesion) at the initial visit as determined by a fluorescein angiogram (FA). Subsequent follow-up visits will require either an optical coherence tomography (OCT) or an FA to access treatment response. OPT with verteporfin is covered for the above indication and will remain non-covered for all other indications related to AMD (see section 80.2). OPT with Verteporfin for use in non-AMD conditions is eligible for coverage through individual contractor discretion.

## 100-03, 80.3.1

### Verteporfin-Effective April 3, 2013

#### A. General

Verteporfin, a benzoporphyrin derivative, is an intravenous lipophilic photosensitive drug with an absorption peak of 690 nm. Verteporfin was first approved by the Food and Drug Administration on April 12, 2000, and subsequently approved for inclusion in the United States Pharmacopoeia on July 18, 2000, meeting Medicare's definition of a drug as defined under Sec. 1861(t)(1) of the Social Security Act. Verteporfin is only covered when used in conjunction with ocular photodynamic therapy OPT) when furnished intravenously incident to a physician's service.

#### B. Nationally Covered Indications

Effective April 1, 2004, OPT with verteporfin is covered for patients with a diagnosis of neovascular age-related macular degeneration (AMD) with:

- Predominately classic subfoveal choroidal neovascularization (CNV) lesions (where the area of classic CNV occupies = 50% of the area of the entire lesion) at the initial visit as determined by a fluorescein angiogram. (CNV lesions are comprised of classic and/or occult components.) Subsequent follow-up visits require either an optical coherence tomography (OCT) (effective April 3, 2013) or a fluorescein angiogram (FA) (effective April 1, 2004) to access treatment response.

There are no requirements regarding visual acuity, lesion size, and number of retreatments when treating predominantly classic lesions.

- Subfoveal occult with no classic associated with AMD.

© 2016 Optum360, LLC

- Subfoveal minimally classic CNV CNV (where the area of classic CNV occupies <50% of the area of the entire lesion) associated with AMD.

The above 2 indications are considered reasonable and necessary only when:

1. The lesions are small (4 disk areas or less in size) at the time of initial treatment or within the 3 months prior to initial treatment; and,

2. The lesions have shown evidence of progression within the 3 months prior to initial treatment. Evidence of progression must be documented by deterioration of visual acuity (at least 5 letters on a standard eye examination chart), lesion growth (an increase in at least 1 disk area), or the appearance of blood associated with the lesion.

### C. Nationally Non-Covered Indications

Other uses of OPT with verteporfin to treat AMD not already addressed by the Centers for Medicare & Medicaid Services will continue to be non-covered. These include, but are not limited to, the following AMD indications: juxtafoveal or extrafoveal CNV lesions (lesions outside the fovea), inability to obtain an FA, or atrophic or "dry" AMD.

### D. Other

The OPT with verteporfin for other ocular indications, such as pathologic myopia or presumed ocular histoplasmosis syndrome, continue to be eligible for local coverage determinations through individual contractor discretion.

## 100-03, 90.1

### Pharmacogenomic Testing to Predict Warfarin Responsiveness (Effective August 3, 2009)

#### A. General

Warfarin sodium is an orally administered anticoagulant drug that is marketed most commonly as Coumadin(R). (The Food and Drug Administration (FDA) approved labeling for Coumadin(R) includes a Black Box Warning dating back to 2007.) Anticoagulant drugs are sometimes referred to as blood thinners by the lay public. Warfarin affects the vitamin K-dependent clotting factors II, VII, IX, and X. Warfarin is thought to interfere with clotting factor synthesis by inhibition of the C1 subunit of the vitamin K epoxide reductase (VKORC1) enzyme complex, thereby reducing the regeneration of vitamin K1 epoxide. The elimination of warfarin is almost entirely by metabolic conversion to inactive metabolites by cytochrome P450 (CYP) enzymes in liver cells. CYP2C9 is the principal cytochrome P450 enzyme that modulates the anticoagulant activity of warfarin. From results of clinical studies, genetic variation in the CYP2C9 and/or VKORC1 genes can, in concert with clinical factors, predict how each individual responds to warfarin

Pharmacogenomics denotes the study of how an individual's genetic makeup, or genotype, affects the body's response to drugs. Pharmacogenomics as a science examines associations among variations in genes with individual responses to a drug or medication. In application, pharmacogenomic results (i.e., information on the patient's genetic variations) can contribute to predicting a patient's response to a given drug: good, bad, or none at all. Pharmacogenomic testing of CYP2C9 or VKORC1 alleles to predict a patient's response to warfarin occurs ideally prior to initiation of the drug. This would be an once-in-a-lifetime test, absent any reason to believe that the patient's personal genetic characteristics would change over time. Although such pharmacogenomic testing would be used to attempt to better approximate the best starting dose of warfarin, it would not eliminate the need for periodic PT/INR testing, a standard diagnostic test for coagulation activity and for assessing how a patient is reacting to a warfarin dose.

#### Nationally Covered Indications

Effective August 3, 2009, the Centers for Medicare & Medicaid Services (CMS) believes that the available evidence supports that coverage with evidence development (CED) under Sec.1862(a)(1)(E) of the Social Security Act (the Act) is appropriate for pharmacogenomic testing of CYP2C9 or VKORC1 alleles to predict warfarin responsiveness by any method, and is therefore covered only when provided to Medicare beneficiaries who are candidates for anticoagulation therapy with warfarin who:

1. Have not been previously tested for CYP2C9 or VKORC1 alleles; and

2. Have received fewer than five days of warfarin in the anticoagulation regimen for which the testing is ordered; and

3. Are enrolled in a prospective, randomized, controlled clinical study when that study meets the following standards. A clinical study seeking Medicare payment for pharmacogenomic testing of CYP2C9 or VKORC1 alleles to predict warfarin responsiveness provided to the Medicare beneficiary who is a candidate for anticoagulation therapy with warfarin pursuant to CED must address one or more aspects of the following question:

Prospectively, in Medicare-aged subjects whose warfarin therapy management includes pharmacogenomic testing of CYP2C9 or VKORC1 alleles to predict warfarin response, what is the frequency and severity of the following outcomes, compared to subjects whose warfarin therapy management does not include pharmacogenomic testing?

    Major hemorrhage

    Minor hemorrhage

    Thromboembolism related to the primary indication for anticoagulation

    Other thromboembolic event

    Mortality

The study must adhere to the following standards of scientific integrity and relevance to the Medicare population:

a. The principal purpose of the research study is to test whether a particular intervention potentially improves the participants' health outcomes.

b. The research study is well-supported by available scientific and medical information or it is intended to clarify or establish the health outcomes of interventions already in common clinical use.

c. The research study does not unjustifiably duplicate existing studies.

d. The research study design is appropriate to answer the research question being asked in the study.

e. The research study is sponsored by an organization or individual capable of executing the proposed study successfully.

f. The research study is in compliance with all applicable Federal regulations concerning the protection of human subjects found in the Code of Federal Regulations (CFR) at 45 CFR Part 46. If a study is regulated by the FDA, it also must be in compliance with 21 CFR Parts 50 and 56.

g. All aspects of the research study are conducted according to the appropriate standards of scientific integrity.

h. The research study has a written protocol that clearly addresses, or incorporates by reference, the Medicare standards.

i. The clinical research study is not designed to exclusively test toxicity or disease pathophysiology in healthy individuals. Trials of all medical technologies measuring therapeutic outcomes as one of the objectives meet this standard only if the disease or condition being studied is life-threatening as defined in 21 CFR Sec. 312.81(a) and the patient has no other viable treatment options.

j. The clinical research study is registered on the www.ClinicalTrials.gov website by the principal sponsor/investigator prior to the enrollment of the first study subject.

k. The research study protocol specifies the method and timing of public release of all pre-specified outcomes to be measured including release of outcomes if outcomes are negative or study is terminated early. The results must be made public within 24 months of the end of data collection. If a report is planned to be published in a peer-reviewed journal, then that initial release may be an abstract that meets the requirements of the International Committee of Medical Journal Editors. However, a full report of the outcomes must be made public no later than 3 years after the end of data collection.

l. The research study protocol must explicitly discuss subpopulations affected by the treatment under investigation, particularly traditionally underrepresented groups in clinical studies, how the inclusion and exclusion criteria affect enrollment of these populations, and a plan for the retention and reporting of said populations on the trial. If the inclusion and exclusion criteria are expected to have a negative effect on the recruitment or retention of underrepresented populations, the protocol must discuss why these criteria are necessary.

m. The research study protocol explicitly discusses how the results are or are not expected to be generalizable to the Medicare population to infer whether Medicare patients may benefit from the intervention. Separate discussions in the protocol may be necessary for populations eligible for Medicare due to age, disability or Medicaid eligibility. Consistent with section 1142 of the Act, the Agency for Healthcare Research and Quality (AHRQ) supports clinical research studies that CMS determines meet the above-listed standards and address the above-listed research questions.

#### B. Nationally Non-Covered Indications

The CMS believes that the available evidence does not demonstrate that pharmacogenomic testing of CYP2C9 or VKORC1 alleles to predict warfarin responsiveness improves health outcomes in Medicare beneficiaries outside the context of CED, and is therefore not reasonable and necessary under Sec.1862(a)(1)(A) of the Act.

© 2016 Optum360, LLC

## C. Other

This NCD does not determine coverage to identify CYP2C9 or VKORC1 alleles for other purposes, nor does it determine national coverage to identify other alleles to predict warfarin responsiveness.

(This NCD last reviewed August 2009.)

## 100-03, 110.3

### Anti-Inhibitor Coagulant Complex (AICC)

(Rev. 1, 10-03-03)

CIM 45-24

Anti-inhibitor coagulant complex, AICC, is a drug used to treat hemophilia in patients with factor VIII inhibitor antibodies. AICC has been shown to be safe and effective and has Medicare coverage when furnished to patients with hemophilia A and inhibitor antibodies to factor VIII who have major bleeding episodes and who fail to respond to other, less expensive therapies.

## 100-03, 110.5

### Granulocyte Transfusions

(Rev. 1, 10-03-03)

CIM 45-18

Granulocyte transfusions to patients suffering from severe infection and granulocytopenia are a covered service under Medicare. Granulocytopenia is usually identified as fewer than 500 granulocytes/mm3 whole blood. Accepted indications for granulocyte transfusions include:

- Granulocytopenia with evidence of gram negative sepsis; and
- Granulocytopenia in febrile patients with local progressive infections unresponsive to appropriate antibiotic therapy, thought to be due to gram negative organisms.

## 100-03, 110.10

### Intravenous Iron Therapy

Iron deficiency is a common condition in end stage renal disease (ESRD) patients undergoing hemodialysis. Iron is a critical structural component of hemoglobin, a key protein found in normal red blood cells (RBCs) that transports oxygen. Without this important building block, anemic patients experience difficulty in restoring adequate, healthy RBCs that improve hematocrit levels. Clinical management of iron deficiency involves treating patients with iron replacement products while they undergo hemodialysis. Body iron stores can be supplemented with either oral or intravenous (IV) iron products. The available evidence suggests that the mode of intravenous administration is perhaps the most effective treatment for iron deficiency in hemodialysis patients. Unlike oral iron products which must be absorbed through the GI tract, IV iron products are infused directly into the bloodstream in a form that is readily available to the bone marrow for RBC synthesis, resulting in an earlier correction of iron deficiency and anemia.

Effective December 1, 2000, Medicare covers sodium ferric gluconate complex in sucrose injection as a first line treatment of iron deficiency anemia when furnished intravenously to patients undergoing chronic hemodialysis who are receiving supplemental erythropoeitin therapy.

Effective October 1, 2001, Medicare also covers iron sucrose injection as a first line treatment of iron deficiency anemia when furnished intravenously to patients undergoing chronic hemodialysis who are receiving supplemental erythropoeitin therapy.

## 100-03, 110.17

### Anti-Cancer Chemotherapy for Colorectal Cancer (Effective January 28, 2005)

Anti-Cancer Chemotherapy for Colorectal Cancer (Effective January 28, 2005)

### A. General

Oxaliplatin (Eloxatin™), irinotecan (Camptosar®), cetuximab (Erbitux™), and bevacizumab (Avastin™) are anti-cancer chemotherapeutic agents approved by the Food and Drug Administration (FDA) for the treatment of colorectal cancer. Anti-cancer chemotherapeutic agents are eligible for coverage when used in accordance with FDA-approved labeling (see section 1861(t)(2)(B) of the Social Security Act (the Act)), when the off-label use is supported in one of the authoritative drug compendia listed in section 1861(t)(2)(B)(ii)(I) of the Act, or when the Medicare Administrative Contractor (MAC) determines an off-label use is medically accepted based on guidance provided by the Secretary (section 1861(t)(2)(B)(ii)(II).

### B. Nationally Covered Indications

Pursuant to this national coverage determination (NCD), the off-label use of clinical items and services, including the use of the studied drugs oxaliplatin, irinotecan, cetuximab, or bevacizumab, are covered in specific clinical trials identified by the Centers for Medicare & Medicaid Services (CMS). The clinical trials identified by CMS for coverage of clinical items and services are sponsored by the National Cancer Institute (NCI) and study the use of one or more off-label uses of these four drugs in colorectal cancer and in other cancer types. The list of identified trials is on the CMS Web site at: http://www.cms.hhs.gov/coverage/download/id90b.pdf.

### C. Other

This policy does not alter Medicare coverage for items and services that may be covered or non-covered according to the existing national coverage policy for Routine Costs in a Clinical Trial (NCD Manual section 310.1). Routine costs will continue to be covered as well as other items and services provided as a result of coverage of these specific trials in this policy. The basic requirements for enrollment in a trial remain unchanged.

The existing requirements for coverage of oxaliplatin, irinotecan, cetuximab, bevacizumab, or other anticancer chemotherapeutic agents for FDA-approved indications or for indications listed in an approved compendium are not modified.

MACs shall continue to make reasonable and necessary coverage determinations under section 1861(t)(2)(B)(ii)(II) of the Act based on guidance provided by the Secretary for medically accepted uses of off-label indications of oxaliplatin, irinotecan, cetuximab, bevacizumab, or other anticancer chemotherapeutic agents provided outside of the identified clinical trials appearing on the CMS website noted above.

## 100-03, 110.18

### NCD for Aprepitant for Chemotherapy-Induced Emesis (110.18)

#### A. General

Chemotherapy-induced nausea and vomiting (CINV) can range from mild to severe, with the most severe cases resulting in dehydration, malnutrition, metabolic imbalances, and potential withdrawal from future chemotherapy treatments. The incidence and severity of CINV are influenced by the specific chemotherapeutic agent(s) used; dosage, schedule and route of administration; and drug combinations. Patient specific risk factors such as gender, age, history of motion sickness, and prior `exposure to chemotherapeutic agents can also have an effect on CINV incidence and severity. Progress has been made in reducing CINV, although it can still be hard to control symptoms that occur more than a day after chemotherapy, during repeat cycles of chemotherapy, and when chemotherapy is given on more than one day or in very high doses. No single antiemetic agent is completely effective in all patients. As noted above, many factors influence the incidence and severity of CINV, with the specific chemotherapeutic agent as the primary factor to consider when deciding which antiemetic to administer. Aprepitant (Emend®) is the first Food and Drug Administration-approved drug of its type. Aprepitant has been proposed to function in combination with other oral antiemetics for a specified population of Medicare patients receiving highly emetogenic chemotherapy and/or moderately emetogenic chemotherapy.

CMS is defining highly emetogenic chemotherapy and moderately emetogenic chemotherapy as those anticancer agents so designated in at least two of three guidelines published by the National Comprehensive Cancer Network (NCCN), American Society of Clinical Oncology (ASCO), and European Society of Medical Oncology (ESMO)/Multinational Association of Supportive Care in Cancer (MASCC). The inclusive examples are: NCCN plus ASCO, NCCN plus ESMO/MASCC, or ASCO plus ESMO/MASCC.

#### B. Nationally Covered Indications

Effective for services performed between April 4, 2005, and May 29, 2013, the Centers for Medicare & Medicaid Services makes the following determinations regarding the use of aprepitant in the treatment of reducing chemotherapy-induced emesis:

The evidence is adequate to conclude that the use of the oral antiemetic three-drug combination of oral aprepitant (Emend®), an oral 5HT3 antagonist, and oral dexamethasone is reasonable and necessary for a specified patient population. We have defined the patient population for which the use of the oral antiemetic three-drug combination of oral aprepitant (Emend®), an oral 5HT3 antagonist, and oral dexamethasone is reasonable and necessary as only those patients who are receiving one or more of the following anti-cancer chemotherapeutic agents:

- Carmustine
- Cisplatin
- Cyclophosphamide
- Dacarbazine
- Mechlorethamine
- Streptozocin
- Doxorubicin
- Epirubicin

Appendix 4 — Internet-only Manuals (IOMs)

- Lomustine

Effective for services performed on or after May 29, 2013, the oral three-drug regimen of oral aprepitant, an oral 5HT3 antagonist and oral dexamethasone is reasonable and necessary for beneficiaries receiving, either singularly or in combination with other drugs the following anticancer chemotherapeutic agents:

- Alemtuzumab
- Azacitidine
- Bendamustine
- Carboplatin
- Carmustine
- Cisplatin
- Clofarabine
- Cyclophosphamide
- Cytarabine
- Dacarbazine
- Daunorubicin
- Doxorubicin
- Epirubicin
- Idarubicin
- Ifosfamide
- Irinotecan
- Lomustine
- Mechlorethamine
- Oxaliplatin
- Streptozocin

The oral three drug regimen must be administered immediately before and within 48 hours after the administration of these chemotherapeutic agents.

### C. Nationally Noncovered Indications

The evidence is adequate to conclude that aprepitant cannot function alone as a full replacement for intravenously administered antiemetic agents for patients who are receiving highly emetogenic chemotherapy and/or moderately emetogenic chemotherapy. Medicare does not cover under Part B for oral antiemetic drugs in antiemetic drug combination regimens that are administered in part, via an oral route and in part, via an intravenous route. Medicare does not cover under Part B aprepitant when it is used alone for anticancer chemotherapy related nausea and vomiting.

### D. Other

Medicare Administrative Contractors may determine coverage for other all-oral three-drug antiemesis regimens of aprepitant or any other FDA approved oral NK-1 antagonist in combination with an oral 5HT3 antagonist and oral dexamethasone with the chemotherapeutic agents listed above, or any other anticancer chemotherapeutic agents that are FDA approved and are defined as highly or moderately emetogenic.

(Last revised May 2013)

## 100-03, 110.21

### Erythropoiesis Stimulating Agents (ESAs) in Cancer and Related Neoplastic Conditions

### A. General

Erythropoiesis stimulating agents (ESAs) stimulate the bone marrow to make more red blood cells and are United States Food and Drug Administration (FDA) approved for use in reducing the need for blood transfusion in patients with specific clinical indications. The FDA has issued alerts and warnings for ESAs administered for a number of clinical conditions, including cancer. Published studies report a higher risk of serious and life-threatening events associated with oncologic uses of ESAs.

### B. Nationally Covered Indications

ESA treatment for the anemia secondary to myelosuppressive anticancer chemotherapy in solid tumors, multiple myeloma, lymphoma, and lymphocytic leukemia is only reasonable and necessary under the following specified conditions:

- The hemoglobin level immediately prior to initiation or maintenance of ESA treatment is <10 g/dL (or the hematocrit is <30%).
- The starting dose for ESA treatment is the recommended FDA label starting dose, no more than 150 U/kg/3 times weekly for epoetin and 2.25 mcg/kg/1 time weekly for darbepoetin alpha. Equivalent doses may be given over other approved time periods.

- Maintenance of ESA therapy is the starting dose if the hemoglobin level remains below 10g/dL (or hematocrit is <30%) 4 weeks after initiation of therapy and the rise in hemoglobin is >1g/dL (hematocrit >3%);
- For patients whose hemoglobin rises <1g/dl (hematocrit rise <3%) compared to pretreatment baseline over 4 weeks of treatment and whose hemoglobin level remains <10g/dL after the 4 weeks of treatment (or the hematocrit is <30%), the recommended FDA label starting dose may be increased once by 25%. Continued use of the drug is not reasonable and necessary if the hemoglobin rises <1g/dl (hematocrit rise <3%) compared to pretreatment baseline by 8 weeks of treatment.
- Continued administration of the drug is not reasonable and necessary if there is a rapid rise in hemoglobin >1g/dl (hematocrit >3%) over 2 weeks of treatment unless the hemoglobin remains below or subsequently falls to <10g/dL (or the hematocrit is <30%). Continuation and reinstitution of ESA therapy must include a dose reduction of 25% from the previously administered dose.
- ESA treatment duration for each course of chemotherapy includes the 8 weeks following the final dose of myelosuppressive chemotherapy in a chemotherapy regimen.

### C. Nationally Non-Covered Indications

ESA treatment is not reasonable and necessary for beneficiaries with certain clinical conditions, either because of a deleterious effect of the ESA on their underlying disease or because the underlying disease increases their risk of adverse effects related to ESA use. These conditions include:

- Any anemia in cancer or cancer treatment patients due to folate deficiency, B-12 deficiency, iron deficiency, hemolysis, bleeding, or bone marrow fibrosis;
- The anemia associated with the treatment of acute and chronic myelogenous leukemias (CML, AML), or erythroid cancers;
- The anemia of cancer not related to cancer treatment;
- Any anemia associated only with radiotherapy;
- Prophylactic use to prevent chemotherapy-induced anemia;
- Prophylactic use to reduce tumor hypoxia;
- Patients with erythropoietin-type resistance due to neutralizing antibodies; and
- Anemia due to cancer treatment if patients have uncontrolled hypertension.

### D. Other

Local Medicare Administrative Contractors may continue to make reasonable and necessary determinations on all other uses of ESAs not specified in this National Coverage Determination.

See the Medicare Benefit Policy Manual, chapter 11, section 90 and chapter 15, section 50.5.2 for coverage of ESAs for end-stage renal disease-related anemia. 100-03,1121

## 100-03, 110.22

### Autologous Cellular Immunotherapy Treatment (Effective June 30, 2011)

### A. General

Prostate cancer is the most common non-cutaneous cancer in men in the United States. In 2009, an estimated 192,280 new cases of prostate cancer were diagnosed and an estimated 27,360 deaths were reported. The National Cancer Institute states that prostate cancer is predominantly a cancer of older men; the median age at diagnosis is 72 years. Once the patient has castration-resistant, metastatic prostate cancer the median survival is generally less than two years.

In 2010 the Food and Drug Administration (FDA) approved sipuleucel-T (PROVENGE®; APC8015), for patients with castration-resistant, metastatic prostate cancer. The posited mechanism of action, immunotherapy, is different from that of anti-cancer chemotherapy such as docetaxel. This is the first immunotherapy for prostate cancer to receive FDA approval.

The goal of immunotherapy is to stimulate the body's natural defenses (such as the white blood cells called dendritic cells, T-lymphocytes and mononuclear cells) in a specific manner so that they attack and destroy, or at least prevent, the proliferation of cancer cells. Specificity is attained by intentionally exposing a patient's white blood cells to a particular protein (called an antigen) associated with the prostate cancer. This exposure "trains" the white blood cells to target and attack the prostate cancer cells. Clinically, this is expected to result in a decrease in the size and/or number of cancer sites, an increase in the time to cancer progression, and/or an increase in survival of the patient.

Sipuleucel-T differs from other infused anti-cancer therapies. Most such anti-cancer therapies are manufactured and sold by a biopharmaceutical company and then purchased by and dispensed from a pharmacy. In contrast, once the decision is made

© 2016 Optum360, LLC

to treat with sipuleucel-T, a multi-step process is used to produce sipuleucel-T. Sipuleucel-T is made individually for each patient with his own white blood cells. The patient's white blood cells are removed via a procedure called leukapheresis. In a laboratory the white blood cells are exposed to PA2024, which is a molecule created by linking prostatic acid phosphatase (PAP) with granulocyte/macrophage-colony stimulating factor (GM-CSF). PAP is an antigen specifically associated with prostate cancer cells; GM-CSF is a protein that targets a receptor on the surface of white blood cells. Hence, PAP serves to externally manipulate the immunological functioning of the patient's white blood cells while GM-CSF serves to stimulate the white blood cells into action. As noted in the FDA's clinical review, each dose of sipuleucel-T contains a minimum of 40 million treated white blood cells, however there is "high inherent variability" in the yield of sipuleucel-T from leukapheresis to leukapheresis in the same patient as well as from patient to patient. The treated white blood cells are then infused back into the same patient. The FDA-approved dosing regimen is three doses with each dose administered two weeks apart.

**Indications and Limitations of Coverage**

**B. Nationally Covered Indications**

Effective for services performed on or after June 30, 2011, The Centers for Medicare and Medicaid Services (CMS) proposes that the evidence is adequate to conclude that the use of autologous cellular immunotherapy treatment - sipuleucel-T; PROVENGE® improves health outcomes for Medicare beneficiaries with asymptomatic or minimally symptomatic metastatic castrate-resistant (hormone refractory) prostate cancer, and thus is reasonable and necessary for this on-label indication under 1862(a)(1)(A) of the Social Security Act.

**C. Nationally Non-Covered Indications**

N/A

**D. Other**

Effective for services performed on or after June 30, 2011, coverage of all off-label uses of autologous cellular immunotherapy treatment —sipuleucel-T; PROVENGE® for the treatment of prostate cancer is left to the discretion of the local Medicare Administrative Contractors.

(NCD last reviewed June 2011.)

## 100-03, 150.12

**Collagen Meniscus Implant (Effective May 25, 2010)**

**A. General**

The knee menisci are wedge-shaped, semi-lunar discs of fibrous tissue located in the knee joint between the ends of the femur and the tibia and fibula. There is a lateral and medial meniscus in each knee. It is known now that the menisci provide mechanical support, localized pressure distribution, and lubrication of the knee joint. Initially, meniscal tears were treated with total meniscectomy; however, as knowledge of the function of the menisci and the potential long term effects of total meniscectomy on the knee joint evolved, treatment of symptomatic meniscal tears gravitated to repair of the tear, when possible, or partial meniscectomy.

The collagen meniscus implant (also referred to as collagen scaffold (CS), CMI or MenaflexTM meniscus implant throughout the published literature) is used to fill meniscal defects that result from partial meniscectomy. The collagen meniscus implant is not intended to replace the entire meniscus at it requires a meniscal rim for attachment. The literature describes the placement of the collagen meniscus implant through an arthroscopic procedure with an additional incision for capture of the repair needles and tying of the sutures. After debridement of the damaged meniscus, the implant is trimmed to the size of meniscal defect and sutured into place. The collagen meniscus implant is described as a tissue engineered scaffold to support the generation of new meniscus-like tissue. The collagen meniscus implant is manufactured from bovine collagen and should not be confused with the meniscus transplant which involves the replacement of the meniscus with a transplant meniscus from a cadaver donor. The meniscus transplant is not addressed under this national coverage determination.

**B. Nationally Covered Indications**

N/A

**C. Nationally Non-Covered Indications**

Effective for claims with dates of service performed on or after May 25, 2010, the Centers for Medicare & Medicaid Services has determined that the evidence is adequate to conclude that the collagen meniscus implant does not improve health outcomes and, therefore, is not reasonable and necessary for the treatment of meniscal injury/tear under section 1862(a)(1)(A) of the Social Security Act. Thus, the collagen meniscus implant is non-covered by Medicare.

**D. Other**

N/A

(This NCD last reviewed May 2010.)

## 100-03, 160.13

**NCD for Supplies Used in the Delivery of Transcutaneous Electrical Nerve Stimulation (TENS) and Neuromuscular Electrical Stimulation (NMES)**

Transcutaneous Electrical Nerve Stimulation (TENS) and/or Neuromuscular Electrical Stimulation (NMES) can ordinarily be delivered to patients through the use of conventional electrodes, adhesive tapes and lead wires. There may be times, however, where it might be medically necessary for certain patients receiving TENS or NMES treatment to use, as an alternative to conventional electrodes, adhesive tapes and lead wires, a form-fitting conductive garment (i.e., a garment with conductive fibers which are separated from the patients' skin by layers of fabric).

A form-fitting conductive garment (and medically necessary related supplies) may be covered under the program only when:

1. It has received permission or approval for marketing by the Food and Drug Administration;

2. It has been prescribed by a physician for use in delivering covered TENS or NMES treatment; and

3. One of the medical indications outlined below is met:

   • The patient cannot manage without the conductive garment because there is such a large area or so many sites to be stimulated and the stimulation would have to be delivered so frequently that it is not feasible to use conventional electrodes, adhesive tapes and lead wires;

   • The patient cannot manage without the conductive garment for the treatment of chronic intractable pain because the areas or sites to be stimulated are inaccessible with the use of conventional electrodes, adhesive tapes and lead wires;

   • The patient has a documented medical condition such as skin problems that preclude the application of conventional electrodes, adhesive tapes and lead wires;

   • The patient requires electrical stimulation beneath a cast either to treat disuse atrophy, where the nerve supply to the muscle is intact, or to treat chronic intractable pain; or

   • The patient has a medical need for rehabilitation strengthening (pursuant to a written plan of rehabilitation) following an injury where the nerve supply to the muscle is intact.

A conductive garment is not covered for use with a TENS device during the trial period specified in §160.3 unless:

4. The patient has a documented skin problem prior to the start of the trial period; and

5. The carrier's medical consultants are satisfied that use of such an item is medically necessary for the patient.

(See conditions for coverage of the use of TENS in the diagnosis and treatment of chronic intractable pain in §§160.3,160.13 and 160.27 and the use of NMES in the treatment of disuse atrophy in §150.4.)

## 100-03,160.27

**NCD for Transcutaneous Electrical Nerve Stimulation (TENS) for Chronic Low Back Pain (CLBP)**

The TENS is a type of electrical nerve stimulator that is employed to treat chronic intractable pain. This stimulator is attached to the surface of the patient's skin over the peripheral nerve to be stimulated. It may be applied in a variety of settings (in the patient's home, a physician's office, or in an outpatient clinic). Payment for TENS may be made under the durable medical equipment benefit.

**A. General**

For the purposes of this decision chronic low back pain (CLBP) is defined as:

1. an episode of low back pain that has persisted for three months or longer; and

2. is not a manifestation of a clearly defined and generally recognizable primary disease entity. For example, there are cancers that, through metastatic spread to the spine or pelvis, may elicit pain in the lower back as a symptom; and certain systemic diseases such as rheumatoid arthritis and multiple sclerosis manifest many debilitating symptoms of which low back pain is not the primary focus. B. Nationally Covered Indications Effective June 8, 2012, the Centers for Medicare & Medicaid Services (CMS) will allow coverage for Transcutaneous Electrical Nerve Stimulation (TENS) for CLBP only when all of the following conditions are met.

In order to support additional research on the use of TENS for CLBP, we will cover this item under section 1862(a)(1)(E) of the Social Security Act (the Act) subject to all of the following conditions:

1. Coverage under this section expires three years after the publication of this decision on the CMS website.

© 2016 Optum360, LLC

**Appendix 4 — Internet-only Manuals (IOMs)**

2. The beneficiary is enrolled in an approved clinical study meeting all of the requirements below. The study must address one or more aspects of the following questions in a randomized, controlled design using validated and reliable instruments. This can include randomized crossover designs when the impact of prior TENS use is appropriately accounted for in the study protocol.

   i. Does the use of TENS provide clinically meaningful reduction in pain in Medicare beneficiaries with CLBP?

   ii. Does the use of TENS provide a clinically meaningful improvement of function in Medicare beneficiaries with CLBP?

   iii. Does the use of TENS impact the utilization of other medical treatments or services used in the medical management of CLBP?

These studies must be designed so that the patients in the control and comparison groups receive the same concurrent treatments and either sham (placebo) TENS or active TENS intervention.

The study must adhere to the following standards of scientific integrity and relevance to the Medicare population:

   a. The principal purpose of the research study is to test whether a particular intervention potentially improves the participants' health outcomes.

   b. The research study is well supported by available scientific and medical information or it is intended to clarify or establish the health outcomes of interventions already in common clinical use.

   c. The research study does not unjustifiably duplicate existing studies.

   d. The research study design is appropriate to answer the research question being asked in the study.

   e. The research study is sponsored by an organization or individual capable of executing the proposed study successfully. f. The research study is in compliance with all applicable Federal regulations concerning the protection of human subjects found at 45 CFR Part 46. If a study is regulated by the Food and Drug Administration (FDA), it must be in compliance with 21 CFR parts 50 and 56.

   g. All aspects of the research study are conducted according to appropriate standards of scientific integrity (see http://www.icmje.org).

   h. The research study has a written protocol that clearly addresses, or incorporates by reference, the standards listed here as Medicare requirements for CED coverage.

   i. The clinical research study is not designed to exclusively test toxicity or disease pathophysiology in healthy individuals. Trials of all medical technologies measuring therapeutic outcomes as one of the objectives meet this standard only if the disease or condition being studied is life threatening as defined in 21 CFR § 312.81(a) and the patient has no other viable treatment options.

   j. The clinical research study is registered on the ClinicalTrials.gov website by the principal sponsor/investigator prior to the enrollment of the first study subject.

   k. The research study protocol specifies the method and timing of public release of all prespecified outcomes to be measured including release of outcomes if outcomes are negative or study is terminated early. The results must be made public within 24 months of the end of data collection. If a report is planned to be published in a peer reviewed journal, then that initial release may be an abstract that meets the requirements of the International Committee of Medical Journal Editors (http://www.icmje.org).

   l. The research study protocol must explicitly discuss subpopulations affected by the treatment under investigation, particularly traditionally underrepresented groups in clinical studies, how the inclusion and exclusion criteria effect enrollment of these populations, and a plan for the retention and reporting of said populations on the trial. If the inclusion and exclusion criteria are expected to have a negative effect on the recruitment or retention of underrepresented populations, the protocol must discuss why these criteria are necessary

   m. The research study protocol explicitly discusses how the results are or are not expected to be generalizable to the Medicare population to infer whether Medicare patients may benefit from the intervention. Separate discussions in the protocol may be necessary for populations eligible for Medicare due to age, disability or Medicaid eligibility. .

**C. Nationally Non-Covered Indications**

TENS is not reasonable and necessary for the treatment of CLBP under section 1862(a)(1)(A) of the Act.

**D. Other**

See §160.13 for an explanation of coverage of medically necessary supplies for the effective use of TENS. See §160.7.1 for an explanation of coverage for assessing patients suitability for electrical nerve stimulation therapy. See §10.2 for an explanation of coverage of transcutaneous electrical nerve stimulation (TENS) for acute post-operative pain. Please note, §280.13Transcutaneous Electrical Nerve Stimulators (TENS) NCD has been removed from the NCD manual and incorporated into NCD 160.27.

(This NCD last reviewed June 2012

## 100-03,160.7.1

### Assessing Patients Suitability for Electrical Nerve Stimulation Therapy

**B. Percutaneous Electrical Nerve Stimulation (PENS)**

This diagnostic procedure which involves stimulation of peripheral nerves by a needle electrode inserted through the skin is performed only in a physician's office, clinic, or hospital outpatient department. Therefore, it is covered only when performed by a physician or incident to physician's service. If pain is effectively controlled by percutaneous stimulation, implantation of electrodes is warranted.

As in the case of TENS (described in subsection A), generally the physician should be able to determine whether the patient is likely to derive a significant therapeutic benefit from continuing use of an implanted nerve stimulator within a trial period of 1 month. In a few cases, this determination may take longer to make. The medical necessity for such diagnostic services which are furnished beyond the first month must be documented.

NOTE: Electrical nerve stimulators do not prevent pain but only alleviate pain as it occurs. A patient can be taught how to employ the stimulator, and once this is done, can use it safely and effectively without direct physician supervision. Consequently, it is inappropriate for a patient to visit his/her physician, physical therapist, or an outpatient clinic on a continuing basis for treatment of pain with electrical nerve stimulation. Once it is determined that electrical nerve stimulation should be continued as therapy and the patient has been trained to use the stimulator, it is expected that a stimulator will be implanted or the patient will employ the TENS on a continual basis in his/her home. Electrical nerve stimulation treatments furnished by a physician in his/her office, by a physical therapist or outpatient clinic are excluded from coverage by §1862(a)(1) of the Act. (See §160.7 for an explanation of coverage of the therapeutic use of implanted peripheral nerve stimulators under the prosthetic devices benefit.) See §160.27 for an explanation of coverage of the therapeutic use of TENS under the durable medical equipment benefit.

## 100-03, 180.2

### Enteral and Parenteral Nutritional Therapy

**Covered As Prosthetic Device**

There are patients who, because of chronic illness or trauma, cannot be sustained through oral feeding. These people must rely on either enteral or parenteral nutritional therapy, depending upon the particular nature of their medical condition.

Coverage of nutritional therapy as a Part B benefit is provided under the prosthetic device benefit provision which requires that the patient must have a permanently inoperative internal body organ or function thereof. Therefore, enteral and parenteral nutritional therapy are normally not covered under Part B in situations involving temporary impairments.

Coverage of such therapy, however, does not require a medical judgment that the impairment giving rise to the therapy will persist throughout the patient's remaining years. If the medical record, including the judgment of the attending physician, indicates that the impairment will be of long and indefinite duration, the test of permanence is considered met.

If the coverage requirements for enteral or parenteral nutritional therapy are met under the prosthetic device benefit provision, related supplies, equipment and nutrients are also covered under the conditions in the following paragraphs and the Medicare Benefit Policy Manual, Chapter 15, "Covered Medical and Other Health Services," §120.

Parenteral Nutrition Therapy Daily parenteral nutrition is considered reasonable and necessary for a patient with severe pathology of the alimentary tract which does not allow absorption of sufficient nutrients to maintain weight and strength commensurate with the patient's general condition.

Since the alimentary tract of such a patient does not function adequately, an indwelling catheter is placed percutaneously in the subclavian vein and then advanced into the superior vena cava where intravenous infusion of nutrients is given for part of the day. The catheter is then plugged by the patient until the next infusion. Following a period of hospitalization, which is required to initiate parenteral nutrition and to train the patient in catheter care, solution preparation, and infusion technique, the parenteral nutrition can be provided safely and effectively in the patient's home by nonprofessional persons who have undergone special training. However, such persons cannot be paid for their services, nor is payment available for any services furnished by non-physician professionals except as services furnished incident to a physician's service.

For parenteral nutrition therapy to be covered under Part B, the claim must contain a physician's written order or prescription and sufficient medical documentation to permit an independent conclusion that the requirements of the prosthetic device benefit are met and that parenteral nutrition therapy is medically necessary. An example of a condition that typically qualifies for coverage is a massive small bowel resection resulting in severe nutritional deficiency in spite of adequate oral intake. However, coverage of parenteral nutrition therapy for this and any other condition must be approved on an individual, case-by-case basis initially and at periodic intervals of no more than three months by the Medicare Administrative Contractor (A/B MAC (B)) medical consultant or specially trained staff, relying on such medical and other documentation as the A/B MAC (B) may require. If the claim involves an infusion pump, sufficient evidence must be provided to support a determination of medical necessity for the pump. Program payment for the pump is based on the reasonable charge for the simplest model that meets the medical needs of the patient as established by medical documentation.

Nutrient solutions for parenteral therapy are routinely covered. However, Medicare pays for no more than one month's supply of nutrients at any one time. Payment for the nutrients is based on the reasonable charge for the solution components unless the medical record, including a signed statement from the attending physician, establishes that the beneficiary, due to his/her physical or mental state, is unable to safely or effectively mix the solution and there is no family member or other person who can do so. Payment will be on the basis of the reasonable charge for more expensive premixed solutions only under the latter circumstances.

**Enteral Nutrition Therapy**

Enteral nutrition is considered reasonable and necessary for a patient with a functioning gastrointestinal tract who, due to pathology to, or non-function of, the structures that normally permit food to reach the digestive tract, cannot maintain weight and strength commensurate with his or her general condition. Enteral therapy may be given by nasogastric, jejunostomy, or gastrostomy tubes and can be provided safely and effectively in the home by nonprofessional persons who have undergone special training. However, such persons cannot be paid for their services, nor is payment available for any services furnished by non-physician professionals except as services furnished incident to a physician's service.

Typical examples of conditions that qualify for coverage are head and neck cancer with reconstructive surgery and central nervous system disease leading to interference with the neuromuscular mechanisms of ingestion of such severity that the beneficiary cannot be maintained with oral feeding. However, claims for Part B coverage of enteral nutrition therapy for these and any other conditions must be approved on an individual, case-by-case basis. Each claim must contain a physician's written order or prescription and sufficient medical documentation (e.g., hospital records, clinical findings from the attending physician) to permit an independent conclusion that the patient's condition meets the requirements of the prosthetic device benefit and that enteral nutrition therapy is medically necessary. Allowed claims are to be reviewed at periodic intervals of no more than 3 months by the A/B MAC (B) medical consultant or specially trained staff, and additional medical documentation considered necessary is to be obtained as part of this review.

Medicare pays for no more than one month's supply of enteral nutrients at any one time.

If the claim involves a pump, it must be supported by sufficient medical documentation to establish that the pump is medically necessary, i.e., gravity feeding is not satisfactory due to aspiration, diarrhea, dumping syndrome. Program payment for the pump is based on the reasonable charge for the simplest model that meets the medical needs of the patient as established by medical documentation.

Nutritional Supplementation

Some patients require supplementation of their daily protein and caloric intake. Nutritional supplements are often given as a medicine between meals to boost protein-caloric intake or the mainstay of a daily nutritional plan. Nutritional supplementation is not covered under Medicare Part B.

## 100-03, 190.9

### NCD for Serologic Testing for Acquired Immunodeficiency Syndrome (AIDS) (190.9)

These tests may be covered when performed to help determine a diagnosis for symptomatic patients. They are not covered when furnished as part of a screening program for asymptomatic persons.

Note: Two enzyme-linked immunosorbent assay (ELISA) tests that were conducted on the same specimen must both be positive before Medicare will cover the Western blot test.

## 100-03, 190.11

### NCD for Home Prothrombin Time International Normalized Ratio (INR) Monitoring for Anticoagulation Management (190.11)

#### A. General

Use of the International Normalized Ratio (INR) or prothrombin time (PT) - standard measurement for reporting the blood's clotting time) - allows physicians to determine the level of anticoagulation in a patient independent of the laboratory reagents used. The INR is the ratio of the patient's PT (extrinsic or tissue-factor dependent coagulation pathway) compared to the mean PT for a group of normal individuals. Maintaining patients within his/her prescribed therapeutic range minimizes adverse events associated with inadequate or excessive anticoagulation such as serious bleeding or thromboembolic events. Patient self-testing and self-management through the use of a home INR monitor may be used to improve the time in therapeutic rate (TTR) for select groups of patients. Increased TTR leads to improved clinical outcomes and reductions in thromboembolic and hemorrhagic events.

Warfarin (also prescribed under other trade names, e.g., Coumadin(R)) is a self-administered, oral anticoagulant (blood thinner) medication that affects the vitamin K- dependent clotting factors II, VII, IX and X. It is widely used for various medical conditions, and has a narrow therapeutic index, meaning it is a drug with less than a 2-fold difference between median lethal dose and median effective dose. For this reason, since October 4, 2006, it falls under the category of a Food and Drug administration (FDA) "black-box" drug whose dosage must be closely monitored to avoid serious complications. A PT/INR monitoring system is a portable testing device that includes a finger-stick and an FDA-cleared meter that measures the time it takes for a person's blood plasma to clot.

#### B. Nationally Covered Indications

For services furnished on or after March 19, 2008, Medicare will cover the use of home PT/INR monitoring for chronic, oral anticoagulation management for patients with mechanical heart valves, chronic atrial fibrillation, or venous thromboembolism (inclusive of deep venous thrombosis and pulmonary embolism) on warfarin. The monitor and the home testing must be prescribed by a treating physician as provided at 42 CFR 410.32(a), and all of the following requirements must be met:

1.  The patient must have been anticoagulated for at least 3 months prior to use of the home INR device; and,

2.  The patient must undergo a face-to-face educational program on anticoagulation management and must have demonstrated the correct use of the device prior to its use in the home; and,

3.  The patient continues to correctly use the device in the context of the management of the anticoagulation therapy following the initiation of home monitoring; and,

4.  Self-testing with the device should not occur more frequently than once a week.

#### C. Nationally Non-Covered Indications

N/A

#### D. Other

1.  All other indications for home PT/INR monitoring not indicated as nationally covered above remain at local Medicare contractor discretion.

2.  This national coverage determination (NCD) is distinct from, and makes no changes to, the PT clinical laboratory NCD at section 190.17 of Publication 100-03 of the NCD Manual.

## 100-03,190.14

### NCD for Human Immunodeficiency Virus (HIV) Testing (Diagnosis) (190.14)

#### Indications and Limitations of Coverage

#### Indications

Diagnostic testing to establish HIV infection may be indicated when there is a strong clinical suspicion supported by one or more of the following clinical findings:

The patient has a documented, otherwise unexplained, AIDS-defining or AIDS-associated opportunistic infection.

The patient has another documented sexually transmitted disease which identifies significant risk of exposure to HIV and the potential for an early or subclinical infection.

The patient has documented acute or chronic hepatitis B or C infection that identifies a significant risk of exposure to HIV and the potential for an early or subclinical infection.

The patient has a documented AIDS-defining or AIDS-associated neoplasm.

The patient has a documented AIDS-associated neurologic disorder or otherwise unexplained dementia.

The patient has another documented AIDS-defining clinical condition, or a history of other severe, recurrent, or persistent conditions which suggest an underlying immune deficiency (for example, cutaneous or mucosal disorders).

The patient has otherwise unexplained generalized signs and symptoms suggestive of a chronic process with an underlying immune deficiency (for example, fever, weight loss, malaise, fatigue, chronic diarrhea, failure to thrive, chronic cough, hemoptysis, shortness of breath, or lymphadenopathy).

The patient has otherwise unexplained laboratory evidence of a chronic disease process with an underlying immune deficiency (for example, anemia, leukopenia, pancytopenia, lymphopenia, or low CD4+ lymphocyte count).

The patient has signs and symptoms of acute retroviral syndrome with fever, malaise, lymphadenopathy, and skin rash.

The patient has documented exposure to blood or body fluids known to be capable of transmitting HIV (for example, needlesticks and other significant blood exposures) and antiviral therapy is initiated or anticipated to be initiated.

The patient is undergoing treatment for rape. (HIV testing is a part of the rape treatment protocol.)

### Limitations

HIV antibody testing in the United States is usually performed using HIV-1 or HIV-¬¾ combination tests. HIV-2 testing is indicated if clinical circumstances suggest HIV-2 is likely (that is, compatible clinical findings and HIV-1 test negative). HIV-2 testing may also be indicated in areas of the country where there is greater prevalence of HIV-2 infections.

The Western Blot test should be performed only after documentation that the initial EIA tests are repeatedly positive or equivocal on a single sample.

The HIV antigen tests currently have no defined diagnostic usage.

Direct viral RNA detection may be performed in those situations where serologic

testing does not establish a diagnosis but strong clinical suspicion persists (for example, acute retroviral syndrome, nonspecific serologic evidence of HIV, or perinatal HIV infection).

If initial serologic tests confirm an HIV infection, repeat testing is not indicated.

If initial serologic tests are HIV EIA negative and there is no indication for confirmation of infection by viral RNA detection, the interval prior to retesting is 3-6 months.

Testing for evidence of HIV infection using serologic methods may be medically appropriate in situations where there is a risk of exposure to HIV. However, in the absence of a documented AIDS defining or HIV- associated disease, an HIV associated sign or symptom, or documented exposure to a known HIV-infected source, the testing is considered by Medicare to be screening and thus is not covered by Medicare (for example, history of multiple blood component transfusions, exposure to blood or body fluids not resulting in consideration of therapy, history of transplant, history of illicit drug use, multiple sexual partners, same-sex encounters, prostitution, or contact with prostitutes).

The CPT Editorial Panel has issued a number of codes for infectious agent detection by direct antigen or nucleic acid probe techniques that have not yet been developed or are only being used on an investigational basis. Laboratory providers are advised to remain current on FDA-approval status for these tests.

## 100-03, 200.1

### Nesiritide for Treatment of Heart Failure Patients (Effective March 2, 2006)

#### A. General
Nesiritide (Natrecor®) is Food and Drug Administration (FDA)-approved for the intravenous treatment of patients with acutely decompensated congestive heart failure (CHF) who have dyspnea (shortness of breath) at rest or with minimal activity. Nesiritide is not self-administered.

#### B. Nationally Covered Indications
N/A

#### C. Nationally Non-Covered Indications
Effective for dates of service on or after March 2, 2006, the Centers for Medicare & Medicaid Services has determined that there is sufficient evidence to conclude that

the use of Nesiritide for the treatment of CHF is not reasonable and necessary for Medicare beneficiaries in any setting.

#### D. Other
Effective for dates of service on or after March 2, 2006, this determination applies only to the treatment of CHF and does not change Medicare Administrative Contractor discretion to cover other off-label uses of Nesiritide or use consistent with the current FDA indication for intravenous treatment of patients with acutely decompensated CHF who have dyspnea at rest or with minimal activity.

## 100-03, 200.2

### Nebulized Beta Adrenergic Agonist Therapy for Lung Diseases – (Effective September 10, 2007)

Nebulized Beta Adrenergic Agonist Therapy for Lung Diseases – (Effective September 10, 2007)

#### A. General
Lung diseases such as chronic obstructive pulmonary disease (COPD) and asthma are characterized by airflow limitation that may be partially or completely reversible. Pharmacologic treatment with bronchodilators is used to prevent and/or control daily symptoms that may cause disability for persons with these diseases. These medications are intended to improve the movement of air into and from the lungs by relaxing and dilating the bronchial passageways. Beta adrenergic agonists are a commonly prescribed class of bronchodilator drug. They can be administered via nebulizer, metered dose inhaler, orally, or dry powdered inhaler.

Nebulized beta adrenergic agonist with racemic albuterol has been used for many years. More recently, levalbuterol, the (R) enantiomer of racemic albuterol, has been used in some patient populations. There are concerns regarding the appropriate use of nebulized beta adrenergic agonist therapy for lung disease.

#### B. Nationally Covered Indications
N/A

#### C. Nationally Non-Covered Indications
N/A

#### D. Other
After examining the available medical evidence, the Centers for Medicare & Medicaid Services determines that no national coverage determination is appropriate at this time. Section 1862(a)(1)(A) of the Social Security Act decisions should be made by local Medicare Administrative Contractors through a local coverage determination process or case-by-case adjudication. See Heckler v. Ringer, 466 U.S. 602, 617 (1984) (Recognizing that the Secretary has discretion to either establish a generally applicable rule or to allow individual adjudication.). See also, 68 Fed. Reg. 63692, 63693 (November 7, 2003).

## 100-03, 210.2

### NCD for Screening Pap Smears and Pelvic Examinations for Early Detection of Cervical or Vaginal Cancer (210.2)

#### Screening Pap Smear
A screening pap smear and related medically necessary services provided to a woman for the early detection of cervical cancer (including collection of the sample of cells and a physician's interpretation of the test results) and pelvic examination (including clinical breast examination) are covered under Medicare Part B when ordered by a physician (or authorized practitioner) under one of the following conditions:

She has not had such a test during the preceding two years or is a woman of childbearing age (§1861(nn) of the Social Security Act (the Act).

There is evidence (on the basis of her medical history or other findings) that she is at high risk of developing cervical cancer and her physician (or authorized practitioner) recommends that she have the test performed more frequently than every two years.

High risk factors for cervical and vaginal cancer are:

- Early onset of sexual activity (under 16 years of age)
- Multiple sexual partners (five or more in a lifetime)
- History of sexually transmitted disease (including HIV infection)
- Fewer than three negative or any pap smears within the previous seven years; and
- DES (diethylstilbestrol) - exposed daughters of women who took DES during pregnancy.

NOTE: Claims for pap smears must indicate the beneficiary's low or high risk status by including the appropriate diagnosis code on the line item (Item 24E of the Form CMS-1500).

**Definitions**

A woman as described in §1861(nn) of the Act is a woman who is of childbearing age and has had a pap smear test during any of the preceding 3 years that indicated the presence of cervical or vaginal cancer or other abnormality, or is at high risk of developing cervical or vaginal cancer.

A woman of childbearing age is one who is premenopausal and has been determined by a physician or other qualified practitioner to be of childbearing age, based upon the medical history or other findings.

Other qualified practitioner, as defined in 42 CFR 410.56(a) includes a certified nurse midwife (as defined in §1861(gg) of the Act), or a physician assistant, nurse practitioner, or clinical nurse specialist (as defined in §1861(aa) of the Act) who is authorized under State law to perform the examination.

**Screening Pelvic Examination**

Section 4102 of the Balanced Budget Act of 1997 provides for coverage of screening pelvic examinations (including a clinical breast examination) for all female beneficiaries, subject to certain frequency and other limitations. A screening pelvic examination (including a clinical breast examination) should include at least seven of the following eleven elements:

Inspection and palpation of breasts for masses or lumps, tenderness, symmetry, or nipple discharge.

Digital rectal examination including sphincter tone, presence of hemorrhoids, and rectal masses. Pelvic examination (with or without specimen collection for smears and cultures) including:

- External genitalia (for example, general appearance, hair distribution, or lesions).
- Urethral meatus (for example, size, location, lesions, or prolapse).
- Urethra (for example, masses, tenderness, or scarring).
- Bladder (for example, fullness, masses, or tenderness).
- Vagina (for example, general appearance, estrogen effect, discharge lesions, pelvic support, cystocele, or rectocele).
- Cervix (for example, general appearance, lesions, or discharge).
- Uterus (for example, size, contour, position, mobility, tenderness, consistency, descent, or support).
- Adnexa/parametria (for example, masses, tenderness, organomegaly, or nodularity).
- Anus and perineum.

This description is from Documentation Guidelines for Evaluation and Management Services, published in May 1997 and was developed by the Centers for Medicare & Medicaid Services and the American Medical Association.

## 100-03, 210.2.1

**Screening for Cervical Cancer with Human Papillomavirus (HPV) Testing**

**A. General**

Medicare covers a screening pelvic examination and Pap test for all female beneficiaries at 12 or 24 month intervals, based on specific risk factors. See 42 C.F.R. §410.56; Medicare National Coverage Determinations Manual, §210.2.1 Current Medicare coverage does not include the HPV testing. Pursuant to §1861(ddd) of the Social Security Act, the Secretary may add coverage of "additional preventive services" if certain statutory requirements are met.

**B. Nationally Covered Indications**

Effective for services performed on or after July 9, 2015, CMS has determined that the evidence is sufficient to add Human Papillomavirus (HPV) testing once every five years as an additional preventive service benefit under the Medicare program for asymptomatic beneficiaries aged 30 to 65 years in conjunction with the Pap smear test. CMS will cover screening for cervical cancer with the appropriate U.S. Food and Drug Administration (FDA) approved/cleared laboratory tests, used consistent with FDA approved labeling and in compliance with the Clinical Laboratory Improvement Act (CLIA) regulations.

**C. Nationally Non-Covered Indications**

Unless specifically covered in this NCD, any other NCD, by statute or regulation, preventive services are non-covered by Medicare.

**D. Other**

(This NCD last reviewed July 2015.)

## 100-03, 210.4

**NCD for Smoking and Tobacco-Use Cessation Counseling (210.4)**

**A. General**

Tobacco use continues to be the leading cause of preventable death in the United States. In 1964, the Surgeon General of the U.S. Public Health Service (PHS) issued the report of his Advisory Committee on Smoking and Health, officially recognizing that cigarette smoking is a cause of cancer and other serious diseases. Though smoking rates have significantly declined, 9.3% of the population age 65 and older smokes cigarettes. Approximately 440,000 people die annually from smoking related disease, with 68% (300,000) age 65 or older. Many more people of all ages suffer from serious illness caused from smoking, leading to disability and decreased quality of life. Reduction in smoking prevalence is a national objective in Healthy People 2010.

**B. Nationally Covered Indications**

Effective March 22, 2005, the Centers for Medicare and Medicaid Services (CMS) has determined that the evidence is adequate to conclude that smoking and tobacco use cessation counseling, based on the current PHS Guideline, is reasonable and necessary for a patient with a disease or an adverse health effect that has been found by the U.S. Surgeon General to be linked to tobacco use, or who is taking a therapeutic agent whose metabolism or dosing is affected by tobacco use as based on FDA-approved information.

Patients must be competent and alert at the time that services are provided. Minimal counseling is already covered at each evaluation and management (E&M) visit. Beyond that, Medicare will cover 2 cessation attempts per year. Each attempt may include a maximum of 4 intermediate or intensive sessions, with the total annual benefit covering up to 8 sessions in a 12-month period. The practitioner and patient have flexibility to choose between intermediate or intensive cessation strategies for each attempt.

Intermediate and intensive smoking cessation counseling services will be covered for outpatient and hospitalized beneficiaries who are smokers and who qualify as above, as long as those services are furnished by qualified physicians and other Medicare-recognized practitioners.

**C. Nationally Non-Covered Indications**

Inpatient hospital stays with the principal diagnosis of Tobacco Use Disorder are not reasonable and necessary for the effective delivery of tobacco cessation counseling services. Therefore, we will not cover tobacco cessation services if tobacco cessation is the primary reason for the patient's hospital stay.

**D. Other**

N/A

(This NCD last reviewed May 2005.)

## 100-03, 210.7

**NCD for Screening for the Human Immunodeficiency Virus (HIV) Infection (210.7)**

**A. General**

Infection with the human immunodeficiency virus (HIV) is a continuing, worldwide pandemic described by the World Health Organization as "the most serious infectious disease challenge to global public health". Acquired immunodeficiency syndrome (AIDS) is diagnosed when a HIV-infected person's immune system becomes severely compromised and/or a person becomes ill with a HIV-related opportunistic infection. Without treatment, AIDS usually develops within 8-10 years after a person's initial HIV infection. While there is presently no cure for HIV, an infected individual can be recognized by screening, and subsequent access to skilled care plus vigilant monitoring and adherence to continuous antiretroviral therapy may delay the onset of AIDS and increase quality of life for many years.

Significantly, more than half of new HIV infections are estimated to be sexually transmitted from infected individuals who are unaware of their HIV status. Consequently, improved secondary disease prevention and wider availability of screening linked to HIV care and treatment would not only delay disease progression and complications in untested or unaware older individuals, but could also decrease the spread of disease to those living with or partnered with HIV-infected individuals.

HIV antibody testing first became available in 1985. These commonly used, Food and Drug Administration (FDA)-approved HIV antibody screening tests – using serum or plasma from a venipuncture or blood draw – are known as EIA (enzyme immunoassay) or ELISA (enzyme-linked immunosorbent assay) tests.

Developed for point-of-care testing using alternative samples, six rapid HIV-1 and/or HIV-2 antibody tests – using fluid obtained from the oral cavity or using whole blood, serum, or plasma from a blood draw or fingerstick – were approved by the FDA from 2002-2006.

Effective January 1, 2009, the Centers for Medicare & Medicaid Services (CMS) is allowed to add coverage of "additional preventive services" through the national coverage determination (NCD) process if certain statutory requirements are met, as provided under section 101(a) of the Medicare Improvements for Patients and Providers Act. One of those requirements is that the service(s) be categorized as a grade A (strongly recommends) or grade B (recommends) rating by the US Preventive Services Task Force (USPSTF). The USPSTF strongly recommends screening for all adolescents and adults at risk for HIV infection, as well as all pregnant women.

### B. Nationally Covered Indications

Effective for claims with dates of service on and after December 8, 2009, CMS determines that the evidence is adequate to conclude that screening for HIV infection is reasonable and necessary for early detection of HIV and is appropriate for individuals entitled to benefits under

Part A or enrolled under Part B. Therefore, CMS proposes to cover both standard and FDA-approved HIV rapid screening tests for:

1. A maximum of one, annual voluntary HIV screening of Medicare beneficiaries at increased risk for HIV infection per USPSTF guidelines as follows:

   - Men who have had sex with men after 1975
   - Men and women having unprotected sex with multiple [more than one] partners
   - Past or present injection drug users
   - Men and women who exchange sex for money or drugs, or have sex partners who do
   - Individuals whose past or present sex partners were HIV-infected, bisexual or injection drug users
   - Persons being treated for sexually transmitted diseases
   - Persons with a history of blood transfusion between 1978 and 1985
   - Persons who request an HIV test despite reporting no individual risk factors, since this group is likely to include individuals not willing to disclose high-risk behaviors; and,

2. A maximum of three, voluntary HIV screenings of pregnant Medicare beneficiaries: (1) when the diagnosis of pregnancy is known, (2) during the third trimester, and (3) at labor, if ordered by the woman's clinician.

### C. Nationally Non-Covered Indications

Effective for claims with dates of service on and after December 8, 2009, Medicare beneficiaries with any known diagnosis of a HIV-related illness are not eligible for this screening test.

Medicare beneficiaries (other than those who are pregnant) who have had a prior HIV screening test within one year are not eligible (11 full months must have elapsed following the month in which the previous test was performed in order for the subsequent test to be covered).

Pregnant Medicare beneficiaries who have had three screening tests within their respective term of pregnancy are not eligible (beginning with the date of the first test).

### D. Other

N/A

(This NCD last reviewed November 2009.)

## 100-03, 210.8

### Screening and Behavioral Counseling Interventions in Primary Care to Reduce Alcohol Misuse (Effective October 14, 2011)

#### A. General

Based upon authority to cover "additional preventive services" for Medicare beneficiaries if certain statutory requirements are met, the Centers for Medicare & Medicaid Services (CMS) initiated a new national coverage analysis on annual screening and brief behavioral counseling in primary care to reduce alcohol misuse in adults, including pregnant women. Annual screening and behavioral counseling for alcohol misuse in adults is recommended with a grade of B by the U.S. Preventive Services Task Force (USPSTF) and is appropriate for individuals entitled to benefits under Part A and Part B.

CMS will cover annual alcohol screening and up to four, brief face-to-face behavioral counseling in primary care settings to reduce alcohol misuse. CMS does not identify specific alcohol misuse screening tools. Rather, the decision to use a specific tool is at the discretion of the clinician in the primary care setting. Various screening tools are available for screening for alcohol misuse.

#### B. Nationally Covered Indications

Effective for claims with dates of service on or after October 14, 2011, CMS will cover annual alcohol screening, and for those that screen positive, up to four brief, face-to-

face, behavioral counseling interventions per year for Medicare beneficiaries, including pregnant women:

- Who misuse alcohol, but whose levels or patterns of alcohol consumption do not meet criteria for alcohol dependence (defined as at least three of the following: tolerance, withdrawal symptoms, impaired control, preoccupation with acquisition and/or use, persistent desire or unsuccessful efforts to quit, sustains social, occupational, or recreational disability, use continues despite adverse consequences); and

- Who are competent and alert at the time that counseling is provided; and,

- Whose counseling is furnished by qualified primary care physicians or other primary care practitioners in a primary care setting.

Each of the behavioral counseling interventions should be consistent with the 5A' approach that has been adopted by the USPSTF to describe such services. They are:

1. Assess: Ask about/assess behavioral health risk(s) and factors affecting choice of behavior change goals/methods.

2. Advise: Give clear, specific, and personalized behavior change advice, including information about personal health harms and benefits.

3. Agree: Collaboratively select appropriate treatment goals and methods based on the patient's interest in and willingness to change the behavior.

4. Assist: Using behavior change techniques (self-help and/or counseling), aid the patient in achieving agreed upon goals by acquiring the skills, confidence, and social/environmental supports for behavior change, supplemented with adjunctive medical treatments when appropriate.

5. Arrange: Schedule follow-up contacts (in person or by telephone) to provide ongoing assistance/support and to adjust the treatment plan as needed, including referral to more intensive or specialized treatment. For the purposes of this policy, a primary care setting is defined as one in which there is provision of integrated, accessible health care services by clinicians who are accountable for addressing a large majority of personal health care needs, developing a sustained partnership with patients, and practicing in the context of family and community. Emergency departments, inpatient hospital settings, ambulatory surgical centers, independent diagnostic testing facilities, skilled nursing facilities, inpatient rehabilitation facilities and hospices are not considered primary care settings under this definition.

For the purposes of this policy a "primary care physician" and "primary care practitioner" are to be defined based on two existing sections of the Social Security Act, §1833(u)(6), §1833(x)(2)(A)(i)(I) and §1833(x)(2)(A)(i)(II):

§1833(u)

(6)Physician Defined.—For purposes of this paragraph, the term "physician" means a physician described in section 1861(r)(1) and the term "primary care physician" means a physician who is identified in the available data as a general practitioner, family practice practitioner, general internist, or obstetrician or gynecologist.

§1833(x)(2)(A)(i)

(I) is a physician (as described in section 1861(r)(1)) who has a primary specialty designation of family medicine, internal medicine, geriatric medicine, or pediatric medicine; or

(II) is a nurse practitioner, clinical nurse specialist, or physician assistant (as those terms are defined in section 1861(aa)(5)).

#### C. Nationally Non-Covered Indications

1. Alcohol screening is non-covered when performed more than one time in a 12-month period.

2. Brief face-to-face behavioral counseling interventions are non-covered when performed more than once a day; that is, two counseling interventions on the same day are non-covered.

3. Brief face-to-face behavioral counseling interventions are non-covered when performed more than four times in a 12-month period

#### D. Other

Medicare coinsurance and Part B deductible are waived for this preventive service

(This NCD last reviewed October 2011.)

## 100-03, 210.10

### Screening for Sexually Transmitted Infections (STIs) and High Intensity Behavioral Counseling (HIBC) to Prevent STIs

#### A. General

Sexually transmitted infections (STIs) are infections that are passed from one person to another through sexual contact. STIs remain an important cause of morbidity in the United States and have both health and economic consequences. Many of the

© 2016 Optum360, LLC

complications of STIs are borne by women and children Often, STIs do not present any symptoms so can go untreated for long periods of time The presence of an STI during pregnancy may result in significant health complications for the woman and infant. In fact, any person who has an STI may develop health complications. Screening tests for the STIs in this national coverage determination (NCD) are laboratory tests.

Under §1861(ddd) of the Social Security Act (the Act), the Centers for Medicare & Medicaid Services (CMS) has the authority to add coverage of additional preventive services if certain statutory requirements are met. The regulations provide:

§410.64 Additional preventive services

(a) Medicare Part B pays for additional preventive services not described in paragraph (1) or (3) of the definition of "preventive services" under §410.2, that identify medical conditions or risk factors for individuals if the Secretary determines through the national coverage determination process (as defined in section 1869(f)(1)(B) of the Act) that these services are all of the following: (1) reasonable and necessary for the prevention or early detection of illness or disability.(2) recommended with a grade of A or B by the United States Preventive Services Task Force, (3) appropriate for individuals entitled to benefits under Part A or enrolled under Part B.

(b) In making determinations under paragraph (a) of this section regarding the coverage of a new preventive service, the Secretary may conduct an assessment of the relation between predicted outcomes and the expenditures for such services and may take into account the results of such an assessment in making such national coverage determinations.

The scope of the national coverage analysis for this NCD evaluated the evidence for the following STIs and high intensity behavioral counseling (HIBC) to prevent STIs for which the United States Preventive Services Task Force (USPSTF) has issued either an A or B recommendation:

- Screening for chlamydial infection for all sexually active non-pregnant young women aged 24 and younger and for older non-pregnant women who are at increased risk,
- Screening for chlamydial infection for all pregnant women aged 24 and younger and for older pregnant women who are at increased risk,
- Screening for gonorrhea infection in all sexually active women, including those who are pregnant, if they are at increased risk,
- Screening for syphilis infection for all pregnant women and for all persons at increased risk,
- Screening for hepatitis B virus (HBV) infection in pregnant women at their first prenatal visit,
- HIBC for the prevention of STIs for all sexually active adolescents, and for adults at increased risk for STIs.

**B. Nationally Covered Indications**

CMS has determined that the evidence is adequate to conclude that screening for chlamydia, gonorrhea, syphilis, and hepatitis B, as well as HIBC to prevent STIs, consistent with the grade A and B recommendations by the USPSTF, is reasonable and necessary for the early detection or prevention of an illness or disability and is appropriate for individuals entitled to benefits under Part A or enrolled under Part B.

Therefore, effective for claims with dates of services on or after November 8, 2011, CMS will cover screening for these USPSTF-indicated STIs with the appropriate Food and Drug Administration (FDA)-approved/cleared laboratory tests, used consistent with FDA-approved labeling, and in compliance with the Clinical Laboratory Improvement Act (CLIA) regulations, when ordered by the primary care physician or practitioner, and performed by an eligible Medicare provider for these services.

Screening for chlamydia and gonorrhea:

- Pregnant women who are 24 years old or younger when the diagnosis of pregnancy is known, and then repeat screening during the third trimester if high-risk sexual behavior has occurred since the initial screening test.
- Pregnant women who are at increased risk for STIs when the diagnosis of pregnancy is known, and then repeat screening during the third trimester if high-risk sexual behavior has occurred since the initial screening test.
- Women at increased risk for STIs annually.

Screening for syphilis:

- Pregnant women when the diagnosis of pregnancy is known, and then repeat screening during the third trimester and at delivery if high-risk sexual behavior has occurred since the previous screening test.
- Men and women at increased risk for STIs annually.

Screening for hepatitis B:

- Pregnant women at the first prenatal visit when the diagnosis of pregnancy is known, and then rescreening at time of delivery for those with new or continuing risk factors. In addition, effective for claims with dates of service on or after November 8, 2011, CMS will cover up to two individual 20- to 30-minute, face-to-face counseling sessions annually for Medicare beneficiaries for HIBC to prevent STIs, for all sexually active adolescents, and for adults at increased risk for STIs, if referred for this service by a primary care physician or practitioner, and provided by a Medicare eligible primary care provider in a primary care setting. Coverage of HIBC to prevent STIs is consistent with the USPSTF recommendation.

HIBC is defined as a program intended to promote sexual risk reduction or risk avoidance, which includes each of these broad topics, allowing flexibility for appropriate patient-focused elements:

- education,
- skills training,
- guidance on how to change sexual behavior.

The high/increased risk individual sexual behaviors, based on the USPSTF guidelines, include any of the following:

- Multiple sex partners
- Using barrier protection inconsistently
- Having sex under the influence of alcohol or drugs
- Having sex in exchange for money or drugs
- Age (24 years of age or younger and sexually active for women for chlamydia and gonorrhea)
- Having an STI within the past year
- IV drug use (for hepatitis B only)

In addition for men

- men having sex with men (MSM) and engaged in high risk sexual behavior, but no regard to age

In addition to individual risk factors, in concurrence with the USPSTF recommendations, community social factors such as high prevalence of STIs in the community populations should be considered in determining high/increased risk for chlamydia, gonorrhea, syphilis, and for recommending HIBC.

High/increased risk sexual behavior for STIs is determined by the primary care provider by assessing the patient's sexual history which is part of any complete medical history, typically part of an annual wellness visit or prenatal visit and considered in the development of a comprehensive prevention plan. The medical record should be a reflection of the service provided.

For the purposes of this NCD, a primary care setting is defined as the provision of integrated, accessible health care services by clinicians who are accountable for addressing a large majority of personal health care needs, developing a sustained partnership with patients, and practicing in the context of family and community. Emergency departments, inpatient hospital settings, ambulatory surgical centers, independent diagnostic testing facilities, skilled nursing facilities, inpatient rehabilitation facilities, clinics providing a limited focus of health care services, and hospice are examples of settings not considered primary care settings under this definition.

For the purposes of this NCD, a "primary care physician" and "primary care practitioner" will be defined based on existing sections of the Social Security Act (§1833(u)(6), §1833(x)(2)(A)(i)(I) and §1833(x)(2)(A)(i)(II)).

§1833(u)

(6) Physician Defined.?or purposes of this paragraph, the term "physician" means a physician described in section 1861(r)(1) and the term "primary care physician" means a physician who is identified in the available data as a general practitioner, family practice practitioner, general internist, or obstetrician or gynecologist.

§1833(x)(2)(A)(i)

(I) is a physician (as described in section 1861(r)(1)) who has a primary specialty designation of family medicine, internal medicine, geriatric medicine, or pediatric medicine; or

(II) is a nurse practitioner, clinical nurse specialist, or physician assistant (as those terms are defined in section 1861(aa)(5));

**C. Nationally Non-Covered Indications**

Unless specifically covered in this NCD, any other NCD, or in statute, preventive services are non-covered by Medicare.

**D. Other**

Medicare coinsurance and Part B deductible are waived for these preventive services.

HIBC to prevent STIs may be provided on the same date of services as an annual wellness visit, evaluation and management (E&M) service, or during the global billing period for obstetrical car, but only one HIBC may be provided on any one date of service. See the claims processing manual for further instructions on claims processing.

For services provided on an annual basis, this is defined as a 12-month period.

(This NCD last reviewed November 2011.)

## 100-03, 210.11

### Intensive Behavioral Therapy for Cardiovascular Disease (CVD) (Effective November 8, 2011

#### A. General

Cardiovascular disease (CVD) is the leading cause of mortality in the United States. CVD, which is comprised of hypertension, coronary heart disease (such as myocardial infarction and angina pectoris), heart failure and stroke, is also the leading cause of hospitalizations. Although the overall adjusted mortality rate from heart disease has declined over the past decade, opportunities for improvement still exist. Risk factors for CVD include being overweight, obesity, physical inactivity, diabetes, cigarette smoking, high blood pressure, high blood cholesterol, family history of myocardial infarction, and older age.

Under §1861(ddd) of the Social Security Act (the Act), the Centers for Medicare & Medicaid Services (CMS) has the authority to add coverage of additional preventive services through the National Coverage Determination (NCD) process if certain statutory requirements are met. Following its review, CMS has determined that the evidence is adequate to conclude that intensive behavioral therapy for CVD is reasonable and necessary for the prevention or early detection of illness or disability, is appropriate for individuals entitled to benefits under Part A or enrolled under Part B, and is comprised of components that are recommended with a grade of A or B by the U.S. Preventive Services Task Force (USPSTF).

#### B. Nationally Covered Indications

Effective for claims with dates of service on or after November 8, 2011, CMS covers intensive behavioral therapy for CVD (referred to below as a CVD risk reduction visit), which consists of the following three components:

- encouraging aspirin use for the primary prevention of CVD when the benefits outweigh the risks for men age 45-79 years and women 55-79 years;
- screening for high blood pressure in adults age 18 years and older; and
- intensive behavioral counseling to promote a healthy diet for adults with hyperlipidemia, hypertension, advancing age, and other known risk factors for cardiovascular- and diet-related chronic disease.

We note that only a small proportion (about 4%) of the Medicare population is under 45 years (men) or 55 years (women), therefore the vast majority of beneficiaries should receive all three components. Intensive behavioral counseling to promote a healthy diet is broadly recommended to cover close to 100% of the population due to the prevalence of known risk factors.

Therefore, CMS covers one, face-to-face CVD risk reduction visit per year for Medicare beneficiaries who are competent and alert at the time that counseling is provided, and whose counseling is furnished by a qualified primary care physician or other primary care practitioner in a primary care setting.

The behavioral counseling intervention for aspirin use and healthy diet should be consistent with the Five As approach that has been adopted by the USPSTF to describe such services:

- Assess: Ask about/assess behavioral health risk(s) and factors affecting choice of behavior change goals/methods.
- Advise: Give clear, specific, and personalized behavior change advice, including information about personal health harms and benefits.
- Agree: Collaboratively select appropriate treatment goals and methods based on the patient's interest in and willingness to change the behavior.
- Assist: Using behavior change techniques (self-help and/or counseling), aid the patient in achieving agreed-upon goals by acquiring the skills, confidence, and social/environmental supports for behavior change, supplemented with adjunctive medical treatments when appropriate.
- Arrange: Schedule follow-up contacts (in person or by telephone) to provide ongoing assistance/support and to adjust the treatment plan as needed, including referral to more intensive or specialized treatment. For the purpose of this NCD, a primary care setting is defined as the provision of integrated, accessible health care services by clinicians who are accountable for addressing a large majority of personal health care needs, developing a sustained partnership with patients, and practicing in the context of family and community. Emergency departments, inpatient hospital settings, ambulatory

surgical centers, independent diagnostic testing facilities, skilled nursing facilities, inpatient rehabilitation facilities, and hospices are not considered primary care settings under this definition.

For the purpose of this NCD, a "primary care physician" and "primary care practitioner" are defined consistent with existing sections of the Act (§1833(u)(6), §1833(x)(2)(A)(i)(I) and §1833(x)(2)(A)(i)(II)).

§1833(u)

(6) Physician Defined.?or purposes of this paragraph, the term "physician" means a physician described in section 1861(r)(1) and the term "primary care physician" means a physician who is identified in the available data as a general practitioner, family practice practitioner, general internist, or obstetrician or gynecologist.

§1833(x)(2)

(A) Primary care practitioner. he term "primary care practitioner" means an individual—

(i) who—

(I) is a physician (as described in section 1861(r)(1)) who has a primary specialty designation of family medicine, internal medicine, geriatric medicine, or pediatric medicine; or

(II) is a nurse practitioner, clinical nurse specialist, or physician assistant (as those terms are defined in section 1861(aa)(5)).

#### C. Nationally Non-Covered Indications

Unless specifically covered in this NCD, any other NCD, or in statute, preventive services are non-covered by Medicare.

#### D. Other

Medicare coinsurance and Part B deductible are waived for this preventive service.

(This NCD last reviewed November 2011.)

## 100-03, 210.12

#### A. General

Based upon authority to cover "additional preventive services" for Medicare beneficiaries if certain statutory requirements are met, the Centers for Medicare & Medicaid Services (CMS) initiated a new national coverage analysis on intensive behavioral therapy for obesity. Screening for obesity in adults is recommended with a grade of B by the U.S. Preventive Services Task Force (USPSTF) and is appropriate for individuals entitled to benefits under Part A and Part B.

The Centers for Disease Control (CDC) reported that "obesity rates in the U.S. have increased dramatically over the last 30 years, and obesity is now epidemic in the United States." In the Medicare population over 30% of men and women are obese. Obesity is directly or indirectly associated with many chronic diseases including cardiovascular disease, musculoskeletal conditions and diabetes.

#### B. Nationally Covered Indications

Effective for claims with dates of service on or after November 29, 2011, CMS covers intensive behavioral therapy for obesity, defined as a body mass index (BMI) >= 30 kg/m2, for the prevention or early detection of illness or disability.

Intensive behavioral therapy for obesity consists of the following:

1. Screening for obesity in adults using measurement of BMI calculated by dividing weight in kilograms by the square of height in meters (expressed kg/m2);
2. Dietary (nutritional) assessment; and
3. Intensive behavioral counseling and behavioral therapy to promote sustained weight loss through high intensity interventions on diet and exercise.

The intensive behavioral intervention for obesity should be consistent with the 5-A framework that has been highlighted by the USPSTF:

1. Assess: Ask about/assess behavioral health risk(s) and factors affecting choice of behavior change goals/methods.
2. Advise: Give clear, specific, and personalized behavior change advice, including information about personal health harms and benefits.
3. Agree: Collaboratively select appropriate treatment goals and methods based on the patient's interest in and willingness to change the behavior.
4. Assist: Using behavior change techniques (self-help and/or counseling), aid the patient in achieving agreed-upon goals by acquiring the skills, confidence, and social/environmental supports for behavior change, supplemented with adjunctive medical treatments when appropriate. 5. Arrange: Schedule follow-up contacts (in person or by telephone) to provide ongoing assistance/support and to adjust the treatment plan as needed, including referral to more intensive or specialized treatment. For Medicare beneficiaries with obesity, who are competent and alert at the time that counseling is provided and whose

counseling is furnished by a qualified primary care physician or other primary care practitioner and in a primary care setting, CMS covers:

- One face-to-face visit every week for the first month;
- One face-to-face visit every other week for months 2-6;
- One face-to-face visit every month for months 7-12, if the beneficiary meets the 3kg weight loss requirement during the first six months as discussed below.

At the six month visit, a reassessment of obesity and a determination of the amount of weight loss must be performed. To be eligible for additional face-to-face visits occurring once a month for an additional six months, beneficiaries must have achieved a reduction in weight of at least 3kg over the course of the first six months of intensive therapy. This determination must be documented in the physician office records for applicable beneficiaries consistent with usual practice. For beneficiaries who do not achieve a weight loss of at least 3kg during the first six months of intensive therapy, a reassessment of their readiness to change and BMI is appropriate after an additional six month period.

For the purposes of this decision memorandum, a primary care setting is defined as one in which there is provision of integrated, accessible health care services by clinicians who are accountable for addressing a large majority of personal health care needs, developing a sustained partnership with patients, and practicing in the context of family and community. Emergency departments, inpatient hospital settings, ambulatory surgical centers, independent diagnostic testing facilities, skilled nursing facilities, inpatient rehabilitation facilities and hospices are not considered primary care settings under this definition.

For the purposes of this decision memorandum a "primary care physician" and "primary care practitioner" will be defined consistent with existing sections of the Social Security Act (§1833(u)(6), §1833(x)(2)(A)(i)(I) and §1833(x)(2)(A)(i)(II)).

§1833(u)

(6) Physician Defined.—For purposes of this paragraph, the term "physician" means a physician described in section 1861(r)(1) and the term "primary care physician" means a physician who is identified in the available data as a general practitioner, family practice practitioner, general internist, or obstetrician or gynecologist.

§1833(x)(2)(A)

Primary care practitioner—The term "primary care practitioner" means an individual—

(i) who—

(I) is a physician (as described in section 1861(r)(1)) who has a primary specialty designation of family medicine, internal medicine, geriatric medicine, or pediatric medicine; or

(II) is a nurse practitioner, clinical nurse specialist, or physician assistant (as those terms are defined in section 1861(aa)(5))

### C. Nationally Non-Covered Indications
All other indications remain non-covered.

### D. Other
Medicare coinsurance and Part B deductible are waived for this service

(This NCD last reviewed November 2011)

## 100-03, 210.13

### Screening for Hepatitis C Virus (HCV) in Adults

#### A. General
Hepatitis C Virus (HCV) is an infection that attacks the liver and leads to inflammation. The infection is often asymptomatic and can go undiagnosed for decades. It is difficult for the human immune system to eliminate the HCV and it is a major cause of chronic liver disease. The presence of HCV in the liver initiates a response from the immune system which in turn causes inflammation. Inflammation over long periods of time (usually decades) can cause scarring, called cirrhosis. A cirrhotic liver fails to perform the normal functions of the liver which leads to liver failure. Cirrhotic livers are more prone to become cancerous and liver failure leads to serious complications, even death. HCV is reported to be the leading cause of chronic hepatitis, cirrhosis and liver cancer and a primary indication for liver transplant in the Western World.

Under §1861(ddd) of the Social Security Act (the Act), the Centers for Medicare & Medicaid Services (CMS) has the authority to add coverage of additional preventive services if certain statutory requirements are met. The regulations provide:

42 CFR §410.64 Additional preventive services

(a) Medicare Part B pays for additional preventive services not described in paragraph (1) or (3) of the definition of "preventive services" under 42 CFR §410.2, that identify medical conditions or risk factors for individuals if the Secretary determines through the national coverage determination process (as defined in

section 1869(f)(1)(B) of the Act) that these services are all of the following: (1) reasonable and necessary for the prevention or early detection of illness or disability,(2) recommended with a grade of A or B by the United States Preventive Services Task Force (USPSTF), (3) appropriate for individuals entitled to benefits under Part A or enrolled under Part B.

(b) In making determinations under paragraph (a) of this section regarding the coverage of a new preventive service, the Secretary may conduct an assessment of the relation between predicted outcomes and the expenditures for such services and may take into account the results of such an assessment in making such national coverage determinations.

The scope of the review for this national coverage determination (NCD) evaluated and determined if the existing body of evidence was sufficient for Medicare coverage for screening for HCV in adults at high risk for HCV infection and one-time screening for HCV infection for adults born between 1945 and 1965, which is recommended with a grade B by the USPSTF.

#### B. Nationally Covered Indications
Effective for services performed on or after June 2, 2014, CMS has determined the following:

The evidence is adequate to conclude that screening for HCV, consistent with the grade B recommendations by the USPSTF, is reasonable and necessary for the prevention or early detection of an illness or disability and is appropriate for individuals entitled to benefits under Part A or enrolled under Part B, as described below.

Therefore, CMS will cover screening for HCV with the appropriate U.S. Food and Drug Administration (FDA)-approved/cleared laboratory tests, used consistent with FDA-approved labeling and in compliance with the Clinical Laboratory Improvement Act regulations, when ordered by the beneficiary's primary care physician or practitioner within the context of a primary care setting, and performed by an eligible Medicare provider for these services, for beneficiaries who meet either of the following conditions:

1. A screening test is covered for adults at high risk for HCV infection. "High risk" is defined as persons with a current or past history of illicit injection drug use; and persons who have a history of receiving a blood transfusion prior to 1992. Repeat screening for high risk persons is covered annually only for persons who have had continued illicit injection drug use since the prior negative screening test.

2. A single screening test is covered for adults who do not meet the high risk definition above, but who were born from 1945 through 1965.

The determination of "high risk for HCV" is identified by the primary care physician or practitioner who assesses the patient's history, which is part of any complete medical history, typically part of an annual wellness visit and considered in the development of a comprehensive prevention plan. The medical record should be a reflection of the service provided.

A primary care setting is defined by the provision of integrated, accessible health care services by clinicians who are accountable for addressing a large majority of personal health care needs, developing a sustained partnership with patients, and practicing in the context of family and community. Emergency departments, inpatient hospital settings, ambulatory surgical centers, independent diagnostic testing facilities, skilled nursing facilities, inpatient rehabilitation facilities, clinics providing a limited focus of health care services, and hospice are examples of settings not considered primary care settings under this definition.

A "primary care physician" and "primary care practitioner" will be defined consistent with existing sections of the Act (§1833(u)(6), §1833(x)(2)(A)(i)(I) and §1833(x)(2)(A)(i)(II)).

§1833(u)

(6) Physician Defined.—For purposes of this paragraph, the term "physician" means a physician described in section 1861(r)(1) and the term "primary care physician" means a physician who is identified in the available data as a general practitioner, family practice practitioner, general internist, or obstetrician or gynecologist.

§1833(x)(2)(A)(i)

(I) is a physician (as described in section 1861(r)(1)) who has a primary specialty designation of family medicine, internal medicine, geriatric medicine, or pediatric medicine; or

(II) is a nurse practitioner, clinical nurse specialist, or physician assistant (as those terms are defined in section 1861(aa)(5)).

#### C. Nationally Non-Covered Indications
Unless specifically covered in this NCD, any other NCD, or in statute, preventive services are non-covered by Medicare.

**D. Other**

N/A

(This NCD last reviewed June 2014.)

## 100-03, 220.6.1

### NCD for PET for Perfusion of the Heart (220.6.1)

**Indications and Limitations of Coverage**

1. Rubidium 82 (Effective March 14, 1995)

   Effective for services performed on or after March 14, 1995, PET scans performed at rest or with pharmacological stress used for noninvasive imaging of the perfusion of the heart for the diagnosis and management of patients with known or suspected coronary artery disease using the FDA-approved radiopharmaceutical Rubidium 82 (Rb 82) are covered, provided the requirements below are met:

   The PET scan, whether at rest alone, or rest with stress, is performed in place of, but not in addition to, a single photon emission computed tomography (SPECT); or

   The PET scan, whether at rest alone or rest with stress, is used following a SPECT that was found to be inconclusive. In these cases, the PET scan must have been considered necessary in order to determine what medical or surgical intervention is required to treat the patient. (For purposes of this requirement, an inconclusive test is a test(s) whose results are equivocal, technically uninterpretable, or discordant with a patient's other clinical data and must be documented in the beneficiary's file.)

   For any PET scan for which Medicare payment is claimed for dates of services prior to July 1, 2001, the claimant must submit additional specified information on the claim form (including proper codes and/or modifiers), to indicate the results of the PET scan. The claimant must also include information on whether the PET scan was performed after an inconclusive noninvasive cardiac test. The information submitted with respect to the previous noninvasive cardiac test must specify the type of test performed prior to the PET scan and whether it was inconclusive or unsatisfactory. These explanations are in the form of special G codes used for billing PET scans using Rb 82. Beginning July 1, 2001, claims should be submitted with the appropriate codes.

2. Ammonia N-13 (Effective October 1, 2003)

   Effective for services performed on or after October 1, 2003, PET scans performed at rest or with pharmacological stress used for noninvasive imaging of the perfusion of the heart for the diagnosis and management of patients with known or suspected coronary artery disease using the FDA-approved radiopharmaceutical ammonia N-13 are covered, provided the requirements below are met:

   The PET scan, whether at rest alone, or rest with stress, is performed in place of, but not in addition to, a SPECT; or

   The PET scan, whether at rest alone or rest with stress, is used following a SPECT that was found to be inconclusive. In these cases, the PET scan must have been considered necessary in order to determine what medical or surgical intervention is required to treat the patient. (For purposes of this requirement, an inconclusive test is a test whose results are equivocal, technically uninterpretable, or discordant with a patient's other clinical data and must be documented in the beneficiary's file.)

(This NCD last reviewed March 2005.)

## 100-03, 220.6.12

### FDG PET for Soft Tissue Sarcoma (Various Effective Dates Below)

(Replaced with Section 220.6.17)

(Rev. 120; Issued: 05-06-10; Effective Date: 04-03-09; Implementation Date: 10-30-09)

## 100-03, 220.6.13

### Positron Emission Tomography (PET) for Dementia and Neurodegenerative Diseases

**A. General**

Medicare covers FDG Positron Emission Tomography (PET) scans for either the differential diagnosis of fronto-temporal dementia (FTD) and Alzheimer's disease (AD) under specific requirements; OR, its use in a Centers for Medicare & Medicaid Services (CMS)-approved practical clinical trial focused on the utility of FDG PET in the diagnosis or treatment of dementing neurodegenerative diseases. Specific requirements for each indication are clarified below:

**B. Nationally Covered Indications**

1. FDG PET Requirements for Coverage in the Differential Diagnosis of AD and FTD

An FDG PET scan is considered reasonable and necessary in patients with a recent diagnosis of dementia and documented cognitive decline of at least 6 months, who meet diagnostic criteria for both AD and FTD. These patients have been evaluated for specific alternate neurodegenerative diseases or other causative factors, but the cause of the clinical symptoms remains uncertain.

The following additional conditions must be met before an FDG PET scan will be covered:

a. The patient's onset, clinical presentation, or course of cognitive impairment is such that FTD is suspected as an alternative neurodegenerative cause of the cognitive decline. Specifically, symptoms such as social disinhibition, awkwardness, difficulties with language, or loss of executive function are more prominent early in the course of FTD than the memory loss typical of AD;

b. The patient has had a comprehensive clinical evaluation (as defined by the American Academy of Neurology encompassing a medical history from the patient and a well-acquainted informant (including assessment of activities of daily living), physical and mental status examination (including formal documentation of cognitive decline occurring over at least 6 months) aided by cognitive scales or neuropsychological testing, laboratory tests, and structural imaging such as magnetic resonance imaging (MRI) or computed tomography (CT);

c. The evaluation of the patient has been conducted by a physician experienced in the diagnosis and assessment of dementia;

d. The evaluation of the patient did not clearly determine a specific neurodegenerative disease or other cause for the clinical symptoms, and information available through FDG PET is reasonably expected to help clarify the diagnosis between FTD and AD and help guide future treatment;

e. The FDG PET scan is performed in a facility that has all the accreditation necessary to operate nuclear medicine equipment. The reading of the scan should be done by an expert in nuclear medicine, radiology, neurology, or psychiatry, with experience interpreting such scans in the presence of dementia;

f. A brain single photon emission computed tomography (SPECT) or FDG PET scan has not been obtained for the same indication. (The indication can be considered to be different in patients who exhibit important changes in scope or severity of cognitive decline, and meet all other qualifying criteria listed above and below (including the judgment that the likely diagnosis remains uncertain.) The results of a prior SPECT or FDG PET scan must have been inconclusive or, in the case of SPECT, difficult to interpret due to immature or inadequate technology. In these instances, an FDG PET scan may be covered after one year has passed from the time the first SPECT or FDG PET scan was performed.)

g. The referring and billing provider(s) have documented the appropriate evaluation of the Medicare beneficiary. Providers should establish the medical necessity of an FDG PET scan by ensuring that the following information has been collected and is maintained in the beneficiary medical record:

   – Date of onset of symptoms;

   – Diagnosis of clinical syndrome (normal aging; mild cognitive impairment (MCI); mild, moderate or severe dementia);

   – Mini mental status exam (MMSE) or similar test score;

   – Presumptive cause (possible, probable, uncertain AD);

   – Any neuropsychological testing performed;

   – Results of any structural imaging (MRI or CT) performed;

   – Relevant laboratory tests (B12, thyroid hormone); and,

   – Number and name of prescribed medications.

The billing provider must furnish a copy of the FDG PET scan result for use by CMS and its Medicare Administrative Contractors upon request. These verification requirements are consistent with Federal requirements set forth in 42 Code of Federal Regulations section 410.32 generally for diagnostic x-ray tests, diagnostic laboratory tests, and other tests. In summary, section 410.32 requires the billing physician and the referring physician to maintain information in the medical record of each patient to demonstrate medical necessity [410.32(d) (2)] and submit the information demonstrating medical necessity to CMS and/or its agents upon request [410.32(d)(3)(I)] (OMB number 0938-0685).

2. FDG PET Requirements for Coverage in the Context of a CMS-approved Practical Clinical Trial Utilizing a Specific Protocol to Demonstrate the Utility of FDG PET in the Diagnosis, and Treatment of Neurodegenerative Dementing Diseases

An FDG PET scan is considered reasonable and necessary in patients with MCI or early dementia (in clinical circumstances other than those specified in subparagraph 1) only in the context of an approved clinical trial that contains patient safeguards and protections to ensure proper administration, use and evaluation of the FDG PET scan.

The clinical trial must compare patients who do and do not receive an FDG PET scan and have as its goal to monitor, evaluate, and improve clinical outcomes. In addition, it must meet the following basic criteria:

– Written protocol on file;

– Institutional Review Board review and approval;

– Scientific review and approval by two or more qualified individuals who are not part of the research team; and,

Certification that investigators have not been disqualified.

### C. Nationally Non- Covered Indications

All other uses of FDG PET for patients with a presumptive diagnosis of dementia-causing neurodegenerative disease (e.g., possible or probable AD, clinically typical FTD, dementia of Lewy bodies, or Creutzfeld-Jacob disease) for which CMS has not specifically indicated coverage continue to be noncovered.

### D. Other

Not applicable.

(This NCD last reviewed September 2004.)

## 100-03, 220.6.17

### Positron Emission Tomography (FDG PET) for Oncologic Conditions
(Effective June 11, 2013)

(Rev. 173, Issued: 09-04-14, Effective: Upon Implementation: of ICD-10, Implementation: Upon Implementation of ICD-10)

### A. General

FDG (2-[F18] fluoro-2-deoxy-D-glucose) Positron Emission Tomography (PET) is a minimally-invasive diagnostic imaging procedure used to evaluate glucose metabolism in normal tissue as well as in diseased tissues in conditions such as cancer, ischemic

heart disease, and some neurologic disorders. FDG is an injected radionuclide (or radiopharmaceutical) that emits sub-atomic particles, known as positrons, as it decays. FDG PET uses a positron camera (tomograph) to measure the decay of FDG. The rate of FDG decay provides biochemical information on glucose metabolism in the tissue being studied. As malignancies can cause abnormalities of metabolism and blood flow, FDG PET evaluation may indicate the probable presence or absence of a malignancy based upon observed differences in biologic activity compared to adjacent tissues.

The Centers for Medicare and Medicaid Services (CMS) was asked by the National Oncologic PET Registry (NOPR) to reconsider section 220.6 of the National Coverage Determinations (NCD) Manual to end the prospective data collection requirements under Coverage with Evidence Development (CED) across all oncologic indications of FDG PET imaging. The CMS received public input indicating that the current coverage framework of prospective data collection under CED be ended for all oncologic uses of FDG PET imaging.

1. Framework

   Effective for claims with dates of service on and after June 11, 2013, CMS is adopting a coverage framework that ends the prospective data collection requirements by NOPR under CED for all oncologic uses of FDG PET imaging. CMS is making this change for all NCDs that address coverage of FDG PET for oncologic uses addressed in this decision. This decision does not change coverage for any use of PET imaging using radiopharmaceuticals NaF-18 (fluorine-18 labeled sodium fluoride), ammonia N-13, or rubidium-82 (Rb-82).

2. Initial Anti-Tumor Treatment Strategy

   CMS continues to believe that the evidence is adequate to determine that the results of FDG PET imaging are useful in determining the appropriate initial anti-tumor treatment strategy for beneficiaries with suspected cancer and improve health outcomes and thus are reasonable and necessary under §1862(a)(1)(A) of the Social Security Act (the Act).

   Therefore, CMS continues to nationally cover one FDG PET study for beneficiaries who have cancers that are biopsy proven or strongly suspected based on other diagnostic testing when the beneficiary's treating physician determines that the FDG PET study is needed to determine the location and/or extent of the tumor for the following therapeutic purposes related to the initial anti-tumor treatment strategy:

   – To determine whether or not the beneficiary is an appropriate candidate for an invasive diagnostic or therapeutic procedure; or

   – To determine the optimal anatomic location for an invasive procedure; or

– To determine the anatomic extent of tumor when the recommended anti-tumor treatment reasonably depends on the extent of the tumor.

See the table at the end of this section for a synopsis of all nationally covered and non-covered oncologic uses of FDG PET imaging.

### B.1. Initial Anti-Tumor Treatment Strategy Nationally Covered Indications

a. CMS continues to nationally cover FDG PET imaging for the initial anti-tumor treatment strategy for male and female breast cancer only when used in staging distant metastasis.

b. CMS continues to nationally cover FDG PET to determine initial anti-tumor treatment strategy for melanoma other than for the evaluation of regional lymph nodes.

c. CMS continues to nationally cover FDG PET imaging for the detection of pre-treatment metastasis (i.e., staging) in newly diagnosed cervical cancers.

d. C.1 Initial Anti-Tumor Treatment Strategy Nationally Non-Covered Indications

a. CMS continues to nationally non-cover initial anti-tumor treatment strategy in Medicare beneficiaries who have adenocarcinoma of the prostate.

b. CMS continues to nationally non-cover FDG PET imaging for diagnosis of breast cancer and initial staging of axillary nodes.

c. CMS continues to nationally non-cover FDG PET imaging for initial anti-tumor treatment strategy for the evaluation of regional lymph nodes in melanoma.

d. CMS continues to nationally non-cover FDG PET imaging for the diagnosis of cervical cancer related to initial anti-tumor treatment strategy.

3. Subsequent Anti-Tumor Treatment Strategy
   B.2. Subsequent Anti-Tumor Treatment Strategy Nationally Covered Indications

   Three FDG PET scans are nationally covered when used to guide subsequent management of anti-tumor treatment strategy after completion of initial anti-cancer therapy. Coverage of more than three FDG PET scans to guide subsequent management of anti-tumor treatment strategy after completion of initial anti-cancer therapy shall be determined by the local Medicare Administrative Contractors.

4. Synopsis of Coverage of FDG PET for Oncologic Conditions

   Effective for claims with dates of service on and after June 11, 2013, the chart below summarizes national FDG PET coverage for oncologic conditions:

| FDG PET for Cancers Tumor Type | Initial Treatment Strategy (formerly "diagnosis" & "staging") | Subsequent Treatment Strategy (formerly "restaging" & "monitoring response to treatment") |
|---|---|---|
| Colorectal | Cover | Cover |
| Esophagus | Cover | Cover |
| Head and Neck (not thyroid, CNS) | Cover | Cover |
| Lymphoma | Cover | Cover |
| Non-small cell lung | Cover | Cover |
| Ovary | Cover | Cover |
| Brain | Cover | Cover |
| Cervix | Cover with exceptions * | Cover |
| Small cell lung | Cover | Cover |
| Soft tissue sarcoma | Cover | Cover |
| Pancreas | Cover | Cover |
| Testes | Cover | Cover |
| Prostate | Non-cover | Cover |
| Thyroid | Cover | Cover |
| Breast (male and female) | Cover with exceptions * | Cover |
| Melanoma | Cover with exceptions * | Cover |
| All other solid tumors | Cover | Cover |
| Myeloma | Cover | Cover |

| FDG PET for Cancers Tumor Type | Initial Treatment Strategy (formerly "diagnosis" & "staging" | Subsequent Treatment Strategy (formerly "restaging" & "monitoring response to treatment" |
|---|---|---|
| All other cancers not listed | Cover | Cover |

\* Cervix: Nationally non-covered for the initial diagnosis of cervical cancer related to initial anti-tumor treatment strategy. All other indications for initial anti-tumor treatment strategy for cervical cancer are nationally covered.
\* Breast: Nationally non-covered for initial diagnosis and/or staging of axillary lymph nodes. Nationally covered for initial staging of metastatic disease. All other indications for initial anti-tumor treatment strategy for breast cancer are nationally covered.
\* Melanoma: Nationally non-covered for initial staging of regional lymph nodes. All other indications for initial anti-tumor treatment strategy for melanoma are nationally covered.

### D. Other
N/A

## 100-03, 220.6.19

### Positron Emission Tomography NaF-18 (NaF-18 PET) to Identify Bone Metastasis of Cancer (Effective February 26, 2010)

#### A. General
Positron Emission Tomography (PET) is a non-invasive, diagnostic imaging procedure that assesses the level of metabolic activity and perfusion in various organ systems of the body. A positron camera (tomograph) is used to produce cross-sectional tomographic images, which are obtained from positron-emitting radioactive tracer substances (radiopharmaceuticals) such as

F-18 sodium fluoride. NaF-18 PET has been recognized as an excellent technique for imaging areas of altered osteogenic activity in bone. The clinical value of detecting and assessing the initial extent of metastatic cancer in bone is attested by a number of professional guidelines for oncology. Imaging to detect bone metastases is also recommended when a patient, following completion of initial treatment, is symptomatic with bone pain suspicious for metastases from a known primary tumor.

#### B. Nationally Covered Indications
Effective February 26, 2010, the Centers for Medicare & Medicaid Services (CMS) will cover NaF-18 PET imaging when the beneficiary's treating physician determines that the NaF-18 PET study is needed to inform to inform the initial antitumor treatment strategy or to guide subsequent antitumor treatment strategy after the completion of initial treatment, and when the beneficiary is enrolled in, and the NaF-18 PET provider is participating in, the following type of prospective clinical study:

A NaF-18 PET clinical study that is designed to collect additional information at the time of the scan to assist in initial antitumor treatment planning or to guide subsequent treatment strategy by the identification, location and quantification of bone metastases in beneficiaries in whom bone metastases are strongly suspected based on clinical symptoms or the results of other diagnostic studies. Qualifying clinical studies must ensure that specific hypotheses are addressed; appropriate data elements are collected; hospitals and providers are qualified to provide the PET scan and interpret the results; participating hospitals and providers accurately report data on all enrolled patients not included in other qualifying trials through adequate auditing mechanisms; and all patient confidentiality, privacy, and other Federal laws must be followed.

The clinical studies for which Medicare will provide coverage must answer one or more of the following questions:

Prospectively, in Medicare beneficiaries whose treating physician determines that the NaF-18 PET study results are needed to inform the initial antitumor treatment strategy or to guide subsequent antitumor treatment strategy after the completion of initial treatment, does the addition of NaF-18 PET imaging lead to:

A change in patient management to more appropriate palliative care; or A change in patient management to more appropriate curative care; or Improved quality of life; or Improved survival?

The study must adhere to the following standards of scientific integrity and relevance to the Medicare population:

a. The principal purpose of the research study is to test whether a particular intervention potentially improves the participants' health outcomes.

b. The research study is well-supported by available scientific and medical information or it is intended to clarify or establish the health outcomes of interventions already in common clinical use.

c. The research study does not unjustifiably duplicate existing studies.

d. The research study design is appropriate to answer the research question being asked in the study.

e. The research study is sponsored by an organization or individual capable of executing the proposed study successfully.

f. The research study is in compliance with all applicable Federal regulations concerning the protection of human subjects found in the Code of Federal Regulations (CFR) at 45 CFR Part 46. If a study is regulated by the Food and Drug Administration (FDA), it also must be in compliance with 21 CFR Parts 50 and 56.

g. All aspects of the research study are conducted according to the appropriate standards of scientific integrity.

h. The research study has a written protocol that clearly addresses, or incorporates by reference, the Medicare standards.

i. The clinical research study is not designed to exclusively test toxicity or disease pathophysiology in healthy individuals. Trials of all medical technologies measuring therapeutic outcomes as one of the objectives meet this standard only if the disease or condition being studied is life-threatening as defined in 21 CFR Sec.312.81(a) and the patient has no other viable treatment options.

j. The clinical research study is registered on the www.ClinicalTrials.gov Web site by the principal sponsor/investigator prior to the enrollment of the first study subject.

k. The research study protocol specifies the method and timing of public release of all pre-specified outcomes to be measured including release of outcomes if outcomes are negative or study is terminated early. The results must be made public within 24 months of the end of data collection. If a report is planned to be published in a peer-reviewed journal, then that initial release may be an abstract that meets the requirements of the International Committee of Medical Journal Editors. However, a full report of the outcomes must be made public no later than three (3) years after the end of data collection.

l. The research study protocol must explicitly discuss subpopulations affected by the treatment under investigation, particularly traditionally underrepresented groups in clinical studies, how the inclusion and exclusion criteria affect enrollment of these populations, and a plan for the retention and reporting of said populations on the trial. If the inclusion and exclusion criteria are expected to have a negative effect on the recruitment or retention of underrepresented populations, the protocol must discuss why these criteria are necessary.

m. The research study protocol explicitly discusses how the results are or are not expected to be generalizable to the Medicare population to infer whether Medicare patients may benefit from the intervention. Separate discussions in the protocol may be necessary for populations eligible for Medicare due to age, disability or Medicaid eligibility.

Consistent with section 1142 of the Social Security Act (the Act), the Agency for Healthcare Research and Quality (AHRQ) supports clinical research studies that the Centers for Medicare and Medicaid Services (CMS) determines meet the above-listed standards and address the above-listed research questions.

#### C. Nationally Non-Covered Indications
Effective February 26, 2010, CMS determines that the evidence is not sufficient to determine that the results of NaF-18 PET imaging to identify bone metastases improve health outcomes of beneficiaries with cancer and is not reasonable and necessary under Sec.1862(a)(1)(A) of the Act unless it is to inform initial antitumor treatment strategy or to guide subsequent antitumor treatment strategy after completion of initial treatment, and then only under CED. All other uses and clinical indications of NaF-18 PET are nationally non-covered.

#### D. Other
The only radiopharmaceutical diagnostic imaging agents covered by Medicare for PET cancer imaging are 2-[F-18] Fluoro-D-Glucose (FDG) and NaF-18 (sodium fluoride-18). All other PET radiopharmaceutical diagnostic imaging agents are non-covered for this indication.

(This NCD was last reviewed in February 2010.)

## 100-03, 220.6.2

### NCD for PET (FDG) for Lung Cancer (220.6.2)
220.6.2 - FDG PET for Lung Cancer (Replaced with Section 220.6.17)

## 100-03, 220.6.3

### NCD for PET (FDG) for Esophageal Cancer (220.6.3)
220.6.3 - FDG PET for Esophageal Cancer (Replaced with Section 220.6.17)

## 100-03, 220.6.4

### NCD for PET (FDG) for Colorectal Cancer (220.6.4)
220.6.4 - FDG PET for Colorectal Cancer (Replaced with Section 220.6.17

© 2016 Optum360, LLC

## 100-03, 220.6.5

### NCD for PET (FDG) for Lymphoma (220.6.5)
220.6.5 - FDG PET for Lymphoma (Replaced with Section 220.6.17)

## 100-03, 220.6.6

### NCD for PET (FDG) for Melanoma (220.6.6)
220.6.6 - FDG PET for Melanoma (Replaced with Section 220.6.17)

## 100-03, 220.6.7

### NCD for PET (FDG) for Head and Neck Cancers (220.6.7)
220.6.7 - FDG PET for Head and Neck Cancers (Replaced with Section 220.6.17)

## 100-03, 220.6.9

### FDG PET for Refractory Seizures (Effective July 1, 2001)
Beginning July 1, 2001, Medicare covers FDG PET for pre-surgical evaluation for the purpose of localization of a focus of refractory seizure activity.

Limitations: Covered only for pre-surgical evaluation.

Documentation that these conditions are met should be maintained by the referring physician in the beneficiary's medical record, as is normal business practice.

(This NCD last reviewed June 2001.)

## 100-03, 230.6

### NCD for Vabra Aspirator (230.6)

#### Item/Service Description
The VABRA aspirator is a sterile, disposable, vacuum aspirator which is used to collect uterine tissue for study to detect endometrial carcinoma. The use of this device is indicated where the patient exhibits clinical symptoms or signs suggestive of endometrial disease, such as irregular or heavy vaginal bleeding.

Indications and Limitations of Coverage

Program payment cannot be made for the aspirator or the related diagnostic services when furnished in connection with the examination of an asymptomatic patient. Payment for routine physical checkups is precluded under the statute (§1862(a)(7) of the Act).

## 100-03, 240.4

### NCD for Continuous Positive Airway Pressure (CPAP) Therapy For Obstructive Sleep Apnea (OSA) (240.4)

#### B. Nationally Covered Indications
Effective for claims with dates of service on and after March 13, 2008, the Centers for Medicare & Medicaid Services (CMS) determines that CPAP therapy when used in adult patients with OSA is considered reasonable and necessary under the following situations:

1. The use of CPAP is covered under Medicare when used in adult patients with OSA. Coverage of CPAP is initially limited to a 12-week period to identify beneficiaries diagnosed with OSA as subsequently described who benefit from CPAP. CPAP is subsequently covered only for those beneficiaries diagnosed with OSA who benefit from CPAP during this 12-week period.

2. The provider of CPAP must conduct education of the beneficiary prior to the use of the CPAP device to ensure that the beneficiary has been educated in the proper use of the device. A caregiver, for example a family member, may be compensatory, if consistently available in the beneficiary's home and willing and able to safely operate the CPAP device.

3. A positive diagnosis of OSA for the coverage of CPAP must include a clinical evaluation and a positive:

    a. attended PSG performed in a sleep laboratory; or

    b. unattended HST with a Type II home sleep monitoring device; or

    c. unattended HST with a Type III home sleep monitoring device; or

    d. unattended HST with a Type IV home sleep monitoring device that measures at least 3 channels.

4. The sleep test must have been previously ordered by the beneficiary?s treating physician and furnished under appropriate physician supervision.

5. An initial 12-week period of CPAP is covered in adult patients with OSA if either of the following criterion using the AHI or RDI are met:

    a. AHI or RDI greater than or equal to 15 events per hour, or

    b. AHI or RDI greater than or equal to 5 events and less than or equal to 14 events per hour with documented symptoms of excessive daytime sleepiness, impaired cognition, mood disorders or insomnia, or documented hypertension, ischemic heart disease, or history of stroke.

6. The AHI or RDI is calculated on the average number of events of per hour. If the AHI or RDI is calculated based on less than 2 hours of continuous recorded sleep, the total number of recorded events to calculate the AHI or RDI during sleep testing must be at a minimum the number of events that would have been required in a 2-hour period.

7. Apnea is defined as a cessation of airflow for at least 10 seconds. Hypopnea is defined as an abnormal respiratory event lasting at least 10 seconds with at least a 30% reduction in thoracoabdominal movement or airflow as compared to baseline, and with at least a 4% oxygen desaturation.

8. Coverage with Evidence Development (CED): Medicare provides the following limited coverage for CPAP in adult beneficiaries who do not qualify for CPAP coverage based on criteria 1-7 above. A clinical study seeking Medicare payment for CPAP provided to a beneficiary who is an enrolled subject in that study must address one or more of the following questions:

    a. In Medicare-aged subjects with clinically identified risk factors for OSA, how does the diagnostic accuracy of a clinical trial of CPAP compare with PSG and Type II, III & IV HST in identifying subjects with OSA who will respond to CPAP?

    b. In Medicare-aged subjects with clinically identified risk factors for OSA who have not undergone confirmatory testing with PSG or Type II, III & IV HST, does CPAP cause clinically meaningful harm?

    The study must meet the following additional standards:

    c. The principal purpose of the research study is to test whether a particular intervention potentially improves the participants? health outcomes.

    d. The research study is well-supported by available scientific and medical information or it is intended to clarify or establish the health outcomes of interventions already in common clinical use.

    e. The research study does not unjustifiably duplicate existing studies.

    f. The research study design is appropriate to answer the research question being asked in the study.

    g. The research study is sponsored by an organization or individual capable of executing the proposed study successfully.

    h. The research study is in compliance with all applicable Federal regulations concerning the protection of human subjects found at 45 CFR Part 46. If a study is Food and Drug Administration-regulated, it also must be in compliance with 21 CFR Parts 50 and 56.

    i. All aspects of the research study are conducted according to the appropriate standards of scientific integrity.

    j. The research study has a written protocol that clearly addresses, or incorporates by reference, the Medicare standards.

    k. The clinical research study is not designed to exclusively test toxicity or disease pathophysiology in healthy individuals. Trials of all medical technologies measuring therapeutic outcomes as one of the objectives meet this standard only if the disease or condition being studied is life-threatening as defined in 21 CFR ? 312.81(a) and the patient has no other viable treatment options.

    l. The clinical research study is registered on the ClinicalTrials.gov Web site by the principal sponsor/investigator prior to the enrollment of the first study subject.

    m. The research study protocol specifies the method and timing of public release of all pre-specified outcomes to be measured, including release of outcomes if outcomes are negative or study is terminated early. The results must be made public within 24 months of the end of data collection. If a report is planned for publication in a peer-reviewed journal, then that initial release may be an abstract that meets the requirements of the International Committee of Medical Journal Editors. However, a full report of the outcomes must be made public no later than 3 years after the end of data collection.

    n. The research study protocol must explicitly discuss subpopulations affected by the treatment under investigation, particularly traditionally underrepresented groups in clinical studies, how the inclusion and exclusion criteria affect enrollment of these populations, and a plan for the retention and reporting of said populations in the trial. If the inclusion and exclusion criteria are expected to have a negative effect on the recruitment or retention of underrepresented populations, the protocol must discuss why these criteria are necessary.

    o. The research study protocol explicitly discusses how the results are or are not expected to be generalizable to the Medicare population to infer whether Medicare patients may benefit from the intervention. Separate discussions in the protocol may be necessary for populations eligible for Medicare due to age, disability, or Medicaid eligibility.

**C. Nationally Non-covered Indications**

Effective for claims with dates of services on and after March 13, 2008, other diagnostic tests for the diagnosis of OSA, other than those noted above for prescribing CPAP, are not sufficient for the coverage of CPAP.

**D. Other**

N/A

(This NCD last reviewed March 2008.)

## 100-03, 250.5

**Dermal Injections for the Treatment of Facial Lipodystrophy Syndrome (LDS) - Effective March 23, 2010**

**A. General**

Treatment of persons infected with the human immunodeficiency virus (HIV) or persons who have Acquired Immune Deficiency Syndrome (AIDS) may include highly active antiretroviral therapy (HAART). Drug reactions commonly associated with long-term use of HAART include metabolic complications such as, lipid abnormalities, e.g., hyperlipidemia, hyperglycemia, diabetes, lipodystrophy, and heart disease. Lipodystrophy is characterized by abnormal fat distribution in the body.

The LDS is often characterized by a loss of fat that results in a facial abnormality such as severely sunken cheeks. The patient's physical appearance may contribute to psychological conditions (e.g., depression) or adversely impact a patient's adherence to antiretroviral regimens (therefore jeopardizing their health) and both of these are important health-related outcomes of interest in this population. Therefore, improving a patient's physical appearance through the use of dermal injections could improve these health-related outcomes.

**B. Nationally Covered Indications**

Effective for claims with dates of service on and after March 23, 2010, dermal injections for LDS are only reasonable and necessary using dermal fillers approved by the Food and Drug Administration (FDA) for this purpose, and then only in HIV-infected beneficiaries when LDS caused by antiretroviral HIV treatment is a significant contributor to their depression.

**C. Nationally Non-Covered Indications**

1. Dermal fillers that are not approved by the FDA for the treatment of LDS.

2. Dermal fillers that are used for any indication other than LDS in HIV-infected individuals who manifest depression as a result of their antiretroviral HIV treatments.

**D. Other**

N/A

(This NCD last reviewed March 2010.)

## 100-03, 270.3

**NCD for Blood-Derived Products for Chronic Non-Healing Wounds (270.3)**

**A. General**

Wound healing is a dynamic, interactive process that involves multiple cells and proteins. There are three progressive stages of normal wound healing, and the typical wound healing duration is about 4 weeks. While cutaneous wounds are a disruption of the normal, anatomic structure and function of the skin, subcutaneous wounds involve tissue below the skin? surface. Wounds are categorized as either acute, in where the normal wound healing stages are not yet completed but it is presumed they will be, resulting in orderly and timely wound repair, or chronic, in where a wound has failed to progress through the normal wound healing stages and repair itself within a sufficient time period.

Platelet-rich plasma (PRP) is produced in an autologous or homologous manner. Autologous PRP is comprised of blood from the patient who will ultimately receive the PRP. Alternatively, homologous PRP is derived from blood from multiple donors.

Blood is donated by the patient and centrifuged to produce an autologous gel for treatment of chronic, non-healing cutaneous wounds that persists for 30 days or longer and fail to properly complete the healing process. Autologous blood derived products for chronic, non-healing wounds includes both: (1) platelet derived growth factor (PDGF) products (such as Procuren), and (2) PRP (such as AutoloGel).

The PRP is different from previous products in that it contains whole cells including white cells, red cells, plasma, platelets, fibrinogen, stem cells, macrophages, and fibroblasts.

The PRP is used by physicians in clinical settings in treating chronic, non-healing wounds, open, cutaneous wounds, soft tissue, and bone. Alternatively, PDGF does not contain cells and was previously marketed as a product to be used by patients at home.

**B. Nationally Covered Indications**

Effective August 2, 2012, upon reconsideration, The Centers for Medicare and Medicaid Services (CMS) has determined that platelet-rich plasma (PRP) ?an autologous blood-derived product, will be covered only for the treatment of chronic non-healing diabetic, venous and/or pressure wounds and only when the following conditions are met:

The patient is enrolled in a clinical trial that addresses the following questions using validated and reliable methods of evaluation. Clinical study applications for coverage pursuant to this National coverage Determination (NCD) must be received by August 2, 2014.

The clinical research study must meet the requirements specified below to assess the effect of PRP for the treatment of chronic non-healing diabetic, venous and/or pressure wounds. The clinical study must address:

Prospectively, do Medicare beneficiaries that have chronic non-healing diabetic, venous and/or pressure wounds who receive well-defined optimal usual care along with PRP therapy, experience clinically significant health outcomes compared to patients who receive well-defined optimal usual care for chronic non-healing diabetic, venous and/or pressure wounds as indicated by addressing at least one of the following:

a. Complete wound healing

b. Ability to return to previous function and resumption of normal activities

c. Reduction of wound size or healing trajectory which results in the patient's ability to return to previous function and resumption of normal activities

The required clinical trial of PRP must adhere to the following standards of scientific integrity and relevance to the Medicare population:

a. The principal purpose of the CLINICAL STUDY is to test whether PRP improves the participants?health outcomes.

b. The CLINICAL STUDY is well supported by available scientific and medical information or it is intended to clarify or establish the health outcomes of interventions already in common clinical use.

c. The CLINICAL STUDY does not unjustifiably duplicate existing studies.

d. The CLINICAL STUDY design is appropriate to answer the research question being asked in the study.

e. The CLINICAL STUDY is sponsored by an organization or individual capable of executing the proposed study successfully.

f. The CLINICAL STUDY is in compliance with all applicable Federal regulations concerning the protection of human subjects found at 45 CFR Part 46.

g. All aspects of the CLINICAL STUDY are conducted according to appropriate standards of scientific integrity set by the International Committee of Medical Journal Editors (http://www.icmje.org).

h. The CLINICAL STUDY has a written protocol that clearly addresses, or incorporates by reference, the standards listed here as Medicare requirements for coverage with evidence development (CED).

i. The CLINICAL STUDY is not designed to exclusively test toxicity or disease pathophysiology in healthy individuals. Trials of all medical technologies measuring therapeutic outcomes as one of the objectives meet this standard only if the disease or condition being studied is life threatening as defined in 21 CFR ?312.81(a) and the patient has no other viable treatment options.

j. The CLINICAL STUDY is registered on the ClinicalTrials.gov website by the principal sponsor/investigator prior to the enrollment of the first study subject.

k. The CLINICAL STUDY protocol specifies the method and timing of public release of all pre-specified outcomes to be measured including release of outcomes if outcomes are negative or study is terminated early. The results must be made public within 24 months of the end of data collection. If a report is planned to be published in a peer reviewed journal, then that initial release may be an abstract that meets the requirements of the International Committee of Medical Journal Editors (http://www.icmje.org). However a full report of the outcomes must be made public no later than three (3) years after the end of data collection.

l. The CLINICAL STUDY protocol must explicitly discuss subpopulations affected by the treatment under investigation, particularly traditionally underrepresented groups in clinical studies, how the inclusion and exclusion criteria effect enrollment of these populations, and a plan for the retention and reporting of said populations on the trial. If the inclusion and exclusion criteria are expected to have a negative effect on the recruitment or retention of underrepresented populations, the protocol must discuss why these criteria are necessary.

© 2016 Optum360, LLC

m. The CLINICAL STUDY protocol explicitly discusses how the results are or are not expected to be generalizable to the Medicare population to infer whether Medicare patients may benefit from the intervention. Separate discussions in the protocol may be necessary for populations eligible for Medicare due to age, disability or Medicaid eligibility. Consistent with ?1142 of the Social Security Act (the Act), the Agency for Healthcare Research and Quality (AHRQ) supports clinical research studies that CMS determines meet the above-listed standards and address the above-listed research questions.

Any clinical study undertaken pursuant to this NCD must be approved no later than August 2, 2014. If there are no approved clinical studies on or before August 2, 2014, this CED will expire. Any clinical study approved will adhere to the timeframe designated in the approved clinical study protocol.

### C. Nationally Non-Covered Indications

1. Effective December 28, 1992, the Centers for Medicare & Medicaid Services (CMS) issued a national non-coverage determination for platelet-derived wound-healing formulas intended to treat patients with chronic, non-healing wounds. This decision was based on a lack of sufficient published data to determine safety and efficacy, and a public health service technology assessment.

## 100-04, 1, 10.1.4.1

### Physician and Ambulance Services Furnished in Connection With Covered Foreign Inpatient Hospital Services

Payment is made for necessary physician and ambulance services that meet the other coverage requirements of the Medicare program, and are furnished in connection with and during a period of covered foreign hospitalization.

### A. Coverage of Physician and Ambulance Services Furnished Outside the U.S.

- Where inpatient services in a foreign hospital are covered, payment may also be made for
- Physicians' services furnished to the beneficiary while he/she is an inpatient,
- Physicians' services furnished to the beneficiary outside the hospital on the day of his/her admission as an inpatient, provided the services were for the same condition for which the beneficiary was hospitalized (including the services of a Canadian ship's physician who furnishes emergency services in Canadian waters on the day the patient is admitted to a Canadian hospital for a covered emergency stay and,
- Ambulance services, where necessary, for the trip to the hospital in conjunction with the beneficiary's admission as an inpatient. Return trips from a foreign hospital are not covered.

In cases involving foreign ambulance services, the general requirements in Chapter 15 are also applicable, subject to the following special rules:

- If the foreign hospitalization was determined to be covered on the basis of emergency services, the medical necessity requirements outlined in Chapter 15 are considered met.
- The definition of "physician," for purposes of coverage of services furnished outside the U.S., is expanded to include a foreign practitioner, provided the practitioner is legally licensed to practice in the country in which the services are furnished.
- Only the enrollee can file for Part B benefits; the assignment method may not be used.
- Where the enrollee is deceased, the rules for settling Part B underpayments are applicable. Payment is made to the foreign physician or foreign ambulance company on an unpaid bill provided the physician or ambulance company accepts the payment as the full charge for the service, or payment an be made to a person who has agreed to assume legal liability to pay the physician or supplier. Where the bill is paid, payment may be made in accordance with Medicare regulations. The regular deductible and coinsurance requirements apply to physicians' and ambulance services furnished outside the U.S.

## 100-04, 1, 30.3.5

### Effect of Assignment Upon Purchase of Cataract Glasses From Participating Physician or Supplier on Claims Submitted to Carriers
B3-3045.4

A pair of cataract glasses is comprised of two distinct products: a professional product (the prescribed lenses) and a retail commercial product (the frames). The frames serve not only as a holder of lenses but also as an article of personal apparel. As such, they are usually selected on the basis of personal taste and style. Although Medicare will pay only for standard frames, most patients want deluxe frames. Participating physicians and suppliers cannot profitably furnish such deluxe frames unless they can make an extra (noncovered) charge for the frames even though they accept assignment.

Therefore, a participating physician or supplier (whether an ophthalmologist, optometrist, or optician) who accepts assignment on cataract glasses with deluxe frames may charge the Medicare patient the difference between his/her usual charge to private pay patients for glasses with standard frames and his/her usual charge to such patients for glasses with deluxe frames, in addition to the applicable deductible and coinsurance on glasses with standard frames, if all of the following requirements are met:

A. The participating physician or supplier has standard frames available, offers them for sale to the patient, and issues and ABN to the patient that explains the price and other differences between standard and deluxe frames. Refer to Chapter 30.

B. The participating physician or supplier obtains from the patient (or his/her representative) and keeps on file the following signed and dated statement:

_____

Name of Patient                                        Medicare Claim Number

Having been informed that an extra charge is being made by the physician or supplier for deluxe frames, that this extra charge is not covered by Medicare, and that standard frames are available for purchase from the physician or supplier at no extra charge, I have chosen to purchase deluxe frames.

_____

Signature                                              Date

C. The participating physician or supplier itemizes on his/her claim his/her actual charge for the lenses, his/her actual charge for the standard frames, and his/her actual extra charge for the deluxe frames (charge differential). Once the assigned claim for deluxe frames has been processed, the carrier will follow the ABN instructions as described in Sec.60.

## 100-04, 3, 40.2.2

### Charges to Beneficiaries for Part A Services

The hospital submits a bill even where the patient is responsible for a deductible which covers the entire amount of the charges for non-PPS hospitals, or in PPS hospitals, where the DRG payment amount will be less than the deductible.

A hospital receiving payment for a covered hospital stay (or PPS hospital that includes at least one covered day, or one treated as covered under guarantee of payment or limitation on liability) may charge the beneficiary, or other person, for items and services furnished during the stay only as described in subsections A through H. If limitation of liability applies, a beneficiary's liability for payment is governed by the limitation on liability notification rules in Chapter 30 of this manual. For related notices for inpatient hospitals, see CMS Transmittal 594, Change Request 3903, dated June 24, 2005.

### A. Deductible and Coinsurance

The hospital may charge the beneficiary or other person for applicable deductible and coinsurance amounts. The deductible is satisfied only by charges for covered services. The FI deducts the deductible and coinsurance first from the PPS payment. Where the deductible exceeds the PPS amount, the excess will be applied to a subsequent payment to the hospital. (See Chapter 3 of the Medicare General Information, Eligibility, and Entitlement Manual for specific policies.)

### B. Blood Deductible

The Part A blood deductible provision applies to whole blood and red blood cells, and reporting of the number of pints is applicable to both PPS and non-PPS hospitals. (See Chapter 3 of the Medicare General Information, Eligibility, and Entitlement Manual for specific policies.) Hospitals shall report charges for red blood cells using revenue code 381, and charges for whole blood using revenue code 382.

### C. Inpatient Care No Longer Required

The hospital may charge for services that are not reasonable and necessary or that constitute custodial care. Notification may be required under limitation of liability. See CMS Transmittal 594, Change Request 3903, dated June 24, 2005, section V. of the attachment, for specific notification requirements. Note this transmittal will be placed in Chapter 30 of this manual at a future point. Chapter 1, section 150 of this manual also contains related billing information in addition to that provided below.

In general, after proper notification has occurred, and assuming an expedited decision is received from a Quality Improvement Organization (QIO), the following entries are required on the bill the hospital prepares:

- Occurrence code 31 (and date) to indicate the date the hospital notified the patient in accordance with the first bullet above;
- Occurrence span code 76 (and dates) to indicate the period of noncovered care for which it is charging the beneficiary;

- Occurrence span code 77 (and dates) to indicate the period of noncovered care for which the provider is liable, when it is aware of this prior to billing; and

- Value code 3l (and amount) to indicate the amount of charges it may bill the beneficiary for days for which inpatient care was no longer required. They are included as noncovered charges on the bill.

### D. Change in the Beneficiary's Condition

If the beneficiary remains in the hospital after receiving notice as described in subsection C, and the hospital, the physician who concurred in the hospital's determination, or the QIO, subsequently determines that the beneficiary again requires inpatient hospital care, the hospital may not charge the beneficiary or other person for services furnished after the beneficiary again required inpatient hospital care until proper notification occurs (see subsection C).

If a patient who needs only a SNF level of care remains in the hospital after the SNF bed becomes available, and the bed ceases to be available, the hospital may continue to charge the beneficiary. It need not provide the beneficiary with another notice when the patient chose not to be discharged to the SNF bed.

### E. Admission Denied

If the entire hospital admission is determined to be not reasonable or necessary, limitation of liability may apply. See 2005 CMS transmittal 594, section V. of the attachment, for specific notification requirements.

NOTE: This transmittal will be placed in Chapter 30 of this manual at a future point.

In such cases the following entries are required on the bill:

- Occurrence code 3l (and date) to indicate the date the hospital notified the beneficiary.

- Occurrence span code 76 (and dates) to indicate the period of noncovered care for which the hospital is charging the beneficiary.

- Occurrence span code 77 (and dates) to indicate any period of noncovered care for which the provider is liable (e.g., the period between issuing the notice and the time it may charge the beneficiary) when the provider is aware of this prior to billing.

- Value code 3l (and amount) to indicate the amount of charges the hospital may bill the beneficiary for hospitalization that was not necessary or reasonable. They are included as noncovered charges on the bill.

### F. Procedures, Studies and Courses of Treatment That Are Not Reasonable or Necessary

If diagnostic procedures, studies, therapeutic studies and courses of treatment are excluded from coverage as not reasonable and necessary (even though the beneficiary requires inpatient hospital care) the hospital may charge the beneficiary or other person for the services or care according the procedures given in CMS Transmittal 594, Change Request3903, dated June 24, 2005.

The following bill entries apply to these circumstances:

- Occurrence code 32 (and date) to indicate the date the hospital provided the notice to the beneficiary.

- Value code 3l (and amount) to indicate the amount of such charges to be billed to the beneficiary. They are included as noncovered charges on the bill.

### G. Nonentitlement Days and Days after Benefits Exhausted

If a hospital stay exceeds the day outlier threshold, the hospital may charge for some, or all, of the days on which the patient is not entitled to Medicare Part A, or after the Part A benefits are exhausted (i.e., the hospital may charge its customary charges for services furnished on those days). It may charge the beneficiary for the lesser of:

- The number of days on which the patient was not entitled to benefits or after the benefits were exhausted; or

- The number of outlier days. (Day outliers were discontinued at the end of FY 1997.)

If the number of outlier days exceeds the number of days on which the patient was not entitled to benefits, or after benefits were exhausted, the hospital may charge for all days on which the patient was not entitled to benefits or after benefits were exhausted. If the number of days on which the beneficiary was not entitled to benefits, or after benefits were exhausted, exceeds the number of outlier days, the hospital determines the days for which it may charge by starting with the last day of the stay (i.e., the day before the day of discharge) and identifying and counting off in reverse order, days on which the patient was not entitled to benefits or after the benefits were exhausted, until the number of days counted off equals the number of outlier days. The days counted off are the days for which the hospital may charge.

### H. Contractual Exclusions

In addition to receiving the basic prospective payment, the hospital may charge the beneficiary for any services that are excluded from coverage for reasons other than, or in addition to, absence of medical necessity, provision of custodial care, non-

entitlement to Part A, or exhaustion of benefits. For example, it may charge for most cosmetic and dental surgery.

### I. Private Room Care

Payment for medically necessary private room care is included in the prospective payment. Where the beneficiary requests private room accommodations, the hospital must inform the beneficiary of the additional charge. (See the Medicare Benefit Policy Manual, Chapter 1.) When the beneficiary accepts the liability, the hospital will supply the service, and bill the beneficiary directly. If the beneficiary believes the private room was medically necessary, the beneficiary has a right to a determination and may initiate a Part A appeal.

### J. Deluxe Item or Service

Where a beneficiary requests a deluxe item or service, i.e., an item or service which is more expensive than is medically required for the beneficiary's condition, the hospital may collect the additional charge if it informs the beneficiary of the additional charge. That charge is the difference between the customary charge for the item or service most commonly furnished by the hospital to private pay patients with the beneficiary's condition, and the charge for the more expensive item or service requested. If the beneficiary believes that the more expensive item or service was medically necessary, the beneficiary has a right to a determination and may initiate a Part A appeal.

### K - Inpatient Acute Care Hospital Admission Followed By a Death or Discharge Prior To Room Assignment

A patient of an acute care hospital is considered an inpatient upon issuance of written doctor's orders to that effect. If a patient either dies or is discharged prior to being assigned and/or occupying a room, a hospital may enter an appropriate room and board charge on the claim. If a patient leaves of their own volition prior to being assigned and/or occupying a room, a hospital may enter an appropriate room and board charge on the claim as well as a patient status code 07 which indicates they left against medical advice. A hospital is not required to enter a room and board charge, but failure to do so may have a minimal impact on future DRG weight calculations.

## 100-04, 4, 20.6.4

### Use of Modifiers for Discontinued Services

#### A. General

Modifiers provide a way for hospitals to report and be paid for expenses incurred in preparing a patient for a procedure and scheduling a room for performing the procedure where the service is subsequently discontinued. This instruction is applicable to both outpatient hospital departments and to ambulatory surgical centers.

Modifier -73 is used by the facility to indicate that a procedure requiring anesthesia was terminated due to extenuating circumstances or to circumstances that threatened the well being of the patient after the patient had been prepared for the procedure (including procedural pre-medication when provided), and been taken to the room where the procedure was to be performed, but prior to administration of anesthesia. For purposes of billing for services furnished in the hospital outpatient department, anesthesia is defined to include local, regional block(s), moderate sedation/analgesia ("conscious sedation"), deep sedation/analgesia, or general anesthesia. This modifier code was created so that the costs incurred by the hospital to prepare the patient for the procedure and the resources expended in the procedure room and recovery room (if needed) could be recognized for payment even though the procedure was discontinued.

Modifier -74 is used by the facility to indicate that a procedure requiring anesthesia was terminated after the induction of anesthesia or after the procedure was started (e.g., incision made, intubation started, scope inserted) due to extenuating circumstances or circumstances that threatened the well being of the patient. This modifier may also be used to indicate that a planned surgical or diagnostic procedure was discontinued, partially reduced or cancelled at the physician's discretion after the administration of anesthesia. For purposes of billing for services furnished in the hospital outpatient department, anesthesia is defined to include local, regional block(s), moderate sedation/analgesia ("conscious sedation"), deep sedation/analgesia, and general anesthesia. This modifier code was created so that the costs incurred by the hospital to initiate the procedure (preparation of the patient, procedure room, recovery room) could be recognized for payment even though the procedure was discontinued prior to completion.

Coinciding with the addition of the modifiers -73 and -74, modifiers -52 and -53 were revised. Modifier -52 is used to indicate partial reduction, cancellation, or discontinuation of services for which anesthesia is not planned. The modifier provides a means for reporting reduced services without disturbing the identification of the basic service. Modifier -53 is used to indicate discontinuation of physician services and is not approved for use for outpatient hospital services.

The elective cancellation of a procedure should not be reported.

Modifiers -73 and -74 are only used to indicate discontinued procedures for which anesthesia is planned or provided.

### B. Effect on Payment

Procedures that are discontinued after the patient has been prepared for the procedure and taken to the procedure room but before anesthesia is provided will be paid at 50 percent of the full OPPS payment amount. Modifier -73 is used for these procedures.

Procedures that are discontinued, partially reduced or cancelled after the procedure has been initiated and/or the patient has received anesthesia will be paid at the full OPPS payment amount. Modifier -74 is used for these procedures.

Procedures for which anesthesia is not planned that are discontinued, partially reduced or cancelled after the patient is prepared and taken to the room where the procedure is to be performed will be paid at 50 percent of the full OPPS payment amount. Modifier -52 is used for these procedures.

### C. Termination Where Multiple Procedures Planned

When one or more of the procedures planned is completed, the completed procedures are reported as usual. The other(s) that were planned, and not started, are not reported. When none of the procedures that were planned are completed, and the patient has been prepared and taken to the procedure room, the first procedure that was planned, but not completed is reported with modifier -73. If the first procedure has been started (scope inserted, intubation started, incision made, etc.) and/or the patient has received anesthesia, modifier -74 is used. The other procedures are not reported.

If the first procedure is terminated prior to the induction of anesthesia and before the patient is wheeled into the procedure room, the procedure should not be reported. The patient has to be taken to the room where the procedure is to be performed in order to report modifier -73 or -74.

### 100-04, 4, 160

#### Clinic and Emergency Visits

CMS has acknowledged from the beginning of the OPPS that CMS believes that CPT Evaluation and Management (E/M) codes were designed to reflect the activities of physicians and do not describe well the range and mix of services provided by hospitals during visits of clinic and emergency department patients. While awaiting the development of a national set of facility-specific codes and guidelines, providers should continue to apply their current internal guidelines to the existing CPT codes. Each hospital's internal guidelines should follow the intent of the CPT code descriptors, in that the guidelines should be designed to reasonably relate the intensity of hospital resources to the different levels of effort represented by the codes. Hospitals should ensure that their guidelines accurately reflect resource distinctions between the five levels of codes.

Effective January 1, 2007, CMS is distinguishing between two types of emergency departments: Type A emergency departments and Type B emergency departments.

A Type A emergency department is defined as an emergency department that is available 24 hours a day, 7 days a week and is either licensed by the State in which it is located under applicable State law as an emergency room or emergency department or it is held out to the public (by name, posted signs, advertising, or other means) as a place that provides care for emergency medical conditions on an urgent basis without requiring a previously scheduled appointment.

A Type B emergency department is defined as an emergency department that meets the definition of a "dedicated emergency department" as defined in 42 CFR 489.24 under the EMTALA regulations. It must meet at least one of the following requirements: (1) It is licensed by the State in which it is located under applicable State law as an emergency room or emergency department; (2) It is held out to the public (by name, posted signs, advertising, or other means) as a place that provides care for emergency medical conditions on an urgent basis without requiring a previously scheduled appointment; or (3) During the calendar year immediately preceding the calendar year in which a determination under 42 CFR 489.24 is being made, based on a representative sample of patient visits that occurred during that calendar year, it provides at least one-third of all of its outpatient visits for the treatment of emergency medical conditions on an urgent basis without requiring a previously scheduled appointment.

Hospitals must bill for visits provided in Type A emergency departments using CPT emergency department E/M codes. Hospitals must bill for visits provided in Type B emergency departments using the G-codes that describe visits provided in Type B emergency departments.

Hospitals that will be billing the new Type B ED visit codes may need to update their internal guidelines to report these codes.

Emergency department and clinic visits are paid in some cases separately and in other cases as part of a composite APC payment. See section 10.2.1 of this chapter for further details.

### 100-04, 4, 160.1

#### Critical Care Services

Hospitals should separately report all HCPCS codes in accordance with correct coding principles, CPT code descriptions, and any additional CMS guidance, when available. Specifically with respect to CPT code 99291 (Critical care, evaluation and management of the critically ill or critically injured patient; first 30-74 minutes), hospitals must follow the CPT instructions related to reporting that CPT code. Prior to January 1, 2011, any services that CPT indicates are included in the reporting of CPT code 99291 (including those services that would otherwise be reported by and paid to hospitals using any of the CPT codes specified by CPT) should not be billed separately by the hospital. Instead, hospitals should report charges for any services provided as part of the critical care services. In establishing payment rates for critical care services, and other services, CMS packages the costs of certain items and services separately reported by HCPCS codes into payment for critical care services and other services, according to the standard OPPS methodology for packaging costs.

Beginning January 1, 2011, in accordance with revised CPT guidance, hospitals that report in accordance with the CPT guidelines will begin reporting all of the ancillary services and their associated charges separately when they are provided in conjunction with critical care. CMS will continue to recognize the existing CPT codes for critical care services and will establish payment rates based on historical data, into which the cost of the ancillary services is intrinsically packaged. The I/OCE conditionally packages payment for the ancillary services that are reported on the same date of service as critical care services in order to avoid overpayment. The payment status of the ancillary services does not change when they are not provided in conjunction with critical care services. Hospitals may use HCPCS modifier -59 to indicate when an ancillary procedure or service is distinct or independent from critical care when performed on the same day but in a different encounter.

Beginning January 1, 2007, critical care services will be paid at two levels, depending on the presence or absence of trauma activation. Providers will receive one payment rate for critical care without trauma activation and will receive additional payment when critical care is associated with trauma activation.

To determine whether trauma activation occurs, follow the National Uniform Billing Committee (NUBC) guidelines in the Claims Processing Manual, Pub 100-04, Chapter 25, §75.4 related to the reporting of the trauma revenue codes in the 68x series. The revenue code series 68x can be used only by trauma centers/hospitals as licensed or designated by the state or local government authority authorized to do so, or as verified by the American College of Surgeons. Different subcategory revenue codes are reported by designated Level 1-4 hospital trauma centers. Only patients for whom there has been prehospital notification based on triage information from prehospital caregivers, who meet either local, state or American College of Surgeons field triage criteria, or are delivered by inter-hospital transfers, and are given the appropriate team response can be billed a trauma activation charge.

When critical care services are provided without trauma activation, the hospital may bill CPT code 99291, Critical care, evaluation and management of the critically ill or critically injured patient; first 30-74 minutes (and 99292, if appropriate). If trauma activation occurs under the circumstances described by the NUBC guidelines that would permit reporting a charge under 68x, the hospital may also bill one unit of code G0390, which describes trauma activation associated with hospital critical care services. Revenue code 68x must be reported on the same date of service. The OCE will edit to ensure that G0390 appears with revenue code 68x on the same date of service and that only one unit of G0390 is billed. CMS believes that trauma activation is a one-time occurrence in association with critical care services, and therefore, CMS will only pay for one unit of G0390 per day.

The CPT code 99291 is defined by CPT as the first 30-74 minutes of critical care. This 30 minute minimum has always applied under the OPPS. The CPT code 99292, Critical care, evaluation and management of the critically ill or critically injured patient; each additional 30 minutes, remains a packaged service under the OPPS, so that hospitals do not have the ongoing administrative burden of reporting precisely the time for each critical service provided. As the CPT guidelines indicate, hospitals that provide less than 30 minutes of critical care should bill for a visit, typically an emergency department visit, at a level consistent with their own internal guidelines.

Under the OPPS, the time that can be reported as critical care is the time spent by a physician and/or hospital staff engaged in active face-to-face critical care of a critically ill or critically injured patient. If the physician and hospital staff or multiple hospital staff members are simultaneously engaged in this active face-to-face care, the time involved can only be counted once.

Appendix 4 — Internet-only Manuals (IOMs)

- Beginning in CY 2007 hospitals may continue to report a charge with RC 68x without any HCPCS code when trauma team activation occurs. In order to receive additional payment when critical care services are associated with trauma activation, the hospital must report G0390 on the same date of service as RC 68x, in addition to CPT code 99291 (or 99292, if appropriate.)

- Beginning in CY 2007 hospitals should continue to report 99291 (and 99292 as appropriate) for critical care services furnished without trauma team activation. CPT 99291 maps to APC 0617 (Critical Care). (CPT 99292 is packaged and not paid separately, but should be reported if provided.)

Critical care services are paid in some cases separately and in other cases as part of a composite APC payment. See Section 10.2.1 of this chapter for further details.

Future updates will be issued in a Recurring Update Notification.

## 100-04, 4, 200.1

### Billing for Corneal Tissue

Corneal tissue will be paid on a cost basis, not under OPPS. To receive cost based reimbursement hospitals must bill charges for corneal tissue using HCPCS code V2785.

## 100-04, 4, 200.2

### Hospital Dialysis Services For Patients with and without End Stage Renal Disease (ESRD)

Effective with claims with dates of service on or after August 1, 2000, hospital-based End Stage Renal Disease (ESRD) facilities must submit services covered under the ESRD benefit in 42 CFR 413.174 (maintenance dialysis and those items and services directly related to dialysis such as drugs, supplies) on a separate claim from services not covered under the ESRD benefit. Items and services not covered under the ESRD benefit must be billed by the hospital using the hospital bill type and be paid under the Outpatient Prospective Payment System (OPPS) (or to a CAH at reasonable cost). Services covered under the ESRD benefit in 42 CFR 413.174 must be billed on the ESRD bill type and must be paid under the ESRD PPS. This requirement is necessary to properly pay only unrelated ESRD services (those not covered under the ESRD benefit) under OPPS (or to a CAH at reasonable cost).

Medicare does not allow payment for routine or related dialysis treatments, which are covered and paid under the ESRD PPS, when furnished to ESRD patients in the outpatient department of a hospital. However, in certain medical situations in which the ESRD outpatient cannot obtain her or his regularly scheduled dialysis treatment at a certified ESRD facility, the OPPS rule for 2003 allows payment for non-routine dialysis treatments (which are not covered under the ESRD benefit) furnished to ESRD outpatients in the outpatient department of a hospital. Payment for unscheduled dialysis furnished to ESRD outpatients and paid under the OPPS is limited to the following circumstances:

- Dialysis performed following or in connection with a dialysis-related procedure such as vascular access procedure or blood transfusions;

- Dialysis performed following treatment for an unrelated medical emergency; e.g., if a patient goes to the emergency room for chest pains and misses a regularly scheduled dialysis treatment that cannot be rescheduled, CMS allows the hospital to provide and bill Medicare for the dialysis treatment; or

- Emergency dialysis for ESRD patients who would otherwise have to be admitted as inpatients in order for the hospital to receive payment.

In these situations, non-ESRD certified hospital outpatient facilities are to bill Medicare using the Healthcare Common Procedure Coding System (HCPCS) code G0257 (Unscheduled or emergency dialysis treatment for an ESRD patient in a hospital outpatient department that is not certified as an ESRD facility).

HCPCS code G0257 may only be reported on type of bill 13X (hospital outpatient service) or type of bill 85X (critical access hospital) because HCPCS code G0257 only reports services for hospital outpatients with ESRD and only these bill types are used to report services to hospital outpatients. Effective for services on and after October 1, 2012, claims containing HCPCS code G0257 will be returned to the provider for correction if G0257 is reported with a type of bill other than 13X or 85X (such as a 12x inpatient claim).

HCPCS code 90935 (Hemodialysis procedure with single physician evaluation) may be reported and paid only if one of the following two conditions is met:

1) The patient is a hospital inpatient with or without ESRD and has no coverage under Part A, but has Part B coverage. The charge for hemodialysis is a charge for the use of a prosthetic device. See Benefits Policy Manual 100-02 Chapter 15 section 120. A. The service must be reported on a type of bill 12X or type of bill 85X. See the Benefits Policy Manual 100-02 Chapter 6 section 10 (Medical and Other Health Services Furnished to Inpatients of Participating Hospitals) for the criteria that must be met for services to be paid when a hospital inpatient has Part B coverage but does not have coverage under Part A; or 2) A hospital outpatient does not have ESRD and is

receiving hemodialysis in the hospital outpatient department. The service is reported on a type of bill 13X or type of bill 85X. CPT code 90945 (Dialysis procedure other than hemodialysis (e.g. peritoneal dialysis, hemofiltration, or other continuous replacement therapies)), with single physician evaluation, may be reported by a hospital paid under the OPPS or CAH method I or method II on type of bill 12X, 13X or 85X.

## 100-04, 4, 200.4

### Billing for Amniotic Membrane

Hospitals should report HCPCS code V2790 (Amniotic membrane for surgical reconstruction, per procedure) to report amniotic membrane tissue when the tissue is used. A specific procedure code associated with use of amniotic membrane tissue is CPT code 65780 (Ocular surface reconstruction; amniotic membrane transplantation).

Payment for the amniotic membrane tissue is packaged into payment for CPT code 65780 or other procedures with which the amniotic membrane is used.

## 100-04, 4, 200.6

### Billing and Payment for Alcohol and/or Substance Abuse Assessment and Intervention Services

For CY 2008, the CPT Editorial Panel has created two new Category I CPT codes for reporting alcohol and/or substance abuse screening and intervention services. They are CPT code 99408 (Alcohol and/or substance (other than tobacco) abuse structured screening (e.g., AUDIT, DAST), and brief intervention (SBI) services; 15 to 30 minutes); and CPT code 99409 (Alcohol and/or substance (other than tobacco) abuse structured screening (e.g., AUDIT, DAST), and brief intervention (SBI) services; greater than 30 minutes). However, screening services are not covered by Medicare without specific statutory authority, such as has been provided for mammography, diabetes, and colorectal cancer screening. Therefore, beginning January 1, 2008, the OPPS recognizes two parallel G-codes (HCPCS codes G0396 and G0397) to allow for appropriate reporting and payment of alcohol and substance abuse structured assessment and intervention services that are not provided as screening services, but that are performed in the context of the diagnosis or treatment of illness or injury.

Contractors shall make payment under the OPPS for HCPCS code G0396 (Alcohol and/or substance (other than tobacco) abuse structured assessment (e.g., AUDIT, DAST) and brief intervention, 15 to 30 minutes) and HCPCS code G0397, (Alcohol and/or substance(other than tobacco) abuse structured assessment (e.g., AUDIT, DAST) and intervention greater than 30 minutes), only when reasonable and necessary (i.e., when the service is provided to evaluate patients with signs/symptoms of illness or injury) as per section 1862(a)(1)(A) of the Act.

HCPCS codes G0396 and G0397 are to be used for structured alcohol and/or substance (other than tobacco) abuse assessment and intervention services that are distinct from other clinic and emergency department visit services performed during the same encounter. Hospital resources expended performing services described by HCPCS codes G0396 and G0397 may not be counted as resources for determining the level of a visit service and vice versa (i.e., hospitals may not double count the same facility resources in order to reach a higher level clinic or emergency department visit). However, alcohol and/or substance structured assessment or intervention services lasting less than 15 minutes should not be reported using these HCPCS codes, but the hospital resources expended should be included in determining the level of the visit service reported.

## 100-04, 4, 200.7.2

### Cardiac Echocardiography With Contrast

Hospitals are instructed to bill for echocardiograms with contrast using the applicable HCPCS code(s) included in Table 200.7.2 below. Hospitals should also report the appropriate units of the HCPCS codes for the contrast agents used in the performance of the echocardiograms.

Table 200.7.2 - HCPCS Codes For Echocardiograms With Contrast

| PCS | Long Descriptor |
|---|---|
| C8921 | Transthoracic echocardiography with contrast, or without contrast followed by with contrast, for congenital cardiac anomalies; complete |
| C8922 | Transthoracic echocardiography with contrast, or without contrast followed by with contrast, for congenital cardiac anomalies; follow-up or limited study |
| C8923 | Transthoracic echocardiography with contrast, or without contrast followed by with contrast, real-time with image documentation (2D), includes M-mode recording, when performed, complete, without spectral or color Doppler echocardiography |

© 2016 Optum360, LLC

| PCS | Long Descriptor |
|---|---|
| C8924 | Transthoracic echocardiography with contrast, or without contrast followed by with contrast, real-time with image documentation (2D), includes M-mode recording, when performed, follow-up or limited study |
| C8925 | Transesophageal echocardiography (TEE) with contrast, or without contrast followed by with contrast, real time with image documentation (2D) (with or without M-mode recording); including probe placement, image acquisition, interpretation and report |
| C8926 | Transesophageal echocardiography (TEE) with contrast, or without contrast followed by with contrast, for congenital cardiac anomalies; including probe placement, image acquisition, interpretation and report |
| C8927 | Transesophageal echocardiography (TEE) with contrast, or without contrast followed by with contrast, for monitoring purposes, including probe placement, real time 2-dimensional image acquisition and interpretation leading to ongoing (continuous) assessment of (dynamically changing) cardiac pumping function and to therapeutic measures on an immediate time basis |
| C8928 | Transthoracic echocardiography with contrast, or without contrast followed by with contrast, real-time with image documentation (2D), includes M-mode recording, when performed, during rest and cardiovascular stress test using treadmill, bicycle exercise and/or pharmacologically induced stress, with interpretation and report |
| C8929 | Transthoracic echocardiography with contrast, or without contrast followed by with contrast, real-time with image documentation (2D), includes M-mode recording, when performed, complete, with spectral Doppler echocardiography, and with color flow Doppler echocardiography |
| C8930 | Transthoracic echocardiography, with contrast, or without contrast followed by with contrast, real-time with image documentation (2D), includes M-mode recording, when performed, during rest and cardiovascular stress test using treadmill, bicycle exercise and/or pharmacologically induced stress, with interpretation and report; including performance of continuous electrocardiographic monitoring, with physician supervision |

## 100-04, 4, 230.2

### Coding and Payment for Drug Administration
Coding and Payment for Drug Administration

#### A. Overview
Drug administration services furnished under the Hospital Outpatient Prospective Payment System (OPPS) during CY 2005 were reported using CPT codes 90780, 90781, and 96400-96459.

Effective January 1, 2006, some of these CPT codes were replaced with more detailed CPT codes incorporating specific procedural concepts, as defined and described by the CPT manual, such as initial, concurrent, and sequential.

Hospitals are instructed to use the full set of CPT codes, including those codes referencing concepts of initial, concurrent, and sequential, to bill for drug administration services furnished in the hospital outpatient department beginning January 1, 2007. In addition, hospitals are instructed to continue billing the HCPCS codes that most accurately describe the service(s) provided.

Hospitals are reminded to bill a separate Evaluation and Management code (with modifier 25) only if a significant, separately identifiable E/M service is performed in the same encounter with OPPS drug administration services.

#### B. Billing for Infusions and Injections
Beginning in CY 2007, hospitals were instructed to use the full set of drug administration CPT codes (90760-90779; 96401-96549), (96413-96523 beginning in CY 2008) (96360-96549 beginning in CY 2009) when billing for drug administration services provided in the hospital outpatient department. In addition, hospitals are to continue to bill HCPCS code C8957 (Intravenous infusion for therapy/diagnosis; initiation of prolonged infusion (more than 8 hours), requiring use of portable or implantable pump) when appropriate. Hospitals are expected to report all drug administration CPT codes in a manner consistent with their descriptors, CPT instructions, and correct coding principles. Hospitals should note the conceptual changes between CY 2006 drug administration codes effective under the OPPS and the CPT codes in effect beginning January 1, 2007, in order to ensure accurate billing under the OPPS. Hospitals should report all HCPCS codes that describe the drug administration services provided, regardless of whether or not those services are separately paid or their payment is packaged.

Medicare's general policy regarding physician supervision within hospital outpatient departments meets the physician supervision requirements for use of CPT codes 90760-90779, 96401-96549, (96413-96523 beginning in CY 2008). (Reference: Pub.100-02, Medicare Benefit Policy Manual, Chapter 6, §20.4.)

Drug administration services are to be reported with a line item date of service on the day they are provided. In addition, only one initial drug administration service is to be reported per vascular access site per encounter, including during an encounter where observation services span more than 1 calendar day.

#### C. Payments For Drug Administration Services
For CY 2007, OPPS drug administration APCs were restructured, resulting in a six-level hierarchy where active HCPCS codes have been assigned according to their clinical coherence and resource use. Contrary to the CY 2006 payment structure that bundled payment for several instances of a type of service (non-chemotherapy, chemotherapy by infusion, non-infusion chemotherapy) into a per-encounter APC payment, structure introduced in CY 2007 provides a separate APC payment for each reported unit of a separately payable HCPCS code.

Hospitals should note that the transition to the full set of CPT drug administration codes provides for conceptual differences when reporting, such as those noted below.

- In CY 2006, hospitals were instructed to bill for the first hour (and any additional hours) by each type of infusion service (non-chemotherapy, chemotherapy by infusion, non-infusion chemotherapy). Beginning in CY 2007, the first hour concept no longer exists. CPT codes in CY 2007 and beyond allow for only one initial service per encounter, for each vascular access site, no matter how many types of infusion services are provided; however, hospitals will receive an APC payment for the initial service and separate APC payment(s) for additional hours of infusion or other drug administration services provided that are separately payable.

- In CY 2006, hospitals providing infusion services of different types (non-chemotherapy, chemotherapy by infusion, non-infusion chemotherapy) received payment for the associated per-encounter infusion APC even if these infusions occurred during the same time period. Beginning in CY 2007, hospitals should report only one initial drug administration service, including infusion services, per encounter for each distinct vascular access site, with other services through the same vascular access site being reported via the sequential, concurrent or additional hour codes. Although new CPT guidance has been issued for reporting initial drug administration services, Medicare contractors shall continue to follow the guidance given in this manual.

(NOTE: This list above provides a brief overview of a limited number of the conceptual changes between CY 2006 OPPS drug administration codes and CY 2007 OPPS drug administration codes - this list is not comprehensive and does not include all items hospitals will need to consider during this transition)

For APC payment rates, refer to the most current quarterly version of Addendum B on the CMS Web site at http://www.cms.hhs.gov/HospitalOutpatientPPS/.

#### D. Infusions Started Outside the Hospital
Hospitals may receive Medicare beneficiaries for outpatient services who are in the process of receiving an infusion at their time of arrival at the hospital (e.g., a patient who arrives via ambulance with an ongoing intravenous infusion initiated by paramedics during transport). Hospitals are reminded to bill for all services provided using the HCPCS code(s) that most accurately describe the service(s) they provided. This includes hospitals reporting an initial hour of infusion, even if the hospital did not initiate the infusion, and additional HCPCS codes for additional or sequential infusion services if needed.

## 100-04, 4, 230.2.1

### Administration of Drugs Via Implantable or Portable Pumps
for Implantable or Portable Pumps 2005 CPT Final CY 2006 OPPS 2005 CPT 2005 Description Code Description SI APC n/a n/a C8957 Intravenous infusion for therapy/diagnosis; initiation of prolonged infusion (more than 8 hours), requiring use of portable or implantable pump S 0120 96414 Chemotherapy administration, intravenous; infusion technique, initiation of prolonged infusion (more than 8 hours), requiring the use of a portable or implantable pump 96416 Chemotherapy administration, intravenous infusion technique; initiation of prolonged chemotherapy infusion (more than 8 hours), requiring use of portable or implantable pump S 0117 96425 Chemotherapy administration, infusion technique, initiation of prolonged infusion (more than 8 hours), requiring the use of a portable or implantable pump) 96425 Chemotherapy administration, intra-arterial; infusion technique, initiation of prolonged infusion (more than 8 hours), requiring the use of a portable or implantable pump S 0117 96520 Refilling and maintenance of portable

pump 96521 Refilling and maintenance of portable pump T 0125 2005 CPT Final CY 2006 OPPS 2005 CPT 2005 Description Code Description SI APC 96530 Refilling and maintenance of implantable pump or reservoir for drug delivery, systemic [e.g. Intravenous, intra-arterial] 96522 Refilling and maintenance of implantable pump or reservoir for drug delivery, systemic (e.g., intravenous, intra-arterial) T 0125 n/a n/a 96523 Irrigation of implanted venous access device for drug delivery systems N - Hospitals are to report HCPCS code C8957 and CPT codes 96416 and 96425 to indicate the initiation of a prolonged infusion that requires the use of an implantable or portable pump. CPT codes 96521, 92522, and 96523 should be used by hospitals to indicate refilling and maintenance of drug delivery systems or irrigation of implanted venous access devices for such systems, and may be reported for the servicing of devices used for therapeutic drugs other than chemotherapy.

## 100-04, 4, 231.4

### Billing for Split Unit of Blood

HCPCS code P9011 was created to identify situations where one unit of blood or a blood product is split and some portion of the unit is transfused to one patient and the other portions are transfused to other patients or to the same patient at other times. When a patient receives a transfusion of a split unit of blood or blood product, OPPS providers should bill P9011 for the blood product transfused, as well as CPT 86985 (Splitting, blood products) for each splitting procedure performed to prepare the blood product for a specific patient.

Providers should bill split units of packed red cells and whole blood using Revenue Code 389 (Other blood), and should not use Revenue Codes 381 (Packed red cells) or 382 (Whole blood). Providers should bill split units of other blood products using the applicable revenue codes for the blood product type, such as 383 (Plasma) or 384 (Platelets), rather than 389. Reporting revenue codes according to these specifications will ensure the Medicare beneficiary's blood deductible is applied correctly.

EXAMPLE: OPPS provider splits off a 100cc aliquot from a 250 cc unit of leukocytereduced red blood cells for a transfusion to Patient X. The hospital then splits off an 80cc aliquot of the remaining unit for a transfusion to Patient Y. At a later time, the remaining 70cc from the unit is transfused to Patient Z.

In billing for the services for Patient X and Patient Y, the OPPS provider should report the charges by billing P9011 and 86985 in addition to the CPT code for the transfusion service, because a specific splitting service was required to prepare a split unit for transfusion to each of those patients. However, the OPPS provider should report only P9011 and the CPT code for the transfusion service for Patient Z because no additional splitting was necessary to prepare the split unit for transfusion to Patient Z. The OPPS provider should bill Revenue Code 0389 for each split unit of the leukocyte-reduced red blood cells that was transfused.

## 100-04, 4, 260.5

Hospitals other than CAHs are required to report line item dates of service per revenue code line for partial hospitalization claims. Where services are provided on more than one day included in the billing period, the date of service must be identified. Each service (revenue code) provided must be repeated on a separate line item along with the specific date the service was provided for every occurrence. See examples below of reporting line item dates of service. These examples are for group therapy services provided twice during a billing period.

For the claims, report as follows:

| Revenue Code | HCPCS | Dates of Service | Units | Total Charges |
|---|---|---|---|---|
| 0915 | G0176 | 20090505 | 1 | $80.00 |
| 0915 | G0176 | 20090529 | 2 | $160.00 |

NOTE: Information regarding the Form CMS-1450 form locators that correspond with these fields is found in Chapter 25 of this manual. See the ASC X12 837 Institutional Claim Implementation Guide for related guidelines for the electronic claim.

The A/B MAC (A) must return to the hospital (RTP) claims where a line item date of service is not entered for each HCPCS code reported, or if the line item dates of service reported are outside of the statement covers period. Line item date of service reporting is effective for claims with dates of service on or after June 5, 2000.

## 100-04, 4, 290.1

### Observation Services Overview

Observation care is a well-defined set of specific, clinically appropriate services, which include ongoing short term treatment, assessment, and reassessment, that are furnished while a decision is being made regarding whether patients will require further treatment as hospital inpatients or if they are able to be discharged from the hospital. Observation status is commonly assigned to patients who present to the emergency department and who then require a significant period of treatment or monitoring in order to make a decision concerning their admission or discharge.

Observation services are covered only when provided by the order of a physician or another individual authorized by State licensure law and hospital staff bylaws to admit patients to the hospital or to order outpatient services.

Observation services must also be reasonable and necessary to be covered by Medicare. In only rare and exceptional cases do reasonable and necessary outpatient observation services span more than 48 hours. In the majority of cases, the decision whether to discharge a patient from the hospital following resolution of the reason for the observation care or to admit the patient as an inpatient can be made in less than 48 hours, usually in less than 24 hours.

## 100-04, 4, 290.2.2

### Reporting Hours of Observation

Observation time begins at the clock time documented in the patient's medical record, which coincides with the time the patient is placed in a bed for the purpose of initiating observation care in accordance with a physician's order. Hospitals should round to the nearest hour. For example, a patient who was placed in an observation bed at 3:03 p.m. according to the nurses' notes and discharged to home at 9:45 p.m. should have a "7" placed in the units field of the reported observation HCPCS code.

General standing orders for observation services following all outpatient surgery are not recognized. Hospitals should not report as observation care, services that are part of another Part B service, such as postoperative monitoring during a standard recovery period (e.g., 4-6 hours), which should be billed as recovery room services. Similarly, in the case of patients who undergo diagnostic testing in a hospital outpatient department, routine preparation services furnished prior to the testing and recovery afterwards are included in the payments for those diagnostic services. Observation services should not be billed concurrently with diagnostic or therapeutic services for which active monitoring is a part of the procedure (e.g., colonoscopy, chemotherapy). In situations where such a procedure interrupts observation services, hospitals would record for each period of observation services the beginning and ending times during the hospital outpatient encounter and add the length of time for the periods of observation services together to reach the total number of units reported on the claim for the hourly observation services HCPCS code G0378 (Hospital observation service, per hour).

Observation time ends when all medically necessary services related to observation care are completed. For example, this could be before discharge when the need for observation has ended, but other medically necessary services not meeting the definition of observation care are provided (in which case, the additional medically necessary services would be billed separately or included as part of the emergency department or clinic visit). Alternatively, the end time of observation services may coincide with the time the patient is actually discharged from the hospital or admitted as an inpatient.

Observation time may include medically necessary services and follow-up care provided after the time that the physician writes the discharge order, but before the patient is discharged. However, reported observation time would not include the time patients remain in the observation area after treatment is finished for reasons such as waiting for transportation home.

If a period of observation spans more than 1 calendar day, all of the hours for the entire period of observation must be included on a single line and the date of service for that line is the date that observation care begins.

## 100-04, 4, 290.4.1

### Billing and Payment for All Hospital Observation Services Furnished Between January 1, 2006 and December 31, 2007

Since January 1, 2006, two G-codes have been used to report observation services and direct referral for observation care. For claims for dates of service January 1, 2006 through December 31, 2007, the Integrated Outpatient Code Editor (I/OCE) determines whether the observation care or direct referral services are packaged or separately payable. Thus, hospitals provide consistent coding and billing under all circumstances in which they deliver observation care.

Beginning January 1, 2006, hospitals should not report CPT codes 99217-99220 or 99234-99236 for observation services. In addition, the following HCPCS codes were discontinued as of January 1, 2006: G0244 (Observation care by facility to patient), G0263 (Direct Admission with congestive heart failure, chest pain or asthma), and G0264 (Assessment other than congestive heart failure, chest pain, or asthma).

The three discontinued G-codes and the CPT codes that were no longer recognized were replaced by two new G-codes to be used by hospitals to report all observation services, whether separately payable or packaged, and direct referral for observation care, whether separately payable or packaged:

G0378- Hospital observation service, per hour; and

G0379- Direct admission of patient for hospital observation care.

© 2016 Optum360, LLC

The I/OCE determines whether observation services billed as units of G0378 are separately payable under APC 0339 (Observation) or whether payment for observation services will be packaged into the payment for other services provided by the hospital in the same encounter. Therefore, hospitals should bill HCPCS code G0378 when observation services are ordered and provided to any patient regardless of the patient's condition. The units of service should equal the number of hours the patient receives observation services.

Hospitals should report G0379 when observation services are the result of a direct referral for observation care without an associated emergency room visit, hospital outpatient clinic visit, critical care service, or hospital outpatient surgical procedure (status indicator T procedure) on the day of initiation of observation services. Hospitals should only report HCPCS code G0379 when a patient is referred directly for observation care after being seen by a physician in the community (see Sec.290.4.2 below)

Some non-repetitive OPPS services provided on the same day by a hospital may be billed on different claims, provided that all charges associated with each procedure or service being reported are billed on the same claim with the HCPCS code which describes that service. See chapter 1, section 50.2.2 of this manual. It is vitally important that all of the charges that pertain to a non-repetitive, separately paid procedure or service be reported on the same claim with that procedure or service. It should also be emphasized that this relaxation of same day billing requirements for some non-repetitive services does not apply to non-repetitive services provided on the same day as either direct referral to observation care or observation services because the OCE claim-by-claim logic cannot function properly unless all services related to the episode of observation care, including diagnostic tests, lab services, hospital clinic visits, emergency department visits, critical care services, and status indicator T procedures, are reported on the same claim. Additional guidance can be found in chapter 1, section 50.2.2 of this manual.

## 100-04, 4, 290.4.2

**Separate and Packaged Payment for Direct Admission to Observation**

In order to receive separate payment for a direct referral for observation care (APC 0604), the claim must show:

1. Both HCPCS codes G0378 (Hourly Observation) and G0379 (Direct Admit to Observation) with the same date of service;

2. That no services with a status indicator T or V or Critical care (APC 0617) were provided on the same day of service as HCPCS code G0379; and

3. The observation care does not qualify for separate payment under APC 0339.

Only a direct referral for observation services billed on a 13X bill type may be considered for a separate APC payment.

Separate payment is not allowed for HCPCS code G0379, direct admission to observation care, when billed with the same date of service as a hospital clinic visit, emergency room visit, critical care service, or "T" status procedure.

If a bill for the direct referral for observation services does not meet the three requirements listed above, then payment for the direct referral service will be packaged into payments for other separately payable services provided to the beneficiary in the same encounter.

## 100-04, 4, 290.4.3

**Separate and Packaged Payment for Observation Services Furnished Between January 1, 2006 and December 31, 2007**

Separate payment may be made for observation services provided to a patient with congestive heart failure, chest pain, or asthma. The list of ICD-9-CM diagnosis codes eligible for separate payment is reviewed annually. Any changes in applicable ICD-9-CM diagnosis codes are included in the October quarterly update of the OPPS and also published in the annual OPPS Final Rule. The list of qualifying ICD-9-CM diagnosis codes is also published on the OPPS Web page.

All of the following requirements must be met in order for a hospital to receive a separate APC payment for observation services through APC 0339:

1. Diagnosis Requirements

   a. The beneficiary must have one of three medical conditions: congestive heart failure, chest pain, or asthma.

   b. Qualifying ICD-9-CM diagnosis codes must be reported in Form Locator (FL) 76, Patient Reason for Visit, or FL 67, principal diagnosis, or both in order for the hospital to receive separate payment for APC 0339. If a qualifying ICD-9-CM diagnosis code(s) is reported in the secondary diagnosis field, but is not reported in either the Patient Reason for Visit field (FL 76) or in the principal diagnosis field (FL 67), separate payment for APC 0339 is not allowed.

2. Observation Time

   a. Observation time must be documented in the medical record.

   b. Hospital billing for observation services begins at the clock time documented in the patient's medical record, which coincides with the time that observation services are initiated in accordance with a physician's order for observation services.

   c. A beneficiary's time receiving observation services (and hospital billing) ends when all clinical or medical interventions have been completed, including follow-up care furnished by hospital staff and physicians that may take place after a physician has ordered the patient be released or admitted as an inpatient.

   d. The number of units reported with HCPCS code G0378 must equal or exceed 8 hours.

3. Additional Hospital Services

   a. The claim for observation services must include one of the following services in addition to the reported observation services. The additional services listed below must have a line item date of service on the same day or the day before the date reported for observation:

   > An emergency department visit (APC 0609, 0613, 0614, 0615, 0616) or
   >
   > A clinic visit (APC 0604, 0605, 0606, 0607, 0608); or
   >
   > Critical care (APC 0617); or
   >
   > Direct referral for observation care reported with HCPCS code G0379 (APC 0604); must be reported on the same date of service as the date reported for observation services.

   b. No procedure with a T status indicator can be reported on the same day or day before observation care is provided.

4. Physician Evaluation

   a. The beneficiary must be in the care of a physician during the period of observation, as documented in the medical record by outpatient registration, discharge, and other appropriate progress notes that are timed, written, and signed by the physician.

   b. The medical record must include documentation that the physician explicitly assessed patient risk to determine that the beneficiary would benefit from observation care.

Only observation services that are billed on a 13X bill type may be considered for a separate APC payment.

Hospitals should bill all of the other services associated with the observation care, including direct referral for observation, hospital clinic visits, emergency room visits, critical care services, and T status procedures, on the same claim so that the claims processing logic may appropriately determine the payment status (either packaged or separately payable) of HCPCS codes G0378 and G0379.

If a bill for observation care does not meet all of the requirements listed above, then payment for the observation care will be packaged into payments for other separately payable services provided to the beneficiary in the same encounter.

## 100-04, 4, 290.5.1

**Billing and Payment for Observation Services Beginning January 1, 2008**

Observation services are reported using HCPCS code G0378 (Hospital observation service, per hour). Beginning January 1, 2008, HCPCS code G0378 for hourly observation services is assigned status indicator N, signifying that its payment is always packaged. No separate payment is made for observation services reported with HCPCS code G0378, and APC 0339 is deleted as of January 1, 2008. In most circumstances, observation services are supportive and ancillary to the other services provided to a patient. Beginning January 1, 2014, in certain circumstances when observation care is billed in conjunction with a clinic visit, high level Type A emergency department visit (Level 4 or 5), high level Type B emergency department visit (Level 5), critical care services, or a direct referral as an integral part of a patient's extended encounter of care, payment may be made for the entire extended care encounter through APC 8009 (Extended Assessment and Management Composite) when certain criteria are met. Prior to January 1, 2014, in certain circumstances when observation care was billed in conjunction with a high level clinic visit (Level 5), high level Type A emergency department visit (Level 4 or 5), high level Type B emergency department visit (Level 5), critical care services, or a direct referral as an integral part of a patient's extended encounter of care, payment could be made for the entire extended care encounter through one of two composite APCs (APCs 8002 and 8003) when certain criteria were met. APCs 8002 and 8003 are deleted as of January 1, 2014. For information about payment for extended assessment and management composite APC, see §10.2.1 (Composite APCs) of this chapter.

There is no limitation on diagnosis for payment of APC 8009; however, composite APC payment will not be made when observation services are reported in association with a surgical procedure (T status procedure) or the hours of observation care reported are less than 8. The I/OCE evaluates every claim received to determine if payment through a composite APC is appropriate. If payment through a composite APC is inappropriate, the I/OCE, in conjunction with the Pricer, determines the appropriate status indicator, APC, and payment for every code on a claim.

All of the following requirements must be met in order for a hospital to receive an APC payment for an extended assessment and management composite APC:

1.  Observation Time

    a.  Observation time must be documented in the medical record.

    b.  Hospital billing for observation services begins at the clock time documented in the patient's medical record, which coincides with the time that observation services are initiated in accordance with a physician's order for observation services.

    c.  A beneficiary's time receiving observation services (and hospital billing) ends when all clinical or medical interventions have been completed, including follow-up care furnished by hospital staff and physicians that may take place after a physician has ordered the patient be released or admitted as an inpatient.

    d.  The number of units reported with HCPCS code G0378 must equal or exceed 8 hours.

2.  Additional Hospital Services

    a.  The claim for observation services must include one of the following services in addition to the reported observation services. The additional services listed below must have a line item date of service on the same day or the day before the date reported for observation:

        A Type A or B emergency department visit (CPT codes 99284 or 99285 or HCPCS code G0384); or

        A clinic visit (CPT code 99205 or 99215); or

        Critical care (CPT code 99291); or

        Direct referral for observation care reported with HCPCS code G0379 (APC 0604) must be reported on the same date of service as the date reported for observation services.

    b.  No procedure with a T status indicator can be reported on the same day or day before observation care is provided.

3.  Physician Evaluation

    a.  The beneficiary must be in the care of a physician during the period of observation, as documented in the medical record by outpatient registration, discharge, and other appropriate progress notes that are timed, written, and signed by the physician.

    b.  The medical record must include documentation that the physician explicitly assessed patient risk to determine that the beneficiary would benefit from observation care.

Criteria 1 and 3 related to observation care beginning and ending time and physician evaluation apply regardless of whether the hospital believes that the criteria will be met for payment of the extended encounter through extended assessment and management composite payment.

Only visits, critical care and observation services that are billed on a 13X bill type may be considered for a composite APC payment.

Non-repetitive services provided on the same day as either direct referral for observation care or observation services must be reported on the same claim because the OCE claim-by-claim logic cannot function properly unless all services related to the episode of observation care, including hospital clinic visits, emergency department visits, critical care services, and T status procedures, are reported on the same claim. Additional guidance can be found in chapter 1, section 50.2.2 of this manual.

If a claim for services provided during an extended assessment and management encounter including observation care does not meet all of the requirements listed above, then the usual APC logic will apply to separately payable items and services on the claim; the special logic for direct admission will apply, and payment for the observation care will be packaged into payments for other separately payable services provided to the beneficiary in the same encounter.

## 100-04, 4, 290.5.2

### Billing and Payment for Direct Referral for Observation Care Furnished Beginning January 1, 2008

Direct referral for observation care continues to be reported using HCPCS code G0379 (Direct admission of patient for hospital observation care). Hospitals should report G0379 when observation services are the result of a direct referral for observation care without an associated emergency room visit, hospital outpatient clinic visit, or critical care service on the day of initiation of observation services. Hospitals should only report HCPCS code G0379 when a patient is referred directly to observation care after being seen by a physician in the community.

Payment for direct referral for observation care will be made either separately as a low level hospital clinic visit under APC 0604 or packaged into payment for composite APC 8002 (Level I Prolonged Assessment and Management Composite) or packaged into the payment for other separately payable services provided in the same encounter. For information about payment for extended assessment and management composite APCs, see, Sec.10.2.1 (Composite APCs) of this chapter.

The criteria for payment of HCPCS code G0379 under either APC 0604 or APC 8002 include:

1.  Both HCPCS codes G0378 (Hospital observation services, per hr) and G0379 (Direct admission of patient for hospital observation care) are reported with the same date of service.

2.  No service with a status indicator of T or V or Critical Care (APC 0617) is provided on the same day of service as HCPCS code G0379.

If either of the above criteria is not met, HCPCS code G0379 will be assigned status indicator N and will be packaged into payment for other separately payable services provided in the same encounter.

Only a direct referral for observation services billed on a 13X bill type may be considered for a composite APC payment.

## 100-04, 4, 290.5.3

### Billing and Payment for Observation Services Furnished Beginning January 1, 2016

Observation services are reported using HCPCS code G0378 (Hospital observation service, per hour). Beginning January 1, 2008, HCPCS code G0378 for hourly observation services is assigned status indicator N, signifying that its payment is always packaged. No separate payment is made for observation services reported with HCPCS APCs, see §10.2.3 (Comprehensive APCs) of this chapter.

There is no limitation on diagnosis for payment of APC 8011; however, comprehensive APC payment will not be made when observation services are reported in association with a surgical procedure (T status procedure) or the hours of observation care reported are less than 8. The I/OCE evaluates every claim received to determine if payment through a comprehensive APC is appropriate. If payment through a comprehensive APC is inappropriate, the I/OCE, in conjunction with the Pricer, determines the appropriate status indicator, APC, and payment for every code on a claim.

All of the following requirements must be met in order for a hospital to receive a comprehensive APC payment through the Comprehensive Observation Services APC (APC 8011):

1.  Observation Time

    a.  Observation time must be documented in the medical record.

    b.  Hospital billing for observation services begins at the clock time documented in the patient's medical record, which coincides with the time that observation services are initiated in accordance with a physician's order for observation services.

    c.  A beneficiary's time receiving observation services (and hospital billing) ends when all clinical or medical interventions have been completed, including follow-up care furnished by hospital staff and physicians that may take place after a physician has ordered the patient be released or admitted as an inpatient.

    d.  The number of units reported with HCPCS code G0378 must equal or exceed 8 hours.

2.  Additional Hospital Services

    a.  The claim for observation services must include one of the following services in addition to the reported observation services. The additional services listed below must have a line item date of service on the same day or the day before the date reported for observation:

    •   A Type A or B emergency department visit (CPT codes 99281 through 99285 or HCPCS codes G0380 through G0384); or

- A clinic visit (HCPCS code G0463); or
- Critical care (CPT code 99291); or
- Direct referral for observation care reported with HCPCS code G0379 (APC 5013) must be reported on the same date of service as the date reported for observation services.

    b. No procedure with a T status indicator or a J1 status indicator can be reported on the claim.

3. Physician Evaluation

    a. The beneficiary must be in the care of a physician during the period of observation, as documented in the medical record by outpatient registration, discharge, and other appropriate progress notes that are timed, written, and signed by the physician.

    b. The medical record must include documentation that the physician explicitly assessed patient risk to determine that the beneficiary would benefit from observation care.

Criteria 1 and 3 related to observation care beginning and ending time and physician evaluation apply regardless of whether the hospital believes that the criteria will be met for payment of the extended encounter through the Comprehensive Observation Services APC (APC 8011).

Only visits, critical care and observation services that are billed on a 13X bill type may be considered for a comprehensive APC payment through the Comprehensive Observation Services APC (APC 8011).

Non-repetitive services provided on the same day as either direct referral for observation care or observation services must be reported on the same claim because the OCE claim-by-claim logic cannot function properly unless all services related to the episode of observation care, including hospital clinic visits, emergency department visits, critical care services, and T status procedures, are reported on the same claim. Additional guidance can be found in chapter 1, section 50.2.2 of this manual.

If a claim for services provided during an extended assessment and management encounter including observation care does not meet all of the requirements listed above, then the usual APC logic will apply to separately payable items and services on the claim; the special logic for direct admission will apply, and payment for the observation care will be packaged into payments for other separately payable services provided to the beneficiary in the same encounter.

## 100-04, 4, 300.6

### Common Working File (CWF) Edits

The CWF edit will allow 3 hours of therapy for MNT in the initial calendar year. The edit will allow more than 3 hours of therapy if there is a change in the beneficiary's medical condition, diagnosis, or treatment regimen and this change must be documented in the beneficiary's medical record. Two new G codes have been created for use when a beneficiary receives a second referral in a calendar year that allows the beneficiary to receive more than 3 hours of therapy. Another edit will allow 2 hours of follow up MNT with another referral in subsequent years.

### Advance Beneficiary Notice (ABN)

The beneficiary is liable for services denied over the limited number of hours with referrals for MNT. An ABN should be issued in these situations. In absence of evidence of a valid ABN, the provider will be held liable.

An ABN should not be issued for Medicare-covered services such as those provided by hospital dietitians or nutrition professionals who are qualified to render the service in their state but who have not obtained Medicare provider numbers.

### Duplicate Edits

Although beneficiaries are allowed to receive training and therapy during the same time period Diabetes Self-Management and Training (DSMT) and Medical Nutrition Therapy (MNT) services may not be provided on the same day to the same beneficiary. Effective April 1, 2010 CWF shall implement a new duplicate crossover edit to identify and prevent claims for DSMT/MNT services from being billed with the same dates of services for the same beneficiaries submitted from institutional providers and from a professional provider.

## 100-04, 4, 320.1

### HCPCS Coding for OIVIT

HCPCS code G9147, effective with the April IOCE and MPFSDB updates, is to be used on claims with dates of service on and after December 23, 2009, billing for non-covered OIVIT and any services comprising an OIVIT regimen.

NOTE: HCPCS codes 99199 or 94681(with or without diabetes related conditions 250.00-250.93) are not to be used on claims billing for non-covered OIVIT and any services comprising an OIVIT regimen when furnished pursuant to an OIVIT regimen.

Claims billing for HCPCS codes 99199 and 94681 for non-covered OIVIT are to be returned to provider/returned as unprocessable.

## 100-04, 4, 320.2

### Outpatient Intravenous Insulin Treatment (OIVIT)

Effective for claims with dates of service on and after December 23, 2009, the Centers for Medicare and Medicaid Services (CMS) determines that the evidence does not support a conclusion that OIVIT improves health outcomes in Medicare beneficiaries. Therefore, CMS has determined that OIVIT is not reasonable and necessary for any indication under section 1862(a)(1)(A) of the Social Security Act. Services comprising an OIVIT regimen are nationally non-covered under Medicare when furnished pursuant to an OIVIT regimen.

See Pub. 100-03, Medicare National Coverage Determinations Manual, Section 40.7, Outpatient Intravenous Insulin Treatment (Effective December 23, 2009), for general information and coverage indications.

## 100-04, 5, 10.6

### Functional Reporting

#### A. General

Section 3005(g) of the Middle Class Tax Relief and Jobs Creation Act (MCTRJCA) amended Section 1833(g) of the Act to require a claims-based data collection system for outpatient therapy services, including physical therapy (PT), occupational therapy (OT) and speech-language pathology (SLP) services. 42 CFR 410.59, 410.60, 410.61, 410.62 and 410.105 implement this requirement. The system will collect data on beneficiary function during the course of therapy services in order to better understand beneficiary conditions, outcomes, and expenditures.

Beneficiary unction information is reported using 42 nonpayable functional G-codes and seven severity/complexity modifiers on claims for PT, OT, and SLP services. Functional reporting on one functional limitation at a time is required periodically throughout an entire PT, OT, or SLP therapy episode of care.

The nonpayable G-codes and severity modifiers provide information about the beneficiary's functional status at the outset of the therapy episode of care, including projected goal status, at specified points during treatment, and at the time of discharge. These G-codes, along with the associated modifiers, are required at specified intervals on all claims for outpatient therapy services – not just those over the cap.

#### B. Application of New Coding Requirements

This functional data reporting and collection system is effective for therapy services with dates of service on and after January 1, 2013. A testing period will be in effect from January 1, 2013, until July 1, 2013, to allow providers and practitioners to use the new coding requirements to assure that systems work. Claims for therapy services furnished on and after July 1, 2013, that do not contain the required functional G-code/modifier information will be returned or rejected, as applicable.

#### C. Services Affected

These requirements apply to all claims for services furnished under the Medicare Part B outpatient therapy benefit and the PT, OT, and SLP services furnished under the CORF benefit. They also apply to the therapy services furnished personally by and incident to the service of a physician or a nonphysician practitioner (NPP), including a nurse practitioner (NP), a certified nurse specialist (CNS), or a physician assistant (PA), as applicable.

#### D. Providers and Practitioners Affected.

The functional reporting requirements apply to the therapy services furnished by the following providers: hospitals, CAHs, SNFs, CORFs, rehabilitation agencies, and HHAs (when the beneficiary is not under a home health plan of care). It applies to the following practitioners: physical therapists, occupational therapists, and speech-language pathologists in private practice (TPPs), physicians, and NPPs as noted above. The term "clinician" is applied to these practitioners throughout this manual section. (See definition section of Pub. 100-02, chapter 15, section 220.)

#### E. Function-related G-codes

There are 42 functional G-codes, 14 sets of three codes each. Six of the G-code sets are generally for PT and OT functional limitations and eight sets of G-codes are for SLP functional limitations.

The following G-codes are for functional limitations typically seen in beneficiaries receiving PT or OT services. The first four of these sets describe categories of functional limitations and the final two sets describe "other" functional limitations, which are to be used for functional limitations not described by one of the four categories.

**Appendix 4 — Internet-only Manuals (IOMs)**

## NONPAYABLE G-CODES FOR FUNCTIONAL LIMITATIONS

| | Long Descriptor | Short Descriptor |
|---|---|---|
| **Mobility G-code Set** | | |
| G8978 | Mobility: walking & moving around functional limitation, current status, at therapy episode outset and at reporting intervals | Mobility current status |
| G8979 | Mobility: walking & moving around functional limitation, projected goal status, at therapy episode outset, at reporting intervals, and at discharge or to end reporting | Mobility goal status |
| G8980 | Mobility: walking & moving around functional limitation, discharge status, at discharge from therapy or to end reporting | Mobility D/C status |
| **Changing & Maintaining Body Position G-code Set** | | |
| G8981 | Changing & maintaining body position functional limitation, current status, at therapy episode outset and at reporting intervals | Body pos current status |
| G8982 | Changing & maintaining body position functional limitation, projected goal status, at therapy episode outset, at reporting intervals, and at discharge or to end reporting | Body pos goal status |
| G8983 | Changing & maintaining body position functional limitation, discharge status, at discharge from therapy or to end reporting | Body pos D/C status |
| **Carrying, Moving & Handling Objects G-code Set** | | |
| G8984 | Carrying, moving & handling objects functional limitation, current status, at therapy episode outset and at reporting intervals | Carry current status |
| G8985 | Carrying, moving & handling objects functional limitation, projected goal status, at therapy episode outset, at reporting intervals, and at discharge or to end reporting | Carry goal status |
| G8986 | Carrying, moving & handling objects functional limitation, discharge status, at discharge from therapy or to end reporting | Carry D/C status |
| **Self Care G-code Set** | | |
| G8987 | Self care functional limitation, current status, at therapy episode outset and at reporting intervals | Self care current status |
| G8988 | Self care functional limitation, projected goal status, at therapy episode outset, at reporting intervals, and at discharge or to end reporting | Self care goal status |
| G8989 | Self care functional limitation, discharge status, at discharge from therapy or to end reporting | Self care D/C status |

- The following "other PT/OT" functional G-codes are used to report:
- a beneficiary's functional limitation that is not defined by one of the above four categories;
- a beneficiary whose therapy services are not intended to treat a functional limitation;
- or a beneficiary's functional limitation when an overall, composite or other score from a functional assessment too is used and it does not clearly represent a functional limitation defined by one of the above four code sets.

| | Long Descriptor | Short Descriptor |
|---|---|---|
| **Other PT/OT Primary G-code Set** | | |
| G8990 | Other physical or occupational therapy primary functional limitation, current status, at therapy episode outset and at reporting intervals | Other PT/OT current status |
| G8991 | Other physical or occupational therapy primary functional limitation, projected goal status, at therapy episode outset, at reporting intervals, and at discharge or to end reporting | Other PT/OT goal status |
| G8992 | Other physical or occupational therapy primary functional limitation, discharge status, at discharge from therapy or to end reporting | Other PT/OT D/C status |

| | Long Descriptor | Short Descriptor |
|---|---|---|
| **Other PT/OT Subsequent G-code Set** | | |
| G8993 | Other physical or occupational therapy subsequent functional limitation, current status, at therapy episode outset and at reporting intervals | Sub PT/OT current status |
| G8994 | Other physical or occupational therapy subsequent functional limitation, projected goal status, at therapy episode outset, at reporting intervals, and at discharge or to end reporting | Sub PT/OT goal status |

The following G-codes are for functional limitations typically seen in beneficiaries receiving SLP services. Seven are for specific functional communication measures, which are modeled after the National Outcomes Measurement System (NOMS), and one is for any "other" measure not described by one of the other seven.

| | Long Descriptor | Short Descriptor |
|---|---|---|
| **Swallowing G-code Set** | | |
| G8996 | Swallowing functional limitation, current status, at therapy episode outset and at reporting intervals | Swallow current status |
| G8997 | Swallowing functional limitation, projected goal status, at therapy episode outset, at reporting intervals, and at discharge or to end reporting | Swallow goal status |
| G8998 | Swallowing functional limitation, discharge status, at discharge from therapy or to end reporting | Swallow D/C status |
| **Motor Speech G-code Set (Note: These codes are not sequentially numbered)** | | |
| G8999 | Motor speech functional limitation, current status, at therapy episode outset and at reporting intervals | Motor speech current status |
| G9186 | Motor speech functional limitation, projected goal status at therapy episode outset, at reporting intervals, and at discharge or to end reporting | Motor speech goal status |
| G9158 | Motor speech functional limitation, discharge status, at discharge from therapy or to end reporting | Motor speech D/C status |
| **Spoken Language Comprehension G-code Set** | | |
| G9159 | Spoken language comprehension functional limitation, current status, at therapy episode outset and at reporting intervals | Lang comp current status |
| G9160 | Spoken language comprehension functional limitation, projected goal status, at therapy episode outset, at reporting intervals, and at discharge or to end reporting | Lang comp goal status |
| G9161 | Spoken language comprehension functional limitation, discharge status, at discharge from therapy or to end reporting | Lang comp D/C status |
| **Spoken Language Expressive G-code Set** | | |
| G9162 | Spoken language expression functional limitation, current status, at therapy episode outset and at reporting intervals | Lang express current status |
| G9163 | Spoken language expression functional limitation, projected goal status, at therapy episode outset, at reporting intervals, and at discharge or to end reporting | Lang press goal status |
| G9164 | Spoken language expression functional limitation, discharge status, at discharge from therapy or to end reporting | Lang express D/C status |
| **Attention G-code Set** | | |
| G9165 | Attention functional limitation, current status, at therapy episode outset and at reporting intervals | Atten current status |
| G9166 | Attention functional limitation, projected goal status, at therapy episode outset, at reporting intervals, and at discharge or to end reporting | Atten goal status |

© 2016 Optum360, LLC

| | Long Descriptor | Short Descriptor |
|---|---|---|
| G9167 | Attention functional limitation, discharge status, at discharge from therapy or to end reporting | Atten D/C status |

**Memory G-code Set**

| | Long Descriptor | Short Descriptor |
|---|---|---|
| G9168 | Memory functional limitation, current status, at therapy episode outset and at reporting intervals | Memory current status |
| G9169 | Memory functional limitation, projected goal status, at therapy episode outset, at reporting intervals, and at discharge or to end reporting | Memory goal status |
| G9170 | Memory functional limitation, discharge status, at discharge from therapy or to end reporting | Memory D/C status |

**Voice G-code Set**

| | Long Descriptor | Short Descriptor |
|---|---|---|
| G9171 | Voice functional limitation, current status, at therapy episode outset and at reporting intervals | Voice current status |
| G9172 | Voice functional limitation, projected goal status, at therapy episode outset, at reporting intervals, and at discharge or to end reporting | Voice goal status |
| G9173 | Voice functional limitation, discharge status, at discharge from therapy or to end reporting | Voice D/C status |

The following "other SLP" G-code set is used to report:

- on one of the other eight NOMS-defined functional measures not described by the above code sets; or
- to report an overall, composite or other score from assessment tool that does not clearly represent one of the above seven categorical SLP functional measures.

| | Long Descriptor | Short Descriptor |
|---|---|---|
| **Other Speech Language Pathology G-code Set** | | |
| G9174 | Other speech language pathology functional limitation, current status, at therapy episode outset and at reporting intervals | Speech lang current status |
| G9175 | Other speech language pathology functional limitation, projected goal status, at therapy episode outset, at reporting intervals, and at discharge or to end reporting | Speech lang goal status |
| G9176 | Other speech language pathology functional limitation, discharge status, at discharge from therapy or to end reporting | Speech lang D/C status |

### F. Severity/Complexity Modifiers

For each nonpayable functional G-code, one of the modifiers listed below must be used to report the severity/complexity for that functional limitation.

| Modifier | Impairment Limitation Restriction |
|---|---|
| CH | 0 percent impaired, limited or restricted |
| CI | At least 1 percent but less than 20 percent impaired, limited or restricted |
| CJ | At least 20 percent but less than 40 percent impaired, limited or restricted |
| CK | At least 40 percent but less than 60 percent impaired, limited or restricted |
| CL | At least 60 percent but less than 80 percent impaired, limited or restricted |
| CM | At least 80 percent but less than 100 percent impaired, limited or restricted |
| CN | 100 percent impaired, limited or restricted |

The severity modifiers reflect the beneficiary's percentage of functional impairment as determined by the clinician furnishing the therapy services.

### G. Required Reporting of Functional G-codes and Severity Modifiers

The functional G-codes and severity modifiers listed above are used in the required reporting on therapy claims at certain specified points during therapy episodes of care. Claims containing these functional G-codes must also contain another billable and separately payable (non-bundled) service. Only one functional limitation shall be reported at a given time for each related therapy plan of care (POC).

Functional reporting using the G-codes and corresponding severity modifiers is required reporting on specified therapy claims. Specifically, they are required on claims:

- At the outset of a therapy episode of care (i.e., on the claim for the date of service (DOS) of the initial therapy service);
- At least once every 10 treatment days, which corresponds with the progress reporting period;
- When an evaluative procedure, including a re-evaluative one, ( HCPCS/CPT codes 92506, 92597, 92607, 92608, 92610, 92611, 92612, 92614, 92616, 96105, 96125, 97001, 97002, 97003, 97004) is furnished and billed;
- At the time of discharge from the therapy episode of care–(i.e., on the date services related to the discharge [progress] report are furnished); and
- At the time reporting of a particular functional limitation is ended in cases where the need for further therapy is necessary.
- At the time reporting is begun for a new or different functional limitation within the same episode of care (i.e., after the reporting of the prior functional limitation is ended)

Functional reporting is required on claims throughout the entire episode of care. When the beneficiary has reached his or her goal or progress has been maximized on the initially selected functional limitation, but the need for treatment continues, reporting is required for a second functional limitation using another set of G-codes. In these situations two or more functional limitations will be reported for a beneficiary during the therapy episode of care. Thus, reporting on more than one functional limitation may be required for some beneficiaries but not simultaneously.

When the beneficiary stops coming to therapy prior to discharge, the clinician should report the functional information on the last claim. If the clinician is unaware that the beneficiary is not returning for therapy until after the last claim is submitted, the clinician cannot report the discharge status.

When functional reporting is required on a claim for therapy services, two G-codes will generally be required.

Two exceptions exist:

1. Therapy services under more than one therapy POC. Claims may contain more than two nonpayable functional G-codes when in cases where a beneficiary receives therapy services under multiple POCs (PT, OT, and/or SLP) from the same therapy provider.

2. One-Time Therapy Visit. When a beneficiary is seen and future therapy services are either not medically indicated or are going to be furnished by another provider, the clinician reports on the claim for the DOS of the visit, all three G-codes in the appropriate code set (current status, goal status and discharge status), along with corresponding severity modifiers. Each reported functional G-code must also contain the following line of service information:

   - Functional severity modifier
   - Therapy modifier indicating the related discipline/POC -- GP, GO or GN -- for PT, OT, and SLP services, respectively
   - Date of the related therapy service
   - Nominal charge, e.g., a penny, for institutional claims submitted to the FIs and A/MACs. For professional claims, a zero charge is acceptable for the service line. If provider billing software requires an amount for professional claims, a nominal charge, e.g., a penny, may be included. Note: The KX modifier is not required on the claim line for nonpayable G-codes, but would be required with the procedure code for medically necessary therapy services furnished once the beneficiary's annual cap has been reached.

The following example demonstrates how the G-codes and modifiers are used. In this example, the clinician determines that the beneficiary's mobility restriction is the most clinically relevant functional limitation and selects the Mobility G-code set (G8978 – G8980) to represent the beneficiary's functional limitation. The clinician also determines the severity/complexity of the beneficiary's functional limitation and selects the appropriate modifier. In this example, the clinician determines that the beneficiary has a 75 percent mobility restriction for which the CL modifier is applicable. The clinician expects that at the end of therapy the beneficiaries will have only a 15 percent mobility restriction for which the CI modifier is applicable. When the beneficiary attains the mobility goal, therapy continues to be medically necessary to addresss a functional limitation for which there is no categorical G-code. The clinician reports this using (G8990 – G8992).

At the outset of therapy. On the DOS for which the initial evaluative procedure is furnished or the initial treatment day of a therapy POC, the claim for the service will also include two G-codes as shown below.

- G8978-CL to report the functional limitation (Mobility with current mobility limitation of "at least 60 percent but less than 80 percent impaired, limited or restricted")

- G8979-CI to report the projected goal for a mobility restriction of "at least 1 percent but less than 20 percent impaired, limited or restricted."

At the end of each progress reporting period. On the claim for the DOS when the services related to the progress report (which must be done at least once each 10 treatment days) are furnished, the clinician will report the same two G-codes but the modifier for the current status may be different.

- G8978 with the appropriate modifier are reported to show the beneficiary's current status as of this DOS. So if thebeneficiary has made no progress, this claim will include G8978-CL. If the beneficiary made progress and now has a mobility restriction of 65 percent CL would still be the appropriate modifier for 65 percent, and G8978-CL would be reported in this case. If the beneficiary now has a mobility restriction of 45 percent, G8978-CK would be reported.

- G8979-CI would be reported to show the projected goal. This severity modifier would not change unless the clinician adjusts the beneficiary's goal. This step is repeated as necessary and clinically appropriate, adjusting the current status modifier used as the beneficiary progresses through therapy.

- At the time the beneficiary is discharged from the therapy episode. The final claim for therapy episode will include two G-codes.

- G8979-CI would be reported to show the projected goal. G8980-CI would be reported if the beneficiary attained the 15 percent mobility goal. Alternatively, if the beneficiary's mobility restriction only reached 25 percent; G8980-CJ would be reported. To end reporting of one functional limitation. As noted above, functional reporting is required to continue throughout the entire episode of care. Accordingly, when further therapy is medically necessary after the beneficiary attains the goal for the first reported functional limitation, the clinician would end reporting of the first functional limitation by using the same G-codes and modifiers that would be used at the time of discharge. Using the mobility example, to end reporting of the mobility functional limitation, G8979-CI and G8980-CI would be reported on the same DOS that coincides with end of that progress reporting period.

To begin reporting of a second functional limitation. At the time reporting is begun for a new and different functional limitation, within the same episode of care (i.e., after the reporting of the prior functional limitation is ended). Reporting on the second functional limitation, however, is not begun until the DOS of the next treatment day -- which is day one of the new progress reporting period. When the next functional limitation to be reported is NOT defined by one of the other three PT/OT categorical codes, the G-code set (G8990 - G8992) for the "other PT/OT primary" functional limitation is used, rather than the G-code set for the "other PT/OT subsequent" ? because it is the first reported "other PT/OT" functional limitation. This reporting begins on the DOS of the first treatment day following the mobility "discharge" reporting, which is counted as the initial service for the "other PT/OT primary" functional limitation and the first treatment day of the new progress reporting period. In this case, G8990 and G8991, along with the corresponding modifiers, are reported on the claim for therapy services.

The table below illustrates when reporting is required using this example and what G-codes would be used.

Example of Required Reporting

| Key: Reporting Period (RP) | Begin RP #1 for Mobility at Episode Outset | End RP#1 for Mobility at Progress Report | Mobility RP #2 Begins Next Treatment Day | End RP#2 for Mobility at Progress Report | Mobility RP #3 Begins Next Treatment Day | D/C or End Reporting for \Mobility | Begin RP #1 for Other PT/OT Primary |
|---|---|---|---|---|---|---|---|
| **Mobility: Walking & Moving Around** | | | | | | | |
| G8978 – Current Status | X | X | | X | | | |
| G 8979– Goal Status | X | X | | X | | X | |
| G8980 – Discharge Status | | | | | | X | |
| Other PT/OT Primary | | | | | | | |
| G8990 – Current Status | | | | | | | X |
| G8991 – Goal Status | | | | | | | X |
| G8992 – Discharge Status | | | | | | | |

| No Functional Reporting Req'd | | | X | | X | | |
|---|---|---|---|---|---|---|---|

## H. Required Tracking and Documentation of Functional G-codes and Severity Modifiers

The clinician who furnishes the services must not only report the functional information on the therapy claim, but, he/she must track and document the G-codes and severity modifiers used for this reporting in the beneficiary's medical record of therapy services.

For details related to the documentation requirements, refer to Pub. 100-02, Medicare Benefit Policy Manual, chapter 15, section 220.4, - MCTRJCA-required Functional Reporting. For coverage rules related to MCTRJCA and therapy goals, refer to Pub. 100-02: a) for outpatient therapy services, see chapter 15, section 220.1.2 B and b) for instructions specific to PT, OT, and SLP services in the CORF, see chapter 12, section 10.

## 100-04, 5, 20.4

### Coding Guidance for Certain CPT Codes - All Claims

The following provides guidance about the use of codes 96105, 97026, 97150, 97545, 97546, and G0128.

### CPT Codes 96105, 97545, and 97546.

Providers report code 96105, assessment of aphasia with interpretation and report in 1-hour units. This code represents formal evaluation of aphasia with an instrument such as the Boston Diagnostic Aphasia Examination. If this formal assessment is performed during treatment, it is typically performed only once during treatment and its medical necessity should be documented. If the test is repeated during treatment, the medical necessity of the repeat administration of the test must also be documented. It is common practice for regular assessment of a patient's progress in therapy to be documented in the chart, and this may be done using test items taken from the formal examinations. This is considered to be part of the treatment and should not be billed as 96105 unless a full, formal assessment is completed.

Other timed physical medicine codes are 97545 and 97546. The interval for code 97545 is 2 hours and for code 97546, 1 hour. These are specialized codes to be used in the context of rehabilitating a worker to return to a job. The expectation is that the entire time period specified in the codes 97545 or 97546 would be the treatment period, since a shorter period of treatment could be coded with another code such as codes 97110, 97112, or 97537. (Codes 97545 and 97546 were developed for reporting services to persons in the worker's compensation program, thus we do not expect to see them reported for Medicare patients except under very unusual circumstances. Further, we would not expect to see code 97546 without also seeing code 97545 on the same claim. Code 97546, when used, is used in conjunction with 97545.)

### CPT Code 97026

Effective for services performed on or after October 24, 2006, the Centers for Medicare & Medicaid Services announce a NCD stating the use of infrared and/or near-infrared light and/or heat, including monochromatic infrared energy (MIRE), is non-covered for the treatment, including symptoms such as pain arising from these conditions, of diabetic and/or non-diabetic peripheral sensory neuropathy, wounds and/or ulcers of the skin and/or subcutaneous tissues in Medicare beneficiaries. Further coverage guidelines can be found in the National Coverage Determination Manual (Publication 100-03), section 270.6.

Contractors shall deny claims with CPT 97026 (infrared therapy incident to or as a PT/OT benefit) and HCPCS E0221 or A4639, if the claim contains any of the following ICD-9 codes: 250.60-250.63, 354.4, 354.5, 354.9, 355.1-355.4, 355.6-355.9, 356.0, 356.2-356.4, 356.8-356.9, 357.0-357.7, 674.10, 674.12, 674.14, 674.20, 674.22, 674.24, 707.00-707.07, 707.09-707.15, 707.19, 870.0-879.9, 880.00-887.7, 890.0-897.7, 998.31-998.32. Contractors can use the following messages when denying the service:

- Medicare Summary Notice # 21.11 "This service was not covered by Medicare at the time you received it."

- Reason Claim Adjustment Code #50 "These are noncovered services because this is not deemed a medical necessity by the payer."

Advanced Beneficiary Notice (ABN): Physicians, physical therapists, occupational therapists, outpatient rehabilitation facilities (ORFs), comprehensive outpatient rehabilitation facilities (CORFs), home health agencies (HHA), and hospital outpatient departments are liable if the service is performed, unless the beneficiary signs an ABN.

Similarly, DME suppliers and HHA are liable for the devices when they are supplied, unless the beneficiary signs an ABN.

## 100-04, 5, 100.3

### Proper Reporting of Nursing Services by CORFs - A/B MAC (A)

(Rev. 1459; Issued: 02-22-08; Effective: 07-01-08; Implementation: 07-07-08)

Nursing services performed in the CORF shall be billed utilizing the following HCPCS code:

G0128 – Direct (Face to Face w/ patient) skilled nursing services of a registered nurse provided in a CORF, each 10 minutes beyond the first 5 minutes.

In addition, HCPCS G0128 is billable with revenue codes 0550 and 0559 only.

## 100-04, 5, 100.4

### Outpatient Mental Health TreatmentLimitation

The Outpatient Mental Health Treatment Limitation (the limitation) is not applicable to CORF services because CORFs do not provide services to treat mental, psychoneurotic and personality disorders that are subject to the limitation in section 1833(c) of the Act. For dates of service on or after October 1, 2012, HCPCS code G0409 is the only code allowed for social work and psychological services furnished in a CORF. This service is not subject to the limitation because it is not a psychiatric mental health treatment service.

For additional information on the limitation, see Publication 100-01, Chapter 3, section 30 and Publication 100-02, Chapter 12, sections 50-50.5.

## 100-04, 5, 100.11

### Billing for Social Work and Psychological Services in a CORF

The CORF providers shall only bill social work and psychological services with the following HCPCS code:

G0409 Social work and psychological services, directly relating to and/or the patient's rehabilitation goals, each 15 minutes, face-to-face; individual (services provided by a CORF-qualified social worker or psychologist in a CORF).

In addition, HCPCS code G0409 shall only be billed with revenue code 0569 or 0911.

## 100-04, 6, 20.1.1.2

### Hospital's "Facility Charge" in Connection with Clinic Services of a Physician

(Rev. 3230, Issued: 04-03-15, Effective: 06-15-15, Implementation: 06-15-15)

As noted above in section 20.1.1, physician services are excluded from Part A PPS payment and the requirement for consolidated billing. When a beneficiary receives clinic services from a hospital-based physician, the physician in this situation would bill his or her own professional services directly to the Part B MAC and would be reimbursed at the facility rate of the Medicare physician fee schedule--which does not include overhead expenses. The hospital historically has submitted a separate Part B "facility charge" for the associated overhead expenses to its Part A MAC. The hospital's facility charge does not involve a separate service (such as a diagnostic test) furnished in addition to the physician's professional service; rather, it represents solely the overhead expenses associated with furnishing the professional service itself. Accordingly, hospitals bill for "facility charges" under the physician evaluation and management (E&M) codes in the range of 99201-99245 and G0463 (for hospitals paid under the Outpatient Prospective Payment System).

E&M codes, representing the hospital's "facility charge" for the overhead expenses associated with furnishing the professional service itself, are excluded from SNF CB. Effective for claims with dates of service on or after January 1, 2006, the CWF will bypass CB edits when billed with revenue code 0510 (clinic visit) with an E&M HCPCS code in the range of 99201-99245 and, effective January 1, 2014 with HCPCS code G0463.

NOTE: Unless otherwise excluded in one of the Five Major Categories for billing services to FIs, physician services codes are to be billed to the carrier by the physician. Facility charges associated with the physician's clinic visit must be reported as explained above.

## 100-04, 7, 80.2

### Mammography Screening

Section 4163 of the Omnibus Budget Reconciliation Act of 1990 added §1834(c) of the Act to provide for Part B coverage of mammography screening for certain women entitled to Medicare for screenings performed on or after January 1, 1991. The term "screening mammography" means a radiologic procedure provided to an asymptomatic woman for the purpose of early detection of breast cancer and includes a physician's interpretation of the results of the procedure. Unlike diagnostic mammographies, there do not need to be signs, symptoms, or history of breast disease in order for the exam to be covered.

The technical component portion of the screening mammography should be billed on the the ASC X12 837 institutional claim format or if permissible Form CMS-1450

under bill type 22X for SNF Part A and Part B inpatients or 23X for SNF outpatients. Claims for mammography screening should include only the charges for the screening mammography.

## 100-04, 8, 60.2.1.1

### Separately Billable ESRD Drugs

The following categories of drugs (including but not limited to) are separately billable when used to treat the patient's renal condition:

- Antibiotics;
- Analgesics;
- Anabolics;
- Hematinics;
- Muscle relaxants;
- Sedatives;
- Tranquilizers; and
- Thrombolytics: used to declot central venous catheters. **Note:** Thrombolytics were removed from the separately billable drugs for claims with dates of service on or after January 1, 2013.

For claims with dates of service on or after July 1, 2013, when these drugs are administered through the dialysate the provider must append the modifier JE (Administered via Dialysate).

These separately billable drugs may only be billed by an ESRD facility if they are actually administered in the facility by the facility staff. Staff time used to administer separately billable drugs is covered under the composite rate and may not be billed separately. However, the supplies used to administer these drugs may be billed in addition to the composite rate.

Effective January 1, 2011, section 153b of the MIPPA requires that all ESRD-related drugs and biologicals be billed by the renal dialysis facility. When a drug or biological is billed by providers other than the ESRD facility and the drug or biological furnished is designated as a drug or biological that is included in the ESRD PPS (ESRD-related), the claim will be rejected or denied. In the event that an ESRD-related drug or biological was furnished to an ESRD beneficiary for reasons other than for the treatment of ESRD, the provider may submit a claim for separate payment using modifier AY.

All drugs reported on the renal dialysis facility claim are considered included in the ESRD PPS. The list of drugs and biologicals for consolidated billing are designated as always ESRD-related and therefore not allowing separate payment to be made to ESRD facilities. However, CMS has determined that some of these drugs may warrant separate payment.

**Exceptions to "Always ESRD Related" Drugs:**

The following drugs have been approved for separate payment consideration when billed with the AY modifier attesting to the drug not being used for the treatment of ESRD. The ESRD facility is required to indicate (in accordance with ICD-9 guidelines) the diagnosis code for which the drug is indicated.

- Vancomycin, effective January 1, 2012
- Daptomycin, effective January 1, 2013

Items and services subject to the consolidated billing requirements for the ESRD PPS can be found on the CMS website at:

http://www.cms.gov/ESRDPayment/50_Consolidated_Billing.asp#TopOfPage.

Other drugs and biologicals may be considered separately payable to the dialysis facility if the drug was not for the treatment of ESRD. The facility must include the modifier AY to indicate it was not for the treatment of ESRD.

Drugs are assigned HCPCS codes. If no HCPCS code is listed for a drug (e.g., a new drug) the facility bills using HCPCS code J3490, "Unclassified Drugs," and submits documentation identifying the drug. To establish a code for the drug, the FI checks HCPCS to verify that there is no acceptable HCPCS code for billing and if a code is not found checks with the local carrier, which may have a code and price that is appropriate. If no code is found the drug is processed under HCPCS code J3490. See Chapter 17 for a complete description of drug pricing.

## 100-04, 8, 60.2.4.2

### Physician Billing Requirements to the A/B MAC (B)

#### A. Sodium Ferric Gluconate Complex in Sucrose Injection

Sodium Ferric Gluconate Complex in sucrose injection may be payable for claims with dates of service on or after December 1, 2000 when furnished intravenously, for first line treatment of iron deficiency anemia in patients undergoing chronic hemodialysis who are receiving supplemental erythropoietin therapy. Physicians bill and A/B MACs (B) pay for HCPCS code J1756 when submitted with a primary diagnosis for chronic renal failure and a secondary diagnosis for iron deficiency anemia.

These diagnoses are listed below. Use ICD-9-CM or ICD-10-CM as applicable for the service date.

Chronic Renal Failure (Primary Diagnosis):

- ICD-9-CM – 585
- ICD-10-CM – N18.3, N18.4, N18.5, N18.6,

Iron Deficiency Anemia (Secondary Diagnosis):

- ICD-9-CM – 280.0, 280.1, 280.8, or 280.9
- ICD-10-CM – D50.0, D50.1, D50.8, D50.9,D63.1

This benefit is subject to the Part B deductible and coinsurance and should be paid per current Medicare drug payment reimbursement rules. A/B MACs (B) may cover other uses of this drug at their discretion.

**B. Iron Sucrose Injection**

Iron Sucrose injections are payable for claims with dates of service on or after October 1, 2001, when furnished intravenously, for first line treatment of iron deficiency anemia in patients undergoing chronic hemodialysis who are receiving supplemental erythropoeitin therapy. Until a specific code for iron sucrose injection is developed, providers must submit HCPCS code J1756, with the appropriate explanation of drug name and dosage entered on the claim. The primary diagnosis code for chronic renal failure and one of the following secondary diagnosis codes for iron deficiency must be entered.

These diagnoses are listed below. Use ICD-9-CM or ICD-10-CM as applicable for the service date.

- Chronic Renal Failure (Primary Diagnosis)
- ICD-9-CM - 585
- ICD-10-CM - N18.3, N18.4, N18.5, N18.6, Iron Deficiency Anemia (Secondary Diagnosis)
- ICD-9-CM – 280.0, 280.1, 280.8, or 280.9
- ICD-10-CM – D50.0, D50.1, D50.8, D50.9,D63.1

Iron sucrose injection is subject to the Part B deductible and coinsurance and should be paid per current Medicare drug payment reimbursement rules. A/B MACs (B) may cover other uses of this drug at their discretion.

**C. Messages for Use with Denials**

The following denial messages should be used to deny claims for sodium ferric gluconate complex in sucrose injection or iron sucrose injection due to a missing diagnosis code.

Remittance Advice: Claim adjustment reason code 16, Claim/service lacks information which is needed for adjudication, along with remark code M76, Incomplete/invalid patient's diagnosis(es) and condition (s).

Explanation of Medicare Benefits: 9.8, Medicare cannot pay for this service because the claim is missing information/documentation.

Medicare Summary Notice: 9.2, This item or service was denied because information required to make payment was missing.

## 100-04, 8, 60.4

**Erythropoietin Stimulating Agents (ESAs)**

Coverage rules for ESAs are explained in the Medicare Benefit Policy Manual, Publication 100-02, chapter 11.

Fiscal intermediaries (FIs) pay for ESAs, to end-stage renal disease (ESRD) facilities as separately billable drugs to the composite rate. No additional payment is made to administer an ESA, whether in a facility or a home. Effective January 1, 2005, the cost of supplies to administer EPO may be billed to the FI. HCPCS A4657 and Revenue Code 270 should be used to capture the charges for syringes used in the administration of EPO.

ESAs and their administration supplies are included in the payment for the ESRD Prospective Payment System effective January 1, 2011. Providers must continue to report ESAs on the claim as ESAs are subject to a national claims monitoring program and are entitled to outlier payment consideration. The Medicare allowed payment (MAP) amount for outlier includes the ESA rate provided on the Average Sale Price (ASP) list, subject to reduction based on the ESA monitoring policy.

Medicare has an established national claims monitoring policy for erythropoietin stimulating agents for the in-facility dialysis population as outlined in the sections below.

## 100-04, 8, 60.4.1

**ESA Claims Monitoring Policy**

Effective for services provided on or after April 1, 2006, Medicare has implemented a national claims monitoring policy for ESAs administered in Medicare renal dialysis

facilities. This policy does not apply to claims for ESAs for patients who receive their dialysis at home and self-administer their ESA.

While Medicare is not changing its coverage policy on erythropoietin use to maintain a target hematocrit level between 30% and 36%, we believe the variability in response to ESAs warrants postponing requiring monitoring until the hematocrit reaches higher levels. For dates of services April 1, 2006, and later, the Centers for Medicare & Medicaid Services (CMS) claims monitoring policy applies when the hematocrit level exceeds 39.0% or the hemoglobin level exceeds 13.0g/dL. This does not preclude the contractors from performing medical review at lower levels.

Effective for services provided on or after April 1, 2006, for claims reporting hematocrit or hemoglobin levels exceeding the monitoring threshold, the dose shall be reduced by 25% over the preceding month. Providers may report that a dose reduction did occur in response to the reported elevated hematocrit or hemoglobin level by adding a GS modifier on the claim. The definition of the GS modifier is defined as: "Dosage of ESA has been reduced and maintained in response to hematocrit or hemoglobin level." Thus, for claims reporting a hematocrit level or hemoglobin level exceeding the monitoring threshold without the GS modifier, CMS will reduce the covered dosage reported on the claim by 25%. The excess dosage is considered to be not reasonable and necessary. Providers are reminded that the patient's medical records should reflect hematocrit/hemoglobin levels and any dosage reduction reported on the claim during the same time period for which the claim is submitted.

Effective for dates of service provided on and after January 1, 2008, requests for payments or claims for ESAs for ESRD patients receiving dialysis in renal dialysis facilities reporting a hematocrit level exceeding 39.0% (or hemoglobin exceeding 13.0g/dL) shall also include modifier ED and EE. Claims reporting neither modifier or both modifiers will be returned to the provider for correction.

The definition of modifier ED is "The hematocrit level has exceeded 39.0% (or hemoglobin 1evel has exceeded 13.0g/dL) 3 or more consecutive billing cycles immediately prior to and including the current billing cycle." The definition of modifier EE is "The hematocrit level has exceeded 39.0% (or hemoglobin level has exceeded 13.0g/dL) less than 3 consecutive billing cycles immediately prior to and including the current billing cycle." The GS modifier continues to be defined as stated above.

Providers may continue to report the GS modifier when the reported hematocrit or hemoglobin levels exceed the monitoring threshold for less than 3 months and a dose reduction has occurred. When both modifiers GS and EE are included, no reduction in the covered dose will occur. Claims reporting a hematocrit or hemoglobin level exceeding the monitoring threshold and the ED modifier shall have an automatic 50% reduction in the covered dose applied, even if the claim also reports the GS modifier.

Below is a chart illustrating the resultant claim actions under all possible reporting scenarios:

| Hct Exceeds 39.0% or Hgb Exceeds 13.0g/dL | ED Modifier? (Hct >39% or Hgb >13g/dL =3 cycles) | EE Modifier? Hct >39% or Hgb >13g/dL <3 cycles) | GS Modifier? (Dosage reduced and maintained) | Claim Action |
|---|---|---|---|---|
| No | N/A | N/A | N/A | Do not reduce reported dose. |
| Yes | No | No | No | Return to provider for correction. Claim must report either modifier ED or EE. |
| Yes | No | No | Yes | Return to provider for correction. Claim must report either modifier ED or EE. |
| Yes | No | Yes | Yes | Do not reduce reported dose. |
| Yes | No | Yes | No | Reduce reported dose 25%. |
| Yes | Yes | No | Yes | Reduce reported dose 50%. |
| Yes | Yes | No | No | Reduce reported dose 50%. |

In some cases, physicians may believe there is medical justification to maintain a hematocrit above 39.0% or hemoglobin above 13.0g/dL. Beneficiaries, physicians, and/or renal facilities may submit additional medical documentation to justify this belief under the routine appeal process. You may reinstate any covered dosage reduction amounts under this first level appeal process when you believe the documentation supports a higher hematocrit/hemoglobin level.

Providers are reminded that, in accordance with FDA labeling, CMS expects that as the hematocrit approaches 36.0% (hemoglobin 12.0g/dL), a dosage reduction occurs. Providers are expected to maintain hematocrit levels between 30.0 to 36.0% (hemoglobin 10.0-12.0g/dL). Hematocrit levels that remain below 30.0% (hemoglobin levels below 10.0g/dL) despite dosage increases, should have causative factors evaluated. The patient's medical record should reflect the clinical reason for dose changes and hematocrit levels outside the range of 30.0-36.0% (hemoglobin levels 10.0-12.0g/dL). Medicare contractors may review medical records to assure appropriate dose reductions are applied and maintained and hematological target ranges are maintained.

These hematocrit requirements apply only to ESAs furnished as an ESRD benefit under §1881(b) of the Social Security Act.

### Medically Unlikely Edits (MUE)

For dates of service on and after January 1, 2008, the MUE for claims billing for Epogen® is reduced to 400,000 units from 500,000. The MUE for claims for Aranesp® is reduced to 1200 mcg from 1500 mcg.

For dates of service on and after April 1, 2013, the MUE for claims billing for peginesatide is applicable when units billed are equal to or greater than 26 mg.

It is likely that claims reporting doses exceeding the threshold reflect typographical errors and will be returned to providers for correction.

## 100-04, 8, 60.4.2

### 60.4.2 - Facility Billing Requirements for ESAs

#### Hematocrit and Hemoglobin Levels

Renal dialysis facilities are required to report hematocrit or hemoglobin levels for their Medicare patients receiving erythropoietin products. Hematocrit levels are reported in value code 49 and reflect the most recent reading taken before the start of the billing period. Hemoglobin readings before the start of the billing period are reported in value code 48.

To report a hemoglobin or hematocrit reading for a new patient on or after January 1, 2006, the provider should report the reading that prompted the treatment of epoetin alfa. The provider may use results documented on form CMS 2728 or the patient's medical records from a transferring facility.

Effective January 1, 2012, ESRD facilities are required to report hematocrit or hemoglobin levels on all ESRD claims. Reporting the value 99.99 is not permitted when billing for an ESA.

The revenue codes for reporting Epoetin Alfa are 0634 and 0635. All other ESAs are reported using revenue code 0636. The HCPCS code for the ESA must be included: HCPCS

| HCPCS | HCPCS Description | Dates of Service |
|-------|-------------------|------------------|
| Q4055 | Injection, Epoetin Alfa, 1,000 units (for ESRD on Dialysis) | 1/1/2004 through 12/31/2005 |
| J0886 | Injection, Epoetin Alfa, 1,000 units (for ESRD on Dialysis) | 1/1/2006 through 12/31/2006 |
| Q4081 | Injection, Epoetin alfa, 100 units (for ESRD on Dialysis) | 1/1/2007 to present |
| Q4054 | Injection, Darbepoetin Alfa, 1mcg (for ESRD on Dialysis) | 1/1/2004 through 12/31/2005 |
| J0882 | Injection, Darbepoetin Alfa, | 1/1/2006 to present |

Each administration of an ESA is reported on a separate line item with the units reported used as a multiplier by the dosage description in the HCPCS to arrive at the dosage per administration.

#### Route of Administration Modifiers

Patients with end stage renal disease (ESRD) receiving administrations of erythropoiesis stimulating agents (ESA) for the treatment of anemia may receive intravenous administration or subcutaneous administrations of the ESA. Effective for claims with dates of services on or after January 1, 2012, all facilities billing for injections of ESA for ESRD beneficiaries must include the modifier JA on the claim to indicate an intravenous administration or modifier JB to indicate a subcutaneous administration. ESRD claims containing ESA administrations that are submitted without the route of administration modifiers will be returned to the provider for correction. Renal dialysis facilities claim including charges for administrations of the ESA by both methods must report separate lines to identify the number of administration provided using each method.

Effective July 1, 2013, providers must identify when a drug is administered via the dialysate by appending the modifier JE (administered via dialysate).

### ESA Monitoring Policy Modifiers

Append modifiers ED, EE and GS as applicable, see instructions in section 60.4.1.

### Maximum Allowable Administrations

The maximum number of administrations of EPO for a billing cycle is 13 times in 30 days and 14 times in 31 days.

The maximum number of administrations of Aranesp for a billing cycle is 5 times in 30/ 31days.

The maximum number of administrations of Peginesatide is 1 time in 30/ 31days.

## 100-04, 8, 60.4.4

### Payment Amount for Epoetin Alfa (EPO)

~Dates of service prior to January 1, 2005, the Medicare contractor pays the facility $10 per 1,000 units of EPO administered, rounded to the nearest 100 units (i.e., $1.00 per 100 units). Effective January 1, 2005, EPO will be paid based on the ASP Pricing File. Also effective January 1, 2005, the cost of supplies to administer EPO may be billed to the Medicare contractor. HCPCS A4657 and Revenue Code 270 should be used to capture the charges for syringes used in the administration of EPO. Where EPO is furnished by a supplier that is not a facility, the DMERC pays at the same rate.

Physician payment is calculated through the drug payment methodology described in Chapter 17 of the Claims Processing Manual.

**EXAMPLE:** The billing period is 2/1/94 - 2/28/94.

The facility provides the following:

| Date | Units | Date | Units |
|------|-------|------|-------|
| 2/1 | 3000 | 2/15 | 2500 |
| 2/4 | 3000 | 2/18 | 2500 |
| 2/6 | 3000 | 2/20 | 2560 |
| 2/8 | 3000 | 2/22 | 2500 |
| 2/11 | 2500 | 2/25 | 2000 |
| 2/13 | 2500 | 2/27 | 2000 |

Total 31,060 units

For value code 68, the facility enters 31,060. The 31,100 are used to determine the rate payable. This is 31,060 rounded to the nearest 100 units. The amount payable is 31.1 x $10 =$311.00. In their systems, FIs have the option of setting up payment of $1.00 per 100 units. Effective January 1, 2005, EPO will be paid based on the ASP Pricing File.

Effective January 1, 2008, payment is calculated on a renal dialysis facility claim at the line level by multiplying the rate from the ASP pricing file by the number of units reported on the line billing for EPO.

**EXAMPLE:** 311 x $1.00 = $311.00

If an ESRD beneficiary requires 10,000 units or more of EPO per administration, special documentation must be made in the medical records. It must consist of a narrative report that addresses the following:

- Iron deficiency. Most patients need supplemental iron therapy while being treated, even if they do not start out iron deficient;
- Concomitant conditions such as infection, inflammation, or malignancy. These conditions must be addressed to assure that EPO has maximum effect;
- Unrecognized blood loss. Patients with kidney disease and anemia may easily have chronic blood loss (usually gastrointestinal) as a major cause of anemia. In those circumstances, EPO is limited in effectiveness;
- Concomitant hemolysis, bone morrow dysplasia, or refractory anemia for a reason other than renal disease, e.g., aluminum toxicity;
- Folic acid or vitamin B12 deficiencies;
- Circumstances in which the bone morrow is replaced with other tissue, e.g., malignancy or osteitis fibrosa cystica; and

Patient's weight, the current dose required, a historical record of the amount that has been given, and the hematocrit response to date.

Payment for ESRD-related EPO is included in the ESRD PPS for claims with dates of service on or after January 1, 2011.

## 100-04, 8, 60.4.4.1

### Payment for Epoetin Alfa (EPO) in Other Settings

~With the implementation of the ESRD PPS, ESRD-related EPO is included in ESRD PPS payment amount and is not separately payable on Part B claims with dates of service on or after January 1, 2011 for other providers with the exception of a hospital billing for an emergency or unscheduled dialysis session.

In the hospital inpatient setting, payment under Part A is included in the DRG.

In the hospital inpatient setting, payment under Part B is made on bill type 12x. Hospitals report the drug units based on the units defined in the HCPCS description. Hospitals do not report value code 68 for units of EPO. For dates of service prior to April 1, 2006, report EPO under revenue code 0636. For dates of service from April 1, 2006 report EPO under the respective revenue code 0634 for EPO less than 10,000 units and revenue code 0635 for EPO over 10,000 units. Payment will be based on the ASP Pricing File.

In a skilled nursing facility (SNF), payment for EPO covered under the Part B EPO benefit is not included in the prospective payment rate for the resident's Medicare-covered SNF stay.

In a hospice, payment is included in the hospice per diem rate.

For a service furnished by a physician or incident to a physician's service, payment is made to the physician by the carrier in accordance with the rules for 'incident to' services. When EPO is administered in the renal facility, the service is not an "incident to" service and not under the "incident to" provision.

## 100-04, 8, 60.4.4.2

### Epoetin Alfa (EPO) Provided in the Hospital Outpatient Departments

When ESRD patients come to the hospital for an unscheduled or emergency dialysis treatment they may also require the administration of EPO. Effective January 1, 2005, EPO will be paid based on the ASP Pricing File.

Hospitals use type of bill 13X (or 85X for Critical Access Hospitals) and report charges under the respective revenue code 0634 for EPO less than 10,000 units and revenue code 0635 for EPO over 10,000 units. Hospitals report the drug units based on the units defined in the HCPCS description. Hospitals do not report value code 68 for units of EPO. Value code 49 must be reported with the hematocrit value for the hospital outpatient visits prior to January 1, 2006, and for all claims with dates of service on or after January 1, 2008.

## 100-04, 8, 60.4.5.1

### Self Administered ESA Supply

Initially, facilities may bill for up to a 2-month supply of an ESA for Method I beneficiaries who meet the criteria for selection for self-administration. After the initial two months' supply, the facility will bill for one month's supply at a time. Condition code 70 is used to indicate payment requested for a supply of an ESA furnished a beneficiary. Usually, revenue code 0635 would apply to EPO since the supply would be over 10,000 units. Facilities leave FL 46, Units of Service, blank since they are not administering the drug.

For claims with dates of service on or after January 1, 2008, supplies of an ESA for self administration should be billed according to the pre-determined plan of care schedule provided to the beneficiary. Submit a separate line item for each date an administration is expected to be performed with the expected dosage. In the event that the schedule was changed, the provider should note the changes in the medical record and bill according to the revised schedule. For patients beginning to self administer an ESA at home receiving an extra month supply of the drug, bill the one month reserve supply on one claim line and include modifier EM defined as "Emergency Reserve Supply (for ESRD benefit only)".

When billing for drug wastage in accordance with the policy in chapter 17 of this manual, section 40.1 the provider must show the wastage on a separate line item with the modifier JW. The line item date of service should be the date of the last covered administration according to the plan of care or if the patient dies use the date of death.

Condition code 70 should be reported on claims billing for home dialysis patients that self administer anemia management drugs including ESAs.

## 100-04, 8, 60.4.6.3

### Payment Amount for Darbepoetin Alfa (Aranesp)

For Method I patients, the FI pays the facility per one mcg of Aranesp administered, in accordance with the MMA Drug Payment Limits Pricing File rounded up to the next highest whole mcg. Effective January 1, 2005, Aranesp will be paid based on the ASP Pricing File. Effective January 1, 2005, the cost of supplies to administer Aranesp may be billed to the FI. HCPCS A4657 and Revenue Code 270 should be used to capture the charges for syringes used in the administration of Aranesp.

Physician payment is calculated through the drug payment methodology described in Chapter 17, of the Claims Processing Manual.

The coinsurance and deductible are based on the Medicare allowance payable, not on the provider's charges. The provider may not charge the beneficiary more than 20 percent of the Medicare Aranesp allowance. This rule applies to independent and hospital based renal facilities.

Payment for ESRD-related Aranesp is included in the ESRD PPS for claims with dates of service on or after January 1, 2011.

## 100-04, 8, 60.4.6.4

### Payment for Darbepoetin Alfa (Aranesp) in Other Settings

In the hospital inpatient setting, payment under Part A for Aranesp is included in the DRG.

In the hospital inpatient setting, payment under Part B is made on bill type 12x when billed with revenue code 0636. The total number of units as a multiple of 1mcg is placed in the unit field. Reimbursement is based on the payment allowance limit for Medicare Part B drugs as found in the ASP pricing file.

In a skilled nursing facility (SNF), payment for Aranesp covered under the Part B EPO benefit is not included in the prospective payment rate for the resident's Medicare-covered SNF stay.

In a hospice, payment is included in the hospice per diem rate.

For a service furnished by a physician or incident to a physician's service, payment is made to the physician by the carrier in accordance with the rules for 'incident to' services. When Aranesp is administered in the renal facility, the service is not an "incident to" service and not under the "incident to" provision.

With the implementation of the ESRD PPS, ESRD-related Aranesp is included in the ESRD PPS payment amount and is not separately payable on Part B claims with dates of service on or after January 1,2011 for other providers, with the exception of a hospital billing for an emergency or unscheduled dialysis session.

## 100-04, 8, 60.4.6.5

### Payment for Darbepoetin Alfa (Aranesp) in the Hospital Outpatient Department

When ESRD patients come to the hospital for an unscheduled or emergency dialysis treatment they may also require the administration of Aranesp. For patients with ESRD who are on a regular course of dialysis, Aranesp administered in a hospital outpatient department is paid the MMA Drug Pricing File rate. Effective January 1, 2005, Aranesp will be paid based on the ASP Pricing File.

Hospitals use bill type 13X (or 85X for Critical Access Hospitals) and report charges under revenue code 0636. The total number of units as a multiple of 1mcg is placed in the unit field. Value code 49 must be reported with the hematocrit value for the hospital outpatient visits prior to January 1, 2006, and for all claims with dates of service on or after January 1, 2008.

## 100-04, 8, 60.4.7

### Payment for Peginesatide in the Hospital Outpatient Department

When ESRD patients come to the hospital for an unscheduled or emergency dialysis treatment they may also require the administration of an ESA, such as peginesatide. When hospitals bill for an unscheduled or emergency outpatient dialysis session (G0257) they may include the administration of an ESA.

## 100-04, 8, 60.7

### Darbepoetin Alfa (Aranesp) for ESRD Patients

Coverage rules for Aranesp® are explained in the Medicare Benefit Policy Manual, Publication 100-02, chapter 11. For an explanation of Method I and Method II reimbursement for patients dialyzing at home see section 40.1.

Fiscal intermediaries (FIs) pay for Aranesp® to end-stage renal disease (ESRD) facilities as a separately billable drug to the composite rate. No additional payment is made to administer Aranesp®, whether in a facility or a home. Effective January 1, 2005, the cost of supplies to administer Aranesp® may be billed to the FI. HCPCS A4657 and Revenue Code 270 should be used to capture the charges for syringes used in the administration of Aranesp®.

If the beneficiary obtains Aranesp® from a supplier for self-administration, the supplier bills the durable medical equipment regional carrier (DMERC), and the DMERC pays in accordance with MMA Drug Payment Limits Pricing File.

Program payment may not be made to a physician for self-administration of Aranesp®. When Aranesp® is furnished by a physician as "incident to services," the carrier processes the claim.

For ESRD patients on maintenance dialysis treated in a physician's office, code J0882, "injection, darbepoetin alfa, 1 mcg (for ESRD patients)," should continue to be used with the hematocrit included on the claim. (For ANSI 837 transactions, the hematocrit (HCT) value is reported in 2400 MEA03 with a qualifier of R2 in 2400 MEA02.) Claims without this information will be denied due to lack of documentation. Physicians who provide Aranesp® for ESRD patients on maintenance dialysis must bill using code J0882.

### Darbepoetin Alfa Payment Methodology

| Type of Provider | Separately Billable | DMERC Payment | No payment |
|---|---|---|---|
| In-facility freestanding and hospital-based ESRD facility | X | | |
| Self-administer Home Method I | X | | |
| Self-administer Home Method II | | X | |
| Incident to physician in facility or for self-administration * | | | X |

Medicare pays for a drug if self-administered by a dialysis patient. When Aranesp® is administered in a dialysis facility, the service is not an "incident to" service, and not under the "incident to" provision.

Renal dialysis facilities are required to report hematocrit or hemoglobin levels for their Medicare patients receiving erythropoietin products. Hematocrit levels are reported in value code 49 and reflect the most recent reading taken before the start of the billing period. Hemoglobin readings before the start of the billing period are reported in value code 48. See ?60.4.1.

Effective January 1, 2012, ESRD facilities are required to report hematocrit or hemoglobin levels on all ESRD claims irrespective of ESA administration. Reporting the value 99.99 is not permitted when billing for an ESA.

Effective January 1, 2012, renal dialysis facilities are required to report hematocrit or hemoglobin levels on all ESRD claims irrespective of ESA administration. Reporting the value 99.99 is not permitted when billing for an ESA.

Effective for services provided on or after April 1, 2006, Medicare has implemented a national claims monitoring policy for Aranesp® administered in Medicare renal dialysis facilities. This policy does not apply to claims for Aranesp® for patients who receive their dialysis at home and self-administer their Aranesp®.

While Medicare is not changing its coverage policy on erythropoietin use to maintain a target hematocrit level between 30% and 36%, we believe the variability in response to EPO warrants postponing requiring monitoring until the hematocrit reaches higher levels. For dates of services on and after April 1, 2006, the Centers for Medicare & Medicaid Services (CMS) will not initiate monitoring until the hematocrit level exceeds 39.0% or the hemoglobin level exceeds 13.0g/dL. This does not preclude the contractors from performing medical review at lower levels. The Food and Drug Administration (FDA) labeling for Aranesp® notes that as the hematocrit approaches a reading of 36.0% (or hemoglobin 12.0g/dL), the dose of the drug should be reduced by 25%.

Effective for dates of service provided on or after April 1, 2006, for claims reporting hematocrit or hemoglobin levels exceeding the monitoring threshold, the dose shall be reduced by 25% over the preceding month. Providers may report that a dose reduction did occur in response to the reported elevated hematocrit or hemoglobin level by adding a GS modifier on the claim. The definition of the GS modifier continues to be defined as: "Dosage of EPO or Darbepoetin Alfa has been reduced and maintained in response to hematocrit or hemoglobin level." Thus, for claims reporting a hematocrit level or hemoglobin level exceeding the monitoring threshold without the GS modifier, CMS shall reduce the dosage reported on the claim by 25%. The excess dosage is considered to be not reasonable and necessary. Providers are reminded that the patient? medical records should reflect hematocrit/hemoglobin levels and any dosage reduction reported on the claim during the same time period for which the claim is submitted.

Effective for dates of service provided on an after January 1, 2008, requests for payments or claims for Aranesp® for ESRD patients receiving dialysis in renal dialysis facilities reporting a hematocrit level exceeding 39.0% (or hemoglobin exceeding 13.0g/dL) shall also include modifier ED or EE. Claims reporting neither modifier or both modifiers will be returned to the provider for correction.

The definition of modifier ED is "The hematocrit level has exceeded 39.0% (or hemoglobin 1evel has exceeded 13.0g/dL) 3 or more consecutive billing cycles immediately prior to and including the current billing cycle." The definition of modifier EE is "The hematocrit level has exceeded 39.0% (or hemoglobin level has exceeded 13.0g/dL) less than 3 consecutive billing cycles immediately prior to and including the current billing cycle." The GS modifier continues to be defined as stated above.

Providers may continue to report the GS modifier when the reported hematocrit or hemoglobin levels exceed the monitoring threshold for less than 3 months and a dose reduction has occurred. When both modifiers GS and EE are included, no reduction in the reported dose will occur. Claims reporting a hematocrit or hemoglobin level exceeding the monitoring threshold and the ED modifier shall have an automatic 50% reduction in the reported dose applied, even if the claim also reports the GS modifier.

Below is a chart illustrating the resultant claim actions under all possible reporting scenarios.

| Hct Exceeds 39.0% or Hgb Exceeds 13.0g/dL | ED Modifier? (Hct >39% or Hgb >13g/dL =3 cycles) | EE Modifier? (Hct >39% or Hgb >13g/dL <3 cycles) | GS Modifier? (Dosage reduced and maintained) | Claim Action |
|---|---|---|---|---|
| No | N/A | N/A | N/A | Do not reduce reported dose. |
| Yes | No | No | No | Return to provider for correction. Claim must report either ED or EE. |
| Yes | No | No | Yes | Return to provider for correction. Claim must report either ED or EE. |
| Yes | No | Yes | Yes | Do not reduce reported dose. |
| Yes | No | Yes | No | Reduce reported dose 25%. |
| Yes | Yes | No | Yes | Reduce reported dose 50%. |
| Yes | Yes | No | No | Reduce reported dose 50%. |

These hematocrit requirements apply only to Aranesp® furnished as an ESRD benefit under ?1881(b) of the Social Security Act. Aranesp® furnished incident to a physician? service is not included in this policy. Carriers have discretion for local policy for Aranesp® furnished as "incident to service."

## 100-04, 8, 60.7.3

### Payment Amount for Darbepoetin Alfa (Aranesp)

For Method I patients, the FI pays the facility per one mcg of Aranesp administered, in accordance with the MMA Drug Payment Limits Pricing File rounded up to the next highest whole mcg. Effective January 1, 2005, Aranesp will be paid based on the ASP Pricing File. Effective January 1, 2005, the cost of supplies to administer Aranesp may be billed to the FI. HCPCS A4657 and Revenue Code 270 should be used to capture the charges for syringes used in the administration of Aranesp.

Physician payment is calculated through the drug payment methodology described in Chapter 17, of the Claims Processing Manual.

The coinsurance and deductible are based on the Medicare allowance payable, not on the provider‚Äüs charges. The provider may not charge the beneficiary more than 20 percent of the Medicare Aranesp allowance. This rule applies to independent and hospital based renal facilities.

Payment for ESRD-related Aranesp is included in the ESRD PPS for claims with dates of service on or after January 1, 2011.

## 100-04, 9, 150

### Initial Preventive Physical Examination (IPPE)

Effective for services furnished on or after January 1, 2005, Section 611 of the Medicare Prescription Drug Improvement and Modernization Act of 2003 (MMA) provides for coverage under Part B of one initial preventive physical examination (IPPE) for new beneficiaries only, subject to certain eligibility and other limitations. For RHCs the Part B deductible for IPPE is waived for services provided on or after January 1, 2009. FQHC services are always exempt from the Part B deductible. Coinsurance is applicable.

Payment for the professional services will be made under the all-inclusive rate. Encounters with more than one health professional and multiple encounters with the same health professionals that take place on the same day and at a single location generally constitute a single visit. However, in rare circumstances an RHC/FQHC can receive a separate payment for an encounter in addition to the payment for the IPPE when they are performed on the same day.

RHCs and FQHCs must HCPCS code for IPPE for the following reasons:

- To avoid application of deductible (on RHC claims);
- To assure payment for this service in addition to another encounter on the same day if they are both separate, unrelated, and appropriate; and
- To update the CWF record to track this once in a lifetime benefit.

Beginning with dates of service on or after January 1, 2009 if an IPPE is provided in an RHC or FQHC, the professional portion of the service is billed to the FI or Part A MAC using TOBs 71X and 73X, respectively, and the appropriate site of service revenue code in the 052X revenue code series, and must include HCPCS G0402. Additional information on IPPE can be found in Chapter 18, section 80 of this manual.

NOTE: The technical component of an EKG performed at a clinic/center is not a Medicare-covered RHC/FQHC service and is not billed by the independent RHC/FQHC. Rather, it is billed to Medicare carriers or Part B MACs on professional claims (Form CMS-1500 or 837P) under the practitioner's ID following instructions for submitting practitioner claims. Likewise, the technical component of the EKG performed at a provider-based clinic/center is not a Medicare-covered RHC/FQHC service and is not billed by the provider-based RHC\FQHC. Instead, it is billed on the applicable TOB and submitted to the FI or Part A MAC using the base provider's ID following instructions for submitting claims to the FI/Part A MAC from the base provider. For the professional component of the EKG, there is no separate payment and no separate billing of it. The IPPE is the only HCPCS for which the deductible is waived under this benefit. For more information on billing for a screening EKG see chapter 18 section 80 of this manual.

## 100-04, 9, 181

### 181 - Diabetes Self-Management Training (DSMT) Services Provided by RHCs and FQHCs

A - FQHCs  Previously, DSMT type services rendered by qualified registered dietitians or nutrition professionals were considered incident to services under the FQHC benefit, if all relevant program requirements were met. Therefore, separate all-inclusive encounter rate payment could not be made for the provision of DSMT services. With passage of DRA, effective January 1, 2006, FQHCs are eligible for a separate payment under Part B for these services provided they meet all program requirements. See Pub. 100-04, chapter 18, section 120. Payment is made at the all-inclusive encounter rate to the FQHC. This payment can be in addition to payment for any other qualifying visit on the same date of service as the beneficiary received qualifying DSMT services.

For FQHCs to qualify for a separate visit payment for DSMT services, the services must be a one-on-one face-to-face encounter. Group sessions don't constitute a billable visit for any FQHC services. Rather, the cost of group sessions is included in the calculation of the all-inclusive FQHC visit rate. To receive separate payment for DSMT services, the DSMT services must be billed on TOB 73X with HCPCS code G0108 and the appropriate site of service revenue code in the 052X revenue code series. This payment can be in addition to payment for any other qualifying visit on the same date of service that the beneficiary received qualifying DSMT services as long as the claim for DSMT services contains the appropriate coding specified above. Additional information on DSMT can be found in Chapter 18, section 120 of this manual.

NOTE: DSMT is not a qualifying visit on the same day that MNT is provided.

Group services (G0109) do not meet the criteria for a separate qualifying encounter. All line items billed on TOBs 73x with HCPCS codes for DSMT services will be denied.

B - RHCs  Separate payment to RHCs for these practitioners/services continues to be precluded as these services are not within the scope of Medicare-covered RHC benefits. Note that the provision of the services by registered dietitians or nutritional professionals, might be considered incident to services in the RHC setting, provided all applicable conditions are met. However, they do not constitute an RHC visit, in and of themselves. All line items billed on TOB 71x with HCPCS code G0108 or G0109 will be denied.

## 100-04, 9, 182

### Medical Nutrition Therapy (MNT) Services

#### A - FQHCs

Previously, MNT type services were considered incident to services under the FQHC benefit, if all relevant program requirements were met. Therefore, separate all-inclusive encounter rate payment could not be made for the provision of MNT services. With passage of DRA, effective January 1, 2006, FQHCs are eligible for a separate payment under Part B for these services provided they meet all program requirements. Payment is made at the all-inclusive encounter rate to the FQHC. This payment can be in addition to payment for any other qualifying visit on the same date of service as the beneficiary received qualifying MNT services.

For FQHCs to qualify for a separate visit payment for MNT services, the services must be a one-on-one face-to-face encounter. Group sessions don't constitute a billable visit for any FQHC services. Rather, the cost of group sessions is included in the calculation of the all-inclusive FQHC visit rate. To receive payment for MNT services, the MNT services must be billed on TOB 73X with the appropriate individual MNT HCPCS code (codes 97802, 97803, or G0270) and with the appropriate site of service revenue code in the 052X revenue code series. This payment can be in addition to payment for any other qualifying visit on the same date of service as the beneficiary received qualifying MNT services as long as the claim for MNT services contain the appropriate coding specified above.

NOTE: MNT is not a qualifying visit on the same day that DSMT is provided.

Additional information on MNT can be found in Chapter 4, section 300 of this manual.

Group services (HCPCS 97804 or G0271) do not meet the criteria for a separate qualifying encounter. All line items billed on TOB 73x with HCPCS code 97804 or G0271 will be denied.

#### B - RHCs

Separate payment to RHCs for these practitioners/services continues to be precluded as these services are not within the scope of Medicare-covered RHC benefits. All line items billed on TOB 71x with HCPCS codes for MNT services will be denied.

## 100-04, 10, 40.2

### HH PPS Claims

The following data elements are required to submit a claim under home health PPS. For billing of home health claims not under an HH plan of care (not under HH PPS), see §90. Home health services under a plan of care are paid based on a 60-day episode of care. Payment for this episode will usually be made in two parts. After an RAP has been paid and a 60-day episode has been completed, or the patient has been discharged, the HHA submits a claim to receive the balance of payment due for the episode.

HH PPS claims will be processed in Medicare claims processing systems as debit/credit adjustments against the record created by the RAP, except in the case of "No-RAP" LUPA claims (see §40.3). As the claim is processed the payment on the RAP will be reversed in full and the full payment due for the episode will be made on the claim. Both the debit and credit actions will be reflected on the remittance advice (RA) so the net payment on the claim can be easily understood. Detailed RA information is contained in chapter 22.

### Billing Provider Name, Address, and Telephone Number

Required – The HHA's minimum entry is the agency's name, city, State, and ZIP Code. The post office box number or street name and number may be included. The State may be abbreviated using standard post office abbreviations. Five or nine-digit ZIP Codes are acceptable. Medicare contractors use this information in connection with the provider identifier to verify provider identity.

### Patient Control Number and Medical/Health Record Number

Required - The patient's control number may be shown if the patient is assigned one and the number is needed for association and reference purposes.

The HHA may enter the number assigned to the patient's medical/health record. If this number is entered, the Medicare contractor must carry it through their system and return it on the remittance record.

### Type of Bill

Required - This 3-digit alphanumeric code gives three specific pieces of information. The first digit identifies the type of facility. The second classifies the type of care. The third indicates the sequence of this bill in this particular episode of care. It is referred to as a "frequency" code. The types of bill accepted for HH PPS claims are any combination of the codes listed below:

Code Structure (only codes used to bill Medicare are shown).

lst Digit-Type of Facility

    3 - Home Health

2nd Digit-Bill Classification (Except Clinics and Special Facilities)

    2 - Hospital Based or Inpatient (Part B) (includes HHA visits under a Part B plan of treatment).

NOTE: While the bill classification of 3, defined as "Outpatient (includes HHA visits under a Part A plan of treatment and use of HHA DME under a Part A plan of treatment)" may also be appropriate to an HH PPS claim, Medicare encourages HHAs to submit all claims with bill classification 2. Medicare claims systems determine whether an HH claim should be paid from the Part A or Part B trust fund and will change the bill classification digit on the electronic claim record as necessary to reflect this.

3rd Digit-Frequency - Definition

7 - Replacement of Prior Claim - HHAs use to correct a previously submitted bill. Apply this code for the corrected or "new" bill. These adjustment claims must be accepted at any point within the timely filing period after the payment of the original claim.

8 - Void/Cancel of a Prior Claim - HHAs use this code to indicate this bill is an exact duplicate of an incorrect bill previously submitted. A replacement RAP or claim must be submitted for the episode to be paid.

9 - Final Claim for an HH PPS Episode - This code indicates the HH bill should be processed as a debit/credit adjustment to the RAP. This code is specific to home health and does not replace frequency codes 7, or 8.

HHAs must submit HH PPS claims with the frequency of "9." These claims may be adjusted with frequency "7" or cancelled with frequency "8." Medicare contractors do not accept late charge bills, submitted with frequency "5," on HH PPS claims. To add services within the period of a paid HH claim, the HHA must submit an adjustment.

**Statement Covers Period**
Required - The beginning and ending dates of the period covered by this claim. The "from" date must match the date submitted on the RAP for the episode. For continuous care episodes, the "through" date must be 59 days after the "from" date. The patient status code must be 30 in these cases.

In cases where the beneficiary has been discharged or transferred within the 60-day episode period, HHAs will report the date of discharge in accordance with internal discharge procedures as the "through" date. If the beneficiary has died, the HHA reports the date of death in the "through date."

Any NUBC approved patient status code may be used in these cases. The HHA may submit claims for payment immediately after the claim "through" date. It is not required to hold claims until the end of the 60-day episode unless the beneficiary continues under care.

**Patient Name/Identifier**
Required – The HHA enters the patient's last name, first name, and middle initial.

**Patient Address**
Required - The HHA enters the patient's full mailing address, including street number and name, post office box number or RFD, City, State, and ZIP Code.

**Patient Birth Date**
Required - The HHA enters the month, day, and year of birth of patient. If the full correct date is not known, leave blank.

**Patient Sex**
Required - "M" for male or "F" for female must be present. This item is used in conjunction with diagnoses and surgical procedures to identify inconsistencies.

**Admission/Start of Care Date**
Required - The HHA enters the same date of admission that was submitted on the RAP for the episode.

**Point of Origin for Admission or Visit**
Required - The HHA enters the same point of origin code that was submitted on the RAP for the episode.

**Patient Discharge Status**
Required - The HHA enters the code that most accurately describes the patient's status as of the "Through" date of the billing period. Any applicable NUBC approved code may be used.

Patient status code 06 should be reported in all cases where the HHA is aware that the episode will be paid as a partial episode payment (PEP) adjustment. These are cases in which the agency is aware that the beneficiary has transferred to another HHA within the 60-day episode, or the agency is aware that the beneficiary was discharged with the goals of the original plan of care met and has been readmitted within the 60-day episode. Situations may occur in which the HHA is unaware at the time of billing the discharge that these circumstances exist. In these situations, Medicare claims processing systems will adjust the discharge claim automatically to reflect the PEP adjustment, changing the patient status code on the paid claims record to 06.

In cases where an HHA is changing the Medicare contractor to which they submit claims, the service dates on the claims must fall within the provider's effective dates at each contractor. To ensure this, RAPs for all episodes with "from" dates before the provider's termination date must be submitted to the contractor the provider is leaving. The resulting episode must be resolved by the provider submitting claims for shortened periods, with "through" dates on or before the termination date. The provider must indicate that these claims will be PEP adjustments by using patient status code 06. Billing for the beneficiary is being "transferred" to the new contractor.

In cases where the ownership of an HHA is changing and the CMS certification number (CCN) also changes, the service dates on the claims must fall within the

effective dates of the terminating CCN. To ensure this, RAPs for all episodes with "from" dates before the termination date of the CCN must be resolved by the provider submitting claims for shortened periods, with "through" dates on or before the termination date. The provider must indicate that these claims will be PEP adjustments by using patient status 06. Billing for the beneficiary is being "transferred" to the new agency ownership. In changes of ownership which do not affect the CCN, billing for episodes is also unaffected.

In cases where an HHA is aware in advance that a beneficiary will become enrolled in a Medicare Advantage (MA) Organization as of a certain date, the provider should submit a claim for the shortened period prior to the MA Organization enrollment date. The claim should be coded with patient status 06. Payment responsibility for the beneficiary is being "transferred" from Medicare fee-for-service to MA Organization, since HH PPS applies only to Medicare fee-for-service.

If HHAs require guidance on OASIS assessment procedures in these cases, they should contact the appropriate state OASIS education coordinator.

**Condition Codes**
Conditional – The HHA enters any NUBC approved code to describe conditions that apply to the claim.

If the RAP is for an episode in which the patient has transferred from another HHA, the HHA enters condition code 47.

HHAs that are adjusting previously paid claims enter one of the condition codes representing Claim Change Reasons (code values D0 through E0). If adjusting the claim to correct a HIPPS code, HHAs use condition code D2 and enter "Remarks" indicating the reason for the HIPPS code change. HHAs use D9 if multiple changes are necessary.

When submitting a HH PPS claim as a demand bill, HHAs use condition code 20. See §50 for more detailed instructions regarding demand billing.

When submitting a HH PPS claim for a denial notice, HHAs use condition code 21. See §60 for more detailed instructions regarding no-payment billing.

Required - If canceling the claim (TOB 0328), HHAs report the condition codes D5 or D6 and enter "Remarks" indicating the reason for cancellation of the claim.

**Occurrence Codes and Dates**
Conditional - The HHA enters any NUBC approved code to describe occurrences that apply to the claim.

**Occurrence Span Code and Dates**
Conditional - The HHA enters any NUBC approved Occurrence Span code to describe occurrences that apply to the claim. Reporting of occurrence span code 74 is not required to show the dates of an inpatient admission during an episode.

**Value Codes and Amounts**
Required - Home health episode payments must be based upon the site at which the beneficiary is served. For episodes in which the beneficiary's site of service changes from one CBSA to another within the episode period, HHAs should submit the CBSA code corresponding to the site of service at the end of the episode on the claim.

NOTE: Contractor-entered value codes. The Medicare contractor enters codes 17 and 62 - 65 on the claim in processing. They may be visible in the Medicare contractor's online claim history and on remittances.

| Code | Title | Definition |
|---|---|---|
| 17 | Outlier Amount | The amount of any outlier payment returned by the Pricer with this code. (Contractors always place condition code 61 on the claim along with this value code.) |
| 61 | Location Where Service is Furnished (HHA and Hospice) | HHAs report the MSA number or Core Based Statistical Area (CBSA) number (or rural state code) of the location where the home health or hospice service is delivered. The HHA reports the number in dollar portion of the form locator right justified to the left of the dollar/cents delimiter, add two zeros to the cents field if no cents. |
| 62 | HH Visits - Part A | The number of visits determined by Medicare to be payable from the Part A trust fund to reflect the shift of payments from the Part A to the Part B trust fund as mandated by §1812 (a)(3) of the Social Security Act. |
| 63 | HH Visits - Part B | The number of visits determined by Medicare to be payable from the Part B trust fund to reflect the shift of payments from the Part A to the Part B trust fund as mandated by §1812 (a)(3) of the Social Security Act. |

| Code | Title | Definition |
|------|-------|------------|
| 64 | HH Reimbursement - Part A | The dollar amounts determined to be associated with the HH visits identified in a value code 62 amount. This Part A payment reflects the shift of payments from the Part A to the Part B trust fund as mandated by §1812 (a)(3) of the Social Security Act. |
| 65 | HH Reimbursement - Part B | The dollar amounts determined to be associated with the HH visits identified in a value code 63 amount. This Part B payment reflects the shift of payments from the Part A to the Part B trust fund as mandated by §1812 (a)(3) of the Social Security Act. |

If information returned from the Common Working File (CWF) indicates all visits on the claim are Part A, the shared system must place value codes 62 and 64 on the claim record, showing the total visits and total PPS payment amount as the values, change the TOB on the claim record to 33X, and send the claim to CWF with RIC code V.

If information returned from CWF indicates all visits on the claim are Part B, the shared system must place value codes 63 and 65 on the claim record, showing the total visits and total PPS payment amount as the values, change the TOB on the claim record to 32X, and send the claim to CWF with RIC code W.

If information returned from CWF indicates certain visits on the claim are payable from both Part A and Part B, the shared system must place value codes 62, 63, 64, and 65 on the claim record. The shared system also must populate the values for code 62 and 63 based on the numbers of visits returned from CWF and prorate the total PPS reimbursement amount based on the numbers of visits to determine the dollars amounts to be associated with value codes 64 and 65. The shared system will not change the TOB and will return the claim to CWF with RIC code U.

### Revenue Code and Revenue Description

### Required

HH PPS claims must report a 0023 revenue code line on which the first four positions of the HIPPS code match the code submitted on the RAP. The fifth position of the code represents the non-routine supply (NRS) severity level. This fifth position may differ to allow the HHA to change a code that represents that supplies were provided to a code that represents that supplies were not provided, or vice versa. However, the fifth position may only change between the two values that represent the same NRS severity level. Section 10.1.9 of this chapter contains the pairs of corresponding values. If these criteria are not met, Medicare claims processing systems will return the claim.

HHAs enter only one 0023 revenue code per claim in all cases.

Unlike RAPs, claims must also report all services provided to the beneficiary within the episode. Each service must be reported in line item detail. Each service visit (revenue codes 042x, 043x, 044x, 055x, 056x and 057x) must be reported as a separate line. Any of the following revenue codes may be used:

| 027X | Medical/Surgical Supplies (Also see 062X, an extension of 027X) |
|------|------------------------------------------------------------------|
| | Required detail: With the exception of revenue code 0274 (prosthetic and orthotic devices), only service units and a charge must be reported with this revenue code. If also reporting revenue code 0623 to separately identify specific wound care supplies, not just supplies for wound care patients, ensure that the charge amounts for revenue code 0623 lines are mutually exclusive from other lines for supply revenue codes reported on the claim. Report only nonroutine supply items in this revenue code or in 0623. |
| | Revenue code 0274 requires an HCPCS code, the date of service units and a charge amount. |
| | NOTE: Revenue Codes 0275 through 0278 are not used for Medicare billing on HH PPS types of bills |
| 042X | Physical Therapy |
| | Required detail: One of the physical therapy HCPCS codes defined below in the instructions for the HCPCS code field, the date of service, service units which represent the number of 15 minute increments that comprised the visit, and a charge amount. |
| 043X | Occupational Therapy |
| | Required detail: One of the occupational therapy HCPCS codes defined below in the instructions for the HCPCS code field, the date of service, service units which represent the number of 15 minute increments that comprised the visit, and a charge amount. |

| 044X | Speech-Language Pathology |
|------|---------------------------|
| | Required detail: One of the speech-language pathology HCPCS codes defined below in the instructions for the HCPCS code field, the date of service, service units which represent the number of 15 minute increments that comprised the visit, and a charge amount. |
| 055X | Skilled Nursing |
| | Required detail: One of the skilled nursing HCPCS codes defined below in the instructions for the HCPCS code field, the date of service, service units which represent the number of 15 minute increments that comprised the visit, and a charge amount. |
| 056X | Medical Social Services |
| | Required detail: The medical social services HCPCS code defined below in the instructions for the HCPCS code field, the date of service, service units which represent the number of 15 minute increments that comprised the visit, and a charge amount. |
| 057X | Home Health Aide (Home Health) |
| | Required detail: The home health aide HCPCS code defined below in the instructions for the HCPCS code field, the date of service, service units which represent the number of 15 minute increments that comprised the visit, and a charge amount. |

NOTE: Contractors do not accept revenue codes 058X or 059X when submitted with covered charges on Medicare home health claims under HH PPS. They also do not accept revenue code 0624, investigational devices, on HH claims under HH PPS.

| 029X | Durable Medical Equipment (DME) (Other Than Renal) |
|------|----------------------------------------------------|
| | Required detail: the applicable HCPCS code for the item, a date of service indicating the purchase date or the beginning date of a monthly rental, a number of service units, and a charge amount. Monthly rental items should be reported with a separate line for each month's rental and service units of one. |
| | Revenue code 0294 is used to bill drugs/supplies for the effective use of DME. |
| 060X | Oxygen (Home Health) |
| | Required detail: the applicable HCPCS code for the item, a date of service, a number of service units, and a charge amount. |

### Revenue Codes for Optional Billing of DME

Billing of Durable Medical Equipment (DME) provided in the episode is not required on the HH PPS claim. Home health agencies retain the option to bill these services to their Medicare contractor processing home health claims or to have the services provided under arrangement with a supplier that bills these services to the DME MAC. Agencies that choose to bill DME services on their HH PPS claims must use the revenue codes below. These services will be paid separately in addition to the HH PPS amount, based on the applicable Medicare fee schedule. For additional instructions for billing DME services see chapter 20.

| 0274 | Prosthetic/Orthotic Devices |
|------|------------------------------|
| | Required detail: the applicable HCPCS code for the item, a date of service, a number of service units, and a charge amount. |
| 029X | Durable Medical Equipment (DME) (Other Than Renal) |
| | Required detail: the applicable HCPCS code for the item, a date of service indicating the purchase date or the beginning date of a monthly rental, a number of service units, and a charge amount. Monthly rental items should be reported with a separate line for each month's rental and service units of one. |
| | Revenue code 0294 is used to bill drugs/supplies for the effective use of DME. |
| 060X | Oxygen (Home Health) |
| | Required detail: the applicable HCPCS code for the item, a date of service, a number of service units, and a charge amount. |

                                          © 2016 Optum360, LLC

**Revenue Code for Optional Reporting of Wound Care Supplies**

| 0623 | Medical/Surgical Supplies - Extension of 027X |
|------|-----------------------------------------------|
|      | Required detail: Only service units and a charge must be reported with this revenue code. If also reporting revenue code 027x to identify nonroutine supplies other than those used for wound care, the HHA must ensure that the charge amounts for the two revenue code lines are mutually exclusive. |

HHAs may voluntarily report a separate revenue code line for charges for nonroutine wound care supplies, using revenue code 0623. Notwithstanding the standard abbreviation "surg dressings," HHAs use this code to report charges for ALL nonroutine wound care supplies, including but not limited to surgical dressings.

Pub. 100-02, Medicare Benefit Policy Manual, chapter 7, defines routine vs. nonroutine supplies. HHAs use that definition to determine whether any wound care supply item should be reported in this line because it is nonroutine.

HHAs can assist Medicare's future refinement of payment rates if they consistently and accurately report their charges for nonroutine wound care supplies under revenue center code 0623. HHAs should ensure that charges reported under revenue code 027x for nonroutine supplies are also complete and accurate.

**Validating Required Reporting of Supply Revenue Code**
The HH PPS includes a separate case-mix adjustment for non-routine supplies. Nonroutine supply severity levels are indicated on HH PPS claims through a code value in the 5th position of the HIPPS code. The 5th position of the HIPPS code can contain two sets of values. One set of codes (the letters S through X) indicate that supplies were provided. The second set of codes (the numbers 1 through 6) indicate the HHA is intentionally reporting that they did not provide supplies during the episode. See section 10.1.9 for the complete composition of HIPPS under the HH PPS.

HHAs must ensure that if they are submitting a HIPPS code with a 5th position containing the letters S through X, the claim must also report a non-routine supply revenue with covered charges. This revenue code may be either revenue code 27x, excluding 274, or revenue code 623, consistent with the instructions for optional separate reporting of wound care supplies.

Medicare systems will return the claim to the HHA if the HIPPS code indicates nonroutine supplies were provided and supply charges are not reported on the claim. When the HHA receives a claim returned for this reason, the HHA must review their records regarding the supplies provided to the beneficiary. The HHA may take one of the following actions, based on the review of their records:

- If non-routine supplies were provided, the supply charges must be added to the claim using the appropriate supply revenue code.
- If non-routine supplies were not provided, the HHA must indicate that on the claim by changing the 5th position of the HIPPS code to the appropriate numeric value in the range 1 through 6.

After completing one of these actions, the HHA may return the claim to the Medicare contractor for continued adjudication.

**HCPCS/Accommodation Rates/HIPPS Rate Codes**
Required - On the 0023 revenue code line, the HHA must report the HIPPS code that was reported on the RAP. The first four positions of the code must be identical to the value reported on the RAP. The fifth position may vary from the letter value reported on the RAP to the corresponding number which represents the same non-routine supply severity level but which reports that non-routine supplies were not provided.

HHAs enter only one HIPPS code per claim in all cases. Claims submitted with additional HIPPS codes will be returned to the provider.

Medicare may change the HIPPS used for payment of the claim in the course of claims processing, but the HIPPS code submitted by the provider in this field is never changed or replaced. If the HIPPS code is changed, the code used for payment is recorded in the APC-HIPPS field of the electronic claim record.

For revenue code lines other than 0023, the HHA reports HCPCS codes as appropriate to that revenue code.

To report HH visits on episodes beginning before January 1, 2011, the HHA reports a single HCPCS code to represent each HH care discipline. These codes are:

G0151 Services of physical therapist in home health or hospice setting, each 15 minutes.

G0152 Services of an occupational therapist in home health or hospice setting, each 15 minutes.

G0153 Services of a speech language pathologist in home health or hospice setting, each 15 minutes.

G0154 Services of skilled nurse in the home health or hospice settings, each 15 minutes.

G0155 Services of a clinical social worker under a home health plan of care, each 15 minutes.

G0156 Services of a home health aide under a home health plan of care, each 15 minutes.

To report HH visits on episodes beginning on or after January 1, 2011, the HHA reports one of the following HCPCS code to represent each HH care discipline:

Physical Therapy (revenue code 042x)

G0151 Services performed by a qualified physical therapist in the home health or hospice setting, each 15 minutes.

G0157 Services performed by a qualified physical therapist assistant in the home health or hospice setting, each 15 minutes.

G0159 Services performed by a qualified physical therapist, in the home health setting, in the establishment or delivery of a safe and effective physical therapy maintenance program, each 15 minutes.

Occupational Therapy (revenue code 043x)

G0152 Services performed by a qualified occupational therapist in the home health or hospice setting, each 15 minutes.

G0158 Services performed by a qualified occupational therapist assistant in the home health or hospice setting, each 15 minutes.

G0160 Services performed by a qualified occupational therapist, in the home health setting, in the establishment or delivery of a safe and effective occupational therapy maintenance program, each 15 minutes.

Speech-Language Pathology (revenue code 044x)

G0153 Services performed by a qualified speech-language pathologist in the home health or hospice setting, each 15 minutes.

G0161 Services performed by a qualified speech-language pathologist, in the home health setting, in the establishment or delivery of a safe and effective speech-language pathology maintenance program, each 15 minutes.

Note that modifiers indicating services delivered under a therapy plan of care (modifiers GN, GO or GP) are not required on HH PPS claims.

Skilled Nursing (revenue code 055x)

G0154 Direct skilled services of a licensed nurse (LPN or RN) in the home health or hospice setting, each 15 minutes.

G0162 Skilled services by a licensed nurse (RN only) for management and evaluation of the plan of care, each 15 minutes (the patient's underlying condition or complication requires an RN to ensure that essential non-skilled care achieves its purpose in the home health or hospice setting).

G0163 Skilled services of a licensed nurse (LPN or RN) for the observation and assessment of the patient's condition, each 15 minutes (the change in the patient's condition requires skilled nursing personnel to identify and evaluate the patient's need for possible modification of treatment in the home health or hospice setting).

G0164 Skilled services of a licensed nurse (LPN or RN), in the training and/or education of a patient or family member, in the home health or hospice setting, each 15 minutes.

Medical Social Services (revenue code 056x)

G0155 Services of a clinical social worker under a home health plan of care, each 15 minutes.

Home Health Aide (revenue code 057x)

G0156 Services of a home health aide under a home health plan of care, each 15 minutes.

Regarding all skilled nursing and skilled therapy visits

In the course of a single visit, a nurse or qualified therapist may provide more than one of the nursing or therapy services reflected in the codes above. HHAs must not report more than one G-code for each visit regardless of the variety of services provided during the visit. In cases where more than one nursing or therapy service is provided in a visit, the HHA must report the G-code which reflects the service for which the clinician spent most of his/her time.

For instance, if direct skilled nursing services are provided, and the nurse also provides training/education of a patient or family member during that same visit, we would expect the HHA to report the G-code which reflects the service for which most of the time was spent during that visit. Similarly, if a qualified therapist is performing a therapy service and also establishes a maintenance program during the same visit, the HHA should report the G-code which reflects the service for which most of the time was spent during that visit. In all cases, however, the number of 15-minute increments reported for the visit should reflect the total time of the visit.

### Service Date

Required - On the 0023 revenue code line, the HHA reports the date of the first service provided under the HIPPS code. For other line items detailing all services within the episode period, it reports service dates as appropriate to that revenue code. Coding detail for each revenue code under HH PPS is defined above under Revenue Codes. For service visits that begin in 1 calendar day and span into the next calendar day, report one visit using the date the visit ended as the service date.

When the claim Admission Date matches the Statement Covers "From" Date, Medicare systems ensure that the Service Date on the 0023 revenue code line also matches these dates.

### Service Units

Required - Transaction standards require the reporting of a number greater than zero as the units on the 0023 revenue code line. However, Medicare systems will disregard the submitted units in processing the claim. For line items detailing all services within the episode period, the HHA reports units of service as appropriate to that revenue code. Coding detail for each revenue code under HH PPS is defined above under Revenue Codes.

For the revenue codes that represent home health visits (042x, 043x, 044x, 055x, 056x, and 057x), the HHA reports as service units a number of 15 minute increments that comprise the time spent treating the beneficiary. Time spent completing the OASIS assessment in the home as part of an otherwise covered and billable visit and time spent updating medical records in the home as part of such a visit may also be reported. Visits of any length are to be reported, rounding the time to the nearest 15-minute increment. Visits cannot be split into multiple lines. Report covered and noncovered increments of the same visit on the same line.

### Total Charges

Required - The HHA must report zero charges on the 0023 revenue code line (the field must contain zero).

For line items detailing all services within the episode period, the HHA reports charges as appropriate to that revenue code. Coding detail for each revenue code under HH PPS is defined above under Revenue Codes. Charges may be reported in dollars and cents (i.e., charges are not required to be rounded to dollars and zero cents). Medicare claims processing systems will not make any payments based upon submitted charge amounts.

### Non-covered Charges

Required – The HHA reports the total non-covered charges pertaining to the related revenue code here. Examples of non-covered charges on HH PPS claims may include:

- Visits provided exclusively to perform OASIS assessments
- Visits provided exclusively for supervisory or administrative purposes
- Therapy visits provided prior to the required re-assessments

### Payer Name

Required - See chapter 25.

### Release of Information Certification Indicator

Required - See chapter 25.

### National Provider Identifier – Billing Provider

Required - The HHA enters their provider identifier.

### Insured's Name

Required only if MSP involved. See Pub. 100-05, Medicare Secondary Payer Manual.

### Patient's Relationship To Insured

Required only if MSP involved. See Pub. 100-05, Medicare Secondary Payer Manual.

### Insured's Unique Identifier

Required only if MSP involved. See Pub. 100-05, Medicare Secondary Payer Manual.

### Insured's Group Name

Required only if MSP involved. See Pub. 100-05, Medicare Secondary Payer Manual.

### Insured's Group Number

Required only if MSP involved. See Pub. 100-05, Medicare Secondary Payer Manual.

### Treatment Authorization Code

Required - The HHA enters the claim-OASIS matching key output by the Grouper software. This data element enables historical claims data to be linked to individual OASIS assessments supporting the payment of individual claims for research purposes. It is also used in recalculating payment group codes in the HH Pricer (see section 70).

The format of the treatment authorization code is shown here:

| Position | Definition | Format |
|---|---|---|
| 1-2 | M0030 (Start-of-care date) —2 digit year | 99 |
| 3-4 | M0030 (Start-of-care date) —alpha code for date | XX |
| 5-6 | M0090 (Date assessment completed) —2 digit year | 99 |
| 7-8 | M0090 (Date assessment completed) —alpha code for date | XX |
| 9 | M0100 (Reason for assessment) | 9 |
| 10 | M0110 (Episode Timing) —Early = 1, Late = 2 | 9 |
| 11 | Alpha code for Clinical severity points —under Equation 1 | X |
| 12 | Alpha code for Functional severity points —under Equation 1 | X |
| 13 | Alpha code for Clinical severity points —under Equation 2 | X |
| 14 | Alpha code for Functional severity points —under Equation 2 | X |
| 15 | Alpha code for Clinical severity points —under Equation 3 | X |
| 16 | Alpha code for Functional severity points —under Equation 3 | X |
| 17 | Alpha code for Clinical severity points —under Equation 4 | X |
| 18 | Alpha code for Functional severity points —under Equation 4 | X |

NOTE: The dates in positions 3-4 and 7-8 are converted to 2 position alphabetic values using a hexavigesimal coding system. The 2 position numeric point scores in positions 11 – 18 are converted to a single alphabetic code using the same system. Tables defining these conversions are included in the documentation for the Grouper software that is available on the CMS Web site. This is an example of a treatment authorization code created using this format:

| Position | Definition | Actual Value | Resulting Code |
|---|---|---|---|
| 1-2 | M0030 (Start-of-care date) —2 digit year | 2007 | 07 |
| 3-4 | M0030 (Start-of-care date) —code for date | 09/01 | JK |
| 5-6 | M0090 (Date assessment completed) —2 digit year | 2008 | 08 |
| 7-8 | M0090 (Date assessment completed) —code for date | 01/01 | AA |
| 9 | M0100 (Reason for assessment) | 04 | 4 |
| 10 | M0110 (Episode Timing) | 01 | 1 |
| 11 | Clinical severity points —under Equation 1 | 7 | G |
| 12 | Functional severity points —under Equation 1 | 2 | B |
| 13 | Clinical severity points —under Equation 2 | 13 | M |
| 14 | Functional severity points —under Equation 2 | 4 | D |
| 15 | Clinical severity points —under Equation 3 | 3 | C |
| 16 | Functional severity points —under Equation 3 | 4 | D |
| 17 | Clinical severity points —under Equation 4 | 12 | L |
| 18 | Functional severity points —under Equation 4 | 7 | G |

The treatment authorization code that would appear on the claim would be, in this example: 07JK08AA41GBMDCDLG.

In cases of billing for denial notice, using condition code 21, this code may be filled with a placeholder value as defined in section 60.

The investigational device (IDE) revenue code, 0624, is not allowed on HH PPS claims. Therefore, treatment authorization codes associated with IDE items must never be submitted in this field.

The claims-OASIS matching key on the claim will match that submitted on the RAP.

### Document Control Number (DCN)

Required - If submitting an adjustment (TOB 0327) to a previously paid HH PPS claim, the HHA enters the control number assigned to the original HH PPS claim here.

Since HH PPS claims are processed as adjustments to the RAP, Medicare claims processing systems will match all HH PPS claims to their corresponding RAP and populate this field on the electronic claim record automatically. Providers do not need to submit a DCN on all HH PPS claims, only on adjustments to paid claims.

**Employer Name**
Required only if MSP involved. See Pub. 100-05, Medicare Secondary Payer Manual.

**Principal Diagnosis Code**
Required - The HHA enters the ICD-CM code for the principal diagnosis. The code must be reported according to Official ICD Guidelines for Coding and Reporting, as required by the Health Insurance Portability and Accountability Act (HIPAA). The code must be the full diagnosis code, including all five digits for ICD-9-CM or all seven digits for ICD-10 CM where applicable. Where the proper code has fewer than the maximum number of digits, the HHA does not fill it with zeros.

The code and principle diagnosis reported must match the primary diagnosis code reported on the OASIS form item M1020 (Primary Diagnosis).

The principal diagnosis code on the claim will match that submitted on the RAP.

**Other Diagnosis Codes**
Required - The HHA enters the full diagnosis codes for up to eight additional conditions if they coexisted at the time of the establishment of the plan of care. These codes may not duplicate the principal diagnosis as an additional or secondary diagnosis.

For other diagnoses, the diagnoses and codes reported on the claim must match the additional diagnoses reported on the OASIS, form item M1022 (Other Diagnoses). In listing the diagnoses, the HHA places them in order to best reflect the seriousness of the patient's condition and to justify the disciplines and services provided in accordance with the Official ICD Guidelines for Coding and Reporting. The sequence of codes should follow ICD guidelines for reporting manifestation codes. Therefore, if a manifestation code is part of the primary diagnosis, the first two diagnoses should match and appear in the same sequence on both forms. Medicare does not have any additional requirements regarding the reporting or sequence of the codes beyond those contained in ICD guidelines.

Diagnosis codes in OASIS form item M1024, which reports Payment Diagnoses, are not directly reported in any field of the claim form. If under ICD coding guidelines the codes reported in these OASIS items must be reported as Other Diagnoses, the codes may be repeated in OASIS form item M1022 and will be reported on the claim. In other circumstances, the codes reported in payment diagnosis fields in OASIS may not appear on the claim form at all.

**Attending Provider Name and Identifiers**
Required - The HHA enters the name and national provider identifier of the attending physician who signed the plan of care.

**Other Provider (Individual) Names and Identifiers**
Required - The HHA enters the name and NPI of the physician who certified/re-certified the patient's eligibility for home health services.

NOTE: Both the attending physician and other provider fields should be completed unless the patient's designated attending physician is the same as the physician who certified/re-certified the patient's eligibility. When the attending physician is also the certifying/re-certifying physician, only the attending physician is required to be reported.

**Remarks**
Conditional - Remarks are required only in cases where the claim is cancelled or adjusted.

## 100-04, 10, 90.1

### Osteoporosis Injections as HHA Benefit

#### A - Billing Requirements
The administration of the drug is included in the charge for the skilled nursing visit billed using TOB 032x. The cost of the drug is billed using TOB 034x, using revenue code 0636. Drugs that have the ingredient calcitonin are billed using HCPCS code J0630. Drugs that have the ingredient teriparatide may be billed using HCPCS code J3110, if all existing guidelines for coverage under the home health benefit are met. All other osteoporosis drugs that are FDA approved and are awaiting a HCPCS code must use the miscellaneous code of J3490 until a specific HCPCS code is approved for use.

HCPCS code J0630 is defined as up to 400 units. Therefore, the provider must calculate units for the bill as follows:

| Units Furnished During Billing Period | Units of Service Entry on Bill |
| --- | --- |
| 100-400 | 1 |
| 401-800 | 2 |
| 801-1200 | 3 |
| 1201-1600 | 4 |
| 1601-2000 | 5 |
| 2001-2400 | 6 |

HCPCS code J3110 is defined as 10 mcg. Providers should report 1 unit for each 10 mcg dose provided during the billing period.

These codes are paid on a reasonable cost basis, using the provider's submitted charges to make initial payments, which are subject to annual cost settlement.

Coverage requirements for osteoporosis drugs are found in Pub. 100-02, Medicare Benefit Policy Manual, chapter 7, section 50.4.3. Coverage requirements for the home health benefit in general are found in Pub. 100-02, Medicare Benefit Policy Manual, chapter 7, section 30.

#### B - Edits
Medicare system edits require that the date of service on a 034x claim for covered osteoporosis drugs falls within the start and end dates of an existing home health PPS episode. Once the system ensures the service dates on the 034x claim fall within an HH PPS episode that is open for the beneficiary on CWF, CWF edits to assure that the provider number on the 034x claim matches the provider number on the episode file. This is to reflect that although the osteoporosis drug is paid separately from the HH PPS episode rate it is included in consolidated billing requirements (see §10.1.25 regarding consolidated billing).

Claims are also edited to assure that if the claim is an HH claim (TOB 034x), the beneficiary is female and that the diagnosis code for post-menopausal osteoporosis is present.

## 100-04, 11, 10

### Overview
(Rev. 304, Issued: 09-24-04, Effective: 12-08-03, Implementation: 06-28-04)

Medicare beneficiaries entitled to hospital insurance (Part A) who have terminal illnesses and a life expectancy of six months or less have the option of electing hospice benefits in lieu of standard Medicare coverage for treatment and management of their terminal condition. Only care provided by a Medicare certified hospice is covered under the hospice benefit provisions.

Hospice care is available for two 90-day periods and an unlimited number of 60-day periods during the remainder of the hospice patient's lifetime. However, a beneficiary may voluntarily terminate his hospice election period. Election/termination dates are retained on CWF.

When hospice coverage is elected, the beneficiary waives all rights to Medicare Part B payments for services that are related to the treatment and management of his/her terminal illness during any period his/her hospice benefit election is in force, except for professional services of an attending physician, which may include a nurse practitioner. If the attending physician, who may be a nurse practitioner, is an employee of the designated hospice, he or she may not receive compensation from the hospice for those services under Part B. These physician professional services are billed to Medicare Part A by the hospice.

To be covered, hospice services must be reasonable and necessary for the palliation or management of the terminal illness and related conditions. The individual must elect hospice care and a certification that the individual is terminally ill must be completed by the patient's attending physician (if there is one), and the Medical Director (or the physician member of the Interdisciplinary Group (IDG)). Nurse practitioners serving as the attending physician may not certify or re-certify the terminal illness. A plan of care must be established before services are provided. To be covered, services must be consistent with the plan of care. Certification of terminal illness is based on the physician's or medical director's clinical judgment regarding the normal course of an individual's illness. It should be noted that predicting life expectancy is not always exact.

See the Medicare Benefit Policy Manual, Chapter 9, for additional general information about the Hospice benefit.

See Chapter 29 of this manual for information on the appeals process that should be followed when an entity is dissatisfied with the determination made on a claim.

See Chapter 9 of the Medicare Benefit Policy Manual for hospice eligibility requirements and election of hospice care.

## 100-04, 11, 10.1

### Hospice Pre-Election Evaluation and Counseling Services
Effective January 1, 2005, Medicare allows payment to a hospice for specified hospice pre-election evaluation and counseling services when furnished by a physician who is either the medical director of or employee of the hospice.

Medicare covers a one- time only payment on behalf of a beneficiary who is terminally ill, (defined as having a prognosis of 6 months or less if the disease follows its normal course), has no previous hospice elections, and has not previously received hospice pre-election evaluation and counseling services.

HCPCS code G0337 "Hospice Pre-Election Evaluation and Counseling Services" is used to designate that these services have been provided by the medical director or a physician employed by the hospice. Hospice agencies bill their Medicare contractor with home health and hospice jurisdiction directly using HCPCS G0337 with Revenue Code 0657. No other revenue codes may appear on the claim.

Claims for "Hospice Pre-Election and Counseling Services", HCPCS code G0337, are not subject to the editing usually required on hospice claims to match the claim to an established hospice period. Further, contractors do not apply payments for hospice pre-election evaluation and counseling consultation services to the overall hospice cap amount.

Medicare must ensure that this counseling service occurs only one time per beneficiary by imposing safeguards to detect and prevent duplicate billing for similar services. If "new patient" physician services (HCPCS codes 99201-99205) are submitted by a Medicare contractor to CWF for payment authorization but HCPCS code G0337 (Hospice Pre-Election Evaluation and Counseling Services) has already been approved for a hospice claim for the same beneficiary, for the same date of service, by the same physician, the physician service will be rejected by CWF and the service shall be denied as a duplicate. Medicare contractors use the following messages in this case:

HCPCS code G0337 is only payable when billed on a hospice claim. Contractors shall not make payment for HCPCS code G0337 on professional claims. Contractors shall deny line items on professional claims for HCPCS code G0337 and use the following messages:

## 100-04, 11, 100.1

### Billing for Denial of Hospice Room and Board Charges
Hospice providers wishing to receive a line item denial for room and board charges may submit the charges as non-covered using revenue code 0659 with HCPCS A9270 and modifier GY on an otherwise covered hospice claim.

## 100-04, 12, 30.6.15.4

### Power Mobility Devices (PMDs) (Code G0372)
Section 302(a)(2)(E)(iv) of the Medicare Prescription Drug, Improvement, and Modernization Act of 2003 (MMA) sets forth revised conditions for Medicare payment of Power Mobility Devices (PMDs). This section of the MMA states that payment for motorized or power wheelchairs may not be made unless a physician (as defined in §1861(r)(1) of the Act), a physician assistant, nurse practitioner, or a clinical nurse specialist (as those terms are defined in §1861(aa)(5)) has conducted a face-to-face examination of the beneficiary and written a prescription for the PMD.

Payment for the history and physical examination will be made through the appropriate evaluation and management (E&M) code corresponding to the history and physical examination of the patient. Due to the MMA requirement that the physician or treating practitioner create a written prescription and a regulatory requirement that the physician or treating practitioner prepare pertinent parts of the medical record for submission to the durable medical equipment supplier, code G0372 (physician service required to establish and document the need for a power mobility device)has been established to recognize additional physician services and resources required to establish and document the need for the PMD.

The G code indicates that all of the information necessary to document the PMD prescription is included in the medical record, and the prescription and supporting documentation is delivered to the PMD supplier within 30 days after the face-to-face examination.

Effective October 25, 2005, G0372 will be used to recognize additional physician services and resources required to establish and document the need for the PMD and will be added to the Medicare physician fee schedule.

## 100-04, 12, 80.1

### Healthcare Common Procedure Coding System (HCPCS) Coding for the IPPE
The HCPCS codes listed below were developed for the IPPE benefit effective January 1, 2005, for individuals whose initial enrollment is on or after January 1, 2005.

G0344: Initial preventive physical examination; face-to-face visit, services limited to new beneficiary during the first 6 months of Medicare enrollment

Short Descriptor: Initial Preventive Exam

G0366: Electrocardiogram, routine ECG with 12 leads; performed as a component of the initial preventive examination with interpretation and report

Short Descriptor: EKG for initial prevent exam

G0367: tracing only, without interpretation and report, performed as a component of the initial preventive examination

Short Descriptor: EKG tracing for initial prev

G0368: interpretation and report only, performed as a component of the initial preventive examination

Short Descriptor: EKG interpret & report preve

The following new HCPCS codes were developed for the IPPE benefit effective January 1, 2009, and replaced codes G0344, G0366, G0367, and G0368 shown above beginning with dates of service on or after January 1, 2009:

G0402: Initial preventive physical examination; face-to-face visit, services limited to new beneficiary during the first 12 months of Medicare enrollment

Short Descriptor: Initial Preventive exam

G0403: Electrocardiogram, routine ECG with 12 leads; performed as a screening for the initial preventive physical examination with interpretation and report

Short Descriptor: EKG for initial prevent exam

G0404: Electrocardiogram, routine ECG with 12 leads; tracing only, without interpretation and report, performed as a screening for the initial preventive physical examination

Short Descriptor: EKG tracing for initial prev

G0405: Electrocardiogram, routine ECG with 12 leads; interpretation and report only, performed as a screening for the initial preventive physical examination

Short Descriptor: EKG interpret & report preve

## 100-04, 12, 100.1.1

### Evaluation and Management (E/M) Services

#### A. General Documentation Instructions and Common Scenarios
Evaluation and Management (E/M) Services -- For a given encounter, the selection of the appropriate level of E/M service should be determined according to the code definitions in the American Medical Association's Current Procedural Terminology (CPT) and any applicable documentation guidelines.

For purposes of payment, E/M services billed by teaching physicians require that they personally document at least the following:

- That they performed the service or were physically present during the key or critical portions of the service when performed by the resident; and
- The participation of the teaching physician in the management of the patient.

When assigning codes to services billed by teaching physicians, reviewers will combine the documentation of both the resident and the teaching physician.

Documentation by the resident of the presence and participation of the teaching physician is not sufficient to establish the presence and participation of the teaching physician.

On medical review, the combined entries into the medical record by the teaching physician and the resident constitute the documentation for the service and together must support the medical necessity of the service.

Following are four common scenarios for teaching physicians providing E/M services:

Scenario 1:

The teaching physician personally performs all the required elements of an E/M service without a resident. In this scenario the resident may or may not have performed the E/M service independently.

In the absence of a note by a resident, the teaching physician must document as he/she would document an E/M service in a nonteaching setting.

Where a resident has written notes, the teaching physician's note may reference the resident's note. The teaching physician must document that he/she performed the critical or key portion(s) of the service, and that he/she was directly involved in the management of the patient. For payment, the composite of the teaching physician's entry and the resident's entry together must support the medical necessity of the billed service and the level of the service billed by the teaching physician.

Scenario 2:

The resident performs the elements required for an E/M service in the presence of, or jointly with, the teaching physician and the resident documents the service. In this case, the teaching physician must document that he/she was present during the performance of the critical or key portion(s) of the service and that he/she was directly involved in the

management of the patient. The teaching physician's note should reference the resident's note. For payment, the composite of the teaching physician's entry and the

© 2016 Optum360, LLC

resident's entry together must support the medical necessity and the level of the service billed by the teaching physician.

Scenario 3:

The resident performs some or all of the required elements of the service in the absence of the teaching physician and documents his/her service. The teaching physician independently performs the critical or key portion(s) of the service with or without the resident present and, as appropriate, discusses the case with the resident. In this instance, the teaching physician must document that he/she personally saw the patient, personally performed critical or key portions of the service, and participated in the management of the patient. The teaching physician's note should reference the resident's note. For payment, the composite of the teaching physician's entry and the resident's entry together must support the medical necessity of the billed service and the level of the service billed by the teaching physician.

Scenario 4:

When a medical resident admits a patient to a hospital late at night and the teaching physician does not see the patient until later, including the next calendar day:

- The teaching physician must document that he/she personally saw the patient and participated in the management of the patient. The teaching physician may reference the resident's note in lieu of re-documenting the history of present illness, exam, medical decision-making, review of systems and/or past family/social history provided that the patient's condition has not changed, and the teaching physician agrees with the resident's note.

- The teaching physician's note must reflect changes in the patient's condition and clinical course that require that the resident's note be amended with further information to address the patient's condition and course at the time the patient is seen personally by the teaching physician.

- The teaching physician's bill must reflect the date of service he/she saw the patient and his/her personal work of obtaining a history, performing a physical, and participating in medical decision-making regardless of whether the combination of the teaching physician's and resident's documentation satisfies criteria for a higher level of service. For payment, the composite of the teaching physician's entry and the resident's entry together must support the medical necessity of the billed service and the level of the service billed by the teaching physician.

Following are examples of minimally acceptable documentation for each of these scenarios:

Scenario 1:

Admitting Note: "I performed a history and physical examination of the patient and discussed his management with the resident. I reviewed the resident's note and agree with the documented findings and plan of care."

Follow-up Visit: "Hospital Day #3. I saw and evaluated the patient. I agree with the findings and the plan of care as documented in the resident's note."

Follow-up Visit: "Hospital Day #5. I saw and examined the patient. I agree with the resident's note except the heart murmur is louder, so I will obtain an echo to evaluate."

(NOTE: In this scenario if there are no resident notes, the teaching physician must document as he/she would document an E/M service in a non-teaching setting.)

Scenario 2:

Initial or Follow-up Visit: "I was present with the resident during the history and exam. I discussed the case with the resident and agree with the findings and plan as documented in the resident's note."

Follow-up Visit: "I saw the patient with the resident and agree with the resident's findings and plan."

Scenarios 3 and 4:

Initial Visit: "I saw and evaluated the patient. I reviewed the resident's note and agree, except that picture is more consistent with pericarditis than myocardial ischemia. Will begin NSAIDs."

Initial or Follow-up Visit: "I saw and evaluated the patient. Discussed with resident and agree with resident's findings and plan as documented in the resident's note."

Follow-up Visit: "See resident's note for details. I saw and evaluated the patient and agree with the resident's finding and plans as written."

Follow-up Visit: "I saw and evaluated the patient. Agree with resident's note but lower extremities are weaker, now 3/5; MRI of L/S Spine today."

Following are examples of unacceptable documentation:

"Agree with above.", followed by legible countersignature or identity;

"Rounded, Reviewed, Agree.", followed by legible countersignature or identity;

"Discussed with resident. Agree.", followed by legible countersignature or identity;

"Seen and agree.", followed by legible countersignature or identity;

"Patient seen and evaluated.", followed by legible countersignature or identity; and

A legible countersignature or identity alone.

Such documentation is not acceptable, because the documentation does not make it possible to determine whether the teaching physician was present, evaluated the patient, and/or had any involvement with the plan of care.

**B. E/M Service Documentation Provided By Students**

Any contribution and participation of a student to the performance of a billable service (other than the review of systems and/or past family/social history which are not separately billable, but are taken as part of an E/M service) must be performed in the physical presence of a teaching physician or physical presence of a resident in a service meeting the requirements set forth in this section for teaching physician billing.

Students may document services in the medical record. However, the documentation of an E/M service by a student that may be referred to by the teaching physician is limited to documentation related to the review of systems and/or past family/social history. The teaching physician may not refer to a student's documentation of physical exam findings or medical decision making in his or her personal note. If the medical student documents E/M services, the teaching physician must verify and redocument the history of present illness as well as perform and redocument the physical exam and medical decision making activities of the service.

**C. Exception for E/M Services Furnished in Certain Primary Care Centers**

Teaching physicians providing E/M services with a GME program granted a primary care exception may bill Medicare for lower and mid-level E/M services provided by residents. For the E/M codes listed below, teaching physicians may submit claims for services furnished by residents in the absence of a teaching physician:

| New Patient | Established Patient |
|---|---|
| 99201 | 99211 |
| 99202 | 99212 |
| 99203 | 99213 |

Effective January 1, 2005, the following code is included under the primary care exception: HCPCS code G0402 (Initial preventive physical examination; face-to-face visit services limited to new beneficiary during the first 12 months of Medicare enrollment).

Effective January 1, 2011, the following codes are included under the primary care exception: HCPCS codes G0438 (Annual wellness visit, including personal preventive plan service, first visit) and G0439 (Annual wellness visit, including personal preventive plan service, subsequent visit).

If a service other than those listed above needs to be furnished, then the general teaching physician policy set forth in §100.1 applies. For this exception to apply, a center must attest in writing that all the following conditions are met for a particular residency program. Prior approval is not necessary, but centers exercising the primary care exception must maintain records demonstrating that they qualify for the exception.

The services must be furnished in a center located in the outpatient department of a hospital or another ambulatory care entity in which the time spent by residents in patient care activities is included in determining direct GME payments to a teaching hospital by the hospital's FI. This requirement is not met when the resident is assigned to a physician's office away from the center or makes home visits. In the case of a nonhospital entity, verify with the FI that the entity meets the requirements of a written agreement between the hospital and the entity set forth at 42 CFR 413.78(e)(3)(ii).

Under this exception, residents providing the billable patient care service without the physical presence of a teaching physician must have completed at least 6 months of a GME approved residency program. Centers must maintain information under the provisions at 42 CFR 413.79(a)(6).

Teaching physicians submitting claims under this exception may not supervise more than four residents at any given time and must direct the care from such proximity as to constitute immediate availability. Teaching physicians may include residents with less than 6 months in a GME approved residency program in the mix of four residents under the teaching physician's supervision. However, the teaching physician must be physically present for the critical or key portions of services furnished by the residents with less than 6 months in a GME approved residency program. That is, the primary care exception does not apply in the case of residents with less than 6 months in a GME approved residency program.

Teaching physicians submitting claims under this exception must:

- Not have other responsibilities (including the supervision of other personnel) at the time the service was provided by the resident;
- Have the primary medical responsibility for patients cared for by the residents;
- Ensure that the care provided was reasonable and necessary;
- Review the care provided by the resident during or immediately after each visit. This must include a review of the patient's medical history, the resident's findings on physical examination, the patient's diagnosis, and treatment plan (i.e., record of tests and therapies); and
- Document the extent of his/her own participation in the review and direction of the services furnished to each patient.

Patients under this exception should consider the center to be their primary location for health care services. The residents must be expected to generally provide care to the same group of established patients during their residency training. The types of services furnished by residents under this exception include:

- Acute care for undifferentiated problems or chronic care for ongoing conditions including chronic mental illness;
- Coordination of care furnished by other physicians and providers; and,
- Comprehensive care not limited by organ system or diagnosis.

Residency programs most likely qualifying for this exception include family practice, general internal medicine, geriatric medicine, pediatrics, and obstetrics/gynecology.

Certain GME programs in psychiatry may qualify in special situations such as when the program furnishes comprehensive care for chronically mentally ill patients. These would be centers in which the range of services the residents are trained to furnish, and actually do furnish, include comprehensive medical care as well as psychiatric care. For example, antibiotics are being prescribed as well as psychotropic drugs.

## 100-04, 12, 180

### Care Plan Oversight Services

The Medicare Benefit Policy Manual, Chapter 15, contains requirements for coverage for medical and other health services including those of physicians and non-physician practitioners.

Care plan oversight (CPO) is the physician supervision of a patient receiving complex and/or multidisciplinary care as part of Medicare-covered services provided by a participating home health agency or Medicare approved hospice.

CPO services require complex or multidisciplinary care modalities involving: Regular physician development and/or revision of care plans; Review of subsequent reports of patient status; Review of related laboratory and other studies; Communication with other health professionals not employed in the same practice who are involved in the patient's care; Integration of new information into the medical treatment plan; and/or Adjustment of medical therapy.

The CPO services require recurrent physician supervision of a patient involving 30 or more minutes of the physician's time per month. Services not countable toward the 30 minutes threshold that must be provided in order to bill for CPO include, but are not limited to: Time associated with discussions with the patient, his or her family or friends to adjust medication or treatment; Time spent by staff getting or filing charts; Travel time; and/or Physician's time spent telephoning prescriptions into the pharmacist unless the telephone conversation involves discussions of pharmaceutical therapies.

Implicit in the concept of CPO is the expectation that the physician has coordinated an aspect of the patient's care with the home health agency or hospice during the month for which CPO services were billed. The physician who bills for CPO must be the same physician who signs the plan of care.

Nurse practitioners, physician assistants, and clinical nurse specialists, practicing within the scope of State law, may bill for care plan oversight. These non-physician practitioners must have been providing ongoing care for the beneficiary through evaluation and management services. These non-physician practitioners may not bill for CPO if they have been involved only with the delivery of the Medicare-covered home health or hospice service.

### A. Home Health CPO

Non-physician practitioners can perform CPO only if the physician signing the plan of care provides regular ongoing care under the same plan of care as does the NPP billing for CPO and either: The physician and NPP are part of the same group practice; or If the NPP is a nurse practitioner or clinical nurse specialist, the physician signing the plan of care also has a collaborative agreement with the NPP; or If the NPP is a physician assistant, the physician signing the plan of care is also the physician who provides general supervision of physician assistant services for the practice.

Billing may be made for care plan oversight services furnished by an NPP when: The NPP providing the care plan oversight has seen and examined the patient; The NPP

providing care plan oversight is not functioning as a consultant whose participation is limited to a single medical condition rather than multidisciplinary coordination of care; and The NPP providing care plan oversight integrates his or her care with that of the physician who signed the plan of care.

NPPs may not certify the beneficiary for home health care.

### B. Hospice CPO

The attending physician or nurse practitioner (who has been designated as the attending physician) may bill for hospice CPO when they are acting as an "attending physician".

An "attending physician" is one who has been identified by the individual, at the time he/she elects hospice coverage, as having the most significant role in the determination and delivery of their medical care. They are not employed nor paid by the hospice. The care plan oversight services are billed using Form CMS-1500 or electronic equivalent.

For additional information on hospice CPO, see Chapter 11, 40.1.3.1 of this manual.

## 100-04, 12, 180.1

### Care Plan Oversight Billing Requirements

#### A. Codes for Which Separate Payment May Be Made

Effective January 1, 1995, separate payment may be made for CPO oversight services for 30 minutes or more if the requirements specified in the Medicare Benefits Policy Manual, Chapter 15 are met.

Providers billing for CPO must submit the claim with no other services billed on that claim and may bill only after the end of the month in which the CPO services were rendered. CPO services may not be billed across calendar months and should be submitted (and paid) only for one unit of service.

Physicians may bill and be paid separately for CPO services only if all the criteria in the Medicare Benefit Policy Manual, Chapter 15 are met.

#### B. Physician Certification and Recertification of Home Health Plans of Care

Effective 2001, two new HCPCS codes for the certification and recertification and development of plans of care for Medicare-covered home health services were created.

See the Medicare General Information, Eligibility, and Entitlement Manual, Pub. 100-01, Chapter 4, "Physician Certification and Recertification of Services," 10-60, and the Medicare Benefit Policy Manual, Pub. 100-02, Chapter 7, "Home Health Services", 30.

The home health agency certification code can be billed only when the patient has not received Medicare-covered home health services for at least 60 days. The home health agency recertification code is used after a patient has received services for at least 60 days (or one certification period) when the physician signs the certification after the initial certification period. The home health agency recertification code will be reported only once every 60 days, except in the rare situation when the patient starts a new episode before 60 days elapses and requires a new plan of care to start a new episode.

#### C. Provider Number of Home Health Agency (HHA) or Hospice

For claims for CPO submitted on or after January 1, 1997, physicians must enter on the Medicare claim form the 6-character Medicare provider number of the HHA or hospice providing Medicare-covered services to the beneficiary for the period during which CPO services was furnished and for which the physician signed the plan of care. Physicians are responsible for obtaining the HHA or hospice Medicare provider numbers.

Additionally, physicians should provide their UPIN to the HHA or hospice furnishing services to their patient.

NOTE: There is currently no place on the HIPAA standard ASC X12N 837 professional format to specifically include the HHA or hospice provider number required for a care plan oversight claim. For this reason, the requirement to include the HHA or hospice provider number on a care plan oversight claim is temporarily waived until a new version of this electronic standard format is adopted under HIPAA and includes a place to provide the HHA and hospice provider numbers for care plan oversight claims.

## 100-04, 12, 190.3

### List of Medicare Telehealth Services

The use of a telecommunications system may substitute for an in-person encounter for professional consultations, office visits, office psychiatry services, and a limited number of other physician fee schedule (PFS) services. The various services and corresponding current procedure terminology (CPT) or Healthcare Common Procedure Coding System (HCPCS) codes are listed below.

- Consultations (CPT codes 99241 - 99275) - Effective October 1, 2001 – December 31, 2005;

- Consultations (CPT codes 99241 - 99255) - Effective January 1, 2006 – December 31, 2009;
- Telehealth consultations, emergency department or initial inpatient (HCPCS codes G0425 – G0427) - Effective January 1, 2010;
- Follow-up inpatient telehealth consultations (HCPCS codes G0406, G0407, and G0408) - Effective January 1, 2009;
- Office or other outpatient visits (CPT codes 99201 - 99215);
- Subsequent hospital care services, with the limitation of one telehealth visit every 3 days (CPT codes 99231, 99232, and 99233) – Effective January 1, 2011;
- Subsequent nursing facility care services, with the limitation of one telehealth visit every 30 days (CPT codes 99307, 99308, 99309, and 99310) – Effective January 1, 2011;
- Pharmacologic management (CPT code 90862) – Effective March 1, 2003 – December 31, 2012;
- Individual psychotherapy (CPT codes 90804 - 90809); Psychiatric diagnostic interview examination (CPT code 90801) – Effective March 1, 2003 – December 31, 2012;
- Individual psychotherapy (CPT codes 90832 – 90834, 90836 – 90838); Psychiatric diagnostic interview examination (CPT codes 90791 -- 90792) – Effective January 1, 2013.
- Neurobehavioral status exam (CPT code 96116) - Effective January 1, 2008;
- End Stage Renal Disease (ESRD) related services (HCPCS codes G0308, G0309, G0311, G0312, G0314, G0315, G0317, and G0318) – Effective January 1, 2005 – December 31, 2008;
- End Stage Renal Disease (ESRD) related services (CPT codes 90951, 90952, 90954, 90955, 90957, 90958, 90960, and 90961) – Effective January 1, 2009;
- Individual and group medical nutrition therapy (HCPCS codes G0270, 97802, 97803, and 97804) – Individual effective January 1, 2006; group effective January 1, 2011;
- Individual and group health and behavior assessment and intervention (CPT codes 96150 – 96154) – Individual effective January 1, 2010; group effective January 1, 2011.
- Individual and group kidney disease education (KDE) services (HCPCS codes G0420 and G0421) – Effective January 1, 2011; and
- Individual and group diabetes self-management training (DSMT) services, with a minimum of 1 hour of in-person instruction to be furnished in the initial year training period to ensure effective injection training (HCPCS codes G0108 and G0109) - Effective January 1, 2011.
- Smoking Cessation Services (CPT codes 99406 and 99407and HCPCS codes G0436 and G0437) – Effective January 1, 2012.
- Alcohol and/or substance (other than tobacco) abuse structured assessment and intervention services (HCPCS codes G0396 and G0397) – Effective January 1, 2013.
- Annual alcohol misuse screening (HCPCS code G0442) – Effective January 1, 2013.
- Brief face-to-face behavioral counseling for alcohol misuse (HCPCS code G0443) – Effective January 1, 2013.
- Annual Depression Screening (HCPCS code G0444) – Effective January 1, 2013.
- High-intensity behavioral counseling to prevent sexually transmitted infections (HCPCS code G0445) – Effective January 1, 2013.
- Annual, face-to-face Intensive behavioral therapy for cardiovascular disease (HCPCS code G0446) – Effective January 1, 2013.
- Face-to-face behavioral counseling for obesity (HCPCS code G0447) – Effective January 1, 2013.
- Transitional Care Management Services (CPT codes 99495 -99496) – Effective January 1, 2014.

NOTE: Beginning January 1, 2010, CMS eliminated the use of all consultation codes, except for inpatient telehealth consultation G-codes. CMS no longer recognizes office/outpatient or inpatient consultation CPT codes for payment of office/outpatient or inpatient visits. Instead, physicians and practitioners are instructed to bill a new or established patient office/outpatient visit CPT code or appropriate hospital or nursing facility care code, as appropriate to the particular patient, for all office/outpatient or inpatient visits.

## 100-04, 12, 190.3.1

### Telehealth Consultation Services, Emergency Department or Initial Inpatient versus Inpatient Evaluation and Management (E/M) Visits

A consultation service is an evaluation and management (E/M) service furnished to evaluate and possibly treat a patient's problem(s). It can involve an opinion, advice, recommendation, suggestion, direction, or counsel from a physician or qualified nonphysician practitioner (NPP) at the request of another physician or appropriate source.

Section 1834(m) of the Social Security Act includes "professional consultations" in the definition of telehealth services. Inpatient or emergency department consultations furnished via telehealth can facilitate the provision of certain services and/or medical expertise that might not otherwise be available to a patient located at an originating site.

The use of a telecommunications system may substitute for an in-person encounter for emergency department or initial and follow-up inpatient consultations.

Medicare contractors pay for reasonable and medically necessary inpatient or emergency department telehealth consultation services furnished to beneficiaries in hospitals or SNFs when all of the following criteria for the use of a consultation code are met:

- An inpatient or emergency department consultation service is distinguished from other inpatient or emergency department evaluation and management (E/M) visits because it is provided by a physician or qualified nonphysician practitioner (NPP) whose opinion or advice regarding evaluation and/or management of a specific problem is requested by another physician or other appropriate source. The qualified NPP may perform consultation services within the scope of practice and licensure requirements for NPPs in the State in which he/she practices;
- A request for an inpatient or emergency department telehealth consultation from an appropriate source and the need for an inpatient or emergency department telehealth consultation (i.e., the reason for a consultation service) shall be documented by the consultant in the patient's medical record and included in the requesting physician or qualified NPP's plan of care in the patient's medical record; and
- After the inpatient or emergency department telehealth consultation is provided, the consultant shall prepare a written report of his/her findings and recommendations, which shall be provided to the referring physician.

The intent of an inpatient or emergency department telehealth consultation service is that a physician or qualified NPP or other appropriate source is asking another physician or qualified NPP for advice, opinion, a recommendation, suggestion, direction, or counsel, etc. in evaluating or treating a patient because that individual has expertise in a specific medical area beyond the requesting professional's knowledge.

Unlike inpatient or emergency department telehealth consultations, the majority of subsequent inpatient hospital, emergency department and nursing facility care services require in-person visits to facilitate the comprehensive, coordinated, and personal care that medically volatile, acutely ill patients require on an ongoing basis.

Subsequent hospital care services are limited to one telehealth visit every 3 days. Subsequent nursing facility care services are limited to one telehealth visit every 30 days.

## 100-04, 12, 190.3.2

### Telehealth Consultation Services, Emergency Department or Initial Inpatient Defined

Emergency department or initial inpatient telehealth consultations are furnished to beneficiaries in hospitals or SNFs via telehealth at the request of the physician of record, the attending physician, or another appropriate source. The physician or practitioner who furnishes the emergency department or initial inpatient consultation via telehealth cannot be the physician of record or the attending physician, and the emergency department or initial inpatient telehealth consultation would be distinct from the care provided by the physician of record or the attending physician. Counseling and coordination of care with other providers or agencies is included as well, consistent with the nature of the problem(s) and the patient's needs. Emergency department or initial inpatient telehealth consultations are subject to the criteria for emergency department or initial inpatient telehealth consultation services, as described in section 190.3.1 of this chapter.

Payment for emergency department or initial inpatient telehealth consultations includes all consultation related services furnished before, during, and after communicating with the patient via telehealth. Pre-service activities would include, but would not be limited to, reviewing patient data (for example, diagnostic and imaging studies, interim labwork) and communicating with other professionals or family members. Intra-service activities must include the three key elements described below for each procedure code. Post-service activities would include, but would not be limited to, completing medical records or other documentation and communicating results of the consultation and further care plans to other health care professionals. No additional E/M service could be billed for work related to an emergency department or initial inpatient telehealth consultation.

Emergency department or initial inpatient telehealth consultations could be provided at various levels of complexity:

- Practitioners taking a problem focused history, conducting a problem focused examination, and engaging in medical decision making that is straightforward, would bill HCPCS code G0425 (Telehealth consultation, emergency department or initial inpatient, typically 30 minutes communicating with the patient via telehealth).

- Practitioners taking a detailed history, conducting a detailed examination, and engaging in medical decision making that is of moderate complexity, would bill HCPCS code G0426 (Telehealth consultation, emergency department or initial inpatient, typically 50 minutes communicating with the patient via telehealth).

- Practitioners taking a comprehensive history, conducting a comprehensive examination, and engaging in medical decision making that is of high complexity, would bill HCPCS code G0427 (Telehealth consultation, emergency department or initial inpatient, typically 70 minutes or more communicating with the patient via telehealth).

Although emergency department or initial inpatient telehealth consultations are specific to telehealth, these services must be billed with either the -GT or -GQ modifier to identify the telehealth technology used to provide the service. See section 190.6 of this chapter for instructions on how to use these modifiers.

## 100-04, 12, 190.3.3

### Follow-Up Inpatient Telehealth Consultations Defined

Follow-up inpatient telehealth consultations are furnished to beneficiaries in hospitals or SNFs via telehealth to follow up on an initial consultation, or subsequent consultative visits requested by the attending physician. The initial inpatient consultation may have been provided in person or via telehealth.

Follow-up inpatient telehealth consultations include monitoring progress, recommending management modifications, or advising on a new plan of care in response to changes in the patient's status or no changes on the consulted health issue. Counseling and coordination of care with other providers or agencies is included as well, consistent with the nature of the problem(s) and the patient's needs.

The physician or practitioner who furnishes the inpatient follow-up consultation via telehealth cannot be the physician of record or the attending physician, and the follow-up inpatient consultation would be distinct from the follow-up care provided by the physician of record or the attending physician. If a physician consultant has initiated treatment at an initial consultation and participates thereafter in the patient's ongoing care management, such care would not be included in the definition of a follow-up inpatient consultation and is not appropriate for delivery via telehealth. Follow-up inpatient telehealth consultations are subject to the criteria for inpatient telehealth consultation services, as described in Sec.190.3.1

Payment for follow-up inpatient telehealth consultations includes all consultation related services furnished before, during, and after communicating with the patient via telehealth. Pre-service activities would include, but would not be limited to, reviewing patient data (for example, diagnostic and imaging studies, interim labwork) and communicating with other professionals or family members. Intra-service activities must include at least two of the three key elements described below for each procedure code. Post-service activities would include, but would not be limited to, completing medical records or other documentation and communicating results of the consultation and further care plans to other health care professionals. No additional evaluation and management service could be billed for work related to a follow-up inpatient telehealth consultation.

Follow-up inpatient telehealth consultations could be provided at various levels of complexity:

Practitioners taking a problem focused interval history, conducting a problem focused examination, and engaging in medical decision making that is straightforward or of low complexity, would bill a limited service, using HCPCS G0406, Follow-up inpatient telehealth consultation, limited. At this level of service, practitioners would typically spend 15 minutes communicating with the patient via telehealth.

Practitioners taking an expanded focused interval history, conducting an expanded problem focused examination, and engaging in medical decision making that is of moderate complexity, would bill an intermediate service using HCPCS G0407, Follow-up inpatient telehealth consultation, intermediate. At this level of service, practitioners would typically spend 25 minutes communicating with the patient via telehealth.

Practitioners taking a detailed interval history, conducting a detailed examination, and engaging in medical decision making that is of high complexity, would bill a complex service, using HCPCS G0408, Follow-up inpatient telehealth consultation, complex. At this level of service, practitioners would typically spend 35 minutes or more communicating with the patient via telehealth.

Although follow-up inpatient telehealth consultations are specific to telehealth, these services must be billed with either the "GT" or "GQ" modifier to identify the telehealth technology used to provide the service. (See Sec.190.6 et. al. for instructions on how to use these modifiers.)

## 100-04, 12, 190.6

### 1. Originating site defined

The term originating site means the location of an eligible Medicare beneficiary at the time the service being furnished via a telecommunications system occurs. For asynchronous, store and forward telecommunications technologies, an originating site is only a Federal telemedicine demonstration program conducted in Alaska or Hawaii.

### 2. Facility fee for originating site

The originating site facility fee is a separately billable Part B payment. The contractor pays it outside of other payment methodologies. This fee is subject to post payment verification.

For telehealth services furnished from October 1, 2001, through December 31, 2002, the originating site facility fee is the lesser of $20 or the actual charge. For services furnished on or after January 1 of each subsequent year, the originating site facility fee is updated by the Medicare Economic Index. The updated fee is included in the Medicare Physician Fee Schedule (MPFS) Final Rule, which is published by November 1 prior to the start of the calendar year for which it is effective. The updated fee for each calendar year is also issued annually in a Recurring Update Notification instruction for January of each year.

### 3. Payment amount:

The originating site facility fee is a separately billable Part B payment. The payment amount to the originating site is the lesser of 80 percent of the actual charge or 80 percent of the originating site facility fee, except CAHs. The beneficiary is responsible for any unmet deductible amount and Medicare coinsurance.

The originating site facility fee payment methodology for each type of facility is clarified below.

Hospital outpatient department. When the originating site is a hospital outpatient department, payment for the originating site facility fee must be made as described above and not under the outpatient prospective payment system (OPPS). Payment is not based on the OPPS payment methodology.

Hospital inpatient. For hospital inpatients, payment for the originating site facility fee must be made outside the diagnostic related group (DRG) payment, since this is a Part B benefit, similar to other services paid separately from the DRG payment, (e.g., hemophilia blood clotting factor).

Critical access hospitals. When the originating site is a critical access hospital, make payment separately from the cost-based reimbursement methodology. For CAH's, the payment amount is 80 percent of the originating site facility fee.

Federally qualified health centers (FQHCs) and rural health clinics (RHCs). The originating site facility fee for telehealth services is not an FQHC or RHC service. When an FQHC or RHC serves as the originating site, the originating site facility fee must be paid separately from the center or clinic all-inclusive rate.

Physicians' and practitioners' offices. When the originating site is a physician's or practitioner's office, the payment amount, in accordance with the law, is the lesser of 80 percent of the actual charge or 80 percent of the originating site facility fee, regardless of geographic location. The carrier shall not apply the geographic practice cost index (GPCI) to the originating site facility fee. This fee is statutorily set and is not subject to the geographic payment adjustments authorized under the MPFS.

Hospital-based or critical access-hospital based renal dialysis center (or their satellites). When a hospital-based or critical access hospital-based renal dialysis center (or their satellites) serves as the originating site, the originating site facility fee is covered in addition to any composite rate or MCP amount.

Skilled nursing facility (SNF). The originating site facility fee is outside the SNF prospective payment system bundle and, as such, is not subject to SNF consolidated billing. The originating site facility fee is a separately billable Part B payment.

Community Mental Health Center (CMHC). The originating site facility fee is not a partial hospitalization service. The originating site facility fee does not count towards the number of services used to determine payment for partial hospitalization services. The originating site facility fee is not bundled in the per diem payment for partial hospitalization. The originating site facility fee is a separately billable Part B payment.

To receive the originating facility site fee, the provider submits claims with HCPCS code "Q3014, telehealth originating site facility fee"; short description "telehealth facility fee." The type of service for the telehealth originating site facility fee is "9, other items and services." For carrier-processed claims, the "office" place of service (code 11) is the only payable setting for code Q3014. There is no participation payment differential for code Q3014. Deductible and coinsurance rules apply to Q3014. By submitting Q3014 HCPCS code, the originating site authenticates they are located in either a rural HPSA or non-MSA county.

This benefit may be billed on bill types 12X, 13X, 22X, 23X, 71X, 72X, 73X, 76X, and 85X. Unless otherwise applicable, report the originating site facility fee under revenue code 078X and include HCPCS code "Q3014, telehealth originating site facility fee."

Hospitals and critical access hospitals bill their intermediary for the originating site facility fee. Telehealth bills originating in inpatient hospitals must be submitted on a 12X TOB using the date of discharge as the line item date of service.

Independent and provider-based RHCs and FQHCs bill the appropriate intermediary using the RHC or FQHC bill type and billing number. HCPCS code Q3014 is the only non-RHC/FQHC service that is billed using the clinic/center bill type and provider number. All RHCs and FQHCs must use revenue code 078X when billing for the originating site facility fee. For all other non-RHC/FQHC services, provider based RHCs and FQHCs must bill using the base provider's bill type and billing number. Independent RHCs and FQHCs must bill the carrier for all other non-RHC/FQHC services. If an RHC/FQHC visit occurs on the same day as a telehealth service, the RHC/FQHC serving as an originating site must bill for HCPCS code Q3014 telehealth originating site facility fee on a separate revenue line from the RHC/FQHC visit using revenue code 078X.

Hospital-based or CAH-based renal dialysis centers (including satellites) bill their local FIs and/or Part A MACs for the originating site facility fee. Telehealth bills originating in renal dialysis centers must be submitted on a 72X TOB. All hospital-based or CAH-based renal dialysis centers (including satellites) must use revenue code 078X when billing for the originating site facility fee. The renal dialysis center serving as an originating site must bill for HCPCS code Q3014, telehealth originating site facility fee, on a separate revenue line from any other services provided to the beneficiary.

Skilled nursing facilities (SNFs) bill their local FIs and/or Part A MACs for the originating site facility fee. Telehealth bills originating in SNFs must be submitted on TOB 22X or 23X. For SNF inpatients in a covered Part A stay, the originating site facility fee must be submitted on a 22X TOB. All SNFs must use revenue code 078X when billing for the originating site facility fee. The SNF serving as an originating site must bill for HCPCS code Q3014, telehealth originating site facility fee, on a separate revenue line from any other services provided to the beneficiary.

Community mental health centers (CMHCs) bill their local FIs and/or Part A MACs for the originating site facility fee. Telehealth bills originating in CMHCs must be submitted on a 76X TOB. All CMHCs must use revenue code 078X when billing for the originating site facility fee. The CMHC serving as an originating site must bill for HCPCS code Q3014, telehealth originating site facility fee, on a separate revenue line from any other services provided to the beneficiary. Note that Q3014 does not count towards the number of services used to determine per diem payments for partial hospitalization services.

The beneficiary is responsible for any unmet deductible amount and Medicare coinsurance.

## 100-04, 12, 190.7

### Contractor Editing of Telehealth Claims

Medicare telehealth services (as listed in section 190.3) are billed with either the "GT" or "GQ" modifier. The contractor shall approve covered telehealth services if the physician or practitioner is licensed under State law to provide the service. Contractors must familiarize themselves with licensure provisions of States for which they process claims and disallow telehealth services furnished by physicians or practitioners who are not authorized to furnish the applicable telehealth service under State law. For example, if a nurse practitioner is not licensed to provide individual psychotherapy under State law, he or she would not be permitted to receive payment for individual psychotherapy under Medicare. The contractor shall install edits to ensure that only properly licensed physicians and practitioners are paid for covered telehealth services.

If a contractor receives claims for professional telehealth services coded with the "GQ" modifier (representing "via asynchronous telecommunications system"), it shall approve/pay for these services only if the physician or practitioner is affiliated with a Federal telemedicine demonstration conducted in Alaska or Hawaii. The contractor may require the physician or practitioner at the distant site to document his or her participation in a Federal telemedicine demonstration program conducted in Alaska or Hawaii prior to paying for telehealth services provided via asynchronous, store and forward technologies.

If a contractor denies telehealth services because the physician or practitioner may not bill for them, the contractor uses MSN message 21.18: "This item or service is not covered when performed or ordered by this practitioner." The contractor uses remittance advice message 52 when denying the claim based upon MSN message 21.18.

If a service is billed with one of the telehealth modifiers and the procedure code is not designated as a covered telehealth service, the contractor denies the service using MSN message 9.4: "This item or service was denied because information required to make payment was incorrect." The remittance advice message depends on what is incorrect, e.g., B18 if procedure code or modifier is incorrect, 125 for submission billing errors, 4-12 for difference inconsistencies. The contractor uses B18 as the explanation for the denial of the claim.

The only claims from institutional facilities that FIs shall pay for telehealth services at the distant site, except for MNT services, are for physician or practitioner services when the distant site is located in a CAH that has elected Method II, and the physician or practitioner has reassigned his/her benefits to the CAH. The CAH bills its regular FI for the professional services provided at the distant site via a telecommunications system, in any of the revenue codes 096x, 097x or 098x. All requirements for billing distant site telehealth services apply.

Claims from hospitals or CAHs for MNT services are submitted to the hospital's or CAH's regular FI. Payment is based on the non-facility amount on the Medicare Physician Fee Schedule for the particular HCPCS codes.

## 100-04, 13, 30.1.3.1

### A/B MAC (A) Payment for Low Osmolar Contrast Material (LOCM) (Radiology)

The LOCM is paid on a reasonable cost basis when rendered by a SNF to its Part B patients (in addition to payment for the radiology procedure) when it is used in one of the situations listed below.

The following HCPCS are used when billing for LOCM.

| HCPCS Code | Description (January 1. 1994, and later) |
|---|---|
| A4644 | Supply of low osmolar contrast material (100-199 mgs of iodine); |
| A4645 | Supply of low osmolar contrast material (200-299 mgs of iodine); or |
| A4646 | Supply of low osmolar contrast material (300-399 mgs of iodine). |

When billing for LOCM, SNFs use revenue code 0636. If the SNF charge for the radiology procedure includes a charge for contrast material, the SNF must adjust the charge for the radiology procedure to exclude any amount for the contrast material.

NOTE: LOCM is never billed with revenue code 0255 or as part of the radiology procedure.

The A/B MAC (A) will edit for the intrathecal procedure codes and the following codes to determine if payment for LOCM is to be made. If an intrathecal procedure code is not present, or one of the ICD codes is not present to indicate that a required medical condition is met, the A/B MAC (A) will deny payment for LOCM. In these instances, LOCM is not covered and should not be billed to Medicare.

When LOCM Is Separately Billable and Related Coding Requirements

- In all intrathecal injections. HCPCS codes that indicate intrathecal injections are:

  – 70010  70015  72240  72255  72265  72270  72285  72295

One of these must be included on the claim; or

- In intravenous and intra-arterial injections only when certain medical conditions are present in an outpatient. The SNF must verify the existence of at least one of the following medical conditions, and report the applicable diagnosis code(s) either as a principal diagnosis code or other diagnosis codes on the claim:

  – A history of previous adverse reaction to contrast material. The applicable ICD-9-CM codes are V14.8 and V14.9. The applicable ICD-10-CM codes are Z88.8 and Z88.9. The conditions which should not be considered adverse reactions are a sensation of heat, flushing, or a single episode of nausea or vomiting. If the adverse reaction occurs on that visit with the induction of contrast material, codes describing hives, urticaria, etc. should also be present, as well as a code describing the external cause of injury and poisoning, ICD-9-CM code E947.8. The applicable ICD-10 CM codes are: T50.8X5A Adverse effect of diagnostic agents, initial encounter, T50.8X5S Adverse effect of diagnostic agents, sequela , T50.995A Adverse effect of other drugs, medicaments and biological substances, initial encounter, or

T50.995S Adverse effect of other drugs, medicaments and biological substances, sequela;

– A history or condition of asthma or allergy. The applicable ICD-9-CM codes are V07.1, V14.0 through V14.9, V15.0, 493.00, 493.01, 493.10, 493.11, 493.20, 493.21, 493.90, 493.91, 495.0, 495.1, 495.2, 495.3, 495.4, 495.5, 495.6, 495.7, 495.8, 495.9, 995.0, 995.1, 995.2, and 995.3. The applicable ICD-10-CM codes are in the table below:

## ICD-10-CM Codes

| | | | | |
|---|---|---|---|---|
| J44.0 | J44.9 | J45.20 | J45.22 | J45.30 |
| J45.32 | J45.40 | J45.42 | J45.50 | J45.52 |
| J45.902 | J45.909 | J45.998 | J67.0 | J67.1 |
| JJ67.2 | J67.3 | J67.4 | J67.5 | J67.6 |
| J67.7 | J67.8 | J67.9 | J96.00 | J96.01 |
| J96.02 | J96.90 | J96.91 | J96.92 | T36.0X5A |
| T36.1X5A | T36.2X5A | T36.3X5A | T36.4X5A | T36.5X5A |
| T36.6X5A | T36.7X5A | T36.8X5A | T36.95XA | T37.0X5A |
| T37.1X5A | T37.2X5A | T37.3X5A | T37.8X5A | T37.95XA |
| T38.0X5A | T38.1X5A | T38.2X5A | T38.3X5A | T38.4X5A |
| T38.6X5A | T38.7X5A | T38.805A | T38.815A | T38.895A |
| T38.905A | T38.995A | T39.015A | T39.095A | T39.1X5A |
| T39.2X5A | T39.2X5A | T39.315A | T39.395A | T39.4X5A |
| T39.8X5A | T39.95XA | T40.0X5A | T40.1X5A | T40.2X5A |
| T40.3X5A | T40.4X5A | T40.5X5A | T40.605A | T40.695A |
| T40.7X5A | T40.8X5A | T40.905A | T40.995A | T41.0X5A |
| T41.1X5A | T41.205A | T41.295A | T41.3X5A | T41.4X5A |
| T41.X5A | T41.5X5A | T42.0X5A | T42.1X5A | T42.2X5A |
| T42.3X5A | T42.4X5A | T42.5X5A | T42.6X5A | 427.5XA |
| 428.X5A | T43.015A | T43.025A | T43.1X5A | T43.205A |
| T43.215A | T43.225A | T43.295A | T43.3X5A | T43.4X5A |
| T43.505A | T43.595A | T43.605A | T43.615A | T43.625A |
| T43.635A | T43.695A | T43.8X5A | T43.95XA | T44.0X5A |
| T44.1X5A | T44.2X5A | T44.3X5A | T44.6X5A | T44.7X5A |
| T44.8X5A | T44.905A | T44.995A | T45.0X5A | T45.1X5A |
| T45.2X5A | T45.3X5A | T45.4X5A | T45.515A | T45.525A |
| T45.605A | T45.615A | T45.625A | T45.695A | T45.7X5A |
| T45.8X5A | T45.95XA | T46.0X5A | T46.1X5A | T46.2X5A |
| T46.3X5A | T46.4X5A | T46.5X5A | T46.6X5A | T46.7X5A |
| T46.8X5A | T46.905A | T46.995A | T47.0X5A | T47.1X5A |
| T47.2X5A | T47.3X5A | T47.4X5A | T47.5X5A | T47.6X5A |
| T47.7X5A | T47.8X5A | T47.95XA | T48.0X5A | T48.1X5A |
| T48.205A | T48.295A | T48.3X5A | T48.4X5A | T48.5X5A |
| T48.6X5A | T48.905A | T48.995A | T49.0X5A | T49.1X5A |
| T49.2X5A | T49.3X5A | T49.4X5A | T49.5X5A | T49.6X5A |
| T49.6X5A | T47.X5A9 | T49.8X5A | T49.95XA | T50.0X5A |
| T50.1X5A | T50.2X5A | T50.3X5A | T50.4X5A | T50.5X5A |
| T50.6X5A | T50.7X5A | T50.8X5A | T50.905a | T50.995A |
| T50.A15A | T50.A25A | T50.A95A | T50.B15A | T50.B95A |
| T50.Z15A | T50.Z95A | T78.2XXA | T78.3XXA | T78.40XA |
| T78.41XA | T88.52XA | T88.59XA | T88.6XXA | Z51.89 |
| Z88.0 | Z88.1 | Z88.2 | Z88.3 | Z88.4 |
| Z88.5 | Z88.6 | Z88.7 | Z88.8 | Z88.9 |
| Z91.010 | | | | |

– Significant cardiac dysfunction including recent or imminent cardiac decompensation, severe arrhythmia, unstable angina pectoris, recent

myocardial infarction, and pulmonary hypertension. The applicable ICD-9-CM codes are:

## ICD-9-CM

| | | | | |
|---|---|---|---|---|
| 402.00 | 402.01 | 402.10 | 402.11 | 402.90 |
| 402.91 | 404.00 | 404.01 | 404.02 | 404.03 |
| 404.10 | 404.11 | 404.12 | 404.13 | 404.90 |
| 404.91 | 404.92 | 404.93 | 410.00 | 410.01 |
| 410.02 | 410.10 | 410.11 | 410.12 | 410.20 |
| 410.21 | 410.22 | 410.30 | 410.31 | 410.32 |
| 410.40 | 410.41 | 410.42 | 410.50 | 410.51 |
| 410.52 | 410.60 | 410.61 | 410.62 | 410.70 |
| 410.71 | 410.72 | 410.80 | 410.81 | 410.82 |
| 410.90 | 410.91 | 410.92 | 411.1 | 415.0 |
| 416.0 | 416.1 | 416.8 | 416.9 | 420.0 |
| 420.90 | 420.91 | 420.99 | 424.90 | 424.91 |
| 424.99 | 427.0 | 427.1 | 427.2 | 427.31 |
| 427.32 | 427.41 | 427.42 | 427.5 | 427.60 |
| 427.61 | 427.69 | 427.81 | 427.89 | 427.9 |
| 428.0 | 428.1 | 428.9 | 429.0 | 429.1 |
| 429.2 | 429.3 | 429.4 | 429.5 | 429.6 |
| 429.71 | 429.79 | 429.81 | 429.82 | 429.89 |
| 429.9 | 785.50 | 785.51 | 785.59 | |

– The applicable ICD-10-CM codes are in the table below:

## ICD-10-CM Codes

| | | | | |
|---|---|---|---|---|
| A18.84 | I11.0 | I11.9 | I13.0 | I13.10 |
| I13.11 | I13.2 | I20.0 | I21.01 | I21.02 |
| I21.09 | I21.11 | I21.19 | I21.21 | I21.29 |
| I21.3 | I21.4 | I22.1 | I22.2 | I22.8 |
| I23.0 | I23.1 | I23.2 | I23.3 | I23.4 |
| I23.5 | I23.6 | I23.7 | I23.8 | I25.10 |
| I25.110 | I25.700 | I25.710 | I25.720 | I25.730 |
| I25.750 | I25.760 | I25.790 | I26.01 | I26.02 |
| I26.09 | I27.0 | I27.1 | I27.2 | I27.81 |
| I27.89 | I27.9 | I30.0 | I30.1 | I30.8 |
| I30.9 | I32 | I38 | I39 | I46.2 |
| I46.8 | I46.9 | I47.0 | I471 | I472 |
| I47.9 | I48.0 | I48.1 | I48.1 | I48.2 |
| I48.3 | I48.4 | I48.91 | I48.92 | I49.01 |
| I49.02 | I49.1 | I49.2 | I49.3 | I49.40 |
| I49.49 | I49.5 | I49.8 | I49.9 | I50.1 |
| I50.20 | I50.21 | I50.22 | I50.23 | I50.30 |
| I50.31 | I50.32 | I50.33 | I50.40 | I50.41 |
| I50.42 | I50.43 | I50.9 | I51 | I51.0 |
| I51.1 | I51.2 | I51.3 | I51.4 | I51.5 |
| I51.7 | I51.89 | I51.9 | I52 | I97.0 |
| I97.110 | I97.111 | I97.120 | I97.121 | I97.130 |
| I97.131 | I97.190 | I97.191 | M32.11 | M32.12 |
| R00.1 | R57.0 | R57.8 | R57.9 | |

– Generalized severe debilitation. The applicable ICD-9-CM codes are: 203.00, 203.01, all codes for diabetes mellitus, 518.81, 585, 586, 799.3, 799.4, and V46.1. The applicable ICD-10-CM codes are: J96.850, J96.00 through J96.02, J96.90 through J96.91, N18.1 through N19, R53.81, R64, and Z99.11 through Z99.12. Or

– Sickle Cell disease. The applicable ICD-9-CM codes are 282.4, 282.60, 282.61, 282.62, 282.63, and 282.69. The applicable ICD-10-CM codes are D56.0

© 2016 Optum360, LLC

through D56.3, D56.5 through D56.9, D57.00 through D57.1, D57.20, D57.411 through D57.419, and D57.811 through D57.819.

## 100-04, 13, 40.1.1

### Magnetic Resonance Angiography (MRA) Coverage Summary

Section 1861(s)(2)(C) of the Social Security Act provides for coverage of diagnostic testing. Coverage of magnetic resonance angiography (MRA) of the head and neck, and MRA of the peripheral vessels of the lower extremities is limited as described in Publication (Pub.) 100-03, the Medicare National Coverage Determinations (NCD) Manual. This instruction has been revised as of July 1, 2003, based on a determination that coverage is reasonable and necessary in additional circumstances. Under that instruction, MRA is generally covered only to the extent that it is used as a substitute for contrast angiography, except to the extent that there are documented circumstances consistent with that instruction that demonstrates the medical necessity of both tests. Prior to June 3, 2010, there was no coverage of MRA outside of the indications and circumstances described in that instruction.

Effective for claims with dates of service on or after June 3, 2010, contractors have the discretion to cover or not cover all indications of MRA (and magnetic resonance imaging (MRI)) that are not specifically nationally covered or nationally non-covered as stated in section 220.2 of the NCD Manual.

Because the status codes for HCPCS codes 71555, 71555-TC, 71555-26, 74185, 74185-TC, and 74185-26 were changed in the Medicare Physician Fee Schedule Database from 'N' to 'R' on April 1, 1998, any MRA claims with those HCPCS codes with dates of service between April 1, 1998, and June 30, 1999, are to be processed according to the contractor's discretionary authority to determine payment in the absence of national policy.

Effective for claims with dates of service on or after February 24, 2011, Medicare will provide coverage for MRIs for beneficiaries with implanted cardiac pacemakers or implantable cardioverter defibrillators if the beneficiary is enrolled in an approved clinical study under the Coverage with Study Participation form of Coverage with Evidence Development that meets specific criteria per Pub. 100-03, the NCD Manual, chapter 1, section 220.2.C.1

## 100-04, 13, 40.1.2

### HCPCS Coding Requirements

Providers must report HCPCS codes when submitting claims for MRA of the chest, abdomen, head, neck or peripheral vessels of lower extremities. The following HCPCS codes should be used to report these services:

| | |
|---|---|
| MRA of head | 70544, 70544-26, 70544-TC |
| MRA of head | 70545, 70545-26, 70545-TC |
| MRA of head | 70546, 70546-26, 70546-TC |
| MRA of neck | 70547, 70547-26, 70547-TC |
| MRA of neck | 70548, 70548-26, 70548-TC |
| MRA of neck | 70549, 70549-26, 70549-TC |
| MRA of chest | 71555, 71555-26, 71555-TC |
| MRA of pelvis | 72198, 72198-26, 72198-TC |

MRA of abdomen (dates of service 74185, 74185-26, 74185-TC on or after July 1, 2003)—see below.

| | |
|---|---|
| MRA of peripheral vessels of lower extremities | 73725, 73725-26, 73725-TC |

## 100-04, 13, 60

### Positron Emission Tomography (PET) Scans - General Information

Positron emission tomography (PET) is a noninvasive imaging procedure that assesses perfusion and the level of metabolic activity in various organ systems of the human body. A positron camera (tomograph) is used to produce cross-sectional tomographic images which are obtained by detecting radioactivity from a radioactive tracer substance radiopharmaceutical) that emits a radioactive tracer substance (radiopharmaceutical FDG) such as 2 -[F-18] flouro-D-glucose FDG, that is administered intravenously to the patient.

The Medicare National Coverage Determinations (NCD) Manual, Chapter 1, Sec.220.6, contains additional coverage instructions to indicate the conditions under which a PET scan is performed.

### A. Definitions

For all uses of PET, excluding Rubidium 82 for perfusion of the heart, myocardial viability and refractory seizures, the following definitions apply:

**Diagnosis:** PET is covered only in clinical situations in which the PET results may assist in avoiding an invasive diagnostic procedure, or in which the PET results may assist in determining the optimal anatomical location to perform an invasive

diagnostic procedure. In general, for most solid tumors, a tissue diagnosis is made prior to the performance of PET scanning. PET scans following a tissue diagnosis are generally performed for the purpose of staging, rather than diagnosis. Therefore, the use of PET in the diagnosis of lymphoma, esophageal and colorectal cancers, as well as in melanoma, should be rare. PET is not covered for other diagnostic uses, and is not covered for screening (testing of patients without specific signs and symptoms of disease).

**Staging:** PET is covered in clinical situations in which (1) (a) the stage of the cancer remains in doubt after completion of a standard diagnostic workup, including conventional imaging (computed tomography, magnetic resonance imaging, or ultrasound) or, (b) the use of PET would also be considered reasonable and necessary if it could potentially replace one or more conventional imaging studies when it is expected that conventional study information is insufficient for the clinical management of the patient and, (2) clinical management of the patient would differ depending on the stage of the cancer identified.

NOTE: Effective for services on or after April 3, 2009, the terms "diagnosis" and "staging" will be replaced with "Initial Treatment Strategy." For further information on this new term, refer to Pub. 100-03, NCD Manual, section 220.6.17.

**Restaging:** PET will be covered for restaging: (1) after the completion of treatment for the purpose of detecting residual disease, (2) for detecting suspected recurrence, or metastasis, (3) to determine the extent of a known recurrence, or (4) if it could potentially replace one or more conventional imaging studies when it is expected that conventional study information is to determine the extent of a known recurrence, or if study information is insufficient for the clinical management of the patient. Restaging applies to testing after a course of treatment is completed and is covered subject to the conditions above.

**Monitoring:** Use of PET to monitor tumor response to treatment during the planned course of therapy (i.e., when a change in therapy is anticipated).

NOTE: Effective for services on or after April 3, 2009, the terms "restaging" and "monitoring" will be replaced with "Subsequent Treatment Strategy." For further information on this new term, refer to Pub. 100-03, NCD Manual, section 220.6.17.

### B. Limitations

For staging and restaging: PET is covered in either/or both of the following circumstances:

The stage of the cancer remains in doubt after completion of a standard diagnostic workup, including conventional imaging (computed tomography, magnetic resonance imaging, or ultrasound); and/or

The clinical management of the patient would differ depending on the stage of the cancer identified. PET will be covered for restaging after the completion of treatment for the purpose of detecting residual disease, for detecting suspected recurrence, or to determine the extent of a known recurrence. Use of PET would also be considered reasonable and necessary if it could potentially replace one or more conventional imaging studies when it is expected that conventional study information is insufficient for the clinical management of the patient.

The PET is not covered for other diagnostic uses, and is not covered for screening (testing of patients without specific symptoms). Use of PET to monitor tumor response during the planned course of therapy (i.e. when no change in therapy is being contemplated) is not covered.

## 100-04, 13, 60.3

### PET Scan Qualifying Conditions and HCPCS Code Chart

Below is a summary of all covered PET scan conditions, with effective dates.

NOTE: The G codes below except those a # can be used to bill for PET Scan services through January 27, 2005. Effective for dates of service on or after January 28, 2005, providers must bill for PET Scan services using the appropriate CPT codes. See section 60.3.1. The G codes with a # can continue to be used for billing after January 28, 2005 and these remain non-covered by Medicare. (NOTE: PET Scanners must be FDA-approved.)

| Conditions | Coverage Effective Date | ****HCPCS/CPT |
|---|---|---|
| *Myocardial perfusion imaging (following previous PET G0030-G0047) single study, rest or stress (exercise and/or pharmacologic) | 3/14/95 | G0030 |
| *Myocardial perfusion imaging (following previous PET G0030-G0047) multiple studies, rest or stress (exercise and/or pharmacologic) | 3/14/95 | G0031 |

| Conditions | Coverage Effective Date | ****HCPCS/CPT |
|---|---|---|
| *Myocardial perfusion imaging (following rest SPECT, 78464); single study, rest or stress (exercise and/or pharmacologic) | 3/14/95 | G0032 |
| *Myocardial perfusion imaging (following rest SPECT 78464); multiple studies, rest or stress (exercise and/or pharmacologic) | 3/14/95 | G0033 |
| *Myocardial perfusion (following stress SPECT 78465); single study, rest or stress (exercise and/or pharmacologic) | 3/14/95 | G0034 |
| *Myocardial Perfusion Imaging (following stress SPECT 78465); multiple studies, rest or stress (exercise and/or pharmacologic) | 3/14/95 | G0035 |
| *Myocardial Perfusion Imaging (following coronary angiography 93510-93529); single study, rest or stress (exercise and/or pharmacologic) | 3/14/95 | G0036 |
| *Myocardial Perfusion Imaging, (following coronary angiography), 93510-93529); multiple studies, rest or stress (exercise and/or pharmacologic) | 3/14/95 | G0037 |
| *Myocardial Perfusion Imaging (following stress planar myocardial perfusion, 78460); single study, rest or stress (exercise and/or pharmacologic) | 3/14/95 | G0038 |
| *Myocardial Perfusion Imaging (following stress planar myocardial perfusion, 78460); multiple studies, rest or stress (exercise and/or pharmacologic) | 3/14/95 | G0039 |
| *Myocardial Perfusion Imaging (following stress echocardiogram 93350); single study, rest or stress (exercise and/or pharmacologic) | 3/14/95 | G0040 |
| *Myocardial Perfusion Imaging (following stress echocardiogram, 93350); multiple studies, rest or stress (exercise and/or pharmacologic) | 3/14/95 | G0041 |
| *Myocardial Perfusion Imaging (following stress nuclear ventriculogram 78481 or 78483); single study, rest or stress (exercise and/or pharmacologic) | 3/14/95 | G0042 |
| *Myocardial Perfusion Imaging (following stress nuclear ventriculogram 78481 or 78483); multiple studies, rest or stress (exercise and/or pharmacologic) | 3/14/95 | G0043 |
| *Myocardial Perfusion Imaging (following stress ECG, 93000); single study, rest or stress (exercise and/or pharmacologic) | 3/14/95 | G0044 |
| *Myocardial perfusion (following stress ECG, 93000), multiple studies; rest or stress (exercise and/or pharmacologic) | 3/14/95 | G0045 |
| *Myocardial perfusion (following stress ECG, 93015), single study; rest or stress (exercise and/or pharmacologic) | 3/14/95 | G0046 |
| *Myocardial perfusion (following stress ECG, 93015); multiple studies, rest or stress (exercise and/or pharmacologic) | 3/14/95 | G0047 |
| PET imaging regional or whole body; single pulmonary nodule | 1/1/98 | G0125 |
| Lung cancer, non-small cell (PET imaging whole body) Diagnosis, Initial Staging, Restaging | 7/1/01 | G0210 G0211 G0212 |
| Colorectal cancer (PET imaging whole body) Diagnosis, Initial Staging, Restaging | 7/1/01 | G0213 G0214 G0215 |

| Conditions | Coverage Effective Date | ****HCPCS/CPT |
|---|---|---|
| Melanoma (PET imaging whole body) Diagnosis, Initial Staging, Restaging | 7/1/01 | G0216 G0217 G0218 |
| Melanoma for non-covered indications Lymphoma (PET imaging whole body) | 7/1/01 | #G0219 |
| Diagnosis, Initial Staging, Restaging | 7/1/01 | G0220 G0221 G0222 |
| Head and neck cancer; excluding thyroid and CNS cancers (PET imaging whole body or regional) Diagnosis, Initial Staging, Restaging | 7/1/01 | G0223 G0224 G0225 |

## 100-04, 13, 60.3.1

### Appropriate CPT Codes Effective for PET Scans for Services Performed on or After January 28, 2005

NOTE: All PET scan services require the use of a radiopharmaceutical diagnostic imaging agent (tracer). The applicable tracer code should be billed when billing for a PET scan service. See section 60.3.2 below for applicable tracer codes.

| CPT Code | Description |
|---|---|
| 78459 | Myocardial imaging, positron emission tomography (PET), metabolic evaluation |
| 78491 | Myocardial imaging, positron emission tomography (PET), perfusion, single study at rest or stress |
| 78492 | Myocardial imaging, positron emission tomography (PET), perfusion, multiple studies at rest and/or stress |
| 78608 | Brain imaging, positron emission tomography (PET); metabolic evaluation |
| 78811 | Tumor imaging, positron emission tomography (PET); limited area (eg, chest, head/neck) |
| 78812 | Tumor imaging, positron emission tomography (PET); skull base to mid-thigh |
| 78813 | Tumor imaging, positron emission tomography (PET); whole body |
| 78814 | Tumor imaging, positron emission tomography (PET) with concurrently acquired computed tomography (CT) for attenuation correction and anatomical localization; limited area (eg, chest, head/neck) |
| 78815 | Tumor imaging, positron emission tomography (PET) with concurrently acquired computed tomography (CT) for attenuation correction and anatomical localization; skull base to mid-thigh |
| 78816 | Tumor imaging, positron emission tomography (PET) with concurrently acquired computed tomography (CT) for attenuation correction and anatomical localization; whole body |

## 100-04, 13, 60.3.2

### Tracer Codes Required for PET Scans

The following tracer codes are applicable only to CPT 78491 and 78492. They can not be reported with any other code.

Institutional providers billing the fiscal intermediary

| HCPCS | Description |
|---|---|
| *A9555 | Rubidium Rb-82, Diagnostic, Per study dose, Up To 60 Millicuries |
| * Q3000 (Deleted effective 12/31/05) | Supply of Radiopharmaceutical Diagnostic Imaging Agent, Rubidium Rb-82, per dose |
| A9526 | Nitrogen N-13 Ammonia, Diagnostic, Per study dose, Up To 40 Millicuries |

NOTE: For claims with dates of service prior to 1/01/06, providers report Q3000 for supply of radiopharmaceutical diagnostic imaging agent, Rubidium Rb-82. For claims with dates of service 1/01/06 and later, providers report A9555 for radiopharmaceutical diagnostic imaging agent, Rubidium Rb-82 in place of Q3000.

© 2016 Optum360, LLC

Physicians / practitioners billing the carrier:

| | |
|---|---|
| *A4641 | Supply of Radiopharmaceutical Diagnostic Imaging Agent, Not Otherwise Classified |
| A9526 | Nitrogen N-13 Ammonia, Diagnostic, Per study dose, Up To 40 Millicuries |
| A9555 | Rubidium Rb-82, Diagnostic, Per study dose, Up To 60 Millicuries |

\* NOTE: Effective January 1, 2008, tracer code A4641 is not applicable for PET Scans.

The following tracer codes are applicable only to CPT 78459, 78608, 78811-78816. They can not be reported with any other code:

Institutional providers billing the fiscal intermediary:

| | |
|---|---|
| * A9552 | Fluorodeoxyglucose F18, FDG, Diagnostic, Per study dose, Up to 45 Millicuries |
| *C1775 (Deleted effective 12/31/05) | Supply of Radiopharmaceutical Diagnostic Imaging Agent, Fluorodeoxyglucose F18, (2-Deoxy-2-18F Fluoro-D-Glucose), Per dose (4-40 Mci/Ml) |
| **A4641 | Supply of Radiopharmaceutical Diagnostic Imaging Agent, Not Otherwise Classified |
| A9580 | Sodium Fluoride F-18, Diagnostic, per study dose, up to 30 Millicuries |

\*\* NOTE: Effective January 1, 2008, tracer code A4641 is not applicable for PET Scans.
\*\*\* NOTE: Effective for claims with dates of service February 26, 2010 and later, tracer code A9580 is applicable for PET Scans.

NOTE: For claims with dates of service prior to 1/01/06, OPPS hospitals report C1775 for supply of radiopharmaceutical diagnostic imaging agent, Fluorodeoxyglucose F18. For claims with dates of service January 1, 2006 and later, providers report A9552 for radiopharmaceutical diagnostic imaging agent, Fluorodeoxyglucose F18 in place of C1775.

Physicians / practitioners billing the carrier:

| | |
|---|---|
| A9552 | Fluorodeoxyglucose F18, FDG, Diagnostic, Per study dose, Up to 45 Millicuries |
| *A4641 | Supply of Radiopharmaceutical Diagnostic Imaging Agent, Not Otherwise Classified |
| A9580 | Sodium Fluoride F-18, Diagnostic, per study dose, up to 30 Millicuries |

\* NOTE: Effective January 1, 2008, tracer code A4641 is not applicable for PET Scans.
\*\*\* NOTE: Effective for claims with dates of service February 26, 2010 and later, tracer code A9580 is applicable for PET Scans.

Positron Emission Tomography Reference Table

| CPT | Short Descriptor | Tracer/ Code | or | Tracer/ Code | Comment |
|---|---|---|---|---|---|
| 78459 | Myocardial imaging, positron emission tomography (PET), metabolic imaging | FDG A9552 | -- | -- | N/A |
| 78491 | Myocardial imaging, positron emission tomography (PET), perfusion; single study at rest or stress | N-13 A9526 | or | Rb-82 A9555 | N/A |
| 78492 | Myocardial imaging, positron emission tomography (PET), perfusion; multiple studies at rest and/or stress | N-13 A9526 | or | Rb-82 A9555 | N/A |

| CPT | Short Descriptor | Tracer/ Code | or | Tracer/ Code | Comment |
|---|---|---|---|---|---|
| 78608 | Brain imaging, positron emission tomography (PET); metabolic evaluation | FDG A9552 | -- | -- | Covered indications: Alzheimer's disease/dementias, intractable seizures Note: This code is also covered for dedicated PET brain tumor imaging. |
| 78609 | Brain imaging, positron emission tomography (PET); perfusion evaluation | -- | -- | -- | Nationally noncovered |
| 78811 | Positron emission tomography (PET) imaging; limited area (e.g, chest, head/neck) | FDG A9552 | or | NaF-18 A9580 | NaF-18 PET is covered only to identify bone metastasis of cancer. |

## 100-04, 13, 60.7.1

### Darbepoetin Alfa (Aranesp) Facility Billing Requirements

Revenue code 0636 is used to report Aranesp.

The HCPCS code for aranesp must be included: HCPCS HCPCS Description Dates of Service Q4054 Injection, darbepoetin alfa, 1mcg (for ESRD on Dialysis) 1/1/2004 through 12/31/2005 J0882 Injection, darbepoetin alfa, 1mcg (for ESRD on Dialysis) 1/1/2006 to present The hematocrit reading taken prior to the last administration of Aranesp during the billing period must also be reported on the UB-92/Form CMS-1450 with value code 49. For claims with dates of service on or after April 1, 2006, a hemoglobin reading may be reported on Aranesp claims using value code 48.

Effective January 1, 2006 the definition of value code 48 and 49 used to report the hemoglobin and hematocrit readings are changed to indicate the patient's most recent reading taken before the start of the billing period.

To report a hematocrit or hemoglobin reading for a new patient on or after January 1, 2006, the provider should report the reading that prompted the treatment of darbepoetin alfa. The provider may use results documented on form CMS 2728 or the patient's medical records from a transferring facility.

The payment allowance for Aranesp is the only allowance for the drug and its administration when used for ESRD patients. Effective January 1, 2005, the cost of supplies to administer Aranesp may be billed to the FI. HCPCS A4657 and Revenue Code 270 should be used to capture the charges for syringes used in the administration of Aranesp. The maximum number of administrations of Aranesp for a billing cycle is 5 times in 30/ 31days.

## 100-04, 13, 60.12

### Coverage for PET Scans for Dementia and Neurodegenerative Diseases
(Rev. 3227, Issued: 04-02-15, Effective; ASC-X12: January 1, 2012

Fluorodeoxyglucose (FDG) Positron Emission Tomography (PET) for Solid Tumors: June 11, 2013, ICD-10: Upon Implementation of ICD-10

Implementation: ASC X12: November 10, 2014 Fluorodeoxyglucose (FDG) Positron Emission Tomography (PET) for Solid Tumors: May 19, 2014 - MAC Non-Shared System Edits; July 7, 2014 - CWF development/testing, FISS requirement development; October 6, 2014 - CWF, FISS, MCS Shared System Edits), ICD-10: Upon Implementation of ICD-10)

Effective for dates of service on or after September 15, 2004, Medicare will cover FDG PET scans for a differential diagnosis of fronto-temporal dementia (FTD) and Alzheimer's disease OR; its use in a CMS-approved practical clinical trial focused on the utility of FDG-PET in the diagnosis or treatment of dementing neurodegenerative diseases. Refer to Pub. 100-03, NCD Manual, section 220.6.13, for complete coverage conditions and clinical trial requirements and section 60.15 of this manual for claims processing information.

© 2016 Optum360, LLC

## A. A/B MAC (A and B) Billing Requirements for PET Scan Claims for FDG-PET for the Differential Diagnosis of Fronto-temporal Dementia and Alzheimer's Disease:

### CPT Code for PET Scans for Dementia and Neurodegenerative Diseases

Contractors shall advise providers to use the appropriate CPT code from section 60.3.1 for dementia and neurodegenerative diseases for services performed on or after January 28, 2005.

Diagnosis Codes for PET Scans for Dementia and Neurodegenerative Diseases

The contractor shall ensure one of the following appropriate diagnosis codes is present on claims for PET Scans for AD:

- If ICD-9-CM is applicable, ICD-9 codes are: 290.0, 290.10 - 290.13, 290.20 - 290, 21, 290.3, 331.0, 331.11, 331.19, 331.2, 331.9, 780.93
- If ICD-10-CM is applicable, ICD-10 codes are: F03.90, F03.90 plus F05, G30.9, G31.01, G31.9, R41.2 or R41.3

Medicare contractors shall use an appropriate Medicare Summary Notice (MSN) message such as 16.48, "Medicare does not pay for this item or service for this condition" to deny claims when submitted with an appropriate CPT code from section 60.3.1 and with a diagnosis code other than the range of codes listed above. Also, contractors shall use an appropriate Remittance Advice (RA) such as 11, "The diagnosis is inconsistent with the procedure."

Medicare contractors shall instruct providers to issue an Advanced Beneficiary Notice to beneficiaries advising them of potential financial liability prior to delivering the service if one of the appropriate diagnosis codes will not be present on the claim.

### Provider Documentation Required with the PET Scan Claim

Medicare contractors shall inform providers to ensure the conditions mentioned in the NCD Manual, section 220.6.13, have been met. The information must also be maintained in the beneficiary's medical record:

- Date of onset of symptoms;
- Diagnosis of clinical syndrome (normal aging, mild cognitive impairment or MCI: mild, moderate, or severe dementia);
- Mini mental status exam (MMSE) or similar test score;
- Presumptive cause (possible, probably, uncertain AD);
- Any neuropsychological testing performed;
- Results of any structural imaging (MRI, CT) performed;
- Relevant laboratory tests (B12, thyroid hormone); and,
- Number and name of prescribed medications.

## B. Billing Requirements for Beta Amyloid Positron Emission Tomography (PET) in Dementia and Neurodegenerative Disease:

Effective for claims with dates of service on and after September 27, 2013, Medicare will only allow coverage with evidence development (CED) for Positron Emission Tomography (PET) beta amyloid (also referred to as amyloid-beta (Aβ)) imaging (HCPCS A9586)or (HCPCS A9599) (one PET Aβ scan per patient).

NOTE: Please note that effective January 1, 2014 the following code A9599 will be updated in the IOCE and HCPCS update. This code will be contractor priced.

Medicare Summary Notices, Remittance Advice Remark Codes, and Claim Adjustment Reason Codes

Effective for dates of service on or after September 27, 2013, contractors shall return as unprocessable/return to provider claims for PET Aβ imaging, through CED during a clinical trial, not containing the following:

- Condition code 30, (FI only)
- Modifier Q0 and/or modifier Q1 as appropriate
- ICD-9 dx code V70.7/ICD-10 dx code Z00.6 (on either the primary/secondary position)
- A PET HCPCS code (78811 or 78814)
- At least, one Dx code from the table below,

| ICD-9 Codes | Corresponding ICD-10 Codes |
|---|---|
| 290.0 Senile dementia, uncomplicated | F03.90 Unspecified dementia without behavioral disturbance |
| 290.10 Presenile dementia, uncomplicated | F03.90 Unspecified dementia without behavioral disturbance |
| 290.11 Presenile dementia with delirium | F03.90 Unspecified dementia without behavioral disturbance |
| 290.12 Presenile dementia with delusional features | F03.90 Unspecified dementia without behavioral disturbance |

| ICD-9 Codes | Corresponding ICD-10 Codes |
|---|---|
| 290.13 Presenile dementia with depressive features | F03.90 Unspecified dementia without behavioral disturbance |
| 290.20 Senile dementia with delusional features | F03.90 Unspecified dementia without behavioral disturbance |
| 290.21 Senile dementia with depressive features | F03.90 Unspecified dementia without behavioral disturbance |
| 290.3 Senile dementia with delirium | F03.90 Unspecified dementia without behavioral disturbance |
| 290.40 Vascular dementia, uncomplicated | F01.50 Vascular dementia without behavioral disturbance |
| 290.41 Vascular dementia with delirium | F01.51 Vascular dementia with behavioral disturbance |
| 290.42 Vascular dementia with delusions | F01.51 Vascular dementia with behavioral disturbance |
| 290.43 Vascular dementia with depressed mood | F01.51 Vascular dementia with behavioral disturbance |
| 294.10 Dementia in conditions classified elsewhere without behavioral disturbance | F02.80 Dementia in other diseases classified elsewhere without behavioral disturbance |
| 294.11 Dementia in conditions classified elsewhere with behavioral disturbance | F02.81 Dementia in other diseases classified elsewhere with behavioral disturbance |
| 294.20 Dementia, unspecified, without behavioral disturbance | F03.90 Unspecified dementia without behavioral disturbance |
| 294.21 Dementia, unspecified, with behavioral disturbance | F03.91 Unspecified dementia with behavioral disturbance |
| 331.11 Pick's Disease | G31.01 Pick's disease |
| 331.19 Other Frontotemporal dementia | G31.09 Other frontotemporal dementia |
| 331.6 Corticobasal degeneration | G31.85 Corticobasal degeneration |
| 331.82 Dementia with Lewy Bodies | G31.83 Dementia with Lewy bodies |
| 331.83 Mild cognitive impairment, so stated | G31.84 Mild cognitive impairment, so stated |
| 780.93 Memory LossR41.1 Anterograde amnesia | R41.2 Retrograde amnesia<br>R41.3 Other amnesia (Amnesia NOS, Memory loss NOS) |
| V70.7 Examination for normal comparison or control in clinical | Z00.6 Encounter for examination for normal comparison and control in clinical research program |

and

- Aβ HCPCS code A9586 or A9599

Contractors shall return as unprocessable claims for PET Aβ imaging using the following messages:

- Claim Adjustment Reason Code 4 – the procedure code is inconsistent with the modifier used or a required modifier is missing.

  Note: Refer to the 835 Healthcare Policy Identification Segment (loop 2110 Service Payment Information REF), if present.

- Remittance Advice Remark Code N517 - Resubmit a new claim with the requested information.
- Remittance Advice Remark Code N519 - Invalid combination of HCPCS modifiers.

Contractors shall line-item deny claims for PET Aβ , HCPCS code A9586 or A9599 , where a previous PET Aβ, HCPCS code A9586 or A9599 is paid in history using the following messages:

- CARC 149: "Lifetime benefit maximum has been reached for this service/benefit category."
- RARC N587: "Policy benefits have been exhausted".
- MSN 20.12: "This service was denied because Medicare only covers this service once a lifetime."
- Spanish Version: "Este servicio fue negado porque Medicare sólo cubre este servicio una vez en la vida."
- Group Code: PR, if a claim is received with a GA modifier
- Group Code: CO, if a claim is received with a GZ modifier

© 2016 Optum360, LLC

## 100-04, 13, 60.13

### Billing Requirements for PET Scans for Specific Indications of Cervical Cancer for Services Performed on or After January 28, 2005

Contractors shall accept claims for these services with the appropriate CPT code listed in section 60.3.1. Refer to Pub. 100-03, section 220.6.17, for complete coverage guidelines for this new PET oncology indication. The implementation date for these CPT codes will be April 18, 2005. Also see section 60.17, of this chapter for further claims processing instructions for cervical cancer indications.

## 100-04, 13, 60.14

### Billing Requirements for PET Scans for Non-Covered Indications

For services performed on or after January 28, 2005, contractors shall accept claims with the following HCPCS code for non-covered PET indications: - G0235: PET imaging, any site not otherwise specified Short Descriptor: PET not otherwise specified Type of Service: 4

NOTE: This code is for a non-covered service.

## 100-04, 13, 60.15

### Billing Requirements for CMS - Approved Clinical Trials and Coverage With Evidence Development Claims for PET Scans for Neurodegenerative Diseases, Previously Specified Cancer Indications, and All Other Cancer Indications Not Previously Specified

#### Parts A and B Medicare Administrative Contractors (MACs)

Effective for services on or after January 28, 2005, contractors shall accept and pay for claims for Positron Emission Tomography (PET) scans for lung cancer, esophageal cancer, colorectal cancer, lymphoma, melanoma, head & neck cancer, breast cancer, thyroid cancer, soft tissue sarcoma, brain cancer, ovarian cancer, pancreatic cancer, small cell lung cancer, and testicular cancer, as well as for neurodegenerative diseases and all other cancer indications not previously mentioned in this chapter, if these scans were performed as part of a Centers for Medicare & Medicaid (CMS)-approved clinical trial. (See Pub. 100-03, National Coverage Determinations (NCD) Manual, sections 220.6.13 and 220.6.17.)

Contractors shall also be aware that PET scans for all cancers not previously specified at Pub. 100-03, NCD Manual, section 220.6.17, remain nationally non-covered unless performed in conjunction with a CMS-approved clinical trial.

Effective for dates of service on or after June 11, 2013, Medicare has ended the coverage with evidence development (CED) requirement for FDG (2-[F18] fluoro-2-deoxy-D-glucose) PET and PET/computed tomography (CT) and PET/magnetic resonance imaging (MRI) for all oncologic indications contained in section 220.6.17 of the NCD Manual. Modifier -Q0 (Investigational clinical service provided in a clinical research study that is in an approved clinical research study) or -Q1 (routine clinical service provided in a clinical research study that is in an approved clinical research study) is no longer mandatory for these services when performed on or after June 11, 2013.

#### Part B MACs Only

Part B MACs shall pay claims for PET scans for beneficiaries participating in a CMS-approved clinical trial submitted with an appropriate current procedural terminology (CPT) code from section 60.3.1 of this chapter and modifier -Q0/-Q1 for services performed on or after January 1, 2008, through June 10, 2013. (NOTE: Modifier -QR (Item or service provided in a Medicare specified study) and -QA (FDA investigational device exemption) were replaced by modifier -Q0 effective January 1, 2008.) Modifier -QV (item or service provided as routine care in a Medicare qualifying clinical trial) was replaced by modifier -Q1 effective January 1, 2008.) Beginning with services performed on or after June 11, 2013, modifier -Q0/-Q1 is no longer required for PET FDG services.

#### Part A MACs Only

In order to pay claims for PET scans on behalf of beneficiaries participating in a CMS-approved clinical trial, Part A MACs require providers to submit claims with ICD-9/ICD-10 code V70.7/Z00.6 in the primary/secondary diagnosis position on the CMS-1450 (UB-04), or the electronic equivalent, with the appropriate principal diagnosis code and an appropriate CPT code from section 60.3.1. Effective for PET scan claims for dates of service on or after January 28, 2005, through December 31, 2007, FIs shall accept claims with the -QR, -QV, or -QA modifier on other than inpatient claims. Effective for services on or after January 1, 2008, through June 10, 2013, modifier -Q0 replaced the -QR and -QA modifier, modifier -Q1 replaced the -QV modifier. Modifier -Q0/-Q1 is no longer required for services performed on or after June 11, 2013.

## 100-04, 13, 60.16

### Billing and Coverage Changes for PET Scans Effective for Services on or After April 3, 2009

#### A. Summary of Changes

Effective for services on or after April 3, 2009, Medicare will not cover the use of FDG PET imaging to determine initial treatment strategy in patients with adenocarcinoma of the prostate.

Medicare will also not cover FDG PET imaging for subsequent treatment strategy for tumor types other than breast, cervical, colorectal, esophagus, head and neck (non-CNS/thyroid), lymphoma, melanoma, myeloma, non-small cell lung, and ovarian, unless the FDG PET is provided under the coverage with evidence development (CED) paradigm (billed with modifier -Q0, see section 60.15 of this chapter).

Last, Medicare will cover FDG PET imaging for initial treatment strategy for myeloma.

For further information regarding the changes in coverage, refer to Pub.100-03, NCD Manual, section 220.6.17.

#### B. New Modifiers for PET Scans

Effective for claims with dates of service on or after April 3, 2009, the following modifiers have been created for use to inform for the initial treatment strategy of biopsy-proven or strongly suspected tumors or subsequent treatment strategy of cancerous tumors:

PI -Positron Emission Tomography (PET) or PET/Computed Tomography (CT) to inform the initial treatment strategy of tumors that are biopsy proven or strongly suspected of being cancerous based on other diagnostic testing.

Short descriptor: PET tumor init tx strat

PS - Positron Emission Tomography (PET) or PET/Computed Tomography (CT) to inform the subsequent treatment strategy of cancerous tumors when the beneficiary's treatment physician determines that the PET study is needed to inform subsequent anti-tumor strategy.

Short descriptor: PS - PET tumor subsq tx strategy

#### C. Billing Changes for A/B MACs, FIs and Carriers

Effective for claims with dates of service on or after April 3, 2009, contractors shall accept FDG PET claims billed to inform initial treatment strategy with the following CPT codes AND modifier -PI: 78608, 78811, 78812, 78813, 78814, 78815, 78816.

Effective for claims with dates of service on or after April 3, 2009, contractors shall accept FDG PET claims with modifier -PS for the subsequent treatment strategy for solid tumors using a CPT code above AND a cancer diagnosis code.

Contractors shall also accept FDG PET claims billed to inform initial treatment strategy or subsequent treatment strategy when performed under CED with one of the PET or PET/CT CPT codes above AND modifier -PI OR modifier -PS AND and a cancer diagnosis code AND modifier -Q0 (Investigational clinical service provided in a clinical research study that is in an approved clinical research study).

NOTE: For institutional claims providers report condition code 30 and ICD-9 CM diagnosis V70.7 or ICD-10-CM diagnosis code Z006 on the claim.

#### D. Medicare Summary Notices, Remittance Advice Remark Codes, and Claim Adjustment Reason Codes

Effective for dates of service on or after April 3, 2009, contractors shall return as unprocessable/return to provider claims that do not include the -PI modifier with one of the PET/PET/CT CPT codes listed in subsection C. above when billing for the initial treatment strategy for solid tumors in accordance with Pub.100-03, NCD Manual, section 220.6.17.

In addition, contractors shall return as unprocessable/return to provider claims that do not include the -PS modifier with one of the CPT codes listed in subsection C. above when billing for the subsequent treatment strategy for solid tumors in accordance with Pub.100-03, NCD Manual, section 220.6.17.

The following messages apply:

- Claim Adjustment Reason Code 4 – the procedure code is inconsistent with the modifier used or a required modifier is missing.
- Remittance Advice Remark Code MA-130 - Your claim contains incomplete and/or invalid information, and no appeal rights are afforded because the claim is unprocessable. Submit a new claim with the complete/correct information.
- Remittance Advice Remark Code M16 - Alert: See our Web site, mailings, or bulletins for more details concerning this policy/procedure/decision.

Also, effective for claims with dates of service on or after April 3, 2009, contractors shall return as unprocessable/return to provider FDG PET claims billed to inform initial treatment strategy or subsequent treatment strategy when performed under

CED without one of the PET/PET/CT CPT codes listed in subsection C. above AND modifier –PI OR modifier –PS AND an ICD-9 cancer diagnosis code AND modifier –Q0.

The following messages apply to return as unprocessable claims:

- Claim Adjustment Reason Code 4 – the procedure code is inconsistent with the modifier used or a required modifier is missing.
- Remittance Advice Remark Code MA-130 - Your claim contains incomplete and/or invalid information, and no appeal rights are afforded because the claim is unprocessable. Submit a new claim with the complete/correct information.
- Remittance Advice Remark Code M16 - Alert: See our Web site, mailings, or bulletins for more details concerning this policy/procedure/decision.

Effective April 3, 2009, contractors shall deny claims with ICD-9 diagnosis code 185 or ICD-10 diagnosis code C61 for FDG PET imaging for the initial treatment strategy of patients with adenocarcinoma of the prostate.

Contractors shall also deny claims for FDG PET imaging for subsequent treatment strategy for tumor types other than breast, cervical, colorectal, esophagus, head and neck (non-CNS/thyroid), lymphoma, melanoma, myeloma, non-small cell lung, and ovarian, unless the FDG PET is provided under CED (submitted with the -Q0 modifier) and use the following messages:

- Medicare Summary Notice 15.4 - Medicare does not support the need for this service or item
- Claim Adjustment Reason Code 50 - These are non-covered services because this is not deemed a 'medical necessity' by the payer.
- Contractors shall use Group Code CO (Contractual Obligation)

If an ABN is provided with a GA modifier indicating there is a signed ABN on file, contractors shall use Group Code PR (Patient Responsibility) and the liability falls to the beneficiary.

If an ABN is provided with a GZ modifier indicating no ABN was provided, contractors shall use Group Code CO (Contractual Obligation) and the liability falls to the provider.

Medicare will also not cover FDG PET imaging for subsequent treatment strategy for tumor types other than breast, cervical, colorectal, esophagus, head and neck (non-CNS/thyroid), lymphoma, melanoma, myeloma, non-small cell lung, and ovarian, unless the FDG PET is provided under the coverage with evidence development (CED) paradigm (billed with modifier -Q0, see section 60.15 of this chapter).

Last, Medicare will cover FDG PET imaging for initial treatment strategy for myeloma.

For further information regarding the changes in coverage, refer to Pub.100-03, NCD Manual, section 220.6.17.

**B. New Modifiers for PET Scans**
Effective for claims with dates of service on or after April 3, 2009, the following modifiers have been created for use to inform for the initial treatment strategy of biopsy-proven or strongly suspected tumors or subsequent treatment strategy of cancerous tumors:

PI -Positron Emission Tomography (PET) or PET/Computed Tomography (CT) to inform the initial treatment strategy of tumors that are biopsy proven or strongly suspected of being cancerous based on other diagnostic testing.

Short descriptor: PET tumor init tx strat

PS - Positron Emission Tomography (PET) or PET/Computed Tomography (CT) to inform the subsequent treatment strategy of cancerous tumors when the beneficiary's treatment physician determines that the PET study is needed to inform subsequent anti-tumor strategy.

Short descriptor: PS - PET tumor subsq tx strategy

**C. Billing Changes for A/B MACs, FIs and Carriers**
Effective for claims with dates of service on or after April 3, 2009, contractors shall accept FDG PET claims billed to inform initial treatment strategy with the following CPT codes AND modifier –PI: 78608, 78811, 78812, 78813, 78814, 78815, 78816.

Effective for claims with dates of service on or after April 3, 2009, contractors shall accept FDG PET claims with modifier –PS for the subsequent treatment strategy for solid tumors using a CPT code above AND an ICD-9 cancer diagnosis code.

Contractors shall also accept FDG PET claims billed to inform initial treatment strategy or subsequent treatment strategy when performed under CED with one of the PET or PET/CT CPT codes above AND modifier -PI OR modifier -PS AND an ICD-9 cancer diagnosis code AND modifier -Q0 (Investigational clinical service provided in a clinical research study that is in an approved clinical research study).

**NOTE:** For institutional claims continue to use diagnosis code V70.7 and condition code 30 on the claim.

**D. Medicare Summary Notices, Remittance Advice Remark Codes, and Claim Adjustment Reason Codes**
Effective for dates of service on or after April 3, 2009, contractors shall return as unprocessable/return to provider claims that do not include the -PI modifier with one of the PET/PET/CT CPT codes listed in subsection C. above when billing for the initial treatment strategy for solid tumors in accordance with Pub.100-03, NCD Manual, section 220.6.17.

In addition, contractors shall return as unprocessable/return to provider claims that do not include the -PS modifier with one of the CPT codes listed in subsection C. above when billing for the subsequent treatment strategy for solid tumors in accordance with Pub.100-03, NCD Manual, section 220.6.17.

The following messages apply:

- -Claim Adjustment Reason Code 4 – the procedure code is inconsistent with the modifier used or a required modifier is missing.
- -Remittance Advice Remark Code MA-130 - Your claim contains incomplete and/or invalid information, and no appeal rights are afforded because the claim is unprocessable. Submit a new claim with the complete/correct information.
- Remittance Advice Remark Code M16 - Alert: See our Web site, mailings, or bulletins for more details concerning this policy/procedure/decision.

Also, effective for claims with dates of service on or after April 3, 2009, contractors shall return as unprocessable/return to provider FDG PET claims billed to inform initial treatment strategy or subsequent treatment strategy when performed under CED without one of the PET/PET/CT CPT codes listed in subsection C. above AND modifier –PI OR modifier –PS AND an ICD-9 cancer diagnosis code AND modifier –Q0.

The following messages apply to return as unprocessable claims:

- Claim Adjustment Reason Code 4 – the procedure code is inconsistent with the modifier used or a required modifier is missing.
- Remittance Advice Remark Code MA-130 - Your claim contains incomplete and/or invalid information, and no appeal rights are afforded because the claim is unprocessable. Submit a new claim with the complete/correct information.
- Remittance Advice Remark Code M16 - Alert: See our Web site, mailings, or bulletins for more details concerning this policy/procedure/decision.

Effective April 3, 2009, contractors shall deny claims with ICD-9 diagnosis code 185 for FDG PET imaging for the initial treatment strategy of patients with adenocarcinoma of the prostate.

Contractors shall also deny claims for FDG PET imaging for subsequent treatment strategy for tumor types other than breast, cervical, colorectal, esophagus, head and neck (non-CNS/thyroid), lymphoma, melanoma, myeloma, non-small cell lung, and ovarian, unless the FDG PET is provided under CED (submitted with the -Q0 modifier) and use the following messages:

- Medicare Summary Notice 15.4 - Medicare does not support the need for this service or item
- Claim Adjustment Reason Code 50 - These are non-covered services because this is not deemed a 'medical necessity' by the payer.
- Contractors shall use Group Code CO (Contractual Obligation)

If an ABN is provided with a GA modifier indicating there is a signed ABN on file, contractors shall use Group Code PR (Patient Responsibility) and the liability falls to the beneficiary.

If an ABN is provided with a GZ modifier indicating no ABN was provided, contractors shall use Group Code CO (Contractual Obligation) and the liability falls to the provider.

## 100-04, 13, 60.17

### Billing and Coverage Changes for PET Scans for Cervical Cancer Effective for Services on or After November 10, 2009

**A. Billing Changes for A/B MACs, FIs, and Carriers**
Effective for claims with dates of service on or after November 10, 2009, contractors shall accept FDG PET oncologic claims billed to inform initial treatment strategy; specifically for staging in beneficiaries who have biopsy-proven cervical cancer when the beneficiary's treating physician determines the FDG PET study is needed to determine the location and/or extent of the tumor as specified in Pub. 100-03, section 220.6.17.

EXCEPTION: CMS continues to non-cover FDG PET for initial diagnosis of cervical cancer related to initial treatment strategy.

NOTE: Effective for claims with dates of service on and after November 10, 2009, the –Q0 modifier is no longer necessary for FDG PET for cervical cancer.

© 2016 Optum360, LLC

**B. Medicare Summary Notices, Remittance Advice Remark Codes, and Claim Adjustment Reason Codes**

Additionally, contractors shall return as unprocessable /return to provider for FDG PET for cervical cancer for initial treatment strategy billed without the following: one of the PET/PET/ CT CPT codes listed in 60.16 C above AND modifier –PI AND a cervical cancer diagnosis code.

Use the following messages:

- Claim Adjustment Reason Code 4 – the procedure code is inconsistent with the modifier used or a required modifier is missing.
- Remittance Advice Remark Code MA-130 - Your claim contains incomplete and/or invalid information, and no appeal rights are afforded because the claim is unprocessable. Submit a new claim with the complete/correct information.
- Remittance Advice Remark Code M16 - Alert: See our Web site, mailings, or bulletins for more details concerning this policy/procedure/decision.

## 100-04, 13, 60.18

**Billing and Coverage Changes for PET (NaF-18) Scans to Identify Bone Metastasis of Cancer Effective for Claims With Dates of Services on or After February 26, 2010**

**A. Billing Changes for A/B MACs, FIs, and Carriers**

Effective for claims with dates of service on and after February 26, 2010, contractors shall pay for NaF-18 PET oncologic claims to inform of initial treatment strategy (PI) or subsequent treatment strategy (PS) for suspected or biopsy proven bone metastasis ONLY in the context of a clinical study and as specified in Pub. 100-03, section 220.6. All other claims for NaF-18 PET oncology claims remain non-covered.

**B. Medicare Summary Notices, Remittance Advice Remark Codes, and Claim Adjustment Reason Codes**

Effective for claims with dates of service on or after February 26, 2010, contractors shall return as unprocessable NaF-18 PET oncologic claims billed with modifier TC or globally (for FIs modifier TC or globally does not apply) and HCPCS A9580 to inform the initial treatment strategy or subsequent treatment strategy for bone metastasis that do not include ALL of the following:

- PI or –PS modifier AND
- PET or PET/CT CPT code (78811, 78812, 78813, 78814, 78815, 78816) AND
- Cancer diagnosis code AND
- Q0 modifier – Investigational clinical service provided in a clinical research study, are present on the claim.

NOTE: For institutional claims, continue to include ICD-9 diagnosis code V70.7 or ICD-10 diagnosis code Z006 and condition code 30 to denote a clinical study.

Use the following messages:

- Claim Adjustment Reason Code 4 – The procedure code is inconsistent with the modifier used or a required modifier is missing. Note: Refer to the 835 Healthcare Policy Identification Segment (loop 2110 Service Payment Information REF), if present.
- Remittance Advice Remark Code MA-130 - Your claim contains incomplete and/or invalid information, and no appeal rights are afforded because the claim is unprocessable. Submit a new claim with the complete/correct information.
- Remittance Advice Remark Code M16 - Alert: See our Web site, mailings, or bulletins for more details concerning this policy/procedure/decision.
- Claim Adjustment Reason Code 167 – This (these) diagnosis(es) is (are) not covered.

Effective for claims with dates of service on or after February 26, 2010, contractors shall accept PET oncologic claims billed with modifier 26 and modifier KX to inform the initial treatment strategy or strategy or subsequent treatment strategy for bone metastasis that include the following:

- PI or –PS modifier AND
- PET or PET/CT CPT code (78811, 78812, 78813, 78814, 78815, 78816) AND
- Cancer diagnosis code AND
- Q0 modifier – Investigational clinical service provided in a clinical research study, are present on the claim.

NOTE: If modifier KX is present on the professional component service, Contractors shall process the service as PET NaF-18 rather than PET with FDG.

Contractors shall also return as unprocessable NaF-18 PET oncologic professional component claims (i.e., claims billed with modifiers 26 and KX) to inform the initial

treatment strategy or strategy or subsequent treatment strategy for bone metastasis billed with HCPCS A9580 and use the following message:

Claim Adjustment Reason Code 97 – The benefit for this service is included in the payment/allowance for another service/procedure that has already been adjudicated.

NOTE: Refer to the 835 Healthcare Policy identification Segment (loop 2110 Service Payment Information REF), if present.

## 100-04, 13, 90.3

**Transportation Component (HCPCS Codes R0070 - R0076)**
(Rev. 3387, Issued: 10-30-15, Effective: 01-01-16, Implementation: 01-01-16)

This component represents the transportation of the equipment to the patient. Establish local RVUs for the transportation R codes based on Medicare Administrative Contractor (MAC) knowledge of the nature of the service furnished. The MACs shall allow only a single transportation payment for each trip the portable x-ray supplier makes to a particular location. When more than one patient is x-rayed at the same location, e.g., a nursing home, prorate the single fee schedule transportation payment among all patients (Medicare Parts A and B, and non-Medicare) receiving the portable x-ray services during that trip, regardless of their insurance status. For example, for portable x-ray services furnished at a Skilled Nursing Facility (SNF), the transportation fee should be allocated among all patients receiving portable x-ray services at the same location in a single trip irrespective of whether the patient is in a Part A stay, a Part B patient, or not a Medicare beneficiary at all. If the patient is in a Part A SNF stay, the transportation and set up costs are subject to consolidated billing and not separately billable to Medicare Part B. For a privately insured patient, it would be the responsibility of that patient's insurer. For a Medicare Part B patient, payment would be made under Part B for the share of the transportation fee attributable to that patient.

R0075 must be billed in conjunction with the CPT radiology codes (7000 series) and only when the x-ray equipment used was actually transported to the location where the x-ray was taken. R0075 would not apply to the x-ray equipment stored in the location where the x-ray was done (e.g., a nursing home) for use as needed.

Below are the definitions for each modifier that must be reported with R0075. Only one of these five modifiers shall be reported with R0075. NOTE: If only one patient is served, R0070 should be reported with no modifier since the descriptor for this code reflects only one patient seen.

    UN - Two patients served
    UP - Three patients served
    UQ - Four patients served
    UR - Five Patients served
    US - Six or more patients served

Payment for the above modifiers must be consistent with the definition of the modifiers. Therefore, for R0075 reported with modifiers, -UN, -UP, -UQ, and –UR, the total payment for the service shall be divided by 2, 3, 4, and 5 respectively. For modifier –US, the total payment for the service shall be divided by 6 regardless of the number of patients served. For example, if 8 patients were served, R0075 would be reported with modifier –US and the total payment for this service would be divided by 6.

The units field for R0075 shall always be reported as "1" except in extremely unusual cases. The number in the units field should be completed in accordance with the provisions of 100-04, chapter 23, section 10.2 item 24 G which defines the units field as the number of times the patient has received the itemized service during the dates listed in the from/to field. The units field must never be used to report the number of patients served during a single trip. Specifically, the units field must reflect the number of services that the specific beneficiary received, not the number of services received by other beneficiaries.

As a contractor priced service, MACs must initially determine a payment rate for portable x-ray transportation services that is associated with the cost of providing the service. In order to determine an appropriate cost, the MAC should, at a minimum, cost out the vehicle, vehicle modifications, gasoline and the staff time involved in only the transportation for a portable x-ray service. A review of the pricing of this service should be done every five years.

Direct costs related to the vehicle carrying the x-ray machine are fully allocable to determining the payment rate. This includes the cost of the vehicle using a recognized depreciation method, the salary and fringe benefits associated with the staff who drive the vehicle, the communication equipment used between the vehicle and the home office, the salary and fringe benefits of the staff who determine the vehicles route (this could be proportional of office staff), repairs and maintenance of the vehicle(s), insurance for the vehicle(s), operating expenses for the vehicles and any other reasonable costs associated with this service as determined by the MAC. The MAC will have discretion for allocating indirect costs (those costs that cannot be directly attributed to portable x-ray transportation) between the transportation service and the technical component of the x-ray tests.

Suppliers may send MACs unsolicited cost information. The MACs may use this cost data as a comparison to its contractor priced determination. The data supplied should reflect a year's worth (either calendar or corporate fiscal) of information. Each provider who submits such data is to be informed that the data is subject to verification and will be used to supplement other information that is used to determine Medicare's payment rate.

The MACs are required to update the rate on an annual basis using independently determined measures of the cost of providing the service. A number of readily available measures (e.g., ambulance inflation factor, the Medicare economic index) that are used by the Medicare program to adjust payment rates for other types of services may be appropriate to use to update the rate for years that the MAC does not recalibrate the payment. Each MAC has the flexibility to identify the index it will use to update the rate. In addition, the MAC can consider locally identified factors that are measured independently of CMS as an adjunct to the annual adjustment.

NOTE: No transportation charge is payable unless the portable x-ray equipment used was actually transported to the location where the x-ray was taken. For example, MACs do not allow a transportation charge when the x-ray equipment is stored in a nursing home for use as needed. However, a set-up payment (see §90.4, below) is payable in such situations. Further, for services furnished on or after January 1, 1997, MACs may not make separate payment under HCPCS code R0076 for the transportation of EKG equipment by portable x-ray suppliers or any other entity.

## 100-04, 13, 90.4

### Set-Up Component (HCPCS Code Q0092)

(Rev. 1, 10-01-03)

Carriers must pay a set-up component for each radiologic procedure (other than retakes of the same procedure) during both single patient and multiple patient trips under Level II HCPCS code Q0092. Carriers do not make the set-up payment for EKG services furnished by the portable x-ray supplier.

## 100-04, 14, 40.8

### 40.8 - Payment When a Device is Furnished With No Cost or With Full or Partial Credit Beginning January 1, 2008

Contractors pay ASCs a reduced amount for certain specified procedures when a specified device is furnished without cost or for which either a partial or full credit is received (e.g., device recall). For specified procedure codes that include payment for a device, ASCs are required to include modifier -FB on the procedure code when a specified device is furnished without cost or for which full credit is received. If the ASC receives a partial credit of 50 percent or more of the cost of a specified device, the ASC is required to include modifier -FC on the procedure code if the procedure is on the list of specified procedures to which the -FC reduction applies. A single procedure code should not be submitted with both modifiers -FB and -FC. The pricing determination related to modifiers -FB and -FC is made prior to the application of multiple procedure payment reductions. Contractors adjust beneficiary coinsurance to reflect the reduced payment amount. Tables listing the procedures and devices to which the payment adjustments apply, and the full and partial adjustment amounts, are available on the CMS Web site.

In order to report that the receipt of a partial credit of 50 percent or more of the cost of a device, ASCs have the option of either: 1) Submitting the claim for the procedure to their Medicare contractor after the procedure's performance but prior to manufacturer acknowledgement of credit for a specified device, and subsequently contacting the contractor regarding a claims adjustment once the credit determination is made; or 2) holding the claim for the procedure until a determination is made by the manufacturer on the partial credit and submitting the claim with modifier -FC appended to the implantation procedure HCPCS code if the partial credit is 50 percent or more of the cost of the device. If choosing the first billing option, to request a claims adjustment once the credit determination is made, ASCs should keep in mind that the initial Medicare payment for the procedure involving the device is conditional and subject to adjustment.

## 100-04, 15, 20.1.4

### Components of the Ambulance Fee Schedule

The mileage rates provided in this section are the base rates that are adjusted by the yearly ambulance inflation factor (AIF). The payment amount under the fee schedule is determined as follows:

- For ground ambulance services, the fee schedule amount includes:
  1. A money amount that serves as a nationally uniform base rate, called a "conversion factor" (CF), for all ground ambulance services;
  2. A relative value unit (RVU) assigned to each type of ground ambulance service;
  3. A geographic adjustment factor (GAF) for each ambulance fee schedule locality area (geographic practice cost index (GPCI));
  4. A nationally uniform loaded mileage rate;
  5. An additional amount for certain mileage for a rural point-of-pickup; and
  6. For specified temporary periods, certain additional payment amounts as described in section 20.1.4A, below.

- For air ambulance services, the fee schedule amount includes:
  1. A nationally uniform base rate for fixed wing and a nationally uniform base rate for rotary wing;
  2. A geographic adjustment factor (GAF) for each ambulance fee schedule locality area (GPCI);
  3. A nationally uniform loaded mileage rate for each type of air service; and
  4. A rural adjustment to the base rate and mileage for services furnished for a rural point-of-pickup.

### A. Ground Ambulance Services

1. Conversion Factor

The conversion factor (CF) is a money amount used to develop a base rate for each category of ground ambulance service. The CF is updated annually by the ambulance inflation factor and for other reasons as necessary.

2. Relative Value Units

Relative value units (RVUs) set a numeric value for ambulance services relative to the value of a base level ambulance service. Since there are marked differences in resources necessary to furnish the various levels of ground ambulance services, different levels of payment are appropriate for the various levels of service. The different payment amounts are based on level of service. An RVU expresses the constant multiplier for a particular type of service (including, where appropriate, an emergency response). An RVU of 1.00 is assigned to the BLS of ground service, e.g., BLS has an RVU of 1; higher RVU values are assigned to the other types of ground ambulance services, which require more service than BLS.

The RVUs are as follows:

| Service Level | RVU |
|---|---|
| BLS | 1.00 |
| BLS - Emergency | 1.60 |
| ALS1 | 1.20 |
| ALS1- Emergency | 1.90 |
| ALS2 | 2.75 |
| SCT | 3.25 |
| PI | 1.75 |

3. Geographic Adjustment Factor (GAF)

The GAF is one of two factors intended to address regional differences in the cost of furnishing ambulance services. The GAF for the ambulance FS uses the non-facility practice expense (PE) of the geographic practice cost index (GPCI) of the Medicare physician fee schedule to adjust payment to account for regional differences. Thus, the geographic areas applicable to the ambulance FS are the same as those used for the physician fee schedule.

The location where the beneficiary was put into the ambulance (POP) establishes which GPCI applies. For multiple vehicle transports, each leg of the transport is separately evaluated for the applicable GPCI. Thus, for the second (or any subsequent) leg of a transport, the POP establishes the applicable GPCI for that portion of the ambulance transport.

For ground ambulance services, the applicable GPCI is multiplied by 70 percent of the base rate. Again, the base rate for each category of ground ambulance services is the CF multiplied by the applicable RVU. The GPCI is not applied to the ground mileage rate.

4. Mileage

In the context of all payment instructions, the term "mileage" refers to loaded mileage. The ambulance FS provides a separate payment amount for mileage. The mileage rate per statute mile applies for all types of ground ambulance services, except Paramedic Intercept, and is provided to all Medicare contractors electronically by CMS as part of the ambulance FS. Providers and suppliers must report all medically necessary mileage, including the mileage subject to a rural adjustment, in a single line item.

© 2016 Optum360, LLC

5. Adjustment for Certain Ground Mileage for Rural Points of Pickup (POP)
The payment rate is greater for certain mileage where the POP is in a rural area to account for the higher costs per ambulance trip that are typical of rural operations where fewer trips are made in any given period.

If the POP is a rural ZIP Code, the following calculations should be used to determine the rural adjustment portion of the payment allowance. For loaded miles 1-17, the rural adjustment for ground mileage is 1.5 times the rural mileage allowance.

For services furnished during the period July 1, 2004 through December 31, 2008, a 25 percent increase is applied to the appropriate ambulance FS mileage rate to each mile of a transport (both urban and rural POP) that exceeds 50 miles (i.e., mile 51 and greater).

The following chart summarizes the above information:

| Service | Dates of Service | Bonus | Calculation |
|---|---|---|---|
| Loaded miles 1-17, Rural POP | Beginning 4/1/02 | 50% | FS Rural mileage * 1.5 |
| Loaded miles 18-50, Rural POP | 4/1/02 – 12/31/03 | 25% | FS Rural mileage * 1.25 |
| All loaded miles (Urban or Rural POP) 51+ | 7/1/04 – 12/31/08 | 25% | FS Urban or Rural mileage * 1.25 |

The POP, as identified by ZIP Code, establishes whether a rural adjustment applies to a particular service. Each leg of a multi-leg transport is separately evaluated for a rural adjustment application. Thus, for the second (or any subsequent) leg of a transport, the ZIP Code of the POP establishes whether a rural adjustment applies to such second (or subsequent) transport.

For the purpose of all categories of ground ambulance services except paramedic intercept, a rural area is defined as a U.S. Postal Service (USPS) ZIP Code that is located, in whole or in part, outside of either a Metropolitan Statistical Area (MSA) or in New England, a New England County Metropolitan Area (NECMA), or is an area wholly within an MSA or NECMA that has been identified as rural under the "Goldsmith modification." (The Goldsmith modification establishes an operational definition of rural areas within large counties that contain one or more metropolitan areas. The Goldsmith areas are so isolated by distance or physical features that they are more rural than urban in character and lack easy geographic access to health services.)

For Paramedic Intercept, an area is a rural area if:

- It is designated as a rural area by any law or regulation of a State;
- It is located outside of an MSA or NECMA; or
- It is located in a rural census tract of an MSA as determined under the most recent Goldsmith modification.

See IOM Pub. 100-02, Medicare Benefit Policy Manual, chapter 10 – Ambulance Services, section 30.1.1 – Ground Ambulance Services for coverage requirements for the Paramedic Intercept benefit. Presently, only the State of New York meets these requirements.

Although a transport with a POP located in a rural area is subject to a rural adjustment for mileage, Medicare still pays the lesser of the billed charge or the applicable FS amount for mileage. Thus, when rural mileage is involved, the contractor compares the calculated FS rural mileage payment rate to the provider's/supplier's actual charge for mileage and pays the lesser amount.

The CMS furnishes the ambulance FS files to claims processing contractors electronically. A version of the Ambulance Fee Schedule is also posted to the CMS website (http://www.cms.hhs.gov/AmbulanceFeeSchedule/02_afspuf.asp) for public consumption. To clarify whether a particular ZIP Code is rural or urban, please refer to the most recent version of the Medicare supplied ZIP Code file.

6. Regional Ambulance FS Payment Rate Floor for Ground Ambulance Transports
For services furnished during the period July 1, 2004 through December 31, 2009, the base rate portion of the payment under the ambulance FS for ground ambulance transports is subject to a minimum amount. This minimum amount depends upon the area of the country in which the service is furnished. The country is divided into 9 census divisions and each of the census divisions has a regional FS that is constructed using the same methodology as the national FS. Where the regional FS is greater than the national FS, the base rates for ground ambulance transports are determined by a blend of the national rate and the regional rate in accordance with the following schedule:

| Year | National FS Percentage | Regional FS Percentage |
|---|---|---|
| 7/1/04 - 12/31/04 | 20% | 80% |
| CY 2005 | 40% | 60% |
| CY 2006 | 60% | 40% |
| CY 2007 – CY 2009 | 80% | 20% |
| CY 2010 and thereafter | 100% | 0% |

Where the regional FS is not greater than the national FS, there is no blending and only the national FS applies. Note that this provision affects only the FS portion of the blended transition payment rate. This floor amount is calculated by CMS centrally and is incorporated into the FS amount that appears in the FS file maintained by CMS and downloaded by CMS contractors. There is no calculation to be done by the Medicare B/MAC or A/MAC in order to implement this provision.

7. Adjustments for FS Payment Rate for Certain Rural Ground Ambulance Transports
For services furnished during the period July 1, 2004 through December 31, 2010, the base rate portion of the payment under the FS for ground ambulance transports furnished in certain rural areas is increased by a percentage amount determined by CMS . Section 3105 (c) and 10311 (c) of the Affordable Care Act amended section 1834 (1) (13) (A) of the Act to extend this rural bonus for an additional year through December 31, 2010. This increase applies if the POP is in a rural county (or Goldsmith area) that is comprised by the lowest quartile by population of all such rural areas arrayed by population density. CMS will determine this bonus amount and the designated POP rural ZIP Codes in which the bonus applies. Beginning on July 1, 2004, rural areas qualifying for the additional bonus amount will be identified with a "B" indicator on the national ZIP Code file. Contractors must apply the additional rural bonus amount as a multiplier to the base rate portion of the FS payment for all ground transports originating in the designated POP ZIP Codes.

Subsequently, section of 106 (c) of the MMEA again amended section 1843 (l) (13) (A) of the Act to extend the rural bonus an additional year, through December 31, 2011.

8. Adjustments for FS Payment Rates for Ground Ambulance Transports
The payment rates under the FS for ground ambulance transports (both the fee schedule base rates and the mileage amounts) are increased for services furnished during the period July 1, 2004 through December 31, 2006 as well as July 1, 2008 through December 31, 2010. For ground ambulance transport services furnished where the POP is urban, the rates are increased by 1 percent for claims with dates of service July 1, 2004 through December 31, 2006 in accordance with Section 414 of the Medicare Modernization Act (MMA) of 2004 and by 2 percent for claims with dates of service July 1, 2008 through December 31, 2010 in accordance with Section 146(a) of the Medicare Improvements for Patients and Providers Act of 2008 and Sections 3105(a) and 10311(a) of the Patient Protection and Affordable Care Act (ACA) of

2010. For ground ambulance transport services furnished where the POP is rural, the rates are increased by 2 percent for claims with dates of service July 1, 2004 through December 31, 2006 in accordance with Section 414 of the Medicare Modernization Act (MMA) of 2004 and by 3 percent for claims with dates of service July 1, 2008 through December 31, 2010 in accordance with Section 146(a) of the Medicare Improvements for Patients and Providers Act of 2008 and Sections 3105(a) and 10311(a) of the Patient Protection and Affordable Care Act (ACA) of 2010. Subsequently, section 106 (a) of the Medicare and Medicaid Extenders Act of 2010 (MMEA) again amended section 1834 (1) (12) (A) of the Act to extend the payment increases for an additional year, through December 31, 2011. These amounts are incorporated into the fee schedule amounts that appear in the Ambulance FS file maintained by CMS and downloaded by CMS contractors. There is no calculation to be done by the Medicare carrier or intermediary in order to implement this provision.

The following chart summarizes the Medicare Prescription Drug, Improvement, and Modernization Act (MMA) of 2003 payment changes for ground ambulance services that became effective on July 1, 2004 as well as the Medicare Improvement for Patients and Providers Act (MIPPA) of 2008 changes that became effective July 1, 2008 and were extended by the Patient Protection and Affordable Care Act of 2010 and the Medicare and Medicaid Extenders Act of 2010 (MMEA).

Summary Chart of Additional Payments for Ground Ambulance Services Provided by MMA, MIPPA and MMEA

| Service | Effective Dates | Payment Increase* |
|---|---|---|
| All rural miles | 7/1/04 - 12/31/06 | 2% |
| All rural miles | 7/1/08 – 12/31/11 | 3% |
| Rural miles 51+ | 7/1/04 - 12/31/08 | 25% ** |
| All urban miles | 7/1/04 - 12/31/06 | 1% |
| All urban miles | 7/1/08 – 12/31/11 | 2% |

© 2016 Optum360, LLC

| Service | Effective Dates | Payment Increase* |
|---|---|---|
| Urban miles 51+ | 7/1/04 - 12/31/08 | 25% ** |
| All rural base rates | 7/1/04 - 12/31/06 | 2% |
| All rural base rates | 7/1/08 – 12/31/11 | 3% |
| Rural base rates (lowest quartile) | 7/1/04 - 12/31/11 | 22.6%** |
| All urban base rates | 7/1/04 - 12/31/06 | 1% |
| All urban base rates | 7/1/08 – 12/31/11 | 2% |
| All base rates (regional fee schedule blend) | 7/1/04 - 12/31/09 | Floor |

NOTES: * All payments are percentage increases and all are cumulative.

**Contractor systems perform this calculation. All other increases are incorporated into the CMS Medicare Ambulance FS file.

### B. Air Ambulance Services

1. Base Rates
   Each type of air ambulance service has a base rate. There is no conversion factor (CF) applicable to air ambulance services.

2. Geographic Adjustment Factor (GAF)
   The GAF, as described above for ground ambulance services, is also used for air ambulance services. However, for air ambulance services, the applicable GPCI is applied to 50 percent of each of the base rates (fixed and rotary wing).

3. Mileage
   The FS for air ambulance services provides a separate payment for mileage.

4. Adjustment for Services Furnished in Rural Areas
   The payment rates for air ambulance services where the POP is in a rural area are greater than in an urban area. For air ambulance services (fixed or rotary wing), the rural adjustment is an increase of 50 percent to the unadjusted FS amount, e.g., the applicable air service base rate multiplied by the GAF plus the mileage amount or, in other words, 1.5 times both the applicable air service base rate and the total mileage amount.

The basis for a rural adjustment for air ambulance services is determined in the same manner as for ground services. That is, whether the POP is within a rural ZIP Code as described above for ground services.

## 100-04, 15, 20.2

### Payment for Mileage Charges
B3-5116.3, PM AB-00-131

Charges for mileage must be based on loaded mileage only, e.g., from the pickup of a patient to his/her arrival at destination. It is presumed that all unloaded mileage costs are taken into account when a supplier establishes his basic charge for ambulance services and his rate for loaded mileage. Suppliers should be notified that separate charges for unloaded mileage will be denied.

Instructions on billing mileage are found in Sec.30.

## 100-04, 15, 20.3

### Air Ambulance
PHs AB-01-165, AB-02-036, and AB-02-131; B3-5116.5, B3-5205 partial

Refer to IOM Pub. 100-02, Medicare Benefit Policy Manual, chapter 10 - Ambulance Services, section 10.4 - Air Ambulance Services, for additional information on the coverage of air ambulance services. Under certain circumstances, transportation by airplane or helicopter may qualify as covered ambulance services. If the conditions of coverage are met, payment may be made for the air ambulance services.

Air ambulance services are paid at different rates according to two air ambulance categories:

- AIR ambulance service, conventional air services, transport, one way, fixed wing (FW) (HCPCS code A0430)
- AIR ambulance service, conventional air services, transport, one way, rotary wing (RW) (HCPCS code A0431)

Covered air ambulance mileage services are paid when the appropriate HCPCS code is reported on the claim:

HCPCS code A0435 identifies FIXED WING AIR MILEAGE

HCPCS code A0436 identifies ROTARY WING AIR MILEAGE

Air mileage must be reported in whole numbers of loaded statute miles flown. Contractors must ensure that the appropriate air transport code is used with the appropriate mileage code.

Air ambulance services may be paid only for ambulance services to a hospital. Other destinations e.g., skilled nursing facility, a physician's office, or a patient's home may not be paid air ambulance. The destination is identified by the use of an appropriate modifier as defined in Section 30(A) of this chapter.

Claims for air transports may account for all mileage from the point of pickup, including where applicable: ramp to taxiway, taxiway to runway, takeoff run, air miles, roll out upon landing, and taxiing after landing. Additional air mileage may be allowed by the contractor in situations where additional mileage is incurred, due to circumstances beyond the pilot's control. These circumstances include, but are not limited to, the following:

Military base and other restricted zones, air-defense zones, and similar FAA restrictions and prohibitions;

Hazardous weather; or

Variances in departure patterns and clearance routes required by an air traffic controller.

If the air transport meets the criteria for medical necessity, Medicare pays the actual miles flown for legitimate reasons as determined by the Medicare contractor, once the Medicare beneficiary is loaded onto the air ambulance.

IOM Pub. 100-08, Medicare Program Integrity Manual, chapter 6 - Intermediary MR Guidelines for Specific Services contains instructions for Medical Review of Air Ambulance Services.

## 100-04, 15, 20.6

### Payment for Non-Emergency Trips to/from ESRD Facilities
Section 637 of the American Taxpayer Relief Act of 2012 requires that, effective for transports occurring on and after October 1, 2013, fee schedule payments for non-emergency basic life support (BLS) transports of individuals with end-stage renal disease (ESRD) to and from renal dialysis treatment be reduced by 10%. The payment reduction affects transports (base rate and mileage) to and from hospital-based and freestanding renal dialysis treatment facilities for dialysis services provided on a non-emergency basis. Non-emergency BLS ground transports are identified by Healthcare Common Procedure Code System (HCPCS) code A0428. Ambulance transports to and from renal dialysis treatment are identified by modifier codes "G" (hospital-based ESRD) and "J" (freestanding ESRD facility) in either the first position (origin code) or second position (destination code) within the two-digit ambulance modifier. (See Section 30 (A) for information regarding modifiers specific to ambulance.)

Effective for claims with dates of service on and after October 1, 2013, the 10% reduction will be calculated and applied to HCPCS code A0428 when billed with modifier code "G" or "J". The reduction will also be applied to any mileage billed in association with a non-emergency transport of a beneficiary with ESRD to and from renal dialysis treatment. BLS mileage is identified by HCPCS code A0425.

The 10% reduction will be taken after calculation of the normal fee schedule payment amount, including any add-on or bonus payments, and will apply to transports in rural and urban areas as well as areas designated as "super rural".

Payment for emergency transports is not affected by this reduction. Payment for non-emergency BLS transports to other destinations is also not affected. This reduction does not affect or change the Ambulance Fee Schedule.

Note: The 10% reduction applies to beneficiaries with ESRD that are receiving non-emergency BLS transport to and from renal dialysis treatment. While it is possible that a beneficiary who is not diagnosed with ESRD will require routine transport to and from renal dialysis treatment, it is highly unlikely. However, contractors have discretion to override or reverse the reduction on appeal if they deem it appropriate based on supporting documentation.

## 100-04, 15, 30

### General Billing Guidelines
(Rev. 3076, Issued: 09-24-14, Effective: Upon Implementation of ICD-10 ASC X12: 01-01-12, Implementation: ICD-10: Upon Implementation of ICD-10 ASC X12: 09-16-14)

Independent ambulance suppliers may bill on the ASC X12 837 professional claim transaction or the CMS-1500 form. These claims are processed using the Multi-Carrier System (MCS).

Institution based ambulance providers may bill on the ASC X12 837 institutional claim transaction or Form CMS 1450. These claims are processed using the Fiscal Intermediary Shared System (FISS).

### A. Modifiers Specific to Ambulance Service Claims
For ambulance service claims, institutional-based providers and suppliers must report an origin and destination modifier for each ambulance trip provided in HCPCS/Rates. Origin and destination modifiers used for ambulance services are created by combining two alpha characters. Each alpha character, with the exception

of "X", represents an origin code or a destination code. The pair of alpha codes creates one modifier. The first position alpha code equals origin; the second position alpha code equals destination. Origin and destination codes and their descriptions are listed below:

D= Diagnostic or therapeutic site other than P or H when these are used as origin codes;

E = Residential, domiciliary, custodial facility (other than 1819 facility);

G = Hospital based ESRD facility;

H = Hospital;

I = Site of transfer (e.g. airport or helicopter pad) between modes of ambulance transport;

J = Freestanding ESRD facility;

N = Skilled nursing facility;

P = Physician's office;

R = Residence;

S = Scene of accident or acute event;

X = Intermediate stop at physician's office on way to hospital (destination code only)

In addition, institutional-based providers must report one of the following modifiers with every HCPCS code to describe whether the service was provided under arrangement or directly:

QM - Ambulance service provided under arrangement by a provider of services; or

QN - Ambulance service furnished directly by a provider of services.

While combinations of these items may duplicate other HCPCS modifiers, when billed with an ambulance transportation code, the reported modifiers can only indicate origin/destination.

### B. HCPCS Codes

The following codes and definitions are effective for billing ambulance services on or after January 1, 2001.

### AMBULANCE HCPCS CODES AND DEFINITIONS

| Code | Description |
| --- | --- |
| A0425 | BLS mileage (per mile) |
| A0425 | ALS mileage (per mile) |
| A0426 | Ambulance service, Advanced Life Support (ALS), non-emergency transport, Level 1 |
| A0427 | Ambulance service, ALS, emergency transport, Level 1 |
| A0428 | Ambulance service, Basic Life Support (BLS), non-emergency transport |
| A0429 | Ambulance service, basic life support (BLS), emergency transport |
| A0430 | Ambulance service, conventional air services, transport, one way, fixed wing (FW) |
| A0431 | Ambulance service, conventional air services, transport, one way, rotary wing (RW) |
| A0432 | Paramedic ALS intercept (PI), rural area transport furnished by a volunteer ambulance company, which is prohibited by state law from billing third party payers. |
| A0433 | Ambulance service, advanced life support, level 2 (ALS2) |
| A0434 | Ambulance service, specialty care transport (SCT) |
| A0435 | Air mileage; FW, (per statute mile) |
| A0436 | Air mileage; RW, (per statute mile) |

NOTE: PI, ALS2, SCT, FW, and RW assume an emergency condition and do not require an emergency designator.

Refer to IOM Pub. 100-02, Medicare Benefit Policy Manual, Chapter 10 – Ambulance Service, section 30.1 – Definitions of Ambulance Services, for the definitions of levels of ambulance services under the fee schedule.

## 100-04, 15, 30.1.2

### Coding Instructions for Paper and Electronic Claim Forms

Except as otherwise noted, beginning with dates of service on or after January 1, 2001, the following coding instructions must be used.

In item 23 of the CMS-1500 Form, billers shall code the 5-digit ZIP Code of the point of pickup.

Electronic billers using ANSI X12N 837 should refer to the Implementation Guide to determine how to report the origin information (e.g., the ZIP Code of the point of pickup).

Since the ZIP Code is used for pricing, more than one ambulance service may be reported on the same paper claim for a beneficiary if all points of pickup have the same ZIP Code. Suppliers must prepare a separate paper claim for each trip if the points of pickup are located in different ZIP Codes.

Claims without a ZIP Code in item 23 on CMS-1500 Form item 23, or with multiple ZIP Codes in item 23, must be returned as unprocessable. Carriers use message N53 on the remittance advice in conjunction with reason code 16.

ZIP Codes must be edited for validity.

The format for a ZIP Code is five numerics. If a nine-digit ZIP Code is submitted, the last four digits are ignored. If the data submitted in the required field does not match that format, the claim is rejected.

Generally, each ambulance trip will require two lines of coding, e.g., one line for the service and one line for the mileage. Suppliers who do not bill mileage would have one line of code for the service.

Beginning with dates of service on or after January 1, 2011, if mileage is billed it must be reported as fractional units in Item 24G of the Form CMS-1500 paper claim or the corresponding loop and segment of the ANSI X12N 837P electronic claim for trips totaling up to 100 covered miles. When reporting fractional mileage, suppliers must round the total miles up to the nearest tenth of a mile and report the resulting number

with the appropriate HCPCS code for ambulance mileage. The decimal must be used in the appropriate place (e.g., 99.9).

For trips totaling 100 covered miles and greater, suppliers must report mileage rounded up to the next whole number mile without the use of a decimal (e.g., 998.5 miles should be reported as 999).

For trips totaling less than 1 mile, enter a "0" before the decimal (e.g., 0.9).

Fractional mileage reporting applies only to ambulance services billed on a Form CMS-1500 paper claim, ANSI X12N 837P, or 837I electronic claims. It does not apply to providers billing on the Form CMS-1450.

For mileage HCPCS billed on a Form CMS-1500 or ANSI X12N 837P only, contractors shall automatically default to "0.1" units when the total mileage units are missing in Item 24G.

## 100-04, 15, 30.2

### Intermediary Guidelines

For SNF Part A, the cost of transportation to receive most services included in the RUG rate is included in the cost for the service. This includes transportation in an ambulance. Payment for the SNF claim is based on the RUGs, and recalibration for future years takes into account the cost of transportation to receive the ancillary services.

If the services are excluded from the SNF PPS rate, the ambulance service may be billed separately as can the excluded service.

Refer to section 10.5, of chapter 3, of the Medicare Claims Processing Manual, for additional information on hospital inpatient bundling of ambulance services.

In general, the intermediary processes claims for Part B ambulance services provided by an ambulance supplier under arrangements with hospitals or SNFs. These providers bill intermediaries using only Method 2.

The provider must furnish the following data in accordance with intermediary instructions. The intermediary will make arrangements for the method and media for submitting the data: A detailed statement of the condition necessitating the ambulance service; A statement indicating whether the patient was admitted as an inpatient. If yes the name and address of the facility must be shown; Name and address of certifying physician; Name and address of physician ordering service if other than certifying physician; Point of pickup (identify place and completed address); Destination (identify place and complete address); Number of loaded miles (the number of miles traveled when the beneficiary was in the ambulance); Cost per mile; Mileage charge; Minimum or base charge; and Charge for special items or services. Explain.

### A. General

The reasonable cost per trip of ambulance services furnished by a provider of services may not exceed the prior year's reasonable cost per trip updated by the ambulance inflation factor. This determination is effective with services furnished during Federal Fiscal Year (FFY) 1998 (between October 1, 1997, and September 30, 1998).

Providers are to bill for Part B ambulance services using the billing method of base rate including supplies, with mileage billed separately as described below.

The following instructions provide billing procedures implementing the above provisions.

### B. Applicable Bill Types

The appropriate type of bill (13X, 22X, 23X, 83X, and 85X) must be reported. For SNFs, ambulance cannot be reported on a 21X type of bill.

### C. Value Code Reporting

For claims with dates of service on or after January 1, 2001, providers must report on every Part B ambulance claim value code A0 (zero) and the related ZIP code of the geographic location from which the beneficiary was placed on board the ambulance in FLs 39-41 "Value Codes." The value code is defined as "ZIP Code of the location from which the beneficiary is initially placed on board the ambulance." Providers report the number in dollar portion of the form location right justified to the left to the dollar/cents delimiter. Providers utilizing the UB-92 flat file use Record Type 41 fields 16-39. On the X-12 institutional claims transactions, providers show HI*BE:A0:::12345, 2300 Loop, HI segment.

More than one ambulance trip may be reported on the same claim if the ZIP code of all points of pickup are the same. However, since billing requirements do not allow for value codes (ZIP codes) to be line item specific and only one ZIP code may be reported per claim, providers must prepare a separate claim for a beneficiary for each trip if the points of pickup are located in different ZIP codes.

### D. Revenue Code/HCPCS Code Reporting

Providers must report revenue code 054X and, for services provided before January 1, 2001, one of the following CMS HCPCS codes in FL 44 "HCPCS/Rates" for each ambulance trip provided during the billing period: A0030 (discontinued 12/31/2000); A0040 (discontinued 12/31/2000); A0050 (discontinued 12/31/2000); A0320 (discontinued 12/31/2000); A0322 (discontinued 12/31/2000); A0324 (discontinued 12/31/2000); A0326 (discontinued 12/31/2000); A0328, (discontinued 12/31/2000); or A0330 (discontinued 12/31/2000).

In addition, providers report one of A0380 or A0390 for mileage HCPCS codes. No other HCPCS codes are acceptable for reporting ambulance services and mileage.

Providers report one of the following revenue codes: 0540; 0542; 0543; 0545; 0546; or 0548.

Do not report revenue codes 0541, 0544, or 0547.

For claims with dates of service on or after January 1, 2001, providers must report revenue code 540 and one of the following HCPCS codes in FL 44 "HCPCS/Rates" for each ambulance trip provided during the billing period: A0426; A0427; A0428; A0429; A0430; A0431; A0432; A0433; or A0434.

Providers using an ALS vehicle to furnish a BLS level of service report HCPCS code, A0426 (ALS1) or A0427 (ALS1 emergency), and are paid accordingly.

In addition, all providers report one of the following mileage HCPCS codes: A0380; A0390; or A0436.

Since billing requirements do not allow for more than one HCPCS code to be reported for per revenue code line, providers must report revenue code 0540 (ambulance) on two separate and consecutive lines to accommodate both the Part B ambulance service and the mileage HCPCS codes for each ambulance trip provided during the billing period. Each loaded (e.g., a patient is onboard) 1-way ambulance trip must be reported with a unique pair of revenue code lines on the claim. Unloaded trips and mileage are NOT reported.

However, in the case where the beneficiary was pronounced dead after the ambulance is called but before the ambulance arrives at the scene: Payment may be made for a BLS service if a ground vehicle is dispatched or at the fixed wing or rotary wing base rate, as applicable, if an air ambulance is dispatched. Neither mileage nor a rural adjustment would be paid. The blended rate amount will otherwise apply. Providers report the A0428 (BLS) HCPCS code. Providers report modifier QL (Patient pronounced dead after ambulance called) in Form Locator (FL) 44 "HCPCS/Rates" instead of the origin and destination modifier. In addition to the QL modifier, providers report modifier QM or QN.

### E. Modifier Reporting

Providers must report an origin and destination modifier for each ambulance trip provided in FL 44 "HCPCS/Rates." Origin and destination modifiers used for ambulance services are created by combining two alpha characters. Each alpha character, with the exception of x, represents an origin code or a destination code. The pair of alpha codes creates one modifier. The first position alpha code equals origin; the second position alpha code equals destination. Origin and destination codes and their descriptions are listed below: D - Diagnostic or therapeutic site other than "P" or "H" when these are used as origin codes; E - Residential, Domiciliary, Custodial Facility (other than an 1819 facility); H - Hospital; I - Site of transfer (e.g. airport or helicopter pad) between modes of ambulance transport; J - Nonhospital based dialysis facility; N - Skilled Nursing Facility (SNF) (1819 facility); P - Physician's

office (Includes HMO nonhospital facility, clinic, etc.); R - Residence; S - Scene of accident or acute event; or X - (Destination Code Only) intermediate stop at physician's office enroute to the hospital. (Includes HMO nonhospital facility, clinic, etc.) In addition, providers must report one of the following modifiers with every HCPCS code to describe whether the service was provided under arrangement or directly: QM - Ambulance service provided under arrangement by a provider of services; or QN - Ambulance service furnished directly by a provider of services.

### F. Line-Item Dates of Service Reporting

Providers are required to report line-item dates of service per revenue code line. This means that they must report two separate revenue code lines for every ambulance trip provided during the billing period along with the date of each trip. This includes situations in which more than one ambulance service is provided to the same beneficiary on the same day. Line-item dates of service are reported on the hard copy UB-92 in FL 45 "Service Date" (MMDDYY), and on RT 61, field 13, "Date of Service" (YYYYMMDD) on the UB-92 flat file.

### G. Service Units Reporting

For line items reflecting HCPCS code A0030, A0040, A0050, A0320, A0322, A0324, A0326, A0328, or A0330 (services before January 1, 2001) or code A0426, A0427, A0428, A0429, A0430, A0431, A0432, A0433, or A0434 (services on and after January 1, 2001), providers are required to report in FL 46 "Service Units" each ambulance trip provided during the billing period. Therefore, the service units for each occurrence of these HCPCS codes are always equal to one. In addition, for line items reflecting HCPCS code A0380 or A0390, the number of loaded miles must be reported. (See examples below.) Therefore, the service units for each occurrence of these HCPCS codes are always equal to one.

In addition, for line items reflecting HCPCS code A0380, A0390, A0435, or A0436, the number of loaded miles must be reported.

### H. Total Charges Reporting

For line items reflecting HCPCS code: A0030, A0040, A0050, A0320, A0322, A0324, A0326, A0328, or A0330 (services before January 1, 2001); OR HCPCS code A0426, A0427, A0428, A0429, A0430, A0431, A0432, A0433, or A0434 (on or after January 1, 2001); Providers are required to report in FL 47 "Total Charges" the actual charge for the ambulance service including all supplies used for the ambulance trip but excluding the charge for mileage.

For line items reflecting HCPCS code A0380, A0390, A0435, or A0436, report the actual charge for mileage.

NOTE:There are instances where the provider does not incur any cost for mileage, e.g., if the beneficiary is pronounced dead after the ambulance is called but before the ambulance arrives at the scene. In these situations, providers report the base rate ambulance trip and mileage as separate revenue code lines. Providers report the base rate ambulance trip in accordance with current billing requirements. For purposes of reporting mileage, they must report the appropriate HCPCS code, modifiers, and units as a separate line item. For the related charges, providers report $1.00 in FL48 for noncovered charges. Intermediaries should assign ANSI Group Code OA to the $1.00 noncovered mileage line, which in turn informs the beneficiaries and providers that they each have no liability.

Prior to submitting the claim to CWF, the intermediary will remove the entire revenue code line containing the mileage amount reported in FL 48 "Noncovered Charges" to avoid nonacceptance of the claim.

EXAMPLES:The following provides examples of how bills for Part B ambulance services should be completed based on the reporting requirements above. These examples reflect ambulance services furnished directly by providers. Ambulance services provided under arrangement between the provider and an ambulance company are reported in the same manner except providers report a QM modifier instead of a QN modifier. The following examples are for claims submitted with dates of service on or after January 1, 2001.

**EXAMPLE 1:**Claim containing only one ambulance trip:

For the UB-92 Flat File, providers report as follows:

| Modifier Record Type | Revenue Code | HCPCS Modifier | Date of Service | Units | Total Charges |
|---|---|---|---|---|---|
| 61 | 0540 | A0428RHQN | 082701 | 1 (trip) | 100.00 |
| 61 | 0540 | A0380RHQN | 082701 | 4 (mileage) | 8.00 |

For the hard copy UB-92 (Form CMS-1450), providers report as follows:

| Modifier Record Type | Revenue Code | HCPCS Modifier | Date of Service | Units | Total Charges |
|---|---|---|---|---|---|
| FL 42, FL 44 | 0540 | A0428RHQN | 082701 | 1 (trip) | 100.00 |
| FL 45, FL 46 FL 47 | 0540 | A0380RHQN | 082701 | 4 (mileage) | 8.00 |

**EXAMPLE 2:** Claim containing multiple ambulance trips:
For the UB-92 Flat File, providers report as follows:

| Modifier Record Type | Revenue Code | HCPCS Code | Modifiers #1 | #2 | Date of Service | Units | Total Charges |
|---|---|---|---|---|---|---|---|
| 61 | 0540 | A0429 | RH | QN | 082801 | 1 (trip) | 100.00 |
| 61 | 0540 | A0380 | RH | QN | 082801 | 2 (mileage) | 4.00 |
| 61 | 0540 | A0330 | RH | QN | 082901 | 1 (trip) | 400.00 |
| 61 | 0540 | A0390 | RH | QN | 082901 | 3 (mileage) | 6.00 |
| 61 | 0540 | A0426 | RH | QN | 083001 | 1 (trip) | 500.00 |
| 61 | 0540 | A0390 | RH | QN | 083001 | 5 (mileage) | 10.00 |
| 61 | 0540 | A0390 | RH | QN | 082901 | 3 (mileage) | 6.00 |
| 61 | 0540 | A0426 | RH | QN | 083001 | 1 (trip) | 500.00 |

For the hard copy UB-92 (Form CMS-1450), providers report as follows:

| Modifier | Revenue Code | HCPCS Code | #1 | #2 | Date of Service | Units | Total Charges |
|---|---|---|---|---|---|---|---|
| FL42, FL 44, FL 45, FL 46, FL 47 | 0540 | A0429 | RH | QN | 082801 | 1 (trip) | 100.00 |
| | 0540 | A0380 | RH | QN | 082801 | 2 (mileage) | 4.00 |

**EXAMPLE 3:** Claim containing more than one ambulance trip provided on the same day: For the UB-92 Flat File, providers report as follows:

| Modifier Record Type | Revenue Code | HCPCS Code | #1 | #2 | Date of Service | Units | Total Charges |
|---|---|---|---|---|---|---|---|
| 61 | 0540 | A0429 | RH | QN | 090201 | 1 (trip) | 100.00 |
| 61 | 0540 | A0380 | RH | QN | 090201 | 2 (mileage) | 4.00 |
| 61 | 0540 | A0429 | HR | QN | 090201 | 1 (trip) | 100.00 |
| 61 | 0540 | A0380 | HR | QN | 090201 | 2 (mileage) | 4.00 |

For the hard copy UB-92 (Form CMS-1450), providers report as follows:

| Modifier | Revenue Code | HCPCS Code | #1 | #2 | Date of Service | Units | Total Charges |
|---|---|---|---|---|---|---|---|
| FL42, FL 44, FL 45, FL 46, FL 47 | 0540 | A0429 | RH | QN | 090201 | 1 (trip) | 100.00 |
| | 0540 | A0380 | RH | QN | 090201 | 2 (mileage) | 4.00 |
| | 0540 | A0429 | HR | QN | 090201 | 1 (trip) | 100.00 |
| | 0540 | A0380 | HR | QN | 090201 | 2 (mileage) | 4.00 |

**I. Edits Intermediaries edit to assure proper reporting as follows:**
For claims with dates of service before January 1, 2001, each pair of revenue codes 0540 must have one of the following ambulance trip HCPCS codes - A0030, A0040, A0050, A0320, A0322, A0324, A0326, A0328 or A0330; and one of the following mileage HCPCS codes - A0380 or A0390; For claims with dates of service on or after January 1, 2001, each pair of revenue codes 0540 must have one of the following ambulance HCPCS codes - A0426, A0427, A0428, A0429, A0430, A0431, A0432, A0433, or A0434; and one of the following mileage HCPCS codes - A0435, A0436 or for claims with dates of service before April 1, 2002, A0380, or A0390, or for claims with dates of service on or after April 1, 2002, A0425; For claims with dates of service on or after January 1, 2001, the presence of an origin and destination modifier and a QM or QN modifier for every line item containing revenue code 0540; The units field is completed for every line item containing revenue code 0540; For claims with dates of service on or after January 1, 2001, the units field is completed for every line item containing revenue code 0540; Service units for line items containing HCPCS codes A0030, A0040, A0050, A0320, A0322, A0324, A0326, A0328, A0330, A0426, A0427, A0428, A0429, A0430, A0431, A0432, A0433, or A0434 always equal "1" For claims

with dates of service on or after July 1, 2001, each 1-way ambulance trip, line-item dates of service for the ambulance service, and corresponding mileage are equal.

## 100-04, 15, 30.2.1

**A/MAC Bill Processing Guidelines Effective April 1, 2002, as a Result of Fee Schedule Implementation**
For SNF Part A, the cost of medically necessary ambulance transportation to receive most services included in the RUG rate is included in the cost for the service. Payment for the SNF claim is based on the RUGs, which takes into account the cost of such transportation to receive the ancillary services.

Refer to IOM Pub. 100-04, Medicare Claims Processing Manual, chapter 6—SNF Inpatient Part A Billing, Section 20.3.1—Ambulance Services for additional information on SNF consolidated billing and ambulance transportation.

Refer to IOM Pub. 100-04, Medicare Claims Processing Manual, chapter 3—Inpatient Hospital Billing, section 10.5—Hospital Inpatient Bundling, for additional information on hospital inpatient bundling of ambulance services.

In general, the A/MAC processes claims for Part B ambulance services provided by an ambulance supplier under arrangements with hospitals or SNFs. These providers bill A/MACs using only Method 2.

The provider must furnish the following data in accordance with A/MAC instructions. The A/MAC will make arrangements for the method and media for submitting the data:

- A detailed statement of the condition necessitating the ambulance service;
- A statement indicating whether the patient was admitted as an inpatient. If yes the name and address of the facility must be shown;
- Name and address of certifying physician;
- Name and address of physician ordering service if other than certifying physician;
- Point of pickup (identify place and completed address);
- Destination (identify place and complete address);
- Number of loaded miles (the number of miles traveled when the beneficiary was in the ambulance);
- Cost per mile;
- Mileage charge;
- Minimum or base charge; and
- Charge for special items or services. Explain.

**A. Revenue Code Reporting**
Providers report ambulance services under revenue code 540 in FL 42 "Revenue Code."

**B. HCPCS Codes Reporting**
Providers report the HCPCS codes established for the ambulance fee schedule. No other HCPCS codes are acceptable for the reporting of ambulance services and mileage. The HCPCS code must be used to reflect the type of service the beneficiary received, not the type of vehicle used.

Providers must report one of the following HCPCS codes in FL 44 "HCPCS/Rates" for each base rate ambulance trip provided during the billing period:

A0426; A0427; A0428; A0429; A0430; A0431; A0432; A0433; or A0434.

These are the same codes required effective for services January 1, 2001.

In addition, providers must report one of HCPCS mileage codes:

A0425; A0435; or A0436.

Since billing requirements do not allow for more than one HCPCS code to be reported per revenue code line, providers must report revenue code 540 (ambulance) on two separate and consecutive line items to accommodate both the ambulance service and the mileage HCPCS codes for each ambulance trip provided during the billing period. Each loaded (e.g., a patient is onboard) 1-way ambulance trip must be reported with a unique pair of revenue code lines on the claim. Unloaded trips and mileage are NOT reported.

For UB-04 hard copy claims submission prior to August 1, 2011, providers code one mile for trips less than a mile. Miles must be entered as whole numbers. If a trip has a fraction of a mile, round up to the nearest whole number.

Beginning with dates of service on or after January 1, 2011, for UB-04 hard copy claims submissions August 1, 2011 and after, mileage must be reported as fractional units. When reporting fractional mileage, providers must round the total miles up to the nearest tenth of a mile and the decimal must be used in the appropriate place (e.g., 99.9).

For trips totaling less than 1 mile, enter a "0" before the decimal (e.g., 0.9).

For electronic claims submissions prior to January 1, 2011, providers code one mile for trips less than a mile. Miles must be entered as whole numbers. If a trip has a fraction of a mile, round up to the nearest whole number.

Beginning with dates of service on or after January 1, 2011, for electronic claim submissions only, mileage must be reported as fractional units in the ANSI X12N 837I element SV205 for trips totaling up to 100 covered miles. When reporting fractional mileage, providers must round the total miles up to the nearest tenth of a mile and the decimal must be used in the appropriate place (e.g., 99.9).

For trips totaling 100 covered miles and greater, providers must report mileage rounded up to the nearest whole number mile (e.g., 999) and not use a decimal when reporting whole number miles over 100 miles.

For trips totaling less than 1 mile, enter a "0" before the decimal (e.g., 0.9).

### C. Modifier Reporting
Providers must report an origin and destination modifier for each ambulance trip provided and either a QM (Ambulance service provided under arrangement by a provider of services) or QN (Ambulance service furnished directly by a provider of services) modifier in FL 44 "HCPCS/Rates".

### D. Service Units Reporting
For line items reflecting HCPCS codes A0426, A0427, A0428, A0429, A0430, A0431, A0432, A0433, or A0434, providers are required to report in FL 46 "Service Units" for each ambulance trip provided. Therefore, the service units for each occurrence of these HCPCS codes are always equal to one. In addition, for line items reflecting HCPCS code A0425, A0435, or A0436, providers must also report the number of loaded miles.

### E. Total Charges Reporting
For line items reflecting HCPCS codes A0426, A0427, A0428, A0429, A0430, A0431, A0432, A0433, or A0434, providers are required to report in FL 47, "Total Charges," the actual charge for the ambulance service including all supplies used for the ambulance trip but excluding the charge for mileage. For line items reflecting HCPCS codes A0425, A0435, or A0436, providers are to report the actual charge for mileage.

NOTE: There are instances where the provider does not incur any cost for mileage, e.g., if the beneficiary is pronounced dead after the ambulance is called but before the ambulance arrives at the scene. In these situations, providers report the base rate ambulance trip and mileage as separate revenue code lines. Providers report the base rate ambulance trip in accordance with current billing requirements. For purposes of reporting mileage, they must report the appropriate HCPCS code, modifiers, and units. For the related charges, providers report $1.00 in non-covered charges. A/MACs should assign ANSI Group Code OA to the $1.00 non-covered mileage line, which in turn informs the beneficiaries and providers that they each have no liability.

### F. Edits (A/MAC Claims with Dates of Service On or After 4/1/02)
For claims with dates of service on or after April 1, 2002, A/MACs perform the following edits to assure proper reporting:

Edit to assure each pair of revenue codes 540 have one of the following ambulance HCPCS codes - A0426, A0427, A0428, A0429, A0430, A0431, A0432, A0433, or A0434; and one of the following mileage HCPCS codes - A0425, A0435, or A0436.

Edit to assure the presence of an origin, destination modifier, and a QM or QN modifier for every line item containing revenue code 540;

Edit to assure that the unit's field is completed for every line item containing revenue code 540;

Edit to assure that service units for line items containing HCPCS codes A0426, A0427, A0428, A0429, A0430, A0431, A0432, A0433, or A0434 always equal "1"; and

Edit to assure on every claim that revenue code 540, a value code of A0 (zero), and a corresponding ZIP Code are reported. If the ZIP Code is not a valid ZIP Code in accordance with the USPS assigned ZIP Codes, intermediaries verify the ZIP Code to determine if the ZIP Code is a coding error on the claim or a new ZIP Code from the USPS not on the CMS supplied ZIP Code File.

Beginning with dates of service on or after April 1, 2012, edit to assure that only non-emergency trips (i.e., HCPCS A0426, A0428 [when A0428 is billed without modifier QL]) require an NPI in the Attending Physician field. Emergency trips do not require an NPI in the Attending Physician field (i.e., A0427, A0429, A0430, A0431, A0432, A0433, A0434 and A0428 [when A0428 is billed with modifier QL])

### G. CWF (A/MACs)
A/MACs report the procedure codes in the financial data section (field 65a-65j). They include revenue code, HCPCS code, units, and covered charges in the record. Where more than one HCPCS code procedure is applicable to a single revenue code, the provider reports each HCPCS code and related charge on a separate line, and the A/MAC reports this to CWF. Report the payment amount before adjustment for beneficiary liability in field 65g "Rate" and the actual charge in field 65h, "Covered Charges."

## 100-04, 15, 30.2.4

### 30.2.4 - Non-covered Charges on Institutional Ambulance Claims
Medicare law contains a restriction that miles beyond the closest available facility cannot be billed to Medicare. Non-covered miles beyond the closest facility are billed with HCPCS procedure code A0888 ("non-covered ambulance mileage per mile, e.g., for miles traveled beyond the closest appropriate facility"). These non-covered line items can be billed on claims also containing covered charges. Ambulance claims may use the -GY modifier on line items for such non-covered mileage, and liability for the service will be assigned correctly to the beneficiary.

The method of billing all miles for the same trip, with covered and non-covered portions, on the same claim is preferable in this scenario. However, billing the non-covered mileage using condition code 21 claims is also permitted, if desired, as long as all line items on the claims are non-covered and the beneficiary is liable. Additionally, unless requested by the beneficiary or required by specific Medicare policy, services excluded by statute do not have to be billed to Medicare.

When the scenario is point of pick up outside the United States, including U.S. territories but excepting some points in Canada and Mexico in some cases, mileage is also statutorily excluded from Medicare coverage. Such billings are more likely to be submitted on entirely non-covered claims using condition code 21. This scenario requires the use of a different message on the Medicare Summary Notice (MSN) sent to beneficiaries.

Another scenario in which billing non-covered mileage to Medicare may occur is when the beneficiary dies after the ambulance has been called but before the ambulance arrives. The -QL modifier should be used on the base rate line in this scenario, in place of origin and destination modifiers, and the line is submitted with covered charges. The -QL modifier should also be used on the accompanying mileage line, if submitted, with non-covered charges. Submitting this non-covered mileage line is optional for providers.

Non-covered charges may also apply is if there is a subsidy of mileage charges that are never charged to Medicare. Because there are no charges for Medicare to share in, the only billing option is to submit non-covered charges, if the provider bills Medicare at all (it is not required in such cases). These non-covered charges are unallowable, and should not be considered in settlement of cost reports. However, there is a difference in billing if such charges are subsidized, but otherwise would normally be charged to Medicare as the primary payer. In this latter case, CMS examination of existing rules relating to grants policy since October 1983, supported by Federal regulations (42CFR 405.423), generally requires providers to reduce their costs by the amount of grants and gifts restricted to pay for such costs. Thereafter, section 405.423 was deleted from the regulations.

Thus, providers were no longer required to reduce their costs for restricted grants and gifts, and charges tied to such grants/gifts/subsidies should be submitted as covered charges. This is in keeping with Congress's intent to encourage hospital philanthropy, allowing the provider receiving the subsidy to use it, and also requiring Medicare to share in the unreduced cost. Treatment of subsidized charges as non-covered Medicare charges serves to reduce Medicare payment on the Medicare cost report contrary to the 1983 change in policy.

Medicare requires the use of the -TQ modifier so that CMS can track the instances of the subsidy scenario for non-covered charges. The -TQ should be used whether the subsidizing entity is governmental or voluntary. The -TQ modifier is not required in the case of covered charges submitted when a subsidy has been made, but charges are still normally made to Medicare as the primary payer.

If providers believe they have been significantly or materially penalized in the past by the failure of their cost reports to consider covered charges occurring in the subsidy case, since Medicare had previous billing instructions that stated all charges in the case of a subsidy, not just charges when the entity providing the subsidy never charges another entity/primary payer, should be submitted as non-covered charges, they may contact their FI about reopening the reports in question for which the time period in 42 CFR 405.1885 has not expired. FIs have the discretion to determine if the amount in question warrants reopening. The CMS does not expect many such cases to occur.

Billing requirements for all these situations, including the use of modifiers, are presented in the chart below:

| Mileage Scenario | HCPCS | Modifiers* | Liability | Billing | Remit. Requirements | MSN Message |
|---|---|---|---|---|---|---|
| STATUTE: Miles beyond closest facility, OR **Pick up point outside of U.S. | A0888 on line item for the non-covered mileage | -QM or -QN, origin/destination modifier, and -GY unless condition code 21 claim used | Beneficiary | Bill mileage line item with A0888 - GY and other modifiers as needed to establish liability, line item will be denied; OR bill service on condition code 21 claim, no -GY required, claim will be denied | Group code PR, reason code 96 | 16.10 "Medicare does not pay for this item or service"; OR, "Medicare no paga por este artículo o servicio" |
| Beneficiary dies after ambulance is called | Most appropriate ambulance HCPCS mileage code (i.e., ground, air) | -QL unless condition code -21 claim | Provider | Bill mileage line item with -QL as non-covered, line item will be denied | Group Code CO, reason code 96 | 16.58 "The provider billed this charge as non-covered. You do not have to pay this amount."; OR, "El proveedor facuró este cargo como no cubierto. Usted no tiene que pagar ests cantidad." |
| Subsidy or government owned Ambulance, Medicare NEVER billed*** | A0888 on line item for the non-covered mileage | -QM or -QN, origin/ destination modifier, and -TQ must be used for policy purposes | Provider | Bill mileage line item with A0888, and modifiers as non-covered, line item will be denied | Group Code CO, reason code 96 | 16.58 "The provider billed this charge as non-covered. You do not have to pay this amount."; OR, "El proveedor facuró este cargo como no cubierto. Usted no tiene que pagar ests cantidad." |

\* Current ambulance billing requirements state that either the -QM or -QN modifier must be used on services. The -QM is used when the "ambulance service is provided under arrangement by a provider of services," and the -QN when the "ambulance service is provided directly by a provider of services." Line items using either the -QM or -QN modifiers are not subject to the FISS edit associated with FISS reason code 31322 so that these lines items will process to completion. Origin/destination modifiers, also required by current instruction, combine two alpha characters: one for origin, one for destination, and are not non-covered by definition.

\*\* This is the one scenario where the base rate is not paid in addition to mileage, and there are certain exceptions in Canada and Mexico where mileage is covered as described in existing ambulance instructions.

\*\*\* If Medicare would normally have been billed, submit mileage charges as covered charges despite subsidies.

Medicare systems may return claims to the provider if they do not comply with the requirements in the table.

## 100-04, 15, 40

### Medical Conditions List and Instructions
(Rev. 3240, Issued: 04-24-15, Effective: 07-27-15, Implementation: 07-27-15)

See http://www.cms.gov/Center/Provider-Type/Ambulances-Services-Center.html for a medical conditions list and instructions to assist ambulance providers and suppliers to communicate the

patient's condition to Medicare contractors, as reported by the dispatch center and as observed by the ambulance crew. Use of the medical conditions list does not guarantee payment of the claim or payment for a certain level of service.

In addition to reporting one of the medical conditions on the claim, one of the transportation indicators may be included on the claim to indicate why it was necessary for the patient to be transported in a particular way or circumstance. The provider or supplier will place the transportation indicator in the "narrative" field on the claim. Information on the appropriate use of transportation indicators is also available at http://www.cms.gov/Center/Provider-Type/Ambulances-Services-Center.html.

## 100-04, 16, 60.1.4

### Coding Requirements for Specimen Collection
The following HCPCS codes and terminology must be used:

- 36415 – Collection of venous blood by venipuncture.
- G0471 – Collection of venous blood by venipuncture or urine sample by catheterization from an individual in a skilled nursing facility (SNF) or by a laboratory on behalf of a home health agency (HHA)
- P9615 – Catheterization for collection of specimen(s).

The allowed amount for specimen collection in each of the above circumstances is included in the laboratory fee schedule distributed annually by CMS.

## 100-04, 16, 70.8

### Certificate of Waiver
Effective September 1, 1992, all laboratory testing sites (except as provided in 42 CFR 493.3(b)) must have either a CLIA certificate of waiver, certificate for provider-performed microscopy procedures, certificate of registration, certificate of compliance, or certificate of accreditation to legally perform clinical laboratory testing on specimens from individuals in the United States.

The Food and Drug Administration approves CLIA waived tests on a flow basis. The CMS identifies CLIA waived tests by providing an updated list of waived tests to the

Medicare contractors on a quarterly basis via a Recurring Update Notification. To be recognized as a waived test, some CLIA waived tests have unique HCPCS procedure codes and some must have a QW modifier included with the HCPCS code.

For a list of specific HCPCS codes subject to CLIA see http://www.cms.hhs.gov/CLIA/downloads/waivetbl.pdf

## 100-04, 17, 80.1.1

### HCPCS Service Coding for Oral Cancer Drugs
(Rev. 1, 10-01-03)

The following codes may be used for drugs other than Prodrugs, when covered:

| Generic/Chemical Name | How Supplied | HCPCS |
|---|---|---|
| Busulfan | 2 mg/ORAL | J8510 |
| Capecitabine | 150mg/ORAL | J8520 |
| Capecitabine | 500mg/ORAL | J8521 |
| Methotrexate | 2.5 mg/ORAL | J8610 |
| Cyclophosphamide * | 25 mg/ORAL | J8530 |
| Cyclophosphamide * | (Treat 50 mg. as 2 units 50 mg/ORAL | J8530 |
| Etoposide | 50 mg/ORAL | J8560 |
| Melphalan | 2 mg/ORAL | J8600 |
| Prescription Drug chemotherapeutic NOC | ORAL | J8999 |

Each tablet or capsule is equal to one unit, except for 50 mg./ORAL of cyclophosphamide (J8530), which is shown as 2 units. The 25m and 50 mg share the same code.

NOTE: HIPAA requires that drug claims submitted to DMERCs be identified by NDC.

## 100-04, 17, 80.1.2

### HCPCS and NDC Reporting for Prodrugs
(Rev. 136, 04-09-04)

#### FI claims
For oral anti-cancer Prodrugs HCPCS code J8999 is reported with revenue code 0636.

#### DMERC claims
The supplier reports the NDC code on the claim. The DMERC converts the NDC code to a "WW" HCPCS code for CWF. As new "WW" codes are established for oral anti-cancer drugs they will be communicated in a Recurring Update Notification.

## 100-04, 17, 80.2.1

The physician/supplier bills for these drugs on Form CMS-1500 or its electronic equivalent, the 837P. The facility bills for these drugs on Form CMS-1450 or its electronic equivalent, the 837I. The following HCPCS codes are assigned:

**J8501** APREPITANT, oral, 5 mg

(Note: HCPCS code is effective January 1, 2005, but coverage for aprepitant is effective April 4, 2005. Aprepitant is only covered in combination with a 5HT3 antagonist, and dexamethasone for beneficiaries who have received one or more of the specified anti-cancer chemotherapeutic agents.)

**Q0161** CHLORPROMAZINE HYDROCHLORIDE 5mg, oral, FDA-approved prescription anti-emetic, for use as a complete therapeutic substitute for an IV anti-emetic at the time of chemotherapy treatment, not to exceed a 48-hour dosage regimen.

**Q0162** ONDANSETRON 1mg, oral, FDA-approved prescription anti-emetic, for use as a complete therapeutic substitute for an IV anti-emetic at the time of chemotherapy treatment, not to exceed a 48-hour dosage regimen.

**Q0163** DIPHENHYDRAMINE HYDROCHLORIDE, 50mg, oral, FDA-approved prescription anti-emetic, for use as a complete therapeutic substitute for an IV anti-emetic at time of chemotherapy treatment not to exceed a 48-hour dosage regimen.

**Q0164** PROCHLORPERAZINE MALEATE, 5mg, oral, FDA-approved prescription anti-emetic, for use as a complete therapeutic substitute for an IV anti-emetic at the time of chemotherapy treatment, not to exceed a 48-hour dosage regimen.

**Q0165** PROCHLORPERAZINE MALEATE, 10mg, oral, FDA-approved prescription anti-emetic, for use as a complete therapeutic substitute for an IV anti-emetic at the time of chemotherapy treatment, not to exceed a 48-hour dosage regimen.

**Q0166** GRANISETRON HYDROCHLORIDE, 1mg, oral, FDA-approved prescription anti-emetic, for use as a complete therapeutic substitute for an IV anti-emetic at the time of chemotherapy treatment, not to exceed a 24-hour dosage regimen.

**Q0167** DRONABINOL 2.5mg, oral, FDA-approved prescription anti-emetic, for use as a complete therapeutic substitute for an IV anti-emetic at the time of chemotherapy treatment, not to exceed a 48-hour dosage regimen.

**Q0168** DRONABINOL 5mg, oral, FDA-approved prescription anti-emetic, for use as a complete therapeutic substitute for an IV anti-emetic at the time of chemotherapy treatment, not to exceed a 48-hour dosage regimen.

**Q0169** PROMETHAZINE HYDROCHLORIDE, 12.5mg, oral, FDA-approved prescription anti-emetic, for use as a complete therapeutic substitute for an IV anti-emetic at the time of chemotherapy treatment, not to exceed a 48-hour dosage regimen.

**Q0170** PROMETHAZINE HYDROCHLORIDE, 25mg, oral, FDA-approved prescription anti-emetic, for use as a complete therapeutic substitute for an IV anti-emetic at the time of chemotherapy treatment, not to exceed a 48-hour dosage regimen.

**Q0171** CHLORPROMAZINE HYDROCHLORIDE, 10mg, oral, FDA-approved prescription anti-emetic, for use as a complete therapeutic substitute for an IV anti-emetic at the time of chemotherapy treatment, not to exceed a 48-hour dosage regimen.

**Q0172** CHLORPROMAZINE HYDROCHLORIDE, 25mg, oral, FDA-approved prescription anti-emetic, for use as a complete therapeutic substitute for an IV anti-emetic at the time of chemotherapy treatment, not to exceed a 48-hour dosage regimen.

**Q0173** TRIMETHOBENZAMIDE HYDROCHLORIDE, 250mg, oral, FDA-approved prescription anti-emetic, for use as a complete therapeutic substitute for an IV anti-emetic at the time of chemotherapy treatment, not to exceed a 48-hour dosage regimen.

**Q0174** THIETHYLPERAZINE MALEATE, 10mg, oral, FDA-approved prescription anti-emetic, for use as a complete therapeutic substitute for an IV anti-emetic at the time of chemotherapy treatment, not to exceed a 48-hour dosage regimen.

**Q0175** PERPHENAZINE, 4mg, oral, FDA-approved prescription anti-emetic, for use as a complete therapeutic substitute for an IV anti-emetic at the time of chemotherapy treatment, not to exceed a 48-hour dosage regimen.

**Q0176** PERPHENAZINE, 8mg, oral, FDA-approved prescription anti-emetic, for use as a complete therapeutic substitute for an IV anti-emetic at the time of chemotherapy treatment, not to exceed a 48-hours dosage regimen.

**Q0177** HYDROXYZINE PAMOATE, 25mg, oral, FDA-approved prescription anti-emetic, for use as a complete therapeutic substitute for an IV anti-emetic at the time of chemotherapy treatment, not to exceed a 48-hour dosage regimen.

**Q0178** HYDROXYZINE PAMOATE, 50mg, oral, FDA-approved prescription anti-emetic, for use as a complete therapeutic substitute for an IV anti-emetic at the time of chemotherapy treatment, not to exceed a 48-hour dosage regimen.

**Q0179** ONDANSETRON mg, oral, FDA-approved prescription anti-emetic, for use as a complete therapeutic substitute for an IV anti-emetic at the time of chemotherapy treatment, not to exceed a 48-hour dosage regimen.

**Q0180** DOLASETRON MESYLATE, 100mg, oral, FDA-approved prescription anti-emetic, for use as a complete therapeutic substitute for an IV anti-emetic at the time of chemotherapy treatment, not to exceed a 24-hour dosage regimen.

**Q0181** UNSPECIFIED ORAL DOSAGE FORM, FDA-approved prescription anti-emetic, for use as a complete therapeutic substitute for an IV anti-emetic at the time of chemotherapy treatment, not to exceed a 48-hour dosage regimen.

NOTE: The 24-hour maximum drug supply limitation on dispensing, for HCPCS Codes Q0166 and Q0180, has been established to bring the Medicare benefit as it applies to these two therapeutic entities in conformity with the "Indications and Usage" section of currently FDA-approved product labeling for each affected drug product.

## 100-04, 17, 80.2.4

**Billing and Payment Instructions for A/B MACs (A)**

(Rev. 3085, Issued: 10-03-14, Effective: ICD-10: Upon Implementation of ICD-10; ASC X12: January 1, 2012, Implementation: ICD-10: Upon Implementation of ICD-10; ASC X12: November 4, 2014)

Claims for the oral anti-emetic drug aprepitant, either as a 3-day supply dispensed in a Tri-Pak or as the first day supply (not dispensed in a Tri-Pak), must be billed to the A/B MAC (A) on the ASC 837 institutional claim format or on hard copy Form CMS-1450 with the appropriate cancer diagnosis and HCPCS code or Current Procedural Terminology (CPT) code.

Claims for the second and third dose of the oral anti-emetic drug aprepitant not dispensed in a Tri-Pak must be billed to the DME MAC.

The following payment methodologies apply when hospital and SNF outpatient claims are processed by the A/B MAC (A):

- Based on APC for hospitals subject to the outpatient prospective payment system (OPPS);
- Under current payment methodologies for hospitals not subject to OPPS; or
- On a reasonable cost basis for SNFs.

Institutional providers bill for aprepitant under Revenue Code 0636 (Drugs requiring detailed coding).

NOTE: Inpatient claims submitted for oral anti-emetic drugs are processed under the current payment methodologies.

Medicare contractors shall pay claims submitted for services provided by a CAH as follows: Method I technical services are paid at 101% of reasonable cost; Method II technical services are paid at 101% of reasonable cost; and, Professional services are paid at 115% of the Medicare Physician Fee Schedule Data Base.

## 100-04, 17, 80.3

**Billing for Immunosuppressive Drugs**

(Rev. 1448; Issued: 02-15-08; Effective: 07-01-08; Implementation: 07-07-08)

Beginning January 1, 1987, Medicare pays for FDA approved immunosuppressive drugs and for drugs used in immunosuppressive therapy. (See the Medicare Benefit Policy Manual, Chapter 15 for detailed coverage requirements.) Generally, contractors pay for self-administered immunosuppressive drugs that are specifically labeled and approved for marketing as such by the FDA, or identified in FDA-approved labeling for use in conjunction with immunosuppressive drug therapy. This benefit is subject to the Part B deductible and coinsurance provision.

Contractors are expected to keep informed of FDA additions to the list of the immunosuppressive drugs and notify providers. Prescriptions for immunosuppressive drugs generally should be nonrefillable and limited to a 30-day supply. The 30-day guideline is necessary because dosage frequently diminishes over

© 2016 Optum360, LLC

a period of time, and further, it is not uncommon for the physician to change the prescription from one drug to another. Also, these drugs are expensive and the coinsurance liability on unused drugs could be a financial burden to the beneficiary. Unless there are special circumstances, contractors will not consider a supply of drugs in excess of 30 days to be reasonable and necessary and should deny payment accordingly.

Entities that normally bill the carrier bill the DME MAC. Entities that normally bill the FI continue to bill the FI, except for hospitals subject to OPPS, which must bill the DME MAC.

Prior to December 21, 2000 coverage was limited to immunosuppressive drugs received within 36 months of a transplant. ESRD beneficiaries continue to be limited to 36 months of coverage after a Medicare covered kidney transplant. For all other beneficiaries, BBA '97 increased the length of time a beneficiary could receive immunosuppressives by a sliding method. So for the period 8/97 thru 12/00 a longer period of time MAY apply for a transplant. Effective with immunosuppressive drugs furnished on or after December 21, 2000, there is no time limit, but an organ transplant must have occurred for which immunosuppressive therapy is appropriate. That is, the time limit for immunosuppressive drugs was eliminated for transplant beneficiaries that will continue Medicare coverage after 36 months based on disability or age. The date of transplant is reported to the FI with occurrence code 36.

CWF will edit claim records to determine if a history of a transplant is on record. If not an error will be returned. See Chapter 27 for edit codes and resolution.

For claims filed on and after July 1, 2008, suppliers that furnish an immunosuppressive drug to a Medicare beneficiary, when such drug has been prescribed due to the beneficiary having undergone an organ transplant, shall: 1) secure from the prescriber the date of such organ transplant, 2) retain documentation of such transplant date in its files, and 3) annotate the Medicare claim for such drug with the "KX" modifier to signify both that the supplier retains such documentation of the beneficiary's transplant date and that such transplant date precedes the Date of Service (DOS) for furnishing the drug.

For claims received on and after July 1, 2008, contractors shall accept claims for immunosuppressive drugs without a KX modifier but shall deny such claims unless a query of the Master Beneficiary Record (MBR) shows that Medicare has made payment for an organ transplant on a date that precedes the DOS of the immunosuppressive drug claim.

In the context of a claim for an immunosuppressive drug that is submitted to Medicare in order to receive payment, the use of the KX modifier signifies that the supplier has documentation on file to the effect that the beneficiary has undergone an organ transplant on a date certain and that the immunosuppressive drug has been prescribed incident to such transplant.

If a supplier has not determined (or does not have documentation on file to support a determination) that either the beneficiary did not receive an organ transplant or that the beneficiary was not enrolled in Medicare Part A as of the date of the transplant, then the supplier may not, with respect to furnishing an immunosuppressive drug: 1) bill Medicare, 2) bill or collect any amount from the beneficiary, or 3) issue an Advance Beneficiary Notice (ABN) to the beneficiary.

## 100-04, 17, 80.4

### Billing for Hemophilia Clotting Factors

(Rev. 1564, Issued: 07-25-08, Effective: 04-01-08, Implementation: 01-05-09)

Blood clotting factors not paid on a cost or prospective payment system basis are priced as a drug/biological under the drug pricing fee schedule effective for the specific date of service. As of January 1, 2005, the average sales price (ASP) plus 6 percent shall be used.

If a beneficiary is in a covered part A stay in a PPS hospital, the clotting factors are paid in addition to the DRG/HIPPS payment. For FY 2005, this payment is based on 95 percent of AWP. For FY 2006, the add-on payment for blood clotting factor administered to hemophilia inpatients is based on average sales price (ASP) + 6 percent and a furnishing fee. The furnishing fee is updated each calendar year. For a SNF subject to SNF/PPS, the payment is bundled into the SNF/PPS rate.

For hospitals subject to OPPS, the clotting factors, when paid under Part B, are paid the APC. For SNFs the clotting factors, when paid under Part B, are paid based on cost.

Local carriers and Part B MACs shall process non-institutional blood clotting factor claims.

The FIs and Part A MACs shall process institutional blood clotting factor claims (Part A and Part B institutional).

## 100-04, 17, 80.4.1

(Rev. 3340, Issued: 08-21-15, Effective: 01-01-16, Implementation: 01-04-16)

### Clotting Factor Furnishing Fee

The Medicare Modernization Act section 303(e)(1) added section 1842(o)(5)(C) of the Social Security Act which requires that, beginning January 1, 2005, a furnishing fee will be paid for items and services associated with clotting factor.

Beginning January 1, 2005, a clotting factor furnishing fee is separately payable to entities that furnish clotting factor unless the costs associated with furnishing the clotting factor is paid through another payment system.

The clotting factor furnishing fee is updated each calendar year based on the percentage increase in the consumer price index (CPI) for medical care for the 12-month period ending with June of the previous year. The clotting factor furnishing fees applicable for dates of service in each calendar year (CY) are listed below:

CY 2005 - 0.140 per unit

CY 2006 - 0.146 per unit

CY 2007 - 0.152 per unit

CY 2008 - 0.158 per unit

CY 2009 - 0.164 per unit

CY 2010 - 0.170 per unit

CY 2011 - 0.176 per unit

CY 2012 - 0.181 per unit

CY 2013 - 0.188 per unit

CY 2014 - 0.192 per unit

CY 2015 - 0.197 per unit

CY 2016 - $0.202 per unit

Annual updates to the clotting factor furnishing fee are subsequently communicated by a Recurring Update Notification.

CMS includes this clotting factor furnishing fee in the nationally published payment limit for clotting factor billing codes. When the clotting factor is not included on the Average Sales Price (ASP) Medicare Part B Drug Pricing File or Not Otherwise Classified (NOC) Pricing File, the contractor must make payment for the clotting factor as well as make payment for the furnishing fee.

## 100-04, 17, 80.6

### Intravenous Immune Globulin

(Rev. 3085, Issued: 10-03-14, Effective: ICD-10: Upon Implementation of ICD-10; ASC X12: January 1, 2012, Implementation: ICD-10: Upon Implementation of ICD-10; ASC X12: November 4, 2014)

Beginning for dates of service on or after January 1, 2004, Medicare pays for intravenous immune globulin administered in the home. (See the Medicare Benefit Policy Manual, Chapter 15 for coverage requirements.) Contractors pay for the drug, but not the items or services related to the administration of the drug when administered in the home, if deemed medically appropriate.

Contractors may pay any entity licensed in the State to furnish intravenous immune globulin. Payment will be furnished to the entity with the authority to furnish the drug. Beneficiaries are ineligible to receive payment for the drug.

Pharmacies and hospitals dispensing intravenous immune globulin for home use would bill the DME MAC. If the beneficiary is receiving treatment in an outpatient hospital, the bill must be sent to the A/B MAC (A). If the beneficiary is receiving treatment in a physician's office, the bill must be sent to the A/B MAC (B). Home Health Agencies dispensing intravenous immune globulin would bill the A/B MAC (HHH). Physicians furnishing intravenous immune globulin for the refilling of an external pump for home infusion would bill the DME MAC.

Effective January 1, 2006, Medicare makes an additional payment once per day per beneficiary for preadministration-related services whenever a beneficiary receives intravenous immune globulin.

## 100-04, 17, 80.12

### Claims Processing Rules for ESAs Administered to Cancer Patients for Anti-Anemia Therapy

(Rev. 3085, Issued: 10-03-14, Effective: ICD-10: Upon Implementation of ICD-10; ASC X12: January 1, 2012, Implementation: ICD-10: Upon Implementation of ICD-10; ASC X12: November 4, 2014)

The national coverage determination (NCD) titled, "The Use of ESAs in Cancer and Other Neoplastic Conditions" lists coverage criteria for the use of ESAs in patients who have cancer and experience anemia as a result of chemotherapy or as a result of the cancer itself. The full NCD can be viewed in Publication 100-03 of the NCD Manual, section 110.21.

Effective for claims with dates of service on and after January 1, 2008, non-ESRD ESA services for HCPCS J0881 or J0885 billed with modifier EC (ESA, anemia, non-chemo/radio) shall be denied when any one of the following diagnosis codes is present on the claim:

ICD-9-CM Applicable

- any anemia in cancer or cancer treatment patients due to folate deficiency (281.2),
- B-12 deficiency (281.1, 281.3),
- •ron deficiency (280.0-280.9),
- hemolysis (282.0, 282.2, 282.9, 283.0, 283.2, 283.9-283.10, 283.19), or
- bleeding (280.0, 285.1),
- anemia associated with the treatment of acute and chronic myelogenous leukemias (CML, AML) (205.00-205.21, 205.80-205.91); or
- erythroid cancers (207.00-207.81).

ICD-10-CM Applicable

- any anemia in cancer or cancer treatment patients due to folate deficiency - (D52.0, D52.1, D52.8, or D52.9),
- B-12 deficiency - (D51.1, D51.2, D51.3, D51.8, D51.9, or D53.1),
- iron deficiency - (D50.0, D50.1, D50.8, and D50.9),
- hemolysis - (D55.0, D55.1, D58.0, D58.9, D59.0, D59.1, D59.2, D59 4, D59.5, D59.6, D59.8, or D59.9),
- bleeding - (D50.0, D62),
- anemia associated with the treatment of acute and chronic myelogenous leukemias (CML, AML) - (C92.00, C92.01, C92.02, C92.10, C92.11, C92.12, C92.20, C92.21, C92.40, C92.41, C92.42, C92.50, C92.51, C92.52, C92.60, C92.61, C92.62, C92.90, C92.91, C92.A0, C92.A1, C92.A2, C92Z0, C92Z1, or C92Z2), or
- erythroid cancers - (C94.00, C94.01, C94.02, C94.20, C94.21, C94.22, C94.30, C94.31, C94.80, C94.81, D45).

Effective for claims with dates of service on and after January 1, 2008, contractors shall deny non-ESRD ESA services for HCPCS J0881 or J0885 billed with modifier EC (ESA, anemia, non-chemo/radio) for:

- any anemia in cancer or cancer treatment patients due to bone marrow fibrosis,
- anemia of cancer not related to cancer treatment,
- prophylactic use to prevent chemotherapy-induced anemia,
- prophylactic use to reduce tumor hypoxia,
- patients with erythropoietin-type resistance due to neutralizing antibodies; and
- anemia due to cancer treatment if patients have uncontrolled hypertension.

Effective for claims with dates of service on and after January 1, 2008, non-ESRD ESA services for HCPCS J0881 or J0885 billed with modifier EB (ESA, anemia, radio-induced), shall be denied.

Effective for claims with dates of service on and after January 1, 2008, contractors shall deny non-ESRD ESA services for HCPCS J0881 or J0885 billed with modifier EA (ESA, anemia, chemo-induced) for anemia secondary to myelosuppressive anticancer chemotherapy in solid tumors, multiple myeloma, lymphoma, and lymphocytic leukemia when a hemoglobin 10.0g/dL or greater or hematocrit 30.0% or greater is reported.

NOTE: ESA treatment duration for each course of chemotherapy includes the 8 weeks following the final dose of myelosuppressive chemotherapy in a chemotherapy regime.

Effective for claims with dates of service on and after January 1, 2008, Medicare contractors shall have discretion to establish local coverage policies for those indications not included in NCD 110.21.

Denials of claims for ESAs are based on reasonable and necessary determinations established by NCD 110.21. A provider may have the beneficiary sign an Advanced Beneficiary Notice, making the beneficiary liable for services not deemed reasonable and necessary and thus not covered by Medicare.

Report Medicare Summary Notice message 15.20, "The following policies [NCD 110.21] were used when we made this decision", and remittance reason code 50, "These are non-covered services because this is not deemed a `medical necessity' by the payer" for denied ESA claims.

Medicare contractors have the discretion to conduct medical review of claims and reverse the automated adjudication if the medical review results in a determination of clinical necessity.

## 100-04, 17, 90.3

### Hospital Outpatient Payment Under OPPS for New, Unclassified Drugs and Biologicals After FDA Approval But Before Assignment of a Product-Specific Drug or Biological HCPCS Code

Hospital Outpatient Payment Under OPPS for New, Unclassified Drugs and Biologicals After FDA Approval But Before Assignment of a Product-Specific Drug or Biological HCPCS Code

Section 621(a) of the MMA amends Section 1833(t) of the Social Security Act by adding paragraph (15), Payment for New Drugs and Biologicals Until HCPCS Code Assigned. Under this provision, payment for an outpatient drug or biological that is furnished as part of covered outpatient department services for which a product-specific HCPCS code has not been assigned shall be paid an amount equal to 95 percent of average wholesale price (AWP). This provision applies only to payments under the hospital outpatient prospective payment system (OPPS).

Beginning January 1, 2004, hospital outpatient departments may bill for new drugs and biologicals that are approved by the FDA on or after January 1, 2004, for which a product-specific HCPCS code has not been assigned. Beginning on or after the date of FDA approval, hospitals may bill for the drug or biological using HCPCS code C9399, Unclassified drug or biological.

Hospitals report in the ASC X12 837 institutional claim format in specific locations, or in the "Remarks" section of Form CMS-1450:

1. the National Drug Code (NDC),

2. the quantity of the drug that was administered, expressed in the unit of measure applicable to the drug or biological, and

3. the date the drug was furnished to the beneficiary. Contractors shall manually price the drug or biological at 95 percent of AWP. They shall pay hospitals 80 percent of the calculated price and shall bill beneficiaries 20 percent of the calculated price, after the deductible is met. Drugs and biologicals that are manually priced at 95 percent of AWP are not eligible for outlier payment.

HCPCS code C9399 is only to be reported for new drugs and biologicals that are approved by FDA on or after January 1, 2004, for which there is no HCPCS code that describes the drug.

## 100-04,18,10.1.2

### Influenza Virus Vaccine

Effective for services furnished on or after May 1, 1993, the influenza virus vaccine and its administration is covered when furnished in compliance with any applicable State law. Typically, this vaccine is administered once a flu season. Medicare does not require for coverage purposes that a doctor of medicine or osteopathy order the vaccine. Therefore, the beneficiary may receive the vaccine upon request without a physician's order and without physician supervision. Since there is no yearly limit, contractors determine whether such services are reasonable and allow payment if appropriate.

See Pub. 100-02, Medicare Benefit Policy Manual, Chapter 15, Section 50.4.4.2 for additional coverage requirements for influenza virus vaccine.

| Service | CPT/ HCPCS Code | Long Descriptor | USPSTF Rating | Coins./ Deductible |
|---|---|---|---|---|
| Initial Preventive Physical Examination, IPPE | G0402 | Initial preventive physical examination; face to face visits, services limited to new beneficiary during the first 12 months of Medicare enrollment | *Not Rated | WAIVED |
| | G0403 | Electrocardiogram, routine ECG with 12 leads; performed as a screening for the initial preventive physical examination with interpretation and report | | Not Waived |
| | G0404 | Electrocardiogram, routine ECG with 12 leads; tracing only, without interpretation and report, performed as a screening for the initial preventive physical examination | | Not Waived |

© 2016 Optum360, LLC

| Service | CPT/ HCPCS Code | Long Descriptor | USPSTF Rating | Coins./ Deductible |
|---|---|---|---|---|
| | G0405 | Electrocardiogram, routine ECG with 12 leads; interpretation and report only, performed as a screening for the initial preventive physical examination | | Not Waived |
| Ultrasound Screening for Abdominal Aortic Aneurysm (AAA) | G0389 | Ultrasound, B-scan and /or real time with image documentation; for abdominal aortic aneurysm (AAA) ultrasound screening | B | WAIVED |
| Cardiovascular Disease | 80061 | Lipid panel | A | WAIVED |
| | 82465 | Cholesterol, serum or whole blood, total | | WAIVED |
| | 83718 | Lipoprotein, direct measurement; high density cholesterol (hdl cholesterol) | | WAIVED |
| | 84478 | Triglycerides | | WAIVED |
| Diabetes Screening Tests | 82947 | Glucose; quantitative, blood (except reagent strip) | B | WAIVED |
| | 82950 | Glucose; post glucose dose (includes glucose) | | WAIVED |
| | 82951 | Glucose; tolerance test (gtt), three specimens (includes glucose) | *Not Rated | WAIVED |
| Diabetes Self-Management Training Services (DSMT) | G0108 | Diabetes outpatient self-management training services, individual, per 30 minutes | *Not Rated | Not Waived |
| | G0109 | Diabetes outpatient self-management training services, group session (2 or more), per 30 minutes | | Not Waived |
| Medical Nutrition Therapy (MNT) Services | 97802 | Medical nutrition therapy; initial assessment and intervention, individual, face-to-face with the patient, each 15 minutes | B | WAIVED |
| | 97803 | Medical nutrition therapy; re-assessment and intervention, individual, face-to-face with the patient, each 15 minutes | | WAIVED |
| | 97804 | Medical nutrition therapy; group (2 or more individual(s)), each 30 minutes | | WAIVED |

| Service | CPT/ HCPCS Code | Long Descriptor | USPSTF Rating | Coins./ Deductible |
|---|---|---|---|---|
| | G0270 | Medical nutrition therapy; reassessment and subsequent intervention(s) following second referral in same year for change in diagnosis, medical condition or treatment regimen (including additional hours needed for renal disease), individual, face to face with the patient, each 15 minutes | B | WAIVED |
| | G0271 | Medical nutrition therapy, reassessment and subsequent intervention(s) following second referral in same year for change in diagnosis, medical condition, or treatment regimen (including additional hours needed for renal disease), group (2 or more individuals), each 30 minutes | | WAIVED |
| Screening Pap Test | G0123 | Screening cytopathology, cervical or vaginal (any reporting system), collected in preservative fluid, automated thin layer preparation, screening by cytotechnologist under physician supervision | A | WAIVED |
| | G0124 | Screening cytopathology, cervical or vaginal (any reporting system), collected in preservative fluid, automated thin layer preparation, requiring interpretation by physician | | WAIVED |
| | G0141 | Screening cytopathology smears, cervical or vaginal, performed by automated system, with manual rescreening, requiring interpretation by physician | A | WAIVED |
| | G0143 | Screening cytopathology, cervical or vaginal (any reporting system), collected in preservative fluid, automated thin layer preparation, with manual screening and rescreening by cytotechnologist under physician supervision | A | WAIVED |

| Service | CPT/ HCPCS Code | Long Descriptor | USPSTF Rating | Coins./ Deductible |
|---|---|---|---|---|
| | G0144 | Screening cytopathology, cervical or vaginal (any reporting system), collected in preservative fluid, automated thin layer preparation, with screening by automated system, under physician supervision | A | WAIVED |
| | G0145 | Screening cytopathology, cervical or vaginal (any reporting system), collected in preservative fluid, automated thin layer preparation, with screening by automated system and manual rescreening under physician supervision | A | WAIVED |
| | G0147 | Screening cytopathology smears, cervical or vaginal, performed by automated system under physician supervision | A | WAIVED |
| | G0148 | Screening cytopathology smears, cervical or vaginal, performed by automated system with manual rescreening | A | WAIVED |
| | P3000 | Screening papanicolaou smear, cervical or vaginal, up to three smears, by technician under physician supervision | | WAIVED |
| | P3001 | Screening papanicolaou smear, cervical or vaginal, up to three smears, requiring interpretation by physician | | WAIVED |
| | Q0091 | Screening papanicolaou smear; obtaining, preparing and conveyance of cervical or vaginal smear to laboratory | | WAIVED |
| Screening Pelvic Exam | G0101 | Cervical or vaginal cancer screening; pelvic and clinical breast examination | A | WAIVED |
| Screening Mammography | 77052 | Computer-aided detection (computer algorithm analysis of digital image data for lesion detection) with further physician review for interpretation, with or without digitization of film radiographic images; screening mammography (list separately in addition to code for primary procedure) | B | WAIVED |
| | 77057 | Screening mammography, bilateral (2-view film study of each breast) | B | WAIVED |

| Service | CPT/ HCPCS Code | Long Descriptor | USPSTF Rating | Coins./ Deductible |
|---|---|---|---|---|
| | G0202 | Screening mammography, producing direct digital image, bilateral, all views | | WAIVED |
| Bone Mass Measurement | G0130 | Single energy x-ray absorptiometry (sexa) bone density study, one or more sites; appendicular skeleton (peripheral) (e.g., radius, wrist, heel) | B | WAIVED |
| | 77078 | Computed tomography, bone mineral density study, 1 or more sites; axial skeleton (e.g., hips, pelvis, spine) | | WAIVED |
| | 77079 | Computed tomography, bone mineral density study, 1 or more sites; appendicular skeleton (peripheral) (e.g., radius, wrist, heel) | | WAIVED |
| | 77080 | Dual-energy x-ray absorptiometry (dxa), bone density study, 1 or more sites; axial skeleton (e.g., hips, pelvis, spine) | | WAIVED |
| | 77081 | Dual-energy x-ray absorptiometry (dxa), bone density study, 1 or more sites; appendicular skeleton (peripheral) (e.g., radius, wrist, heel) | | WAIVED |
| | 77083 | Radiographic absorptiometry (e.g., photo densitometry, radiogrammetry), 1 or more sites | | WAIVED |
| | 76977 | Ultrasound bone density measurement and interpretation, peripheral site(s), any method | | WAIVED |
| Colorectal Cancer Screening | G0104 | Colorectal cancer screening; flexible sigmoidoscopy | A | WAIVED |
| | G0105 | Colorectal cancer screening; colonoscopy on individual at high risk | | WAIVED |
| | G0106 | Colorectal cancer screening; alternative to G0104, screening sigmoidoscopy, barium enema | *Not Rated | Coins. Applies & Ded. is waived |
| | G0120 | Colorectal cancer screening; alternative to G0105, screening colonoscopy, barium enema. | | Coins. Applies & Ded. is waived |
| | G0121 | Colorectal cancer screening; colonoscopy on individual not meeting criteria for high risk | A | WAIVED |
| | 82270 | Blood, occult, by peroxidase activity (e.g., guaiac), qualitative; feces, consecutive | | WAIVED |

                                                                          © 2016 Optum360, LLC

| Service | CPT/ HCPCS Code | Long Descriptor | USPSTF Rating | Coins./ Deductible |
|---|---|---|---|---|
| | G0328 | Colorectal cancer screening; fecal occult blood test, immunoassay, 1-3 simultaneous | | WAIVED |
| Prostate Cancer Screening | G0102 | Prostate cancer screening; digital rectal examination | D | Not Waived |
| | G0103 | Prostate cancer screening; prostate specific antigen test (PSA) | | WAIVED |
| Glaucoma Screening | G0117 | Glaucoma screening for high risk patients furnished by an optometrist or ophthalmologist | I | Not Waived |
| | G0118 | Glaucoma screening for high risk patient furnished under the direct supervision of an optometrist or ophthalmologist | | Not Waived |
| Influenza Virus Vaccine | 90654 | Influenza virus vaccine, split virus, preservative free, for intradermal use, for adults ages 18-64 | B | WAIVED |
| | 90654 | Influenza virus vaccine, split virus, preservative free, for intradermal use, for adults ages 18-64 | B | |
| | 90655 | Influenza virus vaccine, split virus, preservative free, when administered to children 6-35 months of age, for intramuscular use | | WAIVED |
| | 90656 | Influenza virus vaccine, split virus, preservative free, when administered to individuals 3 years and older, for intramuscular use | | WAIVED |
| | 90657 | Influenza virus vaccine, split virus, when administered to children 6-35 months of age, for intramuscular use | | WAIVED |
| | 90660 | Influenza virus vaccine, live, for intranasal use | | WAIVED |
| | 90662 | Influenza virus vaccine, split virus, preservative free, enhanced immunogenicity via increased antigen content, for intramuscular use | | WAIVED |
| | Q2034 | Influenza virus vaccine, split virus, for intramuscular use (Agriflu) | | WAIVED |
| | Q2035 | Influenza virus vaccine, split virus, when administered to individuals 3 years of age and older, for intramuscular use (afluria) | | WAIVED |

| Service | CPT/ HCPCS Code | Long Descriptor | USPSTF Rating | Coins./ Deductible |
|---|---|---|---|---|
| | Q2036 | Influenza virus vaccine, split virus, when administered to individuals 3 years of age and older, for intramuscular use (flulaval) | | WAIVED |
| | Q2037 | Influenza virus vaccine, split virus when administered to individuals 3 years of age and older, for intramuscular use (fluvirin) | | WAIVED |
| | Q2038 | Influenza virus vaccine, split virus, when administered to individuals 3 years of age and older, for intramuscular use (fluzone) | | WAIVED |
| | Q2039 | Influenza virus vaccine, split virus, when administered to individuals 3 years of age and older, for intramuscular use (not otherwise specified) | | WAIVED |
| | G0008 | Administration of influenza virus vaccine | | WAIVED |
| | G9141 | Influenza A (H1N1) immunization administration (includes the physician counseling the patient/family) | | WAIVED |
| | G9142 | Influenza A (H1N1) Vaccine, any route of administration | | WAIVED |
| Pneumococcal Vaccine | 90669 | Pneumococcal conjugate vaccine, polyvalent, when administered to children younger than 5 years, for intramuscular use | B | WAIVED |
| | 90670 | Pneumococcal conjugate vaccine, 13 valent, for intramuscular use. | | WAIVED |
| | 90732 | Pneumococcal polysaccharide vaccine, 23-valent, adult or immunosuppressed patient dosage, when administered to individuals 2 years or older, for subcutaneous or intramuscular use | | WAIVED |
| | G0009 | Administration of pneumococcal vaccine | | WAIVED |
| Hepatitis B Vaccine | 90740 | Hepatitis B vaccine, dialysis or immunosuppressed patient dosage (3 dose schedule), for intramuscular use | A | WAIVED |

© 2016 Optum360, LLC

| Service | CPT/ HCPCS Code | Long Descriptor | USPSTF Rating | Coins./ Deductible |
|---|---|---|---|---|
| | 90743 | Hepatitis B vaccine, adolescent (2 dose schedule), for intramuscular use | | WAIVED |
| | 90744 | Hepatitis B vaccine, pediatric/adolescent dosage (3 dose schedule), for intramuscular use | | WAIVED |
| | 90746 | Hepatitis B vaccine, adult dosage, for intramuscular use | | WAIVED |
| | 90747 | Hepatitis B vaccine, dialysis or immunosuppressed patient dosage (4 dose schedule), for intramuscular use | | WAIVED |
| | G0010 | Administration of hepatitis B vaccine | A | WAIVED |
| HIV Screening | G0432 | Infectious agent antigen detection by enzyme immunoassay (EIA) technique, qualitative or semi-qualitative, multiple-step method, HIV-1 or HIV-2, screening | A | WAIVED |
| | G0433 | Infectious agent antigen detection by enzyme-linked immunosorbent assay (ELISA) technique, antibody, HIV-1 or HIV-2, screening | | WAIVED |
| | G0435 | Infectious agent antigen detection by rapid antibody test of oral mucosa transudate, HIV-1 or HIV-2 , screening | | WAIVED |
| Smoking Cessation | G0436 | Smoking and tobacco cessation counseling visit for the asymptomatic patient; intermediate, greater than 3 minutes, up to 10 minutes | A | WAIVED |
| | G0437 | Smoking and tobacco cessation counseling visit for the asymptomatic patient intensive, greater than 10 minutes | | WAIVED |
| Annual Wellness Visit | G0438 | Annual wellness visit, including PPPS, first visit | *Not Rated | WAIVED |
| | G0439 | Annual wellness visit, including PPPS, subsequent visit | | WAIVED |

## 100-04, 18, 10.2.1

### Healthcare Common Procedure Coding System (HCPCS) and Diagnosis Codes

Vaccines and their administration are reported using separate codes. The following codes are for reporting the vaccines only.

| HCPCS | Definition |
|---|---|
| 90653 | Influenza virus vaccine, inactivated, subunit, adjuvanted, for intramuscular use |
| 90654 | Influenza virus vaccine, split virus, preservative-free, for intradermal use, for adults ages 18 – 64; |

| HCPCS | Definition |
|---|---|
| 90655 | Influenza virus vaccine, split virus, preservative free, for children 6-35 months of age, for intramuscular use; |
| 90656 | Influenza virus vaccine, split virus, preservative free, for use in individuals 3 years and above, for intramuscular use; |
| 90657 | Influenza virus vaccine, split virus, for children 6-35 months of age, for intramuscular use; |
| 90660 | Influenza virus vaccine, live, for intranasal use; |
| 90661 | Influenza virus vaccine, derived from cell cultures, subunit, preservative and antibiotic free, for intramuscular use |
| 90662 | Influenza virus vaccine, split virus, preservative free, enhanced immunogenicity via increased antigen content, for intramuscular use |
| 90669 | Pneumococcal conjugate vaccine, polyvalent, for children under 5 years, for intramuscular use |
| 90670 | Pneumococcal conjugate vaccine, 13 valent, for intramuscular use |
| 90672 | Influenza virus vaccine, live, quadrivalent, for intranasal use |
| 90673 | Influenza virus vaccine, trivalent, derived from recombinant DNA (RIV3), hemagglutinin (HA) protein only, preservative and antibiotic free, for intramuscular use |
| 90685 | Influenza virus vaccine, quadrivalent, split virus, preservative free, when administered to children 6-35 months of age, for intramuscular use |
| 90686 | Influenza virus vaccine, quadrivalent, split virus, preservative free, when administered to individuals 3 years of age and older, for intramuscular use |
| 90687 | Influenza virus vaccine, quadrivalent, split virus, when administered to children 6-35 months of age, for intramuscular use |
| 90688 | Influenza virus vaccine, quadrivalent, split virus, when administered to individuals 3 years of age and older, for intramuscular use |
| 90732 | Pneumococcal polysaccharide vaccine, 23-valent, adult or immunosuppressed patient dosage, for use in individuals 2 years or older, for subcutaneous or intramuscular use; |
| 90739 | Hepatitis B vaccine, adult dosage (2 dose schedule), for intramuscular use |
| 90740 | Hepatitis B vaccine, dialysis or immunosuppressed patient dosage (3 dose schedule), for intramuscular use; |
| 90743 | Hepatitis B vaccine, adolescent (2 dose schedule), for intramuscular use; |
| 90744 | Hepatitis B vaccine, pediatric/adolescent dosage (3 dose schedule), for intramuscular use; |
| 90746 | Hepatitis B vaccine, adult dosage, for intramuscular use; and |
| 90747 | Hepatitis B vaccine, dialysis or immunosuppressed patient dosage (4 dose schedule), for intramuscular use. |

G0010. Beginning January 1, 2011, providers should report G0010 for billing under the OPPS rather than 90471 or 90472 to ensure correct waiver of coinsurance and deductible for the administration of hepatitis B vaccine.

One of the following diagnosis codes must be reported as appropriate. If the sole purpose for the visit is to receive a vaccine or if a vaccine is the only service billed on a claim the applicable following diagnosis code may be used.

| Diagnosis Code | Description |
|---|---|
| V03.82 | Pneumococcus |
| V04.81** | Influenza |
| V06.6*** | Pneumococcus and Influenza |
| V05.3 | Hepatitis B |

## 100-04, 18, 10.2.2.1

### FI/AB MAC Payment for Pneumococcal Pneumonia Virus, Influenza Virus, and Hepatitis B Virus Vaccines and Their Administration

Payment for Vaccines

Payment for all of these vaccines is on a reasonable cost basis for hospitals, home health agencies (HHAs), skilled nursing facilities (SNFs), critical access hospitals (CAHs), and hospital-based renal dialysis facilities (RDFs). Payment for comprehensive outpatient rehabilitation facilities (CORFs), Indian Health Service hospitals (IHS), IHS

© 2016 Optum360, LLC

CAHs and independent RDFs is based on 95 percent of the average wholesale price (AWP). Section 10.2.4 of this chapter contains information on payment of these vaccines when provided by RDFs or hospices. See Sec.10.2.2.2 for payment to independent and provider- based Rural Health Centers and Federally Qualified Health Clinics.

Payment for these vaccines is as follows:

| Facility | Type of Bill | Payment |
|---|---|---|
| Hospitals, other than Indian Health Service (IHS) Hospitals and Critical Access Hospitals (CAHs) | 12x, 13x | Reasonable cost |
| IHS Hospitals | 12x, 13x, 83x | 95% of AWP |
| IHS CAHs | 85x | 95% of AWP |
| CAHs Method I and Method II | 85x | Reasonable cost |
| Skilled Nursing Facilities | 22x, 23x | Reasonable cost |
| Home Health Agencies | 34x | Reasonable cost |
| Comprehensive Outpatient Rehabilitation Facilities | 75x | 95% of the AWP |
| Independent Renal Dialysis Facilities | 72x | 95% of the AWP |
| Hospital-based Renal Dialysis Facilities | 72x | Reasonable cost |

Payment for Vaccine Administration

Payment for the administration of influenza virus and pneumococcal vaccines is as follows:

| Facility | Type of Bill | Payment |
|---|---|---|
| Hospitals, other than IHS Hospitals and CAHs | 12x, 13x | Outpatient Prospective Payment System (OPPS) for hospitals subject to OPPS |
| Reasonable cost for hospitals not subject to OPPS IHS Hospitals | 12x, 13x, 83x | MPFS as indicated in guidelines below. |
| IHS CAHs | 85x | MPFS as indicated in guidelines below. |
| CAHs Method I and II | 85x | Reasonable cost |
| Skilled Nursing Facilities | 22x, 23x | MPFS as indicated in the guidelines below |
| Home Health Agencies | 34x | OPPS |
| Comprehensive Outpatient Rehabilitation Facilities | 75x | MPFS as indicated in the guidelines below |
| Independent RDFs | 72x | MPFS as indicated in the guidelines below |
| Hospital-based RDFs | 72x | Reasonable cost |

Guidelines for pricing pneumococcal and influenza virus vaccine administration under the MPFS.

Make reimbursement based on the rate in the MPFS associated with the CPT code 90782 or 90471 as follows:

| HCPCS code | Effective prior to March 1, 2003 | Effective on and after March 1, 2003 |
|---|---|---|
| G0008 | 90782 | 90471 |
| G0009 | 90782 | 90471 |

See Sec.10.2.2.2 for payment to independent and provider based Rural Health Centers and Federally Qualified Health Clinics.

Payment for the administration of hepatitis B vaccine is as follows:

| Facility | Type of Bill | Payment |
|---|---|---|
| Hospitals other than IHS hospitals and CAHs | 12x, 13x | Outpatient Prospective Payment System (OPPS) for hospitals subject to OPPS |
| Reasonable cost for hospitals not subject to OPPS IHS Hospitals | 12x, 13x, 83x | MPFS as indicated in the guidelines below |
| CAHs Method I and II | 85x | Reasonable cost |
| IHS CAHs | 85x | MPFS as indicated in guidelines below. |
| Skilled Nursing Facilities | 22x, 23x | MPFS as indicated in the chart below |
| Home Health Agencies | 34x | OPPS |
| Comprehensive Outpatient Rehabilitation Facilities | 75x | MPFS as indicated in the guidelines below |
| Independent RDFs | 72x | MPFS as indicated in the chart below |
| Hospital-based RDFs | 72x | Reasonable cost |

Guidelines for pricing hepatitis B vaccine administration under the MPFS.

Make reimbursement based on the rate in the MPFS associated with the CPT code 90782 or 90471 as follows:

| HCPCS code | Effective prior to March 1, 2003 | Effective on and after March 1, 2003 |
|---|---|---|
| G0010 | 90782 | 90471 |

See Sec.10.2.2.2 for payment to independent and provider based Rural Health Centers and Federally Qualified Health Clinics.

## 100-04, 18, 10.2.5.2

### Carrier/AB MAC Payment Requirements

Payment for pneumococcal, influenza virus, and hepatitis B vaccines follows the same standard rules that are applicable to any injectable drug or biological. (See chapter 17 for procedures for determining the payment rates for pneumococcal and influenza virus vaccines.) Effective for claims with dates of service on or after February 1, 2001, Sec.114, of the Benefits Improvement and Protection Act of 2000 mandated that all drugs and biologicals be paid based on mandatory assignment. Therefore, all providers of influenza virus and pneumococcal vaccines must accept assignment for the vaccine.

Prior to March 1, 2003, the administration of pneumococcal, influenza virus, and hepatitis B vaccines, (HCPCS codes G0008, G0009, and G0010), though not reimbursed directly through the MPFS, were reimbursed at the same rate as HCPCS code 90782 on the MPFS for the year that corresponded to the date of service of the claim.

Prior to March 1, 2003, HCPCS codes G0008, G0009, and G0010 are reimbursed at the same rate as HCPCS code 90471. Assignment for the administration is not mandatory, but is applicable should the provider be enrolled as a provider type "Mass Immunization Roster Biller," submits roster bills, or participates in the centralized billing program.

Carriers/AB MACs may not apply the limiting charge provision for pneumococcal, influenza virus vaccine, or hepatitis B vaccine and their administration in accordance with Secs.1833(a)(1) and 1833(a)(10)(A) of the Social Security Act (the Act.) The administration of the influenza virus vaccine is covered in the influenza virus vaccine benefit under Sec.1861(s)(10)(A) of the Act, rather than under the physicians' services benefit. Therefore, it is not eligible for the 10 percent Health Professional Shortage Area (HPSA) incentive payment or the 5 percent Physician Scarcity Area (PSA) incentive payment.

No Legal Obligation to Pay  Nongovernmental entities that provide immunizations free of charge to all patients, regardless of their ability to pay, must provide the immunizations free of charge to Medicare beneficiaries and may not bill Medicare. (See Pub. 100-02, Medicare Benefit Policy Manual, chapter 16.) Thus, for example, Medicare may not pay for influenza virus vaccinations administered to Medicare beneficiaries if a physician provides free vaccinations to all non-Medicare patients or where an employer offers free vaccinations to its employees. Physicians also may not charge Medicare beneficiaries more for a vaccine than they would charge non-Medicare patients. (See Sec.1128(b)(6)(A) of the Act.)

When an employer offers free vaccinations to its employees, it must also offer the free vaccination to an employee who is also a Medicare beneficiary. It does not have to offer free vaccinations to its non-Medicare employees.

Nongovernmental entities that do not charge patients who are unable to pay or reduce their charges for patients of limited means, yet expect to be paid if the patient has health insurance coverage for the services provided, may bill Medicare and expect payment.

Governmental entities (such as PHCs) may bill Medicare for pneumococcal, hepatitis B, and influenza virus vaccines administered to Medicare beneficiaries when services are rendered free of charge to non-Medicare beneficiaries.

## 100-04, 18, 10.3.1.1

### Centralized Billing for Influenza Virus and Pneumococcal Vaccines to Medicare Carriers/AB MACs

The CMS currently authorizes a limited number of providers to centrally bill for influenza virus and pneumococcal immunization claims. Centralized billing is an optional program available to providers who qualify to enroll with Medicare as the provider type "Mass Immunization Roster Biller," as well as to other individuals and entities that qualify to enroll as regular Medicare providers. Centralized billers must roster bill, must accept assignment, and must bill electronically.

To qualify for centralized billing, a mass immunizer must be operating in at least three payment localities for which there are three different contractors processing claims. Individuals and entities providing the vaccine and administration must be properly licensed in the State in which the immunizations are given and the contractor must verify this through the enrollment process.

Centralized billers must send all claims for influenza virus and pneumococcal immunizations to a single contractor for payment, regardless of the jurisdiction in which the vaccination was administered. (This does not include claims for the Railroad Retirement Board, United Mine Workers or Indian Health Services. These claims must continue to go to the appropriate processing entity.) Payment is made based on the payment locality where the service was provided. This process is only available for claims for the influenza virus and pneumococcal vaccines and their administration. The general coverage and coding rules still apply to these claims.

This section applies only to those individuals and entities that provide mass immunization services for influenza virus and pneumococcal vaccinations and that have been authorized by CMS to centrally bill. All other providers, including those individuals and entities that provide mass immunization services that are not authorized to centrally bill, must continue to bill for these claims to their regular carrier/AB MAC per the instructions in Sec.10.3.1 of this chapter.

The claims processing instructions in this section apply only to the designated processing contractor. However, all carriers/AB MACs must follow the instructions in Sec.10.3.1.1.J, below, "Provider Education Instructions for All Carriers/AB MACs." A. Processing Contractor  Trailblazers Health Enterprises is designated as the sole contractor for the payment of influenza virus and pneumococcal claims for centralized billers from October 1, 2000, through the length of the contract. The CMS central office will notify centralized billers of the appropriate contractor to bill when they receive their notification of acceptance into the centralized billing program.

### B. Request for Approval
Approval to participate in the CMS centralized billing program is a two part approval process. Individuals and corporations who wish to enroll as a CMS mass immunizer centralized biller must send their request in writing. CMS will complete Part 1 of the approval process by reviewing preliminary demographic information included in the request for participation letter. Completion of Part 1 is not approval to set up vaccination clinics, vaccinate beneficiaries, and bill Medicare for reimbursement. All new  participants must complete Part 2 of the approval process (Form CMS-855 Application) before they may set up vaccination clinics, vaccinate Medicare beneficiaries, and bill Medicare for reimbursement. If an individual or entity's request is approved for centralized billing, the approval is limited to 12 months from September to August 31 of the next year. It is the responsibility of the centralized biller to reapply for approval each year. The designated contractor shall provide in writing to CMS and approved centralized billers notification of completion and approval of Part 2 of the approval process. The designated contractor may not process claims for any centralized biller who has not completed Parts 1 and 2 of the approval process. If claims are submitted by a provider who has not received approval of Parts 1 and 2 of the approval process to participate as a centralized biller, the contractor must return the claims to the provider to submit to the local carrier/AB MAC for payment.

### C. Notification of Provider Participation to the Processing Contractor
Before September 1 of every year, CMS will provide the designated contractor with the names of the entities that are authorized to participate in centralized billing for the 12 month period beginning September 1 and ending August 31 of the next year.

### D. Enrollment
Though centralized billers may already have a Medicare provider number, for purposes of centralized billing, they must also obtain a provider number from the processing contractor for centralized billing through completion of the Form CMS-855 (Provider Enrollment Application). Providers/suppliers are encouraged to apply to enroll as a centralized biller early as possible. Applicants who have not completed the entire enrollment process and received approval from CMS and the designated contractor to participate as a Medicare mass immunizer centralized biller will not be allowed to submit claims to Medicare for reimbursement.

Whether an entity enrolls as a provider type "Mass Immunization Roster Biller" or some other type of provider, all normal enrollment processes and procedures must be followed. Authorization from CMS to participate in centralized billing is dependent upon the entity's ability to qualify as some type of Medicare provider. In addition, as under normal enrollment procedures, the contractor must verify that the entity is fully qualified and certified per State requirements in each State in which they plan to operate.

The contractor will activate the provider number for the 12-month period from September 1 through August 31 of the following year. If the provider is authorized to participate in the centralized billing program the next year, the contractor will extend the activation of the provider number for another year. The entity need not re-enroll with the contractor every year. However, should there be changes in the States in which the entity plans to operate, the contractor will need to verify that the entity meets all State certification and licensure requirements in those new States.

### E. Electronic Submission of Claims on Roster Bills
Centralized billers must agree to submit their claims on roster bills in an Electronic Media Claims standard format using the appropriate version of American National Standards Institute (ANSI) format. Contractors should refer to the appropriate ANSI Implementation Guide to determine the correct location for this information on electronic claims. The processing contractor must provide instructions on acceptable roster billing formats to the approved centralized billers. Paper claims will not be accepted.

### F. Required Information on Roster Bills for Centralized Billing
In addition to the roster billing instructions found in Sec.10.3.1 of this chapter, centralized billers must complete on the electronic format the area that corresponds to Item 32 and 33 on Form CMS 1500 (08-05). The contractor must use the ZIP Code in Item 32 to determine the payment locality for the claim. Item 33 must be completed to report the provider of service/supplier's billing name, address, ZIP Code, and telephone number. In addition, the NPI of the billing provider or group must be appropriately reported.

For electronic claims, the name, address, and ZIP Code of the facility are reported in:

- The HIPAA compliant ANSI X12N 837: Claim level loop 2310D NM101=FA. When implemented, the facility (e.g., hospitals) NPI will be captured in the loop 2310D NM109 (NM108=XX) if one is available. Prior to NPI, enter the tax information in loop 2310D NM109 (NM108=24 or 34) and enter the Medicare legacy facility identifier in loop 2310D REF02 (REF01=1C). Report the address, city, state, and ZIP Code in loop 2310D N301 and N401, N402, and N403. Facility data is not required to be reported at the line level for centralized billing.

### G. Payment Rates and Mandatory Assignment
The payment rates for the administration of the vaccinations are based on the Medicare Physician Fee Schedule (MPFS) for the appropriate year. Payment made through the MPFS is based on geographic locality. Therefore, payments vary based on the geographic locality where the service was performed.

The HCPCS codes G0008 and G0009 for the administration of the vaccines are not paid on the MPFS. However, prior to March 1, 2003, they must be paid at the same rate as HCPCS code 90782, which is on the MPFS. The designated contractor must pay per the correct MPFS file for each calendar year based on the date of service of the claim. Beginning March 1, 2003, HCPCS codes G0008, G0009, and G0010 are to be reimbursed at the same rate as HCPCS code 90471.

In order to pay claims correctly for centralized billers, the designated contractor must have the correct name and address, including ZIP Code, of the entity where the service was provided.

The following remittance advice and Medicare Summary Notice (MSN) messages apply:

- Claim adjustment reason code 16, "Claim/service lacks information which is needed for adjudication. At least one Remark Code must be provided (may be comprised of either the Remittance Advice Remark Code or NCPDP Reject Reason Code.)"  and  Remittance advice remark code MA114, "Missing/incomplete/invalid information on where the services were furnished."  and  MSN 9.4 - "This item or service was denied because information required to make payment was incorrect."  The payment rates for the vaccines must be determined by the standard method used by Medicare for reimbursement of drugs and biologicals. (See chapter 17 for procedures for determining the payment rates for vaccines.) Effective for claims with dates of service on or after February 1, 2001, Sec.114, of the Benefits Improvement and Protection Act of 2000 mandated that all drugs and biologicals be paid based on mandatory assignment. Therefore, all providers of influenza virus and pneumococcal vaccines must accept assignment for the vaccine. In addition, as a requirement for both centralized billing and roster billing, providers must agree to accept assignment for the administration of the vaccines as well. This means that they must agree to accept the amount that Medicare pays for the vaccine and the administration. Also, since there is no coinsurance or deductible for the influenza virus and pneumococcal benefit, accepting assignment means that Medicare beneficiaries cannot be charged for the vaccination.

### H. Common Working File Information

To identify these claims and to enable central office data collection on the project, special processing number 39 has been assigned. The number should be entered on the HUBC claim record to CWF in the field titled Demonstration Number.

### I. Provider Education Instructions for the Processing Contractor

The processing contractor must fully educate the centralized billers on the processes for centralized billing as well as for roster billing. General information on influenza virus and pneumococcal coverage and billing instructions is available on the CMS Web site for providers.

### J. Provider Education Instructions for All Carriers/AB MACs

By April 1 of every year, all carriers/AB MACs must publish in their bulletins and put on their Web sites the following notification to providers. Questions from interested providers should be forwarded to the central office address below. Carriers/AB MACs must enter the name of the assigned processing contractor where noted before sending.

### NOTIFICATION TO PROVIDERS

Centralized billing is a process in which a provider, who provides mass immunization services for influenza virus and pneumococcal pneumonia virus (PPV) immunizations, can send all claims to a single contractor for payment regardless of the geographic locality in which the vaccination was administered. (This does not include claims for the Railroad Retirement Board, United Mine Workers or Indian Health Services. These claims must continue to go to the appropriate processing entity.) This process is only available for claims for the influenza virus and pneumococcal vaccines and their administration. The administration of the vaccinations is reimbursed at the assigned rate based on the Medicare physician fee schedule for the appropriate locality. The vaccines are reimbursed at the assigned rate using the Medicare standard method for reimbursement of drugs and biologicals.

Individuals and entities interested in centralized billing must contact CMS central office, in writing, at the following address by June 1 of the year they wish to begin centrally billing.

Center for Medicare & Medicaid Services  Division of Practitioner Claims Processing  Provider Billing and Education Group  7500 Security Boulevard  Mail Stop C4-10-07  Baltimore, Maryland 21244  By agreeing to participate in the centralized billing program, providers agree to abide by the following criteria.

### CRITERIA FOR CENTRALIZED BILLING

To qualify for centralized billing, an individual or entity providing mass immunization services for influenza virus and pneumococcal vaccinations must provide these services in at least three payment localities for which there are at least three different contractors processing claims.

Individuals and entities providing the vaccine and administration must be properly licensed in the State in which the immunizations are given.

Centralized billers must agree to accept assignment (i.e., they must agree to accept the amount that Medicare pays for the vaccine and the administration).

NOTE: The practice of requiring a beneficiary to pay for the vaccination upfront and to file their own claim for reimbursement is inappropriate. All Medicare providers are required to file claims on behalf of the beneficiary per Sec.1848(g)(4)(A) of the Social Security Act and centralized billers may not collect any payment.

The contractor assigned to process the claims for centralized billing is chosen at the discretion of CMS based on such considerations as workload, user-friendly software developed by the contractor for billing claims, and overall performance. The assigned contractor for this year is [Fill in name of contractor.]

The payment rates for the administration of the vaccinations are based on the Medicare physician fee schedule (MPFS) for the appropriate year. Payment made through the MPFS is based on geographic locality. Therefore, payments received may

vary based on the geographic locality where the service was performed. Payment is made at the assigned rate.

The payment rates for the vaccines are determined by the standard method used by Medicare for reimbursement of drugs and biologicals. Payment is made at the assigned rate.

Centralized billers must submit their claims on roster bills in an approved Electronic Media Claims standard format. Paper claims will not be accepted.

Centralized billers must obtain certain information for each beneficiary including name, health insurance number, date of birth, sex, and signature. [Fill in name of contractor] must be contacted prior to the season for exact requirements. The responsibility lies with the centralized biller to submit correct beneficiary Medicare information (including the beneficiary's Medicare Health Insurance Claim Number) as the contractor will not be able to process incomplete or incorrect claims.

Centralized billers must obtain an address for each beneficiary so that a Medicare Summary Notice (MSN) can be sent to the beneficiary by the contractor. Beneficiaries are sometimes confused when they receive an MSN from a contractor other than the contractor that normally processes their claims which results in unnecessary beneficiary inquiries to the Medicare contractor. Therefore, centralized billers must provide every beneficiary receiving an influenza virus or pneumococcal vaccination with the name of the processing contractor. This notification must be in writing, in the form of a brochure or handout, and must be provided to each beneficiary at the time he or she receives the vaccination.

Centralized billers must retain roster bills with beneficiary signatures at their permanent location for a time period consistent with Medicare regulations. [Fill in name of contractor] can provide this information.

Though centralized billers may already have a Medicare provider number, for purposes of centralized billing, they must also obtain a provider number from [Fill in name of contractor]. This can be done by completing the Form CMS-855 (Provider Enrollment Application), which can be obtained from [Fill in name of contractor].

If an individual or entity's request for centralized billing is approved, the approval is limited to the 12 month period from September 1 through August 31 of the following year. It is the responsibility of the centralized biller to reapply to CMS CO for approval each year by June 1. Claims will not be processed for any centralized biller without permission from CMS.

Each year the centralized biller must contact [Fill in name of contractor] to verify understanding of the coverage policy for the administration of the pneumococcal vaccine, and for a copy of the warning language that is required on the roster bill.

The centralized biller is responsible for providing the beneficiary with a record of the pneumococcal vaccination.

The information in items 1 through 8 below must be included with the individual or entity's annual request to participate in centralized billing:

1. Estimates for the number of beneficiaries who will receive influenza virus vaccinations;

2. Estimates for the number of beneficiaries who will receive pneumococcal vaccinations;

3. The approximate dates for when the vaccinations will be given;

4. A list of the States in which influenza virus and pneumococcal clinics will be held;

5. The type of services generally provided by the corporation (e.g., ambulance, home health, or visiting nurse);

6. Whether the nurses who will administer the influenza virus and pneumococcal vaccinations are employees of the corporation or will be hired by the corporation specifically for the purpose of administering influenza virus and pneumococcal vaccinations;

7. Names and addresses of all entities operating under the corporation's application;

8. Contact information for designated contact person for centralized billing program.

## 100-04, 18, 10.4

### CWF Edits

In order to prevent duplicate payments for influenza virus and pneumococcal vaccination claims by the local contractor/AB MAC and the centralized billing contractor, effective for claims received on or after July 1, 2002, CWF has implemented a number of edits.

NOTE: 90659 was discontinued December 31, 2003.

CWF returns information in Trailer 13 information from the history claim. The following fields are returned to the contractor:

- Trailer Code;
- Contractor Number;
- Document Control Number;
- First Service Date;
- Last Service Date;
- Provider, Physician, Supplier Number;
- Claim Type; Procedure code;
- Alert Code (where applicable); and,
- More history (where applicable.)

## 100-04,18,10.4.1

### CWF Edits on FI/AB MAC Claims

In order to prevent duplicate payment by the same FI/AB MAC, CWF edits by line item on the FI/AB MAC number, the beneficiary Health Insurance Claim (HIC) number, and the date of service, the influenza virus procedure codes 90653, 90654, 90655, 90656, 90657, 90660, 90661, 90662, 90672, 90673, 90685, 90686, 90687, or 90688 and the pneumococcal procedure codes 90669, 90670, or 90732, and the administration codes G0008 or G0009.

If CWF receives a claim with either HCPCS codes 90653, 90654, 90655, 90656, 90657, 90660, 90661, 90662, 90672, 90673, 90685, 90686, 90687, or 90688 and it already has on record a claim with the same HIC number, same FI/AB MAC number, same date of service, and any one of those HCPCS codes, the second claim submitted to CWF rejects.

If CWF receives a claim with HCPCS codes 90669, 90670, or 90732 and it already has on record a claim with the same HIC number, same FI/AB MAC number, same date of service, and the same HCPCS code, the second claim submitted to CWF rejects when all four items match.

If CWF receives a claim with HCPCS administration codes G0008 or G0009 and it already has on record a claim with the same HIC number, same FI/AB MAC number, same date of service, and same procedure code, CWF rejects the second claim submitted when all four items match.

CWF returns to the FI/AB MAC a reject code "7262" for this edit. FIs/AB MACs must deny the second claim and use the same messages they currently use for the denial of duplicate claims.

## 100-04,18,10.4.2

### CWF Edits on Carrier/AB MAC Claims

In order to prevent duplicate payment by the same carrier/AB MAC, CWF will edit by line item on the carrier/AB MAC number, the HIC number, the date of service, the influenza virus procedure codes 90653, 90654, 90655, 90656, 90657, 90660, 90661, 90662, 90672, 90673, 90685, 90686, 90687, or 90688; the pneumococcal procedure codes 90669, 90670, or 90732; and the administration code G0008 or G0009.

If CWF receives a claim with either HCPCS codes 90653, 90654, 90655, 90656, 90657, 90660, 90661, 90662, 90672, 90673, 90685, 90686, 90687, or 90688 and it already has on record a claim with the same HIC number, same carrier/AB MAC number, same date of service, and any one of those HCPCS codes, the second claim submitted to CWF will reject.

If CWF receives a claim with HCPCS codes 90669, 90670, or 90732 and it already has on record a claim with the same HIC number, same carrier/AB MAC number, same date of service, and the same HCPCS code, the second claim submitted to CWF will reject when all four items match.

If CWF receives a claim with HCPCS administration codes G0008 or G0009 and it already has on record a claim with the same HIC number, same carrier/AB MAC number, same date of service, and same procedure code, CWF will reject the second claim submitted.

CWF will return to the carrier/AB MAC a specific reject code for this edit. Carriers/AB MACs must deny the second claim and use the same messages they currently use for the denial of duplicate claims.

In order to prevent duplicate payment by the centralized billing contractor and local carrier/AB MAC, CWF will edit by line item for carrier number, same HIC number, same date of service, the influenza virus procedure codes 90653, 90654, 90655, 90656, 90657, 90660, 90661, 90662, 90672, 90673, 90685, 90686, 90687, or 90688; the pneumococcal procedure codes 90669, 90670, or 90732; and the administration code G0008 or G0009.

If CWF receives a claim with either HCPCS codes 90653, 90654, 90655, 90656, 90657, 90660, 90661, 90662, 90672, 90673, 90685, 90686, 90687, or 90688 and it already has on record a claim with a different carrier/AB MAC number, but same HIC number, same date of service, and any one of those same HCPCS codes, the second claim submitted to CWF will reject.

If CWF receives a claim with HCPCS codes 90669, 90670, or 90732 and it already has on record a claim with the same HIC number, different carrier/AB MAC number, same date of service, and the same HCPCS code, the second claim submitted to CWF will reject.

If CWF receives a claim with HCPCS administration codes G0008 or G0009 and it already has on record a claim with a different carrier/AB MAC number, but the same HIC number, same date of service, and same procedure code, CWF will reject the second claim submitted.

CWF will return a specific reject code for this edit. Carriers/AB MACs must deny the second claim. For the second edit, the reject code should automatically trigger the following Medicare Summary Notice (MSN) and Remittance Advice (RA) messages.

MSN: 7.2 – "This is a duplicate of a claim processed by another contractor. You should receive a Medicare Summary Notice from them."

Claim adjustment reason code 18 – duplicate claim or service

## 100-04,18,10.4.3

### CWF A/B Crossover Edits for FI/AB MAC and Carrier/AB MAC Claims

When CWF receives a claim from the carrier/AB MAC, it will review Part B outpatient claims history to verify that a duplicate claim has not already been posted.

CWF will edit on the beneficiary HIC number; the date of service; the influenza virus procedure codes 90653, 90654, 90655, 90656, 90657, 90660, 90661, 90662, 90672, 90673, 90685, 90686, 90687, or 90688; the pneumococcal procedure codes 90669, 90670, or 90732; and the administration code G0008 or G0009.

CWF will return a specific reject code for this edit. Contractors must deny the second claim and use the same messages they currently use for the denial of duplicate claims.

## 100-04, 18, 20

### Mammography Services (Screening and Diagnostic)

A. Screening Mammography Beginning January 1, 1991, Medicare provides Part B coverage of screening mammographies for women. Screening mammographies are radiologic procedures for early detection of breast cancer and include a physician's interpretation of the results. A doctor's prescription or referral is not necessary for the procedure to be covered.

Whether payment can be made is determined by a woman's age and statutory frequency parameter. See Pub. 100-02, Medicare Benefit Policy Manual, chapter 15, section 280.3 for additional coverage information for a screening mammography.

Section 4101 of the Balanced Budget Act (BBA) of 1997 provides for annual screening mammographies for women over age 39 and waives the Part B deductible. Coverage applies as follows: Age Groups Screening Period Under age 35 No payment allowed for screening mammography.~35-39 Baseline (pay for only one screening mammography performed on a woman between her 35th and 40th birthday) Over age 39 Annual (11 full months have elapsed following the month of last screening NOTE:Count months between screening mammographies beginning the month after the date of the examination. For example, if Mrs. Smith received a screening mammography examination in January 2005, begin counting the next month (February 2005) until 11 months have elapsed. Payment can be made for another screening mammography in January 2006.~B. Diagnostic Mammography A diagnostic mammography is a radiological mammogram and is a covered diagnostic test under the following conditions: A patient has distinct signs and symptoms for which a mammogram is indicated; A patient has a history of breast cancer; or A patient is asymptomatic, but based on the patient's history and other factors the physician considers significant, the physician's judgment is that a mammogram is appropriate.~Beginning January 1, 2005, Medicare Prescription Drug, Improvement, and Modernization Act (MMA) of 2003, Sec. 644, Public Law 108-173 has changed the way Medicare pays for diagnostic mammography. Medicare will pay based on the MPFS in lieu of OPPS or the lower of the actual change.

## 100-04, 18, 20.2

### HCPCS and Diagnosis Codes for Mammography Services

(Rev. 3329, Issued: 08-14-15, Effective: 01-01-12, Implementation: 09-14-15)

The following HCPCS codes are used to bill for mammography services.

| HCPCS Code | Definition |
|---|---|
| 77051* (76082*) | Computer aided detection (computer algorithm analysis of digital image data for lesion detection) with further physician review for interpretation, with or without digitization of film radiographic images, diagnostic mammography (list separately in addition to code for primary procedure). Code 76082 is effective January 1, 2004 thru December 31, 2006. Code 77051 is effective January 1, 2007. |

| HCPCS Code | Definition |
|---|---|
| 77052* (76083*) | Computer aided detection (computer algorithm analysis of digital image data for lesion detection) with further physician review for interpretation, with or without digitization of film radiographic images, screening mammography (list separately in addition to code for primary procedure). Code 76083 is effective January 1, 2004 thru December 31, 2006. Code 77052 is effective January 1, 2007. |
| 77055* (76090*) | Diagnostic mammography, unilateral. |
| 77056* (76091*) | Diagnostic mammography, bilateral. |
| 77057* (76092*) | Screening mammography, bilateral (two view film study of each breast). |
| 77063** | Screening Breast Tomosynthesis; bilateral (list separately in addition to code for primary procedure). |
| G0202 | Screening mammography, producing direct 2-D digital image, bilateral, all views. Code is effective April 1, 2001. This code descriptor effective January 1, 2015. |
| G0204 | Diagnostic mammography, direct 2-D digital image, bilateral, all views. Code is effective April 1, 2001. This code descriptor is effective January 1, 2015. |
| G0206 | Diagnostic mammography, producing direct 2-D digital image, unilateral, all views. Code is effective April 1, 2001. This code descriptor is effective January 1, 2015. |
| G0279** | Diagnostic digital breast tomosynthesis, unilateral or bilateral (List separately in addition to G0204 or G0206) |

** NOTE: HCPCS codes 77063 and G0279 are effective for claims with dates of service on or after January 1, 2015.

* For claims with dates of service prior to January 1, 2007, providers report CPT codes 76082, 76083, 76090, 76091, and 76092. For claims with dates of service January 1, 2007 and later, providers report CPT codes 77051, 77052, 77055, 77056, and 77057 respectively.

**New Modifier "-GG": Performance and payment of a screening mammography and diagnostic mammography on same patient same day** - This is billed with the Diagnostic Mammography code to show the test changed from a screening test to a diagnostic test. Contractors will pay both the screening and diagnostic mammography tests. This modifier is for tracking purposes only. This applies to claims with dates of service on or after January 1, 2002.

**A. Diagnosis for Services On or After January 1, 1998**
The BBA of 1997 eliminated payment based on high-risk indicators. However, to ensure proper coding, one of the following diagnosis codes should be reported on screening mammography claims as appropriate:

ICD-9-CM

V76.11 - "Special screening for malignant neoplasm, screening mammogram for high-risk patients" or;

V76.12 - "Special screening for malignant neoplasm, other screening mammography."

ICD-10-CM

Z12.31 - Encounter for screening mammogram for malignant neoplasm of breast.

Beginning October 1, 2003, A/B MACs (B) are not permitted to plug the code for a screening mammography when the screening mammography claim has no diagnosis code. Screening mammography claims with no diagnosis code must be returned as unprocessable for assigned claims. For unassigned claims, deny the claim.

In general, providers report diagnosis codes in accordance with the instructions in the appropriate ASC X12 837 claim technical report 3 (institutional or professional) and the paper claim form instructions found in chapters 25 (institutional) and 26 (professional).

In addition, for institutional claims, providers report diagnosis code V76.11 or V76.12 (ICD-9-CM) or Z12.31 (if ICD-10-CM is applicable) in "Principal Diagnosis Code" if the screening mammography is the only service reported on the claim. If the claim contains other services in addition to the screening mammography, these diagnostic codes V76.11 or V76.12 (ICD-9-CM) or Z12.31 (ICD-10-CM) are reported, as appropriate, in "Other Diagnostic Codes." NOTE: Information regarding the form locator number that corresponds to the principal and other diagnosis codes is found in chapter 25.

A/B MACs (B) receive this diagnosis in field 21 and field 24E with the appropriate pointer code of Form CMS-1500 or in Loop 2300 of ASC- X12 837 professional claim format.

Diagnosis codes for a diagnostic mammography will vary according to diagnosis.

**B. Diagnoses for Services October 1, 1997 Through December 31, 1997**
On every screening mammography claim where the patient is not a high-risk individual, diagnosis code V76.12 is reported on the claim.

If the screening is for a high risk individual, the provider reports the principal diagnosis code as V76.11 - "Screening mammogram for high risk patient."

In addition, for high-risk individuals, one of the following applicable diagnoses codes is reported as "Other Diagnoses codes":

- V10.3 "Personal history - Malignant neoplasm female breast";
- V16.3 "Family history - Malignant neoplasm breast"; or
- V15.89 "Other specified personal history representing hazards to health."

The following chart indicates the ICD-9-CM diagnosis codes reported for each high-risk category:

| High Risk Category | Appropriate Diagnosis Code |
|---|---|
| A personal history of breast cancer | V10.3 |
| A mother, sister, or daughter who has breast cancer | V16.3 |
| Not given birth prior to age 30 | V15.89 |
| A personal history of biopsy-proven benign breast disease | V15.89 |

## 100-04, 18, 20.2.2

**Screening Digital Breast Tomosynthesis**
(Rev. 3232, Issued: 04-03-15, Effective: 01-01-15, Implementation: 01-05-15)

Effective with claims with dates of service January 1, 2015 and later, HCPCS code 77063, "Screening Digital Breast Tomosynthesis, bilateral, must be billed in conjunction with the primary service mammogram code G0202.

Contractors must assure that claims containing code 77063 also contain HCPCS code G0202. A/B MACs (A) return claims containing code 77063 that do not also contain HCPCS code G0202 with an explanation that payment for code 77063 cannot be made when billed alone. A/B MACs (B) deny payment for 77063 when billed without G0202.

NOTE: When screening digital breast tomosynthesis, code 77063, is billed in conjunction with a screening mammography, code G0202, and the screening mammography G0202 fails the age and frequency edits in CWF, both services will be rejected by CWF.

## 100-04, 18, 20.4

**Billing Requirements - FI/A/B MAC Claims**
Contractors use the weekly-updated MQSA file to verify that the billing facility is certified by the FDA to perform mammography services, and has the appropriate certification to perform the type of mammogram billed (film and/or digital). (See Sec.20.1.) FIs/A/B MACs use the provider number submitted on the claim to identify the facility and use the MQSA data file to verify the facility's certification(s). FIs/A/B MACs complete the following activities in processing mammography claims:

If the provider number on the claim does not correspond with a certified mammography facility on the MQSA file, then intermediaries/A/B MACs deny the claim.

When a film mammography HCPCS code is on a claim, the claim is checked for a "1" film indicator.

If a film mammography HCPCS code comes in on a claim and the facility is certified for film mammography, the claim is paid if all other relevant Medicare criteria are met.

If a film mammography HCPCS code is on a claim and the facility is certified for digital mammography only, the claim is denied.

When a digital mammography HCPCS code is on a claim, the claim is checked for "2" digital indicator.

If a digital mammography HCPCS code is on a claim and the facility is certified for digital mammography, the claim is paid if all other relevant Medicare criteria are met.

If a digital mammography HCPCS code is on a claim and the facility is certified for film mammography only, the claim is denied.

NOTE: The Common Working File (CWF) no longer receives the mammography file for editing purposes.

Except as provided in the following sections for RHCs and FQHCs, the following procedures apply to billing for screening mammographies: The technical component portion of the screening mammography is billed on Form CMS-1450 under bill type 12X, 13X, 14X**, 22X, 23X or 85X using revenue code 0403 and HCPCS code 77057* (76092*).

The technical component portion of the diagnostic mammography is billed on Form CMS-1450 under bill type 12X, 13X, 14X**, 22X, 23X or 85X using revenue code 0401 and HCPCS code 77055* (76090*), 77056* (76091*), G0204 and G0206.

Separate bills are required for claims for screening mammographies with dates of service prior to January 1, 2002. Providers include on the bill only charges for the screening mammography. Separate bills are not required for claims for screening mammographies with dates of service on or after January 1, 2002.

See separate instructions below for rural health clinics (RHCs) and federally qualified health centers (FQHCs).

* For claims with dates of service prior to January 1, 2007, providers report CPT codes 76090, 76091, and 76092. For claims with dates of service January 1, 2007 and later, providers report CPT codes 77055, 77056, and 77057 respectively.

** For claims with dates of service April 1, 2005 and later, hospitals bill for all mammography services under the 13X type of bill or for dates of service April 1, 2007 and later, 12X or 13X as appropriate. The 14X type of bill is no longer applicable. Appropriate bill types for providers other than hospitals are 22X, 23X, and 85X.

In cases where screening mammography services are self-referred and as a result an attending physician NPI is not available, the provider shall duplicate their facility NPI in the attending physician identifier field on the claim.

## 100-04, 18, 20.5

### Billing Requirements - A/B MAC (B) Claims
(Rev. 3329, Issued: 08-14-15, Effective: 01-01-12, Implementation: 09-14-15)

Contractors use the weekly-updated file to verify that the billing facility is certified by the FDA to perform mammography services, and has the appropriate certification to perform the type of mammogram billed (film and/or digital). A/B MACs (B) match the FDA

assigned, 6-digit mammography certification number on the claim to the FDA mammography certification number appearing on the file for the billing facility. A/B MACs (B) complete the following activities in processing mammography claims:

- If the claim does not contain the facility's 6-digit certification number, then A/B MACs (B) return the claim as unprocessable.
- If the claim contains a 6-digit certification number that is reported in the proper field or segment (as specified in the previous bullet) but such number does not correspond to the number specified in the MQSA file for the facility, then A/B MACs (B) deny the claim.
- When a film mammography HCPCS code is on a claim, the claim is checked for a "1" film indicator.
- If a film mammography HCPCS code comes in on a claim and the facility is certified for film mammography, the claim is paid if all other relevant Medicare criteria are met.
- If a film mammography HCPCS code is on a claim and the facility is certified for digital mammography only, the claim is denied.
- When a digital mammography HCPCS code is on a claim, the claim is checked for "2" digital indicator.
- If a digital mammography HCPCS code is on a claim and the facility is certified for digital mammography, the claim is paid if all other relevant Medicare criteria are met.
- Process the claim to the point of payment based on the information provided on the claim and in A/B MAC (B) claims history.
- Identify the claim as a screening mammography claim by the CPT-4 code and diagnosis code(s) listed on the claim.
- Assign physician specialty code 45 to facilities that are certified to perform only screening mammography.
- Ensure that entities that bill globally for screening mammography contain a blank in modifier position #1.
- Ensure that entities that bill for the technical component use only HCPCS modifier "-TC."
- Ensure that physicians who bill the professional component separately use HCPCS modifier "-26."
- Ensure all those who are qualified include the 6-digit FDA-assigned certification number of the screening center on the claim. Providers report this

number in item 32 on the paper 1500 claim form. A/B MACs (B) retain this number in their provider files.

- When a mammography claim contains services subject to the anti-markup payment limitation and the service was acquired from another billing jurisdiction, the provider must submit their own NPI with the name, address, and ZIP code of the performing physician/supplier.
- Refer to Pub. 100-04, chapter 1, section 10.1.1.1., for claims processing instructions for payment jurisdiction.
- Beginning October 1, 2003, A/B MACs (B) are no longer permitted to add the diagnosis code for a screening mammography when the screening mammography claim has no diagnosis code. Screening mammography claims with no diagnosis code must be returned as unprocessable for assigned claims. For unassigned claims, deny the claim.

### A/B MAC (B) Provider Education
- Educate providers that when a screening mammography turns to a diagnostic mammography on the same day for the same beneficiary, add the "-GG" modifier to the diagnostic code and bill both codes on the same claim. Both services are reimbursable by Medicare.
- Educate providers that they cannot bill an add-on code without also billing for the appropriate mammography code. If just the add-on code is billed, the service will be denied. Both the add-on code and the appropriate mammography code should be on the same claim.
- Educate providers to submit their own NPI in place of an attending/referring physician NPI in cases where screening mammography services are self-referred.

## 100-04, 18, 60.1

### Payment
Payment (contractor) is under the MPFS except as follows:

- Fecal occult blood tests (82270* (G0107*) and G0328) are paid under the clinical diagnostic lab fee schedule except reasonable cost is paid to all non-OPPS hospitals, including CAHs, but not IHS hospitals billing on TOB 83x. IHS hospitals billing on TOB 83x are paid the ASC payment amount. Other IHS hospitals (billing on TOB 13x) are paid the OMB approved AIR, or the facility specific per visit amount as applicable. Deductible and coinsurance do not apply for these tests. See section A below for payment to Maryland waiver on TOB 13X. Payment from all hospitals for non-patient laboratory specimens on TOB 14X will be based on the clinical diagnostic fee schedule, including CAHs and Maryland waiver hospitals

Flexible sigmoidoscopy (code G0104) is paid under OPPS for hospital outpatient departments and on a reasonable cost basis for CAHs; or current payment methodologies for hospitals not subject to OPPS.

Colonoscopies (G0105 and G0121) and barium enemas (G0106 and G0120) are paid under OPPS for hospital outpatient departments and on a reasonable costs basis for CAHs or current payment methodologies for hospitals not subject to OPPS. Also colonoscopies may be done in an Ambulatory Surgical Center (ASC) and when done in an ASC the ASC rate applies. The ASC rate is the same for diagnostic and screening colonoscopies. The ASC rate is paid to IHS hospitals when the service is billed on TOB 83x.

Prior to January 1, 2007, deductible and coinsurance apply to HCPCS codes G0104, G0105, G0106, G0120, and G0121. Beginning with services provided on or after January 1, 2007, Section 5113 of the Deficit Reduction Act of 2005 waives the requirement of the annual Part B deductible for these screening services. Coinsurance still applies. Coinsurance and deductible applies to the diagnostic colorectal service codes listed below.

The following screening codes must be paid at rates consistent with the diagnostic codes indicated.

| Screening Code | Diagnostic Code |
| --- | --- |
| G0104 | 45330 |
| G0105 and G0121 | 45378 |
| G0106 and G0120 | 74280 |

### A. Special Payment Instructions for TOB 13X Maryland Waiver Hospitals
For hospitals in Maryland under the jurisdiction of the Health Services Cost Review Commission, screening colorectal services HCPCS codes G0104, G0105, G0106, 82270* (G0107*), G0120, G0121 and G0328 are paid according to the terms of the waiver, that is 94% of submitted charges minus any unmet existing deductible, co-insurance and non-covered charges. Maryland Hospitals bill TOB 13X for outpatient colorectal cancer screenings.

## B. Special Payment Instructions for Non-Patient Laboratory Specimen (TOB 14X) for all hospitals

Payment for colorectal cancer screenings (82270* (G0107*) and G0328) to a hospital for a non-patient laboratory specimen (TOB 14X), is the lesser of the actual charge, the fee schedule amount, or the National Limitation Amount (NLA), (including CAHs and Maryland Waiver hospitals). Part B deductible and coinsurance do not apply.

*NOTE: For claims with dates of service prior to January 1, 2007, physicians, suppliers, and providers report HCPCS code G0107. Effective January 1, 2007, code G0107 is discontinued and replaced with CPT code 82270.

## 100-04, 18, 60.2

### HCPCS Codes, Frequency Requirements, and Age Requirements (If Applicable)

Effective for services furnished on or after January 1, 1998, the following codes are used for colorectal cancer screening services:

- 82270* (G0107*) - Colorectal cancer screening; fecal-occult blood tests, 1-3 simultaneous determinations;
- G0104 - Colorectal cancer screening; flexible sigmoidoscopy;
- G0105 - Colorectal cancer screening; colonoscopy on individual at high risk;
- G0106 - Colorectal cancer screening; barium enema; as an alternative to G0104, screening sigmoidoscopy;
- G0120 - Colorectal cancer screening; barium enema; as an alternative to G0105, screening colonoscopy.

Effective for services furnished on or after July 1, 2001, the following codes are used for colorectal cancer screening services:

- G0121 - Colorectal cancer screening; colonoscopy on individual not meeting criteria for high risk. Note that the description for this code has been revised to remove the term "noncovered."
- G0122 - Colorectal cancer screening; barium enema (noncovered).

Effective for services furnished on or after January 1, 2004, the following code is used for colorectal cancer screening services as an alternative to 82270* (G0107*):

- G0328 - Colorectal cancer screening; immunoassay, fecal-occult blood test, 1-3 simultaneous determinations

*NOTE: For claims with dates of service prior to January 1, 2007, physicians, suppliers, and providers report HCPCS code G0107. Effective January 1, 2007, code G0107 is discontinued and replaced with CPT code 82270.

- G0104 - Colorectal Cancer Screening; Flexible Sigmoidoscopy

Screening flexible sigmoidoscopies (code G0104) may be paid for beneficiaries who have attained age 50, when performed by a doctor of medicine or osteopathy at the frequencies noted below.

For claims with dates of service on or after January 1, 2002, contractors pay for screening flexible sigmoidoscopies (code G0104) for beneficiaries who have attained age 50 when these services were performed by a doctor of medicine or osteopathy, or by a physician assistant, nurse practitioner, or clinical nurse specialist (as defined in Sec.1861(aa)(5) of the Act and in the Code of Federal Regulations at42 CFR 410.74, 410.75, and410.76) at the frequencies noted above. For claims with dates of service prior to January 1, 2002, contractors pay for these services under the conditions noted only when a doctor of medicine or osteopathy performs them.

For services furnished from January 1, 1998, through June 30, 2001, inclusive:

- Once every 48 months (i.e., at least 47 months have passed following the month in which the last covered screening flexible sigmoidoscopy was done).
- For services furnished on or after July 1, 2001:
- Once every 48 months as calculated above unless the beneficiary does not meet the criteria for high risk of developing colorectal cancer (refer to Sec.60.3 of this chapter) and he/she has had a screening colonoscopy (code G0121) within the preceding 10 years. If such a beneficiary has had a screening colonoscopy within the preceding 10 years, then he or she can have covered a screening flexible sigmoidoscopy only after at least 119 months have passed following the month that he/she received the screening colonoscopy (code G0121).

NOTE:If during the course of a screening flexible sigmoidoscopy a lesion or growth is detected which results in a biopsy or removal of the growth; the appropriate diagnostic procedure classified as a flexible sigmoidoscopy with biopsy or removal should be billed and paid rather than code G0104.

G0105 - Colorectal Cancer Screening; Colonoscopy on Individual at High Risk

Screening colonoscopies (code G0105) may be paid when performed by a doctor of medicine or osteopathy at a frequency of once every 24 months for beneficiaries at high risk for developing colorectal cancer (i.e., at least 23 months have passed

following the month in which the last covered G0105 screening colonoscopy was performed). Refer to Sec.60.3of this chapter for the criteria to use in determining whether or not an individual is at high risk for developing colorectal cancer.

NOTE:If during the course of the screening colonoscopy, a lesion or growth is detected which results in a biopsy or removal of the growth, the appropriate diagnostic procedure classified as a colonoscopy with biopsy or removal should be billed and paid rather than code G0105.

### A. Colonoscopy Cannot be Completed Because of Extenuating Circumstances

1   FIs

When a covered colonoscopy is attempted but cannot be completed because of extenuating circumstances, Medicare will pay for the interrupted colonoscopy as long as the coverage conditions are met for the incomplete procedure. However, the frequency standards associated with screening colonoscopies will not be applied by CWF.  When a covered colonoscopy is next attempted and completed, Medicare will pay for that colonoscopy according to its payment methodology for this procedure as long as coverage conditions are met, and the frequency standards will be applied by CWF. This policy is applied to both screening and diagnostic colonoscopies.

When submitting a facility claim for the interrupted colonoscopy, providers are to suffix the colonoscopy HCPCS codes with a modifier of "-73" or" -74" as appropriate to indicate that the procedure was interrupted. Payment for covered incomplete screening colonoscopies shall be consistent with payment methodologies currently in place for complete screening colonoscopies, including those contained in42 CFR 419.44(b). In situations where a critical access hospital (CAH) has elected payment Method II for CAH patients, payment shall be consistent with payment methodologies currently in place as outlined in Chapter 3. As such, instruct CAHs that elect Method II payment to use modifier "-53" to identify an incomplete screening colonoscopy (physician professional service(s) billed in revenue code 096X, 097X, and/or 098X). Such CAHs will also bill the technical or facility component of the interrupted colonoscopy in revenue code 075X (or other appropriate revenue code) using the "-73" or "-74" modifier as appropriate.Note that Medicare would expect the provider to maintain adequate information in the patient's medical record in case it is needed by the contractor to document the incomplete procedure.

2.  Carriers

When a covered colonoscopy is attempted but cannot be completed because of extenuating circumstances (see Chapter 12), Medicare will pay for the interrupted colonoscopy at a rate consistent with that of a flexible sigmoidoscopy as long as coverage conditions are met for the incomplete procedure. When a covered colonoscopy is next attempted and completed, Medicare will pay for that colonoscopy according to its payment methodology for this procedure as long as coverage conditions are met. This policy is applied to both screening and diagnostic colonoscopies.

When submitting a claim for the interrupted colonoscopy, professional providers are to suffix the colonoscopy code with a modifier of "-53" to indicate that the procedure was interrupted.  When submitting a claim for the facility fee associated with this procedure, Ambulatory Surgical Centers (ASCs) are to suffix the colonoscopy code with "-73" or "-74" as appropriate. Payment for covered screening colonoscopies, including that for the associated ASC facility fee when applicable, shall be consistent with payment for diagnostic colonoscopies, whether the procedure is complete or incomplete.Note that Medicare would expect the provider to maintain adequate information in the patient's medical record in case it is needed by the contractor to document the incomplete procedure.

- G0106 - Colorectal Cancer Screening; Barium Enema; as an Alternative to G0104, Screening Sigmoidoscopy

Screening barium enema examinations may be paid as an alternative to a screening sigmoidoscopy (code G0104). The same frequency parameters for screening sigmoidoscopies (see those codes above) apply.  In the case of an individual aged 50 or over, payment may be made for a screening barium enema examination (code G0106) performed after at least 47 months have passed following the month in which the last screening barium enema or screening flexible sigmoidoscopy was performed. For example, the beneficiary received a screening barium enema examination as an alternative to a screening flexible sigmoidoscopy in January 1999. Start counts beginning February 1999. The beneficiary is eligible for another screening barium enema in January 2003. The screening barium enema must be ordered in writing after a determination that the test is the appropriate screening test. Generally, it is expected that this will be a screening double contrast enema unless the individual is unable to withstand such an exam. This means that in the case of a particular individual, the attending physician must determine that the estimated screening potential for the barium enema is equal to or greater than the screening potential that has been estimated for a screening flexible sigmoidoscopy for the same individual. The screening single contrast barium enema also requires a written order from the beneficiary's attending physician in the same manner as described above for the screening double contrast barium enema examination.

- 82270* (G0107*) - Colorectal Cancer Screening; Fecal-Occult Blood Test, 1-3 Simultaneous Determinations

Effective for services furnished on or after January 1, 1998, screening FOBT (code 82270* (G0107*) may be paid for beneficiaries who have attained age 50, and at a frequency of once every 12 months (i.e., at least 11 months have passed following the month in which the last covered screening FOBT was performed). This screening FOBT means a guaiac-based test for peroxidase activity, in which the beneficiary completes it by taking samples from two different sites of three consecutive stools. This screening requires a written order from the beneficiary's attending physician. (The term "attending physician" is defined to mean a doctor of medicine or osteopathy (as defined in Sec.1861(r)(1)of the Act) who is fully knowledgeable about the beneficiary's medical condition, and who would be responsible for using the results of any examination performed in the overall management of the beneficiary's specific medical problem.)

Effective for services furnished on or after January 1, 2004, payment may be made for a immunoassay-based FOBT (G0328, described below) as an alternative to the guaiacbased FOBT, 82270* (G0107*). Medicare will pay for only one covered FOBT per year, either 82270* (G0107*) or G0328, but not both.

*NOTE: For claims with dates of service prior to January 1, 2007, physicians, suppliers, and providers report HCPCS code G0107. Effective January 1, 2007, code G0107 is discontinued and replaced with CPT code 82270.

- G0328 - Colorectal Cancer Screening; Immunoassay, Fecal-Occult Blood Test, 1-3 Simultaneous Determinations

Effective for services furnished on or after January 1, 2004, screening FOBT, (code G0328) may be paid as an alternative to 82270* (G0107*) for beneficiaries who have attained age 50. Medicare will pay for a covered FOBT (either 82270* (G0107*) or G0328, but not both) at a frequency of once every 12 months (i.e., at least 11 months have passed following the month in which the last covered screening FOBT was performed). Screening FOBT, immunoassay, includes the use of a spatula to collect the appropriate number of samples or the use of a special brush for the collection of samples, as determined by the individual manufacturer's instructions. This screening requires a written order from the beneficiary's attending physician. (The term "attending physician" is defined to mean a doctor of medicine or osteopathy (as defined in Sec.1861(r)(1) of the Act) who is fully knowledgeable about the beneficiary's medical condition, and who would be responsible for using the results of any examination performed in the overall management of the beneficiary's specific medical problem.)

- G0120 - Colorectal Cancer Screening; Barium Enema; as an Alternative to or G0105, Screening Colonoscopy

Screening barium enema examinations may be paid as an alternative to a screening colonoscopy (code G0105) examination. The same frequency parameters for screening colonoscopies (see those codes above) apply.  In the case of an individual who is at high risk for colorectal cancer, payment may be made for a screening barium enema examination (code G0120) performed after at least 23 months have passed following the month in which the last screening barium enema or the last screening colonoscopy was performed. For example, a beneficiary at high risk for developing colorectal cancer received a screening barium enema examination (code G0120) as an alternative to a screening colonoscopy (code G0105) in January 2000. Start counts beginning February 2000. The beneficiary is eligible for another screening barium enema examination (code G0120) in January 2002. The screening barium enema must be ordered in writing after a determination that the test is the appropriate screening test. Generally, it is expected that this will be a screening double contrast enema unless the individual is unable to withstand such an exam. This means that in the case of a particular individual, the attending physician must determine that the estimated screening potential for the barium enema is equal to or greater than the screening potential that has been estimated for a screening colonoscopy, for the same individual. The screening single contrast barium enema also requires a written order from the beneficiary's attending physician in the same manner as described above for the screening double contrast barium enema examination.

- G0121 - Colorectal Screening; Colonoscopy on Individual Not Meeting Criteria for High Risk - Applicable On and After July 1, 2001

Effective for services furnished on or after July 1, 2001, screening colonoscopies (code G0121) performed on individuals not meeting the criteria for being at high risk for developing colorectal cancer (refer to Sec.60.3 of this chapter) may be paid under the following conditions:

- At a frequency of once every 10 years (i.e., at least 119 months have passed following the month in which the last covered G0121 screening colonoscopy was performed.)

If the individual would otherwise qualify to have covered a G0121 screening colonoscopy based on the above but has had a covered screening flexible sigmoidoscopy (code G0104), then he or she may have covered a G0121 screening colonoscopy only after at least 47 months have passed following the month in which the last covered G0104 flexible sigmoidoscopy was performed.

NOTE:If during the course of the screening colonoscopy, a lesion or growth is detected which results in a biopsy or removal of the growth, the appropriate diagnostic procedure classified as a colonoscopy with biopsy or removal should be billed and paid rather than code G0121.

- G0122 - Colorectal Cancer Screening; Barium Enema

The code is not covered by Medicare.

## 100-04, 18, 60.1.1

### Deductible and Coinsurance

There is no deductible and no coinsurance or copayment for the FOBTs (HCPCS G0107, G0328), flexible sigmoidoscopies (G0104), colonoscopies on individuals at high risk (HCPCS G0105), or colonoscopies on individuals not meeting criteria of high risk (HCPCS G0121). When a screening colonoscopy becomes a diagnostic colonoscopy anesthesia code 00810 should be submitted with only the -PT modifier and only the deductible will be waived.

Prior to January 1, 2007 deductible and coinsurance apply to other colorectal procedures (HCPCS G0106 and G0120). After January 1, 2007, the deductible is waived for those tests. Coinsurance applies.

Effective January 1, 2015, coinsurance and deductible are waived for anesthesia services CPT 00810, Anesthesia for lower intestinal endoscopic procedures, endoscope introduced distal to duodenum, when performed for screening colonoscopy services and when billed with Modifier 33.

Effective for claims with dates of service on and after October 9, 2014, deductible and coinsurance do not apply to the Cologuard™ multitarget sDNA screening test (HCPCS G0464).

**NOTE:** A 25% coinsurance applies for all colorectal cancer screening colonoscopies (HCPCS G0105 and G0121) performed in ASCs and non-OPPS hospitals effective for services performed on or after January 1, 2007. The 25% coinsurance was implemented in the OPPS PRICER for OPPS hospitals effective for services performed on or after January 1, 1999.

A 25% coinsurance also applies for colorectal cancer screening sigmoidoscopies (HCPCS G0104) performed in non-OPPS hospitals effective for services performed on or after January 1, 2007. Beginning January 1, 2008, colorectal cancer screening sigmoidoscopies (HCPCS G0104) are payable in ASCs, and a 25% coinsurance applies. The 25% coinsurance for colorectal cancer screening sigmoidoscopies was implemented in the OPPS PRICER for OPPS hospitals effective for services performed on or after January 1, 1999.

## 100-04, 18, 60.2.1

### Common Working Files (CWF) Edits

Effective for dates of service January 1, 1998, and later, CWF will edit all colorectal screening claims for age and frequency standards. The CWF will also edit A/B MAC (A) claims for valid procedure codes (HCPCS G0104, G0105, G0106, CPT 82270* (HCPCS G0107*), G0120, G0121, G0122, G0328, and G0464). The CWF currently edits for valid HCPCS codes for A/B/MACs (B). (See §60.6 of this chapter for TOBs.)

**\*NOTE:** For claims with dates of service prior to January 1, 2007, physicians, suppliers, and providers report HCPCS G0107. Effective January 1, 2007, HCPCS G0107 is discontinued and replaced with CPT 82270.

## 100-04, 18, 60.6

### Billing Requirements for Claims Submitted to FIs

(Follow the general bill review instructions in Chapter 25. Hospitals use the ANSI X12N 837I to bill the FI or on the hardcopy Form CMS-1450. Hospitals bill revenue codes and HCPCS codes as follows:

| Screening Test/Procedure | Revenue Code | HCPCS Code | TOB |
|---|---|---|---|
| Fecal Occult blood test | 030X | 82270*** (G0107***), G0328 | 12X, 13X, 14X**, 22X, 23X, 83X, 85X |

| Screening Test/Procedure | Revenue Code | HCPCS Code | TOB |
|---|---|---|---|
| Barium enema | 032X | G0106, G0120, G0122 | 12X, 13X, 22X, 23X, 85X**** |
| Flexible Sigmoidoscopy | * | G0104 | 12X, 13X, 22X, 23X, 83X, 85X**** |
| Colonoscopy-high risk | * | G0105, G0121 | 12X, 13X, 22X, 23X, 83X, 85X**** |

\* The appropriate revenue code when reporting any other surgical procedure.

\** 14X is only applicable for non-patient laboratory specimens.

\*** For claims with dates of service prior to January 1, 2007, physicians, suppliers, and providers report HCPCS code G0107. Effective January 1, 2007, code G0107, is discontinued and replaced with CPT code 82270.

\**** CAHs that elect Method II bill revenue code 096X, 097X, and/or 098X for professional services and 075X (or other appropriate revenue code) for the technical or facility component.

### Special Billing Instructions for Hospital Inpatients

When these tests/procedures are provided to inpatients of a hospital or when Part A benefits have been exhausted, they are covered under this benefit. However, the provider bills on bill type 12X using the discharge date of the hospital stay to avoid editing in the Common Working File (CWF) as a result of the hospital bundling rules.

## 100-04, 18, 70.1.1

### HCPCS and Diagnosis Coding

(Rev. 3329, Issued: 08-14-15, Effective: 01-01-12, Implementation: 09-14-15)

The following HCPCS codes should be reported when billing for screening glaucoma services:

G0117 - Glaucoma screening for high-risk patients furnished by an optometrist (physician for A/B MAC (B)) or ophthalmologist.

G0118 - Glaucoma screening for high-risk patients furnished under the direct supervision of an optometrist (physician for A/B MAC (B) or ophthalmologist.

The A/B MAC (B) claims type of service for the above G codes is: TOS Q.

Glaucoma screening claims should be billed using screening ("V") code V80.1 (Special Screening for Neurological, Eye, and Ear Diseases, Glaucoma), or if ICD-10-CM is applicable, diagnosis code Z13.5 (encounter for screening for eye and ear disorders). Claims submitted without a screening diagnosis code may be returned to the provider as unprocessable (refer to chapter 1 of this manual for more information about incomplete or invalid claims).

## 100-04, 18, 80

### Initial Preventive Physical Examination (IPPE)

(NOTE: For billing and payment requirements for the Annual Wellness Visit, see chapter 18, section 140, of this manual.)

Background: Effective for services furnished on or after January 1, 2005, Section 611 of the Medicare Prescription Drug Improvement and Modernization Act of 2003 (MMA) provides for coverage under Part B of one initial preventive physical examination (IPPE) for new beneficiaries only, subject to certain eligibility and other limitations. CMS amended §§411.15 (a)(1) and 411.15 (k)(11) of the Code of Federal Regulations (CFR) to permit payment for an IPPE as described at 42 CFR §410.16, added by 69 FR 66236, 66420 (November 15, 2004) not later than 6 months after the date the individual's first coverage period begins under Medicare Part B.

Under the MMA of 2003, the IPPE may be performed by a doctor of medicine or osteopathy as defined in section 1861 (r)(1) of the Social Security Act (the Act) or by a qualified mid-level nonphysician practitioner (NPP) (nurse practitioner, physician assistant or clinical nurse specialist), not later than 6 months after the date the individual's first coverage begins under Medicare Part B. (See section 80.3 for a list of bill types of facilities that can bill fiscal intermediaries (FIs) for this service.) This examination will include: (1) review of the individual's medical and social history with attention to modifiable risk factors for disease detection, (2) review of the individual's potential (risk factors) for depression or other mood disorders, (3) review of the individual's functional ability and level of safety; (4) a physical examination to include measurement of the individual's height, weight, blood pressure, a visual acuity screen, and other factors as deemed appropriate by the examining physician or qualified nonphysician practitioner (NPP), (5) performance and interpretation of an electrocardiogram (EKG); (6) education, counseling, and referral, as deemed appropriate, based on the results of the review and evaluation services described in the previous 5 elements, and (7) education, counseling, and referral including a brief written plan (e.g., a checklist or alternative) provided to the individual for obtaining the appropriate screening and other preventive services, which are separately covered under Medicare Part B benefits. The EKG performed as a component of the

IPPE will be billed separately. Medicare will pay for only one IPPE per beneficiary per lifetime. The Common Working File (CWF) will edit for this benefit.

As required by statute under the MMA of 2003, the total IPPE service includes an EKG, but the EKG is billed with its own unique HCPCS code(s). The IPPE does not include other preventive services that are currently separately covered and paid under Section 1861 of the Act under Medicare Part B screening benefits. (That is, pneumococcal, influenza and hepatitis B vaccines and their administration, screening mammography, screening pap smear and screening pelvic examinations, prostate cancer screening tests, colorectal cancer screening tests, diabetes outpatient self-management training services, bone mass measurements, glaucoma screening, medical nutrition therapy for individuals with diabetes or renal disease, cardiovascular screening blood tests, and diabetes screening tests.)

Section 5112 of the Deficit Reduction Act of 2005 allows for one ultrasound screening for Abdominal Aortic Aneurysm (AAA) as a result of a referral from an IPPE effective January 1, 2007. For AAA physician/practitioner billing, correct coding, and payment policy information, refer to section 110 of this chapter.

Effective January 1, 2009, Section 101(b) of the Medicare Improvement for Patients and Providers Act (MIPPA) of 2008 updates the IPPE benefit described under the MMA of 2003. The MIPPA allows the IPPE to be performed not later than 12 months after the date the individual's first coverage period begins under Medicare Part B, requires the addition of the measurement of an individual's body mass index to the IPPE, adds end-of-life planning (upon an individual's consent) to the IPPE, and removes the screening EKG as a mandatory service of the IPPE. The screening EKG is optional effective January 1, 2009, and is permitted as a once-in-a-lifetime screening service as a result of a referral from an IPPE.

The MIPPA of 2008 allows for possible future payment for additional preventive services not otherwise described in Title XVIII of the Act that identify medical conditions or risk factors for eligible individuals if the Secretary determines through the national coverage determination (NCD) process (as defined in section 1869(f)(1)(B) of the Act) that they are: (1) reasonable and necessary for the prevention or early detection of illness or disability, (2) recommended with a grade of A or B by the United States Preventive Services Task Force, and, (3) appropriate for individuals entitled to benefits under Part A or enrolled under Part B, or both. MIPPA requires that there be education, counseling, and referral for additional preventive services, as appropriate, under the IPPE, if the Secretary determines in the future that such services are covered.

For the physician/practitioner billing correct coding and payment policy, refer to chapter 12, section 30.6.1.1, of this manual.

## 100-04, 18, 80.1

### The HCPCS codes listed below were developed for the IPPE benefit effective January 1, 2005, for individuals whose initial enrollment is on or after January 1, 2005.

G0344: Initial preventive physical examination; face-to-face visit, services limited to new beneficiary during the first 6 months of Medicare enrollment

Short Descriptor: Initial Preventive Exam

G0366: Electrocardiogram, routine ECG with 12 leads; performed as a component of the initial preventive examination with interpretation and report

Short Descriptor: EKG for initial prevent exam

G0367: tracing only, without interpretation and report, performed as a component of the initial preventive examination

Short Descriptor: EKG tracing for initial prev

G0368: interpretation and report only, performed as a component of the initial preventive examination

Short Descriptor: EKG interpret & report preve

The following new HCPCS codes were developed for the IPPE benefit effective January 1, 2009, and replaced codes G0344, G0366, G0367, and G0368 shown above beginning with dates of service on or after January 1, 2009:

G0402: Initial preventive physical examination; face-to-face visit, services limited to new beneficiary during the first 12 months of Medicare enrollment

Short Descriptor: Initial Preventive exam

G0403: Electrocardiogram, routine ECG with 12 leads; performed as a screening for the initial preventive physical examination with interpretation and report

Short Descriptor: EKG for initial prevent exam

G0404: Electrocardiogram, routine ECG with 12 leads; tracing only, without interpretation and report, performed as a screening for the initial preventive physical examination

Short Descriptor: EKG tracing for initial prev

G0405: Electrocardiogram, routine ECG with 12 leads; interpretation and report only, performed as a screening for the initial preventive physical examination

Short Descriptor: EKG interpret & report preve

## 100-04, 18, 80.2

### A/B Medicare Administrative Contractor (MAC) and Contractor Billing Requirements

Effective for dates of service on and after January 1, 2005, through December 31, 2008, contractors shall recognize the HCPCS codes G0344, G0366, G0367, and G0368 shown above in §80.1 for an IPPE. The type of service (TOS) for each of these codes is as follows:

G0344: TOS = 1

G0366: TOS = 5

G0367: TOS = 5

G0368: TOS = 5

Contractors shall pay physicians or qualified nonphysician practitioners for only one IPPE performed not later than 6 months after the date the individual's first coverage begins under Medicare Part B, but only if that coverage period begins on or after January 1, 2005.

Effective for dates of service on and after January 1, 2009, contractors shall recognize the HCPCS codes G0402, G0403, G0404, and G0405 shown above in §80.1 for an IPPE. The TOS for each of these codes is as follows:

G0402: TOS = 1

G0403: TOS = 5

G0404: TOS = 5

G0405: TOS = 5

Under the MIPPA of 2008, contractors shall pay physicians or qualified nonphysician practitioners for only one IPPE performed not later than 12 months after the date the individual's first coverage begins under Medicare Part B only if that coverage period begins on or after January 1, 2009.

Contractors shall allow payment for a medically necessary Evaluation and Management (E/M) service at the same visit as the IPPE when it is clinically appropriate. Physicians and qualified nonphysician practitioners shall use CPT codes 99201-99215 to report an E/M with CPT modifier 25 to indicate that the E/M is a significant, separately identifiable service from the IPPE code reported (G0344 or G0402, whichever applies based on the date the IPPE is performed). Refer to chapter 12, § 30.6.1.1, of this manual for the physician/practitioner billing correct coding and payment policy regarding E/M services.

If the EKG performed as a component of the IPPE is not performed by the primary physician or qualified NPP during the IPPE visit, another physician or entity may perform and/or interpret the EKG. The referring physician or qualified NPP needs to make sure that the performing physician or entity bills the appropriate G code for the screening EKG, and not a CPT code in the 93000 series. Both the IPPE and the EKG should be billed in order for the beneficiary to receive the complete IPPE service. Effective for dates of service on and after January 1, 2009, the screening EKG is optional and is no longer a mandated service of an IPPE if performed as a result of a referral from an IPPE.

Should the same physician or NPP need to perform an additional medically necessary EKG in the 93000 series on the same day as the IPPE, report the appropriate EKG CPT code(s) with modifier 59, indicating that the EKG is a distinct procedural service.

Physicians or qualified nonphysician practitioners shall bill the contractor the appropriate HCPCS codes for IPPE on the Form CMS-1500 claim or an approved electronic format. The HCPCS codes for an IPPE and screening EKG are paid under the Medicare Physician Fee Schedule (MPFS). The appropriate deductible and coinsurance applies to codes G0344, G0366, G0367, G0368, G0403, G0404, and G0405. The deductible is waived for code G0402 but the coinsurance still applies.

## 100-04, 18, 80.3.3

### Outpatient Prospective Payment System (OPPS) Hospital Billing

Hospitals subject to OPPS (TOBs 12X and 13X) must use modifier -25 when billing the IPPE G0344 along with the technical component of the EKG, G0367, on the same claim. The same is true when billing IPPE code G0402 along with the technical component of the screening EKG, code G0404. This is due to an OPPS Outpatient Code Editor (OCE) which contains an edit that requires a modifier -25 on any evaluation and management (E/M) HCPCS code if there is also a status "S" or "T" HCPCS procedure code on the claim.

## 100-04, 18, 80.4

### Coinsurance and Deductible

The Medicare deductible and coinsurance apply for the IPPE provided before January 1, 2009.

The Medicare deductible is waived effective for the IPPE provided on or after January 1, 2009. Coinsurance continues to apply for the IPPE provided on or after January 1, 2009.

As a result of the Affordable Care Act, effective for the IPPE provided on or after January 1, 2011, the Medicare deductible and coinsurance (for HCPCS code G0402 only) are waived.

## 100-04, 18, 120.1

### Coding and Payment of DSMT Services

The following HCPCS codes are used to report DSMT: G0108 - Diabetes outpatient self-management training services, individual, per 30 minutes.

G0109 - Diabetes outpatient self-management training services, group session (2 or more), per 30 minutes.

The type of service for these codes is 1.

| Type of Facility | Payment Method | Type of Bill |
|---|---|---|
| Physician (billed to the carrier) | MPFS | NA |
| Hospitals subject to OPPS | MPFS | 12X, 13X |
| Method I and Method II Critical Access Hospitals (CAHs) (technical services) | 101% of reasonable cost | 12X and 85X |
| Indian Health Service (IHS) providers billing hospital outpatient Part B | OMB-approved outpatient per visit all inclusive rate (AIR) | 13X |
| IHS providers billing inpatient Part B | All-inclusive inpatient ancillary per diem rate | 12X |
| IHS CAHs billing outpatient Part B | 101% of the all-inclusive facility specific per visit rate | 85X |
| IHS CAHs billing inpatient Part B | 101% of the all-inclusive facility specific per diem rate | 12X |
| FQHCs* | All-inclusive encounter rate with other qualified services. Separate visit payment available with HCPCS. | 73X |
| Skilled Nursing Facilities ** | MPFS non-facility rate | 22X, 23X |
| Maryland Hospitals under jurisdiction of the Health Services Cost Review Commission (HSCRC) | 94% of provider submitted charges in accordance with the terms of the Maryland Waiver | 12X, 13X |
| Home Health Agencies (can be billed only if the service is provided outside of the treatment plan) | MPFS non-facility rate | 34X |

* Effective January 1, 2006, payment for DSMT provided in an FQHC that meets all of the requirements as above, may be made in addition to one other visit the beneficiary had during the same day, if this qualifying visit is billed on TOB 73X, with HCPCS G0108 or G0109, and revenue codes 0520, 0521, 0522, 0524, 0525, 0527, 0528, or 0900.

** The SNF consolidated billing provision allows separate part B payment for training services for beneficiaries that are in skilled Part A SNF stays, however, the SNF must submit these services on a 22 bill type. Training services provided by other provider types must be reimbursed by X the SNF.

NOTE: An ESRD facility is a reasonable site for this service, however, because it is required to provide dietician and nutritional services as part of the care covered in the composite rate, ESRD facilities are not allowed to bill for it separately and do not receive separate reimbursement. Likewise, an RHC is a reasonable site for this service, however it must be provided in an RHC with other qualifying services and paid at the all-inclusive encounter rate.

Deductible and co-insurance apply.

## 100-04, 18, 130

### Healthcare Common Procedure Coding System (HCPCS) for HIV Screening Tests

Healthcare Common Procedure Coding System (HCPCS) for HIV Screening Tests

Effective for claims with dates of service on and after December 8, 2009, implemented with the April 5, 2010, IOCE, the following HCPCS codes are to be billed for HIV screening:

G0432    Infectious agent antibody detection by enzyme immunoassay (EIA) technique, HIV-1 and/or HIV-2, screening,

G0433    Infectious agent antibody detection by enzyme-linked immunosorbent assay (ELISA) technique, HIV-1 and/or HIV-2, screening, and,

G0435    Infectious agent antibody detection by rapid antibody test, HIV-1 and/or HIV-2, screening

## 100-04, 18, 130.1

### Billing Requirements

Effective for dates of service December 8, 2009, and later, contractors shall recognize the above HCPCS codes for HIV screening.

Medicare contractors shall pay for voluntary HIV screening as follows in accordance with Pub. 100-03, Medicare National Coverage Determinations Manual, sections 190.14 and 210.7:

A maximum of once annually for beneficiaries at increased risk for HIV infection (11 full months must elapse following the month the previous test was performed in order for the subsequent test to be covered), and,

A maximum of three times per term of pregnancy for pregnant Medicare beneficiaries beginning with the date of the first test when ordered by the woman's clinician. Claims that are submitted for HIV screening shall be submitted in the following manner:

For beneficiaries reporting increased risk factors, claims shall contain HCPCS code G0432, G0433, or G0435 with diagnosis code V73.89 (Special screening for other specified viral disease) as primary, and V69.8 (Other problems related to lifestyle), as secondary.

For beneficiaries not reporting increased risk factors, claims shall contain HCPCS code G0432, G0433, or G0435 with diagnosis code V73.89 only.

For pregnant Medicare beneficiaries, claims shall contain HCPCS code G0432, G0433, or G0435 with diagnosis code V73.89 as primary, and one of the following ICD-9 diagnosis codes: V22.0 (Supervision of normal first pregnancy), V22.1 (Supervision of other normal pregnancy), or V23.9 (Supervision of unspecified high-risk pregnancy), as secondary.

## 100-04, 18, 130.4

### Diagnosis Code Reporting

A claim that is submitted for HIV screening shall be submitted with one or more of the following diagnosis codes in the header and pointed to the line item:

a. For claims where increased risk factors are reported: V73.89 as primary and V69.8 as secondary.

b. For claims where increased risk factors are NOT reported: V73.89 as primary only.

c. For claims for pregnant Medicare beneficiaries, the following diagnosis codes shall be submitted in addition to V73.89 to allow for more frequent screening than once per 12-month period:

V22.0 – Supervision of normal first pregnancy, or,

V22.1 – Supervision of other normal pregnancy, or,

V23.9 - Supervision of unspecified high-risk pregnancy).

## 100-04, 18, 140

### Annual Wellness Visit (AWV)

Pursuant to section 4103 of the Affordable Care Act of 2010, the Centers for Medicare & Medicaid Services (CMS) amended section 411.15(a)(1) and 411.15(k)(15) of 42 CFR (list of examples of routine physical examinations excluded from coverage) effective for services furnished on or after January 1, 2011. This expanded coverage is subject to certain eligibility and other limitations that allow payment for an annual wellness visit (AWV), including personalized prevention plan services (PPPS), for an individual who is no longer within 12 months after the effective date of his or her first Medicare Part B coverage period, and has not received either an initial preventive physical examination (IPPE) or an AWV within the past 12 months.

The AWV will include the establishment of, or update to, the individual's medical/family history, measurement of his/her height, weight, body-mass index (BMI) or waist circumference, and blood pressure (BP), with the goal of health

promotion and disease detection and encouraging patients to obtain the screening and preventive services that may already be covered and paid for under Medicare Part B. CMS amended 42 CFR §§411.15(a)(1) and 411.15(k)(15) to allow payment on or after January 1, 2011, for an AWV (as established at 42 CFR 410.15) when performed by qualified health professionals.

Coverage is available for an AWV that meets the following requirements:

1. It is performed by a health professional;

2. It is furnished to an eligible beneficiary who is no longer within 12 months after the effective date of his/her first Medicare Part B coverage period, and he/she has not received either an IPPE or an AWV providing PPPS within the past 12 months.

See Pub. 100-02, Medicare Benefit Policy Manual, chapter 15, section 280.5, for detailed policy regarding the AWV, including definitions of: (1) detection of cognitive impairment, (2) eligible beneficiary, (3) establishment of, or an update to, an individual's medical/family history, (4&5) first and subsequent AWVs providing PPPS, (6) health professional, and, (7) review of an individual's functional ability/level of safety.

## 100-04, 18, 140.1

### Healthcare Common Procedure Coding System (HCPCS) Coding for the AWV

HCPCS codes listed below were developed for the AWV benefit effective January 1, 2011, for individuals whose initial enrollment is on or after January 1, 2011.

G0438 - Annual wellness visit; includes a personalized prevention plan of service (PPPS); first visit

G0439 – Annual wellness visit; includes a personalized prevention plan of service (PPPS); subsequent visit

## 100-04, 18, 140.5

### Coinsurance and Deductible

Sections 4103 and 4104 of the Affordable Care Act provide for a waiver of Medicare coinsurance/copayment and Part B deductible requirements for the AWV effective for services furnished on or after January 1, 2011.

## 100-04, 18, 140.6

### Common Working File (CWF) Edits

Effective for claims with dates of service on and after January 1, 2011, CWF shall reject:

- AWV claims for G0438 when a previous (first) AWV, HCPCS code G0438, is paid in history regardless of when it occurred.

- AWV claims when a previous AWV, G0438 or G0439, is paid in history within the previous 12 months.

- Beginning January 1, 2011, AWV claims when a previous IPPE, HCPCS code G0402, is paid in history within the previous 12 months.

- AWV claims (G0438 and G0439) billed for a date of service within 12 months after the effective date of a beneficiary's first Medicare Part B coverage period.

The following change shall be effective for claims processed on or after April 1, 2013. Typically, when a preventive service is posted to a beneficiary's utilization history, separate entries are posted for a "professional" service (the professional claim for the delivery of the service itself) and a "technical" service (the institutional claims for a facility fee). However, in the case of AWV services, since there is no separate payment for a facility fee, the AWV claim will be posted as the "professional" service only, regardless of whether it is paid on a professional claim or an institutional claim.

## 100-04, 18, 140.8

### Advance Care Planning (ACP) as an Optional Element of an Annual Wellness Visit (AWV)

For services furnished on or after January 1, 2016, Advance Care Planning (ACP) is treated as a preventive service when furnished with an AWV. The Medicare coinsurance and Part B deductible are waived for ACP when furnished as an optional element of an AWV.

The codes for the optional ACP services furnished as part of an AWV are 99497 (Advance care planning including the explanation and discussion of advance directives such as standard forms (with completion of such forms, when performed), by the physician or other qualified health professional; first 30 minutes, face-to-face with the patient, family member(s) and/or surrogate;) and an add-on code 99498 (each additional 30 minutes (List separately in addition to code for primary procedure)). When ACP services are provided as a part of an AWV, practitioners would report CPT code 99497 (and add-on CPT code 99498 when applicable) for the ACP services in addition to either of the AWV codes (G0438 or G0439).

The deductible and coinsurance for ACP will only be waived when billed with modifier 33 on the same day and on the same claim as an AWV (code G0438 or G0439), and must also be furnished by the same provider. Waiver of the deductible and coinsurance for ACP is limited to once per year. Payment for an AWV is limited to once per year. If the AWV billed with ACP is denied for exceeding the once per year limit, the deductible and coinsurance will be applied to the ACP.

Also see Pub. 100-02, Medicare Benefit Policy Manual, chapter 15, section 280.5.1 for more information.

## 100-04, 18, 160

### Intensive Behavioral Therapy (IBT) for Cardiovascular Disease (CVD)

For services furnished on or after November 8, 2011, the Centers for Medicare & Medicaid Services (CMS) covers intensive behavioral therapy (IBT) for cardiovascular disease (CVD). See National Coverage Determinations (NCD) Manual (Pub. 100-03) §210.11 for complete coverage guidelines.

## 100-04, 18, 160.1

### Coding Requirements for IBT for CVD Furnished on or After November 8, 2011

The following is the applicable Healthcare Procedural Coding System (HCPCS) code for IBT for CVD:

G0446: Annual, face-to-face intensive behavioral therapy for cardiovascular disease, individual, 15 minutes

Contractors shall not apply deductibles or coinsurance to claim lines containing HCPCS code G0446.

## 100-04, 18, 160.2.1

### Correct Place of Service (POS) Codes for IBT for CVD on Professional Claims

Contractors shall pay for IBT CVD, G0446 only when services are provided at the following POS:

- 11- Physician's Office
- 22-Outpatient Hospital
- 49- Independent Clinic
- 72-Rural Health Clinic

Claims not submitted with one of the POS codes above will be denied.

The following messages shall be used when Medicare contractors deny professional claims for incorrect POS:

Claim Adjustment Reason Code (CARC) 58: "Treatment was deemed by the payer to have been rendered in an inappropriate or invalid place of service." NOTE: Refer to the 835 Healthcare Policy Identification Segment (loop 2110 Service Payment Information REF), if present.

Remittance Advice Remark Code (RARC) N428: "Not covered when performed in this place of service."

Medicare Summary Notice (MSN) 21.25: "This service was denied because Medicare only covers this service in certain settings."

Spanish Version: El servicio fue denegado porque Medicare solamente lo cubre en ciertas situaciones."

Group Code PR (Patient Responsibility) assigning financial liability to the beneficiary, if a claim is received with a GA modifier indicating a signed ABN is on file.

Group Code CO (Contractual Obligation) assigning financial liability to the provider, if a claim is received with a GZ modifier indicating no signed ABN is on file.

## 100-04, 18, 160.2.2

### Provider Specialty Edits for IBT for CVD on Professional Claims

Contractors shall pay claims for HCPCS code G0446 only when services are submitted by the following provider specialty types found on the provider? enrollment record:

- 01= General Practice
- 08 = Family Practice
- 11= Internal Medicine
- 16 = Obstetrics/Gynecology
- 37= Pediatric Medicine
- 38 = Geriatric Medicine
- 42= Certified Nurse Midwife
- 50 = Nurse Practitioner
- 89 = Certified Clinical Nurse Specialist
- 97= Physician Assistant

Contractors shall deny claim lines for HCPCS code G0446 performed by any other provider specialty type other than those listed above.

The following messages shall be used when Medicare contractors deny IBT for CVD claims billed with invalid provider specialty types:

CARC 185: "The rendering provider is not eligible to perform the service billed."

NOTE: Refer to the 835 Healthcare Policy Identification Segment (loop 2110 Service Payment Information REF), if present.

RARC N95: "This provider type/provider specialty may not bill this service."

MSN 21.18: "This item or service is not covered when performed or ordered by this provider."

Spanish version: "Este servicio no esta cubierto cuando es ordenado o rendido por este proveedor."

Group Code PR (Patient Responsibility) assigning financial liability to the beneficiary, if a claim is received with a GA modifier indicating a signed ABN is on file.

Group Code CO (Contractual Obligation) assigning financial liability to the provider, if a claim is received with a GZ modifier indicating no signed ABN is on file.

## 100-04, 18, 160.3

### Correct Types of Bill (TOB) for IBT for CVD on Institutional Claims

Effective for claims with dates of service on and after November 8, 2011, the following types of bill (TOB) may be used for IBT for CVD: 13X, 71X, 77X, or 85X. All other TOB codes shall be denied.

The following messages shall be used when Medicare contractors deny claims for G0446 when submitted on a TOB other than those listed above:

CARC 170: Payment is denied when performed/billed by this type of provider. Note: Refer to the 835 Healthcare Policy Identification Segment (loop 2110 Service Payment Information REF), if present.

RARC N428: Not covered when performed in this place of service."

MSN 21.25: "This service was denied because Medicare only covers this service in certain settings."

Spanish Version: El servicio fue denegado porque Medicare solamente lo cubre en ciertas situaciones."

Group Code PR (Patient Responsibility) assigning financial liability to the beneficiary, if a claim is received with a GA modifier indicating a signed ABN is on file.

Group Code CO (Contractual Obligation) assigning financial liability to the provider, if a claim is received with a GZ modifier indicating no signed ABN is on file.

## 100-04, 18, 160.4

### Frequency Edits for IBT for CVD Claims

160.4-Frequency Edits for IBT for CVD Claims

(Rev. 2357, Issued: 11-23-11, Effective: 11-08-11, Implementation: 12-27-11 non-shared system edits, 04-02-12 shared system edits, 07-02-12 CWF/HICR/MCS MCDST)

Contractors shall allow claims for G0446 no more than once in a 12-month period.

NOTE: 11 full months must elapse following the month in which the last G0446 IBT for CVD took place.

Contractors shall deny claims IBT for CVD claims that exceed one (1) visit every 12 months.

Contractors shall allow one professional service and one facility fee claim for each visit.

The following messages shall be used when Medicare contractors deny IBT for CVD claims that exceed the frequency limit:

CARC 119: "Benefit maximum for this time period or occurrence has been reached."

RARC N362: "The number of days or units of service exceeds our acceptable maximum."

MSN 20.5: "These services cannot be paid because your benefits are exhausted at this time."

Spanish Version: "Estos servicios no pueden ser pagados porque sus beneficios se han agotado."

Group Code PR (Patient Responsibility) assigning financial liability to the beneficiary, if a claim is received with a GA modifier indicating a signed ABN is on file.

Group Code CO (Contractual Obligation) assigning financial liability to the provider, if a claim is received with a GZ modifier indicating no signed ABN is on file.

© 2016 Optum360, LLC

## 100-04, 18, 160.5

**When applying frequency, CWF shall count 11 full months following the month of the last IBT for CVD, G0446 before allowing subsequent payment of another G0446 screening.**

When applying frequency limitations to G0446, CWF shall allow both a claim for the professional service and a claim for the facility fee. CWF shall identify the following institutional claims as facility fee claims for screening services: TOB 13X, TOB85X when the revenue code is not 096X, 097X, or 098X. CWF shall identify all other claims as professional service claims for screening services.

NOTE: This does not apply to RHCs and FQHCs.

## 100-04, 18, 170.1

### Healthcare Common Procedure Coding System (HCPCS) Codes for Screening for STIs and HIBC to Prevent STIs

Effective for claims with dates of service on and after November 8, 2011, the claims processing instructions for payment of screening tests for STI will apply to the following HCPCS codes:

- Chlamydia: 86631, 86632, 87110, 87270, 87320, 87490, 87491, 87810, 87800 (used for combined chlamydia and gonorrhea testing)
- Gonorrhea: 87590, 87591, 87850, 87800 (used for combined chlamydia and gonorrhea testing)
- Syphilis: 86592, 86593, 86780
- Hepatitis B: (hepatitis B surface antigen): 87340, 87341

Effective for claims with dates of service on and after November 8, 2011, implemented with the January 2, 2012, IOCE, the following HCPCS code is to be billed for HIBC to prevent STIs:

G0445     high-intensity behavioral counseling to prevent sexually transmitted infections, face-to-face, individual, includes: education, skills training, and guidance on how to change sexual behavior, performed semi-annually, 30 minutes.

## 100-04, 18, 170.2

### Diagnosis Code Reporting

A claim that is submitted for screening chlamydia, gonorrhea, syphilis, and/or hepatitis B shall be submitted with one or more of the following diagnosis codes in the header and pointed to the line item:

a.  For claims for screening for chlamydia, gonorrhea, and syphilis in women at increased risk who are not pregnant use the following diagnosis codes:

- V74.5-Screening, bacterial ?sexually transmitted; and
- V69.8 -Other problems related to lifestyle as secondary (This diagnosis code is used to indicate high/increased risk for STIs).

b.  For claims for screening for syphilis in men at increased risk use the following diagnosis codes:

- V74.5-Screening, bacterial ?sexually transmitted; and
- V69.8 -Other problems related to lifestyle as secondary. c. For claims for screening for chlamydia and gonorrhea in pregnant women at increased risk for STIs use the following diagnosis codes:
  -  Screening, bacterial ?sexually transmitted; and
  - V69.8 - Other problems related to lifestyle, and,
  - V22.0 -Supervision of normal first pregnancy, or
  - V22.1 -Supervision of other normal pregnancy, or,
  - V23.9-Supervision of unspecified high-risk pregnancy. d. For claims for screening for syphilis in pregnant women use the following diagnosis codes:
  - V74.5-Screening, bacterial ?sexually transmitted; and
  - V22.0-Supervision of normal first pregnancy, or,
  - V22.1 -Supervision of other normal pregnancy, or,
  - V23.9-Supervision of ?V74.5unspecified high-risk pregnancy.

e.  For claims for screening for syphilis in pregnant women at increased risk for STIs use the following diagnosis codes:

- V74.5-Screening, bacterial ?sexually transmitted; and
- V69.8 -Other problems related to lifestyle, and,
- V22.0-Supervision of normal first pregnancy, or
- V22.1 -Supervision of other normal pregnancy, or,
- V23.9 -Supervision of unspecified high-risk pregnancy. f. For claims for screening for hepatitis B in pregnant women use the following diagnosis codes:

- V73.89-Screening, disease or disorder, viral, specified type NEC; and
- V22.0-Supervision of normal first pregnancy, or,
- V22.1-Supervision of other normal pregnancy, or,
- V23.9-Supervision of unspecified high-risk pregnancy.

g.  For claims for screening for hepatitis B in pregnant women at increased risk for STIs use the following diagnosis codes:

- V73.89-Screening, disease or disorder, viral, specified type NEC; and
- V 69.8 -Other problems related to lifestyle, and,
- V22.0-Supervision of normal first pregnancy, or,
- V22.1-Supervision of other normal pregnancy, or,
- V23.9-Supervision of unspecified high-risk pregnancy.

### ICD-10 Diagnosis Coding:

Contractors shall note the appropriate ICD-10 code(s) that are listed below for future implementation. Contractors shall track the ICD-10 codes and ensure that the updated edit is turned on as part of the ICD-10 implementation effective October 1, 2013.

| ICD-10 | Description |
|--------|-------------|
| Z113 | Encounter for screening for infections with a predominantly sexual mode of transmission |
| Z1159 | Encounter for screening for other viral diseases |
| Z7289 | Other problems related to lifestyle |
| Z3400 | Encounter for supervision of normal first pregnancy, unspecified trimester |
| Z3480 | Encounter for supervision of other normal pregnancy, unspecified trimester |
| O0990 | Supervision of high risk pregnancy, unspecified, unspecified trimester |

## 100-04, 18, 170.3

### Billing Requirements

Effective for dates of service November 8, 2011, and later, contractors shall recognize HCPCS code G0445 for HIBC. Medicare shall cover up to two occurrences of G0445 when billed for HIBC to prevent STIs. A claim that is submitted with HCPCS code G0445 for HIBC shall be submitted with ICD-9 diagnosis code V69.8.

Medicare contractors shall pay for screening for chlamydia, gonorrhea, and syphilis (As indicated by the presence of ICD-9 diagnosis code V74.5); and/or hepatitis B (as indicated by the presence of ICD-9 diagnosis code V73.89) as follows:

- One annual occurrence of screening for chlamydia, gonorrhea, and syphilis (i.e., 1 per 12-month period) in women at increased risk who are not pregnant,
- One annual occurrence of screening for syphilis (i.e., 1 per 12-month period) in men at increased risk,
- Up to two occurrences per pregnancy of screening for chlamydia and gonorrhea in pregnant women who are at increased risk for STIs and continued increased risk for the second screening,
- One occurrence per pregnancy of screening for syphilis in pregnant women,
- Up to an additional two occurrences per pregnancy of screening for syphilis in pregnant women if the beneficiary is at continued increased risk for STIs,
- One occurrence per pregnancy of screening for hepatitis B in pregnant women, and,
- One additional occurrence per pregnancy of screening for hepatitis B in pregnant women who are at continued increased risk for STIs.

## 100-04, 18, 170.4

### Types of Bill (TOBs) and Revenue Codes

The applicable types of bill (TOBs) for HIBC screening, HCPCS code G0445, are: 13X, 71X, 77X, and 85X.

On institutional claims, TOBs 71X and 77X, use revenue code 052X to ensure coinsurance and deductible are not applied.

Critical access hospitals (CAHs) electing the optional method of payment for outpatient services report this service under revenue codes 096X, 097X, or 098X.

## 100-04, 18, 170.4.1

### Payment Method

Payment for HIBC is based on the all-inclusive payment rate for rural health clinics (TOBs 71X) and federally qualified health centers (TOB 77X). Hospital outpatient departments (TOB 13X) are paid based on the outpatient prospective payment system and CAHs (TOB 85X) are paid based on reasonable cost. CAHs electing the optional method of payment for outpatient services are paid based on 115% of the lesser of the Medicare Physician Fee Schedule (MPFS) amount or submitted charge.

Effective for dates of service on and after November 8, 2011, deductible and coinsurance do not apply to claim lines with G0445.

HCPCS code G0445 may be paid on the same date of service as an annual wellness visit, evaluation and management (E&M) code, or during the global billing period for obstetrical care, but only one G0445 may be paid on any one date of service. If billed on the same date of service with an E&M code, the E&M code should have a distinct diagnosis code other than the diagnosis code used to indicate high/increased risk for STIs for the G0445 service. An E&M code should not be billed when the sole reason for the visit is HIBC to prevent STIs.

For Medicare Part B physician and non-practitioner claims, payment for HIBC to prevent STIs is based on the MPFS amount for G0445.

## 100-04, 18, 170.5

### Specialty Codes and Place of Service (POS)

Medicare provides coverage for screening for chlamydià, gonorrhea, syphilis, and/or hepatitis B and HIBC to prevent STIs only when ordered by a primary care practitioner (physician or non-physician) with any of the following specialty codes:

- 01-General Practice
- 08-Family Practice
- 11-Internal Medicine
- 16-Obstetrics/Gynecology
- 37-Pediatric Medicine
- 38-Geriatric Medicine
- 42-Certified Nurse Midwife
- 50-Nurse Practitioner
- 89-Certified Clinical Nurse Specialist
- 97-Physician Assistant

Medicare provides coverage for HIBC to prevent STIs only when provided by a primary care practitioner (physician or non-physician) with any of the specialty codes identified above.

Medicare provides coverage for HIBC to prevent STIs only when the POS billed is 11, 22, 49, or 71.

## 100-04, 18, 180

### Alcohol Screening and Behavioral Counseling Interventions in Primary Care to Reduce Alcohol Misuse

~The United States Preventive Services Task Force (USPSTF) defines alcohol misuse as risky, hazardous, or harmful drinking which places an individual at risk for future problems with alcohol consumption. In the general adult population, alcohol consumption becomes risky or hazardous when consuming:

- Greater than 7 drinks per week or greater than 3drinks per occasion for women and persons greater than 65 years old.
- Greater than 14 drinks per week or greater than 4 drinks per occasion for men 65 years old and younger.

## 100-04, 18, 180.1

### Policy

Claims with dates of service on and after October 14, 2011, the Centers for Medicare & Medicaid Services (CMS) will cover annual alcohol misuse screening (HCPCS code G0442) consisting of 1 screening session, and for those that screen positive, up to 4 brief, face-to-face behavioral counseling sessions (HCPCS code G0443) per 12-month period for Medicare beneficiaries, including pregnant women.

Medicare beneficiaries that may be identified as having a need for behavioral counseling sessions include those:

- Who misuse alcohol, but whose levels or patterns of alcohol consumption do not meet criteria for alcohol dependence (defined as at least three of the following: tolerance, withdrawal symptoms, impaired control, preoccupation with acquisition and/or use, persistent desire or unsuccessful efforts to quit, sustains social, occupational, or recreational disability, use continues despite adverse consequences); and,
- Who are competent and alert at the time that counseling is provided; and,
- Whose counseling is furnished by qualified primary care physicians or other primary care practitioners in a primary care setting.

Once a Medicare beneficiary has agreed to behavioral counseling sessions, the counseling sessions are to be completed based on the 5As approach adopted by the

United States Preventive Services Task Force (USPSTF.) The steps to the 5As approach are listed below.

1. Assess: Ask about/assess behavioral health risk(s) and factors affecting choice of behavior change goals/methods.
2. Advise: Give clear, specific, and personalized behavior change advice, including information about personal health harms and benefits.
3. Agree: Collaboratively select appropriate treatment goals and methods based on the patient? interest in and willingness to change the behavior.
4. Assist: Using behavior change techniques (self-help and/or counseling), aid the patient in achieving agreed-upon goals by acquiring the skills, confidence, and social/environmental supports for behavior change, supplemented with adjunctive medical treatments when appropriate.
5. Arrange: Schedule follow-up contacts (in person or by telephone) to provide ongoing assistance/support and to adjust the treatment plan as needed, including referral to more intensive or specialized treatment.

## 100-04, 18, 180.2

**For claims with dates of service on and after October 14, 2011, Medicare will allow coverage for annual alcohol misuse screening, 15 minutes, G0442, and brief, face-to-face behavioral counseling for alcohol misuse, 15 minutes, G0443 for:**

- Rural Health Clinics (RHCs) - type of bill (TOB) 71X only -based on the all-inclusive payment rate
- Federally Qualified Health Centers (FQHCs) - TOB 77X only-based on the all-inclusive payment rate
- Outpatient hospitals ?TOB 13X - based on Outpatient Prospective Payment System (OPPS)-Critical Access Hospitals (CAHs) - TOB 85X-based on reasonable cost
- CAH Method II-TOB 85X - based on 115% of the lesser of the Medicare Physician Fee Schedule (MPFS) amount or actual charge as applicable with revenue codes 096X, 097X, or 098X.

For RHCs and FQHCs the alcohol screening/counseling is not separately payable with another face-to-face encounter on the same day. This does not apply to the Initial Preventive Physical Examination (IPPE), unrelated services denoted with modifier 59, and 77X claims containing Diabetes Self Management Training (DSMT) and Medical Nutrition Therapy (MNT)services. DSMT and MNT apply to FQHCs only. However, the screening/counseling sessions alone when rendered as a face-to-face visit with a core practitioner do constitute an encounter and is paid based on the all-inclusive payment rate.

Note: For outpatient hospital settings, as in any other setting, services covered under this NCD must be provided by a primary care provider.

Claims submitted with alcohol misuse screening and behavioral counseling HCPCS codes G0442 and G0443 on a TOB other than 13X, 71X, 77X, and 85X will be denied.

Effective October 14, 2011, deductible and co-insurance should not be applied for line items on claims billed for alcohol misuse screening G0442 and behavioral counseling for alcohol misuse G0443.

## 100-04, 18, 180.3

### Professional Billing Requirements

For claims with dates of service on or after October 14, 2011, CMS will allow coverage for annual alcohol misuse screening, 15 minutes, G0442, and behavioral counseling for alcohol misuse, 15 minutes, G0443, only when services are submitted by the following provider specialties found on the provider's enrollment record:

- 01 - General Practice
- 08 - Family Practice
- 11 - Internal Medicine
- 16 - Obstetrics/Gynecology
- 37 - Pediatric Medicine
- 38 - Geriatric Medicine
- 42 - Certified Nurse-Midwife
- 50 - Nurse Practitioner
- 89 - Certified Clinical Nurse Specialist
- 97 - Physician Assistant

Any claims that are not submitted from one of the provider specialty types noted above will be denied.

For claims with dates of service on and after October 14, 2011, CMS will allow coverage for annual alcohol misuse screening, 15 minutes, G0442, and behavioral counseling for alcohol misuse, 15 minutes, G0443, only when submitted with one of the following place of service (POS) codes:

- 11 - Physician's Office
- 22 - Outpatient Hospital
- 49 - Independent Clinic
- 71 - State or local public health clinic or

Any claims that are not submitted with one of the POS codes noted above will be denied.

The alcohol screening/counseling services are payable with another encounter/visit on the same day. This does not apply to RHCs and FQHCs.

## 100-04, 18, 180.4

### Claim Adjustment Reason Codes, Remittance Advice Remark Codes, Group Codes, and Medicare Summary Not

Contractors shall use the appropriate claim adjustment reason codes (CARCs), remittance advice remark codes (RARCs), group codes, or Medicare summary notice (MSN) messages when denying payment for alcohol misuse screening and alcohol misuse behavioral counseling sessions:

- For RHC and FQHC claims that contain screening for alcohol misuse HCPCS code G0442 and alcohol misuse counseling HCPCS code G0443 with another encounter/visit with the same line item date of service, use group code CO and reason code:
  - Claim Adjustment Reason Code (CARC) 97-The benefit for this service is included in the payment/allowance for another service/procedure that has already been adjudicated. Note: Refer to the 835 Healthcare Policy Identification Segment (loop 2110 Service Payment Information REF) if present
- Denying claims containing HCPCS code G0442 and HCPCS code G0443 submitted on a TOB other than 13X, 71X, 77X, and 85X:
  - Claim Adjustment Reason Code (CARC) 5 - The procedure code/bill type is inconsistent with the place of service. Note: Refer to the 835 Healthcare Policy Identification Segment (loop 2110 Service Payment Information REF) if present
  - Remittance Advice Remark Code (RARC) M77 -Missing/incomplete/invalid place of service
  - Group Code PR (Patient Responsibility) assigning financial liability to the beneficiary, if a claim is received with a GA modifier indicating a signed ABN is on file.
  - Group Code CO (Contractual Obligation) assigning financial liability to the provider, if a claim is received with a GZ modifier indicating no signed ABN is on file. NOTE: For modifier GZ, use CARC 50 and MSN 8.81 per instructions in CR 7228/TR 2148.
- Denying claims that contains more than one alcohol misuse behavioral counseling session G0443 on the same date of service:
  - Medicare Summary Notice (MSN) 15.6-The information provided does not support the need for this many services or items within this period of time.
  - Claim Adjustment Reason Code (CARC) 151-Payment adjusted because the payer deems the information submitted does not support this many/frequency of services.
  - Remittance Advice Remark Code (RARC) M86-Service denied because payment already made for same/similar procedure within set time frame.
  - Group Code PR (Patient Responsibility) assigning financial liability to the beneficiary, if a claim is received with a GA modifier indicating a signed ABN is on file.
  - Group Code CO (Contractual Obligation) assigning financial liability to the provider, if a claim is received with a GZ modifier indicating no signed ABN is on file. NOTE: For modifier GZ, use CARC 50 and MSN 8.81 per instructions in CR 7228/TR 2148.
- Denying claims that are not submitted from the appropriate provider specialties:
  - Medicare Summary Notice (MSN) 21.18-This item or service is not covered when performed or ordered by this provider.
  - Claim Adjustment Reason Code (CARC) 185 - The rendering provider is not eligible to perform the service billed. NOTE: Refer to the 835 Healthcare Policy Identification Segment (loop 2110 Service Payment Information REF), if present.
  - Remittance Advice Remark Code (RARC) N95 - This provider type/provider specialty may not bill this service.
  - Group Code PR (Patient Responsibility) assigning financial liability to the beneficiary, if a claim is received with a GA modifier indicating a signed ABN is on file.

- Group Code CO (Contractual Obligation) assigning financial liability to the provider, if a claim is received with a GZ modifier indicating no signed ABN is on file. NOTE: For modifier GZ, use CARC 50 and MSN 8.81 per instructions in CR 7228/TR 2148.
- Denying claims without the appropriate POS code:
  - Medicare Summary Notice (MSN) 21.25-This service was denied because Medicare only covers this service in certain settings.
  - Claim Adjustment Reason Code (CARC) 58 -Treatment was deemed by the payer to have been rendered in an inappropriate or invalid place of service. Note: Refer to the 835 Healthcare Policy Identification Segment (loop 2110 Service Payment Information REF) if present.
  - Remittance Advice Remark Code (RARC) N428-Not covered when performed in this place of service.
  - Group Code PR (Patient Responsibility) assigning financial liability to the beneficiary, if a claim is received with a GA modifier indicating a signed ABN is on file.
  - Group Code CO (Contractual Obligation) assigning financial liability to the provider, if a claim is received with a GZ modifier indicating no signed ABN is on file. NOTE: For modifier GZ, use CARC 50 and MSN 8.81 per instructions in CR 7228/TR 2148.
- Denying claims for alcohol misuse screening HCPCS code G0442 more than once in a 12-month period, and denying alcohol misuse counseling sessions HCPCS code G0443 more than four times in the same 12-month period:
  - Medicare Summary Notice (MSN) 20.5-These services cannot be paid because your benefits are exhausted at this time.
  - Claim Adjustment Reason Code (CARC) 119-Benefit maximum for this time period or occurrence has been reached.
  - Remittance Advice Remark Code (RARC) N362-The number of Days or Units of service exceeds our acceptable maximum.
  - Group Code PR (Patient Responsibility) assigning financial liability to the beneficiary, if a claim is received with a GA modifier indicating a signed ABN is on file.
  - Group Code CO (Contractual Obligation) assigning financial liability to the provider, if a claim is received with a GZ modifier indicating no signed ABN is on file. NOTE: For modifier GZ, use CARC 50 and MSN 8.81 per instructions in CR 7228/TR 2148.

## 100-04, 18, 180.5

### CWF Requirements

When applying frequency, CWF shall count 11 full months following the month of the last alcohol misuse screening visit, G0442, before allowing subsequent payment of another G0442 screening. Additionally, CWF shall create an edit to allow alcohol misuse brief behavioral counseling, HCPCS G0443, no more than 4 times in a 12-month period. CWF shall also count four alcohol misuse counseling sessions HCPCS G0443 in the same 12-month period used for G0442 counting from the date the G0442 screening session was billed.

When applying frequency limitations to G0442 screening on the same date of service as G0443 counseling, CWF shall allow both a claim for the professional service and a claim for a facility fee. CWF shall identify the following institutional claims as facility fee claims for screening services: TOB 13X, TOB 85X when the revenue code is not 096X, 097X, or 098X. CWF shall identify all other claims as professional service claims for screening services (professional claims, and institutional claims with TOB 71X, 77X, and 85X when the revenue code is 096X, 097X, or 098X). NOTE: This does not apply to RHCs and FQHCs.

## 100-04, 18, 190.0

### Screening for Depression in Adults (Effective October 14, 2011)

#### A. Coverage Requirements

Effective October 14, 2011, the Centers for Medicare & Medicaid Services (CMS) will cover annual screening up to 15 minutes for Medicare beneficiaries in primary care settings that have staff-assisted depression care supports in place to assure accurate diagnosis, effective treatment, and follow-up. Various screening tools are available for screening for depression. CMS does not identify specific depression screening tools. Rather, the decision to use a specific tool is at the discretion of the clinician in the primary care setting. Screening for depression is non-covered when performed more than one time in a 12-month period. The Medicare coinsurance and Part B deductible are waived for this preventive service.

Additional information on this National Coverage Determination (NCD) for Screening for Depression in Adults can be found in Publication 100-03, NCD Manual, Section 210.9.

## 100-04, 18, 190.1

### A/B MAC and Carrier Billing Requirements

Effective October 14, 2011, contractors shall recognize new HCPCS G0444, annual depression screening, 15 minutes.

## 100-04, 18, 190.2

### Frequency

Medicare contractors shall pay for annual depression screening, G0444, no more than once in a 12-month period.

NOTE: 11 full months must elapse following the month in which the last annual depression screening took place.

## 100-04, 18, 190.3

### Place of Service (POS)

Contractors shall pay for annual depression screening claims, G0444, only when services are provided at the following places of service (POS):

- 11–Office
- 22–Outpatient Hospital
- 49–Independent Clinic
- 71–State or Local Public Health Clinic

## 100-04, 18, 200

### Intensive Behavioral Therapy for Obesity (Effective November 29, 2011)

The United States Preventive Services Task Force (USPSTF) found good evidence that body mass index (BMI) is a reliable and valid indicator for identifying adults at increased risk for mortality and morbidity due to overweight and obesity. It also good evidence that high intensity counseling combined with behavioral interventions in obese adults (as defined by a BMI =30 kg/m2) produces modest, sustained weight loss.

## 100-04, 18, 200.1

### Policy

For services furnished on or after November 29, 2011, the Centers for Medicare & Medicaid Services (CMS) will cover Intensive Behavioral Therapy for Obesity. Medicare beneficiaries with obesity (BMI =30 kg/m2) who are competent and alert at the time that counseling is provided and whose counseling is furnished by a qualified primary care physician or other primary care practitioner in a primary care setting are eligible for:

- One face-to-face visit every week for the first month;
- One face-to-face visit every other week for months 2-6;
- One face-to-face visit every month for months 7-12, if the beneficiary meets the 3kg (6.6 lbs) weight loss requirement during the first six months as discussed below. The counseling sessions are to be completed based on the 5As approach adopted by the United States Preventive Services Task Force (USPSTF.) The steps to the 5As approach are listed below:

1. Assess: Ask about/assess behavioral health risk(s) and factors affecting choice of behavior change goals/methods.

2. Advise: Give clear, specific, and personalized behavior change advice, including information about personal health harms and benefits.

3. Agree: Collaboratively select appropriate treatment goals and methods based on the patient's interest in and willingness to change the behavior.

4. Assist: Using behavior change techniques (self-help and/or counseling), aid the patient in achieving agreed-upon goals by acquiring the skills, confidence, and social/environmental supports for behavior change, supplemented with adjunctive medical treatments when appropriate.

5. Arrange: Schedule follow-up contacts (in person or by telephone) to provide ongoing assistance/support and to adjust the treatment plan as needed, including referral to more intensive or specialized treatment.

Medicare will cover Face-to-Face Behavioral Counseling for Obesity, 15 minutes, G0447, along with 1 of the ICD-9 codes for BMI 30.0-BMI 70 (V85.30-V85.39 and V85.41-V85.45), up to 22 sessions in a 12-month period for Medicare beneficiaries. The Medicare coinsurance and Part B deductible are waived for this preventive service.

Contractors shall note the appropriate ICD-10 code(s) that are listed below for future implementation. Contractors shall track the ICD-10 codes and ensure that the

updated edit is turned on as part of the ICD-10 implementation effective October 1, 2013.

| ICD-10 | Description |
|--------|-------------|
| Z68.30 | BMI 30.0-30.9, adult |
| Z68.31 | BMI 31.0-31.9, adult |
| Z68.32 | BMI 32.0-32.9, adult |
| Z68.33 | BMI 33.0-33.9, adult |
| Z68.34 | BMI 34.0-34.9, adult |
| Z68.35 | BMI 35.0-35.9, adult |
| Z68.36 | BMI 36.0-36.9, adult |
| Z68.37 | BMI 37.0-37.9, adult |
| Z68.38 | BMI 38.0-38.9, adult |
| Z68.39 | BMI 39.0-39.9, adult |
| Z68.41 | BMI 40.0-44.9, adult |
| Z68.42 | BMI 45.0-49.9, adult |
| Z68.43 | BMI 50.0-59.9, adult |
| Z68.44 | BMI 60.0-69.9, adult |
| Z68.45 | BMI 70 or greater, adult |

See National Coverage Determinations (NCD) Manual (Pub. 100-03) §210.12 for complete coverage guidelines.

## 100-04, 18, 200.2

### Institutional Billing Requirements

Effective for claims with dates of service on and after November 29, 2011, providers may use the following types of bill (TOB) when submitting HCPCS code G0447: 13x, 71X, 77X, or 85X. Service line items on other TOBs shall be denied.

The service shall be paid on the basis shown below:

- Rural Health Clinics (RHCs) - type of bill (TOB) 71X only —based on the all-inclusive payment rate
- Federally Qualified Health Centers (FQHCs) - TOB 77X only —based on the all-inclusive payment rate
- Outpatient hospitals —TOB 13X - based on Outpatient Prospective Payment System (OPPS)
- Critical Access Hospitals (CAHs) - TOB 85X —based on reasonable cost
- CAH Method II —TOB 85X - based on 115% of the lesser of the Medicare Physician Fee Schedule (MPFS) amount or actual charge as applicable with revenue codes 096X, 097X, or 098X.

For RHCs and FQHCs, obesity counseling is not separately payable with another face-to-face encounter on the same day. This does not apply to claims for the Initial Preventive Physical Examination (IPPE), claims with unrelated services denoted with modifier 59, and FQHC claims containing Diabetes Self Management Training (DSMT) and Medical Nutrition Therapy (MNT) services. However, the counseling sessions alone when rendered as a face-to-face visit with a core practitioner do constitute an encounter and are paid based on the all-inclusive payment rate.

Note: For outpatient hospital settings, as in any other setting, services covered under this NCD must be provided by a primary care provider.

## 100-04, 18, 200.3

### Professional Billing Requirements

For claims with dates of service on or after November 29, 2011, CMS will allow coverage for Face-to-Face Behavioral Counseling for Obesity, 15 minutes, G0447, along with 1 of the ICD-9 codes for BMI 30.0-BMI 70 (V85.30-V85.39 and V85.41-V85.45), only when services are submitted by the following provider specialties found on the provider? enrollment record:

- 01 - General Practice
- 08 - Family Practice
- 11 - Internal Medicine
- 16 - Obstetrics/Gynecology
- 37 - Pediatric Medicine
- 38 - Geriatric Medicine
- 50 - Nurse Practitioner
- 89 - Certified Clinical Nurse Specialist
- 97 - Physician Assistant

© 2016 Optum360, LLC

Any claims that are not submitted from one of the provider specialty types noted above will be denied.

For claims with dates of service on or after November 29, 2011, CMS will allow coverage for Face-to-Face Behavioral Counseling for Obesity, 15 minutes, G0447, along with 1 of the ICD-9 codes for BMI 30.0-BMI 70 (V85.30-V85.39 and V85.41-V85.45), only when submitted with one of the following place of service (POS) codes:

- 11- Physician's Office
- 22- Outpatient Hospital
- 49- Independent Clinic
- 71- State or Local Public Health Clinic

Any claims that are not submitted with one of the POS codes noted above will be denied.

## 100-04, 18, 200.4

### Claim Adjustment Reason Codes (CARCs), Remittance Advice Remark Codes (RARCs), Group Codes, and Medicare Summary Notice (MSN) Messages

Contractors shall use the appropriate claim adjustment reason codes (CARCs), remittance advice remark codes (RARCs), group codes, or Medicare summary notice (MSN) messages when denying payment for obesity counseling sessions:

- Denying services submitted on a TOB other than 13X, 71X, 77X, and 85X: CARC 5 - The procedure code/bill type is inconsistent with the place of service.

  – Note: Refer to the 835 Healthcare Policy Identification Segment (loop 2110 Service Payment Information REF), if present.

  – RARC M77 - Missing/incomplete/invalid place of service

  – MSN 21.25: "This service was denied because Medicare only covers this service in certain settings."

  – Group Code PR (Patient Responsibility) assigning financial responsibility to the beneficiary (if a claim is received with a GA modifier indicating a signed ABN is on file).

  – Group Code CO (Contractual Obligation) assigning financial liability to the provider (if a claim is received with a GZ modifier indicating no signed ABN is on file).

  – NOTE: For modifier GZ, use CARC 50 and MSN 8.81 per instructions in CR 7228/TR 2148.

- For RHC and FQHC services that contain HCPCS code G0447 with another encounter/visit with the same line item date of service: Claim Adjustment Reason Code (CARC) 97

  – The benefit for this service is included in the payment/allowance for another service/procedure that has already been adjudicated. Note: Refer to the 835 Healthcare Policy Identification Segment (loop 2110 Service Payment Information REF) if present

  – Group Code CO (Contractual Obligation)

- Denying services for obesity counseling sessions HCPCS code G0447 with 1 of the ICD-9 codes (V85.30-V85.39 or V85.41-V85.45) for more than 22 times in the same 12-month period:

  – CARC 119-Benefit maximum for this time period or occurrence has been reached.

  – RARC N362 - The number of days or units of service exceeds our acceptable maximum.

  – MSN 20.5 - These services cannot be paid because your benefits are exhausted at this time.

  – Group Code PR (Patient Responsibility) assigning financial responsibility to the beneficiary (if a claim is received with a GA modifier indicating a signed ABN is on file).

  – Group Code CO (Contractual Obligation) assigning financial liability to the provider (if a claim is received with a GZ modifier indicating no signed ABN is on file).

  – NOTE: For modifier GZ, use CARC 50 and MSN 8.81 per instructions in CR 7228/TR 2148. -

- Denying claim lines for obesity counseling sessions HCPCS code G0447 without 1 of the appropriate ICD-9 codes (V85.30-V85.39 or V85.41-V85.45):

  – CARC 167 - This (these) diagnosis(es) is (are) not covered.

  – Note: Refer to the 835 Healthcare Policy Identification Segment (loop 2110 Service Payment Information REF), if present.

  – RARC N386 -This decision was based on a National Coverage Determination (NCD). An NCD provides a coverage determination as to whether a particular item or service is covered. A copy of this policy is available at www.cms.gov/mcd/search.asp. If you do not have web access, you may contact the contractor to request a copy of the NCD.

  – MSN 14.9 - Medicare cannot pay for this service for the diagnosis shown on the claim.

  – Group Code PR (Patient Responsibility) assigning financial responsibility to the beneficiary (if a claim is received with a GA modifier indicating a signed ABN is on file).

  – Group Code CO (Contractual Obligation) assigning financial liability to the provider (if a claim is received with a GZ modifier indicating no signed ABN is on file).

  – NOTE: For modifier GZ, use CARC 50 and MSN 8.81 per instructions in CR 7228/TR 2148.

- Denying claim lines without the appropriate POS code: CARC 58 —Treatment was deemed by the payer to have been rendered in an inappropriate or invalid place of service. Note: Refer to the 835 Healthcare Policy Identification Segment (loop 2110 Service Payment Information REF), if present.

  – RARC N428 - Not covered when performed in certain settings.

  – MSN 21.25 - This service was denied because Medicare only covers this service in certain settings.

  – Group Code PR (Patient Responsibility) assigning financial responsibility to the beneficiary (if a claim is received with a GA modifier indicating a signed ABN is on file).

  – Group Code CO (Contractual Obligation) assigning financial liability to the provider (if a claim is received with a GZ modifier indicating no signed ABN is on file).

  – NOTE: For modifier GZ, use CARC 50 and MSN 8.81 per instructions in CR 7228/TR 2148.

- Denying claim lines that are not submitted from the appropriate provider specialties: CARC 185 - The rendering provider is not eligible to perform the service billed. NOTE: Refer to the 835 Healthcare Policy Identification Segment (loop 2110 Service Payment Information REF), if present.

  – RARC N95 - This provider type/provider specialty may not bill this service.

  – MSN 21.18 - This item or service is not covered when performed or ordered by this provider.

  – Group Code PR (Patient Responsibility) assigning financial responsibility to the beneficiary (if a claim is received with a GA modifier indicating a signed ABN is on file).

  – Group Code CO (Contractual Obligation) assigning financial liability to the provider (if a claim is received with a GZ modifier indicating no signed ABN is on file).

  – NOTE: For modifier GZ, use CARC 50 and MSN 8.81 per instructions in CR 7228/TR 2148.

## 100-04, 18, 200.5

### Common Working File (CWF) Edits

When applying frequency, CWF shall count 22 counseling sessions of G0447, along with 1 ICD-9 code from V85.30-V85.39 or V85.41-V85.45 in a 12-month period. When applying frequency limitations to G0447 counseling CWF shall allow both a claim for the professional service and a claim for a facility fee. CWF shall identify the following institutional claims as facility fee claims for this service: TOB 13X, TOB 85X when the revenue code is not 096X, 097X, or 098X. CWF shall identify all other claims as professional service claims. NOTE: This does not apply to RHCs and FQHCs.

## 100-04, 18, 210

### 210 – Screening for Hepatitis C Virus (HCV)

(Rev. 3063, Issued: 09-05-14, Effective: 06-02-14, Implementation: 01-05-15 - For non-shared MAC edits and CWF analysis; 04-06-15 - For remaining shared systems edits)

Effective for services furnished on or after June 2, 2014, an initial screening for hepatitis C virus (HCV) is covered for adults at high risk for HCV infection. "High risk" is defined as persons with a current or past history of illicit injection drug use and persons who have a history of receiving a blood transfusion prior to 1992.

### A. Frequency

A single, one-time screening test is covered for adults who do not meet the high risk definition above, but who were born from 1945 through 1965.

Repeat screening for high risk persons is covered annually only for persons who have had continued illicit injection drug use since the prior negative screening test.

NOTE: Annual means a full 11 months must elapse following the month in which the previous negative screening took place.

### B. Determination of High Risk for Hepatitis C Disease

The determination of "high risk for HCV" is identified by the primary care physician or practitioner who assesses the patient's history, which is part of any complete medical history, typically part of an annual wellness visit, and considered in the development of a comprehensive prevention plan. The medical record should be a reflection of the service provided.

NOTE: See Pub. 100-03, Medicare National Coverage Determinations (NCD) Manual §210.13 for complete coverage guidelines.

NOTE: Beneficiary coinsurance and deductibles do not apply to claim lines containing HCPCS G0472, hepatitis C antibody screening for individual at high risk and other covered indication(s).~Effective for services furnished on or after June 2, 2014, an initial screening for hepatitis C virus (HCV) is covered for adults at high risk for HCV infection. "High risk" is defined as persons with a current or past history of illicit injection drug use and persons who have a history of receiving a blood transfusion prior to 1992.

**A. Frequency**

A single, one-time screening test is covered for adults who do not meet the high risk definition above, but who were born from 1945 through 1965.

Repeat screening for high risk persons is covered annually only for persons who have had continued illicit injection drug use since the prior negative screening test.

NOTE: Annual means a full 11 months must elapse following the month in which the previous negative screening took place.

**B. Determination of High Risk for Hepatitis C Disease**

The determination of "high risk for HCV" is identified by the primary care physician or practitioner who assesses the patient's history, which is part of any complete medical history, typically part of an annual wellness visit, and considered in the development of a comprehensive prevention plan. The medical record should be a reflection of the service provided.

NOTE: See Pub. 100-03, Medicare National Coverage Determinations (NCD) Manual §210.13 for complete coverage guidelines.

NOTE: Beneficiary coinsurance and deductibles do not apply to claim lines containing HCPCS G0472, hepatitis C antibody screening for individual at high risk and other covered indication(s).

Screening for Hepatitis C Virus (HCV)

## 100-04, 18, 210.2

**Professional Billing Requirements**

For claims with dates of service on or after June 2, 2014, Medicare will allow coverage for HCV screening, HCPCS G0472, only when services are ordered by the following provider specialties found on the provider's enrollment record:

- 01 - General Practice
- 08 - Family Practice
- 11 - Internal Medicine
- 16 - Obstetrics/Gynecology
- 37 - Pediatric Medicine
- 38 - Geriatric Medicine
- 42 - Certified Nurse Midwife
- 50 - Nurse Practitioner
- 89 - Certified Clinical Nurse Specialist
- 97 - Physician Assistant

HCV screening services ordered by providers other than the specialty types noted above will be denied.

For claims with dates of service on or after June 2, 2014, Medicare will allow coverage for HCV screening, HCPCS G0472, only when submitted with one of the following place of service (POS) codes:

- 11 - Physician's Office
- 22 - Outpatient Hospital
- 49 - Independent Clinic
- 71 - State or Local Public Health Clinic
- 81 - Independent Laboratory

HCV screening claims submitted without one of the POS codes noted above will be denied.

## 100-04, 18, 210.3

**Claim Adjustment Reason Codes (CARCs), Remittance Advice Remark Codes (RARCs), Group Codes, and Medicare Summary Notice (MSN) Messages**

(Rev. 3285, Issued: 06-19-15, Effective: 06-02-14, Implementation: For FISS shared system edits, split between October 5, 2015, and January 4, 2016, releases; July 20, 2015, - For non-shared MAC edits; October 5, 2015 - For CWF shared systems)

Contractors shall use the appropriate claim adjustment reason codes (CARCs), remittance advice remark codes (RARCs), group codes, or Medicare summary notice (MSN) messages when denying payment for HCV screening, HCPCS G0472:

- Denying services submitted on a TOB other than 13X or 85X:

  CARC 170 - Payment is denied when performed/billed by this type of provider. Note: Refer to the 835 Healthcare Policy Identification Segment (loop 2110 Service Payment Information REF), if present.

  RARC N95 – This provider type/provider specialty may not bill this service.

  MSN 21.25: This service was denied because Medicare only covers this service in certain settings.

  Spanish Version: "El servicio fue denegado porque Medicare solamente lo cubre en ciertas situaciones."

  Group Code CO (Contractual Obligation) assigning financial liability to the provider (if a claim is received with a GZ modifier indicating no signed ABN is on file).

  NOTE: For modifier GZ, use CARC 50 and MSN 8.81.

- Denying services where previous HCV screening, HCPCS G0472, is paid in history for claims with dates of service on and after June 2, 2014, and the patient is not deemed high risk by the presence of ICD-9 diagnosis code V69.8, other problems related to lifestyle/ICD-10 diagnosis code Z72.89, other problems related to lifestyle (once ICD-10 is implemented), and ICD-9 diagnosis code 304.91, unspecified drug dependence, continuous/ICD-10 diagnosis code F19.20, other psychoactive substance dependence, uncomplicated (once ICD-10 is implemented):

  CARC 119 – Benefit maximum for this time period or occurrence has been reached.

  RARC N386 - This decision was based on a National Coverage Determination (NCD). An NCD provides a coverage determination as to whether a particular item or service is covered. A copy of this policy is available at www.cms.gov/mcd/search.asp. If you do not have web access, you may contact the contractor to request a copy of the NCD.

  MSN 15.20 – The following policies NCD210.13 were used when we made this decision.

  Spanish Version – Las siguientes politicas NCD210.13 fueron utilizadas cuando se tomo esta decision.

  MSN 15.19 - Local Coverage Determinations (LCDs) help Medicare decide what is covered. An LCD was used for your claim. You can compare your case to the LCD, and send information from your doctor if you think it could change our decision. Call 1-800-MEDICARE (1-800-633-4227) for a copy of the LCD.

  Spanish Version - Las Determinaciones Locales de Cobertura (LCDs en inglés) le ayudan a decidir a Medicare lo que está cubierto. Un LCD se usó para su reclamación. Usted puede comparar su caso con la determinación y enviar información de su médico si piensa que puede cambiar nuestra decisión. Para obtener una copia del LCD, llame al 1-800-MEDICARE (1-800-633-4227).

  NOTE: Due to system requirement, FISS has combined messages 15.19 and 15.20 so that, when used for the same line item, both messages will appear on the same MSN.

  Group Code CO assigning financial liability to the provider (if a claim is received with a GZ modifier indicating no signed ABN is on file).

  NOTE: For modifier GZ, use CARC 50 and MSN 8.81.

  NOTE: This edit shall be overridable.

- Denying services for HCV screening, HCPCS G0472, for beneficiaries at high risk who have had continued illicit drug use since the prior negative screening test, when claims are not submitted with ICD-9 diagnosis code V69.8/ICD-10 diagnosis code Z72.89 (once ICD-10 is implemented), and ICD-9 diagnosis code 304.91/ICD-10 diagnosis code F19.20 (once ICD-10 is implemented), and/or 11 full months have not passed since the last negative HCV screening test:

CARC 167 – This (these) diagnosis(es) is (are) not covered. Note: Refer to the 835 Healthcare Policy Identification Segment (loop 2110 Service Payment Information REF), if present.

RARC N386 - This decision was based on a National Coverage Determination (NCD). An NCD provides a coverage determination as to whether a particular item or service is covered. A copy of this policy is available at www.cms.gov/mcd/search.asp. If you do not have web access, you may contact the contractor to request a copy of the NCD.

MSN 15.20 – The following policies NCD210.13 were used when we made this decision.

Spanish Version – Las siguientes politicas NCD210.13 fueron utilizadas cuando se tomo esta decision.

MSN 15.19 - Local Coverage Determinations (LCDs) help Medicare decide what is covered. An LCD was used for your claim. You can compare your case to the LCD, and send information from your doctor if you think it could change our decision. Call 1-800-MEDICARE (1-800-633-4227) for a copy of the LCD.

Spanish Version - Las Determinaciones Locales de Cobertura (LCDs en inglés) le ayudan a decidir a Medicare lo que está cubierto. Un LCD se usó para su reclamación. Usted puede comparar su caso con la determinación y enviar información de su médico si piensa que puede cambiar nuestra decisión. Para obtener una copia del LCD, llame al 1-800-MEDICARE (1-800-633-4227).

NOTE: Due to system requirement, FISS has combined messages 15.19 and 15.20 so that, when used for the same line item, both messages will appear on the same MSN.

Group Code CO assigning financial liability to the provider (if a claim is received with a GZ modifier indicating no signed ABN is on file).

NOTE: For modifier GZ, use CARC 50 and MSN 8.81.

NOTE: This edit shall be overridable.

- Denying services for HCV screening, HCPCS G0472, for beneficiaries who do not meet the definition of high risk, but who were born from 1945 through 1965, when claims are submitted more than once in a lifetime:

  CARC 119: "Benefit maximum for this time period or occurrence has been reached."

  RARC N386: "This decision was based on a National Coverage Determination (NCD). An NCD provides a coverage determination as to whether a particular item or service is covered. A copy of this policy is available at www.cms.gov/mcd/search.asp. If you do not have web access, you may contact the contractor to request a copy of the NCD."

  MSN 15.20 – The following policies NCD210.13 were used when we made this decision.

  Spanish Version – Las siguientes politicas NCD210.13 fueron utilizadas cuando se tomo esta decision.

  MSN 15.19 - Local Coverage Determinations (LCDs) help Medicare decide what is covered. An LCD was used for your claim. You can compare your case to the LCD, and send information from your doctor if you think it could change our decision. Call 1-800-MEDICARE (1-800-633-4227) for a copy of the LCD.

  Spanish Version - Las Determinaciones Locales de Cobertura (LCDs en inglés) le ayudan a decidir a Medicare lo que está cubierto. Un LCD se usó para su reclamación. Usted puede comparar su caso con la determinación y enviar información de su médico si piensa que puede cambiar nuestra decisión. Para obtener una copia del LCD, llame al 1-800-MEDICARE (1-800-633-4227).

  NOTE: Due to system requirement, FISS has combined messages 15.19 and 15.20 so that, when used for the same line item, both messages will appear on the same MSN.

  Group Code CO assigning financial liability to the provider (if a claim is received with a GZ modifier indicating no signed ABN is on file).

  NOTE: For modifier GZ, use CARC 50 and MSN 8.81.

  NOTE: This edit shall be overridable.

- Denying claim lines for HCV screening, HCPCS G0472, without the appropriate POS code:

  CARC 171 – Payment is denied when performed by this type of provider on this type of facility. Note: Refer to the 835 Healthcare Policy Identification Segment (loop 2110 Service Payment Information REF), if present.

  RARC N428 - Not covered when performed in certain settings.

  MSN 21.25 - This service was denied because Medicare only covers this service in certain settings.

Spanish Version: "El servicio fue denegado porque Medicare solamente lo cubre en ciertas situaciones."

Group Code CO assigning financial liability to the provider (if a claim is received with a GZ modifier indicating no signed ABN is on file).

NOTE: For modifier GZ, use CARC 50 and MSN 8.81.

- Denying claim lines for HCV screening, HCPCS G0472, that are not ordered by an appropriate provider specialty:

  CARC 184 - The prescribing/ordering provider is not eligible to prescribe/order the service billed. NOTE: Refer to the 835 Healthcare Policy Identification Segment (loop 2110 Service Payment Information REF), if present.

  RARC N574 – Our records indicate the ordering/referring provider is of a type/specialty that cannot order or refer. Please verify that the claim ordering/referring provider information is accurate or contact the ordering/referring provider.

  MSN 21.18 - This item or service is not covered when performed or ordered by this provider.

  Group Code CO assigning financial liability to the provider (if a claim is received with a GZ modifier indicating no signed ABN is on file).

  NOTE: For modifier GZ, use CARC 50 and MSN 8.81.

- Denying claim lines for HCV screening, HCPCS G0472, if beneficiary born prior to 1945 and after 1965 who are not at high risk (absence of V69.8 /ICD-10 diagnosis code Z72.89 (once ICD-10 is implemented) or 304.91/ ICD-10 diagnosis code F19.20 (once ICD-10 is implemented)):

  CARC 96 - Non-covered charge(s). At least one Remark Code must be provided (may be comprised of either the NCPDP Reject Reason [sic] Code, or Remittance Advice Remark Code that is not an ALERT.) Note: Refer to the 835 Healthcare Policy Identification Segment (loop 2110 Service Payment Information REF), if present.

  RARC N386 - This decision was based on a National Coverage Determination (NCD). An NCD provides a coverage determination as to whether a particular item or service is covered. A copy of this policy is available at www.cms.gov/mcd/search.asp. If you do not have web access, you may contact the contractor to request a copy of the NCD.

  MSN 15.19 - Local Coverage Determinations (LCDs) help Medicare decide what is covered. An LCD was used for your claim. You can compare your case to the LCD, and send information from your doctor if you think it could change our decision. Call 1-800-MEDICARE (1-800-633-4227) for a copy of the LCD.

  Spanish Version - Las Determinaciones Locales de Cobertura (LCDs en inglés) le ayudan a decidir a Medicare lo que está cubierto. Un LCD se usó para su reclamación. Usted puede comparar su caso con la determinación y enviar información de su médico si piensa que puede cambiar nuestra decisión. Para obtener una copia del LCD, llame al 1-800-MEDICARE (1-800-633-4227).

  MSN 15.20 – The following policies NCD210.13 were used when we made this decision.

  Spanish Version – Las siguientes politicas NCD210.13 fueron utilizadas cuando se tomo esta decision.

  NOTE: Due to system requirement, FISS has combined messages 15.19 and 15.20 so that, when used for the same line item, both messages will appear on the same MSN.

  Group Code CO assigning financial liability to the provider (if a claim is received with a GZ modifier indicating no signed ABN is on file).

## 100-04, 18, 210.4

### Common Working File (CWF) Edits

(Rev. 3285, Issued: 06-19-15, Effective: 06-02-14, Implementation: For FISS shared system edits, split between October 5, 2015, and January 4, 2016, releases; July 20, 2015, - For non-shared MAC edits; October 5, 2015 - For CWF shared systems)

The common working file (CWF) shall apply the following frequency limitations to HCV screening, HCPCS G0472:

One initial HCV screening, HCPCS G0472, for beneficiaries at high risk, when claims are submitted with ICD-9 diagnosis code V69.8/ICD-10 diagnosis code Z72.89 (once ICD-10 is implemented),

Annual HCV screening, HCPCS G0472, when claims are submitted with ICD-9 diagnosis code V69.8/ICD-10 diagnosis code Z72.89 (once ICD-10 is implemented), and ICD-9 diagnosis code 304.91/ICD-10 diagnosis code F19.20 (once ICD-10 is implemented),

Once in a lifetime HCV screening, HCPCS G0472, for beneficiaries who are not high risk who were born from 1945 through 1965.

NOTE: These edits shall be overridable.

NOTE: HCV screening, HCPCS G0472 is not a covered service for beneficiaries born prior to 1945 and after 1965 who are not at high risk (absence of V69.8/ICD-10 diagnosis code Z72.89 (once ICD-10 is implemented) and/or 304.91/ ICD-10 diagnosis code F19.20 (once ICD-10 is implemented)).

## 100-04, 20, 20

### Calculation and Update of Payment Rates
(Rev. 1, 10-01-03)
B3-5017, PM B-01-54, 2002 PEN Fee Schedule

Section1834 of the Act requires the use of fee schedules under Medicare Part B for reimbursement of durable medical equipment (DME) and for prosthetic and orthotic devices, beginning January 1 1989. Payment is limited to the lower of the actual charge for the equipment or the fee established.

Beginning with fee schedule year 1991, CMS calculates the updates for the fee schedules and national limitation amounts and provides the contractors with the revised payment amounts. The CMS calculates most fee schedule amounts and provides them to the carriers, DMERCs, FIs and RHHIs. However, for some services CMS asks carriers to calculate local fee amounts and to provide them to CMS to include in calculation of national amounts. These vary from update to update, and CMS issues special related instructions to carriers when appropriate.

Parenteral and enteral nutrition services paid on and after January 1, 2002 are paid on a fee schedule. This fee schedule also is furnished by CMS. Prior to 2002, payment amounts for PEN were determined under reasonable charge rules, including the application of the lowest charge level (LCL) restrictions.

The CMS furnishes fee schedule updates (DMEPOS, PEN, etc.) at least 30 days prior to the scheduled implementation. FIs use the fee schedules to pay for covered items, within their claims processing jurisdictions, supplied by hospitals, home health agencies, and other providers. FIs consult with DMERCs and where appropriate with carriers on filling gaps in fee schedules.

The CMS furnishes the fee amounts annually, or as updated if special updates should occur during the year, to carriers and FIs, including DMERCs and RHHIs, and to other interested parties (including the Statistical Analysis DMERC (SADMERC), Railroad Retirement Board (RRB), Indian Health Service, and United Mine Workers).

## 100-04, 20, 20.4

### Contents of Fee Schedule File
(Rev. 1, 10-01-03) PM A-02-090

The fee schedule file provided by CMS contains HCPCS codes and related prices subject to the DMEPOS fee schedules, including application of any update factors and any changes to the national limited payment amounts. The file does not contain fees for drugs that are necessary for the effective use of DME. It also does not include fees for items for which fee schedule amounts are not available. See Chapter 23 for a description of pricing for these. The CMS releases via program issuance, the gap-filled amounts and the annual update factors for the various DMEPOS payment classes:

- IN = Inexpensive/routinely purchased...DME;
- FS = Frequency Service...DME;
- CR = Capped Rental...DME;
- OX = Oxygen and Oxygen Equipment...OXY;
- OS = Ostomy, Tracheostomy and Urologicals...P/O;
- S/D = Surgical Dressings...S/D;
- P/O = Prosthetics and Orthotics...P/O;
- SU = Supplies...DME; and
- TE = TENS...DME

The RHHIs need to retrieve data from all of the above categories. Regular FIs need to retrieve data only from categories P/O, S/D and SU. FIs need to retrieve the SU category in order to be able to price supplies on Part B SNF claims.

## 100-04, 20, 30.1.2

### Transcutaneous Electrical Nerve Stimulator (TENS)
In order to permit an attending physician time to determine whether the purchase of a TENS is medically appropriate for a particular patient, contractors pay 10 percent of the purchase price of the item for each of 2 months. The purchase price and payment for maintenance and servicing are determined under the same rules as any other frequently purchased item, except that there is no reduction in the allowed amount for purchase due to the two months rental.

Effective June 8, 2012, CMS will allow coverage for TENS use in the treatment of chronic low back pain (CLBP) only under specific conditions which are described in the NCD Manual, Pub. 100-03, chapter 1 Section 160.27.

## 100-04, 20, 30.6

### Oxygen and Oxygen Equipment
For oxygen and oxygen equipment, contractors pay a monthly fee schedule amount per beneficiary. Unless otherwise noted below, the fee covers equipment, contents and supplies. Payment is not made for purchases of this type of equipment.

When an inpatient is not entitled to Part A, payment may not be made under Part B for DME or oxygen provided in a hospital or SNF. (See the Medicare Benefit Policy Manual, Chapter 15) Also, for outpatients using equipment or receiving oxygen in the hospital or SNF and not taking the equipment or oxygen system home, the fee schedule does not apply.

There are a number of billing considerations for oxygen claims. The chart in §130.6 indicates what amounts are payable under which situations.

Effective for claims on or after February 14, 2011, payment for the home use of oxygen and oxygen equipment when related to the treatment of cluster headaches is covered under a National Coverage Determination (NCD). For more information, refer to chapter 1, section 240.2.2, Publication 100-03, of the National Coverage Determinations Manual.

## 100-04, 20, 100

### General Documentation Requirements
(Rev. 1, 10-01-03)
B3-4107.1, B3-4107.8, HHA-463, Medicare Handbook for New Suppliers: Getting Started, B-02-31

Benefit policies are set forth in the Medicare Benefit Policy Manual, Chapter 15, §§110-130.

Program integrity policies for DMEPOS are set forth in the Medicare Program Integrity Manual, Chapter 5.

See Chapter 21 for applicable MSN messages.

See Chapter 22 for Remittance Advice coding.

## 100-04, 20, 100.2

### Certificates of Medical Necessity (CMN)
(Rev. 1, 10-01-03)
B3-3312

For certain items or services billed to the DME Regional Carrier (DMERC), the supplier must receive a signed Certificate of Medical Necessity (CMN) from the treating physician. CMNs are not required for the same items when billed by HHAs to RHHIs. Instead, the items must be included in the physician's signed orders on the home health plan of care. See the Medicare Program Integrity Manual, Chapter 6.

The FI will inform other providers (see §01 for definition pf provider) of documentation requirements.

Contractors may ask for supporting documentation beyond a CMN.

Refer to the local DMERC Web site described in §10 for downloadable copies of CMN forms.

See the Medicare Program Integrity Manual, Chapter 5, for specific Medicare policies and instructions on the following topics:

- Requirements for supplier retention of original CMNs
- CMN formats, paper and electronic
- List of currently approved CMNs and items requiring CMNs
- Supplier requirements for submitting CMNs
- Requirements for CMNs to also serve as a physician's order
- Civil monetary penalties for violation of CMN requirements
- Supplier requirements for completing portions of CMNs
- Physician requirements for completing portions of CMNs

## 100-04, 20, 130.2

### Billing for Inexpensive or Other Routinely Purchased DME
(Rev. 1, 10-01-03)
A3-3629, B3-4107.8

This is equipment with a purchase price not exceeding $150, or equipment that the Secretary determines is acquired by purchase at least 75 percent of the time, or equipment that is an accessory used in conjunction with a nebulizer, aspirator, or ventilators that are either continuous airway pressure devices or intermittent assist devices with continuous airway pressure devices. Suppliers and providers other than HHAs bill the DMERC or, in the case of implanted DME only, the local carrier. HHAs bill the RHHI.

Effective for items and services furnished after January 1, 1991, Medicare DME does not include seat lift chairs. Only the seat lift mechanism is defined under Medicare as DME. Therefore, seat lift coverage is limited to the seat lift mechanism. If a seat lift chair is provided to a beneficiary, contractors pay only for the lift mechanism portion of the chair. Some lift mechanisms are equipped with a seat that is considered an integral part of the lift mechanism. Contractors do not pay for chairs (HCPCS code E0620) furnished on or after January 1, 1991. The appropriate HCPCS codes for seat lift mechanisms are E0627, E0628, and E0629.

For TENS, suppliers and providers other than HHAs bill the DMERC. HHAs bill the RHHI using revenue code 0291 for the 2-month rental period (see §30.1.2), billing each month as a separate line item and revenue code 0292 for the actual purchase along with the appropriate HCPCS code.

## 100-04, 20, 130.3

### Billing for Items Requiring Frequent and Substantial Servicing
(Rev. 1, 10-01-03)

A3-3629, B3-4107.8

These are items such as intermittent positive pressure breathing (IPPB) machines and ventilators, excluding ventilators that are either continuous airway pressure devices or intermittent assist devices with continuous airway pressure devices.

Suppliers and providers other than HHAs bill the DMERC. HHAs bill the RHHI.

## 100-04, 20, 130.4

### Billing for Certain Customized Items
(Rev. 1, 10-01-03)

A3-3629, B3-4107.8

Due to their unique nature (custom fabrication, etc.), certain customized DME cannot be grouped together for profiling purposes. Claims for customized items that do not have specific HCPCS codes are coded as E1399 (miscellaneous DME). This includes circumstances where an item that has a HCPCS code is modified to the extent that neither the original terminology nor the terminology of another HCPCS code accurately describes the modified item.

Suppliers and providers other than HHAs bill the DMERC or local carrier. HHAs bill their RHHI, using revenue code 0292 along with the HCPCS.

## 100-04, 20, 130.5

### Billing for Capped Rental Items (Other Items of DME)
(Rev. 1, 10-01-03)

A3-3629, B3-4107.8

These are DME items, other than oxygen and oxygen equipment, not covered by the above categories. Suppliers and providers other than HHAs bill the DMERC. HHAs bill the RHHIs.

## 100-04, 20, 160.2

### 160.2 - Special Considerations for SNF Billing for TPN and EN Under Part B
(Rev. 2993, Effective: ASC X12 – 01-01-12, ICD-10 – Upon Implementation of ICD-10; Implementation: ASC X12 – 08-25-14, ICD-10 – Upon Implementation of ICD-10)

The HCPCS code and any appropriate modifiers are required.

SNFs bill the A/B MAC (B) for TPN and EN under Part B, using the ASC X12 837 professional claim format, or the Form CMS-1500 paper claim if applicable.

The following HCPCS codes apply.

B4034 B4035 B4036 B4081 B4082 B4083 B4084 B4085 B4150 B4151 B4152 B4153 B4154 B4155 B4156 B4164 B4168 B4172 B4176 B4178 B4180 B4184 B4186 B4189 B4193 B4197 B4199 B4216 B4220 B4222 B4224 B5000 B5100 B5200 B9000 B9002 B9004 B9006 E0776XA B9098 B9099

For SNF billing for PEN, a SNF includes the charges for PEN items it supplies beneficiaries under Part A on its Part A bill. The services of SNF personnel who administer the PEN therapy are considered routine and are included in the basic Part A payment for a covered stay. SNF personnel costs to administer PEN therapy are not covered under the Part B prosthetic device benefit.

If TPN supplies, equipment and nutrients qualify as a prosthetic device and the stay is not covered by Part A, they are covered by Part B. Part B coverage applies regardless of whether the TPN items were furnished by the SNF or an outside supplier. The Part B TPN bill must be sent to the DME Medicare Administrative Contractor regardless of whether supplied by the SNF or an outside supplier.

Enteral nutrients provided during a stay that is covered by Part A are classified as food and included in the routine Part A payment sent to the SNF. (See the Medicare Provider Reimbursement Manual, §2203.1E.)

Parenteral nutrient solutions provided during a covered Part A SNF stay are classified as intravenous drugs. The SNF must bill these services as ancillary charges. (See the Medicare Provider Reimbursement Manual, §2203.2.)

## 100-04, 20, 170

### Billing for Splints and Casts
(Rev. 2993, Effective: ASC X12 – 01-01-12, ICD-10 – Upon Implementation of ICD- 10; Implementation: ASC X12 – 08-25-14, ICD-10 – Upon Implementation of ICD- 10)

The cost of supplies used in creating casts are not included in the payment amounts for the CPT codes for fracture management and for casts and splints. Thus, for settings in which CPT codes are used to pay for services that include the provision of a cast or splint, supplies maybe billed with separate CPCS codes. The work and practice expenses involved with the creation of the cast or splint are included in the payment for the code for that service.

For claims with dates of service on or after July 1, 2001, jurisdiction for processing claims for splints transferred from the DME MACs to the A/B MAC (B). The A/B MACs (B) have jurisdiction for processing claims for splints and casts, which includes codes for splints that may have previously been billed to the DME MACs.

Jurisdiction for slings is jointly maintained by the A/B MACs (B) (for physician claims) and the DME MACs (for supplier claims). Notwithstanding the above where the beneficiary receives the service from any of the following providers claims jurisdiction is with the A/B MAC (A). An exception to this is hospital outpatient services and hospital inpatient Part B services, which are included in the OPPS payment and are billed to the A/B MAC (A) using the ASC X12 837 institutional claim format or Form CMS- 1450).

Other providers and suppliers that normally bill the A/B MAC (A) for services bill the A/B MAC (B) for splints and casts.

## 100-04, 23, 60.3
(Rev. 3416, Issued: 11-23-15; Effective: 01-01-16; Implementation: 01-04-16)

The DME MACs and local carriers must gap-fill the DMEPOS fee schedule for items for which charge data were unavailable during the fee schedule data base year using the fee schedule amounts for comparable equipment, using properly calculated fee schedule amounts from a neighboring carrier, or using supplier price lists with prices in effect during the fee schedule data base year. Data base "year" refers to the time period mandated by the statute and/or regulations from which Medicare allowed charge data is to be extracted in order to compute the fee schedule amounts for the various DMEPOS payment categories. For example, the fee schedule base year for inexpensive or routinely purchased durable medical equipment is the 12 month period ending June 30, 1987. Mail order catalogs are particularly suitable sources of price information for items such as urological and ostomy supplies which require constant replacement. DME MACs will gap-fill based on current instructions released each year for implementing and updating the new year's payment amounts.

If the only available price information is from a period other than the base period, apply the deflation factors that are included in the current year implementation instructions against current pricing in order to approximate the base year price for gap-filling purposes.

The deflation factors for gap-filling purposes are:

| Year* | OX | CR | PO | SD | PE |
|---|---|---|---|---|---|
| 1987 | 0.965 | 0.971 | 0.974 | n/a | n/a |
| 1988 | 0.928 | 0.934 | 0.936 | n/a | n/a |
| 1989 | 0.882 | 0.888 | 0.890 | n/a | n/a |
| 1990 | 0.843 | 0.848 | 0.851 | n/a | n/a |
| 1991 | 0.805 | 0.810 | 0.813 | n/a | n/a |
| 1992 | 0.781 | 0.786 | 0.788 | n/a | n/a |
| 1993 | 0.758 | 0.763 | 0.765 | 0.971 | n/a |
| 1994 | 0.740 | 0.745 | 0.747 | 0.947 | n/a |
| 1995 | 0.718 | 0.723 | 0.725 | 0.919 | n/a |
| 1996 | 0.699 | 0.703 | 0.705 | 0.895 | 0.973 |
| 1997 | 0.683 | 0.687 | 0.689 | 0.875 | 0.951 |
| 1998 | 0.672 | 0.676 | 0.678 | 0.860 | 0.936 |
| 1999 | 0.659 | 0.663 | 0.665 | 0.844 | 0.918 |
| 2000 | 0.635 | 0.639 | 0.641 | 0.813 | 0.885 |

| Year* | OX | CR | PO | SD | PE |
|---|---|---|---|---|---|
| 2001 | 0.615 | 0.619 | 0.621 | 0.788 | 0.857 |
| 2002 | 0.609 | 0.613 | 0.614 | 0.779 | 0.848 |
| 2003 | 0.596 | 0.600 | 0.602 | 0.763 | 0.830 |
| 2004 | 0.577 | 0.581 | 0.582 | 0.739 | 0.804 |
| 2005 | 0.563 | 0.567 | 0.568 | 0.721 | 0.784 |
| 2006 | 0.540 | 0.543 | 0.545 | 0.691 | 0.752 |
| 2007 | 0.525 | 0.529 | 0.530 | 0.673 | 0.732 |
| 2008 | 0.500 | 0.504 | 0.505 | 0.641 | 0.697 |
| 2009 | 0.508 | 0.511 | 0.512 | 0.650 | 0.707 |
| 2010 | 0.502 | 0.506 | 0.507 | 0.643 | 0.700 |
| 2011 | 0.485 | 0.488 | 0.490 | 0.621 | 0.676 |
| 2012 | 0.477 | 0.480 | 0.482 | 0.611 | 0.665 |
| 2013 | 0.469 | 0.472 | 0.473 | 0.600 | 0.653 |
| 2014 | 0.459 | 0.462 | 0.464 | 0.588 | 0.640 |
| 2015 | 0.459 | 0.462 | 0.463 | 0.588 | 0.639 |

* Year price in effect

**Payment Category Key:**

OX     Oxygen & oxygen equipment (DME)

CR     Capped rental (DME)

IN     Inexpensive/routinely purchased (DME)

FS     Frequently serviced (DME)

SU     DME supplies

PO     Prosthetics & orthotics

SD     Surgical dressings

OS     Ostomy, tracheostomy, and urological supplies

PE     Parental and enteral nutrition

After deflation, the result must be increased by 1.7 percent and by the cumulative covered item update to complete the gap-filling (e.g., an additional .6 percent for a 2002 DME fee).

Note that when gap-filling for capped rental items, it is necessary to first gap-fill the purchase price then compute the base period fee schedule at 10 percent of the base period purchase price.

For used equipment, establish fee schedule amounts at 75 percent of the fee schedule amount for new equipment.

When gap-filling, for those carrier areas where a sales tax was imposed in the base period, add the applicable sales tax, e.g., five percent, to the gap-filled amount where the gap-filled amount does not take into account the sales tax, e.g., where the gap-filled amount is computed from pre-tax price lists or from another carrier area without a sales tax. Likewise, if the gap-filled amount is calculated from another carrier's fees where a sales tax is imposed, adjust the gap-filled amount to reflect the applicable local sales tax circumstances.

DME MACs and local carriers send their gap-fill information to CMS. After receiving the gap-filled base fees each year, CMS develops national fee schedule floors and ceilings and new fee schedule amounts for these codes and releases them as part of the July update file each year and during the quarterly updates.

**Attachment A**

2012 Fees for Codes K0739, L4205, L7520

| STATE | K0739 | L4205 | L7520 | STATE | K0739 | L4205 | L7520 |
|---|---|---|---|---|---|---|---|
| AK | $26.47 | $30.16 | $35.48 | SC | $14.05 | 20.94 | 28.43 |
| AL | 14.05 | 20.94 | 28.43 | SD | 15.70 | 20.92 | 38.00 |
| AR | 14.05 | 20.94 | 28.43 | TN | 14.05 | 20.94 | 28.43 |
| AZ | 17.37 | 20.92 | 34.98 | TX | 14.05 | 20.94 | 28.43 |
| CA | 21.56 | 34.38 | 40.07 | UT | 14.09 | 20.92 | 44.27 |
| CO | 14.05 | 20.94 | 28.43 | VA | 14.05 | 20.92 | 28.43 |
| CT | 23.47 | 21.41 | 28.43 | VI | 14.05 | 20.94 | 28.43 |

| STATE | K0739 | L4205 | L7520 | STATE | K0739 | L4205 | L7520 |
|---|---|---|---|---|---|---|---|
| DC | 14.05 | 20.92 | 28.43 | VT | 15.08 | 20.92 | 28.43 |
| DE | 25.88 | 20.92 | 28.43 | WA | 22.39 | 30.69 | 36.45 |
| FL | 14.05 | 20.94 | 28.43 | WI | 14.05 | 20.92 | 28.43 |
| GA | 14.05 | 20.94 | 28.43 | WV | 14.05 | 20.92 | 28.43 |
| HI | 17.37 | 30.16 | 35.48 | WY | 19.59 | 27.91 | 39.64 |
| IA | 14.05 | 20.92 | 34.03 | | | | |
| ID | 14.05 | 20.92 | 28.43 | | | | |
| IL | 14.05 | 20.92 | 28.43 | | | | |
| IN | 14.05 | 20.92 | 28.43 | | | | |
| KS | 14.05 | 20.92 | 35.48 | | | | |
| KY | 14.05 | 26.81 | 36.35 | | | | |
| LA | 14.05 | 20.94 | 28.43 | | | | |
| MA | 23.47 | 20.92 | 28.43 | | | | |
| MD | 14.05 | 20.92 | 28.43 | | | | |
| ME | 23.47 | 20.92 | 28.43 | | | | |
| MI | 14.05 | 20.92 | 28.43 | | | | |
| MN | 14.05 | 20.92 | 28.43 | | | | |
| MO | 14.05 | 20.92 | 28.43 | | | | |
| MS | 14.05 | 20.94 | 28.43 | | | | |
| MT | 14.05 | 20.92 | 35.48 | | | | |
| NC | 14.05 | 20.94 | 28.43 | | | | |
| ND | 17.51 | 30.10 | 35.48 | | | | |
| NE | 14.05 | 20.92 | 39.64 | | | | |
| NH | 15.08 | 20.92 | 28.43 | | | | |
| NJ | 18.96 | 20.92 | 28.43 | | | | |
| NM | 14.05 | 20.94 | 28.43 | | | | |
| NV | 22.39 | 20.92 | 38.75 | | | | |
| NY | 25.88 | 20.94 | 28.43 | | | | |
| OH | 14.05 | 20.92 | 28.43 | | | | |
| OK | 14.05 | 20.94 | 28.43 | | | | |
| OR | 14.05 | 20.92 | 40.88 | | | | |
| PA | 15.08 | 21.54 | 28.43 | | | | |
| PR | 14.05 | 20.94 | 28.43 | | | | |
| RI | 16.75 | 21.56 | 28.43 | | | | |

**Attachment B**

HCPCS Codes Selected for the Round One of the DMEPOS Competitive Bidding Program in 2008

**PRODUCT CATEGORY 1**

**Oxygen Supplies and Equipment**

E1390     OXYGEN CONCENTRATOR, SINGLE DELIVERY PORT, CAPABLE OF DELIVERING 85 PERCENT OR GREATER OXYGEN CONCENTRATION AT THE PRESCRIBED FLOW RATE

E1391     OXYGEN CONCENTRATOR, DUAL DELIVERY PORT, CAPABLE OF DELIVERING 85 PERCENT OR GREATER OXYGEN CONCENTRATION AT THE PRESCRIBED FLOW RATE, EACH

E0424     STATIONARY COMPRESSED GASEOUS OXYGEN SYSTEM, RENTAL; INCLUDES CONTAINER, CONTENTS, REGULATOR, FLOWMETER, HUMIDIFIER, NEBULIZER, CANNULA OR MASK, AND TUBING

E0439     STATIONARY LIQUID OXYGEN SYSTEM, RENTAL; INCLUDES CONTAINER, CONTENTS, REGULATOR, FLOWMETER, HUMIDIFIER, NEBULIZER, CANNULA OR MASK, & TUBING

E0431     PORTABLE GASEOUS OXYGEN SYSTEM, RENTAL; INCLUDES PORTABLE CONTAINER, REGULATOR, FLOWMETER, HUMIDIFIER, CANNULA OR MASK, AND TUBING

E0434     PORTABLE LIQUID OXYGEN SYSTEM, RENTAL; INCLUDES PORTABLE CONTAINER, SUPPLY RESERVOIR, HUMIDIFIER, FLOWMETER, REFILL ADAPTOR, CONTENTS GAUGE, CANNULA OR MASK, AND TUBING

A4608     TRANSTRACHEAL OXYGEN CATHETER, EACH

© 2016 Optum360, LLC

| | | |
|---|---|---|
| A4615 | CANNULA, NASAL | |
| A4616 | TUBING (OXYGEN), PER FOOT | |
| A4617 | MOUTH PIECE | |
| A4620 | VARIABLE CONCENTRATION MASK | |
| E0560 | HUMIDIFIER, DURABLE FOR SUPPLEMENTAL HUMIDIFICATION DURING IPPB TREATMENT OR OXYGEN DELIVERY | |
| E0580 | NEBULIZER, DURABLE, GLASS OR AUTOCLAVABLE PLASTIC, BOTTLE TYPE, FOR USE WITH REGULATOR OR FLOWMETER | |
| E1353 | REGULATOR | |
| E1355 | STAND/RACK | |

**PRODUCT CATEGORY 2**

**Standard Power Wheelchairs, Scooters, and Related Accessories**

| | |
|---|---|
| E0950 | WHEELCHAIR ACCESSORY, TRAY, EACH |
| E0951 | HEEL LOOP/HOLDER, ANY TYPE, WITH OR WITHOUT ANKLE STRAP, |

**PRODUCT CATEGORY 1**

**Oxygen Supplies and Equipment**

| | |
|---|---|
| E1390 | OXYGEN CONCENTRATOR, SINGLE DELIVERY PORT, CAPABLE OF DELIVERING 85 PERCENT OR GREATER OXYGEN CONCENTRATION AT THE PRESCRIBED FLOW RATE |
| E1391 | OXYGEN CONCENTRATOR, DUAL DELIVERY PORT, CAPABLE OF DELIVERING 85 PERCENT OR GREATER OXYGEN CONCENTRATION AT THE PRESCRIBED FLOW RATE, EACH |
| E0424 | STATIONARY COMPRESSED GASEOUS OXYGEN SYSTEM, RENTAL; INCLUDES CONTAINER, CONTENTS, REGULATOR, FLOWMETER, HUMIDIFIER, NEBULIZER, CANNULA OR MASK, AND TUBING |
| E0439 | STATIONARY LIQUID OXYGEN SYSTEM, RENTAL; INCLUDES CONTAINER, CONTENTS, REGULATOR, FLOWMETER, HUMIDIFIER, NEBULIZER, CANNULA OR MASK, & TUBING |
| E0431 | PORTABLE GASEOUS OXYGEN SYSTEM, RENTAL; INCLUDES PORTABLE CONTAINER, REGULATOR, FLOWMETER, HUMIDIFIER, CANNULA OR MASK, AND TUBING |
| E0434 | PORTABLE LIQUID OXYGEN SYSTEM, RENTAL; INCLUDES PORTABLE CONTAINER, SUPPLY RESERVOIR, HUMIDIFIER, FLOWMETER, REFILL ADAPTOR, CONTENTS GAUGE, CANNULA OR MASK, AND TUBING |
| A4608 | TRANSTRACHEAL OXYGEN CATHETER, EACH |
| A4615 | CANNULA, NASAL |
| A4616 | TUBING (OXYGEN), PER FOOT |
| A4617 | MOUTH PIECE |
| A4620 | VARIABLE CONCENTRATION MASK |
| E0560 | HUMIDIFIER, DURABLE FOR SUPPLEMENTAL HUMIDIFICATION DURING IPPB TREATMENT OR OXYGEN DELIVERY |
| E0580 | NEBULIZER, DURABLE, GLASS OR AUTOCLAVABLE PLASTIC, BOTTLE TYPE, FOR USE WITH REGULATOR OR FLOWMETER |
| E1353 | REGULATOR |
| E1355 | STAND/RACK |

**PRODUCT CATEGORY 2**

**Standard Power Wheelchairs, Scooters, and Related Accessories**

| | |
|---|---|
| E0950 | WHEELCHAIR ACCESSORY, TRAY, EACH |
| E0951 | HEEL LOOP/HOLDER, ANY TYPE, WITH OR WITHOUT ANKLE STRAP, EACH |
| E0952 | TOE LOOP/HOLDER, ANY TYPE, EACH |
| E0955 | WHEELCHAIR ACCESSORY, HEADREST, CUSHIONED, ANY TYPE, INCLUDING FIXED MOUNTING HARDWARE, EACH |
| E0956 | WHEELCHAIR ACCESSORY, LATERAL TRUNK OR HIP SUPPORT, ANY TYPE, INCLUDING FIXED MOUNTING HARDWARE, EACH |
| E0957 | WHEELCHAIR ACCESSORY, MEDIAL THIGH SUPPORT, ANY TYPE, INCLUDING FIXED MOUNTING HARDWARE, EACH |
| E0960 | WHEELCHAIR ACCESSORY, SHOULDER HARNESS/STRAPS OR CHEST STRAP, INCLUDING ANY TYPE MOUNTING HARDWARE |
| E0973 | WHEELCHAIR ACCESSORY, ADJUSTABLE HEIGHT, DETACHABLE ARMREST, COMPLETE ASSEMBLY, EACH |
| E0978 | WHEELCHAIR ACCESSORY, POSITIONING BELT/SAFETY BELT/PELVIC STRAP, EACH |

| | |
|---|---|
| E0981 | WHEELCHAIR ACCESSORY, SEAT UPHOLSTERY, REPLACEMENT ONLY, EACH |
| E0982 | WHEELCHAIR ACCESSORY, BACK UPHOLSTERY, REPLACEMENT ONLY, EACH |
| E0990 | WHEELCHAIR ACCESSORY, ELEVATING LEG REST, COMPLETE ASSEMBLY, EACH |
| E0995 | WHEELCHAIR ACCESSORY, CALF REST/PAD, EACH |
| E1016 | SHOCK ABSORBER FOR POWER WHEELCHAIR, EACH |
| E1020 | RESIDUAL LIMB SUPPORT SYSTEM FOR WHEELCHAIR |
| E1028 | WHEELCHAIR ACCESSORY, MANUAL SWINGAWAY, RETRACTABLE OR REMOVABLE MOUNTING HARDWARE FOR JOYSTICK, OTHER CONTROL INTERFACE OR POSITIONING ACCESSORY |
| E2208 | WHEELCHAIR ACCESSORY, CYLINDER TANK CARRIER, EACH |
| E2209 | ACCESSORY, ARM TROUGH, WITH OR WITHOUT HAND SUPPORT, EACH |
| E2210 | WHEELCHAIR ACCESSORY, BEARINGS, ANY TYPE, REPLACEMENT ONLY, EACH |
| E2361 | POWER WHEELCHAIR ACCESSORY, 22NF SEALED LEAD ACID BATTERY, EACH, (E.G. GEL CELL, ABSORBED GLASSMAT) |
| E2363 | POWER WHEELCHAIR ACCESSORY, GROUP 24 SEALED LEAD ACID BATTERY, EACH (E.G. GEL CELL, ABSORBED GLASSMAT) |
| E2365 | POWER WHEELCHAIR ACCESSORY, U-1 SEALED LEAD ACID BATTERY, EACH (E.G. GEL CELL, ABSORBED GLASSMAT) |
| E2366 | POWER WHEELCHAIR ACCESSORY, BATTERY CHARGER, SINGLE MODE, FOR USE WITH ONLY ONE BATTERY TYPE, SEALED OR NON-SEALED, EACH |
| E2367 | POWER WHEELCHAIR ACCESSORY, BATTERY CHARGER, DUAL MODE, FOR USE WITH EITHER BATTERY TYPE, SEALED OR NON-SEALED, EACH |
| E2368 | POWER WHEELCHAIR COMPONENT, MOTOR, REPLACEMENT ONLY |
| E2369 | POWER WHEELCHAIR COMPONENT, GEAR BOX, REPLACEMENT ONLY |
| E2370 | POWER WHEELCHAIR COMPONENT, MOTOR AND GEAR BOX COMBINATION, REPLACEMENT ONLY |
| E2371 | POWER WHEELCHAIR ACCESSORY, GROUP 27 SEALED LEAD ACID BATTERY, (E.G. GEL CELL, ABSORBED GLASSMAT), EACH |
| E2381 | POWER WHEELCHAIR ACCESSORY, PNEUMATIC DRIVE WHEEL TIRE, ANY SIZE, REPLACEMENT ONLY, EACH |
| E2382 | POWER WHEELCHAIR ACCESSORY, TUBE FOR PNEUMATIC DRIVE WHEEL TIRE, ANY SIZE, REPLACEMENT ONLY, EACH |
| E2383 | POWER WHEELCHAIR ACCESSORY, INSERT FOR PNEUMATIC DRIVE WHEEL TIRE (REMOVABLE), ANY TYPE, ANY SIZE, REPLACEMENT ONLY, EACH |
| E2384 | POWER WHEELCHAIR ACCESSORY, PNEUMATIC CASTER TIRE, ANY SIZE, REPLACEMENT ONLY, EACH |
| E2385 | POWER WHEELCHAIR ACCESSORY, TUBE FOR PNEUMATIC CASTER TIRE, ANY SIZE, REPLACEMENT ONLY, EACH |
| E2386 | POWER WHEELCHAIR ACCESSORY, FOAM FILLED DRIVE WHEEL TIRE, ANY SIZE, REPLACEMENT ONLY, EACH |
| E2387 | POWER WHEELCHAIR ACCESSORY, FOAM FILLED CASTER TIRE, ANY SIZE, REPLACEMENT ONLY, EACH |
| E2388 | POWER WHEELCHAIR ACCESSORY, FOAM DRIVE WHEEL TIRE, ANY SIZE, REPLACEMENT ONLY, EACH |
| E2389 | POWER WHEELCHAIR ACCESSORY, FOAM CASTER TIRE, ANY SIZE, REPLACEMENT ONLY, EACH |
| E2390 | POWER WHEELCHAIR ACCESSORY, SOLID (RUBBER/PLASTIC) DRIVE WHEEL TIRE, ANY SIZE, REPLACEMENT ONLY, EACH |
| E2391 | POWER WHEELCHAIR ACCESSORY, SOLID (RUBBER/PLASTIC) CASTER TIRE (REMOVABLE), ANY SIZE, REPLACEMENT ONLY, EACH |
| E2392 | POWER WHEELCHAIR ACCESSORY, SOLID (RUBBER/PLASTIC) CASTER TIRE WITH INTEGRATED WHEEL, ANY SIZE, REPLACEMENT ONLY, EACH |
| E2394 | POWER WHEELCHAIR ACCESSORY, DRIVE WHEEL EXCLUDES TIRE, ANY SIZE, REPLACEMENT ONLY, EACH |
| E2395 | POWER WHEELCHAIR ACCESSORY, CASTER WHEEL EXCLUDES TIRE, ANY SIZE, REPLACEMENT ONLY, EACH |
| E2396 | POWER WHEELCHAIR ACCESSORY, CASTER FORK, ANY SIZE, REPLACEMENT ONLY, EACH |

© 2016 Optum360, LLC

| Code | Description |
|------|-------------|
| E2601 | GENERAL USE WHEELCHAIR SEAT CUSHION, WIDTH LESS THAN 22 INCHES, ANY DEPTH |
| E2602 | GENERAL USE WHEELCHAIR SEAT CUSHION, WIDTH 22 INCHES OR GREATER, ANY DEPTH |
| E2603 | SKIN PROTECTION WHEELCHAIR SEAT CUSHION, WIDTH LESS THAN 22 INCHES, ANY DEPTH |
| E2604 | SKIN PROTECTION WHEELCHAIR SEAT CUSHION, WIDTH 22 INCHES OR GREATER, ANY DEPTH |
| E2605 | POSITIONING WHEELCHAIR SEAT CUSHION, WIDTH LESS THAN 22 INCHES, ANY DEPTH |
| E2606 | POSITIONING WHEELCHAIR SEAT CUSHION, WIDTH 22 INCHES OR GREATER, ANY DEPTH |
| E2607 | SKIN PROTECTION AND POSITIONING WHEELCHAIR SEAT CUSHION, WIDTH LESS THAN 22 INCHES, ANY DEPTH |
| E2608 | SKIN PROTECTION AND POSITIONING WHEELCHAIR SEAT CUSHION, WIDTH 22 INCHES OR GREATER, ANY DEPTH |
| E2611 | GENERAL USE WHEELCHAIR BACK CUSHION, WIDTH LESS THAN 22 INCHES, ANY HEIGHT, INCLUDING ANY TYPE MOUNTING HARDWARE |
| E2612 | GENERAL USE WHEELCHAIR BACK CUSHION, WIDTH 22 INCHES OR GREATER, ANY HEIGHT, INCLUDING ANY TYPE MOUNTING HARDWARE |
| E2613 | POSITIONING WHEELCHAIR BACK CUSHION, POSTERIOR, WIDTH LESS THAN 22 INCHES, ANY HEIGHT, INCLUDING ANY TYPE MOUNTING HARDWARE |
| E2614 | POSITIONING WHEELCHAIR BACK CUSHION, POSTERIOR, WIDTH 22 INCHES OR GREATER, ANY HEIGHT, INCLUDING ANY TYPE MOUNTING HARDWARE |
| E2615 | POSITIONING WHEELCHAIR BACK CUSHION, POSTERIOR-LATERAL, WIDTH LESS THAN 22 INCHES, ANY HEIGHT, INCLUDING ANY TYPE MOUNTING HARDWARE |
| E2616 | POSITIONING WHEELCHAIR BACK CUSHION, POSTERIOR-LATERAL, WIDTH 22 INCHES OR GREATER, ANY HEIGHT, INCLUDING ANY TYPE MOUNTING HARDWARE |
| E2619 | REPLACEMENT COVER FOR WHEELCHAIR SEAT CUSHION OR BACK CUSHION, EACH |
| E2620 | POSITIONING WHEELCHAIR BACK CUSHION, PLANAR BACK WITH LATERAL SUPPORTS, WIDTH LESS THAN 22 INCHES, ANY HEIGHT, INCLUDING ANY TYPE MOUNTING HARDWARE |
| E2621 | POSITIONING WHEELCHAIR BACK CUSHION, PLANAR BACK WITH LATERAL SUPPORTS, WIDTH 22 INCHES OR GREATER, ANY HEIGHT, INCLUDING ANY TYPE MOUNTING HARDWARE |
| K0015 | DETACHABLE, NON-ADJUSTABLE HEIGHT ARMREST, EACH |
| K0017 | DETACHABLE, ADJUSTABLE HEIGHT ARMREST, BASE, EACH |
| K0018 | DETACHABLE, ADJUSTABLE HEIGHT ARMREST, UPPER PORTION, EACH |
| K0019 | ARM PAD, EACH |
| K0020 | FIXED, ADJUSTABLE HEIGHT ARMREST, PAIR |
| K0037 | HIGH MOUNT FLIP-UP FOOTREST, EACH |
| K0038 | LEG STRAP, EACH |
| K0039 | LEG STRAP, H STYLE, EACH |
| K0040 | ADJUSTABLE ANGLE FOOTPLATE, EACH |
| K0041 | LARGE SIZE FOOTPLATE, EACH |
| K0042 | STANDARD SIZE FOOTPLATE, EACH |
| K0043 | FOOTREST, LOWER EXTENSION TUBE, EACH |
| K0044 | FOOTREST, UPPER HANGER BRACKET, EACH |
| K0045 | FOOTREST, COMPLETE ASSEMBLY |
| K0046 | ELEVATING LEGREST, LOWER EXTENSION TUBE, EACH |
| K0047 | ELEVATING LEGREST, UPPER HANGER BRACKET, EACH |
| K0050 | RATCHET ASSEMBLY |
| K0051 | CAM RELEASE ASSEMBLY, FOOTREST OR LEGREST, EACH |
| K0052 | SWINGAWAY, DETACHABLE FOOTRESTS, EACH |
| K0053 | ELEVATING FOOTRESTS, ARTICULATING (TELESCOPING), EACH |
| K0098 | DRIVE BELT FOR POWER WHEELCHAIR |
| K0195 | ELEVATING LEG RESTS, PAIR (FOR USE WITH CAPPED RENTAL WHEELCHAIR BASE) |
| K0733 | POWER WHEELCHAIR ACCESSORY, 12 TO 24 AMP HOUR SEALED LEAD ACID BATTERY, EACH (E.G., GEL CELL, ABSORBED GLASSMAT) |
| K0734 | SKIN PROTECTION WHEELCHAIR SEAT CUSHION, ADJUSTABLE, WIDTH LESS THAN 22 INCHES, ANY DEPTH |
| K0735 | SKIN PROTECTION WHEELCHAIR SEAT CUSHION, ADJUSTABLE, WIDTH 22 INCHES OR GREATER, ANY DEPTH |
| K0736 | SKIN PROTECTION AND POSITIONING WHEELCHAIR SEAT CUSHION, ADJUSTABLE, WIDTH LESS THAN 22 INCHES, ANY DEPTH |
| K0737 | SKIN PROTECTION AND POSITIONING WHEELCHAIR SEAT CUSHION, ADJUSTABLE, WIDTH 22 INCHES OR GREATER, ANY DEPTH |
| K0800 | POWER OPERATED VEHICLE, GROUP 1 STANDARD |
| K0801 | POWER OPERATED VEHICLE, GROUP 1 HEAVY DUTY |
| K0802 | POWER OPERATED VEHICLE, GROUP 1 VERY HEAVY DUTY |
| K0806 | POWER OPERATED VEHICLE, GROUP 2 STANDARD |
| K0807 | POWER OPERATED VEHICLE, GROUP 2 HEAVY DUTY |
| K0808 | POWER OPERATED VEHICLE, GROUP 2 VERY HEAVY DUTY |
| K0813 | POWER WHEELCHAIR, GROUP 1 STANDARD, PORTABLE, SLING/SOLID SEAT AND BACK |
| K0814 | POWER WHEELCHAIR, GROUP 1 STANDARD, PORTABLE, CAPTAINS CHAIR |
| K0815 | POWER WHEELCHAIR, GROUP 1 STANDARD, SLING/SOLID SEAT AND BACK |
| K0816 | POWER WHEELCHAIR, GROUP 1 STANDARD, CAPTAINS CHAIR |
| K0820 | POWER WHEELCHAIR, GROUP 2 STANDARD, PORTABLE, SLING/SOLID SEAT/BACK |
| K0821 | POWER WHEELCHAIR, GROUP 2 STANDARD, PORTABLE, CAPTAINS CHAIR |
| K0822 | POWER WHEELCHAIR, GROUP 2 STANDARD, SLING/SOLID SEAT/BACK |
| K0823 | POWER WHEELCHAIR, GROUP 2 STANDARD, CAPTAINS CHAIR |
| K0824 | POWER WHEELCHAIR, GROUP 2 HEAVY DUTY, SLING/SOLID SEAT/BACK |
| K0825 | POWER WHEELCHAIR, GROUP 2 HEAVY DUTY, CAPTAINS CHAIR |
| K0826 | POWER WHEELCHAIR, GROUP 2 VERY HEAVY DUTY, SLING/SOLID SEAT/BACK |
| K0827 | POWER WHEELCHAIR, GROUP 2 VERY HEAVY DUTY, CAPTAINS CHAIR |
| K0828 | POWER WHEELCHAIR, GROUP 2 EXTRA HEAVY DUTY, SLING/SOLID SEAT/BACK |
| K0829 | POWER WHEELCHAIR, GROUP 2 EXTRA HEAVY DUTY, CAPTAINS CHAIR |

**PRODUCT CATEGORY 3**

**Complex Rehabilitative Power Wheelchairs and Related Accessories**

| Code | Description |
|------|-------------|
| E0950 | WHEELCHAIR ACCESSORY, TRAY, EACH |
| E0951 | HEEL LOOP/HOLDER, ANY TYPE, WITH OR WITHOUT ANKLE STRAP, EACH |
| E0952 | TOE LOOP/HOLDER, ANY TYPE, EACH |
| E0955 | WHEELCHAIR ACCESSORY, HEADREST, CUSHIONED, ANY TYPE, INCLUDING FIXED MOUNTING HARDWARE, EACH |
| E0956 | WHEELCHAIR ACCESSORY, LATERAL TRUNK OR HIP SUPPORT, ANY TYPE, INCLUDING FIXED MOUNTING HARDWARE, EACH |
| E0957 | WHEELCHAIR ACCESSORY, MEDIAL THIGH SUPPORT, ANY TYPE, INCLUDING FIXED MOUNTING HARDWARE, EACH |
| E0960 | WHEELCHAIR ACCESSORY, SHOULDER HARNESS/STRAPS OR CHEST STRAP, INCLUDING ANY TYPE MOUNTING HARDWARE |
| E0973 | WHEELCHAIR ACCESSORY, ADJUSTABLE HEIGHT, DETACHABLE ARMREST, COMPLETE ASSEMBLY, EACH |
| E0978 | WHEELCHAIR ACCESSORY, POSITIONING BELT/SAFETY BELT/PELVIC STRAP, EACH |
| E0981 | WHEELCHAIR ACCESSORY, SEAT UPHOLSTERY, REPLACEMENT ONLY, EACH |
| E0982 | WHEELCHAIR ACCESSORY, BACK UPHOLSTERY, REPLACEMENT ONLY, EACH |
| E0990 | WHEELCHAIR ACCESSORY, ELEVATING LEG REST, COMPLETE ASSEMBLY, EACH |
| E0995 | WHEELCHAIR ACCESSORY, CALF REST/PAD, EACH |
| E1002 | WHEELCHAIR ACCESSORY, POWER SEATING SYSTEM, TILT ONLY |

© 2016 Optum360, LLC

E1003    WHEELCHAIR ACCESSORY, POWER SEATING SYSTEM, RECLINE ONLY, WITHOUT SHEAR REDUCTION

E1004    WHEELCHAIR ACCESSORY, POWER SEATING SYSTEM, RECLINE ONLY, WITH MECHANICAL SHEAR REDUCTION

E1005    WHEELCHAIR ACCESSORY, POWER SEATNG SYSTEM, RECLINE ONLY, WITH POWER SHEAR REDUCTION

E1006    WHEELCHAIR ACCESSORY, POWER SEATING SYSTEM, COMBINATION TILT AND RECLINE, WITHOUT SHEAR REDUCTION

E1007    WHEELCHAIR ACCESSORY, POWER SEATING SYSTEM, COMBINATION TILT AND RECLINE, WITH MECHANICAL SHEAR REDUCTION

E1008    WHEELCHAIR ACCESSORY, POWER SEATING SYSTEM, COMBINATION TILT AND RECLINE, WITH POWER SHEAR REDUCTION

E1010    WHEELCHAIR ACCESSORY, ADDITION TO POWER SEATING SYSTEM, POWER LEG ELEVATION SYSTEM, INCLUDING LEG REST, PAIR

E1016    SHOCK ABSORBER FOR POWER WHEELCHAIR, EACH

E1020    RESIDUAL LIMB SUPPORT SYSTEM FOR WHEELCHAIR

E1028    WHEELCHAIR ACCESSORY, MANUAL SWINGAWAY, RETRACTABLE OR REMOVABLE MOUNTING HARDWARE FOR JOYSTICK, OTHER CONTROL INTERFACE OR POSITIONING ACCESSORY

E1029    WHEELCHAIR ACCESSORY, VENTILATOR TRAY, FIXED

E1030    WHEELCHAIR ACCESSORY, VENTILATOR TRAY, GIMBALED

E2208    WHEELCHAIR ACCESSORY, CYLINDER TANK CARRIER, EACH

E2209    ACCESSORY, ARM TROUGH, WITH OR WITHOUT HAND SUPPORT, EACH

E2210    WHEELCHAIR ACCESSORY, BEARINGS, ANY TYPE, REPLACEMENT ONLY, EACH

E2310    POWER WHEELCHAIR ACCESSORY, ELECTRONIC CONNECTION BETWEEN WHEELCHAIR CONTROLLER AND ONE POWER SEATING SYSTEM MOTOR, INCLUDING ALL RELATED ELECTRONICS, INDICATOR FEATURE, MECHANICAL FUNCTION SELECTION SWITCH, AND FIXED MOUNTING HARDWARE

E2311    POWER WHEELCHAIR ACCESSORY, ELECTRONIC CONNECTION BETWEEN WHEELCHAIR CONTROLLER AND TWO OR MORE POWER SEATING SYSTEM MOTORS, INCLUDING ALL RELATED ELECTRONICS, INDICATOR FEATURE, MECHANICAL FUNCTION SELECTION SWITCH, AND FIXED MOUNTING HARDWARE

E2321    POWER WHEELCHAIR ACCESSORY, HAND CONTROL INTERFACE, REMOTE JOYSTICK, NONPROPORTIONAL, INCLUDING ALL RELATED ELECTRONICS, MECHANICAL STOP SWITCH, AND FIXED MOUNTING HARDWARE

E2322    POWER WHEELCHAIR ACCESSORY, HAND CONTROL INTERFACE, MULTIPLE MECHANICAL SWITCHES, NONPROPORTIONAL, INCLUDING ALL RELATED ELECTRONICS, MECHANICAL STOP SWITCH, AND FIXED MOUNTING HARDWARE

E2323    POWER WHEELCHAIR ACCESSORY, SPECIALTY JOYSTICK HANDLE FOR HAND CONTROL INTERFACE, PREFABRICATED

E2324    POWER WHEELCHAIR ACCESSORY, CHIN CUP FOR CHIN CONTROL INTERFACE

E2325    POWER WHEELCHAIR ACCESSORY, SIP AND PUFF INTERFACE, NONPROPORTIONAL, INCLUDING ALL RELATED ELECTRONICS, MECHANICAL STOP SWITCH, AND MANUAL SWINGAWAY MOUNTING HARDWARE

E2326    POWER WHEELCHAIR ACCESSORY, BREATH TUBE KIT FOR SIP AND PUFF INTERFACE

E2327    POWER WHEELCHAIR ACCESSORY, HEAD CONTROL INTERFACE, MECHANICAL, PROPORTIONAL, INCLUDING ALL RELATED ELECTRONICS, MECHANICAL DIRECTION CHANGE SWITCH, AND FIXED MOUNTING HARDWARE

E2328    POWER WHEELCHAIR ACCESSORY, HEAD CONTROL OR EXTREMITY CONTROL INTERFACE, ELECTRONIC, PROPORTIONAL, INCLUDING ALL RELATED ELECTRONICS AND FIXED MOUNTING HARDWARE

E2329    POWER WHEELCHAIR ACCESSORY, HEAD CONTROL INTERFACE, CONTACT SWITCH MECHANISM, NONPROPORTIONAL, INCLUDING ALL RELATED ELECTRONICS, MECHANICAL STOP SWITCH, MECHANICAL DIRECTION CHANGE SWITCH, HEAD ARRAY, AND FIXED MOUNTING HARDWARE

E2330    POWER WHEELCHAIR ACCESSORY, HEAD CONTROL INTERFACE, PROXIMITY SWITCH MECHANISM, NONPROPORTIONAL, INCLUDING ALL RELATED ELECTRONICS, MECHANICAL STOP SWITCH, MECHANICAL DIRECTION CHANGE SWITCH, HEAD ARRAY, AND FIXED MOUNTING HARDWARE

E2351    POWER WHEELCHAIR ACCESSORY, ELECTRONIC INTERFACE TO OPERATE SPEECH GENERATING DEVICE USING POWER WHEELCHAIR CONTROL INTERFACE

E2361    POWER WHEELCHAIR ACCESSORY, 22NF SEALED LEAD ACID BATTERY, EACH, (E.G. GEL CELL, ABSORBED GLASSMAT)

E2363    POWER WHEELCHAIR ACCESSORY, GROUP 24 SEALED LEAD ACID BATTERY, EACH (E.G. GEL CELL, ABSORBED GLASSMAT)

E2365    POWER WHEELCHAIR ACCESSORY, U-1 SEALED LEAD ACID BATTERY, EACH (E.G. GEL CELL, ABSORBED GLASSMAT)

E2366    POWER WHEELCHAIR ACCESSORY, BATTERY CHARGER, SINGLE MODE, FOR USE WITH ONLY ONE BATTERY TYPE, SEALED OR NON-SEALED, EACH

E2367    POWER WHEELCHAIR ACCESSORY, BATTERY CHARGER, DUAL MODE, FOR USE WITH EITHER BATTERY TYPE, SEALED OR NON-SEALED, EACH

E2368    POWER WHEELCHAIR COMPONENT, MOTOR, REPLACEMENT ONLY

E2369    POWER WHEELCHAIR COMPONENT, GEAR BOX, REPLACEMENT ONLY

E2370    POWER WHEELCHAIR COMPONENT, MOTOR AND GEAR BOX COMBINATION, REPLACEMENT ONLY

E2371    POWER WHEELCHAIR ACCESSORY, GROUP 27 SEALED LEAD ACID BATTERY, (E.G. GEL CELL, ABSORBED GLASSMAT), EACH

E2373 KC  POWER WHEELCHAIR ACCESSORY, HAND OR CHIN CONTROL INTERFACE, COMPACT REMOTE JOYSTICK, PROPORTIONAL, INCLUDING FIXED MOUNTING HARDWARE

E2374    POWER WHEELCHAIR ACCESSORY, HAND OR CHIN CONTROL INTERFACE, STANDARD REMOTE JOYSTICK (NOT INCLUDING CONTROLLER), PROPORTIONAL, INCLUDING ALL RELATED ELECTRONICS AND FIXED MOUNTING HARDWARE, REPLACEMENT ONLY

E2375    POWER WHEELCHAIR ACCESSORY, NON-EXPANDABLE CONTROLLER, INCLUDING ALL RELATED ELECTRONICS AND MOUNTING HARDWARE, REPLACEMENT ONLY

E2376    POWER WHEELCHAIR ACCESSORY, EXPANDABLE CONTROLLER, INCLUDING ALL RELATED ELECTRONICS AND MOUNTING HARDWARE, REPLACEMENT ONLY

E2377    POWER WHEELCHAIR ACCESSORY, EXPANDABLE CONTROLLER, INCLUDING ALL RELATED ELECTRONICS AND MOUNTING HARDWARE, UPGRADE PROVIDED AT INITIAL ISSUE

E2381    POWER WHEELCHAIR ACCESSORY, PNEUMATIC DRIVE WHEEL TIRE, ANY SIZE, REPLACEMENT ONLY, EACH

E2382    POWER WHEELCHAIR ACCESSORY, TUBE FOR PNEUMATIC DRIVE WHEEL TIRE, ANY SIZE, REPLACEMENT ONLY, EACH

E2383    POWER WHEELCHAIR ACCESSORY, INSERT FOR PNEUMATIC DRIVE WHEEL TIRE (REMOVABLE), ANY TYPE, ANY SIZE, REPLACEMENT ONLY, EACH

E2384    POWER WHEELCHAIR ACCESSORY, PNEUMATIC CASTER TIRE, ANY SIZE, REPLACEMENT ONLY, EACH

E2385    POWER WHEELCHAIR ACCESSORY, TUBE FOR PNEUMATIC CASTER TIRE, ANY SIZE, REPLACEMENT ONLY, EACH

E2386    POWER WHEELCHAIR ACCESSORY, FOAM FILLED DRIVE WHEEL TIRE, ANY SIZE, REPLACEMENT ONLY, EACH

E2387    POWER WHEELCHAIR ACCESSORY, FOAM FILLED CASTER TIRE, ANY SIZE, REPLACEMENT ONLY, EACH

E2388    POWER WHEELCHAIR ACCESSORY, FOAM DRIVE WHEEL TIRE, ANY SIZE, REPLACEMENT ONLY, EACH

E2389    POWER WHEELCHAIR ACCESSORY, FOAM CASTER TIRE, ANY SIZE, REPLACEMENT ONLY, EACH

E2390    POWER WHEELCHAIR ACCESSORY, SOLID (RUBBER/PLASTIC) DRIVE WHEEL TIRE, ANY SIZE, REPLACEMENT ONLY, EACH

E2391    POWER WHEELCHAIR ACCESSORY, SOLID (RUBBER/PLASTIC) CASTER TIRE (REMOVABLE), ANY SIZE, REPLACEMENT ONLY, EACH

E2392    POWER WHEELCHAIR ACCESSORY, SOLID (RUBBER/PLASTIC) CASTER TIRE WITH INTEGRATED WHEEL, ANY SIZE, REPLACEMENT ONLY, EACH

E2394    POWER WHEELCHAIR ACCESSORY, DRIVE WHEEL EXCLUDES TIRE, ANY SIZE, REPLACEMENT ONLY, EACH

| | | | | |
|---|---|---|---|---|
| E2395 | POWER WHEELCHAIR ACCESSORY, CASTER WHEEL EXCLUDES TIRE, ANY SIZE, REPLACEMENT ONLY, EACH | | K0052 | SWINGAWAY, DETACHABLE FOOTRESTS, EACH |
| E2396 | POWER WHEELCHAIR ACCESSORY, CASTER FORK, ANY SIZE, REPLACEMENT ONLY, EACH | | K0053 | ELEVATING FOOTRESTS, ARTICULATING (TELESCOPING), EACH |
| | | | K0098 | DRIVE BELT FOR POWER WHEELCHAIR |
| E2601 | GENERAL USE WHEELCHAIR SEAT CUSHION, WIDTH LESS THAN 22 INCHES, ANY DEPTH | | K0195 | ELEVATING LEG RESTS, PAIR (FOR USE WITH CAPPED RENTAL WHEELCHAIR BASE) |
| E2602 | GENERAL USE WHEELCHAIR SEAT CUSHION, WIDTH 22 INCHES OR GREATER, ANY DEPTH | | K0733 | POWER WHEELCHAIR ACCESSORY, 12 TO 24 AMP HOUR SEALED LEAD ACID BATTERY, EACH (E.G., GEL CELL, ABSORBED GLASSMAT) |
| E2603 | SKIN PROTECTION WHEELCHAIR SEAT CUSHION, WIDTH LESS THAN 22 INCHES, ANY DEPTH | | K0734 | SKIN PROTECTION WHEELCHAIR SEAT CUSHION, ADJUSTABLE, WIDTH LESS THAN 22 INCHES, ANY DEPTH |
| E2604 | SKIN PROTECTION WHEELCHAIR SEAT CUSHION, WIDTH 22 INCHES OR GREATER, ANY DEPTH | | K0735 | SKIN PROTECTION WHEELCHAIR SEAT CUSHION, ADJUSTABLE, WIDTH 22 INCHES OR GREATER, ANY DEPTH |
| E2605 | POSITIONING WHEELCHAIR SEAT CUSHION, WIDTH LESS THAN 22 INCHES, ANY DEPTH | | K0736 | SKIN PROTECTION AND POSITIONING WHEELCHAIR SEAT CUSHION, ADJUSTABLE, WIDTH LESS THAN 22 INCHES, ANY DEPTH |
| E2606 | POSITIONING WHEELCHAIR SEAT CUSHION, WIDTH 22 INCHES OR GREATER, ANY DEPTH | | K0737 | SKIN PROTECTION AND POSITIONING WHEELCHAIR SEAT CUSHION, ADJUSTABLE, WIDTH 22 INCHES OR GREATER, ANY DEPTH |
| E2607 | SKIN PROTECTION AND POSITIONING WHEELCHAIR SEAT CUSHION, WIDTH LESS THAN 22 INCHES, ANY DEPTH | | K0835 | POWER WHEELCHAIR, GROUP 2 STANDARD, SINGLE POWER OPTION, SLING/SOLID SEAT/BACK, PATIENT WEIGHT CAPACITY UP TO AND INCLUDING 300 POUNDS |
| E2608 | SKIN PROTECTION AND POSITIONING WHEELCHAIR SEAT CUSHION, WIDTH 22 INCHES OR GREATER, ANY DEPTH | | K0836 | POWER WHEELCHAIR, GROUP 2 STANDARD, SINGLE POWER OPTION, CAPTAINS CHAIR, PATIENT WEIGHT CAPACITY UP TO AND INCLUDING 300 POUNDS |
| E2611 | GENERAL USE WHEELCHAIR BACK CUSHION, WIDTH LESS THAN 22 INCHES, ANY HEIGHT, INCLUDING ANY TYPE MOUNTING HARDWARE | | K0837 | POWER WHEELCHAIR, GROUP 2 HEAVY DUTY, SINGLE POWER OPTION, SLING/SOLID SEAT/BACK, PATIENT WEIGHT CAPACITY 301 TO 450 POUNDS |
| E2612 | GENERAL USE WHEELCHAIR BACK CUSHION, WIDTH 22 INCHES OR GREATER, ANY HEIGHT, INCLUDING ANY TYPE MOUNTING HARDWARE | | K0838 | POWER WHEELCHAIR, GROUP 2 HEAVY DUTY, SINGLE POWER OPTION, CAPTAINS CHAIR, PATIENT WEIGHT CAPACITY 301 TO 450 POUNDS |
| E2613 | POSITIONING WHEELCHAIR BACK CUSHION, POSTERIOR, WIDTH LESS THAN 22 INCHES, ANY HEIGHT, INCLUDING ANY TYPE MOUNTING HARDWARE | | K0839 | POWER WHEELCHAIR, GROUP 2 VERY HEAVY DUTY, SINGLE POWER OPTION SLING/SOLID SEAT/BACK, PATIENT WEIGHT CAPACITY 451 TO 600 POUNDS |
| E2614 | POSITIONING WHEELCHAIR BACK CUSHION, POSTERIOR, WIDTH 22 INCHES OR GREATER, ANY HEIGHT, INCLUDING ANY TYPE MOUNTING HARDWARE | | K0840 | POWER WHEELCHAIR, GROUP 2 EXTRA HEAVY DUTY, SINGLE POWER OPTION, SLING/SOLID SEAT/BACK, PATIENT WEIGHT CAPACITY 601 POUNDS OR MORE |
| E2615 | POSITIONING WHEELCHAIR BACK CUSHION, POSTERIOR-LATERAL, WIDTH LESS THAN 22 INCHES, ANY HEIGHT, INCLUDING ANY TYPE MOUNTING HARDWARE | | K0841 | POWER WHEELCHAIR, GROUP 2 STANDARD, MULTIPLE POWER OPTION, SLING/SOLID SEAT/BACK, PATIENT WEIGHT CAPACITY UP TO AND INCLUDING 300 POUNDS |
| E2616 | POSITIONING WHEELCHAIR BACK CUSHION, POSTERIOR-LATERAL, WIDTH 22 INCHES OR GREATER, ANY HEIGHT, INCLUDING ANY TYPE MOUNTING HARDWARE | | K0842 | POWER WHEELCHAIR, GROUP 2 STANDARD, MULTIPLE POWER OPTION, CAPTAINS CHAIR, PATIENT WEIGHT CAPACITY UP TO AND INCLUDING 300 POUNDS |
| E2619 | REPLACEMENT COVER FOR WHEELCHAIR SEAT CUSHION OR BACK CUSHION, EACH | | K0843 | POWER WHEELCHAIR, GROUP 2 HEAVY DUTY, MULTIPLE POWER OPTION, SLING/SOLID SEAT/BACK, PATIENT WEIGHT CAPACITY 301 TO 450 POUNDS |
| E2620 | POSITIONING WHEELCHAIR BACK CUSHION, PLANAR BACK WITH LATERAL SUPPORTS, WIDTH LESS THAN 22 INCHES, ANY HEIGHT, INCLUDING ANY TYPE MOUNTING HARDWARE | | K0848 | POWER WHEELCHAIR, GROUP 3 STANDARD, SLING/SOLID SEAT/BACK, PATIENT WEIGHT CAPACITY UP TO AND INCLUDING 300 POUNDS |
| E2621 | POSITIONING WHEELCHAIR BACK CUSHION, PLANAR BACK WITH LATERAL SUPPORTS, WIDTH 22 INCHES OR GREATER, ANY HEIGHT, INCLUDING ANY TYPE MOUNTING HARDWARE | | K0849 | POWER WHEELCHAIR, GROUP 3 STANDARD, CAPTAINS CHAIR, PATIENT WEIGHT CAPACITY UP TO AND INCLUDING 300 POUNDS |
| K0015 | DETACHABLE, NON-ADJUSTABLE HEIGHT ARMREST, EACH | | K0850 | POWER WHEELCHAIR, GROUP 3 HEAVY DUTY, SLING/SOLID SEAT/BACK, PATIENT WEIGHT CAPACITY 301 TO 450 POUNDS |
| K0017 | DETACHABLE, ADJUSTABLE HEIGHT ARMREST, BASE, EACH | | K0851 | POWER WHEELCHAIR, GROUP 3 HEAVY DUTY, CAPTAINS CHAIR, PATIENT WEIGHT CAPACITY 301 TO 450 POUNDS |
| K0018 | DETACHABLE, ADJUSTABLE HEIGHT ARMREST, UPPER PORTION, EACH | | K0852 | POWER WHEELCHAIR, GROUP 3 VERY HEAVY DUTY, SLING/SOLID SEAT/BACK, PATIENT WEIGHT CAPACITY 451 TO 600 POUNDS |
| K0019 | ARM PAD, EACH | | | |
| K0020 | FIXED, ADJUSTABLE HEIGHT ARMREST, PAIR | | K0853 | POWER WHEELCHAIR, GROUP 3 VERY HEAVY DUTY, CAPTAINS CHAIR, PATIENT WEIGHT CAPACITY 451 TO 600 POUNDS |
| K0037 | HIGH MOUNT FLIP-UP FOOTREST, EACH | | K0854 | POWER WHEELCHAIR, GROUP 3 EXTRA HEAVY DUTY, SLING/SOLID SEAT/BACK, PATIENT WEIGHT CAPACITY 601 POUNDS OR MORE |
| K0038 | LEG STRAP, EACH | | | |
| K0039 | LEG STRAP, H STYLE, EACH | | K0855 | POWER WHEELCHAIR, GROUP 3 EXTRA HEAVY DUTY, CAPTAINS CHAIR, PATIENT WEIGHT CAPACITY 601 POUNDS OR MORE |
| K0040 | ADJUSTABLE ANGLE FOOTPLATE, EACH | | | |
| K0041 | LARGE SIZE FOOTPLATE, EACH | | K0856 | POWER WHEELCHAIR, GROUP 3 STANDARD, SINGLE POWER OPTION, SLING/SOLID SEAT/BACK, PATIENT WEIGHT CAPACITY UP TO AND INCLUDING 300 POUNDS |
| K0042 | STANDARD SIZE FOOTPLATE, EACH | | | |
| K0043 | FOOTREST, LOWER EXTENSION TUBE, EACH | | | |
| K0044 | FOOTREST, UPPER HANGER BRACKET, EACH | | K0857 | POWER WHEELCHAIR, GROUP 3 STANDARD, SINGLE POWER OPTION, CAPTAINS CHAIR, PATIENT WEIGHT CAPACITY UP TO AND INCLUDING 300 POUNDS |
| K0045 | FOOTREST, COMPLETE ASSEMBLY | | | |
| K0046 | ELEVATING LEGREST, LOWER EXTENSION TUBE, EACH | | | |
| K0047 | ELEVATING LEGREST, UPPER HANGER BRACKET, EACH | | | |
| K0050 | RATCHET ASSEMBLY | | | |
| K0051 | CAM RELEASE ASSEMBLY, FOOTREST OR LEGREST, EACH | | | |

© 2016 Optum360, LLC

K0858    POWER WHEELCHAIR, GROUP 3 HEAVY DUTY, SINGLE POWER OPTION, SLING/SOLID SEAT/BACK, PATIENT WEIGHT 301 TO 450 POUNDS

K0859    POWER WHEELCHAIR, GROUP 3 HEAVY DUTY, SINGLE POWER OPTION, CAPTAINS CHAIR, PATIENT WEIGHT CAPACITY 301 TO 450 POUNDS

K0860    POWER WHEELCHAIR, GROUP 3 VERY HEAVY DUTY, SINGLE POWER OPTION, SLING/SOLID SEAT/BACK, PATIENT WEIGHT CAPACITY 451 TO 600 POUNDS

K0861    POWER WHEELCHAIR, GROUP 3 STANDARD, MULTIPLE POWER OPTION, SLING/SOLID SEAT/BACK, PATIENT WEIGHT CAPACITY UP TO AND INCLUDING 300 POUNDS

K0862    POWER WHEELCHAIR, GROUP 3 HEAVY DUTY, MULTIPLE POWER OPTION, SLING/SOLID SEAT/BACK, PATIENT WEIGHT CAPACITY 301 TO 450 POUNDS

K0863    POWER WHEELCHAIR, GROUP 3 VERY HEAVY DUTY, MULTIPLE POWER OPTION, SLING/SOLID SEAT/BACK, PATIENT WEIGHT CAPACITY 451 TO 600 POUNDS

K0864    POWER WHEELCHAIR, GROUP 3 EXTRA HEAVY DUTY, MULTIPLE POWER OPTION, SLING/SOLID SEAT/BACK, PATIENT WEIGHT CAPACITY 601 POUNDS OR MORE

## PRODUCT CATEGORY 4

### Mail-Order Diabetic Supplies

A4233 KL    REPLACEMENT BATTERY, ALKALINE (OTHER THAN J CELL), FOR USE WITH MEDICALLY NECESSARY HOME BLOOD GLUCOSE MONITOR OWNED BY PATIENT, EACH

A4234 KL    REPLACEMENT BATTERY, ALKALINE, J CELL, FOR USE WITH MEDICALLY NECESSARY HOME BLOOD GLUCOSE MONITOR OWNED BY PATIENT, EACH

A4235 KL    REPLACEMENT BATTERY, LITHIUM, FOR USE WITH MEDICALLY NECESSARY HOME BLOOD GLUCOSE MONITOR OWNED BY PATIENT, EACH

A4236 KL    REPLACEMENT BATTERY, SILVER OXIDE, FOR USE WITH MEDICALLY NECESSARY HOME BLOOD GLUCOSE MONITOR OWNED BY PATIENT, EACH

A4253 KL    BLOOD GLUCOSE TEST OR REAGENT STRIPS FOR HOME BLOOD GLUCOSE MONITOR, PER 50 STRIPS

A4256 KL    NORMAL, LOW AND HIGH CALIBRATOR SOLUTION / CHIPS

A4258 KL    SPRING-POWERED DEVICE FOR LANCET, EACH

A4259 KL    LANCETS, PER BOX OF 100

## PRODUCT CATEGORY 5

### Enteral Nutrients, Equipment, and Supplies

B4034    ENTERAL FEEDING SUPPLY KIT; SYRINGE FED, PER DAY

B4035    ENTERAL FEEDING SUPPLY KIT; PUMP FED, PER DAY

B4036    ENTERAL FEEDING SUPPLY KIT; GRAVITY FED, PER DAY

B4081    NASOGASTRIC TUBING WITH STYLET

B4082    NASOGASTRIC TUBING WITHOUT STYLET

B4083    STOMACH TUBE - LEVINE TYPE

B4087    GASTROSTOMY / JEJUNOSTOMY TUBE, ANY MATERIAL, ANY TYPE, (STANDARD), EACH

B4088    GASTROSTOMY / JEJUNOSTOMY TUBE, ANY MATERIAL, ANY TYPE, (LOW PROFILE), EACH

B4149    ENTERAL FORMULA, MANUFACTURED BLENDERIZED NATURAL FOODS WITH INTACT NUTRIENTS, INCLUDES PROTEINS, FATS, CARBOHYDRATES, VITAMINS AND MINERALS, MAY INCLUDE FIBER, ADMINISTERED THROUGH AN ENTERAL FEEDING TUBE, 100 CALORIES = 1 UNIT

B4150    ENTERAL FORMULA, NUTRITIONALLY COMPLETE WITH INTACT NUTRIENTS, INCLUDES PROTEINS, FATS, CARBOHYDRATES, VITAMINS AND MINERALS, MAY INCLUDE FIBER, ADMINISTERED THROUGH AN ENTERAL FEEDING TUBE, 100 CALORIES = 1 UNIT

B4152    ENTERAL FORMULA, NUTRITIONALLY COMPLETE, CALORICALLY DENSE (EQUAL TO OR GREATER THAN 1.5 KCAL/ML) WITH INTACT NUTRIENTS, INCLUDES PROTEINS, FATS, CARBOHYDRATES, VITAMINS AND MINERALS, MAY INCLUDE FIBER, ADMINISTERED THROUGH AN ENTERAL FEEDING TUBE, 100 CALORIES = 1 UNIT

B4153    ENTERAL FORMULA, NUTRITIONALLY COMPLETE, HYDROLYZED PROTEINS (AMINO ACIDS AND PEPTIDE CHAIN), INCLUDES FATS, CARBOHYDRATES, VITAMINS AND MINERALS, MAY INCLUDE FIBER, ADMINISTERED THROUGH AN ENTERAL FEEDING TUBE, 100 CALORIES = 1 UNIT

B4154    ENTERAL FORMULA, NUTRITIONALLY COMPLETE, FOR SPECIAL METABOLIC NEEDS, EXCLUDES INHERITED DISEASE OF METABOLISM, INCLUDES ALTERED COMPOSITION OF PROTEINS, FATS, CARBOHYDRATES, VITAMINS AND/OR MINERALS, MAY INCLUDE FIBER, ADMINISTERED THROUGH AN ENTERAL FEEDING TUBE, 100 CALORIES = 1 UNIT

B4155    ENTERAL FORMULA, NUTRITIONALLY INCOMPLETE/MODULAR NUTRIENTS, INCLUDES SPECIFIC NUTRIENTS, CARBOHYDRATES (E.G. GLUCOSE POLYMERS), PROTEINS/AMINO ACIDS (E.G. GLUTAMINE, ARGININE), FAT (E.G. MEDIUM CHAIN TRIGLYCERIDES) OR COMBINATON, ADMINISTERED THROUGH AN ENTERAL FEEDING TUBE, 100 CALORIES = 1 UNIT NOTE: (SEE J7060, J7070, J7042 FOR SOLUTION CODES FOR OTHER THAN PARENTERAL NUTRITION THERAPY USE)

B9000    ENTERAL NUTRITION INFUSION PUMP - WITHOUT ALARM

B9002    ENTERAL NUTRITION INFUSION PUMP - WITH ALARM

E0776    IV POLE

## PRODUCT CATEGORY 6

### Continuous Positive Airway Pressure Devices, Respiratory Assist Devices, and Related Supplies and Accessories

A4604    TUBING WITH INTEGRATED HEATING ELEMENT FOR USE WITH POSITIVE AIRWAY PRESSURE DEVICE

A7030    FULL FACE MASK USED WITH POSITIVE AIRWAY PRESSURE DEVICE, EACH

A7031    FACE MASK INTERFACE, REPLACEMENT FOR FULL FACE MASK, EACH

A7032    CUSHION FOR USE ON NASAL MASK INTERFACE, REPLACEMENT ONLY, EACH

A7033    PILLOW FOR USE ON NASAL CANNULA TYPE INTERFACE, REPLACEMENT ONLY, PAIR

A7034    NASAL INTERFACE (MASK OR CANNULA TYPE) USED WITH POSITIVE AIRWAY PRESSURE DEVICE, WITH OR WITHOUT HEAD STRAP

A7035    HEADGEAR USED WITH POSITIVE AIRWAY PRESSURE DEVICE

A7036    CHINSTRAP USED WITH POSITIVE AIRWAY PRESSURE DEVICE

A7037    TUBING USED WITH POSITIVE AIRWAY PRESSURE DEVICE

A7038    FILTER, DISPOSABLE, USED WITH POSITIVE AIRWAY PRESSURE DEVICE

A7039    FILTER, NON DISPOSABLE, USED WITH POSITIVE AIRWAY PRESSURE DEVICE

A7044    ORAL INTERFACE USED WITH POSITIVE AIRWAY PRESSURE DEVICE, EACH

A7045    EXHALATION PORT WITH OR WITHOUT SWIVEL USED WITH ACCESSORIES FOR POSITIVE AIRWAY DEVICES, REPLACEMENT ONLY

A7046    WATER CHAMBER FOR HUMIDIFIER, USED WITH POSITIVE AIRWAY PRESSURE DEVICE, REPLACEMENT, EACH

E0470    RESPIRATORY ASSIST DEVICE, BI-LEVEL PRESSURE CAPABILITY, WITHOUT BACKUP RATE FEATURE, USED WITH NONINVASIVE INTERFACE, E.G., NASAL OR FACIAL MASK (INTERMITTENT ASSIST DEVICE WITH CONTINUOUS POSITIVE AIRWAY PRESSURE DEVICE)

E0471    RESPIRATORY ASSIST DEVICE, BI-LEVEL PRESSURE CAPABILITY, WITH BACK-UP RATE FEATURE, USED WITH NONINVASIVE INTERFACE, E.G., NASAL OR FACIAL MASK (INTERMITTENT ASSIST DEVICE WITH CONTINUOUS POSITIVE AIRWAY PRESSURE DEVICE)

E0472    RESPIRATORY ASSIST DEVICE, BI-LEVEL PRESSURE CAPABILITY, WITH BACKUP RATE FEATURE, USED WITH INVASIVE INTERFACE, E.G., TRACHEOSTOMY TUBE (INTERMITTENT ASSIST DEVICE WITH CONTINUOUS POSITIVE AIRWAY PRESSURE DEVICE)

E0561    HUMIDIFIER, NON-HEATED, USED WITH POSITIVE AIRWAY PRESSURE DEVICE

E0562    HUMIDIFIER, HEATED, USED WITH POSITIVE AIRWAY PRESSURE DEVICE

E0601    CONTINUOUS AIRWAY PRESSURE (CPAP) DEVICE

## PRODUCT CATEGORY 7

### Hospital Beds and Related Supplies

E0250    HOSPITAL BED, FIXED HEIGHT, WITH ANY TYPE SIDE RAILS, WITH MATTRESS

E0251    HOSPITAL BED, FIXED HEIGHT, WITH ANY TYPE SIDE RAILS, WITHOUT MATTRESS

E0255    HOSPITAL BED, VARIABLE HEIGHT, HI-LO, WITH ANY TYPE SIDE RAILS, WITH MATTRESS

| | |
|---|---|
| E0256 | HOSPITAL BED, VARIABLE HEIGHT, HI-LO, WITH ANY TYPE SIDE RAILS, WITHOUT MATTRESS |
| E0260 | HOSPITAL BED, SEMI-ELECTRIC (HEAD AND FOOT ADJUSTMENT), WITH ANY TYPE SIDE RAILS, WITH MATTRESS |
| E0261 | HOSPITAL BED, SEMI-ELECTRIC (HEAD AND FOOT ADJUSTMENT), WITH ANY TYPE SIDE RAILS, WITHOUT MATTRESS |
| E0265 | HOSPITAL BED, TOTAL ELECTRIC (HEAD, FOOT AND HEIGHT ADJUSTMENTS), WITH ANY TYPE SIDE RAILS, WITH MATTRESS |
| E0266 | HOSPITAL BED, TOTAL ELECTRIC (HEAD, FOOT AND HEIGHT ADJUSTMENTS), WITH ANY TYPE SIDE RAILS, WITHOUT MATTRESS |
| E0271 | MATTRESS, INNERSPRING |
| E0272 | MATTRESS, FOAM RUBBER |
| E0280 | BED CRADLE, ANY TYPE |
| E0290 | HOSPITAL BED, FIXED HEIGHT, WITHOUT SIDE RAILS, WITH MATTRESS |
| E0291 | HOSPITAL BED, FIXED HEIGHT, WITHOUT SIDE RAILS, WITHOUT MATTRESS |
| E0292 | HOSPITAL BED, VARIABLE HEIGHT, HI-LO, WITHOUT SIDE RAILS, WITH MATTRESS |
| E0293 | HOSPITAL BED, VARIABLE HEIGHT, HI-LO, WITHOUT SIDE RAILS, WITHOUT MATTRESS |
| E0294 | HOSPITAL BED, SEMI-ELECTRIC (HEAD AND FOOT ADJUSTMENT), WITHOUT SIDE RAILS, WITH MATTRESS |
| E0295 | HOSPITAL BED, SEMI-ELECTRIC (HEAD AND FOOT ADJUSTMENT), WITHOUT SIDE RAILS, WITHOUT MATTRESS |
| E0296 | HOSPITAL BED, TOTAL ELECTRIC (HEAD, FOOT AND HEIGHT ADJUSTMENTS). WITHOUT SIDE RAILS, WITH MATTRESS |
| E0297 | HOSPITAL BED, TOTAL ELECTRIC (HEAD, FOOT AND HEIGHT ADJUSTMENTS), WITHOUT SIDE RAILS, WITHOUT MATTRESS |
| E0300 | PEDIATRIC CRIB, HOSPITAL GRADE, FULLY ENCLOSED |
| E0301 | HOSPITAL BED, HEAVY DUTY, EXTRA WIDE, WITH WEIGHT CAPACITY GREATER THAN 350 POUNDS, BUT LESS THAN OR EQUAL TO 600 POUNDS, WITH ANY TYPE SIDE RAILS, WITHOUT MATTRESS |
| E0302 | HOSPITAL BED, EXTRA HEAVY DUTY, EXTRA WIDE, WITH WEIGHT CAPACITY GREATER THAN 600 POUNDS, WITH ANY TYPE SIDE RAILS, WITHOUT MATTRESS |
| E0303 | HOSPITAL BED, HEAVY DUTY, EXTRA WIDE, WITH WEIGHT CAPACITY GREATER THAN 350 POUNDS, BUT LESS THAN OR EQUAL TO 600 POUNDS, WITH ANY TYPE SIDE RAILS, WITH MATTRESS |
| E0304 | HOSPITAL BED, EXTRA HEAVY DUTY, EXTRA WIDE, WITH WEIGHT CAPACITY GREATER THAN 600 POUNDS, WITH ANY TYPE SIDE RAILS, WITH MATTRESS |
| E0305 | BED SIDE RAILS, HALF LENGTH |
| E0310 | BED SIDE RAILS, FULL LENGTH |
| E0316 | SAFETY ENCLOSURE FRAME/CANOPY FOR USE WITH HOSPITAL BED, ANY TYPE |
| E0910 | TRAPEZE BARS, A/K/A PATIENT HELPER, ATTACHED TO BED, WITH GRAB BAR |
| E0911 | TRAPEZE BAR, HEAVY DUTY, FOR PATIENT WEIGHT CAPACITY GREATER THAN 250 POUNDS, ATTACHED TO BED, WITH GRAB BAR |
| E0912 | TRAPEZE BAR, HEAVY DUTY, FOR PATIENT WEIGHT CAPACITY GREATER THAN 250 POUNDS, FREE STANDING, COMPLETE WITH GRAB BAR |
| E0940 | TRAPEZE BAR, FREE STANDING, COMPLETE WITH GRAB BAR |

**PRODUCT CATEGORY 8**

**Negative Pressure Wound Therapy Pumps and Related Supplies and Accessories**

| | |
|---|---|
| A6550 | WOUND CARE SET, FOR NEGATIVE PRESSURE WOUND THERAPY ELECTRICAL PUMP, INCLUDES ALL SUPPLIES AND ACCESSORIES |
| A7000 | CANISTER, DISPOSABLE, USED WITH SUCTION PUMP, EACH |
| E2402 | NEGATIVE PRESSURE WOUND THERAPY ELECTRICAL PUMP, STATIONARY OR PORTABLE |

**PRODUCT CATEGORY 9**

**Walkers and Related Accessories**

| | |
|---|---|
| A4636 | REPLACEMENT, HANDGRIP, CANE, CRUTCH, OR WALKER, EACH |

| | |
|---|---|
| A4637 | REPLACEMENT, TIP, CANE, CRUTCH, WALKER, EACH. |
| E0130 | WALKER, RIGID (PICKUP), ADJUSTABLE OR FIXED HEIGHT |
| E0135 | WALKER, FOLDING (PICKUP), ADJUSTABLE OR FIXED HEIGHT |
| E0140 | WALKER, WITH TRUNK SUPPORT, ADJUSTABLE OR FIXED HEIGHT, ANY TYPE |
| E0141 | WALKER, RIGID, WHEELED, ADJUSTABLE OR FIXED HEIGHT |
| E0143 | WALKER, FOLDING, WHEELED, ADJUSTABLE OR FIXED HEIGHT |
| E0144 | WALKER, ENCLOSED, FOUR SIDED FRAMED, RIGID OR FOLDING, WHEELED WITH POSTERIOR SEAT |
| E0147 | WALKER, HEAVY DUTY, MULTIPLE BRAKING SYSTEM, VARIABLE WHEEL RESISTANCE |
| E0148 | WALKER, HEAVY DUTY, WITHOUT WHEELS, RIGID OR FOLDING, ANY TYPE, EACH |
| E0149 | WALKER, HEAVY DUTY, WHEELED, RIGID OR FOLDING, ANY TYPE |
| E0154 | PLATFORM ATTACHMENT, WALKER, EACH |
| E0155 | WHEEL ATTACHMENT, RIGID PICK-UP WALKER, PER PAIR |
| E0156 | SEAT ATTACHMENT, WALKER |
| E0157 | CRUTCH ATTACHMENT, WALKER, EACH |
| E0158 | LEG EXTENSIONS FOR WALKER, PER SET OF FOUR (4) |
| E0159 | BRAKE ATTACHMENT FOR WHEELED WALKER, REPLACEMENT, EACH |

**PRODUCT CATEGORY 10**

**Support Surfaces**

| | |
|---|---|
| E0193 | POWERED AIR FLOTATION BED (LOW AIR LOSS THERAPY) |
| E0277 | POWERED PRESSURE-REDUCING AIR MATTRESS |
| E0371 | NONPOWERED ADVANCED PRESSURE REDUCING OVERLAY FOR MATTRESS, STANDARD MATTRESS LENGTH AND WIDTH |
| E0372 | POWERED AIR OVERLAY FOR MATTRESS, STANDARD MATTRESS LENGTH AND WIDTH |
| E0373 | NONPOWERED ADVANCED PRESSURE REDUCING MATTRESS |

## 100-04, 32, 11.1

**Electrical Stimulation**

### A. Coding Applicable to Carriers & Fiscal Intermediaries (FIs)

Effective April 1, 2003, a National Coverage Decision was made to allow for Medicare coverage of Electrical Stimulation for the treatment of certain types of wounds. The type of wounds covered are chronic Stage III or Stage IV pressure ulcers, arterial ulcers, diabetic ulcers and venous stasis ulcers. All other uses of electrical stimulation for the treatment of wounds are not covered by Medicare. Electrical stimulation will not be covered as an initial treatment modality.

The use of electrical stimulation will only be covered after appropriate standard wound care has been tried for at least 30 days and there are no measurable signs of healing. If electrical stimulation is being used, wounds must be evaluated periodically by the treating physician but no less than every 30 days by a physician. Continued treatment with electrical stimulation is not covered if measurable signs of healing have not been demonstrated within any 30-day period of treatment. Additionally, electrical stimulation must be discontinued when the wound demonstrates a 100% epithelialzed wound bed.

Coverage policy can be found in Pub. 100-03, Medicare National Coverage Determinations Manual, Chapter 1, Section 270.1 (http://www.cms.hhs.gov/manuals/103_cov_determ/ncd103index.asp)

The applicable Healthcare Common Procedure Coding System (HCPCS) code for Electrical Stimulation and the covered effective date is as follows:

| HCPCS | Definition | Effective Date |
|---|---|---|
| G0281 | Electrical Stimulation, (unattended), to one or more areas for chronic Stage III and Stage IV pressure ulcers, arterial ulcers, diabetic ulcers and venous stasis ulcers not demonstrating measurable signs of healing after 30 days of conventional care as part of a therapy plan of care. | 04/01/2003 |

Medicare will not cover the device used for the electrical stimulation for the treatment of wounds. However, Medicare will cover the service. Unsupervised home use of electrical stimulation will not be covered.

### B. FI Billing Instructions

The applicable types of bills acceptable when billing for electrical stimulation services are 12X, 13X, 22X, 23X, 71X, 73X, 74X, 75X, and 85X. Chapter 25 of this manual provides general billing instructions that must be followed for bills submitted to FIs. FIs pay for electrical stimulation services under the Medicare Physician Fee Schedule for a hospital, Comprehensive Outpatient Rehabilitation Facility (CORF), Outpatient Rehabilitation Facility (ORF), Outpatient Physical Therapy (OPT) and Skilled Nursing Facility (SNF).

Payment methodology for independent Rural Health Clinic (RHC), provider-based RHCs, free-standing Federally Qualified Health Center (FQHC) and provider based FQHCs is made under the all-inclusive rate for the visit furnished to the RHC/FQHC patient to obtain the therapy service. Only one payment will be made for the visit furnished to the

RHC/FQHC patient to obtain the therapy service. As of April 1, 2005, RHCs/FQHCs are no longer required to report HCPCS codes when billing for these therapy services.

Payment Methodology for a Critical Access Hospital (CAH) is on a reasonable cost basis unless the CAH has elected the Optional Method and then the FI pays115% of the MPFS amount for the professional component of the HCPCS code in addition to the technical component.

In addition, the following revenues code must be used in conjunction with the HCPCS code identified:

| Revenue Code | Description |
|---|---|
| 420 | Physical Therapy |
| 430 | Occupational Therapy |
| 520 | Federal Qualified Health Center * |
| 521 | Rural Health Center * |
| 977, 978 | Critical Access Hospital- method II CAH professional services only |

\* NOTE: As of April 1, 2005, RHCs/FQHCs are no longer required to report HCPCS codes when billing for these therapy services.

### C. Carrier Claims

Carriers pay for Electrical Stimulation services billed with HCPCS codes G0281 based on the MPFS. Claims for Electrical Stimulation services must be billed on Form CMS-1500 or the electronic equivalent following instructions in chapter 12 of this manual (http://www.cms.hhs.gov/manuals/104_claims/clm104c12.pdf).

### D. Coinsurance and Deductible

The Medicare contractor shall apply coinsurance and deductible to payments for these therapy services except for services billed to the FI by FQHCs. For FQHCs, only co-insurance applies.

## 100-04, 32, 11.2

### Electromagnetic Therapy

### A. HCPCS Coding Applicable to A/B MACs (A and B)

Effective July 1, 2004, a National Coverage Decision was made to allow for Medicare coverage of electromagnetic therapy for the treatment of certain types of wounds. The type of wounds covered are chronic Stage III or Stage IV pressure ulcers, arterial ulcers, diabetic ulcers and venous stasis ulcers. All other uses of electromagnetic therapy for the treatment of wounds are not covered by Medicare. Electromagnetic therapy will not be covered as an initial treatment modality.

The use of electromagnetic therapy will only be covered after appropriate standard wound care has been tried for at least 30 days and there are no measurable signs of healing. If electromagnetic therapy is being used, wounds must be evaluated periodically by the treating physician but no less than every 30 days. Continued treatment with electromagnetic therapy is not covered if measurable signs of healing have not been demonstrated within any 30-day period of treatment. Additionally, electromagnetic therapy must be discontinued when the wound demonstrates a 100% epithelialzed wound bed.

Coverage policy can be found in Pub. 100-03, Medicare National Coverage Determinations Manual, Chapter 1 section 270.1. (http://www.cms.hhs.gov/manuals/103_cov_determ/ncd103index.asp)

The applicable Healthcare Common Procedure Coding System (HCPCS) code for Electrical Stimulation and the covered effective date is as follows:

| HCPCS | Definition | Effective Date |
|---|---|---|
| G0329 | ElectromagneticTherapy, to one or more areas for chronic Stage III and Stage IV pressure ulcers, arterial ulcers, diabetic ulcers and venous stasis ulcers not demonstrating measurable signs of healing after 30 days of conventional care as part of a therapy plan of care. | 07/01/2004 |

Medicare will not cover the device used for the electromagnetic therapy for the treatment of wounds. However, Medicare will cover the service. Unsupervised home use of electromagnetic therapy will not be covered.

### B. A/B MAC (A) Billing Instructions

The applicable types of bills acceptable when billing for electromagnetic therapy services are 12X, 13X, 22X, 23X, 71X, 73X, 74X, 75X, and 85X. Chapter 25 of this manual provides general billing instructions that must be followed for bills submitted to A/B MACs (A). A/B MACs (A) pay for electromagnetic therapy services under the Medicare Physician Fee Schedule for a hospital, CORF, ORF, and SNF.

Payment methodology for independent (RHC), provider-based RHCs, free-standing FQHC and provider based FQHCs is made under the all-inclusive rate for the visit furnished to the RHC/FQHC patient to obtain the therapy service. Only one payment will be made for the visit furnished to the RHC/FQHC patient to obtain the therapy service. As of April 1, 2005, RHCs/FQHCs are no longer required to report HCPCS codes when billing for the therapy service.

Payment Methodology for a CAH is payment on a reasonable cost basis unless the CAH has elected the Optional Method and then the A/B MAC (A) pays pay 115% of the MPFS amount for the professional component of the HCPCS code in addition to the technical component.

In addition, the following revenues code must be used in conjunction with the HCPCS code identified:

| Revenue Code | Description |
|---|---|
| 420 | Physical Therapy |
| 430 | Occupational Therapy |
| 520 | Federal Qualified Health Center * |
| 521 | Rural Health Center * |
| 977, 978 | Critical Access Hospital- method II CAH professional services only |

\* NOTE: As of April 1, 2005, RHCs/FQHCs are no longer required to report HCPCS codes when billing for the therapy service.

### C. A/B MAC (B) Claims

A/B MACs (B) pay for Electromagnetic Therapy services billed with HCPCS codes G0329 based on the MPFS. Claims for electromagnetic therapy services must be billed using the ASC X12 837 professional claim format or Form CMS-1500 following instructions in chapter 12 of this manual (www.cms.hhs.gov/manuals/104_claims/clm104index.asp).

Payment information for HCPCS code G0329 will be added to the July 2004 update of the Medicare Physician Fee Schedule Database (MPFSD).

### D. Coinsurance and Deductible

The Medicare contractor shall apply coinsurance and deductible to payments for electromagnetic therapy services except for services billed to the A/B MAC (A) by FQHCs. For FQHCs only co-insurance applies.

## 100-04, 32, 11.3.1

### Policy

Effective for claims with dates of service on or after August 2, 2012, contractors shall accept and pay for autologous platelet-rich plasma (PRP) only for the treatment of chronic non-healing diabetic, venous and/or pressure wounds only in the context of an approved clinical study in accordance with the coverage criteria outlined in Pub 100-03, chapter 1, section 270.3, of the NCD Manual.

## 100-04, 32, 11.3.2

### Healthcare Common Procedure Coding System (HCPCS) Codes and Diagnosis Coding

### HCPCS Code

Effective for claims with dates of service on or after August 2, 2012 Medicare providers shall report HCPCS code G0460 for PRP services.

**If ICD-9 Diagnosis coding is applicable**

For claims with dates of service on or after August 2, 2012, PRP, for the treatment of chronic non-healing diabetic, venous and/or pressure wounds only in the context of an approved clinical study must be billed using the following ICD codes:

- V70.7
- ICD-9 code from the approved list of diagnosis codes maintained by the Medicare contractor.

**If ICD-10 Diagnosis coding is applicable**

For claims with dates of service on or after the implementation of ICD-10, ICD-10 CM diagnosis coding is applicable.

- Z00.6
- ICD-10 code from the approved list of diagnosis codes maintained by the Medicare contractor.

**Additional billing requirement:**

The following modifier and condition code shall be reported when billing for PRP services only in the context of an approved clinical study:

- Q0 modifier
- Condition code 30 (for institutional claims only)
- Value Code D4 with an 8-digit clinical trial number. NOTE: This is optional and only applies to Institutional claims.

## 100-04, 32, 11.3.3

The applicable TOBs for PRP services are: 12X, 13X, 22X, 23X, 71X, 75X, 77X, and 85X.

## 100-04, 32, 11.3.4

**Payment Method**

Payment for PRP services is as follows:

- Hospital outpatient departments TOBs 12X and 13X — based on OPPS
- SNFs TOBs 22X and 23X — based on MPFS
- TOB 71X — based on all-inclusive rate — TOB 75X — based on MPFS
- TOB 77X — based on all-inclusive rate
- TOB 85X — based on reasonable cost
- CAHs TOB 85X and revenue codes 096X, 097X, or 098X — based on MPFS

Contractors shall pay for PRP services for hospitals in Maryland under the jurisdiction of the Health Services Cost Review Commission (HSCRC) on an outpatient basis, TOB 13X, in accordance with the terms of the Maryland waiver.

## 100-04, 32, 11.3.5

**Place of Service (POS) for Professional Claims**

Effective for claims with dates of service on or after August 2, 2012, place of service codes 11, 22, and 49 shall be used for PRP services.

## 100-04, 32, 11.3.6

**Medicare Summary Notices (MSNs), Remittance Advice Remark Codes (RARCs), Claim Adjustment Reason Codes (CARCs) and Group Codes**

Contractors shall use the following messages when returning to provider/returning as unprocessable claims when required information is not included on claims for autologous platelet-rich plasma (PRP) for the treatment of chronic non-healing diabetic, venous and/or pressure wounds only in the context of an approved clinical study:

CARC 16 - Claim/service lacks information or has submission/billing error(s) which is (are) needed for adjudication. At least one Remark Code must be provided (may be comprised of either the NCPDP Reject Reason Code, or Remittance Advice Remark Code that is not an ALERT.) NOTE: Refer to the 835 Healthcare Policy Identification Segment (loop 2110 Service Payment Information REF), if present.

RARC MA130 – Your claim contains incomplete and/or invalid information, and no appeal rights are afforded because the claim is unprocessable. Please submit a new claim with the complete/correct information.

Contractors shall deny claims for RPR services, HCPCS code G0460, when services are provided on other than TOBs 12X, 13X, 22X, 23X, 71X, 75X, 77X, and 85X using:

MSN 21.25: "This service was denied because Medicare only covers this service in certain settings."

Spanish Version: "El servicio fue denegado porque Medicare solamente lo cubre en ciertas situaciones."

CARC 58: "Treatment was deemed by the payer to have been rendered in an inappropriate or invalid place of service. NOTE: Refer to the 832 Healthcare Policy Identification Segment (loop 2110 Service payment Information REF), if present.

RARC N428: "Service/procedure not covered when performed in this place of service."

Group Code – CO (Contractual Obligation)

Contractors shall deny claims for PRP services for POS other than 11, 22, or 49 using the following:

MSN 21.25: "This service was denied because Medicare only covers this service in certain settings."

Spanish Version: "El servicio fue denegado porque Medicare solamente lo cubre en ciertas situaciones."

CARC 58: "Treatment was deemed by the payer to have been rendered in an inappropriate or invalid place of service. NOTE; Refer to the 835 Healthcare Policy Identification Segment (loop 2110 Service payment Information REF), if present.

RARC N428: "Service/procedure not covered when performed in this place of service."

Group Code – CO (Contractual Obligation)

## 100-04, 32, 40.1

**Coverage Requirements**

Effective January 1, 2002, sacral nerve stimulation is covered for the treatment of urinary urge incontinence, urgency-frequency syndrome and urinary retention. Sacral nerve stimulation involves both a temporary test stimulation to determine if an implantable stimulator would be effective and a permanent implantation in appropriate candidates. Both the test and the permanent implantation are covered.

The following limitations for coverage apply to all indications:

- Patient must be refractory to conventional therapy (documented behavioral, pharmacologic and/or surgical corrective therapy) and be an appropriate surgical candidate such that implantation with anesthesia can occur.
- Patients with stress incontinence, urinary obstruction, and specific neurologic diseases (e.g., diabetes with peripheral nerve involvement) that are associated with secondary manifestations of the above three indications are excluded.
- Patient must have had a successful test stimulation in order to support subsequent implantation. Before a patient is eligible for permanent implantation, he/she must demonstrate a 50% or greater improvement through test stimulation. Improvement is measured through voiding diaries.
- Patient must be able to demonstrate adequate ability to record voiding diary data such that clinical results of the implant procedure can be properly evaluated.

## 100-04, 32, 60.4.1

**Allowable Covered Diagnosis Codes**

For services furnished on or after July 1, 2002, the applicable ICD-9-CM diagnosis code for this benefit is V43.3, organ or tissue replaced by other means; heart valve.

For services furnished on or after March 19, 2008, the applicable ICD-9-CM diagnosis codes for this benefit are:

V43.3 (organ or tissue replaced by other means; heart valve),

289.81 (primary hypercoagulable state),

451.0-451.9 (includes 451.11, 451.19, 451.2, 451.80-451.84, 451.89) (phlebitis & thrombophlebitis),

453.0-453.3 (other venous embolism & thrombosis),

453.40-453.49 (includes 453.40-453.42, 453.8-453.9) (venous embolism and thrombosis of the deep vessels of the lower extremity, and other specified veins/unspecified sites)

415.11-415.12, 415.19 (pulmonary embolism & infarction) or,

427.31 (atrial fibrillation (established) (paroxysmal)).

## 100-04, 32, 60.12

**Coverage for PET Scans for Dementia and Neurodegenerative DiseasesCoverage for PET Scans for Dementia and Neurodegenerative Diseases**

Effective for dates of service on or after September 15, 2004, Medicare will cover FDG PET scans for a differential diagnosis of fronto-temporal dementia (FTD) and Alzheimer's disease OR; its use in a CMS-approved practical clinical trial focused on the utility of FDG-PET in the diagnosis or treatment of dementing neurodegenerative diseases. Refer to Pub. 100-03, NCD Manual, section 220.6.13, for complete coverage conditions and clinical trial requirements and section 60.15 of this manual for claims processing information.

**A. Carrier and FI Billing Requirements for PET Scan Claims for FDG-PET for the Differential Diagnosis of Fronto-temporal Dementia and Alzheimer's Disease:**
- **CPT Code for PET Scans for Dementia and Neurodegenerative Diseases**

© 2016 Optum360, LLC

Contractors shall advise providers to use the appropriate CPT code from section 60.3.1 for dementia and neurodegenerative diseases for services performed on or after January 28, 2005.

- **Diagnosis Codes for PET Scans for Dementia and Neurodegenerative Diseases**

The contractor shall ensure one of the following appropriate diagnosis codes is present on claims for PET Scans for AD:

- 290.0, 290.10 - 290.13, 290.20 - 290, 21, 290.3, 331.0, 331.11, 331.19, 331.2, 331.9, 780.93

Medicare contractors shall use an appropriate Medicare Summary Notice (MSN) message such as 16.48, "Medicare does not pay for this item or service for this condition" to deny claims when submitted with an appropriate CPT code from section 60.3.1 and with a diagnosis code other than the range of codes listed above. Also, contractors shall use an appropriate Remittance Advice (RA) such as 11, "The diagnosis is inconsistent with the procedure."

Medicare contractors shall instruct providers to issue an Advanced Beneficiary Notice to beneficiaries advising them of potential financial liability prior to delivering the service if one of the appropriate diagnosis codes will not be present on the claim.

- **Provider Documentation Required with the PET Scan Claim**

Medicare contractors shall inform providers to ensure the conditions mentioned in the NCD Manual, section 220.6.13, have been met. The information must also be maintained in the beneficiary's medical record:

- Date of onset of symptoms;
- Diagnosis of clinical syndrome (normal aging, mild cognitive impairment or MCI: mild, moderate, or severe dementia);
- Mini mental status exam (MMSE) or similar test score;
- Presumptive cause (possible, probably, uncertain AD);
- Any neuropsychological testing performed;
- Results of any structural imaging (MRI, CT) performed;
- Relevant laboratory tests (B12, thyroid hormone); and,
- Number and name of prescribed medications.

**B. Billing Requirements for Beta Amyloid Positron Emission Tomography (PET) in Dementia and Neurodegenerative Disease:**

Effective for claims with dates of service on and after September 27, 2013, Medicare will only allow coverage with evidence development (CED) for Positron Emission Tomography (PET) beta amyloid (also referred to as amyloid-beta (Aß)) imaging (HCPCS A9586)or (HCPCS A9599) (one PET Aß scan per patient).

Note: Please note that effective January 1, 2014 the following code A9599 will be updated in the IOCE and HCPCS update. This code will be contractor priced.

**Medicare Summary Notices, Remittance Advice Remark Codes, and Claim Adjustment Reason Codes**

Effective for dates of service on or after September 27, 2013, contractors shall **return as unprocessable/return to provider** claims for PET Aß imaging, through CED during a clinical trial, not containing the following:

- Condition code 30, (FI only)
- Modifier Q0 and/or modifier Q1 as appropriate
- ICD-9 dx code V70.7/ICD-10 dx code Z00.6 (on either the primary/secondary position)
- A PET HCPCS code (78811 or 78814)
- At least, one Dx code from the table below

| ICD-9 Codes | Corresponding ICD-10 Codes |
|---|---|
| 290.0 Senile dementia, uncomplicated | F03.90 Unspecified dementia without behavioral disturbance |
| 290.10 Presenile dementia, uncomplicated | F03.90 Unspecified dementia without behavioral disturbance |
| 290.11 Presenile dementia with delirium | F03.90 Unspecified dementia without behavioral disturbance |
| 290.12 Presenile dementia with delusional features | F03.90 Unspecified dementia without behavioral disturbance |
| 290.13 Presenile dementia with depressive features | F03.90 Unspecified dementia without behavioral disturbance |
| 290.20 Senile dementia with delusional features | F03.90 Unspecified dementia without behavioral disturbance |
| 290.21 Senile dementia with depressive features | F03.90 Unspecified dementia without behavioral disturbance |
| 290.3 Senile dementia with delirium | F03.90 Unspecified dementia without behavioral disturbance |

| ICD-9 Codes | Corresponding ICD-10 Codes |
|---|---|
| 290.40 Vascular dementia, uncomplicated | F01.50 Vascular dementia without behavioral disturbance |
| 290.41 Vascular dementia with delirium | F01.51 Vascular dementia with behavioral disturbance |
| 290.42 Vascular dementia with delusions | F01.51 Vascular dementia with behavioral disturbance |
| 290.43 Vascular dementia with depressed mood | F01.51 Vascular dementia with behavioral disturbance |
| 294.10 Dementia in conditions classified elsewhere without behavioral disturbance | F02.80 Dementia in other diseases classified elsewhere without behavioral disturbance |
| 294.11 Dementia in conditions classified elsewhere with behavioral disturbance | F02.81 Dementia in other diseases classified elsewhere with behavioral disturbance |
| 294.20 Dementia, unspecified, without behavioral disturbance | F03.90 Unspecified dementia without behavioral disturbance |
| 294.21 Dementia, unspecified, with behavioral disturbance | F03.91 Unspecified dementia with behavioral disturbance |
| 331.11 Pick's Disease | G31.01 Pick's disease |
| 331.19 Other Frontotemporal dementia | G31.09 Other frontotemporal dementia |
| 331.6 Corticobasal degeneration | G31.85 Corticobasal degeneration |
| 331.82 Dementia with Lewy Bodies | G31.83 Dementia with Lewy bodies |
| 331.83 Mild cognitive impairment, so stated | G31.84 Mild cognitive impairment, so stated |
| 780.93 Memory Loss | R41.1 Anterograde amnesia |
| | R41.2 Retrograde amnesia |
| | R41.3 Other amnesia (Amnesia NOS, Memory loss NOS) |
| V70.7 Examination for normal comparison or control in clinical | Z00.6 Encounter for examination for normal comparison and control in clinical research program |

and

- Aß HCPCS code A9586 or A9599

Contractors shall return as unprocessable claims for PET Aß imaging using the following messages:

- Claim Adjustment Reason Code 4 ?the procedure code is inconsistent with the modifier used or a required modifier is missing.

Note: Refer to the 835 Healthcare Policy Identification Segment (loop 2110 Service Payment Information REF), if present.

- Remittance Advice Remark Code N517 - Resubmit a new claim with the requested information.
- Remittance Advice Remark Code N519 - Invalid combination of HCPCS modifiers.

Contractors shall line-item deny claims for PET Aß, HCPCS code A9586 or A9599, where a previous PET Aß, HCPCS code A9586 or A9599 is paid in history using the following messages:

- CARC 149: "Lifetime benefit maximum has been reached for this service/benefit category"
- RARC N587: "Policy benefits have been exhausted"
- MSN 20.12: "This service was denied because Medicare only covers this service once a lifetime."
- Spanish Version: "Este servicio fue negado porque Medicare sólo cubre este servicio una vez en la vida."
- Group Code: PR, if a claim is received with a GA modifier
- Group Code: CO, if a claim is received with a GZ modifier

## 100-04, 32, 70

**Billing Requirements for Islet Cell Transplantation for Beneficiaries in a National Institutes of Health (NIH) Clinical Trial**

(Rev. 986, Issued: 06-16-06, Effective: 05-01-06, Implementation: 07-31-06)

For services performed on or after October 1, 2004, Medicare will cover islet cell transplantation for patients with Type I diabetes who are participating in an NIH sponsored clinical trial. See Pub 100-04 (National Coverage Determinations Manual) section 260.3.1 for complete coverage policy.

The islet cell transplant may be done alone or in combination with a kidney transplant. Islet recipients will also need immunosuppressant therapy to prevent

© 2016 Optum360, LLC

rejection of the transplanted islet cells. Routine follow-up care will be necessary for each trial patient. See Pub 100-04, section 310 for further guidance relative to routine care. All other uses for islet cell services will remain non-covered.

## 100-04, 32, 80

### Billing of the Diagnosis and Treatment of Peripheral Neuropathy with Loss of Protective Sensation in People with Diabetes

Coverage Requirements - Peripheral neuropathy is the most common factor leading to amputation in people with diabetes. In diabetes, peripheral neuropathy is an anatomically diffuse process primarily affecting sensory and autonomic fibers; however, distal motor findings may be present in advanced cases. Long nerves are affected first, with symptoms typically beginning insidiously in the toes and then advancing proximally. This leads to loss of protective sensation (LOPS), whereby a person is unable to feel minor trauma from mechanical, thermal, or chemical sources. When foot lesions are present, the reduction in autonomic nerve functions may also inhibit wound healing.

Peripheral neuropathy with LOPS, secondary to diabetes, is a localized illness of the feet and falls within the regulation's exception to the general exclusionary rule (see 42 C.F.R. Sec.411.15(l)(l)(i)). Foot exams for people with diabetic peripheral neuropathy with LOPS are reasonable and necessary to allow for early intervention in serious complications that typically afflict diabetics with the disease.

Effective for services furnished on or after July 1, 2002, Medicare covers, as a physician service, an evaluation (examination and treatment) of the feet no more often than every 6 months for individuals with a documented diagnosis of diabetic sensory neuropathy and LOPS, as long as the beneficiary has not seen a foot care specialist for some other reason in the interim. LOPS shall be diagnosed through sensory testing with the 5.07 monofilament using established guidelines, such as those developed by the National Institute of Diabetes and Digestive and Kidney Diseases guidelines. Five sites should be tested on the plantar surface of each foot, according to the National Institute of Diabetes and Digestive and Kidney Diseases guidelines. The areas must be tested randomly since the loss of protective sensation may be patchy in distribution, and the patient may get clues if the test is done rhythmically. Heavily callused areas should be avoided. As suggested by the American Podiatric Medicine Association, an absence of sensation at two or more sites out of 5 tested on either foot when tested with the 5.07 Semmes-Weinstein monofilament must be present and documented to diagnose peripheral neuropathy with loss of protective sensation.

## 100-04, 32, 80.2

### Applicable HCPCS Codes

G0245 - Initial physician evaluation and management of a diabetic patient with diabetic sensory neuropathy resulting in a loss of protective sensation (LOPS) which must include:

1. The diagnosis of LOPS;

2. A patient history;

3. A physical examination that consists of at least the following elements:

    (a) visual inspection of the forefoot, hindfoot, and toe web spaces,

    (b) evaluation of a protective sensation,

    (c) evaluation of foot structure and biomechanics,

    (d) evaluation of vascular status and skin integrity,

    (e) evaluation and recommendation of footwear, and

4. Patient education.

G0246 - Follow-up physician evaluation and management of a diabetic patient with diabetic sensory neuropathy resulting in a loss of protective sensation (LOPS) to include at least the following:

1. a patient history;

2. a physical examination that includes:

    (a) visual inspection of the forefoot, hindfoot, and toe web spaces,

    (b) evaluation of protective sensation,

    (c) evaluation of foot structure and biomechanics,

    (d) evaluation of vascular status and skin integrity,

    (e) evaluation and recommendation of footwear, and

3. patient education.

G0247 - Routine foot care by a physician of a diabetic patient with diabetic sensory neuropathy resulting in a LOPS to include if present, at least the following:

    (1) local care of superficial (i.e., superficial to muscle and fascia) wounds;

    (2) debridement of corns and calluses; and

    (3) trimming and debridement of nails.

NOTE: Code G0247 must be billed on the same date of service with either G0245 or G0246 in order to be considered for payment.

The short descriptors for the above HCPCS codes are as follows:

    G0245 - INITIAL FOOT EXAM PTLOPS

    G0246 - FOLLOWUP EVAL OF FOOT PT LOP

    G0247 - ROUTINE FOOTCARE PT W LOPS

## 100-04, 32, 80.3

### 80.3 - Diagnosis Codes

(Rev. 2998, Issued: 07-25-14, Effective: Upon implementation of ICD-10; 01-01-12 - ASC X12, Implementation: 08-25-2014 - ASC X12; Upon Implementation of ICD-10)

Diagnosis Codes.--Providers should report one of the following diagnosis codes in conjunction with this benefit:

- If ICD-9-CM is applicable - 250.60, 250.61, 250.62, 250.63, and 357.2.
- If ICD-10-CM is applicable - E08.40, E0.842, E09.40, E09.42, E10.40, E10.41, E10.42, E10.43, E10.44, E10.49, E10.610, E11.40, E11.41, E11.42, E11.43, E11.44, E11.49, E11.610, E13.40, E13.41, E13.42, E13.43, E13.44, E13.49, E13.610

Coverage policy can be found in Pub. 100-03, Medicare National Coverage Determinations Manual, Chapter 1, section 70.2.1 Diabetic neuropathy w/ LOPs. (http://www.cms.hhs.gov/manuals/103_cov_determ/ncd103index.asp

## 100-04, 32, 80.6

### 80.6 - Editing Instructions for A/B MACs (A)

(Rev. 2998, Issued: 07-25-14, Effective: Upon implementation of ICD-10; 01-01-12 - ASC X12, Implementation: 08-25-2014 - ASC X12; Upon Implementation of ICD-10)

Edit 1 - Implement diagnosis to procedure code edits to allow payment only for the LOPS codes, G0245, G0246, and G0247 when submitted with one of the following diagnosis codes

- If ICD-9-CM is applicable: 250.60, 250.61, 250.62, 250.63, or 357.2.
- If ICD-10-CM is applicable: E08.40, E08.42, E09.40, E09.42, E10.40, E10.41, E10.42, E10.43, E10.44, E10.49, E10.610, E11.40, E11.41, E11.42, E11.43, E11.44, E11.49, E11.610, E13.40, E13.41, E13.42, E13.43, E13.44, E13.49, E13.610

Deny these services when submitted without one of the appropriate diagnoses.

Use the same messages you currently use for procedure to diagnosis code denials. Edit 2 – Deny G0247 if it is not submitted on the same claim as G0245 or G0246.

Use MSN 21.21 - This service was denied because Medicare only covers this service under certain circumstances.

Use RA claim adjustment reason code 107 - The related or qualifying claim/service was not identified on this claim. NOTE: Refer to the 835 Healthcare Policy Identification Segment (loop 2110 Service Payment Information REF), if present.

## 100-04, 32, 80.8

### CWF Utilization Edits

Edit 1 - Should CWF receive a claim from an FI for G0245 or G0246 and a second claim from a contractor for either G0245 or G0246 (or vice versa) and they are different dates of service and less than 6 months apart, the second claim will reject. CWF will edit to allow G0245 or G0246 to be paid no more than every 6 months for a particular beneficiary, regardless of who furnished the service. If G0245 has been paid, regardless of whether it was posted as a facility or professional claim, it must be 6 months before G0245 can be paid again or G0246 can be paid. If G0246 has been paid, regardless of whether it was posted as a facility or professional claim, it must be 6 months before G0246 can be paid again or G0245 can be paid. CWF will not impose limits on how many times each code can be paid for a beneficiary as long as there has been 6 months between each service.

The CWF will return a specific reject code for this edit to the contractors and FIs that will be identified in the CWF documentation. Based on the CWF reject code, the contractors and FIs must deny the claims and return the following messages:

MSN 18.4 -- This service is being denied because it has not been __ months since your last examination of this kind (NOTE: Insert 6 as the appropriate number of months.)

RA claim adjustment reason code 96 - Non-covered charges, along with remark code M86 - Service denied because payment already made for same/similar procedure within set time frame.

Edit 2

The CWF will edit to allow G0247 to pay only if either G0245 or G0246 has been submitted and accepted as payable on the same date of service. CWF will return a specific reject code for this edit to the contractors and FIs that will be identified in the CWF documentation. Based on this reject code, contractors and FIs will deny the claims and return the following messages:

MSN 21.21 - This service was denied because Medicare only covers this service under certain circumstances.

RA claim adjustment reason code 107 - The related or qualifying claim/service was not identified on this claim.

Edit 3

Once a beneficiary's condition has progressed to the point where routine foot care becomes a covered service, payment will no longer be made for LOPS evaluation and management services. Those services would be considered to be included in the regular exams and treatments afforded to the beneficiary on a routine basis. The physician or provider must then just bill the routine foot care codes, per Pub 100-02, Chapter 15, Sec.290.

The CWF will edit to reject LOPS codes G0245, G0246, and/or G0247 when on the beneficiary's record it shows that one of the following routine foot care codes were billed and paid within the prior 6 months: 11055, 11056, 11057, 11719, 11720, and/or 11721.

The CWF will return a specific reject code for this edit to the contractors and FIs that will be identified in the CWF documentation. Based on the CWF reject code, the contractors and FIs must deny the claims and return the following messages:

MSN 21.21 - This service was denied because Medicare only covers this service under certain circumstances.

The RA claim adjustment reason code 96 - Non-covered charges, along with remark code M86 - Service denied because payment already made for same/similar procedure within set time frame.

## 100-04, 32, 110.5

### DMERC Billing Instructions

Effective for dates of service on or after April 27, 2005, DMERCs shall allow payment for ultrasonic osteogenic stimulators with the following HCPCS codes:

- E0760 for low intensity ultrasound (include modifier "KF"), or;
- E1399 for other ultrasound stimulation (include modifier "KF")

## 100-04, 32, 120.1

### Payment for Services and Supplies

For an IOL inserted following removal of a cataract in a hospital, on either an outpatient or inpatient basis, that is paid under the hospital Outpatient Prospective Payment System (OPPS) or the Inpatient Prospective Payment System (IPPS), respectively; or in a Medicare-approved ambulatory surgical center (ASC) that is paid under the ASC fee schedule:

Medicare does not make separate payment to the hospital or ASC for an IOL inserted subsequent to extraction of a cataract. Payment for the IOL is packaged into the payment for the surgical cataract extraction/lens replacement procedure.

Any person or ASC, who presents or causes to be presented a bill or request for payment for an IOL inserted during or subsequent to cataract surgery for which payment is made under the ASC fee schedule, is subject to a civil money penalty.

For a P-C IOL or A-C IOL inserted subsequent to removal of a cataract in a hospital, on either an outpatient or inpatient basis, that is paid under the OPPS or the IPPS, respectively; or in a Medicare-approved ASC that is paid under the ASC fee schedule:

The facility shall bill for the removal of a cataract with insertion of a conventional IOL, regardless of whether a conventional, P-C IOL, or A-C IOL is inserted. When a beneficiary receives a P-C or A-C IOL following removal of a cataract, hospitals and ASCs shall report the same CPT code that is used to report removal of a cataract with insertion of a conventional IOL. Physicians, hospitals and ASCs may also report an additional HCPCS code, V2788, to indicate any additional charges that accrue when a P-C IOL or A-C IOL is inserted in lieu of a conventional IOL until Janaury 1, 2008. Effective for A-C IOL insertion services on or after January 1, 2008, physicians, hospitals and ASCs should use V2787 to report any additional charges that accrue. On or after January 1, 2008, physicians, hospitals, and ASCs should continue to report HCPCS code V2788 to indicate any additional charges that accrue for insertion of a P-C IOL. See Section 120.2 for coding guidelines.

There is no Medicare benefit category that allows payment of facility charges for services and supplies required to insert and adjust a P-C or A-C IOL following removal of a cataract that exceed the facility charges for services and supplies required for the insertion and adjustment of a conventional IOL.

There is no Medicare benefit category that allows payment of facility charges for subsequent treatments, services and supplies required to examine and monitor the beneficiary who receives a P-C or A-C IOL following removal of a cataract that exceeds the facility charges for subsequent treatments, services and supplies required to examine and monitor a beneficiary after cataract surgery followed by insertion of a conventional IOL.

### A - For a P-C IOL or A-C IOL inserted in a physician's office

A physician shall bill for a conventional IOL, regardless of a whether a conventional, P-C IOL, or A-C IOL is inserted (see section 120.2, General Billing Requirements)

There is no Medicare benefit category that allows payment of physician charges for services and supplies required to insert and adjust a P-C or A-C IOL following removal of a cataract that exceed the physician charges for services and supplies for the insertion and adjustment of a conventional IOL.

There is no Medicare benefit category that allows payment of physician charges for subsequent treatments, service and supplies required to examine and monitor a beneficiary following removal of a cataract with insertion of a P-C or A-C IOL that exceed physician charges for services and supplies to examine and monitor a beneficiary following removal of a cataract with insertion of a conventional IOL.

### B - For a P-C IOL or A-C IOL inserted in a hospital

A physician may not bill Medicare for a P-C or A-C IOL inserted during a cataract procedure performed in a hospital setting because the payment for the lens is included in the payment made to the facility for the surgical procedure.

There is no Medicare benefit category that allows payment of physician charges for services and supplies required to insert and adjust a P-C or A-C IOL following removal of a cataract that exceed the physician charges for services and supplies required for the insertion of a conventional IOL.

### C - For a P-C IOL or A-C IOL inserted in an Ambulatory Surgical Center

Refer to Chapter 14, Section 40.3 for complete guidance on payment for P-C IOL or A-C IOL in Ambulatory Surgical Centers.

## 100-04, 32, 120.2

### Coding and General Billing Requirements

Physicians and hospitals must report one of the following Current Procedural Terminology (CPT) codes on the claim:

- 66982 - Extracapsular cataract removal with insertion of intraocular lens prosthesis (one stage procedure), manual or mechanical technique (e.g., irrigation and aspiration or phacoemulsification), complex requiring devices or techniques not generally used in routine cataract surgery (e.g., iris expansion device, suture support for intraocular lens, or primary posterior capsulorrhexis) or performed on patients in the amblyogenic development stage.
- 66983 - Intracapsular cataract with insertion of intraocular lens prosthesis (one stage procedure)
- 66984 - Extracapsular cataract removal with insertion of intraocular lens prosthesis (one stage procedure), manual or mechanical technique (e.g., irrigation and aspiration or phacoemulsification)
- 66985 - Insertion of intraocular lens prosthesis (secondary implant), not associated with concurrent cataract extraction
- 66986 - Exchange of intraocular lens

In addition, physicians inserting a P-C IOL or A-C IOL in an office setting may bill code V2632 (posterior chamber intraocular lens) for the IOL. Medicare will make payment for the lens based on reasonable cost for a conventional IOL. Place of Service (POS) = 11.

Effective for dates of service on and after January 1, 2006, physician, hospitals and ASCs may also bill the non-covered charges related to the P-C function of the IOL using HCPCS code V2788. Effective for dates of service on and after January 22, 2007 through January 1, 2008, non-covered charges related to A-C function of the IOL can be billed using HCPCS code V2788. The type of service indicator for the non-covered billed charges is Q. (The type of service is applied by the Medicare carrier and not the provider). Effective for A-C IOL insertion services on or after January 1, 2008, physicians, hospitals and ASCs should use V2787 rather than V2788 to report any additional charges that accrue.

When denying the non-payable charges submitted with V2787 or V2788, contractors shall use an appropriate Medical Summary Notice (MSN) such as 16.10 (Medicare does not pay for this item or service) and an appropriate claim adjustment reason code such as 96 (non-covered charges) for claims submitted with the non-payable charges.

Hospitals and physicians may use the proper CPT code(s) to bill Medicare for evaluation and management services usually associated with services following cataract extraction surgery, if appropriate.

**A - Applicable Bill Types**

The hospital applicable bill types are 12X, 13X, 83X and 85X.

**B - Other Special Requirements for Hospitals**

Hospitals shall continue to pay CAHs method 2 claims under current payment methodologies for conditional IOLs.

## 100-04, 32, 130

### External Counterpulsation (ECP) Therapy

Commonly referred to as enhanced external counterpulsation, is a non-invasive outpatient treatment for coronary artery disease refractory medical and/or surgical therapy. Effective for dates of service July 1, 1999, and after, Medicare will cover ECP when its use is in patients with stable angina (Class III or Class IV, Canadian Cardiovascular Society Classification or equivalent classification) who, in the opinion of a cardiologist or cardiothoracic surgeon, are not readily amenable to surgical intervention, such as PTCA or cardiac bypass, because:

- Their condition is inoperable, or at high risk of operative complications or post-operative failure;
- Their coronary anatomy is not readily amenable to such procedures; or
- They have co-morbid states that create excessive risk.

(Refer to Publication 100-03, section 20.20 for further coverage criteria.)

## 100-04, 32, 130.1

### Billing and Payment Requirements

Effective for dates of service on or after January 1, 2000, use HCPCS code G0166 (External counterpulsation, per session) to report ECP services. The codes for external cardiac assist (92971), ECG rhythm strip and report (93040 or 93041), pulse oximetry (94760 or 94761) and plethysmography (93922 or 93923) or other monitoring tests for examining the effects of this treatment are not clinically necessary with this service and should not be paid on the same day, unless they occur in a clinical setting not connected with the delivery of the ECP. Daily evaluation and management service, e.g., 99201-99205, 99211-99215, 99217-99220, 99241-99245, cannot be billed with the ECP treatments. Any evaluation and management service must be justified with adequate documentation of the medical necessity of the visit. Deductible and coinsurance apply.

## 100-04, 32, 140.2.2.1

### Correct Place of Service (POS) Code for CR and ICR Services on Professional Claims

Effective for claims with dates of service on and after January 1, 2010, place of service (POS) code 11 shall be used for CR and ICR services provided in a physician's office and POS 22 shall be used for services provided in a hospital outpatient setting. All other POS codes shall be denied. Contractors shall adjust their prepayment procedure edits as appropriate.

The following messages shall be used when contractors deny CR and ICR claims for POS:

Claim Adjustment Reason Code (CARC) 171 – Payment is denied when performed/billed by this type of provider in this type of facility.

**NOTE:** Refer to the 832 Healthcare Policy Identification Segment (loop 2110 Service payment Information REF), if present.

Remittance Advice Remark Code (RARC) N428 - Service/procedure not covered when performed in this place of service.

Medicare Summary Notice (MSN) 21.25 - This service was denied because Medicare only covers this service in certain settings.

Group Code PR (Patient Responsibility) - Where a claim is received with the GA modifier indicating that a signed ABN is on file.

Group Code CO (Contractor Responsibility) – Where a claim is received with the GZ modifier indicating that no signed ABN is on file.

## 100-04, 32, 140.2.2.2

### 140.2.2.2 – Requirements for CR and ICR Services on Institutional Claims

(Rev. 2989, Issued: 07-18-14, Effective: 02-18-14, Implementation: 08-18-14)

Effective for claims with dates of service on and after January 1, 2010, contractors shall pay for CR and ICR services when submitted on Types of Bill (TOBs) 13X and 85X only. All other TOBs shall be denied.

The following messages shall be used when contractors deny CR and ICR claims for TOBs 13X and 85X:

Claim Adjustment Reason Code (CARC) 171 – Payment is denied when performed/billed by this type of provider in this type of facility.

Remittance Advice Remark Code (RARC) N428 - Service/procedure not covered when performed in this place of service.

Medicare Summary Notice (MSN) 21.25 - This service was denied because Medicare only covers this service in certain settings.

Group Code PR (Patient Responsibility) – Where a claim is received with the GA modifier indicating that a signed ABN is on file.

Group Code CO (Contractor Responsibility) – Where a claim is received with the GZ modifier indicating that no signed ABN is on file.

## 100-04, 32, 140.3

### Intensive Cardiac Rehabilitation Program Services Furnished On or After January 1, 2010

As specified at 42 CFR 410.49, Medicare covers intensive cardiac rehabilitation items and services for patients who have experienced one or more of the following:

- An acute myocardial infarction within the preceding 12 months; or
- A coronary artery bypass surgery; or
- Current stable angina pectoris; or
- Heart valve repair or replacement; or
- Percutaneous transluminal coronary angioplasty (PTCA) or coronary stenting; or
- A heart or heart-lung transplant or;
- A stable, chronic heart failure defined as patients with left ventricular ejection fraction of 35% or less and New York Heart Association (NYHA) class II to IV symptoms despite being on optimal heart failure therapy for at least 6 weeks (effective February 18, 2014).

Intensive cardiac rehabilitation programs must include the following components:

- Physician-prescribed exercise each day cardiac rehabilitation items and services are furnished;
- Cardiac risk factor modification, including education, counseling, and behavioral intervention at least once during the program, tailored to patients' individual needs;
- Psychosocial assessment;
- Outcomes assessment; and
- An individualized treatment plan detailing how components are utilized for each patient.

Intensive cardiac rehabilitation programs must be approved by Medicare. In order to be approved, a program must demonstrate through peer-reviewed published research that it has accomplished one or more of the following for its patients:

- Positively affected the progression of coronary heart disease;
- Reduced the need for coronary bypass surgery; and
- Reduced the need for percutaneous coronary interventions.

An intensive cardiac rehabilitation program must also demonstrate through peer-reviewed published research that it accomplished a statistically significant reduction in 5 or more of the following measures for patients from their levels before cardiac rehabilitation services to after cardiac rehabilitation services:

- Low density lipoprotein;
- Triglycerides;
- Body mass index;
- Systolic blood pressure;
- Diastolic blood pressure; and
- The need for cholesterol, blood pressure, and diabetes medications.

Intensive cardiac rehabilitation items and services must be furnished in a physician's office or a hospital outpatient setting. All settings must have a physician immediately available and accessible for medical consultations and emergencies at all time items and services are being furnished under the program. This provision is satisfied if the physician meets the requirements for direct supervision of physician office services as specified at 42 CFR 410.26 and for hospital outpatient therapeutic services as specified at 42 CFR 410.27.

As specified at 42 CFR 410.49(f)(2), intensive cardiac rehabilitation program sessions are limited to 72 1-hour sessions, up to 6 sessions per day, over a period of up to 18 weeks.

© 2016 Optum360, LLC

## 100-04, 32, 140.3.1

### Coding Requirements for Intensive Cardiac Rehabilitation Services Furnished On or After January 1, 2010

The following are the applicable HCPCS codes for intensive cardiac rehabilitation services:

G0422     (Intensive cardiac rehabilitation; with or without continuous ECG monitoring, with exercise, per hour, per session)

G0423     (Intensive cardiac rehabilitation; with or without continuous ECG monitoring, without exercise, per hour, per session)

Effective for dates of service on or after January 1, 2010, hospitals and practitioners may report a maximum of 6 1-hour sessions per day. In order to report one session of cardiac rehabilitation services in a day, the duration of treatment must be at least 31 minutes. Additional sessions of intensive cardiac rehabilitation services beyond the first session may only be reported in the same day if the duration of treatment is 31 minutes or greater beyond the hour increment. In other words, in order to report 6 sessions of intensive cardiac rehabilitation services on a given date of service, the first five sessions would account for 60 minutes each and the sixth session would account for at least 31 minutes. If several shorter periods of intensive cardiac rehabilitation services are furnished on a given day, the minutes of service during those periods must be added together for reporting in 1-hour session increments.

Example: If the patient receives 20 minutes of intensive cardiac rehabilitation services in the day, no intensive cardiac rehabilitation session may be reported because less than 31 minutes of services were furnished.

Example: If a patient receives 20 minutes of intensive cardiac rehabilitation services in the morning and 35 minutes of intensive cardiac rehabilitation services in the afternoon of a single day, the hospital or practitioner would report 1 session of intensive cardiac rehabilitation services under 1 unit of the appropriate HCPCS G-code for the total duration of 55 minutes of intensive cardiac rehabilitation services on that day.

Example: If the patient receives 70 minutes of intensive cardiac rehabilitation services in the morning and 25 minutes of intensive cardiac rehabilitation services in the afternoon of a single day, the hospital or practitioner would report two sessions of intensive cardiac rehabilitation services under the appropriate HCPCS G-code(s) because the total duration of intensive cardiac rehabilitation services on that day of 95 minutes exceeds 90 minutes.

Example: If the patient receives 70 minutes of intensive cardiac rehabilitation services in the morning and 85 minutes of intensive cardiac rehabilitation services in the afternoon of a single day, the hospital or practitioner would report three sessions of intensive cardiac rehabilitation services under the appropriate HCPCS G-code(s) because the total duration of intensive cardiac rehabilitation services on that day is 155 minutes, which exceeds 150 minutes and is less than 211 minutes.

## 100-04, 32, 180.4

### Claim Adjustment Reason Codes, Remittance Advice Remark Codes, Group Codes, and Medicare Summary Notice Messages

(Rev 2544, Issued: 09-13-2012, Effective: 10-01-2012, Implementation: 10-01-2012)

Contractors shall use the appropriate claim adjustment reason codes (CARCs), remittance advice remark codes (RARCs), group codes, or Medicare summary notice (MSN) messages when denying payment for alcohol misuse screening and alcohol misuse behavioral counseling sessions:

- For RHC and FQHC claims that contain screening for alcohol misuse HCPCS code G0442 and alcohol misuse counseling HCPCS code G0443 with another encounter/visit with the same line item date of service, use group code CO and reason code:
  - Claim Adjustment Reason Code (CARC) 97 – The benefit for this service is included in the payment/allowance for another service/procedure that has already been adjudicated. Note: Refer to the 835 Healthcare Policy Identification Segment (loop 2110 Service Payment Information REF) if present
- Denying claims containing HCPCS code G0442 and HCPCS code G0443 submitted on a TOB other than 13X, 71X, 77X, and 85X:
  - Claim Adjustment Reason Code (CARC) 5 - The procedure code/bill type is inconsistent with the place of service. Note: Refer to the 835 Healthcare Policy Identification Segment (loop 2110 Service Payment Information REF) if present
  - Remittance Advice Remark Code (RARC) M77 – Missing/incomplete/invalid place of service
  - Group Code PR (Patient Responsibility) assigning financial liability to the beneficiary, if a claim is received with a GA modifier indicating a signed ABN is on file.

- Group Code CO (Contractual Obligation) assigning financial liability to theprovider, if a claim is received with a GZ modifier indicating no signed ABN is on file.

NOTE: For modifier GZ, use CARC 50 and MSN 8.81 per instructions in CR 7228/TR 2148.

- Denying claims that contains more than one alcohol misuse behavioral counseling session G0443 on the same date of service:
  - Medicare Summary Notice (MSN) 15.6 – The information provided does not support the need for this many services or items within this period of time.
  - Claim Adjustment Reason Code (CARC) 151 – Payment adjusted because the payer deems the information submitted does not support this many/frequency of services.
  - Remittance Advice Remark Code (RARC) M86 – Service denied because payment already made for same/similar procedure within set time frame.
  - Group Code PR (Patient Responsibility) assigning financial liability to the beneficiary, if a claim is received with a GA modifier indicating a signed ABN is on file.
  - Group Code CO (Contractual Obligation) assigning financial liability to the provider, if a claim is received with a GZ modifier indicating no signed ABN is on file.

NOTE: For modifier GZ, use CARC 50 and MSN 8.81 per instructions in CR 7228/TR 2148.

- Denying claims that are not submitted from the appropriate provider specialties:
  - Medicare Summary Notice (MSN) 21.18 – This item or service is not covered when performed or ordered by this provider.
  - Claim Adjustment Reason Code (CARC) 185 - The rendering provider is not eligible to perform the service billed. NOTE: Refer to the 835 Healthcare Policy Identification Segment (loop 2110 Service Payment Information REF), if present.
  - Remittance Advice Remark Code (RARC) N95 - This provider type/provider specialty may not bill this service.
  - Group Code PR (Patient Responsibility) assigning financial liability to the beneficiary, if a claim is received with a GA modifier indicating a signed ABN is on file.
  - Group Code CO (Contractual Obligation) assigning financial liability to the provider, if a claim is received with a GZ modifier indicating no signed ABN is on file.

NOTE: For modifier GZ, use CARC 50 and MSN 8.81 per instructions in CR 7228/TR 2148.

- Denying claims without the appropriate POS code:
  - Medicare Summary Notice (MSN) 21.25 – This service was denied because Medicare only covers this service in certain settings.
  - Claim Adjustment Reason Code (CARC) 58 – Treatment was deemed by the payer to have been rendered in an inappropriate or invalid place of service.

Note:  Refer to the 835 Healthcare Policy Identification Segment (loop 2110 Service Payment Information REF) if present.

  - Remittance Advice Remark Code (RARC) N428 – Not covered when performed in this place of service.
  - Group Code PR (Patient Responsibility) assigning financial liability to the beneficiary, if a claim is received with a GA modifier indicating a signed ABN is on file.
  - Group Code CO (Contractual Obligation) assigning financial liability to the provider, if a claim is received with a GZ modifier indicating no signed ABN is on file.

NOTE: For modifier GZ, use CARC 50 and MSN 8.81 per instructions in CR 7228/TR 2148.

- Denying claims for alcohol misuse screening HCPCS code G0442 more than once in a 12-month period, and denying alcohol misuse counseling sessions HCPCS code G0443 more than four times in the same 12-month period:
  - Medicare Summary Notice (MSN) 20.5 – These services cannot be paid because your benefits are exhausted at this time.
  - Claim Adjustment Reason Code (CARC) 119 – Benefit maximum for this time period or occurrence has been reached.
  - Remittance Advice Remark Code (RARC) N362 – The number of Days or Units of service exceeds our acceptable maximum.
  - Group Code PR (Patient Responsibility) assigning financial liability to the beneficiary, if a claim is received with a GA modifier indicating a signed ABN is on file.

– Group Code CO (Contractual Obligation) assigning financial liability to the provider, if a claim is received with a GZ modifier indicating no signed ABN is on file.

NOTE: For modifier GZ, use CARC 50 and MSN 8.81 per instructions in CR 7228/TR 2148.

- Denying claims for alcohol misuse counseling session HCPCS code G0443 when there is no claim in history for the screening service HCPCS code G0442 in the prior 12 months:

  – Medicare Summary Notice (MSN) 16.26 – Medicare does not pay for services or items related to a procedure that has not been approved or billed.

  – Claim Adjustment Reason Code (CARC) B15 – This service/procedure requires that a qualifying service/procedure be received and covered. The qualifying other service/procedure has not been received/adjudicated. Note: Refer to the 835 Healthcare Policy Identification Segment (loop 2110 Service Payment Information REF), if present.

  – Remittance Advice Remark Code (RARC) M16 – Alert: Please see our web site, mailings, or bulletins for more details concerning this policy/procedure/decision.

  – Group Code PR (Patient Responsibility) assigning financial liability to the beneficiary, if a claim is received with a modifier indicating a signed ABN is on file.

  – Group Code CO (Contractual Obligation) assigning financial liability to the provider, if a claim is received without a modifier indicating no signed ABN is on file.

## 100-04, 32, 180.5

### Additional CWF and Contractor Requirements

(Rev 2544, Issued: 09-13-2012, Effective: 10-01-2012, Implementation: 10-01-2012)

- When applying frequency, CWF shall count 11 full months following the month of the last alcohol misuse screening visit, G0442, before allowing subsequent payment of another G0442 screening.

- CWF shall reject incoming claims when G0443 PROF is billed if four G0443 services have been billed and posted to the BEHV auxiliary file within the 12 month period.

- CWF shall continue to reject incoming claims with consistency error code '32#3' when HCPCS code G0442 PROF and HCPCS code G0443 PROF are billed on same day for TOB 71X, 77X, 85X with 096X, 097X and 098X.

- Contractors and CWF shall use the last date of G0442 PROF for counting the 12-month period for G0443 PROF services.

  – Contractors and CWF shall apply all the same TOBs (13x,71x, 77x and 85x with Rev. Code 96, 97 and 98) POS (11, 22, 49 and 71), no deductible/co-insurance and institutional/professional processing for G0443 that was implemented for G0442 in CR 7633.

- If a claim with G0442 is cancelled, CWF shall do a look back for claims with G0443 and create an IUR (Information Unsolicited Response) along with a Trailer '24' back to the contractor to reject the G0443 claim(s) paid within the 12 month period of the G0442 claims.

- CWF shall display the number of counseling sessions remaining for G0443 PROF on all CWF provider query screens (HUQA, HIQA, HIQH, ELGA, ELGB, ELGH).

- CWF shall display the remaining PROF services counting DOWN from four (4) for the HCPCS code 'G0443' on the MBD/NGD extract file.

  – CWF shall calculate a next eligible date for G0442 PROF and G0443 PROF for a given beneficiary.

  – The calculation shall include all applicable factors including beneficiary Part B entitlement status, beneficiary claims history and utilization rules.

  – When there is no next eligible date, the CWF provider query screens shall display an 8-position alpha code in the date field to indicate why there is not a next eligible date.

  – Any change to beneficiary master data or claims data that would result in a change to any next eligible date shall result in an update to the beneficiary's next eligible date.

NOTE: If G0442 is not paid, the beneficiary is not eligible for G0443.

  – CWF shall create a utility to remove previously posted G0442 TECH for the AUX file.

  – CWF shall remove G0442/G0443 TECH from editing, MBD, NGD, Provider Inquiry screens and all other applicable areas (i.e., HICR) previously done under CR 7633.

### Frequency Requirements

When applying frequency, CWF shall count 11 full months following the month of the last alcohol misuse screening visit, G0442, before allowing subsequent payment of

another G0442 screening. Additionally, CWF shall create an edit to allow alcohol misuse brief behavioral counseling, HCPCS G0443, no more than 4 times in a 12-month period. CWF shall also count four alcohol misuse counseling sessions HCPCS G0443 in the same 12- month period used for G0442 counting from the date the G0442 screening session was billed.

When applying frequency limitations to G0442 screening on the same date of service as G0443 counseling, CWF shall allow both a claim for the professional service and a claim for a facility fee. CWF shall identify the following institutional claims as facility fee claims for screening services: TOB 13X, 85X when the revenue code is not 096X, 097X, or 098X. CWF shall identify all other claims as professional service claims for screening services (professional claims, and institutional claims with TOB 71X, 77X, and 85X when the revenue code is 096X, 097X, or 098X).

NOTE: This does not apply to RHCs and FQHCs.

## 100-04, 32, 250.1

### Coverage Requirements

Effective August 3, 2009, pharmacogenomic testing to predict warfarin responsiveness is covered only when provided to Medicare beneficiaries who are candidates for anticoagulation therapy with warfarin; i.e., have not been previously tested for CYP2C9 or VKORC1 alleles; and have received fewer than five days of warfarin in the anticoagulation regimen for which the testing is ordered; and only then in the context of a prospective, randomized, controlled clinical study when that study meets certain criteria as outlined in Pub 100-03, section 90.1, of the NCD Manual.

NOTE: A new temporary HCPCS Level II code effective August 3, 2009, G9143, warfarin responsiveness testing by genetic technique using any method, any number of specimen(s), was developed to enable implementation of CED for this purpose.

## 100-04, 32, 250.2

### Billing Requirements

Institutional clinical trial claims for pharmacogenomic testing for warfarin response are identified through the presence of all of the following elements:

Value Code D4 and 8-digit clinical trial number (when present on the claim) - Refer to Transmittal 310, Change Request 5790, dated January 18, 2008;

ICD-9 diagnosis code V70.7 - Refer to Transmittal 310, Change Request 5790, dated January 18, 2008;

Condition Code 30 - Refer to Transmittal 310, Change Request 5790, dated January 18, 2008;

HCPCS modifier Q0: outpatient claims only - Refer to Transmittal 1418, Change Request 5805, dated January 18, 2008; and,

HCPCS code G9143 (mandatory with the April 2010 Integrated Outpatient Code Editor (IOCE) and the January 2011 Clinical Laboratory Fee Schedule (CLFS) updates. Prior to these times, any trials should bill FIs for this test as they currently do absent these instructions, and the FIs should process and pay those claims accordingly.)

Practitioner clinical trial claims for pharmacogenomic testing for warfarin response are identified through the presence of all of the following elements:

ICD-9 diagnosis code V70.7;

8-digit clinical trial number(when present on the claim);

HCPCS modifier Q0; and HCPCS code G9143 (to be carrier priced for claims with dates of service on and after August 3, 2009, that are processed prior to the January 2011 CLFS update.)

## 100-04, 32, 260.1

### Policy

The Centers for Medicare & Medicaid Services (CMS) received a request for national coverage of treatments for facial lipodystrophy syndrome (LDS) for human immunodeficiency virus (HIV)-infected Medicare beneficiaries. Facial LDS is often characterized by a loss of fat that results in a facial abnormality such as severely sunken cheeks. This fat loss can arise as a complication of HIV and/or highly active antiretroviral therapy. Due to their appearance and stigma of the condition, patients with facial LDS may become depressed, socially isolated, and in some cases may stop their HIV treatments in an attempt to halt or reverse this complication.

Effective for claims with dates of service on and after March 23, 2010, dermal injections for facial LDS are only reasonable and necessary using dermal fillers approved by the Food and Drug Administration for this purpose, and then only in HIV-infected beneficiaries who manifest depression secondary to the physical stigmata of HIV treatment.

## 100-04, 32, 260.2.1

### Hospital Billing Instructions

#### A - Hospital Outpatient Claims

For hospital outpatient claims, hospitals must bill covered dermal injections for treatment of facial LDS by having all of the required elements on the claim:

- A line with HCPCS codes Q2026 or Q2027 with a Line Item Date of service (LIDOS) on or after March 23, 2010,
- A line with HCPCS code G0429 with a LIDOS on or after March 23, 2010,
- If ICD-9-CM is applicable, ICD-9-CM diagnosis codes 042 (HIV) and 272.6 (Lipodystrophy) or, • If ICD-10-CM is applicable, ICD-10-CM diagnosis codes B20 Human Immunodeficiency Virus (HIV) disease and E88.1 Lipodystrophy, not elsewhere classified The applicable NCD is 250.5 Facial Lipodystrophy.

#### B - Outpatient Prospective Payment System (OPPS) Hospitals or Ambulatory Surgical Centers (ASCs):

For line item dates of service on or after March 23, 2010, and until HCPCS codes Q2026 and Q2027 are billable, facial LDS claims shall contain a temporary HCPCS code C9800, instead of HCPCS G0429 and HCPCS Q2026/Q2027, as shown above.

#### C - Hospital Inpatient Claims

Hospitals must bill covered dermal injections for treatment of facial LDS by having all of the required elements on the claim:

- Discharge date on or after March 23, 2010,
- If ICD-9-CM is applicable,
  - ICD-9-CM procedure code 86.99 (other operations on skin and subcutaneous tissue, i.e., injection of filler material), or
  - ICD-9-CM diagnosis codes 042 (HIV) and 272.6 (Lipodystrophy)
- If ICD-10-PCS is applicable, o ICD-10-PCS procedure code 3E00XGC Introduction of Other Therapeutic Substance into Skin and Mucous Membranes, External Approach, or
  - ICD-10-CM diagnosis codes B20 Human Immundodeficiency Virus [HIV] disease and E88.1 Lipodystrophy not elsewhere classified.

A diagnosis code for a comorbidity of depression may also be required for coverage on an outpatient and/or inpatient basis as determined by the individual Medicare contractor's policy.

## 100-04, 32, 260.2.2

### Practitioner Billing Instructions

Practitioners must bill covered claims for dermal injections for treatment of facial LDS by having all of the required elements on the claim:

Performed in a non-facility setting:

- A line with HCPCS codes Q2026 or Q2027 with a LIDOS on or after March 23, 2010,
- A line with HCPCS code G0429 with a LIDOS on or after March 23, 2010,
- If ICD-9-CM applies, diagnosis codes 042 (HIV) and 272.6 (Lipodystrophy) or, • If ICD-10-CM applies, diagnosis codes B20 Human Immunodeficiency Virus (HIV) disease and E88.1 (Lipodystrophy not elsewhere classified).

NOTE: A diagnosis code for a comorbidity of depression may also be required for coverage based on the individual Medicare contractor's policy.

Performed in a facility setting:

- A line with HCPCS code G0429 with a LIDOS on or after March 23, 2010,
- If ICD-9 applies, ICD-9-CM diagnosis codes 042 (HIV) and 272.6 (Lipodystrophy) or • If ICD-10 applies, ICD-10-CM diagnosis codes B20 Human Immundodeficiency Virus (HIV) disease and E88.1 (Lipodystrophy not elsewhere classified).

NOTE: A diagnosis code for a comorbidity of depression may also be required for coverage based on the individual Medicare contractor's policy.

## 100-04, 32, 280.1

### Autologous Cellular Immunotherapy Treatment of Prostate Cancer

Effective for services furnished on or after June 30, 2011, a National Coverage Determination (NCD) provides coverage of sipuleucel-T (PROVENGE®) for patients with asymptomatic or minimally symptomatic metastatic, castrate-resistant (hormone refractory) prostate cancer. Conditions of Medicare Part A and Medicare Part B coverage for sipuleucel-T are located in the Medicare NCD Manual, Publication 100-03, section 110.22.

## 100-04, 32, 280.2

### Healthcare Common Procedure Coding System (HCPCS) Codes and Diagnosis Coding

#### HCPCS Codes

Effective for claims with dates of service on June 30, 2011, Medicare providers shall report one of the following HCPCS codes for PROVENGE®:

- C9273 - Sipuleucel-T, minimum of 50 million autologous CD54+ cells activated with PAP-GM-CSF, including leukapheresis and all other preparatory procedures, per infusion, or
- J3490 - Unclassified Drugs, or
- J3590 - Unclassified Biologics.

NOTE: Contractors shall continue to process claims for HCPCS code C9273, J3490, and J3590, with dates of service June 30, 2011, as they do currently.

Effective for claims with dates of service on and after July 1, 2011, Medicare providers shall report the following HCPCS code:

- Q2043 - Sipuleucel-T, minimum of 50 million autologous CD54+ cells activated with PAP-GM-CSF, including leukapheresis and all other preparatory procedures, per infusion; short descriptor, Sipuleucel-T auto CD54+.

#### ICD-9 Diagnosis Coding

For claims with dates of service on and after July 1, 2011, for PROVENGE®, the on-label indication of asymptomatic or minimally symptomatic metastatic, castrate-resistant (hormone refractory) prostate cancer, must be billed using ICD-9 code 185 (malignant neoplasm of prostate) and at least one of the following ICD-9 codes:

| ICD-9 code | Description |
|---|---|
| 196.1 | Secondary and unspecified malignant neoplasm of intrathoracic lymph nodes |
| 196.2 | Secondary and unspecified malignant neoplasm of intra-abdominal lymph nodes |
| 196.5 | Secondary and unspecified malignant neoplasm of lymph nodes of inguinal region and lower limb |
| 196.6 | Secondary and unspecified malignant neoplasm of intrapelvic lymph nodes |
| 196.8 | Secondary and unspecified malignant neoplasm of lymph nodes of multiple sites |
| 196.9 | Secondary and unspecified malignant neoplasm of lymph node site unspecified – The spread of cancer to and establishment in the lymph nodes. |
| 197.0 | Secondary malignant neoplasm of lung – Cancer that has spread from the original (primary) tumor to the lung. The spread of cancer to the lung. This may be from a primary lung cancer, or from a cancer at a distant site. |
| 197.7 | Malignant neoplasm of liver secondary – Cancer that has spread from the original (primary) tumor to the liver. A malignant neoplasm that has spread to the liver from another (primary) anatomic site. Such malignant neoplasms may be carcinomas (e.g., breast, colon), lymphomas, melanomas, or sarcomas. |
| 198.0 | Secondary malignant neoplasm of kidney – The spread of the cancer to the kidney. This may be from a primary kidney cancer involving the opposite kidney, or from a cancer at a distant site. |
| 198.1 | Secondary malignant neoplasm of other urinary organs |
| 198.5 | Secondary malignant neoplasm of bone and bone marrow —Cancer that has spread from the original (primary) tumor to the bone. The spread of a malignant neoplasm from a primary site to the skeletal system. The majority of metastatic neoplasms to the bone are carcinomas. |
| 198.7 | Secondary malignant neoplasm of adrenal gland |
| 198.82 | Secondary malignant neoplasm of genital organs |

#### Coding for Off-Label PROVENGE® Services

The use of PROVENGE® off-label for the treatment of prostate cancer is left to the discretion of the Medicare Administrative Contractors. Claims with dates of service on and after July 1, 2011, for PROVENGE® paid off-label for the treatment of prostate cancer must be billed using either ICD-9 code 233.4 (carcinoma in situ of prostate), or ICD-9 code 185 (malignant neoplasm of prostate) in addition to HCPCS Q2043. Effective with the implementation date for ICD-10 codes, off-label PROVENGE®

services must be billed with either ICD-10 code D075(carcinoma in situ of prostate), or C61 (malignant neoplasm of prostate) in addition to HCPCS Q2043.

### ICD-10 Diagnosis Coding

Contractors shall note the appropriate ICD-10 code(s) that are listed below for future implementation. Contractors shall track the ICD-10 codes and ensure that the updated edit is turned on as part of the ICD-10 implementation effective October 1, 2013.

| ICD-10 | Description |
|--------|-------------|
| C61 | Malignant neoplasm of prostate (for on-label or off-label indications) |
| D075 | Carcinoma in situ of prostate (for off-label indications only) |
| C77.1 | Secondary and unspecified malignant neoplasm of intrathoracic lymph nodes |
| C77.2 | Secondary and unspecified malignant neoplasm of intra-abdominal lymph nodes |
| C77.4 | Secondary and unspecified malignant neoplasm of inguinal and lower limb lymph nodes |
| C77.5 | Secondary and unspecified malignant neoplasm of intrapelvic lymph nodes |
| C77.8 | Secondary and unspecified malignant neoplasm of lymph nodes of multiple regions |
| C77.9 | Secondary and unspecified malignant neoplasm of lymph node, unspecified |
| C78.00 | Secondary malignant neoplasm of unspecified lung |
| C78.01 | Secondary malignant neoplasm of right lung |
| C78.02 | Secondary malignant neoplasm of left lung |
| C78.7 | Secondary malignant neoplasm of liver |
| C79.00 | Secondary malignant neoplasm of unspecified kidney and renal pelvis |
| C79.01 | Secondary malignant neoplasm of right kidney and renal pelvis |
| C79.02 | Secondary malignant neoplasm of left kidney and renal pelvis |
| C79.10 | Secondary malignant neoplasm of unspecified urinary organs |
| C79.11 | Secondary malignant neoplasm of bladder |
| C79.19 | Secondary malignant neoplasm of other urinary organs |
| C79.51 | Secondary malignant neoplasm of bone |
| C79.52 | Secondary malignant neoplasm of bone marrow |
| C79.70 | Secondary malignant neoplasm of unspecified adrenal gland |
| C79.71 | Secondary malignant neoplasm of right adrenal gland |
| C79.72 | Secondary malignant neoplasm of left adrenal gland |
| C79.82 | Secondary malignant neoplasm of genital organs |

## 100-04, 32, 280.4

### Payment Method

Payment for PROVENGE® is as follows:

- TOBs 12X, 13X, 22X and 23X - based on the Average Sales Price (ASP) + 6%,
- TOB 85X – based on reasonable cost,
- TOBs 71X and 77X – based on all-inclusive rate.

For Medicare Part B practitioner claims, payment for PROVENGE® is based on ASP + 6%.

Contractors shall not pay separately for routine costs associated with PROVENGE®, HCPCS Q2043, except for the cost of administration. (Q2043 is all-inclusive and represents all routine costs except for its cost of administration).

## 100-04, 32, 280.5

### Medicare Summary Notices (MSNs), Remittance Advice Remark Codes (RARCs), Claim Adjustment Reason Codes (CARCs), and Group Codes

Contractors shall use the following messages when denying claims for the on-label indication for PROVENGE®, HCPCS Q2043, submitted without ICD-9-CM diagnosis code 185 and at least one diagnosis code from the ICD-9 table in Section 280.2 above:

MSN 14.9 - Medicare cannot pay for this service for the diagnosis shown on the claim.

Spanish Version - Medicare no puede pagar por este servicio debido al diagn-tico indicado en la reclamaci.

RARC 167 - This (these) diagnosis (es) are not covered. Note: Refer to the 835 Healthcare Policy Identification segment (loop 2110 Service Payment Information REF), if present.

Group Code - Contractual Obligation (CO)

Contractors shall use the following messages when denying claims for the off-label indication for PROVENGE®, HCPCS Q2043, submitted without either ICD-9-CM diagnosis code 233.4 or ICD-9-CM diagnosis code 185:

MSN 14.9 - Medicare cannot pay for this service for the diagnosis shown on the claim.

Spanish Version - Medicare no puede pagar por este servicio debido al diagn?tico indicado en la reclamaci?.

RARC 167 - This (these) diagnosis (es) are not covered. Note: Refer to the 835 Healthcare Policy Identification segment (loop 2110 Service Payment Information REF), if present.

Group Code – CO.

## 100-04, 32, 300

### Billing Requirements for Ocular Photodynamic Therapy (OPT) with Verteporfin

Ocular Photodynamic Therapy (OPT) is used in the treatment of ophthalmologic diseases; specifically, for age-related macular degeneration (AMD), a common eye disease among the elderly. OPT involves the infusion of an intravenous photosensitizing drug called Verteporfin, followed by exposure to a laser. For complete Medical coverage guidelines, see National Coverage Determinations (NCD) Manual (Pub 100-03) ? 80.2 through 80.3.1.

## 100-04, 32, 300.1

### Coding Requirements for OPT with Verteporfin

The following are applicable Current Procedural Terminology (CPT) codes for OPT with Verteporfin:

67221- Destruction of localized lesion of choroid (e.g. choroidal neovascularization); photodynamic therapy (includes intravenous infusion)

67225- Destruction of localized lesion of choroid (e.g. choroidal neovascularization); photodynamic therapy, second eye, at single session (List separately in addition to code for primary eye treatment)

The following are applicable Healthcare Common Procedure Coding System (HCPCS) code for OPT with Verteporfin:

J3396- Injection, Verteporfin, 0.1 mg

## 100-04, 32, 300.2

### Claims Processing Requirements for OPT with Verteporfin Services on Professional Claims and Outpatient Facility Claims

OPT with Verteporfin is a covered service when billed with ICD-9-CM code 362.52 (Exudative Senile Macular Degeneration of Retina (Wet)) or ICD-10-CM code H35.32 (Exudative Age-related Macular Degeneration).

Coverage is denied when billed with either ICD-9-CM code 362.50 (Macular Degeneration (Senile), Unspecified) or 362.51 (Non-exudative Senile Macular Degeneration) or their equivalent ICD-10-CM code H35.30 (Unspecified Macular Degeneration) or H35.31 (Non-exudative Age-Related Macular Degeneration).

OPT with Verteporfin for other ocular indications are eligible for local coverage determinations through individual contractor discretion.

Payment for OPT service (CPT code 67221/67225) must be billed on the same claim as the drug (J3396) for the same date of service.

Claims for OPT with Verteporfin for dates of service prior to April 3, 2013 are covered at the initial visit as determined by a fluorescein angiogram (FA) CPT code 92235 . Subsequent follow-up visits also require a FA prior to treatment.

For claims with dates of service on or after April 3, 2013, contractors shall accept and process claims for subsequent follow-up visits with either a FA, CPT code 92235, or optical coherence tomography (OCT), CPT codes 92133 or 92134, prior to treatment.

Regardless of the date of service of the claim, the FA or OCT is not required to be submitted on the claim for OPT and can be maintained in the patient? file for audit purposes.

## 100-04, 32, 310

### Transesophageal Doppler Used for Cardiac Monitoring

Effective May 17, 2007, Transesophageal Doppler used for cardiac monitoring is covered for ventilated patients in the ICU and operative patients with a need for intra-operative fluid optimization was deemed reasonable and necessary. See National Coverage Determinations Manual (Pub. 100-03) ?220.5, for complete coverage guidelines.

© 2016 Optum360, LLC

A new Healthcare Common Procedure Coding System (HCPCS) code, G9157, Transesophageal Doppler used for cardiac monitoring, will be made effective for use for dates of service on or after January 1, 2013.

## 100-04, 32, 310.10.3

### Correct Place of Service (POS) Code for Transesophageal Doppler Cardiac Monitoring Services on Professional Claims

Contractors shall pay for Transesophageal Doppler cardiac monitoring, G9157, only when services are provided at POS 21.

Contractors shall deny HCPCS G9157 when billed globally in any POS other than 21 for ventilated patients in the ICU or for operative patients with a need for intra-operative fluid optimization using the following messages:

CARC 58: "Treatment was deemed by the payer to have been rendered in an inappropriate or invalid place of service. Note: Refer to the 835 Healthcare Policy Identification Segment (loop 2110 Service Payment Information REF), if present.

MSN 16.2: This service cannot be paid when provided in this location/facility.

Group Code: CO

## 100-04, 32, 310.2

After January 1, 2013, the applicable HCPCS code for Transesophageal Doppler cardiac monitoring is:

HCPCS G9157: Transesophageal Doppler used for cardiac monitoring

Contractors shall allow HCPCS G9157 to be billed when services are provided in POS 21 for ventilated patients in the ICU or for operative patients with a need for intra-operative fluid optimization.

Contractors shall deny HCPCS 76999 when billed for Esophageal Doppler for ventilated patients in the ICU or for operative patients with a need for intra-operative fluid optimization using the following messages:

CARC 189: "'Not otherwise classified' or 'unlisted' procedure code (CPT/HCPCS) was billed when there is a specific procedure code for this procedure/service."

RARC M20: "Missing/incomplete/invalid HCPCS."

MSN 16.13: "The code(s) your provider used is/are not valid for the date of service billed."

(English version) or "El/los código(s) que usó su proveedor no es/son válido(s) en la fecha de servicio facturada." (Spanish version).

Group Code: Contractual Obligation (CO)

## 100-04, 32, 320.3.5

### Replacement Accessories and Supplies for External VADs or Any VAD

Effective April 1, 2013, claims for replacement of accessories and supplies for VADs implanted in patients who were not eligible for coverage under Medicare Part A or had other insurance that paid for the device and hospital stay at the time that the device was implanted, but are now eligible for coverage of the replacement supplies and accessories under Part B, should be submitted using HCPCS code Q0509. Those claims will be manually reviewed. In rare instances it may be appropriate to pay for replacement of supplies and accessories for external VADs used by patient who are discharged from the hospital. In addition, in some rare instances, it may be necessary for a patient to have an emergency back-up controller for an external VAD. Coverage of these items is at the discretion of the contractor. Claims for replacement of supplies and accessories used with an external VAD that are furnished by suppliers should be billed to the B MACs. Claims for replacement of supplies and accessories used with an external VAD that are furnished by hospitals and other providers should be billed to the A MACs. Effective April 1, 2013, these items should be billed using code Q0507 so that the claims can be manually reviewed.

Claims for replacement supplies or accessories used with VADs that do not have specific HCPCS codes and do not meet the criteria of codes Q0507 and Q0509 should be billed using code Q0508.

### Claims Coding

| HCPCS | Definition | Effective Date |
|---|---|---|
| Q0507 | Miscellaneous Supply Or Accessory For Use With An External Ventricular Assist Device | April 1, 2013 |
| Q0508 | Miscellaneous Supply or Accessory For Use With An Implanted Ventricular Assist Device | April 1, 2013 |
| Q0509 | Miscellaneous Supply Or Accessory For Use With Any Implanted Ventricular Assist Device For Which Payment Was Not Made Under Medicare Part A | April 1, 2013 |

## 100-04, 32, 320.5

### Cardiac Pacemaker Claims Without the KX Modifier

**Professional claims**
Contractors shall return claims lines for implanted permanent cardiac pacemakers, single chamber or dual chamber, containing one of the following CPT codes: 33206, 33207, or 33208, as unprocessable when the -KX modifier is not present. Contractors shall use the following messages:

CARC 4 - The procedure code is inconsistent with the modifier used or a required modifier is missing

RARC N517 - Resubmit a new claim with the requested information.

**Institutional claims**
Contractors shall return to providers claims for implanted permanent cardiac pacemakers, single chamber or dual chamber, when the -KX modifier is not present on the claim.

## 100-04, 32, 320.6

### Cardiac Pacemaker Non Covered ICD-9/ICD-10 Diagnosis Codes

For claims with dates of service on and after August 13, 2013, for implanted permanent cardiac pacemakers, single chamber or dual chamber, using one of the following HCPCS and/or CPT codes: C1785, C1786, C2619,C2620, 33206, 33207, or 33208, and at least one of the following ICD-9-CM/ICD-10-CM diagnosis codes, are not covered:

- 426.10 Atrioventricular block, unspecified/ I44.30 Unspecified atrioventricular block
- 426.11 First degree atrioventricular block/ I44.0 Atrioventricular block first degree
- 426.4 Right bundle branch block/ I45.10 Unspecified right bundle-branch block / I45.19 Other right bundle branch block
- 427.0 Paroxysmal supraventricular tachycardia/ I47.1 Supraventricular tachycardia
- 427.31 Atrial fibrillation/ I48.1 Persistent atrial fibrillation/ I48.2 Chronic atrial fibrillation
- 427.32 Atrial flutter/ I48.3 Typical atrial flutter/ I48.4 Atypical atrial flutter
- 427.89 Other specified cardiac dysrhythmias, Other/ I49.8 Other specified cardiac arrhythmias780.2 Syncope and collapse/ R55 Syncope and collapse

The following diagnosis codes are not covered if they are not submitted with at least one of the CPT codes and diagnosis codes listed in section 320.3:

- 426.10 Atrioventricular block, unspecified/ I44.30 Unspecified atrioventricular block
- 426.4 Right bundle branch block/ I45.10 Unspecified right bundle-branch block / I45.19 Other right bundle branch block
- 427.0 Paroxysmal supraventricular tachycardia/ I47.1 Supraventricular tachycardia

## 100-04, 32, 330.1

### Claims Processing Requirements for Percutaneous Image-guided Lumbar Decompression (PILD) for Lumbar Spinal Stenosis (LSS) on Professional Claims

(Rev. 3175, Issued: 01-30-15, Effective: 01-01-15, Implementation: 03-02-15, For Local System edits; July 6, 2015- For Shared Systems edits)

For claims with dates of service on or after January 9, 2014, PILD (procedure code 0275T) is a covered service when billed as part of a clinical trial approved by CMS. The description for CPT 0275T is "Percutaneous laminotomy/laminectomy (intralaminar approach) for decompression of neural elements, (with or without ligamentous resection, discectomy, facetectomy and/or foraminotomy)", any method, under indirect image guidance (e.g., fluoroscopic, CT), with or without the use of an endoscope, single or multiple levels, unilateral or bilateral; lumbar".

For claims with dates of service on or after January 1, 2015, PILD (procedure code G0276) is a covered service when billed as part of a clinical trial approved by CMS. HCPCS G0276 is "Blinded procedure for lumbar stenosis, percutaneous image-guided lumbar decompression (PILD), or placebo control, performed in an approved coverage with evidence development (CED) clinical trial".

The claim may only contain one of these procedure codes, not both. To use G0276, the procedure must be performed in an approved CED clinical trial that is randomized, blinded, and contains a placebo control arm of the trial. CMS will cover procedure code 0275T for PILD only when the procedure is performed within a CED approved randomized and non- blinded clinical trial. Regardless of the type of CED approved clinical trial (e.g. G0276 vs 0275T), PILD is only covered when billed for the

ICD-9 diagnosis of 724.01-724.03 or the ICD-10 diagnosis of M48.05-M48.07, when billed in places of service 22 (Outpatient) or 24 (Ambulatory Surgical Center), when billed along with V70.7 (ICD-9) or Z00.6 (ICD-10) in either the primary/secondary positions, and when billed with modifier Q0.

Additionally, per Transmittal 2805 (Change Request 8401), issued October 30, 2013, all claims for clinical trials must contain the 8 digit clinical trial identifier number.

The following message(s) shall be used to notify providers of return situations that may occur:

### Professional Claims 8-digit Clinical Trial Number

For PILD claims with procedure code 0275T with dates of service on or after January 9, 2014, or for claims with procedure code G0276 with dates of service on or after January 1, 2015, contractors shall pay for PILD only when billed with the numeric, 8-digit clinical trial identifier number preceded by the two alpha characters "CT" when placed in Field 19 of paper Form CMS-1500, or when entered without the "CT" prefix in the electronic 837P in Loop 2300 REF02 (REF01=P4). Claims for PILD which are billed without an 8-digit clinical trial identifier number shall be returned as unprocessable.

The following messages shall be used when Medicare contractors return PILD claims billed without an 8-digit clinical trial identifier number as unprocessable:

Claims Adjustment Reason Code 16: "Claim/service lacks information or has submission/billing error(s) which is needed for adjudication".

Remittance Advice Remark Code N721: "This service is only covered when performed as part of a clinical trial."

Remittance Advice Remark Code MA50: "Missing/incomplete/invalid Investigational Device Exemption number or Clinical Trial number."

Remittance Advice Remark Code N704: "Alert: You may not appeal this decision but can resubmit this claim/service with corrected information if warranted."

### Professional Claims Place of Service – 22 or 24

For PILD claims with procedure code 0275T with dates of service on or after January 9, 2014, or for claims with procedure code G0276 with dates of service on or after January 1, 2015, contractors shall pay for PILD for LSS claims only when billed in place of service 22 or 24. Claims for PILD which are billed in any other place of service shall be returned as unprocessable.

The following messages shall be used when Medicare contractors return PILD claims not billed in place of service 22 or 24:

Claims Adjustment Reason Code 58: "Treatment was deemed by the payer to have been rendered in an inappropriate or invalid place of service."

Remittance Advice Remark Code N704: "Alert: You may not appeal this decision but can resubmit this claim/service with corrected information if warranted."

### Professional Claims Modifier – Q0

For PILD claims with procedure code 0275T with dates of service on or after January 9, 2014, or for claims with procedure code G0276 with dates of service on or after January 1, 2015, contractors shall pay for PILD for LSS claims only when billed with modifier Q0.

Claims for PILD which are billed without modifier Q0 shall be returned as unprocessable.

The following messages shall be used when Medicare contractors return PILD claims billed without modifier Q0 as unprocessable:

Claims Adjustment Reason Code 4: "The procedure code is inconsistent with the modifier used or a required modifier is missing."

Remittance Advice Remark Code N657: "This should be billed with the appropriate code for these services."

Remittance Advice Remark Code N704: "Alert: You may not appeal this decision but can resubmit this claim/service with corrected information if warranted."

### Non-covered Diagnosis

For PILD claims with procedure code 0275T with dates of service on or after January 9, 2014, or for claims with procedure code G0276 with dates of service on or after January 1, 2015, contractors shall pay for PILD for LSS claims only when billed with the ICD-9 diagnosis of 724.01-724.03 or the ICD-10 diagnosis of M48.05-M48.07.

The following messages shall be used when Medicare contractors return PILD claims, billed without the covered diagnosis, as unprocessable:

Claims Adjustment Reason Code B22: "This payment is adjusted based on the diagnosis."

Remittance Advice Remark Code N704: "Alert: You may not appeal this decision but can resubmit this claim/service with corrected information if warranted."

### Clinical Trial Diagnosis

For PILD claims with procedure code 0275T with dates of service on or after January 9, 2014, or for claims with procedure code G0276 with dates of service on or after January 1, 2015, contractors shall pay for PILD only when billed with the ICD-9 diagnosis of V70.7 (ICD-9) or Z00.6 (ICD-10) in either the primary or secondary positions. The following messages shall be used when Medicare contractors return PILD claims, billed without the clinical trial diagnosis, as unprocessable:

Claims Adjustment Reason Code B22: "This payment is adjusted based on the diagnosis."

Remittance Advice Remark Code N704: "Alert: You may not appeal this decision but can resubmit this claim/service with corrected information if warranted."

## 100-04, 32, 330.2

### Claims Processing Requirements for PILD for Outpatient Facilities

(Rev. 3175, Issued: 01-30-15, Effective: 01-01-15, Implementation: 03-02-15, For Local System edits; July 6, 2015- For Shared Systems edits)

Hospital Outpatient facilities shall bill for percutaneous image-guided lumbar decompression (PILD) procedure code 0275T effective on or after January 9, 2014, or procedure code G0276 effective on or after January 1, 2015, for lumbar spinal stenosis (LSS) on a 13X or 85X TOB. Refer to Section 69 of this chapter for further guidance on billing under CED.

Hospital outpatient procedures for PILD shall be covered when billed with:

- ICD-9 V70.7 (ICD-10 Z00.6) and Condition Code 30.
- Modifier Q0
- An 8-digit clinical trial identifier number listed on the CMS Coverage with Evidence Development website

Hospital outpatient procedures for PILD shall be rejected when billed without:

- ICD-9 V70.7 (ICD-10 Z00.6) and Condition Code 30.
- Modifier Q0
- An 8-digit clinical trial identifier number listed on the CMS Coverage with Evidence Development website

Claims billed by hospitals not participating in the trial /registry, shall be rejected with the following message:

CARC: 50 -These are non-covered services because this is not deemed a "medical necessity" by the payer.

RARC N386 - This decision was based on a National Coverage Determination (NCD). An NCD provides a coverage determination as to whether a particular item or service is covered. A copy of this policy is available at http://www.cms.hhs.gov/mcd/search.asp. If you do not have web access, you may contact the contractor to request a copy of the NCD.

### Group Code –Contractual Obligation (CO)

MSN 16.77 – This service/item was not covered because it was not provided as part of a qualifying trial/study. (Este servicio/artículo no fue cubierto porque no estaba incluido como parte de un ensayo clínico/estudio calificado.)

## 100-04, 36, 50.14

### Purchased Accessories & Supplies for Use With Grandfathered Equipment

Purchased Accessories & Supplies for Use With Grandfathered Equipment

Purchased Accessories & Supplies for Use With Grandfathered Equipment

Non-contract grandfathered suppliers must use the KY modifier on claims for CBA-residing beneficiaries with dates of service on or after January 1, 2011, for purchased, covered accessories or supplies furnished for use with rented grandfathered equipment. The following HCPCS codes are the codes for which use of the KY modifier is authorized:

Continuous Positive Airway Pressure Devices, Respiratory Assistive Devices, and Related Supplies and Accessories – A4604, A7030, A7031, A7032, A7033, A7034, A7035, A7036, A7037, A7038, A7039, A7044, A7045, A7046, E0561, and E0562

Hospital Beds and Related Accessories – E0271, E0272, E0280, and E0310

Walkers and Related Accessories – E0154, E0156, E0157 and E0158 Grandfathered suppliers that submit claims for the payment of the aforementioned purchased accessories and supplies for use with grandfathered equipment should submit the applicable single payment amount for the accessory or supply as their submitted charge on the claim. Non-contract grandfathered suppliers should be aware that purchase claims submitted for these codes without the KY modifier will be denied. In addition, claims submitted with the KY modifier for HCPCS codes other than those listed above will be denied.

After the rental payment cap for the grandfathered equipment is reached, the beneficiary must obtain replacement supplies and accessories from a contract supplier. The supplier of the grandfathered equipment is no longer permitted to furnish the supplies and accessories once the rental payment cap is reached.

## 100-04, 36, 50.15

### Hospitals Providing Walkers and Related Accessories to Their Patients on the Date of Discharge

Hospitals may furnish walkers and related accessories to their own patients for use in the home during an admission or on the date of discharge and receive payment at the applicable single payment amount, regardless of whether the hospital is a contract supplier or not. Separate payment is not made for walkers furnished by a hospital for use in the hospital, as payment for these items is included in the Part A payment for inpatient hospital services.

To be paid for walkers as a non-contract supplier, the hospital must use the modifier J4 in combination with the following HCPCS codes: A4636; A4637; E0130; E0135; E0140; E0141; E0143; E0144; E0147; E0148; E0149; E0154; E0155; E0156; E0157; E0158; and E0159. Under this exception, hospitals are advised to submit the claim for the hospital stay before or on the same day that they submit the claim for the walker to ensure timely and accurate claims processing.

Hospitals that are located outside a CBA that furnish walkers and/or related accessories to travelling beneficiaries who live in a CBA must affix the J4 modifier to claims submitted for these items.

The J4 modifier should not be used by contract suppliers.

## 100-08, 10, 2.2.8

### Cardiac Rehabilitation (CR) and Intensive Cardiac Rehabilitation (ICR)

#### A. General Background Information

Effective January 1, 2010, Medicare Part B covers Cardiac Rehabilitation (CR) and Intensive Cardiac Rehabilitation (ICR) program services for beneficiaries who have experienced one or more of the following:

- An acute myocardial infarction within the preceding 12 months;
- A coronary artery bypass surgery;
- Current stable angina pectoris;
- Heart valve repair or replacement;
- Percutaneous transluminal coronary angioplasty or coronary stenting;
- A heart or heart-lung transplant; or,
- Other cardiac conditions as specified through a national coverage determination (NCD) (CR only).

ICR programs must be approved by CMS through the national coverage determination (NCD) process and must meet certain criteria for approval. Individual sites wishing to provide ICR services via an approved ICR program must enroll with their local contractor or MAC as an ICR program supplier.

#### B. ICR Enrollment

In order to enroll as an ICR site, a supplier must complete a Form CMS-855B, with the supplier type of "Other" selected. Contractors shall verify that the ICR program is approved by CMS through the NCD process. A list of approved ICR programs will be identified through the NCD listings, the CMS Web site and the Federal Register. Contractors shall use one of these options to verify that the ICR program has met CMS approval.

ICR suppliers shall be enrolled using specialty code 31. ICR suppliers must separately enroll each of their practice locations. Therefore, each enrolling ICR supplier can only have one practice location on its CMS-855B enrollment application and shall receive its own PTAN.

Contractors shall only accept and process reassignments (855R's) to ICR suppliers for physicians defined in 1861(r)(1) of the Act.

#### C. Additional Information

For more information on ICR suppliers, refer to:

42 CFR Sec.410.49;

Pub. 100-04, Medicare Claims Processing Manual, chapter 32, sections 140.2.2 - 140.2.2.6; and

Pub. 100-02, Medicare Benefit Policy Manual. chapter 15, section 232.

## 100-08, 15, 4.2.8

### Cardiac Rehabilitation (CR) and Intensive Cardiac Rehabilitation (ICR)

#### A. General Background Information

Effective January 1, 2010, Medicare Part B covers Cardiac Rehabilitation (CR) and Intensive Cardiac Rehabilitation (ICR) program services for beneficiaries who have experienced one or more of the following:

- An acute myocardial infarction within the preceding 12 months;

- A coronary artery bypass surgery;
- Current stable angina pectoris;
- Heart valve repair or replacement;
- Percutaneous transluminal coronary angioplasty or coronary stenting;
- A heart or heart-lung transplant; or,
- A stable, chronic heart failure defined as patients with left ventricular ejection fraction of 35% or less and New York Heart Association (NYHA) class II to IV symptoms despite being on optimal heart failure therapy for at least 6 weeks (effective February 18, 2014).

ICR programs must be approved by the Centers for Medicare & Medicaid Services (CMS) through the national coverage determination (NCD) process and must meet certain criteria for approval. Individual sites wishing to provide ICR services via an approved ICR program must enroll with their local Medicare Administrative Contractor (MAC) as an ICR program supplier.

#### B. ICR Enrollment

In order to enroll as an ICR site, a supplier must complete a Form CMS-855B, with the supplier type of "Other" selected. MACs shall verify that the ICR program is approved by CMS through the NCD process. A list of approved ICR programs will be identified through the NCD listings, the CMS Web site and the Federal Register. MACs shall use one of these options to verify that the ICR program has met CMS approval.

ICR suppliers shall be enrolled using specialty code 31. ICR suppliers must separately enroll each of their practice locations. Therefore, each enrolling ICR supplier can only have one practice location on its CMS-855B enrollment application and shall receive its own Provider Transaction Account Number. MACs shall only accept and process reassignments (855R's) to ICR suppliers for physicians defined in 1861(r)(1) of the Social Security Act.

#### C. Additional Information

For more information on ICR suppliers, refer to:

- 42 CFR §410.49
- Pub. 100-04, Medicare Claims Processing Manual, chapter 32, section 140
- Pub. 100-02, Medicare Benefit Policy Manual, chapter 15, section 232
- Pub. 100-03, National Coverage Determinations Manual, chapter 1, part 1, section 20.10

# Appendix 5 — HCPCS Changes for 2017

## NEW CODES

**A4224** Supplies for maintenance of insulin infusion catheter, per week

**A4225** Supplies for external insulin infusion pump, syringe type cartridge, sterile, each

**A4467** Belt, strap, sleeve, garment, or covering, any type

**A4553** Non-disposable underpads, all sizes

**A9285** Inversion/eversion correction device

**A9286** Hygienic item or device, disposable or non-disposable, any type, each

**A9587** Gallium ga-68, dotatate, diagnostic, 0.1 millicurie

**A9588** Fluciclovine f-18, diagnostic, 1 millicurie

**A9597** Positron emission tomography radiopharmaceutical, diagnostic, for tumor identification, not otherwise classified

**A9598** Positron emission tomography radiopharmaceutical, diagnostic, for non-tumor identification, not otherwise classified

**C1889** Implantable/insertable device for device intensive procedure, not otherwise classified

**C9140** Injection, factor VIII (antihemophilic factor, recombinant) (Afstyla), 1 IU

**C9482** Injection, sotalol hydrochloride, 1 mg

**C9483** Injection, atezolizumab, 10 mg

**C9744** Ultrasound, abdominal, with contrast

**G0490** Face-to-face home health nursing visit by a Rural Health Clinic (RHC) or Federally Qualified Health Center (FQHC) in an area with a shortage of home health agencies (services limited to RN or LPN only)

**G0491** Dialysis procedure at a Medicare certified ESRD facility for acute kidney injury without ESRD

**G0492** Dialysis procedure with single evaluation by a physician or other qualified health care professional for acute kidney injury without ESRD

**G0493** Skilled services of a registered nurse (RN) for the observation and assessment of the patient's condition, each 15 minutes (the change in the patient's condition requires skilled nursing personnel to identify and evaluate the patient's need for possible modification of treatment in the home health or hospice setting)

**G0494** Skilled services of a licensed practical nurse (LPN) for the observation and assessment of the patient's condition, each 15 minutes (the change in the patient's condition requires skilled nursing personnel to identify and evaluate the patient's need for possible modification of treatment in the home health or hospice setting)

**G0495** Skilled services of a registered nurse (RN), in the training and/or education of a patient or family member, in the home health or hospice setting, each 15 minutes

**G0496** Skilled services of a licensed practical nurse (LPN), in the training and/or education of a patient or family member, in the home health or hospice setting, each 15 minutes

**G0498** Chemotherapy administration, intravenous infusion technique; initiation of infusion in the office/clinic setting using office/clinic pump/supplies, with continuation of the infusion in the community setting (e.g., home, domiciliary, rest home or assisted living) using a portable pump provided by the office/clinic, includes follow up office/clinic visit at the conclusion of the infusion

**G0499** Hepatitis B screening in non-pregnant, high risk individual includes hepatitis B surface antigen (HBSAG) followed by a neutralizing confirmatory test for initially reactive results, and antibodies to HBSAG (anti-HBS) and hepatitis B core antigen (anti-HBC)

**G0500** Moderate sedation services provided by the same physician or other qualified health care professional performing a gastrointestinal endoscopic service that sedation supports, requiring the presence of an independent trained observer to assist in the monitoring of the patient's level of consciousness and physiological status; initial 15 minutes of intra-service time; patient age 5 years or older (additional time may be reported with 99153, as appropriate)

**G0501** Resource-intensive services for patients for whom the use of specialized mobility-assistive technology (such as adjustable height chairs or tables, patient lift, and adjustable padded leg supports) is medically necessary and used during the provision of an office/outpatient, evaluation and management visit (list separately in addition to primary service)

**G0502** Initial psychiatric collaborative care management, first 70 minutes in the first calendar month of behavioral health care manager activities, in consultation with a psychiatric consultant, and directed by the treating physician or other qualified health care professional, with the following required elements: outreach to and engagement in treatment of a patient directed by the treating physician or other qualified health care professional; initial assessment of the patient, including administration of validated rating scales, with the development of an individualized treatment plan; review by the psychiatric consultant with modifications of the plan if recommended; entering patient in a registry and tracking patient follow-up and progress using the registry, with appropriate documentation, and participation in weekly caseload consultation with the psychiatric consultant; and provision of brief interventions using evidence-based techniques such as behavioral activation, motivational interviewing, and other focused treatment strategies

**G0503** Subsequent psychiatric collaborative care management, first 60 minutes in a subsequent month of behavioral health care manager activities, in consultation with a psychiatric consultant, and directed by the treating physician or other qualified health care professional, with the following required elements: tracking patient follow-up and progress using the registry, with appropriate documentation; participation in weekly caseload consultation with the psychiatric consultant; ongoing collaboration with and coordination of the patient's mental health care with the treating physician or other qualified health care professional and any other treating mental health providers; additional review of progress and recommendations for changes in treatment, as indicated, including medications, based on recommendations provided by the psychiatric consultant; provision of brief interventions using evidence-based techniques such as behavioral activation, motivational interviewing, and other focused treatment strategies; monitoring of patient outcomes using validated rating scales; and relapse prevention planning with patients as they achieve remission of symptoms and/or other treatment goals and are prepared for discharge from active treatment

**G0504** Initial or subsequent psychiatric collaborative care management, each additional 30 minutes in a calendar month of behavioral health care manager activities, in consultation with a psychiatric consultant, and directed by the treating physician or other qualified health care professional (list separately in addition to code for primary procedure); (use G0504 in conjunction with G0502, G0503)

**G0505** Cognition and functional assessment using standardized instruments with development of recorded care plan for the patient with cognitive impairment, history obtained from patient and/or caregiver, in office or other outpatient setting or home or domiciliary or rest home

## NEW CODES (continued)

G0506    Comprehensive assessment of and care planning for patients requiring chronic care management services (list separately in addition to primary monthly care management service)

G0507    Care management services for behavioral health conditions, at least 20 minutes of clinical staff time, directed by a physician or other qualified health care professional, per calendar month, with the following required elements: initial assessment or follow-up monitoring, including the use of applicable validated rating scales; behavioral health care planning in relation to behavioral/psychiatric health problems, including revision for patients who are not progressing or whose status changes; facilitating and coordinating treatment such as psychotherapy, pharmacotherapy, counseling and/or psychiatric consultation; and continuity of care with a designated member of the care team

G0508    Telehealth consultation, critical care, initial, physicians typically spend 60 minutes communicating with the patient and providers via telehealth

G0509    Telehealth consultation, critical care, subsequent, physicians typically spend 50 minutes communicating with the patient and providers via telehealth

G9481    Remote in-home visit for the evaluation and management of a new patient for use only in the Medicare-approved Comprehensive Care for Joint Replacement Model, which requires these 3 key components: A problem focused history; A problem focused examination; Straightforward medical decision making, furnished in real time using interactive audio and video technology. Counseling and coordination of care with other physicians, other qualified health care professionals or agencies are provided consistent with the nature of the problem(s) and the needs of the patient or the family or both. Usually, the presenting problem(s) are self-limited or minor. Typically, 10 minutes are spent with the patient or family or both via real time, audio and video intercommunications technology.

G9482    Remote in-home visit for the evaluation and management of a new patient for use only in the Medicare-approved Comprehensive Care for Joint Replacement Model, which requires these 3 key components: An expanded problem focused history; An expanded problem focused examination; Straightforward medical decision making, furnished in real time using interactive audio and video technology. Counseling and coordination of care with other physicians, other qualified health care professionals or agencies are provided consistent with the nature of the problem(s) and the needs of the patient or the family or both. Usually, the presenting problem(s) are of low to moderate severity. Typically, 20 minutes are spent with the patient or family or both via real time, audio and video intercommunications technology.

G9483    Remote in-home visit for the evaluation and management of a new patient for use only in the Medicare-approved Comprehensive Care for Joint Replacement Model, which requires these 3 key components: A detailed history; A detailed examination; Medical decision making of low complexity, furnished in real time using interactive audio and video technology. Counseling and coordination of care with other physicians, other qualified health care professionals or agencies are provided consistent with the nature of the problem(s) and the needs of the patient or the family or both. Usually, the presenting problem(s) are of moderate severity. Typically, 30 minutes are spent with the patient or family or both via real time, audio and video intercommunications technology.

G9484    Remote in-home visit for the evaluation and management of a new patient for use only in the Medicare-approved Comprehensive Care for Joint Replacement Model, which requires these 3 key components: A comprehensive history; A comprehensive examination; Medical decision making of moderate complexity, furnished in real time using interactive audio and video technology. Counseling and coordination of care with other physicians, other qualified health care professionals or agencies are provided consistent with the nature of the problem(s) and the needs of the patient or the family or both. Usually, the presenting problem(s) are of moderate to high severity. Typically, 45 minutes are spent with the patient or family or both via real time, audio and video intercommunications technology.

G9485    Remote in-home visit for the evaluation and management of a new patient for use only in the Medicare-approved Comprehensive Care for Joint Replacement Model, which requires these 3 key components: A comprehensive history; A comprehensive examination; Medical decision making of high complexity, furnished in real time using interactive audio and video technology. Counseling and coordination of care with other physicians, other qualified health care professionals or agencies are provided consistent with the nature of the problem(s) and the needs of the patient or the family or both. Usually, the presenting problem(s) are of moderate to high severity. Typically, 60 minutes are spent with the patient or family or both via real time, audio and video intercommunications technology.

G9486    Remote in-home visit for the evaluation and management of an established patient for use only in the Medicare-approved Comprehensive Care for Joint Replacement Model, which requires at least 2 of the following 3 key components: A problem focused history; A problem focused examination; Straightforward medical decision making, furnished in real time using interactive audio and video technology. Counseling and coordination of care with other physicians, other qualified health care professionals or agencies are provided consistent with the nature of the problem(s) and the needs of the patient or the family or both. Usually, the presenting problem(s) are self limited or minor. Typically, 10 minutes are spent with the patient or family or both via real time, audio and video intercommunications technology.

G9487    Remote in-home visit for the evaluation and management of an established patient for use only in the Medicare-approved Comprehensive Care for Joint Replacement Model, which requires at least 2 of the following 3 key components: An expanded problem focused history; An expanded problem focused examination; Medical decision making of low complexity, furnished in real time using interactive audio and video technology. Counseling and coordination of care with other physicians, other qualified health care professionals or agencies are provided consistent with the nature of the problem(s) and the needs of the patient or the family or both. Usually, the presenting problem(s) are of low to moderate severity. Typically, 15 minutes are spent with the patient or family or both via real time, audio and video intercommunications technology.

G9488    Remote in-home visit for the evaluation and management of an established patient for use only in the Medicare-approved Comprehensive Care for Joint Replacement Model, which requires at least 2 of the following 3 key components: A detailed history; A detailed examination; Medical decision making of moderate complexity, furnished in real time using interactive audio and video technology. Counseling and coordination of care with other physicians, other qualified health care professionals or agencies are provided consistent with the nature of the problem(s) and the needs of the patient or the family or both. Usually, the presenting problem(s) are of moderate to high severity. Typically, 25 minutes are spent with the patient or family or both via real time, audio and video intercommunications technology.

G9489    Remote in-home visit for the evaluation and management of an established patient for use only in the Medicare-approved Comprehensive Care for Joint Replacement Model, which requires at least 2 of the following 3 key components: A comprehensive history; A comprehensive examination; Medical decision making of high complexity, furnished in real time using interactive audio and video technology. Counseling and coordination of care with other physicians, other qualified health care professionals or agencies are provided consistent with the nature of the problem(s) and the needs of the patient or the family or both. Usually, the presenting problem(s) are of moderate to high severity. Typically, 40 minutes are spent with the patient or family or both via real time, audio and video intercommunications technology.

© 2016 Optum360, LLC

## NEW CODES (continued)

G9490  Comprehensive Care for Joint Replacement Model, home visit for patient assessment performed by clinical staff for an individual not considered homebound, including, but not necessarily limited to patient assessment of clinical status, safety/fall prevention, functional status/ambulation, medication reconciliation/management, compliance with orders/plan of care, performance of activities of daily living, and ensuring beneficiary connections to community and other services (for use only in the Medicare-approved Comprehensive Care for Joint Replacement Model); may not be billed for a 30 day period covered by a transitional care management code.

G9678  Oncology Care Model (OCM) Monthly Enhanced Oncology Services (MEOS) payment for enhanced care management services for OCM beneficiaries. MEOS covers care management services for Medicare beneficiaries in a 6-month OCM Episode of Care triggered by the administration of chemotherapy. Enhanced care management services include services driven by the OCM practice requirements, including: 24/7 clinician access, use of an ONC-certified Electronic Health Record, utilization of data for quality improvement, patient navigation, documentation of care plans, and use of clinical guidelines.

G9679  Onsite acute care treatment of a nursing facility resident with pneumonia. May only be billed once per day per beneficiary

G9680  Onsite acute care treatment of a nursing facility resident with CHF. May only be billed once per day per beneficiary

G9681  Onsite acute care treatment of a nursing facility resident with COPD or asthma. May only be billed once per day per beneficiary

G9682  Onsite acute care treatment of a nursing facility resident with a skin infection. May only be billed once per day per beneficiary

G9683  Onsite acute care treatment of a nursing facility resident with fluid or electrolyte disorder or dehydration (similar pattern). May only be billed once per day per beneficiary

G9684  Onsite acute care treatment of a nursing facility resident for a UTI. May only be billed once per day per beneficiary

G9685  Evaluation and management of a beneficiary's acute change in condition in a nursing facility

G9686  Onsite nursing facility conference, that is separate and distinct from an Evaluation and Management visit, including qualified practitioner and at least one member of the nursing facility interdisciplinary care team

G9687  Hospice services provided to patient any time during the measurement period

G9688  Patients using hospice services any time during the measurement period

G9689  Patient admitted for performance of elective carotid intervention

G9690  Patient receiving hospice services any time during the measurement period

G9691  Patient had hospice services any time during the measurement period

G9692  Hospice services received by patient any time during the measurement period

G9693  Patient use of hospice services any time during the measurement period

G9694  Hospice services utilized by patient any time during the measurement period

G9695  Long-acting inhaled bronchodilator prescribed

G9696  Documentation of medical reason(s) for not prescribing a long-acting inhaled bronchodilator

G9697  Documentation of patient reason(s) for not prescribing a long-acting inhaled bronchodilator

G9698  Documentation of system reason(s) for not prescribing a long-acting inhaled bronchodilator

G9699  Long-acting inhaled bronchodilator not prescribed, reason not otherwise specified

G9700  Patients who use hospice services any time during the measurement period

G9701  Children who are taking antibiotics in the 30 days prior to the date of the encounter during which the diagnosis was established

G9702  Patients who use hospice services any time during the measurement period

G9703  Children who are taking antibiotics in the 30 days prior to the diagnosis of pharyngitis

G9704  AJCC breast cancer stage I: T1 mic or T1a documented

G9705  AJCC breast cancer stage I: T1b (tumor > 0.5 cm but <= 1 cm in greatest dimension) documented

G9706  Low (or very low) risk of recurrence, prostate cancer

G9707  Patient received hospice services any time during the measurement period

G9708  Women who had a bilateral mastectomy or who have a history of a bilateral mastectomy or for whom there is evidence of a right and a left unilateral mastectomy

G9709  Hospice services used by patient any time during the measurement period

G9710  Patient was provided hospice services any time during the measurement period

G9711  Patients with a diagnosis or past history of total colectomy or colorectal cancer

G9712  Documentation of medical reason(s) for prescribing or dispensing antibiotic (e.g., intestinal infection, pertussis, bacterial infection, lyme disease, otitis media, acute sinusitis, acute pharyngitis, acute tonsillitis, chronic sinusitis, infection of the pharynx/larynx/tonsils/adenoids, prostatitis, cellulitis/mastoiditis/bone infections, acute lymphadenitis, impetigo, skin staph infections, pneumonia, gonococcal infections/venereal disease (syphilis, chlamydia, inflammatory diseases [female reproductive organs]), infections of the kidney, cystitis/UTI, acne, HIV disease/asymptomatic HIV, cystic fibrosis, disorders of the immune system, malignancy neoplasms, chronic bronchitis, emphysema, bronchiectasis, extrinsic allergic alveolitis, chronic airway obstruction, chronic obstructive asthma, pneumoconiosis and other lung disease due to external agents, other diseases of the respiratory system, and tuberculosis

G9713  Patients who use hospice services any time during the measurement period

G9714  Patient is using hospice services any time during the measurement period

G9715  Patients who use hospice services any time during the measurement period

G9716  BMI is documented as being outside of normal limits, follow-up plan is not completed for documented reason

G9717  Documentation stating the patient has an active diagnosis of depression or bipolar disorder, therefore screening or follow-up not required

G9718  Hospice services for patient provided any time during the measurement period

G9719  Patient is not ambulatory, bed ridden, immobile, confined to chair, wheelchair bound, dependent on helper pushing wheelchair, independent in wheelchair or minimal help in wheelchair

G9720  Hospice services for patient occurred any time during the measurement period

G9721  Patient not ambulatory, bed ridden, immobile, confined to chair, wheelchair bound, dependent on helper pushing wheelchair, independent in wheelchair or minimal help in wheelchair

G9722  Documented history of renal failure or baseline serum creatinine = 4.0 mg/dl; renal transplant recipients are not considered to have preoperative renal failure, unless, since transplantation the CR has been or is 4.0 or higher

© 2016 Optum360, LLC

## NEW CODES (continued)

G9723 Hospice services for patient received any time during the measurement period

G9724 Patients who had documentation of use of anticoagulant medications overlapping the measurement year

G9725 Patients who use hospice services any time during the measurement period

G9726 Patient refused to participate

G9727 Patient unable to complete the FOTO knee intake PROM at admission and discharge due to blindness, illiteracy, severe mental incapacity or language incompatibility and an adequate proxy is not available

G9728 Patient refused to participate

G9729 Patient unable to complete the FOTO hip intake PROM at admission and discharge due to blindness, illiteracy, severe mental incapacity or language incompatibility and an adequate proxy is not available

G9730 Patient refused to participate

G9731 Patient unable to complete the FOTO foot or ankle intake PROM at admission and discharge due to blindness, illiteracy, severe mental incapacity or language incompatibility and an adequate proxy is not available

G9732 Patient refused to participate

G9733 Patient unable to complete the FOTO lumbar intake PROM at admission and discharge due to blindness, illiteracy, severe mental incapacity or language incompatibility and an adequate proxy is not available

G9734 Patient refused to participate

G9735 Patient unable to complete the FOTO shoulder intake PROM at admission and discharge due to blindness, illiteracy, severe mental incapacity or language incompatibility and an adequate proxy is not available

G9736 Patient refused to participate

G9737 Patient unable to complete the FOTO elbow, wrist or hand intake PROM at admission and discharge due to blindness, illiteracy, severe mental incapacity or language incompatibility and an adequate proxy is not available

G9738 Patient refused to participate

G9739 Patient unable to complete the FOTO general orthopedic intake PROM at admission and discharge due to blindness, illiteracy, severe mental incapacity or language incompatibility and an adequate proxy is not available

G9740 Hospice services given to patient any time during the measurement period

G9741 Patients who use hospice services any time during the measurement period

G9742 Psychiatric symptoms assessed

G9743 Psychiatric symptoms not assessed, reason not otherwise specified

G9744 Patient not eligible due to active diagnosis of hypertension

G9745 Documented reason for not screening or recommending a follow-up for high blood pressure

G9746 Patient has mitral stenosis or prosthetic heart valves or patient has transient or reversible cause of AF (e.g., pneumonia, hyperthyroidism, pregnancy, cardiac surgery)

G9747 Patient is undergoing palliative dialysis with a catheter

G9748 Patient approved by a qualified transplant program and scheduled to receive a living donor kidney transplant

G9749 Patient is undergoing palliative dialysis with a catheter

G9750 Patient approved by a qualified transplant program and scheduled to receive a living donor kidney transplant

G9751 Patient died at any time during the 24-month measurement period

G9752 Emergency surgery

G9753 Documentation of medical reason for not conducting a search for DICOM format images for prior patient CT imaging studies completed at non-affiliated external healthcare facilities or entities within the past 12 months that are available through a secure, authorized, media-free, shared archive (e.g., trauma, acute myocardial infarction, stroke, aortic aneurysm where time is of the essence)

G9754 A finding of an incidental pulmonary nodule

G9755 Documentation of medical reason(s) that follow-up imaging is indicated (e.g., patient has a known malignancy that can metastasize, other medical reason(s)

G9756 Surgical procedures that included the use of silicone oil

G9757 Surgical procedures that included the use of silicone oil

G9758 Patient in hospice and in terminal phase

G9759 History of preoperative posterior capsule rupture

G9760 Patients who use hospice services any time during the measurement period

G9761 Patients who use hospice services any time during the measurement period

G9762 Patient had at least three HPV vaccines on or between the patient's 9th and 13th birthdays

G9763 Patient did not have at least three HPV vaccines on or between the patient's 9th and 13th birthdays

G9764 Patient has been treated with an oral systemic or biologic medication for psoriasis

G9765 Documentation that the patient declined therapy change, has documented contraindications, or has not been treated with an oral systemic or biologic for at least six consecutive months (e.g., experienced adverse effects or lack of efficacy with all other therapy options) in order to achieve better disease control as measured by PGA, BSA, PASI, or DLQI

G9766 Patients who are transferred from one institution to another with a known diagnosis of CVA for endovascular stroke treatment

G9767 Hospitalized patients with newly diagnosed CVA considered for endovascular stroke treatment

G9768 Patients who utilize hospice services any time during the measurement period

G9769 Patient had a bone mineral density test in the past two years or received osteoporosis medication or therapy in the past 12 months

G9770 Peripheral nerve block (PNB)

G9771 At least 1 body temperature measurement equal to or greater than 35.5 degrees celsius (or 95.9 degrees fahrenheit) achieved within the 30 minutes immediately before or the 15 minutes immediately after anesthesia end time

G9772 Documentation of one of the following medical reason(s) for not achieving at least 1 body temperature measurement equal to or greater than 35.5 degrees celsius (or 95.9 degrees fahrenheit) achieved within the 30 minutes immediately before or the 15 minutes immediately after anesthesia end time (e.g., emergency cases, intentional hypothermia, etc.)

G9773 At least 1 body temperature measurement equal to or greater than 35.5 degrees celsius (or 95.9 degrees fahrenheit) not achieved within the 30 minutes immediately before or the 15 minutes immediately after anesthesia end time

G9774 Patients who have had a hysterectomy

G9775 Patient received at least 2 prophylactic pharmacologic anti-emetic agents of different classes preoperatively and/or intraoperatively

© 2016 Optum360, LLC

## NEW CODES (continued)

G9776  Documentation of medical reason for not receiving at least 2 prophylactic pharmacologic anti-emetic agents of different classes preoperatively and/or intraoperatively (e.g., intolerance or other medical reason)

G9777  Patient did not receive at least 2 prophylactic pharmacologic anti-emetic agents of different classes preoperatively and/or intraoperatively

G9778  Patients who have a diagnosis of pregnancy

G9779  Patients who are breastfeeding

G9780  Patients who have a diagnosis of rhabdomyolysis

G9781  Documentation of medical reason(s) for not currently being a statin therapy user or receive an order (prescription) for statin therapy (e.g., patient with adverse effect, allergy or intolerance to statin medication therapy, patients who are receiving palliative care, patients with active liver disease or hepatic disease or insufficiency, and patients with end stage renal disease (ESRD))

G9782  History of or active diagnosis of familial or pure hypercholesterolemia

G9783  Documentation of patients with diabetes who have a most recent fasting or direct LDL- C laboratory test result < 70 mg/dl and are not taking statin therapy

G9784  Pathologists/dermatopathologists providing a second opinion on a biopsy

G9785  Pathology report diagnosing cutaneous basal cell carcinoma or squamous cell carcinoma (to include in situ disease) sent from the pathologist/dermatopathologist to the biopsying clinician for review within 7 business days from the time when the tissue specimen was received by the pathologist

G9786  Pathology report diagnosing cutaneous basal cell carcinoma or squamous cell carcinoma (to include in situ disease) was not sent from the pathologist/dermatopathologist to the biopsying clinician for review within 7 business days from the time when the tissue specimen was received by the pathologist

G9787  Patient alive as of the last day of the measurement year

G9788  Most recent BP is less than or equal to 140/90 mm Hg

G9789  Blood pressure recorded during inpatient stays, emergency room visits, urgent care visits, and patient self-reported BP's (home and health fair BP results)

G9790  Most recent BP is greater than 140/90 mm Hg, or blood pressure not documented

G9791  Most recent tobacco status is tobacco free

G9792  Most recent tobacco status is not tobacco free

G9793  Patient is currently on a daily aspirin or other antiplatelet

G9794  Documentation of medical reason(s) for not on a daily aspirin or other antiplatelet (e.g., history of gastrointestinal bleed or intra-cranial bleed or documentation of active anticoagulant use during the measurement period

G9795  Patient is not currently on a daily aspirin or other antiplatelet

G9796  Patient is currently on a statin therapy

G9797  Patient is not on a statin therapy

G9798  Discharge(s) for AMI between July 1 of the year prior measurement year to June 30 of the measurement period

G9799  Patients with a medication dispensing event indicator of a history of asthma any time during the patient's history through the end of the measure period

G9800  Patients who are identified as having an intolerance or allergy to beta-blocker therapy

G9801  Hospitalizations in which the patient was transferred directly to a non-acute care facility for any diagnosis

G9802  Patients who use hospice services any time during the measurement period

G9803  Patient prescribed a 180-day course of treatment with beta-blockers post discharge for AMI

G9804  Patient was not prescribed a 180-day course of treatment with beta-blockers post discharge for AMI

G9805  Patients who use hospice services any time during the measurement period

G9806  Patients who received cervical cytology or an HPV test

G9807  Patients who did not receive cervical cytology or an HPV test

G9808  Any patients who had no asthma controller medications dispensed during the measurement year

G9809  Patients who use hospice services any time during the measurement period

G9810  Patient achieved a PDC of at least 75% for their asthma controller medication

G9811  Patient did not achieve a PDC of at least 75% for their asthma controller medication

G9812  Patient died including all deaths occurring during the hospitalization in which the operation was performed, even if after 30 days, and those deaths occurring after discharge from the hospital, but within 30 days of the procedure

G9813  Patient did not die within 30 days of the procedure or during the index hospitalization

G9814  Death occurring during hospitalization

G9815  Death did not occur during hospitalization

G9816  Death occurring 30 days post procedure

G9817  Death did not occur 30 days post procedure

G9818  Documentation of sexual activity

G9819  Patients who use hospice services any time during the measurement period

G9820  Documentation of a chlamydia screening test with proper follow-up

G9821  No documentation of a chlamydia screening test with proper follow-up

G9822  Women who had an endometrial ablation procedure during the year prior to the index date (exclusive of the index date)

G9823  Endometrial sampling or hysteroscopy with biopsy and results documented

G9824  Endometrial sampling or hysteroscopy with biopsy and results not documented

G9825  HER2/neu negative or undocumented/unknown

G9826  Patient transferred to practice after initiation of chemotherapy

G9827  HER2-targeted therapies not administered during the initial course of treatment

G9828  HER2-targeted therapies administered during the initial course of treatment

G9829  Breast adjuvant chemotherapy administered

G9830  HER2/neu positive

G9831  AJCC stage at breast cancer diagnosis = II or III

G9832  AJCC stage at breast cancer diagnosis = I (Ia or Ib) and T-stage at breast cancer diagnosis does not equal = T1, T1a, T1b

G9833  Patient transfer to practice after initiation of chemotherapy

G9834  Patient has metastatic disease at diagnosis

G9835  Trastuzumab administered within 12 months of diagnosis

G9836  Reason for not administering trastuzumab documented (e.g., patient declined, patient died, patient transferred, contraindication or other clinical exclusion, neoadjuvant chemotherapy or radiation not complete)

## NEW CODES (continued)

| | |
|---|---|
| G9837 | Trastuzumab not administered within 12 months of diagnosis |
| G9838 | Patient has metastatic disease at diagnosis |
| G9839 | Anti-EGFR monoclonal antibody therapy |
| G9840 | KRAS gene mutation testing performed before initiation of anti-EGFR MoAb |
| G9841 | KRAS gene mutation testing not performed before initiation of anti-EGFR MoAb |
| G9842 | Patient has metastatic disease at diagnosis |
| G9843 | KRAS gene mutation |
| G9844 | Patient did not receive anti-EGFR monoclonal antibody therapy |
| G9845 | Patient received anti-EGFR monoclonal antibody therapy |
| G9846 | Patients who died from cancer |
| G9847 | Patient received chemotherapy in the last 14 days of life |
| G9848 | Patient did not receive chemotherapy in the last 14 days of life |
| G9849 | Patients who died from cancer |
| G9850 | Patient had more than one emergency department visit in the last 30 days of life |
| G9851 | Patient had one or less emergency department visits in the last 30 days of life |
| G9852 | Patients who died from cancer |
| G9853 | Patient admitted to the ICU in the last 30 days of life |
| G9854 | Patient was not admitted to the ICU in the last 30 days of life |
| G9855 | Patients who died from cancer |
| G9856 | Patient was not admitted to hospice |
| G9857 | Patient admitted to hospice |
| G9858 | Patient enrolled in hospice |
| G9859 | Patients who died from cancer |
| G9860 | Patient spent less than three days in hospice care |
| G9861 | Patient spent greater than or equal to three days in hospice care |
| G9862 | Documentation of medical reason(s) for not recommending at least a 10 year follow-up interval (e.g., inadequate prep, familial or personal history of colonic polyps, patient had no adenoma and age is = 66 years old, or life expectancy < 10 years old, other medical reasons) |
| J0883 | Injection, argatroban, 1 mg (for non-ESRD use) |
| J0884 | Injection, argatroban, 1 mg (for ESRD on dialysis) |
| J1942 | Injection, aripiprazole lauroxil, 1 mg |
| J2182 | Injection, mepolizumab, 1 mg |
| J2786 | Injection, reslizumab, 1 mg |
| J7175 | Injection, factor X, (human), 1 IU |
| J7179 | Injection, von Willebrand factor (recombinant), (Vonvendi), 1 IU VWF:RCo |
| J7202 | Injection, factor IX, albumin fusion protein, (recombinant), Idelvion, 1 IU |
| J7207 | Injection, factor VIII, (antihemophilic factor, recombinant), pegylated, 1 IU |
| J7209 | Injection, factor VIII, (antihemophilic factor, recombinant), (Nuwiq), 1 IU |
| J8670 | Rolapitant, oral, 1 mg |
| J9034 | Injection, bendamustine HCl (Bendeka), 1 mg |
| J9145 | Injection, daratumumab, 10 mg |
| J9176 | Injection, elotuzumab, 1 mg |
| J9205 | Injection, irinotecan liposome, 1 mg |
| J9325 | Injection, talimogene laherparepvec, per 1 million plaque forming units |
| J9352 | Injection, trabectedin, 0.1 mg |
| L1851 | Knee orthosis (KO), single upright, thigh and calf, with adjustable flexion and extension joint (unicentric or polycentric), medial-lateral and rotation control, with or without varus/valgus adjustment, prefabricated, off-the-shelf |
| L1852 | Knee orthosis (KO), double upright, thigh and calf, with adjustable flexion and extension joint (unicentric or polycentric), medial-lateral and rotation control, with or without varus/valgus adjustment, prefabricated, off-the-shelf |
| Q4166 | Cytal, per sq cm |
| Q4167 | Truskin, per sq cm |
| Q4168 | AmnioBand, 1 mg |
| Q4169 | Artacent wound, per sq cm |
| Q4170 | Cygnus, per sq cm |
| Q4171 | Interfyl, 1 mg |
| Q4172 | PuraPly or PuraPly AM, per sq cm |
| Q4173 | PalinGen or PalinGen XPlus, per sq cm |
| Q4174 | PalinGen or ProMatrX, 0.36 mg per 0.25 cc |
| Q4175 | Miroderm, per sq cm |
| Q5102 | Injection, infliximab, biosimilar, 10 mg |
| Q9982 | Flutemetamol F18, diagnostic, per study dose, up to 5 millicuries |
| Q9983 | Florbetaben F18, diagnostic, per study dose, up to 8.1 millicuries |
| S0285 | Colonoscopy consultation performed prior to a screening colonoscopy procedure |
| S0311 | Comprehensive management and care coordination for advanced illness, per calendar month |
| T1040 | Medicaid certified community behavioral health clinic services, per diem |
| T1041 | Medicaid certified community behavioral health clinic services, per month |

## CHANGED CODES

| | |
|---|---|
| A4221 | Supplies for maintenance of non-insulin drug infusion catheter, per week (list drugs separately) |
| A9599 | Radiopharmaceutical, diagnostic, for beta-amyloid positron emission tomography (PET) imaging, per study dose, not otherwise specified |
| B9002 | Enteral nutrition infusion pump, any type |
| C1820 | Generator, neurostimulator (implantable), with rechargeable battery and charging system |
| E0627 | Seat lift mechanism, electric, any type |
| E0629 | Seat lift mechanism, non-electric, any type |
| E0740 | Non-implanted pelvic floor electrical stimulator, complete system |
| E0967 | Manual wheelchair accessory, hand rim with projections, any type, replacement only, each |
| E0995 | Wheelchair accessory, calf rest/pad, replacement only, each |
| E2206 | Manual wheelchair accessory, wheel lock assembly, complete, replacement only, each |
| E2220 | Manual wheelchair accessory, solid (rubber/plastic) propulsion tire, any size, replacement only, each |
| E2221 | Manual wheelchair accessory, solid (rubber/plastic) caster tire (removable), any size, replacement only, each |

© 2016 Optum360, LLC

## CHANGED CODES (continued)

**E2222** Manual wheelchair accessory, solid (rubber/plastic) caster tire with integrated wheel, any size, replacement only, each

**E2224** Manual wheelchair accessory, propulsion wheel excludes tire, any size, replacement only, each

**G0202** Screening mammography, bilateral (2-view study of each breast), including computer-aided detection (CAD) when performed

**G0204** Diagnostic mammography, including computer-aided detection (CAD) when performed; bilateral

**G0206** Diagnostic mammography, including computer-aided detection (CAD) when performed; unilateral

**G8427** Eligible clinician attests to documenting in the medical record they obtained, updated, or reviewed the patient's current medications

**G8428** Current list of medications not documented as obtained, updated, or reviewed by the eligible clinician, reason not given

**G8430** Eligible clinician attests to documenting in the medical record the patient is not eligible for a current list of medications being obtained, updated, or reviewed by the eligible clinician

**G8431** Screening for depression is documented as being positive and a follow-up plan is documented

**G8432** Depression screening not documented, reason not given

**G8433** Screening for depression not completed, documented reason

**G8510** Screening for depression is documented as negative, a follow-up plan is not required

**G8511** Screening for depression documented as positive, follow-up plan not documented, reason not given

**G8598** Aspirin or another antiplatelet therapy used

**G8599** Aspirin or another antiplatelet therapy not used, reason not given

**G8649** Risk-adjusted functional status change residual scores for the knee not measured because the patient did not complete FOTO's status survey near discharge, not appropriate

**G8653** Risk-adjusted functional status change residual scores for the hip not measured because the patient did not complete follow up status survey near discharge, patient not appropriate

**G8655** Risk-adjusted functional status change residual score for the foot or ankle successfully calculated and the score was equal to zero (0) or greater than zero (> 0)

**G8656** Risk-adjusted functional status change residual score for the foot or ankle successfully calculated and the score was less than zero (< 0)

**G8657** Risk-adjusted functional status change residual scores for the foot or ankle not measured because the patient did not complete FOTO's status survey near discharge, patient not appropriate

**G8658** Risk-adjusted functional status change residual scores for the foot or ankle not measured because the patient did not complete FOTO's functional intake on admission and/or follow-up status survey near discharge, reason not given

**G8659** Risk-adjusted functional status change residual score for the lumbar impairment successfully calculated and the score was equal to zero (0) or greater than zero (> 0)

**G8660** Risk-adjusted functional status change residual score for the lumbar impairment successfully calculated and the score was less than zero (< 0)

**G8661** Risk-adjusted functional status change residual scores for the lumbar impairment not measured because the patient did not complete FOTO's status survey near discharge, patient not appropriate

**G8662** Risk-adjusted functional status change residual scores for the lumbar impairment not measured because the patient did not complete FOTO's functional intake on admission and/or follow-up status survey near discharge, reason not given

**G8665** Risk-adjusted functional status change residual scores for the shoulder not measured because the patient did not complete FOTO's functional status survey near discharge, patient not appropriate

**G8669** Risk-adjusted functional status change residual scores for the elbow, wrist or hand not measured because the patient did not complete FOTO's functional follow-up status survey near discharge, patient not appropriate

**G8671** Risk-adjusted functional status change residual score for the neck, cranium, mandible, thoracic spine, ribs, or other general orthopaedic impairment successfully calculated and the score was equal to zero (0) or greater than zero (> 0)

**G8672** Risk-adjusted functional status change residual score for the neck, cranium, mandible, thoracic spine, ribs, or other general orthopaedic impairment successfully calculated and the score was less than zero (< 0)

**G8673** Risk-adjusted functional status change residual scores for the neck, cranium, mandible, thoracic spine, ribs, or other general orthopaedic impairment not measured because the patient did not complete FOTO's functional follow-up status survey near discharge, patient not appropriate

**G8674** Risk-adjusted functional status change residual scores for the neck, cranium, mandible, thoracic spine, ribs, or other general orthopaedic impairment not measured because the patient did not complete FOTO's functional intake on admission and/or follow-up status survey near discharge, reason not given

**G8697** Antithrombotic therapy not prescribed for documented reasons (e.g., patient had stroke during hospital stay, patient expired during inpatient stay, other medical reason(s)); (e.g., patient left against medical advice, other patient reason(s))

**G8815** Documented reason in the medical records for why the statin therapy was not prescribed (i.e., lower extremity bypass was for a patient with non-artherosclerotic disease)

**G8924** Spirometry test results demonstrate FEV1/FVC < 70%, FEV < 60% predicted and patient has COPD symptoms (e.g., dyspnea, cough/sputum, wheezing)

**G8925** Spirometry test results demonstrate FEV1 >= 60%, FEV1/FVC >= 70%, predicted or patient does not have COPD symptoms

**G8968** Documentation of medical reason(s) for not prescribing warfarin or another oral anticoagulant that is FDA approved for the prevention of thromboembolism (e.g., allergy, risk of bleeding, other medical reasons)

**G9226** Foot examination performed (includes examination through visual inspection, sensory exam with 10-g monofilament plus testing any one of the following: vibration using 128-hz tuning fork, pinprick sensation, ankle reflexes, or vibration perception threshold, and pulse exam; report when all of the 3 components are completed)

**G9229** Chlamydia, gonorrhea, and syphilis screening results not documented (patient refusal is the only allowed exception)

**G9231** Documentation of end stage renal disease (ESRD), dialysis, renal transplant before or during the measurement period or pregnancy during the measurement period

**G9232** Clinician treating major depressive disorder did not communicate to clinician treating comorbid condition for specified patient reason (e.g., patient is unable to communicate the diagnosis of a comorbid condition; the patient is unwilling to communicate the diagnosis of a comorbid condition; or the patient is unaware of the comorbid condition, or any other specified patient reason)

**G9239** Documentation of reasons for patient initiaiting maintenance hemodialysis with a catheter as the mode of vascular access (e.g., patient has a maturing AVF/AVG, time-limited trial of hemodialysis, other medical reasons, patient declined AVF/AVG, other patient reasons, patient followed by reporting nephrologist for fewer than 90 days, other system reasons)

**G9264** Documentation of patient receiving maintenance hemodialysis for greater than or equal to 90 days with a catheter for documented reasons (e.g., other medical reasons, patient declined AVF/AVG, other patient reasons)

Appendix 5 — HCPCS Changes for 2017

## CHANGED CODES (continued)

G9307 No return to the operating room for a surgical procedure, for complications of the principal operative procedure, within 30 days of the principal operative procedure

G9308 Unplanned return to the operating room for a surgical procedure, for complications of the principal operative procedure, within 30 days of the principal operative procedure

G9326 CT studies performed not reported to a radiation dose index registry that is capable of collecting at a minimum all necessary data elements, reason not given

G9327 CT studies performed reported to a radiation dose index registry that is capable of collecting at a minimum all necessary data elements

G9359 Documentation of negative or managed positive TB screen with further evidence that TB is not active within one year of patient visit

G9361 Medical indication for induction [documentation of reason(s) for elective delivery (c-section) or early induction (e.g., hemorrhage and placental complications, hypertension, preeclampsia and eclampsia, rupture of membranes-premature or prolonged, maternal conditions complicating pregnancy/delivery, fetal conditions complicating pregnancy/delivery, late pregnancy, prior uterine surgery, or participation in clinical trial)]

G9381 Documentation of medical reason(s) for not offering assistance with end of life issues (e.g., patient in hospice care, patient in terminal phase) during the measurement period

G9416 Patient had one tetanus, diphtheria toxoids and acellular pertussis vaccine (TDaP) on or between the patient's 10th and 13th birthdays

G9417 Patient did not have one tetanus, diphtheria toxoids and acellular pertussis vaccine (TDaP) on or between the patient's 10th and 13th birthdays

G9423 Documentation of medical reason for not including PT category, PN category and histologic type [for patient with appropriate exclusion criteria (e.g., metastatic disease, benign tumors, malignant tumors other than carcinomas, inadequate surgical specimens)]

G9424 Specimen site other than anatomic location of lung, or classified as NSCLC-NOS

G9497 Received instruction from the anesthesiologist or proxy prior to the day of surgery to abstain from smoking on the day of surgery

G9500 Radiation exposure indices, or exposure time and number of fluorographic images in final report for procedures using fluoroscopy, documented

G9501 Radiation exposure indices, or exposure time and number of fluorographic images not documented in final report for procedure using fluoroscopy, reason not given

G9519 Patient achieves final refraction (spherical equivalent) +/- 0.5 diopters of their planned refraction within 90 days of surgery

G9520 Patient does not achieve final refraction (spherical equivalent) +/- 0.5 diopters of their planned refraction within 90 days of surgery

G9531 Patient has documentation of ventricular shunt, brain tumor, multisystem trauma, pregnancy, or is currently taking an antiplatelet medication including: ASA/dipyridamole, clopidogrel, prasugrel, ticlopidine, ticagrelor or cilstazol)

G9532 Patient's head injury occurred greater than 24 hours before presentation to the emergency department, or has a GCS score less than 15 or does not have a GCS score documented, or had a head CT for trauma ordered by someone other than an emergency care provider, or was ordered for a reason other than trauma

G9547 Incidental finding: liver lesion <= 0.5 cm, cystic kidney lesion < 1.0 cm or adrenal lesion <= 1.0 cm

G9549 Documentation of medical reason(s) that follow-up imaging is indicated (e.g., patient has a known malignancy that can metastasize, other medical reason(s) such as fever in an immunocompromised patient)

G9551 Final reports for abdominal imaging studies without an incidentally found lesion noted: liver lesion <= 0.5 cm, cystic kidney lesion < 1.0 cm or adrenal lesion <= 1.0 cm noted or no lesion found

G9554 Final reports for CT, CTA, MRI or MRA of the chest or neck or ultrasound of the neck with follow-up imaging recommended

G9555 Documentation of medical reason(s) for recommending follow up imaging (e.g., patient has multiple endocrine neoplasia, patient has cervical lymphadenopathy, other medical reason(s))

G9556 Final reports for CT, CTA, MRI or MRA of the chest or neck or ultrasound of the neck with follow-up imaging not recommended

G9557 Final reports for CT, CTA, MRI or MRA studies of the chest or neck or ultrasound of the neck without an incidentally found thyroid nodule < 1.0 cm noted or no nodule found

G9595 Patient has documentation of ventricular shunt, brain tumor, coagulopathy, including thrombocytopenia

G9596 Pediatric patient's head injury occurred greater than 24 hours before presentation to the emergency department, or has a GCS score less than 15 or does not have a GCS score documented, or had a head CT for trauma ordered by someone other than an emergency care provider, or was ordered for a reason other than trauma

G9607 Documented medical reasons for not performing intraoperative cystoscopy (e.g., urethral pathology precluding cystoscopy, any patient who has a congenital or acquired absence of the urethra)

G9609 Documentation of an order for antiplatelet agents

G9610 Documentation of medical reason(s) in the patient's record for not ordering antiplatelet agents

G9611 Order for antiplatelet agents was not documented in the patient's record, reason not given

G9625 Patient sustained bladder injury at the time of surgery or discovered subsequently up to 1 month postsurgery

G9626 Documented medical reason for not reporting bladder injury (e.g., gynecologic or other pelvic malignancy documented, concurrent surgery involving bladder pathology, injury that occurs during urinary incontinence procedure, patient death from non-medical causes not related to surgery, patient died during procedure without evidence of bladder injury)

G9627 Patient did not sustain bladder injury at the time of surgery nor discovered subsequently up to 1 month postsurgery

G9628 Patient sustained bowel injury at the time of surgery or discovered subsequently up to 1 month postsurgery

G9629 Documented medical reasons for not reporting bowel injury (e.g., gynecologic or other pelvic malignancy documented, planned (e.g., not due to an unexpected bowel injury) resection and/or reanastomosis of bowel, or patient death from nonmedical causes not related to surgery, patient died during procedure without evidence of bowel injury)

G9630 Patient did not sustain a bowel injury at the time of surgery nor discovered subsequently up to 1 month postsurgery

G9632 Documented medical reasons for not reporting ureter injury (e.g., gynecologic or other pelvic malignancy documented, concurrent surgery involving bladder pathology, injury that occurs during a urinary incontinence procedure, patient death from nonmedical causes not related to surgery, patient died during procedure without evidence of ureter injury)

G9633 Patient did not sustain ureter injury at the time of surgery nor discovered subsequently up to 1 month postsurgery

G9642 Current smokers (e.g., cigarette, cigar, pipe, e-cigarette or marijuana)

J0573 Buprenorphine/naloxone, oral, greater than 3 mg, but less than or equal to 6 mg buprenorphine

J1745 Injection, infliximab, excludes biosimilar, 10 mg

J3357 Ustekinumab, for subcutaneous injection, 1 mg

© 2016 Optum360, LLC

## CHANGED CODES (continued)

| | |
|---|---|
| J7201 | Injection, factor IX, Fc fusion protein, (recombinant), Alprolix, 1 IU |
| J7297 | Levonorgestrel-releasing intrauterine contraceptive system (Liletta), 52 mg |
| J7298 | Levonorgestrel-releasing intrauterine contraceptive system (Mirena), 52 mg |
| J7301 | Levonorgestrel-releasing intrauterine contraceptive system (Skyla), 13.5 mg |
| J7340 | Carbidopa 5 mg/levodopa 20 mg enteral suspension, 100 ml |
| J9033 | Injection, bendamustine HCl (Treanda), 1 mg |
| K0019 | Arm pad, replacement only, each |
| K0037 | High mount flip-up footrest, replacement only, each |
| K0042 | Standard size footplate, replacement only, each |
| K0043 | Footrest, lower extension tube, replacement only, each |
| K0044 | Footrest, upper hanger bracket, replacement only, each |
| K0045 | Footrest, complete assembly, replacement only, each |
| K0046 | Elevating legrest, lower extension tube, replacement only, each |
| K0047 | Elevating legrest, upper hanger bracket, replacement only, each |
| K0050 | Ratchet assembly, replacement only |
| K0051 | Cam release assembly, footrest or legrest, replacement only, each |
| K0052 | Swingaway, detachable footrests, replacement only, each |
| K0069 | Rear wheel assembly, complete, with solid tire, spokes or molded, replacement only, each |
| K0070 | Rear wheel assembly, complete, with pneumatic tire, spokes or molded, replacement only, each |
| K0071 | Front caster assembly, complete, with pneumatic tire, replacement only, each |
| K0072 | Front caster assembly, complete, with semipneumatic tire, replacement only, each |
| K0077 | Front caster assembly, complete, with solid tire, replacement only, each |
| K0098 | Drive belt for power wheelchair, replacement only |
| K0552 | Supplies for external non-insulin drug infusion pump, syringe type cartridge, sterile, each |
| L1906 | Ankle foot orthosis, multiligamentous ankle support, prefabricated, off-the-shelf |
| P9072 | Platelets, pheresis, pathogen reduced or rapid bacterial tested, each unit |
| Q2039 | Influenza virus vaccine, not otherwise specified |
| Q4105 | Integra dermal regeneration template (DRT) or Integra Omnigraft dermal regeneration matrix, per sq cm |
| Q4131 | EpiFix or Epicord, per sq cm |

## DELETED CODES

| | | | | | | |
|---|---|---|---|---|---|---|
| A4466 | A9544 | A9545 | B9000 | C9121 | C9137 | C9138 |
| C9139 | C9349 | C9458 | C9459 | C9461 | C9470 | C9471 |
| C9472 | C9473 | C9474 | C9475 | C9476 | C9477 | C9478 |
| C9479 | C9480 | C9481 | C9742 | C9743 | C9800 | E0628 |
| G0163 | G0164 | G0389 | G0436 | G0437 | G3001 | G8401 |
| G8458 | G8460 | G8461 | G8485 | G8486 | G8487 | G8489 |
| G8490 | G8491 | G8494 | G8495 | G8496 | G8497 | G8498 |
| G8499 | G8500 | G8544 | G8545 | G8548 | G8549 | G8551 |
| G8634 | G8645 | G8646 | G8725 | G8726 | G8728 | G8757 |
| G8758 | G8759 | G8761 | G8762 | G8765 | G8784 | G8848 |
| G8853 | G8868 | G8898 | G8899 | G8900 | G8902 | G8903 |
| G8906 | G8927 | G8928 | G8929 | G8940 | G8953 | G8977 |
| G9203 | G9204 | G9205 | G9206 | G9207 | G9208 | G9209 |
| G9210 | G9211 | G9217 | G9219 | G9222 | G9233 | G9234 |
| G9235 | G9236 | G9237 | G9238 | G9244 | G9245 | G9324 |
| G9435 | G9436 | G9437 | G9438 | G9439 | G9440 | G9441 |
| G9442 | G9443 | G9463 | G9464 | G9465 | G9466 | G9467 |
| G9499 | G9572 | G9581 | G9619 | G9650 | G9652 | G9653 |
| G9657 | G9667 | G9669 | G9670 | G9671 | G9672 | G9673 |
| G9677 | J0760 | J1590 | K0901 | K0902 | Q4119 | Q4120 |
| Q4129 | Q9980 | Q9981 | S8032 | | | |

## RECYCLED CODES

| | |
|---|---|
| A9515 | Choline C-11, diagnostic, per study dose up to 20 millicuries |
| J0570 | Buprenorphine implant, 74.2 mg |
| J1130 | Injection, diclofenac sodium, 0.5 mg |
| J2840 | Injection, sebelipase alfa, 1 mg |
| J7320 | Hyaluronan or derivitive, Genvisc 850, for intra-articular injection, 1 mg |
| J7322 | Hyaluronan or derivative, Hymovis, for intra-articular injection, 1 mg |
| J7342 | Installation, ciprofloxacin otic suspension, 6 mg |
| J9295 | Injection, necitumumab, 1 mg |
| S3854 | Gene expression profiling panel for use in the management of breast cancer treatment |

# Appendix 6 — Place of Service and Type of Service

## Place-of-Service Codes for Professional Claims

Listed below are place of service codes and descriptions. These codes should be used on professional claims to specify the entity where service(s) were rendered. Check with individual payers (e.g., Medicare, Medicaid, other private insurance) for reimbursement policies regarding these codes. To comment on a code(s) or description(s), please send your request to posinfo@cms.gov.

| Code | Name | Description |
|---|---|---|
| 01 | Pharmacy | A facility or location where drugs and other medically related items and services are sold, dispensed, or otherwise provided directly to patients. |
| 02 | Telehealth | The location where health services and health related services are provided or received, through telecommunication technology. (Effective January 1, 2016.) |
| 03 | School | A facility whose primary purpose is education. |
| 04 | Homeless shelter | A facility or location whose primary purpose is to provide temporary housing to homeless individuals (e.g., emergency shelters, individual or family shelters). |
| 05 | Indian Health Service freestanding facility | A facility or location, owned and operated by the Indian Health Service, which provides diagnostic, therapeutic (surgical and non-surgical), and rehabilitation services to American Indians and Alaska natives who do not require hospitalization. |
| 06 | Indian Health Service provider-based facility | A facility or location, owned and operated by the Indian Health Service, which provides diagnostic, therapeutic (surgical and nonsurgical), and rehabilitation services rendered by, or under the supervision of, physicians to American Indians and Alaska natives admitted as inpatients or outpatients. |
| 07 | Tribal 638 freestanding facility | A facility or location owned and operated by a federally recognized American Indian or Alaska native tribe or tribal organization under a 638 agreement, which provides diagnostic, therapeutic (surgical and nonsurgical), and rehabilitation services to tribal members who do not require hospitalization. |
| 08 | Tribal 638 Provider-based Facility | A facility or location owned and operated by a federally recognized American Indian or Alaska native tribe or tribal organization under a 638 agreement, which provides diagnostic, therapeutic (surgical and nonsurgical), and rehabilitation services to tribal members admitted as inpatients or outpatients. |
| 09 | Prison/correctional facility | A prison, jail, reformatory, work farm, detention center, or any other similar facility maintained by either federal, state or local authorities for the purpose of confinement or rehabilitation of adult or juvenile criminal offenders. |
| 10 | Unassigned | N/A |
| 11 | Office | Location, other than a hospital, skilled nursing facility (SNF), military treatment facility, community health center, State or local public health clinic, or intermediate care facility (ICF), where the health professional routinely provides health examinations, diagnosis, and treatment of illness or injury on an ambulatory basis. |
| 12 | Home | Location, other than a hospital or other facility, where the patient receives care in a private residence. |
| 13 | Assisted living facility | Congregate residential facility with self-contained living units providing assessment of each resident's needs and on-site support 24 hours a day, 7 days a week, with the capacity to deliver or arrange for services including some health care and other services. |
| 14 | Group home | A residence, with shared living areas, where clients receive supervision and other services such as social and/or behavioral services, custodial service, and minimal services (e.g., medication administration). |
| 15 | Mobile unit | A facility/unit that moves from place-to-place equipped to provide preventive, screening, diagnostic, and/or treatment services. |
| 16 | Temporary lodging | A short-term accommodation such as a hotel, campground, hostel, cruise ship or resort where the patient receives care, and which is not identified by any other POS code. |
| 17 | Walk-in retail health clinic | A walk-in health clinic, other than an office, urgent care facility, pharmacy, or independent clinic and not described by any other place of service code, that is located within a retail operation and provides preventive and primary care services on an ambulatory basis. |
| 18 | Place of employment/worksite | A location, not described by any other POS code, owned or operated by a public or private entity where the patient is employed, and where a health professional provides on-going or episodic occupational medical, therapeutic or rehabilitative services to the individual. |
| 19 | Off campus-outpatient hospital | A portion of an off-campus hospital provider based department which provides diagnostic, therapeutic (both surgical and nonsurgical), and rehabilitation services to sick or injured persons who do not require hospitalization or institutionalization. |
| 20 | Urgent care facility | Location, distinct from a hospital emergency room, an office, or a clinic, whose purpose is to diagnose and treat illness or injury for unscheduled, ambulatory patients seeking immediate medical attention. |

Appendix 6 — Place of Service and Type of Service

| 21 | Inpatient hospital | A facility, other than psychiatric, which primarily provides diagnostic, therapeutic (both surgical and nonsurgical), and rehabilitation services by, or under, the supervision of physicians to patients admitted for a variety of medical conditions. |
|---|---|---|
| 22 | On campus-outpatient hospital | A portion of a hospital's main campus which provides diagnostic, therapeutic (both surgical and nonsurgical), and rehabilitation services to sick or injured persons who do not require hospitalization or institutionalization. |
| 23 | Emergency room— hospital | A portion of a hospital where emergency diagnosis and treatment of illness or injury is provided. |
| 24 | Ambulatory surgical center | A freestanding facility, other than a physician's office, where surgical and diagnostic services are provided on an ambulatory basis. |
| 25 | Birthing center | A facility, other than a hospital's maternity facilities or a physician's office, which provides a setting for labor, delivery, and immediate post-partum care as well as immediate care of new born infants. |
| 26 | Military treatment facility | A medical facility operated by one or more of the uniformed services. Military treatment facility (MTF) also refers to certain former U.S. Public Health Service (USPHS) facilities now designated as uniformed service treatment facilities (USTF). |
| 27-30 | Unassigned | N/A |
| 31 | Skilled nursing facility | A facility which primarily provides inpatient skilled nursing care and related services to patients who require medical, nursing, or rehabilitative services but does not provide the level of care or treatment available in a hospital. |
| 32 | Nursing facility | A facility which primarily provides to residents skilled nursing care and related services for the rehabilitation of injured, disabled, or sick persons, or, on a regular basis, health-related care services above the level of custodial care to other than mentally retarded individuals. |
| 33 | Custodial care facility | A facility which provides room, board, and other personal assistance services, generally on a long-term basis, and which does not include a medical component. |
| 34 | Hospice | A facility, other than a patient's home, in which palliative and supportive care for terminally ill patients and their families are provided. |
| 35-40 | Unassigned | N/A |
| 41 | Ambulance—land | A land vehicle specifically designed, equipped and staffed for lifesaving and transporting the sick or injured. |
| 42 | Ambulance—air or water | An air or water vehicle specifically designed, equipped and staffed for lifesaving and transporting the sick or injured. |
| 43-48 | Unassigned | N/A |
| 49 | Independent clinic | A location, not part of a hospital and not described by any other place-of-service code, that is organized and operated to provide preventive, diagnostic, therapeutic, rehabilitative, or palliative services to outpatients only. |
| 50 | Federally qualified health center | A facility located in a medically underserved area that provides Medicare beneficiaries preventive primary medical care under the general direction of a physician. |
| 51 | Inpatient psychiatric facility | A facility that provides inpatient psychiatric services for the diagnosis and treatment of mental illness on a 24-hour basis, by or under the supervision of a physician. |
| 52 | Psychiatric facility-partial hospitalization | A facility for the diagnosis and treatment of mental illness that provides a planned therapeutic program for patients who do not require full time hospitalization, but who need broader programs than are possible from outpatient visits to a hospital-based or hospital-affiliated facility. |
| 53 | Community mental health center | A facility that provides the following services: outpatient services, including specialized outpatient services for children, the elderly, individuals who are chronically ill, and residents of the CMHC's mental health services area who have been discharged from inpatient treatment at a mental health facility; 24 hour a day emergency care services; day treatment, other partial hospitalization services, or psychosocial rehabilitation services; screening for patients being considered for admission to state mental health facilities to determine the appropriateness of such admission; and consultation and education services. |
| 54 | Intermediate Care Facility/Individuals with Intellectual Disabilities | A facility which primarily provides health-related care and services above the level of custodial care to individuals with Intellectual Disabilities but does not provide the level of care or treatment available in a hospital or SNF. |
| 55 | Residential substance abuse treatment facility | A facility which provides treatment for substance (alcohol and drug) abuse to live-in residents who do not require acute medical care. Services include individual and group therapy and counseling, family counseling, laboratory tests, drugs and supplies, psychological testing, and room and board. |
| 56 | Psychiatric residential treatment center | A facility or distinct part of a facility for psychiatric care which provides a total 24-hour therapeutically planned and professionally staffed group living and learning environment. |
| 57 | Non-residential substance abuse treatment facility | A location which provides treatment for substance (alcohol and drug) abuse on an ambulatory basis. Services include individual and group therapy and counseling, family counseling, laboratory tests, drugs and supplies, and psychological testing. |
| 58-59 | Unassigned | N/A |
| 60 | Mass immunization center | A location where providers administer pneumococcal pneumonia and influenza virus vaccinations and submit these services as electronic media claims, paper claims, or using the roster billing method. This generally takes place in a mass immunization setting, such as, a public health center, pharmacy, or mall but may include a physician office setting. |

© 2016 Optum360, LLC

| 61 | Comprehensive inpatient rehabilitation facility | A facility that provides comprehensive rehabilitation services under the supervision of a physician to inpatients with physical disabilities. Services include physical therapy, occupational therapy, speech pathology, social or psychological services, and orthotics and prosthetics services. |
| 62 | Comprehensive outpatient rehabilitation facility | A facility that provides comprehensive rehabilitation services under the supervision of a physician to outpatients with physical disabilities. Services include physical therapy, occupational therapy, and speech pathology services. |
| 63-64 | Unassigned | N/A |
| 65 | End-stage renal disease treatment facility | A facility other than a hospital, which provides dialysis treatment, maintenance, and/or training to patients or caregivers on an ambulatory or home-care basis. |
| 66-70 | Unassigned | N/A |
| 71 | State or local public health clinic | A facility maintained by either state or local health departments that provides ambulatory primary medical care under the general direction of a physician. |
| 72 | Rural health clinic | A certified facility which is located in a rural medically underserved area that provides ambulatory primary medical care under the general direction of a physician. |
| 73-80 | Unassigned | N/A |
| 81 | Independent laboratory | A laboratory certified to perform diagnostic and/or clinical tests independent of an institution or a physician's office. |
| 82-98 | Unassigned | N/A |
| 99 | Other place of service | Other place of service not identified above. |

## Type of Service

### Common Working File Type of Service (TOS) Indicators

For submitting a claim to the Common Working File (CWF), use the following table to assign the proper TOS. Some procedures may have more than one applicable TOS. CWF will reject alerts on codes with incorrect TOS designations. CWF will produce alerts on codes with incorrect TOS designations.

The only exceptions to this annual update are:

- Surgical services billed for dates of service through December 31, 2007, containing the ASC facility service modifier SG must be reported as TOS F. Effective for services on or after January 1, 2008, the SG modifier is no longer applicable for Medicare services. ASC providers should discontinue applying the SG modifier on ASC facility claims. The indicator F does not appear in the TOS table because its use depends upon claims submitted with POS 24 (ASC facility) from an ASC (specialty 49). This became effective for dates of service January 1, 2008, or after.

- Surgical services billed with an assistant-at-surgery modifier (80-82, AS,) must be reported with TOS 8. The 8 indicator does not appear on the TOS table because its use is dependent upon the use of the appropriate modifier. (See Pub. 100-04 *Medicare Claims Processing Manual,* chapter 12, "Physician/Practitioner Billing," for instructions on when assistant-at-surgery is allowable.)

- Psychiatric treatment services that are subject to the outpatient mental health treatment limitation should be reported with TOS T.

- TOS H appears in the list of descriptors. However, it does not appear in the table. In CWF, "H" is used only as an indicator for hospice. The contractor should not submit TOS H to CWF at this time.

- For outpatient services, when a transfusion medicine code appears on a claim that also contains a blood product, the service is paid under reasonable charge at 80 percent; coinsurance and deductible apply. When transfusion medicine codes are paid under the clinical laboratory fee schedule they are paid at 100 percent; coinsurance and deductible do not apply.

**Note:** For injection codes with more than one possible TOS designation, use the following guidelines when assigning the TOS:

When the choice is L or 1:

- Use TOS L when the drug is used related to ESRD; or
- Use TOS 1 when the drug is not related to ESRD and is administered in the office.

When the choice is G or 1:

- Use TOS G when the drug is an immunosuppressive drug; or
- Use TOS 1 when the drug is used for other than immunosuppression.

When the choice is P or 1:

- Use TOS P if the drug is administered through durable medical equipment (DME); or
- Use TOS 1 if the drug is administered in the office.

The place of service or diagnosis may be considered when determining the appropriate TOS. The descriptors for each of the TOS codes listed in the annual HCPCS update are:

| | |
|---|---|
| 0 | Whole blood |
| 1 | Medical care |
| 2 | Surgery |
| 3 | Consultation |
| 4 | Diagnostic radiology |
| 5 | Diagnostic laboratory |
| 6 | Therapeutic radiology |
| 7 | Anesthesia |
| 8 | Assistant at surgery |
| 9 | Other medical items or services |
| A | Used DME |
| D | Ambulance |
| E | Enteral/parenteral nutrients/supplies |
| F | Ambulatory surgical center (facility usage for surgical services) |
| G | Immunosuppressive drugs |
| J | Diabetic shoes |
| K | Hearing items and services |
| L | ESRD supplies |
| M | Monthly capitation payment for dialysis |
| N | Kidney donor |
| P | Lump sum purchase of DME, prosthetics, orthotics |
| Q | Vision items or services |
| R | Rental of DME |
| S | Surgical dressings or other medical supplies |
| U | Occupational therapy |
| V | Pneumococcal/flu vaccine |
| W | Physical therapy |

## Berenson-Eggers Type of Service (BETOS) Codes

The BETOS coding system was developed primarily for analyzing the growth in Medicare expenditures. The coding system covers all HCPCS codes; assigns a HCPCS code to only one BETOS code; consists of readily understood clinical categories (as opposed to statistical or financial categories); consists of categories that permit objective assignment; is stable over time; and is relatively immune to minor changes in technology or practice patterns.

**BETOS Codes and Descriptions:**

1. **Evaluation and Management**

   1. M1A Office visits—new
   2. M1B Office visits—established
   3. M2A Hospital visit—initial
   4. M2B Hospital visit—subsequent
   5. M2C Hospital visit—critical care
   6. M3 Emergency room visit
   7. M4A Home visit

8.   M4B  Nursing home visit

9.   M5A  Specialist—pathology

10.  M5B  Specialist—psychiatry

11.  M5C  Specialist—ophthalmology

12.  M5D  Specialist—other

13.  M6   Consultations

2.  **Procedures**

1.   P0   Anesthesia

2.   P1A  Major procedure—breast

3.   P1B  Major procedure—colectomy

4.   P1C  Major procedure—cholecystectomy

5.   P1D  Major procedure—TURP

6.   P1E  Major procedure—hysterectomy

7.   P1F  Major procedure—explor/decompr/excis disc

8.   P1G  Major procedure—other

9.   P2A  Major procedure, cardiovascular—CABG

10.  P2B  Major procedure, cardiovascular—aneurysm repair

11.  P2C  Major procedure, cardiovascular—thromboendarterectomy

12.  P2D  Major procedure, cardiovascular—coronary angioplasty (PTCA)

13.  P2E  Major procedure, cardiovascular—pacemaker insertion

14.  P2F  Major procedure, cardiovascular—other

15.  P3A  Major procedure, orthopedic—hip fracture repair

16.  P3B  Major procedure, orthopedic—hip replacement

17.  P3C  Major procedure, orthopedic—knee replacement

18.  P3D  Major procedure, orthopedic—other

19.  P4A  Eye procedure—corneal transplant

20.  P4B  Eye procedure—cataract removal/lens insertion

21.  P4C  Eye procedure—retinal detachment

22.  P4D  Eye procedure—treatment of retinal lesions

23.  P4E  Eye procedure—other

24.  P5A  Ambulatory procedures—skin

25.  P5B  Ambulatory procedures—musculoskeletal

26.  P5C  Ambulatory procedures—inguinal hernia repair

27.  P5D  Ambulatory procedures—lithotripsy

28.  P5E  Ambulatory procedures—other

29.  P6A  Minor procedures—skin

30.  P6B  Minor procedures—musculoskeletal

31.  P6C  Minor procedures—other (Medicare fee schedule)

32.  P6D  Minor procedures—other (non-Medicare fee schedule)

33.  P7A  Oncology—radiation therapy

34.  P7B  Oncology—other

35.  P8A  Endoscopy—arthroscopy

36.  P8B  Endoscopy—upper gastrointestinal

37.  P8C  Endoscopy—sigmoidoscopy

38.  P8D  Endoscopy—colonoscopy

39.  P8E  Endoscopy—cystoscopy

40.  P8F  Endoscopy—bronchoscopy

41.  P8G  Endoscopy—laparoscopic cholecystectomy

42.  P8H  Endoscopy—laryngoscopy

43.  P8I  Endoscopy—other

44.  P9A  Dialysis services (Medicare fee schedule)

45.  P9B  Dialysis services (non-Medicare fee schedule)

3.  **Imaging**

1.   I1A  Standard imaging—chest

2.   I1B  Standard imaging—musculoskeletal

3.   I1C  Standard imaging—breast

4.   I1D  Standard imaging—contrast gastrointestinal

5.   I1E  Standard imaging—nuclear medicine

6.   I1F  Standard imaging—other

7.   I2A  Advanced imaging—CAT/CT/CTA; brain/head/neck

8.   I2B  Advanced imaging—CAT/CT/CTA; other

9.   I2C  Advanced imaging—MRI/MRA; brain/head/neck

10.  I2D  Advanced imaging—MRI/MRA; other

11.  I3A  Echography/ultrasonography—eye

12.  I3B  Echography/ultrasonography—abdomen/pelvis

13.  I3C  Echography/ultrasonography—heart

14.  I3D  Echography/ultrasonography—carotid arteries

15.  I3E  Echography/ultrasonography—prostate, transrectal

16.  I3F  Echography/ultrasonography—other

17.  I4A  Imaging/procedure—heart, including cardiac catheterization

18.  I4B  Imaging/procedure—other

4.  **Tests**

1.   T1A  Lab tests—routine venipuncture (non-Medicare fee schedule)

2.   T1B  Lab tests—automated general profiles

3.   T1C  Lab tests—urinalysis

4.   T1D  Lab tests—blood counts

5.   T1E  Lab tests—glucose

6.   T1F  Lab tests—bacterial cultures

7.   T1G  Lab tests—other (Medicare fee schedule)

8.   T1H  Lab tests—other (non-Medicare fee schedule)

9.   T2A  Other tests—electrocardiograms

10.  T2B  Other tests—cardiovascular stress tests

11.  T2C  Other tests—EKG monitoring

12.  T2D  Other tests—other

5.  **Durable Medical Equipment**

1.   D1A  Medical/surgical supplies

2.   D1B  Hospital beds

3.   D1C  Oxygen and supplies

4.   D1D  Wheelchairs

5.   D1E  Other DME

6.   D1F  Prosthetic/orthotic devices

7.   D1G  Drugs administered through DME

6.  **Other**

1.   O1A  Ambulance

2.   O1B  Chiropractic

3.   O1C  Enteral and parenteral

4.   O1D  Chemotherapy

5.   O1E  Other drugs

6.   O1F  Hearing and speech services

7.   O1G  Immunizations/vaccinations

7.  **Exceptions/Unclassified**

1.   Y1   Other—Medicare fee schedule

2.   Y2   Other—Non-Medicare fee schedule

3.   Z1   Local codes

4.   Z2   Undefined codes

# Appendix 7 — Deleted Code Crosswalk

| Deleted HCPCS 2016 Codes | HCPCS 2017 Codes |
|---|---|
| A4466 | A4467 |
| C9121 | J0883-J0884 |
| C9137 | J7207 |
| C9138 | J7209 |
| C9139 | J7202 |
| C9349 | Q4172 |
| C9458 | Q9983 |
| C9459 | Q9982 |
| C9461 | A9515 |
| C9470 | J1942 |
| C9471 | J7322 |
| C9472 | J9325 |
| C9473 | J2182 |
| C9474 | J9205 |
| C9475 | J9295 |
| C9476 | J9145 |
| C9477 | J9176 |
| C9478 | J2840 |

| Deleted HCPCS 2016 Codes | HCPCS 2017 Codes |
|---|---|
| C9479 | J7342 |
| C9480 | J9352 |
| C9481 | J2786 |
| C9742 | 31573-31574 |
| C9743 | 0438T |
| C9800 | G0429 |
| E0628 | E0627 |
| G0436 | 99406 |
| G0437 | 99407 |
| K0901 | L1851 |
| K0902 | L1852 |
| Q9981 | J8670 |
| S8032 | G0297 |

© 2016 Optum360, LLC

# Appendix 8 — Glossary

**accession.** Process of identifying a specimen and entering a unique specimen identifier into laboratory records.

**alveoplasty.** Procedure in which the physician alters the contours of the alveolus by removing sharp areas or undercuts of alveolar bone.

**angiography.** Radiographic imaging of the arteries. Imaging may be performed to study the vasculature of any given organ, body system, or area of circulation such as the brain, heart, chest, kidneys, limbs, gastrointestinal tract, aorta, and pulmonary circulation to visualize the formation and the function of the blood vessels to detect problems such as a blockage or stricture. A catheter is inserted through an accessible blood vessel and the artery is injected with a radiopaque contrast material after which x-rays are taken.

**apnea.** Absence of breathing or breath.

**apnea monitor.** Device used to monitor breathing during sleep that sounds an alarm if breathing stops for more than the specified amount of time.

**aqueous shunt.** Silicone tube inserted into the anterior chamber of the eye and connected to a reservoir plate behind the pars plana to enhance drainage in the eye's anterior chamber and improve aqueous flow.

**ballistocardiogram.** Graphic recording of the movements of the body caused by cardiac contractions and blood flow, used to evaluate cardiac function.

**BMI.** Body mass index. Tool for calculating weight appropriateness in adults. The Centers for Disease Control and Prevention places adult BMIs in the following categories: below 18.5, underweight; 18.5 to 24.9, normal; 25.0 to 29.9 overweight; 30.0 and above, obese. BMI may be a factor in determining medical necessity for bariatric procedures.

**brace.** Orthotic device that supports, in correct position, any moveable body part, and allows for limited movement. Medicare has a strict definition of a brace that includes only rigid or semirigid devices.

**brachytherapy.** Form of radiation therapy in which radioactive pellets or seeds are implanted directly into the tissue being treated to deliver their dose of radiation in a more directed fashion. Brachytherapy provides radiation to the prescribed body area while minimizing exposure to normal tissue.

**cardiointegram.** Experimental, noninvasive analysis of electrical signals of the heart. Cardiointegram converts analog EKG signals to digital and performs a computer analysis that considers the time element.

**cardiokymography.** Noninvasive test that measures left anterior ventricle segmental wall motion.

**cardioverter-defibrillator.** Device that uses both low energy cardioversion or defibrillating shocks and antitachycardia pacing to treat ventricular tachycardia or ventricular fibrillation.

**cast.** *1)* Rigid encasement or dressing molded to the body from a substance that hardens upon drying to hold a body part immobile during the healing period; a model or reproduction made from an impression or mold. Generally, the supply of a cast is included in the codes describing the reduction. *2)* In dentistry and some other specialties, model or reproduction made from taking an impression or mold.

**catheter.** Flexible tube inserted into an area of the body for introducing or withdrawing fluid.

**cervical cap.** Contraceptive device similar in form and function to the diaphragm but that can be left in place for 48 hours.

**chemotherapy.** Treatment of disease, especially cancerous conditions, using chemical agents.

**CMS.** Centers for Medicare and Medicaid Services. Federal agency that administers the public health programs.

**CMV.** *1)* Controlled mechanical ventilation. *2)* Cytomegalovirus.

**collagen.** Protein based substance of strength and flexibility that is the major component of connective tissue, found in cartilage, bone, tendons, and skin.

**colorectal cancer screening test.** One of the following procedures performed for the purpose of detecting colorectal cancer: screening barium enema, screening fecal-occult blood test, screening flexible sigmoidoscopy, screening colonography, and screening colonoscopy.

**compression sleeve.** Fitted wrap that accelerates recovery in patients with vein disease, lymphedema, or diabetes. Compression sleeves increase circulation and decrease swelling and fluid buildup following surgery.

**contrast material.** Radiopaque substance placed into the body to enable a system or body structure to be visualized, such as nonionic and low osmolar contrast media (LOCM), ionic and high osmolar contrast media (HOCM), barium, and gadolinium.

**covered osteoporosis drug.** Injectable drug approved for treating post-menopausal osteoporosis provided to an individual that has suffered a bone fracture related to post-menopausal osteoporosis.

**CTLSO.** Cervical-thoracic-lumbar-sacral orthosis.

**dermis.** Skin layer found under the epidermis that contains a papillary upper layer and the deep reticular layer of collagen, vascular bed, and nerves.

**dermis graft.** Skin graft that has been separated from the epidermal tissue and the underlying subcutaneous fat, used primarily as a substitute for fascia grafts in plastic surgery.

**dialysis.** Artificial filtering of the blood to remove contaminating waste elements and restore normal balance.

**disarticulation.** Removal of a limb through a joint.

**diskectomy.** Surgical excision of an intervertebral disk.

**DME MAC.** Durable medical equipment Medicare administrative contractor. Entity where claims for specific DMEPOS must be submitted for processing and reimbursement.

**DME PDAC.** Durable Medical Equipment Pricing Data Analysis and Coding. Medicare contractor responsible for maintaining the durable medical equipment classification system (DMECS), including HCPCS coding determinations, and providing durable medical equipment, prosthetics, orthotics, and supplies (DMEPOS) allowables.

**drug eluting stent.** Specialized device placed inside blood vessels for intraluminal support that is coated with a controlled time-release drug that enters the surrounding tissue and helps prevent or slow the growth of plaque or stenotic tissue.

**drug formulary.** List of prescription medications preferred for use by a health plan and dispensed through participating pharmacies to covered persons.

**drugs and biologicals.** Drugs and biologicals included - or approved for inclusion - in the United States Pharmacopoeia, the National Formulary, the United States Homeopathic Pharmacopoeia, in New Drugs or Accepted Dental Remedies, or approved by the pharmacy and drug therapeutics committee of the medical staff of the hospital. Also included are medically accepted and FDA approved drugs used in an anticancer chemotherapeutic regimen. The carrier determines medical acceptance based on supportive clinical evidence.

**dual-lead device.** Implantable cardiac device (pacemaker or implantable cardioverter-defibrillator [ICD]) in which pacing and sensing components are placed in only two chambers of the heart.

**durable medical equipment.** Medical equipment that can withstand repeated use, is not disposable, is used to serve a medical purpose, is generally not useful to a person in the absence of a sickness or injury, and is appropriate for use in the home. Examples of durable medical equipment include hospital beds, wheelchairs, and oxygen equipment.

**Dx.** Diagnosis.

**electrocardiogram.** Recording of the electrical activity of the heart on a moving strip of paper that detects and records the electrical potential of the heart during contraction.

**electroencephalography.** Testing involving amplification, recording, and analysis of the electrical activity of the brain.

**electromyography.** Test that measures muscle response to nerve stimulation determining if muscle weakness is present and if it is related to the muscles themselves or a problem with the nerves that supply the muscles.

**enteral.** Pertaining to the intestines; enteral is often used in the context of nutrition management: formulas, jejunostomy tubes, nasogastric devices, etc.

**epidermis.** Outermost, nonvascular layer of skin that contains four to five differentiated layers depending on its body location: stratum corneum, lucidum, granulosum, spinosum, and basale.

**EPO.** *1)* Epoetin alpha. *2)* Exclusive provider organization. In health care contracting, an organization similar to an HMO, but the member must remain within the provider network to receive benefits. EPOs are regulated under insurance statutes rather than HMO legislation.

**ESRD.** End stage renal disease. Progression of chronic renal failure to lasting and irreparable kidney damage that requires dialysis or renal transplant for survival.

**EVAR.** Endovascular aortic repair. Deployment of a prosthetic stent via a catheter into the site of an abdominal aortic aneurysm (AAA). The stent provides a safe conduit for blood flow to relieve pressure on the aneurysm as the blood flows through the stent instead of continuing to bulge the sac formed by the aorta wall dilation.

**event recorder.** Portable, ambulatory heart monitor worn by the patient that makes electrocardiographic recordings of the length and frequency of aberrant cardiac rhythm to help diagnose heart conditions and to assess pacemaker functioning or programming.

**Food and Drug Administration (FDA).** Federal agency responsible for protecting public health by substantiating the safety, efficacy, and security of human and veterinary drugs, biological products, medical devices, national food supply, cosmetics, and items that give off radiation.

**FOTO.** Focus on therapeutic outcomes.

**gait.** Manner in which a person walks.

**gene.** Basic unit of heredity that contains nucleic acid. Genes are arranged in different and unique sequences or strings that determine the gene's function. Human genes usually include multiple protein coding regions such as exons separated by introns which are nonprotein coding sections.

**genetic test.** Test that is able to detect a gene mutation, either inherited or caused by the environment.

**gingivoplasty.** Repair or reconstruction of the gum tissue, altering the gingival contours by excising areas of gum tissue or making incisions through the gingiva to create a gingival flap.

**glaucoma.** Rise in intraocular pressure, restricting blood flow and decreasing vision.

**halo.** Tool for stabilizing the head and spine.

**health care provider.** Entity that administers diagnostic and therapeutic services.

**hemodialysis.** Cleansing of wastes and contaminating elements from the blood by virtue of different diffusion rates through a semipermeable membrane, which separates blood from a filtration solution that diffuses other elements out of the blood.

**home health services.** Services furnished to patients in their homes under the care of physicians. These services include part-time or intermittent skilled nursing care, physical therapy, medical social services, medical supplies, and some rehabilitation equipment. Home health supplies and services must be prescribed by a physician, and the beneficiary must be confined at home in order for Medicare to pay the benefits in full.

**hospice.** Organization that furnishes inpatient, outpatient, and home health care for the terminally ill. Hospices emphasize support and counseling services for terminally ill people and their families, pain relief, and symptom management. When the Medicare beneficiary chooses hospice benefits, all other Medicare benefits are discontinued, except physician services and treatment of conditions not related to the terminal illness.

**hypertrophic.** Enlarged or overgrown from an increase in cell size of the affected tissue.

**implant.** Material or device inserted or placed within the body for therapeutic, reconstructive, or diagnostic purposes.

**implantable cardioverter-defibrillator.** Implantable electronic cardiac device used to control rhythm abnormalities such as tachycardia, fibrillation, or bradycardia by producing high- or low-energy stimulation and pacemaker functions. It may also have the capability to provide the functions of an implantable loop recorder or implantable cardiovascular monitor.

**in situ.** Located in the natural position or contained within the origin site, not spread into neighboring tissue.

**incontinence.** Inability to control urination or defecation.

**infusion.** Introduction of a therapeutic fluid, other than blood, into the bloodstream.

**infusion pump.** Device that delivers a measured amount of drug or intravenous solution through injection over a period of time.

**intra-arterial.** Within an artery or arteries.

**intramuscular.** Within a muscle.

**intraocular lens.** Artificial lens implanted into the eye to replace a damaged natural lens or cataract.

**intravenous.** Within a vein or veins.

**introducer.** Instrument, such as a catheter, needle, or tube, through which another instrument or device is introduced into the body.

**KAFO.** Knee-ankle-foot orthosis. External apparatus utilized to improve motor control, gait stabilization, and reduce pain. The device is attached to the leg in order to help correct flexible deformities and to halt the progression of fixed deformities.

**keratoprosthesis.** Surgical procedure in which the physician creates a new anterior chamber with a plastic optical implant to replace a severely damaged cornea that cannot be repaired.

**LDS.** Lipodystrophy syndrome. Syndrome which involves the partial or total absence of fat and/or the abnormal deposition and distribution of fat in the body due to a disturbance of the lipid metabolism.

**magnetic resonance angiography.** Diagnostic technique utilizing magnetic fields and radio waves rather than radiation to produce detailed, cross-sectional images of internal body structures.

**multiple-lead device.** Implantable cardiac device (pacemaker or implantable cardioverter-defibrillator [ICD]) in which pacing and sensing components are placed in at least three chambers of the heart.

**mutation.** Alteration in gene function that results in changes to a gene or chromosome. Can cause deficits or disease that can be inherited, can have beneficial effects, or result in no noticeable change.

**nasogastric tube.** Long, hollow, cylindrical catheter made of soft rubber or plastic that is inserted through the nose down into the stomach, and is used for feeding, instilling medication, or withdrawing gastric contents.

**nebulizer.** Latin for mist, a device that converts liquid into a fine spray and is commonly used to deliver medicine to the upper respiratory, bronchial, and lung areas.

**negative pressure dressing.** Adjunctive therapy used to speed wound healing in skin grafts or large wounds. It has been shown to increase blood flow, decrease bacterial count, and increase formation of granulation tissues. A foam pad is placed on the defect and covered with an occlusive drape. A small tube that is non-collapsible is placed into the foam and attached to a disposable pump that provides negative pressure up to -125 mmHg.

**NMES.** Neuromuscular electrical stimulation. Technology that uses percutaneous stimulation to deliver electrical impulses for muscle flexion to trigger action. NMES can, in some cases, create an ability to ambulate among paraplegic patients.

**obturator.** Prosthesis used to close an acquired or congenital opening in the palate that aids in speech and chewing.

**occult blood test.** Chemical or microscopic test to determine the presence of blood in a specimen.

**occupational therapy.** Training, education, and assistance intended to assist a person who is recovering from a serious illness or injury perform the activities of daily life.

                                    © 2016 Optum360, LLC

**ocular implant.** Implant inside muscular cone.

**omnicardiogram.** Method of mathematically interpreting the usual linear form of the electrocardiogram in a different, roughly circular shape. This interpretation is then compared to a normal template and an analysis is performed on two randomly selected cycles from leads I, II, V4, V, and/or V6.

**oral.** Pertaining to the mouth.

**ordering physician.** Physician who orders nonphysician services (e.g., laboratory services, pharmaceutical services, imaging services, or durable medical equipment) for a patient.

**orphan drugs.** Drugs that treat diseases that affect fewer than 200,000 people in the United States, as designated by the FDA. Orphan drugs follow a varied process from other drugs regulated by the FDA.

**orthosis.** Derived from a Greek word meaning "to make straight," it is an artificial appliance that supports, aligns, or corrects an anatomical deformity or improves the use of a moveable body part. Unlike a prosthesis, an orthotic device is always functional in nature.

**orthotic.** Associated with the making and fitting of an orthosis(es).

**osteo-.** Having to do with bone.

**osteogenesis stimulator.** Device used to stimulate the growth of bone by electrical impulses or ultrasound.

**ostomy.** Artificial (surgical) opening in the body used for drainage or for delivery of medications or nutrients.

**pacemaker.** Implantable cardiac device that controls the heart's rhythm and maintains regular beats by artificial electric discharges. This device consists of the pulse generator with a battery and the electrodes, or leads, which are placed in single or dual chambers of the heart, usually transvenously.

**parenteral.** Other than the alimentary canal and is usually used in a method of delivery context: total parenteral nutrition (TPN) and parenteral nutrition therapy (PNT) formulas, kits, and devices.

**parenteral nutrition.** Nutrients provided subcutaneously, intravenously, intramuscularly, or intradermally for patients during the postoperative period and in other conditions, such as shock, coma, and renal failure.

**partial hospitalization.** Situation in which the patient only stays part of each day over a long period. Cardiac, rehabilitation, and chronic pain patients, for example, could use this service.

**passive mobilization.** Pressure, movement, or pulling of a limb or body part utilizing an apparatus or device.

**periradicular.** Surrounding part of the tooth's root.

**peritoneal.** Space between the lining of the abdominal wall, or parietal peritoneum, and the surface layer of the abdominal organs, or visceral peritoneum. It contains a thin, watery fluid that keeps the peritoneal surfaces moist.

**peritoneal dialysis.** Dialysis that filters waste from blood inside the body using the peritoneum, the natural lining of the abdomen, as the semipermeable membrane across which ultrafiltration is accomplished. A special catheter is inserted into the abdomen and a dialysis solution is drained into the abdomen. This solution extracts fluids and wastes, which are then discarded when the fluid is drained. Various forms of peritoneal dialysis include CAPD, CCPD, and NIDP.

**peritoneal effusion.** Persistent escape of fluid within the peritoneal cavity.

**pessary.** Device placed in the vagina to support and reposition a prolapsing or retropositioned uterus, rectum, or vagina.

**photocoagulation.** Application of an intense laser beam of light to disrupt tissue and condense protein material to a residual mass, used especially for treating ocular conditions.

**physician.** Legally authorized practitioners including a doctor of medicine or osteopathy, a doctor of dental surgery or of dental medicine, a doctor of podiatric medicine, a doctor of optometry, and a chiropractor only with respect to treatment by means of manual manipulation of the spine (to correct a subluxation).

**PICC.** Peripherally inserted central catheter. PICC is inserted into one of the large veins of the arm and threaded through the vein until the tip sits in a large vein just above the heart.

**PQRS.** Physician Quality Reporting System. Voluntary CMS reporting mechanism used to measure physician quality that will be mandatory as of January 1, 2015. Eligible providers submit quality data for set measures through approved reporting options.

**prehensile.** Ability to grasp, seize, or hold.

**prodrug.** Inactive drug that goes through a metabolic process when given resulting in a chemical conversion that changes the drug into an active pharmacological agent.

**prophylaxis.** Intervention or protective therapy intended to prevent a disease.

**prostate cancer screening tests.** Test that consists of any (or all) of the procedures provided for the early detection of prostate cancer to a man 50 years of age or older who has not had a test during the preceding year. The procedures are as follows: A digital rectal examination; A prostate-specific antigen blood test. After 2002, the list of procedures may be expanded as appropriate for the early detection of prostate cancer, taking into account changes in technology and standards of medical practice, availability, effectiveness, costs, and other factors.

**prosthetic.** Device that replaces all or part of an internal body organ or body part, or that replaces part of the function of a permanently inoperable or malfunctioning internal body organ or body part.

**pulse generator.** Component of a pacemaker or an implantable cardioverter defibrillator that contains the battery and the electronics for producing the electrical discharge sent to the heart to control cardiac rhythm. Insertion or replacement of the pulse generator may be done alone, not in conjunction with insertion or replacement of the entire pacemaker system.

**residual limb.** Portion of an arm or leg that remains attached to the body after an amputation.

**screening mammography.** Radiologic images taken of the female breast for the early detection of breast cancer.

**screening pap smear.** Diagnostic laboratory test consisting of a routine exfoliative cytology test (Papanicolaou test) provided to a woman for the early detection of cervical or vaginal cancer. The exam includes a clinical breast examination and a physician's interpretation of the results.

**sialodochoplasty.** Surgical repair of a salivary gland duct.

**single-lead device.** Implantable cardiac device (pacemaker or implantable cardioverter-defibrillator [ICD]) in which pacing and sensing components are placed in only one chamber of the heart.

**skin substitute.** Non-autologous human or non-human skin that forms a base for skin growth, often considered a graft dressing.

**speech prosthetic.** Electronic speech aid device for patient who has had a laryngectomy. One operates by placing a vibrating head against the throat; the other amplifies sound waves through a tube which is inserted into the user's mouth.

**splint.** Brace or support. *1)* dynamic splint: brace that permits movement of an anatomical structure such as a hand, wrist, foot, or other part of the body after surgery or injury. *2)* static splint: brace that prevents movement and maintains support and position for an anatomical structure after surgery or injury.

**stent.** Tube to provide support in a body cavity or lumen.

**stereotactic radiosurgery.** Delivery of externally-generated ionizing radiation to specific targets for destruction or inactivation. Most often utilized in the treatment of brain or spinal tumors, high-resolution stereotactic imaging is used to identify the target and then deliver the treatment. Computer-assisted planning may also be employed. Simple and complex cranial lesions and spinal lesions are typically treated in a single planning and treatment session, although a maximum of five sessions may be required. No incision is made for stereotactic radiosurgery procedures.

**subcutaneous.** Below the skin.

**TENS.** Transcutaneous electrical nerve stimulator. TENS is applied by placing electrode pads over the area to be stimulated and connecting the electrodes to a transmitter box, which sends a current through the skin to sensory nerve fibers to help decrease pain in that nerve distribution.

**terminal device.** Addition to an upper limb prosthesis that replaces the function and/or appearance of a missing hand.

**TLSO.** Thoracolumbosacral orthosis.

**tracheostomy.** Formation of a tracheal opening on the neck surface with tube insertion to allow for respiration in cases of obstruction or decreased patency. A tracheostomy may be planned or performed on an emergency basis for temporary or long-term use.

**traction.** Drawing out or holding tension on an area by applying a direct therapeutic pulling force.

**transcutaneous electrical nerve stimulator.** Device that delivers a controlled amount of electricity to an area of the body to stimulate healing and/or to mitigate post-surgical or post-traumatic pain.

**transesophageal echocardiography.** Guidance of a small probe into the esophagus under sedation to closely evaluate the heart and blood vessels within the chest.

**type A emergency department.** Emergency department licensed and advertised to be available to provide emergent care 24 hours a day, seven days a week. Type A emergency departments must meet both the CPT book definition of an emergency department and the EMTALA definition of a dedicated emergency department.

**type B emergency department.** Emergency department licensed and advertised to provide emergent care less than 24 hours a day, seven days a week. Type B emergency departments must meet the EMTALA definition of a dedicated emergency department.

**vascular closure device.** vascular closure devices seal femoral artery punctures caused by invasive or interventional procedures. The closure or seal is achieved by percutaneous delivery of the device's two primary structures, which are usually an anchor and a suture, clip or biologic substance (e.g., collagen, bioabsorbable polymer) or suture through the tissue tract.

© 2016 Optum360, LLC

# Appendix 9 — Physician Quality Reporting System (PQRS)

The Centers for Medicare and Medicare Services (CMS) released the final rule on October 14, 2016 with regards to the Medicare Access and CHIP Reauthorization Act (MACRA), legislation which represents widespread changes for physician payment for services. This legislation replaces the current Medicare Part B Sustainable Growth Rate (SGR) reimbursement formula with a new value-based reimbursement system called the Quality Payment Program (QPP).

The QPP is comprised of two tracks:

*   The Merit-based Incentive Payment System (MIPS)

*   Advanced Alternative Payment Models (Advanced APMs).

MIPS utilizes the existing quality and value reporting systems--Physician Quality Reporting System (PQRS), Medicare Meaningful Use (MU), and Value-Based Modifier (VBM) programs -- to define the following performance categories:

*   Quality (60% for 2017)

*   Advancing Care Information (previously called Meaningful Use) (25% for 2017)

*   Clinical Practice Improvement Activities (CPIA) (15% for 2017)

*   Resource Use (0% for 2017)

Based on the score received, an eligible provider may obtain a composite performance score (CPS) of up to 100 points from these weighted performance categories. This performance score then defines the payment adjustments in the second calendar year after the year the score is obtained. For instance, the score obtained for the 2017 performance year is linked to payment for Medicare Part B services in 2019.

Providers may also choose to participate in Advanced Alternative Payment Models. These providers would not be subject to MIPS payment adjustments, and would also be eligible for a five percent Medicare Part B incentive payment. To be eligible to participate in an advanced alternative Payment Model, providers would need to meet a threshold of a minimum number of patients and other specific requirements.

Even though the MIPS has origins in the PQRS program, CMS will increase and revise existing measures and develop new measures consistent with MIPS. Payment adjustments for PQRS will terminate with the implementation of MIPS payment effective January 1, 2019. Due to the multiple changes anticipated in the coming year due to regulatory changes, Appendix G Physician Quality Reporting System (PQRS) will no longer be included in this publication.

For 2016 diagnostic and procedure information, see www.OptumCoding.com/Product/Updates/PQRS16.